Mosaic of Autoimmunity

Mosaic of Autoimmunity
The Novel Factors of Autoimmune Diseases

Edited by

Carlo Perricone
Rheumatology, Department of Internal Medicine
Sapienza University of Rome
Rome, Italy

Yehuda Shoenfeld
Zabludowicz Center for Autoimmune Diseases
Sheba Medical Center, affiliated to Sackler Faculty of Medicine
Tel Aviv University, Tel Aviv, Israel

Laboratory of the Mosaics of Autoimmunity
Saint-Petersburg University
Saint-Petersburg, Russian Federation

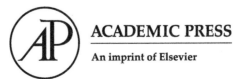

ACADEMIC PRESS
An imprint of Elsevier

Academic Press is an imprint of Elsevier
125 London Wall, London EC2Y 5AS, United Kingdom
525 B Street, Suite 1650, San Diego, CA 92101, United States
50 Hampshire Street, 5th Floor, Cambridge, MA 02139, United States
The Boulevard, Langford Lane, Kidlington, Oxford OX5 1GB, United Kingdom

Notices

Knowledge and best practice in this field are constantly changing. As new research and experience broaden our understanding, changes in research methods, professional practices, or medical treatment may become necessary.

Practitioners and researchers must always rely on their own experience and knowledge in evaluating and using any information, methods, compounds, or experiments described herein. In using such information or methods they should be mindful of their own safety and the safety of others, including parties for whom they have a professional responsibility.

To the fullest extent of the law, neither the Publisher nor the authors, contributors, or editors, assume any liability for any injury and/or damage to persons or property as a matter of products liability, negligence or otherwise, or from any use or operation of any methods, products, instructions, or ideas contained in the material herein.

Library of Congress Cataloging-in-Publication Data
A catalog record for this book is available from the Library of Congress

British Library Cataloguing-in-Publication Data
A catalogue record for this book is available from the British Library

ISBN: 978-0-12-814307-0

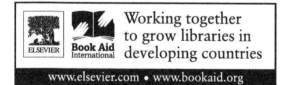

Working together
to grow libraries in
developing countries

www.elsevier.com • www.bookaid.org

Publisher: Mica H. Haley
Acquisition Editor: Linda Versteeg-buschman
Editorial Project Manager: Jennifer Horigan
Production Project Manager: Sreejith Viswanathan
Cover Designer: Mark Rogers

Typeset by TNQ Technologies

Contents

Section III
The Classical Factors Associated with Autoimmunity

Section IV
The Novel Environmental Factors Associated with Autoimmunity

Section V
Classical Autoimmune Diseases

49. Systemic Sclerosis: An Autoimmune Disease Without a Known Pathology and to Be Conquered

Przemyslaw J. Kotyla

50. Sjogren's Syndrome

Barone Francesca and Colafrancesco Serena

51. Autoimmune/Inflammatory Syndrome Induced by Adjuvants (Shoenfeld's Syndrome)

Luis J. Jara, Olga Vera-Lastra, Gabriela Medina, María del Pilar Cruz-Domínguez, Michel A. Martínez-Bencomo, Grettel García-Collinot and Rosa A. Carranza-Muleiro

52. Reproductive Failure

Caterina De Carolis, Paola Triggianese and Roberto Perricone

53. Atherosclerosis in Systemic Autoimmune Rheumatic Diseases

Katarzyna Fischer, Iwona Brzosko and Marek Brzosko

54. A to Z of Some New Autoimmune Diseases: From Alzheimer's to Zinc Deficiency

Zoltán Szekanecz

Section VI
Treatment of Autoimmune Diseases

55. Neuroimmunology

*Maurizio Cutolo and
Amelia Chiara Trombetta*

56. Large-Vessel Vasculitis

*Francesco Muratore, Stefania Croci,
Alessandra Soriano, Nicolò Pipitone
and Carlo Salvarani*

57. Personalized Medicine in Autoimmunity: Rheumatoid Arthritis as a Paradigm

Pier Luigi Meroni and Roberta Gualtierotti

58. Biologics and Biosimilars

*Fabiola Atzeni, Giuseppe Barilaro
and Piercarlo Sarzi-Puttini*

59. Small Molecules

Yoshiya Tanaka

60. Helminthes and Autoimmunity, a Love Story

*Sharon Slomovich, Hanan Guzner-Gur,
Miri Blank and Yehuda Shoenfeld*

List of Contributors

Arnon Afek Zabludowicz Center for Autoimmune Diseases, Sheba Medical Center, Tel-Hashomer, Israel; Sackler Faculty of Medicine, Tel Aviv University, Tel Aviv, Israel

Antonella Afeltra Unit of Allergology, Immunology, Rheumatology, Department of Medicine, Università Campus Bio-Medico di Roma, Rome, Italy

Gabriele Gallo Afflitto Unit of Allergology, Immunology, Rheumatology, Department of Medicine, Università Campus Bio-Medico di Roma, Rome, Italy

Cristiano Alessandri Rheumatology, Department of Internal Medicine, Sapienza University of Rome, Rome, Italy

Stefano Alivernini Institute of Rheumatology, Fondazione Policlinico Universitario A. Gemelli - IRCCS – Catholic University of the Sacred Heart, Rome, Italy

Alessia Alunno Rheumatology Unit, Department of Medicine, University of Perugia, Perugia, Italy

Howard Amital Department of Medicine 'B', Sheba Medical Center, Tel-Hashomer, Israel; Zabludowicz Center for Autoimmune Diseases, Sheba Medical Center, Tel-Hashomer, Israel; Sackler Faculty of Medicine, Tel Aviv University, Tel Aviv, Israel

Laura Andreoli Rheumatology and Clinical Immunology Unit, Spedali Civili, and Department of Clinical and Experimental Sciences, University of Brescia, Brescia, Italy

Alessandro Antonelli Department of Clinical and Experimental Medicine, University of Pisa, Pisa, Italy

Mariachiara Arisi Dermatology Unit, Spedali Civili, and Department of Clinical and Experimental Sciences, University of Brescia, Brescia, Italy

Carolina Artusi Lupus Clinic, Department of Clinical Rheumatology and Medical Sciences, ASST Pini-CTO, Milan, Italy

Fabiola Atzeni Rheumatology Unit, Department of Clinical and Experimental Medicine, University of Messina, Messina, Italy

Eleonora Ballanti Rheumatology, Allergy and Clinical Immunology – University of Rome "Tor Vergata", Rome, Italy

Cristiana Barbati Rheumatology, Department of Internal Medicine, Sapienza University of Rome, Rome, Italy

Giuseppe Barilaro Department of Internal Medicine, ASST Rhodense, Milan, Italy

Elena Bartoloni Rheumatology Unit, Department of Medicine, University of Perugia, Perugia, Italy

Dana Ben-Ami Department of Medicine 'B', Sheba Medical Center, Tel-Hashomer, Israel

Andreia Bettencourt Immunogenetics Laboratory, Abel Salazar Institute of Biomedical Sciences (ICBAS), University of Porto (UP), Porto, Portugal; Unit for Multidisciplinary Research in Biomedicine (UMIB), Abel Salazar Institute of Biomedical Sciences (ICBAS), University of Porto (UP), Porto, Portugal

Nicola Bizzaro Laboratory of Clinical Pathology, Azienda Sanitaria Universitaria Integrata di Udine, San Antonio Hospital, Tolmezzo, Italy; Laboratory of Clinical Pathology, Department of Laboratory Medicine, S. Maria degli Angeli Hospital, Pordenone, Italy

Miri Blank Zabludowicz Center for Autoimmune Diseases, Sheba Medical Center, affiliated to Sackler Faculty of Medicine, Tel Aviv University, Tel Aviv, Israel

Dimitrios P. Bogdanos Department of Rheumatology and Clinical Immunology, Faculty of Medicine, School of Health Sciences, University of Thessaly, Larissa, Greece

Daniela Boleixa Department of Neurology, Centro Hospitalar do Porto-Hospital de Santo António (CHP-HSA), Porto, Portugal; Unidade de Imunologia Clínica (UIC), Centro Hospitalar do Porto-Hospital de Santo António (CHP-HSA)

Vânia Vieira Borba Zabludowicz Center for Autoimmune Diseases, Sheba Medical Center, Tel-Hashomer, Israel; Department 'A' of Internal Medicine, Coimbra University Hospital Centre, Coimbra, Portugal; Faculty of Medicine, University of Coimbra, Coimbra, Portugal

Paola Borgiani Department of Biomedicine and Prevention, Section of Genetics, School of Medicine, University of Rome Tor Vergata, Rome, Italy

Nicola Luigi Bragazzi Postgraduate School of Public Health, Department of Health Sciences (DISSAL), University of Genoa, Genoa, Italy

Iwona Brzosko Independent Laboratory for Rheumatologic Diagnostics, Pomeranian Medical University in Szczecin, Szczecin, Poland

Marek Brzosko Department of Rheumatology, Internal Medicine and Geriatrics, Pomeranian Medical University in Szczecin, Szczecin, Poland

Piergiacomo Calzavara-Pinton Dermatology Unit, Spedali Civili, and Department of Clinical and Experimental Sciences, University of Brescia, Brescia, Italy

Irene Campi Division of Endocrine and Metabolic Diseases, Laboratory of Endocrine and Metabolic Research, IRCCS Istituto Auxologico Italiano, Milan, Italy; Department of Pathophysiology and Transplantation, University of Milan, Milan, Italy

Luca Cantarini Department of Medical Sciences, Surgery and Neurosciences, Research Center of Systemic Autoinflammatory Diseases and Behçet's Disease, Rheumatology Unit, University of Siena, Policlinico Le Scotte, Siena, Italy

Rosa A. Carranza-Muleiro Research Division, Hospital de Especialidades Centro Médico Nacional La Raza, IMSS, Mexico City, Mexico; Instituto Politécnico Nacional, Mexico City, Mexico

Cláudia Carvalho Immunogenetics Laboratory, Abel Salazar Institute of Biomedical Sciences (ICBAS), University of Porto (UP), Porto, Portugal; Unit for Multidisciplinary Research in Biomedicine (UMIB), Abel Salazar Institute of Biomedical Sciences (ICBAS), University of Porto (UP), Porto, Portugal

Francesco Caso Rheumatology Unit, Department of Clinical Medicine and Surgery, School of Medicine and Surgery, University of Naples Federico II, Naples, Italy

Fulvia Ceccarelli Rheumatology, Department of Internal Medicine, Sapienza University of Rome, Rome, Italy

Ricard Cervera Department of Autoimmune Diseases, Hospital Clínic, Barcelona, Spain

Joab Chapman The Department of Neurology, Sheba Medical Center, Tel Hashomer, Ramat-Gan, Israel; The Zabludovich Autoimmune Center, Sheba Medical Center, Tel Hashomer, Ramat-Gan, Israel; Robert and Martha Harden Chair in Mental and Neurological Disease, Sackler Faculty of Medicine, Tel Aviv University, Tel Aviv, Israel

Xian Chen Shenzhen Key Laboratory of Reproductive Immunology for Peri-implantation, Shenzhen Zhongshan Institute for Reproduction and Genetics, Fertility Center, Shenzhen Zhongshan Urology Hospital, Shenzhen, People's Republic of China

Maria Sole Chimenti Rheumatology, Allergy and Clinical Immunology – University of Rome "Tor Vergata", Rome, Italy

Cinzia Ciccacci Department of Biomedicine and Prevention, Section of Genetics, School of Medicine, University of Rome Tor Vergata, Rome, Italy

Enrica Cipriano Rheumatology, Department of Internal Medicine, Sapienza University of Rome, Rome, Italy

Jan Willem Cohen Tervaert Division of Rheumatology, University of Alberta, Edmonton, Canada; Maastricht University, Maastricht, The Netherlands

Tania Colasanti Rheumatology, Department of Internal Medicine, Sapienza University of Rome, Rome, Italy

Paola Conigliaro Rheumatology, Allergy and Clinical Immunology – University of Rome "Tor Vergata", Rome, Italy

Fabrizio Conti Rheumatology, Department of Internal Medicine, Sapienza University of Rome, Rome, Italy

Louis Coplan Sackler Faculty of Medicine, Tel Aviv University, Tel Aviv, Israel

Luisa Costa Rheumatology Unit, Department of Clinical Medicine and Surgery, School of Medicine and Surgery, University of Naples Federico II, Naples, Italy

Stefania Croci Unit of Clinical Immunology, Allergy and Advanced Biotechnologies, Azienda USL-IRCCS di Reggio Emilia, Reggio Emilia, Italy

María del Pilar Cruz-Domínguez Research Division, Hospital de Especialidades Centro Médico Nacional La Raza, IMSS, Mexico City, Mexico; Universidad Nacional Autónoma de México, Mexico City, Mexico

Maurizio Cutolo Research Laboratory and Academic Division of Clinical Rheumatology, Department of Internal Medicine, University of Genova, Polyclinic San Martino Hospital, Genoa, Italy

Shani Dahan Department of medicine "B", Assuta Ashdod Medical Center, Ashdod, Israel; Zabludowicz Center for Autoimmune Diseases, Sheba Medical Center, affiliated to Sackler Faculty of Medicine, Tel Aviv University, Tel Aviv, Israel

Jan Damoiseaux Central Diagnostic Laboratory, Maastricht University Medical Center, Maastricht, The Netherlands

Caterina De Carolis Rheumatology, Allergy and Clinical Immunology – University of Rome "Tor Vergata", Rome, Italy

Antonio Del Puente Rheumatology Unit, Department of Clinical Medicine and Surgery, School of Medicine and Surgery, University of Naples Federico II, Naples, Italy

Vinicius Domingues Florida State University, College of Medicine Daytona Beach, FL, United States

David H. Dreyfus Keren LLC, New Haven CT, United States

Tali Drori The Department of Neurology, Sheba Medical Center, Tel Hashomer, Ramat-Gan, Israel; The Zabludovich Autoimmune Center, Sheba Medical Center, Tel Hashomer, Ramat-Gan, Israel

Michael Ehrenfeld Zabludowicz Center for Autoimmune Diseases, Sheba Medical Center, Tel-Hashomer, Israel

Gerard Espinosa Department of Autoimmune Diseases, Hospital Clínic, Barcelona, Spain

Antonella Farina Department of Experimental Medicine, Sapienza University, Rome, Italy

Giuseppina Alessandra Farina Rheumatology, Boston University School of Medicine, Arthritis Center, Boston, MA, United States

Gianfranco Ferraccioli Institute of Rheumatology, Fondazione Policlinico Universitario A. Gemelli - IRCCS – Catholic University of the Sacred Heart, Rome, Italy

Annacarla Finucci Rheumatology, Department of Internal Medicine, Sapienza University of Rome, Rome, Italy

Antonella Fioravanti Rheumatology Unit, Azienda Ospedaliera Universitaria Senese, Siena, Italy

Katarzyna Fischer Independent Laboratory for Rheumatologic Diagnostics, Pomeranian Medical University in Szczecin, Szczecin, Poland

Giulia Lavinia Fonti Rheumatology, Allergy and Clinical Immunology – University of Rome "Tor Vergata", Rome, Italy

Barone Francesca Centre for Translational Inflammation Research, Institute of Inflammation and Ageing, College of Medical & Dental Sciences, University of Birmingham Research Laboratories, Queen Elizabeth Hospital, Birmingham, United Kingdom

Franco Franceschini Rheumatology and Clinical Immunology Unit, Spedali Civili, and Department of Clinical and Experimental Sciences, University of Brescia, Brescia, Italy

Jozélio Freire de Carvalho Institute for Health Sciences, Federal University of Bahia, Salvador, Brazil; Rheumatology Division, Aliança Medical Center, Salvador, Brazil

Keishi Fujio Department of Allergy and Rheumatology, Graduate School of Medicine, The University of Tokyo, Tokyo, Japan

Grettel García-Collinot Research Division, Hospital de Especialidades Centro Médico Nacional La Raza, IMSS, Mexico City, Mexico; Instituto Politécnico Nacional, Mexico City, Mexico

Elena Generali Division of Rheumatology and Clinical Immunology, Humanitas Research Hospital, Rozzano, Italy

Maria Chiara Gerardi Department of Internal Medicine and Medical Specialties, Rheumatology, Sapienza University of Rome, Rome, Italy

Roberto Gerli Rheumatology Unit, Department of Medicine, University of Perugia, Perugia, Italy

Smadar Gertel Zabludowicz Center for Autoimmune Diseases, Sheba Medical Center, Tel-Hashomer, Israel

Eitan Giat Zabludowicz Center for Autoimmune Diseases, Sheba Medical Center, Tel-Hashomer, Israel

Elisabetta Greco Rheumatology, Allergy and Clinical Immunology – University of Rome "Tor Vergata", Rome, Italy

Elisa Gremese Institute of Rheumatology, Fondazione Policlinico Universitario A. Gemelli - IRCCS – Catholic University of the Sacred Heart, Rome, Italy

Eyal Grunebaum Developmental and Stem Cell Biology Program, Research Institute, Food Allergy and Anaphylaxis Program, Hospital for Sick Children, Toronto, ON, Canada; University of Toronto, Toronto, ON, Canada

Roberta Gualtierotti Lupus Clinic, Department of Clinical Rheumatology and Medical Sciences, ASST Pini-CTO, Milan, Italy; Department of Clinical Sciences and Community Health, University of Milan, Milan, Italy

Maria Domenica Guarino Rheumatology, Allergy and Clinical Immunology – University of Rome "Tor Vergata", Rome, Italy

Hanan Guzner-Gur Zabludowicz Center for Autoimmune Diseases, Sheba Medical Center, Tel-Hashomer, Israel; Sackler Faculty of Medicine, Tel Aviv University, Tel Aviv, Israel

Shu-Gui He Shenzhen Key Laboratory of Reproductive Immunology for Peri-implantation, Shenzhen Zhongshan Institute for Reproduction and Genetics, Fertility Center, Shenzhen Zhongshan Urology Hospital, Shenzhen, People's Republic of China

Cristina Iannuccelli Department of Internal Medicine and Medical Specialties, Rheumatology, Sapienza University of Rome, Rome, Italy

Luis J. Jara Direction of Education and Research, Hospital de Especialidades Centro Médico Nacional La Raza, IMSS, Mexico City, Mexico; Universidad Nacional Autónoma de México, Mexico City, Mexico

Pierre-Yves Jeandel Department of Internal Medicine, Archet-1 Hospital, University of Nice-Sophia-Antipolis, Nice, France

Dr Shaye Kivity Department of Medicine A, Ramat-Gan, Israel; Sackler School of Medicine, Ramat Aviv, Israel; The Zabludowicz Center for Autoimmune Diseases, Ramat-Gan, Israel

Przemysław J. Kotyla Department of Internal Medicine Rheumatology and Clinical Immunology, Medical University of Silesia Katowice, Poland

Alec Krosser Sackler Faculty of Medicine, Tel Aviv University, Tel Aviv, Israel

Andrea Latini Department of Biomedicine and Prevention, Section of Genetics, School of Medicine, University of Rome Tor Vergata, Rome, Italy

Matilde Leon-Ponte Developmental and Stem Cell Biology Program, Research Institute, Food Allergy and Anaphylaxis Program, Hospital for Sick Children, Toronto, ON, Canada

Aaron Lerner B. Rappaport School of Medicine, Technion-Israel Institute of Technology, Haifa, Israel; AESKU. KIPP Institute, Wendelsheim, Germany

Roger Abramino Levy Department of Rheumatology, Hospital Universitário Pedro Ernesto, Universidade do Estado do Rio de Janeiro, Rio de Janeiro, Brazil; Global Medical Expert, GSK, Upper Providence, PA, United States

Benjamin Lichtbroun Zabludowicz Center for Autoimmune Diseases, Sheba Medical Center, Tel-Hashomer, Israel

Ramona Lucchetti Rheumatology, Department of Internal Medicine, Sapienza University of Rome, Rome, Italy

Qianjin Lu Department of Dermatology, Second Xiangya Hospital, Central South University, Hunan Key Laboratory of Medical Epigenomics, Changsha, China

Domenico P.E. Margiotta Unit of Allergology, Immunology, Rheumatology, Department of Medicine, Università Campus Bio-Medico di Roma, Rome, Italy

António Marinho Unidade de Imunologia Clínica (UIC), Centro Hospitalar do Porto-Hospital de Santo António (CHP-HSA); Unit for Multidisciplinary Research in Biomedicine (UMIB), Abel Salazar Institute of Biomedical Sciences (ICBAS), University of Porto (UP), Porto, Portugal

Michel A. Martínez-Bencomo Research Division, Hospital de Especialidades Centro Médico Nacional La Raza, IMSS, Mexico City, Mexico; Universidad Nacional Autónoma de México, Mexico City, Mexico

Torsten Matthias AESKU.KIPP Institute, Wendelsheim, Germany

Gabriela Medina Clinical Research Unit, Hospital de Especialidades Centro Médico Nacional La Raza, IMSS, Mexico City, Mexico; Universidad Nacional Autónoma de México, Mexico City, Mexico

Pier Luigi Meroni Immunorheumatology Research Laboratory, IRCCS Istituto Auxologico Italiano, Milan, Italy

Michael Lichtbroun Zabludowicz Center for Autoimmune Diseases, Sheba Medical Center, Tel-Hashomer, Israel; Sackler Faculty of Medicine, Tel Aviv University, Tel Aviv, Israel

Gustavo Guimarães Moreira Balbi Department of Rheumatology, Hospital Universitário Pedro Ernesto, Universidade do Estado do Rio de Janeiro, Rio de Janeiro, Brazil; Department of Rheumatology, Hospital Universitário, Universidade Federal de Juiz de Fora, Juiz de Fora, Brazil

Francesco Muratore Rheumatology Unit, Azienda USL-IRCCS di Reggio Emilia, Reggio Emilia, Italy; Università di Modena e Reggio Emilia, Modena, Italy

Luca Navarini Unit of Allergology, Immunology, Rheumatology, Department of Medicine, Università Campus Bio-Medico di Roma, Rome, Italy

Giuseppe Novelli Department of Biomedicine and Prevention, Section of Genetics, School of Medicine, University of Rome Tor Vergata, Rome, Italy

Viviana Antonella Pacucci Department of Internal Medicine and Medical Specialties, Rheumatology, Sapienza University of Rome, Rome, Italy

Rosario Peluso Rheumatology Unit, Department of Clinical Medicine and Surgery, School of Medicine and Surgery, University of Naples Federico II, Naples, Italy

Monica Pendolino Department of Internal Medicine and Medical Specialties, Rheumatology, Sapienza University of Rome, Rome, Italy

Dolores Pérez Zabludowitz Center for Autoimmune Diseases, Sheba Medical Center, Tel-Hashomer, Israel

Carlo Perricone Rheumatology, Department of Internal Medicine, Sapienza University of Rome, Rome, Italy

Roberto Perricone Rheumatology, Allergy and Clinical Immunology – University of Rome "Tor Vergata", Rome, Italy

Luca Persani Department of Clinical Sciences and Community Health, University of Milan, Milan, Italy; Division of Endocrine and Metabolic Diseases, Laboratory of Endocrine and Metabolic Research, IRCCS Istituto Auxologico Italiano, Milan, Italy

Luca Petricca Institute of Rheumatology, Fondazione Policlinico Universitario A. Gemelli - IRCCS – Catholic University of the Sacred Heart, Rome, Italy

Nicolò Pipitone Rheumatology Unit, Azienda USL-IRCCS di Reggio Emilia, Reggio Emilia, Italy

Guilherme Ramires de Jesús Department of Obstetrics, Hospital Universitário Pedro Ernesto, Universidade do Estado do Rio de Janeiro, Rio de Janeiro, Brazil

Gustavo Resende Rheumatology Division, Clinical Hospital, Federal University of Minas Gerais, Belo Horizonte, Brazil

Chen Rizenbah Zabludowicz Center for Autoimmune Diseases, Sheba Medical Center, Tel-Hashomer, Israel; Sackler Faculty of Medicine, Tel Aviv University, Tel Aviv, Israel

Ignasi Rodríguez-Pintó Department of Autoimmune Diseases, Hospital Clínic, Barcelona, Spain

Noel R. Rose Department of Pathology, Brigham and Women's Hospital/Harvard Medical School, Boston, MA, United States

Eric Rosenthal Department of Internal Medicine, Archet-1 Hospital, University of Nice-Sophia-Antipolis, Nice, France

Mariateresa Rossi Dermatology Unit, Spedali Civili, and Department of Clinical and Experimental Sciences, University of Brescia, Brescia, Italy

Lazaros I. Sakkas Department of Rheumatology and Clinical Immunology, Faculty of Medicine, School of Health Sciences, University of Thessaly, Larissa, Greece

Carlo Salvarani Rheumatology Unit, Azienda USL-IRCCS di Reggio Emilia, Reggio Emilia, Italy; Università di Modena e Reggio Emilia, Modena, Italy

Piercarlo Sarzi-Puttini Rheumatology Unit, L. Sacco University Hospital, Milan, Italy

Raffaele Scarpa Rheumatology Unit, Department of Clinical Medicine and Surgery, School of Medicine and Surgery, University of Naples Federico II, Naples, Italy

Yahel Segal Zabludowicz Center for Autoimmune Diseases, Sheba Medical Center, affiliated to Sackler Faculty of Medicine, Tel Aviv University, Tel Aviv, Israel

Michael J. Segel Sackler Faculty of Medicine, Tel Aviv University, Tel Aviv, Israel; The Pulmonary Institute, Sheba Medical Center, Tel-Hashomer, Israel

Carlo Selmi Division of Rheumatology and Clinical Immunology, Humanitas Research Hospital, Rozzano, Italy; BIOMETRA Department, University of Milan, Milan, Italy

Dr Lior Seluk Department of Medicine A, Ramat-Gan, Israel

Colafrancesco Serena Department of Internal Medicine and Medical Specialties, Rheumatology Unit, Sapienza University of Rome, Rome, Italy

Amir Sharabi Division of Rheumatology, Beth Israel Deaconess Medical Center, Harvard Medical School, Boston, MA, United States; Department of Clinical Microbiology and Immunology, Sackler School of Medicine, Tel Aviv University, Tel Aviv, Israel

Kassem Sharif Department of Medicine 'B', Sheba Medical Center, Tel-Hashomer, Israel; Zabludowicz Center for Autoimmune Diseases, Sheba Medical Center, Tel-Hashomer, Israel; Sackler Faculty of Medicine, Tel Aviv University, Tel Aviv, Israel

Netta Shoenfeld Sheba Medical Center, Tel-Hashomer, Israel

Yehuda Shoenfeld Zabludowicz Center for Autoimmune Diseases, Sheba Medical Center, affiliated to Sackler Faculty of Medicine, Tel Aviv University, Tel Aviv, Israel; Laboratory of the Mosaics of Autoimmunity, Saint-Petersburg University, Saint-Petersburg, Russian Federation

Flavio Signorelli Department of Rheumatology, Hospital Universitário Pedro Ernesto, Universidade do Estado do Rio de Janeiro, Rio de Janeiro, Brazil; Department of Internal Medicine, Hospital Universitário Clementino Fraga Filho, Universidade Federal do Rio de Janeiro, Rio de Janeiro, Brazil

Ana Martins Silva Department of Neurology, Centro Hospitalar do Porto-Hospital de Santo António (CHP-HSA), Porto, Portugal; Unit for Multidisciplinary Research in Biomedicine (UMIB), Abel Salazar Institute of Biomedical Sciences (ICBAS), University of Porto (UP), Porto, Portugal

Berta Martins Silva Immunogenetics Laboratory, Abel Salazar Institute of Biomedical Sciences (ICBAS), University of Porto (UP), Porto, Portugal; Unit for Multidisciplinary Research in Biomedicine (UMIB), Abel Salazar Institute of Biomedical Sciences (ICBAS), University of Porto (UP), Porto, Portugal

Sharon Slomovich Zabludowicz Center for Autoimmune Diseases, Sheba Medical Center, Tel-Hashomer, Israel

Raz Somech Department of Pediatrics, The Edmond and Lily Safra Children's Hospital, Sheba Medical Center, Tel Hashomer and the Sackler School of Medicine, Tel Aviv University, Tel Aviv, Israel

Alessandra Soriano Unit of Clinical Immunology, Allergy and Advanced Biotechnologies, Azienda USL-IRCCS di Reggio Emilia, Reggio Emilia, Italy

Zoltán Szekanecz Division of Rheumatology, Institute of Internal Medicine, Faculty of Medicine, University of Debrecen, Debrecen, Hungary

Yoshiya Tanaka The First Department of Internal Medicine, School of Medicine, University of Occupational and Environmental Health, Japan, Kitakyushu, Japan

Sara Tenti Department of Medicine, Surgery and Neuroscience, Rheumatology Unit, University of Siena, Policlinico Le Scotte, Siena, Italy

Angela Tincani Rheumatology and Clinical Immunology Unit, Spedali Civili, and Department of Clinical and Experimental Sciences, University of Brescia, Brescia, Italy

Barbara Tolusso Institute of Rheumatology, Fondazione Policlinico Universitario A. Gemelli - IRCCS – Catholic University of the Sacred Heart, Rome, Italy

Jiram Torres-Ruiz Department of Immunology and Rheumatology, Instituto Nacional de Ciencias Médicas y Nutrición Salvador Zubirán, Mexico City, Mexico; Zabludowicz Center for Autoimmune Diseases, Sheba Medical Center, affiliated to Sackler Faculty of Medicine, Tel Aviv University, Tel Aviv, Israel

Elias Toubi Bnai-Zion Medical Center, Faculty of Medicine, Haifa, Israel

Renato Tozzoli Laboratory of Clinical Pathology, Azienda Sanitaria Universitaria Integrata di Udine, San Antonio Hospital, Tolmezzo, Italy; Laboratory of Clinical Pathology, Department of Laboratory Medicine, S. Maria degli Angeli Hospital, Pordenone, Italy

Paola Triggianese Rheumatology, Allergy and Clinical Immunology – University of Rome "Tor Vergata", Rome, Italy

Amelia Chiara Trombetta Research Laboratory and Academic Division of Clinical Rheumatology, Department of Internal Medicine, University of Genova, Polyclinic San Martino Hospital, Genoa, Italy

George C. Tsokos Division of Rheumatology, Beth Israel Deaconess Medical Center, Harvard Medical School, Boston, MA, United States

Yumi Tsuchida Department of Allergy and Rheumatology, Graduate School of Medicine, The University of Tokyo, Tokyo, Japan

Zahava Vadasz The Division of Allergy and Clinical Immunology, Bnai-Zion Medical Center, Faculty of Medicine, Technion, Haifa-Israel

Guido Valesini Rheumatology, Department of Internal Medicine, Sapienza University of Rome, Rome, Italy

Joyce van Beers Central Diagnostic Laboratory, Maastricht University Medical Center, Maastricht, The Netherlands

Pieter van Paassen Department of Internal Medicine, Maastricht University Medical Center, Maastricht, The Netherlands

Guia Maria Vannucchi Division of Endocrine and Metabolic Diseases, Laboratory of Endocrine and Metabolic Research, IRCCS Istituto Auxologico Italiano, Milan, Italy

Carlos Vasconcelos Unidade de Imunologia Clínica (UIC), Centro Hospitalar do Porto-Hospital de Santo António (CHP-HSA); Unit for Multidisciplinary Research in Biomedicine (UMIB), Abel Salazar Institute of Biomedical Sciences (ICBAS), University of Porto (UP), Porto, Portugal

Marina Venturini Dermatology Unit, Spedali Civili, and Department of Clinical and Experimental Sciences, University of Brescia, Brescia, Italy

Olga Vera-Lastra Internal Medicine Department, Hospital de Especialidades Centro Médico Nacional La Raza, IMSS, Mexico City, Mexico; Universidad Nacional Autónoma de México, Mexico City, Mexico

Mathilde Versini Institut Arnault Tzanck, Saint Laurent du Var, France

Marta Vomero Rheumatology, Department of Internal Medicine, Sapienza University of Rome, Rome, Italy

Abdulla Watad Department of Medicine 'B', Sheba Medical Center, Tel-Hashomer, Israel; Zabludowicz Center for Autoimmune Diseases, Sheba Medical Center, Tel-Hashomer, Israel; Sackler Faculty of Medicine, Tel Aviv University, Tel Aviv, Israel

Haijing Wu Department of Dermatology, Second Xiangya Hospital, Central South University, Hunan Key Laboratory of Medical Epigenomics, Changsha, China

Yong Zeng Shenzhen Key Laboratory of Reproductive Immunology for Peri-implantation, Shenzhen Zhongshan Institute for Reproduction and Genetics, Fertility Center, Shenzhen Zhongshan Urology Hospital, Shenzhen, People's Republic of China

Section I

Introduction

FUNDING

This work is supported by the grant of the Government of the Russian Federation for the state support of scientific research carried out under the supervision of leading scientists, agreement 14.W03.31.0009, on the basis of SPbU projects 15.34.3.2017 and 15.64.785.2017.

Chapter 1

The Mosaic of Autoimmunity in History

Noel R. Rose

Department of Pathology, Brigham and Women's Hospital/Harvard Medical School, Boston, MA, United States

INTRODUCTION

The Oxford English dictionary describes mosaic as "the process of producing pictures or patterns by cementing together small pieces of stone, grass etc. of various colors; pictures or patterns thus produced." This is an apt description of the book. Research on autoimmunity and autoimmune disease by its diverse nature involves many colorful little tiles. Each autoimmune disease is an element onto itself. It has its own color and texture conveyed by the clinical signs and symptoms and by its distinct biologic mechanisms. It was the genius of the first edition of *The Mosaic of Autoimmunity* that Yehuda Shoenfeld was able to assemble these different pieces into a coherent image. The pattern was the culmination of three decades of research both in the laboratory and in the clinic that resulted in a portrait of autoimmune diseases as an important component of modern medical science.

PRE-MOSAIC IMMUNOLOGY, 1950–80

Modern day immunology was emerged during the three decades following World War II. The war left science in Europe decimated. In continental Europe, medical scientists were scattered or killed, and the laboratories and medical facilities destroyed. The situation in Great Britain was a bit different from the continent because the country was not actually invaded. Scientists were taken off doing their research and assigned activities to support the war effort. The great names in post–war British immunologic research, Florey, Medawar, Gell, and Humphrey, were able to transition back to fundamental investigation often based on their war time experience.

In Europe, one place where immunology was reborn after the war was Paris. I had the good fortune to spend a sabbatical year at the Pasteur Institute in Paris in 1957 and to experience the renaissance of immunologic research at that distinguished institution. Two units, side by side at the Pasteur Institute, were the nidus from which modern immunology sprang. The molecular biology group under Lwoff defined our understanding of the interaction of genes through the operon. With Monod and Jacob, the group was awarded with the Nobel Prize.

The neighboring unit was headed by Grabar. Although trained as an engineer, Grabar became fascinated by immune reactions in a visit to the United States in the 1930s and established a laboratory after the war with many colleagues who set the stage for what is now referred to as "Immunopathology." The major outcome of the Grabar research was the development of new methods that allowed deeper searching and greater insight into the immune response. This research led to another Nobel Prize given to a past member of a group, Dausset, for discovery of the HLA gene family.

Before World War II, immunology was largely a handmaiden of microbiology and infectious diseases. The major occupation of the immunologist was performing serological tests to aid microbiologic diagnosis. Three tests were available in the laboratory for demonstrating antibodies: agglutination, precipitation, and complement fixation. Each of these tests were greatly expanded and refined in the Grabar laboratory. Precipitation tests performed in an agar gel, for example, made it possible to separate and label the antigens and antibodies that were present in a complex sample. Agglutination was made more versatile and sensitive by devising indirect agglutination methods using particulate carriers of the antigen. Complement fixation was transformed by using defined enzymatic markers, giving raise to ELISA and immunofluorescence as signals. This expanded array of laboratory procedures allowed immunologists to discover worlds that had previously been beyond our vision.

My own year in the Grabar laboratory was occasioned by my studies with Ernest Witebsky of organ-specific or tissue-limited antigens. We discovered that organs with highly restricted antigens, such as the thyroid gland, can relatively easily be induced to develop self-destructive autoimmune responses, something that was previously believed to be impossible. Using Grabar's new methods of separation in agar, I was able to more fully characterize the antibodies to thyroglobulin in both animal and human sera, and to fragment this large antigen into its component epitopes. These studies, which I

Mosaic of Autoimmunity. https://doi.org/10.1016/B978-0-12-814307-0.00001-3

3

described publicly at the first International Symposium on Immunopathology organized by Grabar, were included with a flurry of research papers on possible immunologic causes of human diseases. For example, a young hematologist who was coorganizer of the symposium, Peter Miescher, reported that the LE factor present in most patients with lupus represents antibodies to antigens found in the cell nucleus. Other studies on human diseases of unknown etiology identified many examples associated with, and possibly caused by, an autoantibody response. Autoimmune diseases made their debut on the medical stage at the meeting.

Inspired by these studies on the value of autoantibodies in diagnosis, attention of immunologists was redirected to immune responses in which antibodies played no apparent role. The basis for cell-mediated immunity was demonstrated by Landsteiner and Chase and led to the understanding that much of the injury in an autoimmune disease was due to cytotoxic effects of lymphocytes and other inflammatory cells. Research on cell-mediated immune responses progressed rapidly with the discovery of different families of lymphocytes, T cells and B cells, and of their active mediators, cytokines.

Another turning point in research on autoimmune diseases came from the discovery of my own laboratory that susceptibility to thyroiditis in animals was partly genetically determined, and that the major genes were a part of the major histocompatibility complex (MHC). A similar finding in humans was published soon afterward by McDevitt who described a similar MHC association with lupus. Studies on the genetic regulation of autoimmune disease became a major topic of investigation in the 1970s in both experimental animals and humans. Genetics and immunology merged.

In this era, two concepts of theoretical importance advanced our understanding autoimmune disease: the clonal selection theory propounded mainly by Burnet and specific acquired immunologic tolerance described by Medawar and his colleagues.

As the frequency of the autoimmune immune response was more fully appreciated and the harm that can result from an unregulated autoimmune response were more fully appreciated, investigations of the normal regulation of specific immunity, both antibody-mediated and cell-mediated, became a prominent topic for investigation. The idea that both lymphocytes and antibodies can both initiate and regulate autoimmune responses emerged at this time.

A continuing theme throughout this period was the remarkable specificity of the immune response. Crystallographic and other structure–function studies together with more precise genetic analysis allowed greater understanding of the mechanisms of selection of the receptors on antibodies as well as on T cells. T-cell recognition became an issue because it was clear that unrestrained recognition by T cells of antigen in the blood stream can lead to a storm of devastating cytokine responses. T-cell recognition is therefore circumscribed by MHC-restricted antigen presentation. Studies of T-cell recognition have led to the discovery of the critical importance of cells that prepare antigen for T-cell recognition. The action of antigen-presenting cells depends not only on precise recognition of the cognate antigen but also on nonantigen recognition by other cell surface markers that together help to regulate T-cell responses.

THE DECADE OF THE MOSAICS, 1980–90

By 1980, it became clear that, despite many differences based on their location, all the autoimmune diseases shared a great number of fundamental properties. In my case, it meant getting together with Ian Mackay to produce the first book describing all the then recognized autoimmune diseases. The first part of the book was devoted to the common, underlying mechanisms such as genetics, cytokines, and regulation, whereas the second half described particular diseases with emphasis on applying those common mechanisms. That book, *The Autoimmune Diseases*, is now at its sixth edition.

The Mosaic of Autoimmunity, published in the same decade, approached the issue of the common features of autoimmune disease from a different angle. Shoenfeld took the major topics and trends in modern immunology and illustrated how they contributed to our growing mosaic picture of autoimmune disease. Like a mosaic, the full beauty of the individual pieces can best be appreciated when looked at collectively. Using both clinical features and animal models, the book gave the reader a broad view of the immune system and its many interactions both within and outside of the host, illustrating how each piece of the mosaic can contribute to autoimmunity.

The first edition of *The Mosaic of Autoimmunity* had enormous impact on the direction of future of future research and medical practice with respect to the autoimmune diseases. Journals and review media devoted to autoimmunity disease sprang into existence; regional, national, and international congresses on autoimmunity became regular features of the immunologic calendar. Patients with different autoimmune and related disorders have learned that their voices are much louder when they speak together to the public about the importance of supporting research on the autoimmune diseases.

POST-MOSAIC IMMUNOLOGY 1990–2018

The years following publication of *The Mosaic of Autoimmunity* broadened the concept of autoimmunity and heightened its prominence in human physiology and pathology. For example, investigations of innate immunity gave rise to greater understanding of the invertebrate immune recognition system evolutionarily more primitive than the vertebrate adaptive response.

These studies led to reexamination of the role of innate immunity in shaping the inflammatory response and the subtleties that inflammation played in determining the effector mechanisms of autoimmune disease. The interactions of these two immune systems, innate and adaptive, determine the pathologic or nonpathologic outcome of an autoimmune response. It has led also to a greater appreciation of the critical importance of maintaining the normal homeostasis of the host and of the microbial population, the microbiota, that inhabit the host.

Another overriding issue receiving more appropriate attention is the importance of external as well as internal factors in regulating autoimmunity. Some may operate on the epigenetic level by changing the genetic response. The historic field of infection in induction of autoimmunity found a larger place in the mainstream of immunologic research. New research on such topics as stress and pregnancy dealt with in the first edition shed new light on the darker edges of autoimmunity.

A review of contents of the current edition of *The Mosaic of Autoimmunity* provides an exciting prediction of where the field is likely to go before a future edition of the book. The emphasis clearly is now on translation of the half century of immunologic research to improved treatment and prevention of autoimmune disease. This goal implies earlier intervention. The appearance of antibodies well before clinical signs of disease are evident is only a starting point for understanding that development of autoimmune disease, in many instances, is a long-term process. Early detection of antigen-specific B and T cells and their cytokine products in blood can now be the goal. A part of the risk resides in the inherited traits of the individual patient and requires a personal genetic evaluation. Almost all autoimmune diseases depend on many different genes tied to the regulation of the immune response. Other than MHC, most of these genes individually contribute little to the total heightened risk. Therefore, individual genome-wide studies will have to be applied. Any intervention that can be applied before the disease has become clinically evident and irreversibly destructive requires development of the next generations of benign interventions. They are procedures that can be safely done in a healthy person, particularly a child, that is ethical and will halt the process leading to a pathogenic autoimmune outcome. The goal of early intervention must include assessing environmental factors where immunology has had its greatest successes.

The emphasis on prevention and earlier treatment must be placed on a continuing personal immunologic "mosaic." These programs require assembling huge amounts of data. Methods of handling such information will require greater use of the tools of systemic biology, as this new edition of the book suggests.

As the current edition of the Mosaic book reminds us the immune system is closely integrated with the other major regulatory systems of the body, hormonal and neurologic. A complete systems biology approach is going to include the totality of the physiologic response, not just those classically identified as "immunologic."

A topic of increasing interest is the tracking of regulatory pathways now needed in cancer immunotherapy. The goal of the oncologist is to mobilize the immune system, whereas the "auto-immunologist" is engaged in reducing it. Manipulation of the immune system is best targeted as selectively as possible, an area where the body of immunologic research may contribute.

A final word comes from an omission in the current edition of the Mosaic book. Too many patients are ill-served by our predominantly organ-based medical system because so many autoimmune diseases involve multiple organs. Diagnosis and treatment, therefore, become increasingly difficult as patients move from specialist to specialist. Our medical system must find a way to better serve patients with multiple autoimmune problems. Yehuda Shoenfeld has led the way. His clinic is one of the few in the world where patients with complicated, immune-mediated disorders can be seen by a team of specialists who pool their talents and arrive at a cohesive plan of treatment. Maybe "The Autoimmune Disease Clinic" will be a chapter in the next edition of *The Mosaic of Autoimmunity*.

Chapter 2

The Novel Aspects on the Mosaic of Autoimmunity

Carlo Perricone[1], Yehuda Shoenfeld[2,3]

[1]Rheumatology, Department of Internal Medicine, Sapienza University of Rome, Rome, Italy; [2]Zabludowicz Center for Autoimmune Diseases, Sheba Medical Center, affiliated to Sackler Faculty of Medicine, Tel Aviv University, Tel Aviv, Israel; [3]Laboratory of the Mosaics of Autoimmunity, Saint-Petersburg University, Saint-Petersburg, Russian Federation

Almost 30 years ago, the concept of "Mosaic of Autoimmunity" [1] was introduced to the scientific community, and since then it has continuously evolved adding new tiles to the puzzle [2]. We are looking now at an era in which the players of autoimmunity have changed names and roles.

One of the mainstays of the mosaic concept is that autoimmune diseases (AIDs) occur in genetically predisposed individuals [3]. This concept is now expanded by the evidence of "familial autoimmunity": not only a single AID shows familial aggregation [4,5] but also a familial aggregation of diverse AIDs exists. This was brought to light by the evidences from a systematic review and metaanalysis performed by Cárdenas-Roldán et al. [6]. Physicians should be aware that familial autoimmunity is a frequent event especially in specific disorders, such as autoimmune thyroid disease and systemic lupus erythematosus (SLE), suggesting a stronger shared genetic influence in their development.

To strengthen the theory of a genetic basis, there is the evidence that AIDs occur more often in young people [7]. On the other hand, AIDs were thought to be rare in older persons. Nowadays, this assumption was found to be not always valid, and a tendency to have more severe autoimmunity in older has been noted [8]. The possible explanation of such paradox comes from another branch of the mosaic: the presence of an abnormal immune response. Vadasz et al. [9] indeed suggested that expansion of many protective regulatory mechanisms and especially of peripheral $CD4^+CD25^{high}FoxP3^+$ T-regulatory cells is highly characteristic in the elderly. It is possible that during aging, an imbalance between thymic and peripheral T-regulatory cell output occurs with a *ratio* favoring the peripheral component, possibly allowing a proinflammatory response increasing the susceptibility to autoimmunity. Furthermore, besides adaptive immunity, it has been elucidated that the disruption of the autoimmune response also occurs at the innate immunity system [10].

In this book on the revised concepts of the mosaic of autoimmunity, we will show the main multiple actors that are now on the scene.

If only we consider the cellular and molecular mechanisms, the "old" and well-known cells—B cells, T cells, and so on—have been better characterized and found to play pleiotropic roles in autoimmunity. We will see that B cells are antigen-presenting cells and can have a proinflammatory role [11], and in some instance may produce IL-6 rather than IL-10, generating different immune responses which more likely to associate them to specific autoimmune patterns [12]. B-regulatory cells have been recently described, producing IL-10, but also independently via IL-35 secretion [13].

The counterpart of B cells, T cells have been widely explored and from the CD8 and Th1/Th2 paradigm we are now in an era in which double-negative T cells, Th17 cells, Th9 cells, γδ T cells, T follicular helper (Tfh) cells, and T-regulatory cells have their role in autoimmunity. The imbalance toward any of these population may disrupt the tolerance, leading to the development of an autoimmune disorder, and unveiling such complex pathways will help finding novel targets and biomarkers and, also, develop tools toward personalized medicine [14].

Nevertheless, autoimmunity is not only humoral immunity but innate immunity seems to have a major role. Several studies showed that the number of circulating natural killer cells can be frequently altered, for instance, in multiple sclerosis (MS), rheumatoid arthritis (RA), type 1 diabetes mellitus, Sjögren's syndrome, and miastenia gravis [15], and it was showed that they are detrimental in recurrent spontaneous abortion even when associated with antiphospholipid syndrome (APS) [16].

Dendritic cells are essential in the initiation and perpetuation of inflammation and secrete cytokines that polarize the cooperative immune response toward Th1 and Th17 that have been shown to be important in multiple AIDs, for instance, in

SLE [17]. Even neutrophils take a place in mechanisms leading to autoimmunity: the discovery of the neutrophil extracellular traps (NETs), structures made of chromatin and histones that interact with integrins and toll-like receptors and whose insufficient removal or increased production may be implicated in the pathogenesis of several AIDs including SLE and RA [18].

The "old" complement is a vintage player in autoimmunity: still fundamental in everyday practice, especially in SLE, seems to be a promising therapeutic target in APS, and is implicated in most of the other autoimmune conditions [19].

We have observed in the past decade to an explosion of autoantibodies [20]: over 180 only in SLE and the knowledge that such antibodies often precede the disease of years if not decades. At the same extent, the diagnostic methods to assess such antibodies have improved: besides classical techniques, ELISA and automated tests have improved toward standardization of these tests [21]. When considering the diagnosis of AIDs, the technologic progress has given novel tool to physicians in particular in the assessment of inflammatory arthritides including magnetic resonance and musculoskeletal ultrasonography that permit earlier and more accurate depiction of the inflammatory status as well as of the bone damage in these conditions [22].

Everything is based on the genetic predisposition of the individual: genetic that drives the phenotype, genetic that has evolved in the techniques so that now we have the next generation sequencing allowing to study the whole genome of an individual [23]. Nonetheless, it was shown that epigenetic modifications are detrimental, dramatically changing genetic expression via DNA methylation/demethylation, histone modification, and noncoding RNAs, and thereby play a key role in various biological processes and pathogenesis of disease [24]. In this view, the role of hormones seems now much more an interaction resulting with genetic and epigenetic modifications rather than being detrimental per se [25]. For instance, posttranslational modifications are now part of the mosaic of autoimmunity, citrullination has been discovered, and recently a role for carbamylation has been described, introducing novel classes of autoantibodies frequently linked with the exposure to environmental agents [26]. The families of cytokines and chemokines have enormously increased, the role in each disease better depicted, and several have been identified as therapeutic targets in common clinical practice as well as in future trials [27]. Lysosomal degradation occurring in eukaryotic organisms, namely autophagy, has a crucial role in cell homeostasis by controlling organelles and proteins turnover and sustaining survival in cellular stress conditions such as nutrients deprivation. Dysfunction of this mechanism has been implicated in several autoimmune disorders including SLE, RA, and MS [28]. And another player is microbiota that is the set of microorganisms that cohabit a multicellular organism. Dysbiosis is an event occurring in several autoimmune conditions: specific species seem to become pathogenic by driving the immune response toward an imbalanced status, for instance, toward a Th17 response for segmented filamentous bacteria that proliferate in animal models of arthritis [29]. The counterplayers are infections that are well known to be associated with AID flares and increased disease susceptibility [30]. More recently, parasitic infections have been either associated with or found being protective to certain AIDs, suggesting a possible therapeutic strategy [31].

It is also well known that genetic factors do not explain all of the susceptibility to AIDs, just because of these interactions with epigenetic factors and the environment. The study of the geo-epidemiological factors on big data will allow to identify such data and clarify the pathogenic mechanisms of AIDs [32].

Thus, here we come to the novel factors that have been associated with several autoimmune conditions. Some associations with seasonality have been demonstrated, probably linked with the effects of melatonin [33]. Ultraviolet radiation in some cases can be used as a therapy, for instance, in patients with psoriasis, whereas it is harmful in patients with SLE because of its proapoptotic capacities [34]. Vitamin D has been found to be an immunomodulator by improving the number of T-regulatory cells, and vitamin D supplementation has been suggested as a valid supportive strategy in several conditions besides the treatment of osteoporosis [35]. It has been found that patients with autoimmune disorders have impaired sense of smell, linking the olfactory gene cluster to the major histocompatibility complex located on chromosome 6 [36]. Even breastfeeding (or not breastfeeding) seems to have an influence on future development of autoimmunity [37]. Likewise, prolactin is implicated in a number of autoimmune conditions such as SLE [38].

Vaccination is fundamental in patients with AID because it prevents the onset of infections that trigger disease flares and worsen disease prognosis. It has been found that sporadically, in predisposed individuals, vaccines may trigger autoimmune response and should be avoided in patients with active disease. The role of adjuvants in the vaccines may at least partly explain this effect and rise a question on personalized medicine, notwithstanding that nowadays, vaccine's benefits largely overwhelm the risks, and that vaccines are recommended in patients with AIDs following current recommendations [39]. Chronic silicone stimulation has been for long suspected to trigger autoimmune phenomena [40]. Thus, in 2011, Shoenfeld and Agmon-Levin described five medical conditions with similar complex of symptoms and signs and a common pathogenesis, namely siliconosis, the Gulf War syndrome, the macrophagic myofasciitis syndrome, postvaccination phenomena, and the sick building syndrome, linked with previous exposure to an adjuvant substance. The authors proposed to gather these five entities under a common syndrome denominated "Autoimmune/inflammatory Syndrome Induced by Adjuvants" and suggested a set of diagnostic criteria for this new entity [41].

As we saw that the microbiota can influence the onset of an autoimmune reaction, it is likely that "we are what we eat." Some substances contained in spicy foods, specifically capsaicin, fatty acids, and some beverages such as tea or coffee, can modify our immune system in an anti- or proinflammatory way [42]. Gluten is an important component in wheat whose consumption has dramatically increased over time and that seems to have a proinflammatory effect in predisposed individuals on microbiome and on increasing intestinal permeability, by changing the intestinal tight junctions [43]. It should be not surprising that a proinflammatory state, in which there is an abundance of Th17, such as obesity, is associated with autoimmunity [44]. We have already mentioned smoke, especially cigarette smoke, which has multiple detrimental effects including increase of reactive oxygen species, increased NETosis, increased citrullination especially in the lungs, increased periodontitis, and association with the pathogen *Porphyromonas gingivalis* thus resulting in a destructive arm for predisposed subjects and patients with AIDs [45]. *Cannabis* has been shown to have immunomodulatory and pain relief effects when the endocannabinoids are modulated [46]. Psychological stress and physical activity seem two faces of the same medal leading or rather protecting toward the development of autoimmunity [47]. Living in a polluted environment has been also now recognized as a risk factor for the development of autoimmunity. For instance, it has been shown that diesel exhaust particles induce autophagy and citrullination in normal human bronchial epithelial cells [48]. Another pollutant is bisphenol A, molecule frequently used in the manufacturing of epoxy resins and plastics, which seems to act on estrogens thus driving autoimmunity [49].

Thus, given these premises, it is quite evident that the definitions, management, and treatment of AIDs have changed over the years. There is much more knowledge among the relationships between autoimmunity and cancer: from one side the events linking the development of specific malignant conditions in autoimmune patients, either or not associated with the disease per se rather than with the treatment. On the other side, the novel compounds used treat some neoplasia, the so-called immune checkpoints inhibitors, have been found to have as potential adverse events the development of autoimmune phenomena [50]. In addition, the relationships between allergy and autoimmunity have been better depicted, and some medications are now in development to be effective in both circumstances [51]. A branch, which is neuroimmunology, has been studied and implemented [52], as well as atherosclerosis and autoimmunity have been found to have lots in common starting from a proinflammatory *milieu*.

Novel classification criteria have been developed for SLE, RA, APS, vasculitis, psoriatic arthritis, and Sjögren's syndrome, and novel therapeutic paradigms are now of routine use, including the biologic disease-modifying antirheumatic drugs (bDMARDs) and the targeted synthetic DMARDs. Respectively, we have now monoclonal antibodies and soluble receptors or small molecules, particularly, those inhibiting the JAK-STAT pathway, which represent a giant step forward in the treatment of patients with AIDs. In the past decades, the use of intravenous immunoglobulins has also improved.

We are definitely approaching to a new era: that of personalized medicine, this wind that brings a new hope to the leaves of autoimmunity [53].

REFERENCES

[1] Shoenfeld Y, Isenberg DA. The mosaic of autoimmunity. Immunol Today April 1989;10(4):123–6.

[2] Amital H, Eric Gershwin M, Shoenfeld Y. Reshaping the mosaic of autoimmunity. Semin Arthritis Rheum June 2006;35(6):341–3.

[3] Perricone R, Perricone C, Shoenfeld Y. Autoimmunity: when the immune system becomes the self-ish giant. Autoimmun Rev August 2011;10(10):575–6.

[4] Perricone C, Ceccarelli F, Valesini G. An overview on the genetic of rheumatoid arthritis: a never-ending story. Autoimmun Rev August 2011;10(10):599–608.

[5] Anaya JM. Common mechanisms of autoimmune diseases (the autoimmune tautology). Autoimmun Rev September 2012;11(11):781–4.

[6] Cardenas-Roldan J, Rojas-Villarraga A, Anaya JM. How do autoimmune diseases cluster in families? A systematic review and meta-analysis. BMC Med March 18, 2013;11(1):73.

[7] Anaya JM, Rojas-Villarraga A, García-Carrasco M. The autoimmune tautology: from polyautoimmunity and familial autoimmunity to the autoimmune genes. Autoimmune Dis 2012;2012:297193.

[8] Quintero OL, Rojas-Villarraga A, Mantilla RD, Anaya JM. Autoimmune diseases in the intensive care unit. An update. Autoimmun Rev January 2013;12(3):380–95.

[9] Vadasz Z, Haj T, Kessel A, Toubi E. Age-related autoimmunity. BMC Med April 4, 2013;11.

[10] Chimenti MS, Ballanti E, Perricone C, Cipriani P, Giacomelli R, Perricone R. Immunomodulation in psoriatic arthritis: focus on cellular and molecular pathways. Autoimmun Rev March 2013;12(5):599–606.

[11] Barnett LG, Simkins HM, Barnett BE, Korn LL, Johnson AL, Wherry EJ, et al. B cell antigen presentation in the initiation of follicular helper T cell and germinal center differentiation. J Immunol 2014;192:3607–17.

[12] Taher TE, Ong VH, Bystrom J, Hillion S, Simon Q, Denton CP, et al. Defective regulation of autoreactive IL-6-producing transitional B lymphocytes is associated with disease in patients with systemic sclerosis. Arthritis Rheum March 2018;70(3):450–61.

[13] Shen P, Roch T, Lampropoulou V, O'Connor RA, Stervbo U, Hilgenberg E, Ries S, et al. IL-35-producing B cells are critical regulators of immunity during autoimmune and infectious diseases. Nature March 20, 2014;507(7492):366–70.

[14] Amarilyo G, Lourenço EV, Shi FD, La Cava A. IL-17 promotes murine lupus. J Immunol 2014;193:540–3.

[15] Kastrukoff LF, Morgan NG, Zecchini D, White R, Petkau AJ, Satoh J, Paty DW. A role for natural killer cells in the immunopathogenesis of multiple sclerosis. J Neuroimmunol 1998;86:123–33.

[16] Perricone C, De Carolis C, Giacomelli R, Zaccari G, Cipriani P, Bizzi E, Perricone R. High levels of NK cells in the peripheral blood of patients affected with anti-phospholipid syndrome and recurrent spontaneous abortion: a potential new hypothesis. Rheumatology 2007;46:1574–8.

[17] Kim JM, Park SH, Kim HY, Kwok SK. A plasmacytoid dendritic cells-type I interferon Axis is critically implicated in the pathogenesis of systemic lupus erythematosus. Int J Mol Sci 2015;16(6):14158–70.

[18] Spengler J, Lugonja B, Ytterberg AJ, Zubarev RA, Creese AJ, Pearson MJ, Grant MM, Milward M, Lundberg K, Buckley CD, Filer A, Raza K, Cooper PR, Chapple IL, Scheel-Toellner D. Release of active peptidyl arginine deiminases by neutrophils can explain production of extracellular citrullinated autoantigens in rheumatoid arthritis synovial fluid. Arthritis Rheum 2015;67:3135–45.

[19] Trouw LA, Pickering MC, Blom AM. The complement system as a potential therapeutic target in rheumatic disease. Nat Rev Rheumatol 2017;13(9):538–47.

[20] Yaniv G, Twig G, Shor DB, Furer A, Sherer Y, Mozes O, Komisar O, Slonimsky E, Klang E, Lotan E, Welt M, Marai I, Shina A, Amital H, Shoenfeld Y. A volcanic explosion of autoantibodies in systemic lupus erythematosus: a diversity of 180 different antibodies found in SLE patients. Autoimmun Rev January 2015;14(1):75–9.

[21] Tozzoli R, Villalta D, Bizzaro N. Challenges in the standardization of autoantibody testing: a comprehensive review. Clin Rev Allergy Immunol August 2017;53(1):68–77.

[22] Iagnocco A, Finucci A, Ceccarelli F, Perricone C, Iorgoveanu V, Valesini G. Power Doppler ultrasound monitoring of response to anti-tumour necrosis factor alpha treatment in patients with rheumatoid arthritis. Rheumatology October 2015;54(10):1890–6.

[23] Ceccarelli F, Agmon-Levin N, Perricone C. Genetic factors of autoimmune diseases 2017. J Immunol Res 2017;2017:278924.

[24] Wu H, Zhao M, Tan L, Lu Q. The key culprit in the pathogenesis of systemic lupus erythematosus: aberrant DNA methylation. Autoimmun Rev 2016;15(7):684–9.

[25] Di Comite G, Grazia Sabbadini M, Corti A, Rovere-Querini P, Manfredi AA. Conversation galante: how the immune and the neuroendocrine systems talk to each other. Autoimmun Rev 2007;7(1):23–9.

[26] Valesini G, Gerardi MC, Iannuccelli C, Pacucci VA, Pendolino M, Shoenfeld Y. Citrullination and autoimmunity. Autoimmun Rev June 2015;14(6):490–7.

[27] Akdis M, Aab A, Altunbulakli C, Azkur K, Costa RA, Crameri R, et al. Interleukins (from IL-1 to IL-38), interferons, transforming growth factor beta, and TNF-alpha: receptors, functions, and roles in diseases. J Allergy Clin Immunol 2016;138(4):984–1010.

[28] Vomero M, Barbati C, Colasanti T, Perricone C, Novelli L, Ceccarelli F, Spinelli FR, Di Franco M, Conti F, Valesini G, Alessandri C. Autophagy and rheumatoid arthritis: current knowledges and future perspectives. Front Immunol July 18, 2018;9:1577.

[29] Teng F, Klinger CN, Felix KM, Bradley CP, Wu E, Tran NL, Umesaki Y, Wu HJ. Gut microbiota drive autoimmune arthritis by promoting differentiation and migration of Peyer's patch T follicular helper cells. Immunity April 19, 2016;44(4):875–88.

[30] Sakkas LI, Bogdanos DP. Infections as a cause of autoimmune rheumatic diseases. Auto Immun Highlights 2016;7(1):13.

[31] Segal Y, Blank M, Shoenfeld Y. Tuftsin phosphorylcholine-a novel compound harnessing helminths to fight autoimmunity. Immunol Res 2018 Dec 15.

[32] Theofilopoulos AN, Kono DH, Baccala R. The multiple pathways to autoimmunity. Nat Immunol 2017;18(7):716–24.

[33] Watad A, Azrielant S, Soriano A, Bracco D, Abu Much A, Amital H. Association between seasonal factors and multiple sclerosis. Eur J Epidemiol 2016;31(11):1081–9.

[34] Cohen MR, Isenberg DA. Ultraviolet irradiation in systemic lupus erythematosus: friend or foe? Br J Rheumatol 1996;35(10):1002–7.

[35] Wimalawansa SJ. Non-musculoskeletal benefits of vitamin D. J Steroid Biochem Mol Biol January 2018;175:60–81.

[36] Perricone C, Agmon-Levin N, Shoenfeld N, de Carolis C, Guarino MD, Gigliucci G, et al. Evidence of impaired sense of smell in hereditary angioedema. Allergy 2011;66(1):149–54.

[37] Pannaraj PS, Li F, Cerini C, Bender JM, Yang S, Rollie A, et al. Association between breast milk bacterial communities and establishment and development of the infant gut microbiome. JAMA Pediatr 2017;171(7):647–54.

[38] Vera-Lastra O, Jara LJ, Espinoza LR. Prolactin and autoimmunity. Autoimmun Rev 2002;1(6):360–4.

[39] van Assen S, Agmon-Levin N, Elkayam O, Cervera R, Doran MF, Dougados M, Emery P, Geborek P, Ioannidis JP, Jayne DR, Kallenberg CG, Müller-Ladner U, Shoenfeld Y, Stojanovich L, Valesini G, Wulffraat NM, Bijl M. EULAR recommendations for vaccination in adult patients with autoimmune inflammatory rheumatic diseases. Ann Rheum Dis March 2011;70(3):414–22.

[40] Cohen Tervaert JW, Kappel RM. Silicone implant incompatibility syndrome (SIIS): a frequent cause of ASIA (Shoenfeld's syndrome). Immunol Res 2013;56:293–8.

[41] Shoenfeld Y, Agmon-Levin N. "ASIA" – autoimmune/inflammatory syndrome induced by adjuvants. J Autoimmun 2011;36:4–8.

[42] Dahan S, Segal Y, Shoenfeld Y. Dietary factors in rheumatic autoimmune diseases: a recipe for therapy? Nat Rev Rheumatol June 2017;13(6):348–58.

[43] Lerner A, Matthias T. Changes in intestinal tight junction permeability associated with industrial food additives explain the rising incidence of autoimmune disease. Autoimmun Rev 2015;14(6):479–89.

[44] Versini M, Jeandel PY, Rosenthal E, Shoenfeld Y. Obesity in autoimmune diseases: not a passive bystander. Autoimmun Rev September 2014;13(9):981–1000.

[45] Perricone C, Versini M, Ben-Ami D, Gertel S, Watad A, Segel MJ, Ceccarelli F, Conti F, Cantarini L, Bogdanos DP, Antonelli A, Amital H, Valesini G, Shoenfeld Y. Smoke and autoimmunity: the fire behind the disease. Autoimmun Rev April 2016;15(4):354–74.

[46] Klein TW. Cannabinoid-based drugs as anti-inflammatory therapeutics. Nat Rev Immunol 2005;5(5):400–11.

[47] Di Giuseppe D, Bottai M, Askling J, Wolk A. Physical activity and risk of rheumatoid arthritis in women: a population-based prospective study. Arthritis Res Ther 2015;17.

[48] Colasanti T, Fiorito S, Alessandri C, Serafino A, Andreola F, Barbati C, Morello F, Alfè M, Di Blasio G, Gargiulo V, Vomero M, Conti F, Valesini G. Diesel exhaust particles induce autophagy and citrullination in Normal Human Bronchial Epithelial cells. Cell Death Dis October 19, 2018;9(11):1073.

[49] Mirmira P, Evans-Molina C. Bisphenol A, obesity, and type 2 diabetes mellitus: genuine concern or unnecessary preoccupation? Transl Res 2014;164(1):13–21.

[50] Darvin P, Toor SM, Sasidharan Nair V, Elkord E. Immune checkpoint inhibitors: recent progress and potential biomarkers. Exp Mol Med December 13, 2018;50(12):165.

[51] Fairley JA, Baum CL, Brandt DS, Messingham KA. Pathogenicity of IgE in autoimmunity: successful treatment of bullous pemphigoid with omalizumab. J Allergy Clin Immunol March 2009;123(3):704–5.

[52] Masi A, Bijlsma J, Chikanza I, Pitzalis C, Cutolo M. Neuroendocrine, immunologic, and microvascular systems interactions in rheumatoid arthritis: physiopathogenetic and therapeutic perspectives. Semin Arthritis Rheum 1999;29(2):65–81.

[53] Perricone C, Agmon-Levin N, Shoenfeld Y. Novel pebbles in the mosaic of autoimmunity. BMC Med April 4, 2013;11:101.

Cellular and Molecular Mechanisms

Chapter 3

B Cells: A Main Player in the Development of Autoimmunity

Elias Toubi

Bnai-Zion Medical Center, Faculty of Medicine, Haifa, Israel

B CELLS ARE ANTIGEN-PRESENTING CELLS

The role of B lymphocytes as APCs in activating autoreactive T-cell responses was appreciated almost two decades ago. B cells utilize the specialized major histocompatibility complex class II (MHCII), BCR-bound antigens, and their internalization to present relevant peptides to CD4+ T cells. Effective antigen presentation by B cells involves intracellular and several molecular events. These are: (1) antigen capture and uptake. (2) Creating antigen/BCR complexes with MHCII in cellular compartments. (3) Generation of MHCII/peptide complexes. (4) exocytic transport for presentation of MHCII/ peptide complexes at the surface of B cells. Autoantigen presentation by B cells in autoimmune diseases, such as systemic lupus erythematosus (SLE), is a key step in the activation of autoreactive CD4+ T cells and the production of many pro-inflammatory cytokines [1,2]. T-cell infiltrates in organs such as kidneys and skin were shown to be important features in SLE patients in many early studies. In this respect, the complete absence of T-cell infiltrates in MRL-lpr/lpr mice that lack B cells raised the assumption that B cells are required as APCs for priming autoreactive T cells in SLE. The antigen-presenting function of B cells in autoimmune responses was established by showing that the proliferation of wild-type splenocytes to self-antigens was completely inhibited by blocking the surface Ig-mediated capture by B cells, suggesting again that B cells are required as APCs to induce pathogenic autoimmune T-cell responses [3,4]. In a later study, MHCII-antigen presentation by both B and dendritic cells were shown to be both required (in cooperation) for optimal follicular helper T (Tfh) cells and germinal B-cell differentiation response and the development of high-affinity class-switched antibodies and memory B cells [5]. In line with this, antigen presentation by B cells was shown to be of special importance during germinal center (GC) colonization where B cells engage with Tfh cells leading to their clonal selection and specific antibody affinities. It was well shown that intercellular adhesion molecule 1 (ICAM-1) and ICAM-2 on B cells are essential for long lasting Tfh/B cell interactions and the selection of low-affinity B-cell clones for proliferative clonal expansion. These data suggest that the expression of ICAMs on B cells is important for their effective antigen presentation [6]. In another study, the development of mucosal-associated invariant T (MAIT) cells was shown to be dependent on antigen presentation by B cells. In this case, antigen presentation requires MHC-related protein 1 (MR1) expression as well as commensal bacteria. Treating B cells with toll-like receptor 9 (TLR9) agonists increased MR1 surface expression and related bacterial presentation. This indicates that endosomal TLR9 activation is important for the efficiency of antigen presentation by B cells [7]. Autoantigen presentation by B cells in patients with autoimmune thyroiditis was also studied. In this case, antigen-loaded B cells (by thyroid tissue) have been shown to be capable of inducing the proliferation of auto-specific CD4+ T cells and the development of immune-mediated inflammation [8]. In a very recent study, IgE–immune complexes (IgE-IC) were shown to bind CD23 on B cells leading to their internalization in B cells. Then, B cells recycle IgE-IC in native form to the cell surface followed by the uptake of IgE-IC by DCs in cocultures. Cell-to-cell contact between B cells and DCs was followed by increased upregulation of CD86 and MHCII on DCs. In this study, B cells are shown to act as antigen-presenting cells transferring antigens to more efficient APCs such as DCs. Alternatively, B cells can directly induce DC maturation enhancing by that T-cell stimulation [9].

ACTIVATED B CELLS IN AUTOIMMUNITY

The breakdown of self-tolerance and the development of autoimmune diseases such as SLE is closely related to B-cell hyperactivity and disturbed B-cell homeostasis. The understanding of how B cells are activated in the process of immune-mediated diseases and how memory B cells are switched to become autoreactive is complex. Early studies defined the importance of CD5 and CD95 expression on B cells from SLE patients. It was found that activated B cells are characterized by having increased expression of CD5, and that this expression is in correlation with SLE disease activity. The expression of CD95 on B cells was also evaluated in normal and in SLE patients. In this case, inactive SLE patients were found to have higher proportion of CD95 high B cells being sensitive to undergo apoptosis. This implies that autoantibody-producing B cells are derived from CD95 low B cells thought to be resistant to apoptosis [10]. The differentiation process of naive B cells into IgG-secreting plasma cells is complex, involving many signals and pathways of activation. Looking into one of these, CD27neg B cells with enhanced expression of basal spleen tyrosine kinase (Syk) bright were found to be expanded in patients with SLE. These B cells were characterized as CD38neg but CD20 high and exhibited somatically mutated IgVH rearrangements and showed an enhanced differentiation into IgG-secreting plasma cells in contrast to Syk low B cells. CD27-Syk bright B cells but not Syk low B cells exhibited increased differentiation into CD27 high IgG–secreting cells and were highly inducible when cocultured with IFN-γ or TNF-α. This allows using intracellular markers such as Syk in distinguishing between naïve and memory B-cell subsets and being the source of increased plasma cells in SLE [11]. The role of activated memory B cells in systemic sclerosis (SSc) was also analyzed. Phenotypic characteristics of B cells were assessed in 28 patients with early form of SSc (9 with limited SSc and 19 with diffuse) and in 15 healthy individuals (controls). The following phenotypic subtypes were evaluated: CD19+CD27−IgD+ naïve; CD19+CD27+ memory; CD19+CD27+IgD+ nonswitched memory; CD19+CD27+IgD− switched memory. In addition, CD80+ or CD95+ activated cells were also identified. The proportion of naïve B cells was higher in SSc than in controls, but with decreased numbers of nonswitched memory B cells. In diffuse SSc patients switched memory B cells were found to be significantly higher compared with that in limited SSc. The percentage of CD95+CD27+ memory B cells was also significantly increased in diffused SSc. Increased switched and activated memory B cells are of pathogenic potential role by producing proinflammatory cytokines and autoantibodies [12]. The combination of CpG/TLR9 and IFN-α was shown to increase the differentiation of CD27+IgD+ unswitched memory B cells into CD27 high CD38 high plasmablasts. Whereas, CpG alone induced the differentiation of unswitched memory B cells into B cells with high cytokine production, this differentiation was suppressed by IFN-α. In addition, high m TORC1 activation was noted in CD19+ B cells of patients with SLE and correlated with plasmablasts differentiation and disease activity. The above-described activation pathways of human unswitched memory B cells into plasmablasts seem to be highly important in the pathogenesis of SLE [13]. The identification of human CD43+ B cells and their relation with memory B cells and plasmablasts was recently reported. CD19+CD43+ B cells were found to be of increased proliferating properties than naïve and even memory B cells. Though expressed on both memory B cells and on plasmablasts, CD43+ B cells gave rise to plasmablasts more efficiently than do memory B cells, which suggest that they are closely related to plasmablasts and therefore may be involved in the pathogenesis of autoimmunity [14]. The spontaneous production of IL-10, IL6, and TNF by B cells is minimal. When CD27+ memory B cells are activated with anti-Ig antibodies and CpG, IL-6, and TNF are strongly produced, whereas IL-10 is produced modestly and the capacity of TGF-β production is reduced. Thus, B-cell activation may lead to the development of enhanced immune responses and autoimmunity by decreasing TGF-β production and increasing their proinflammatory properties [15]. The excess of B-cell activating factor (BAFF) leads to the expansion of marginal zone (MZ) B cells and to their capacity in activating T cells. Increased BAFF level has been detected in the serum of many autoimmune diseases such as SLE, RA, and Sjogren's syndrome and in correlation with disease activity. Decreased BAFF receptor expression on peripheral B cells was found to be in association with enhanced disease activity of Sjogren's syndrome (pSS) and SLE. B cells from 20 patients with pSS, 19 with SLE, and 15 controls were analyzed by flow cytometry to assess the expression of BAFF receptor. The expression of BAFF receptor on memory CD27+ B cells was significantly decreased in patients with pSS and SLE. Serum BAFF level is inversely correlated with BAFF receptor expression. Decreased BAFF receptor expression was found to be in correlation with SLE disease activity index. This downregulation is suggested to be the consequence of chronic increase in BAFF. BAFF receptor levels on B cells may serve as a biomarker for assessing autoimmune disease activity [16]. The expression of BAFF receptor 3 (BR3) on B cells from SLE patients was further examined in a later study. Here also, BAFF levels were increased in the serum of these patients and in positive correlation with SLE disease activity but negatively with BR3 expression. Reduced BR3 expression was found to be on CD27− and CD27+ B cells of all SLE patients, but this was more in patients with lupus nephritis. This reduction is again suggested to act as a biomarker for active SLE, namely the occurrence of lupus nephritis [17]. The capacity of endogenous BAFF and IL-21 and exogenous factors such as CpG to induce the production of PR3-ANCA in granulomatosis with polyangiitis (GPA) was studied. Here, the stimulation with BAFF and IL-21 significantly increased ANCA production. This production was further increased by the addition of CpG-ODN. These data demonstrate how toll-like receptor 9 synergizes with IL-21 and with BAFF leading to increased ANCA production [18]. The abovementioned data support the notion that B-cell activation is complex and many signaling pathways are required for the development of autoreactivity and proinflammatory B cells leading to the development of autoimmune diseases.

PROINFLAMMATORY B CELLS AND AUTOIMMUNITY

Humoral immune responses begin when B lymphocytes are activated by antigens followed by the secretion of relevant antibodies. GCs are formed in the follicles of peripheral lymphoid organs when activated B cells migrate into the follicles and proliferate. Antigen-activated B cells are produced in GCs and obtain the ability to survive for long periods. These are memory B cells capable of rapid responses to previously recognized antigens. The production of large quantities of isotype-switched, high-affinity antibodies is increased after second exposure to antigens, usually following the activation of memory cells in GCs and the formation of immune complexes. In addition to their antibody-producing ability, activated B cells via the BCR, CD40 and toll-like receptors are also the source of many proinflammatory cytokines such as IL-10, IL-6, and IFNs.

IL-10-Producing B Cells in Autoimmunity

IL-10 has an important role in the growth, survival, and differentiation of B cells in SLE patients. Increased IL-10 production induces B-cell hyperreactivity resulting in antibody production by switching plasma cells and the development of immune complexes [19]. Increased IL-10 in the serum of SLE patients was suggested in many reports to be associated with SLE disease activity. The loss of B-cell tolerance in the elderly is characterized by the increased prevalence of autoantibodies and rheumatoid factor. The issue of how and which cytokine these B cells produce and how this is related to autoimmunity was assessed. Absolute numbers of circulating B cells were similar in both young and old individuals. However, numbers of transitional B cells (CD19+CD27−CD38hiCD24hi) were decreased in old individuals. Following a short term in vitro stimulation of whole blood, the number of B cells capable of producing TNF-α was similar in young and old individuals, however, IL-10-producing B cells were decreased only in old individuals. Decreased IL-10-producing B cells was mainly noticed in old individuals in which ANA was positive but was retained in those in which RF was positive. These findings suggest that IL-10+ B cells may impact the development of ANAs and RFs in the elderly [20]. When pre-naïve B cells are stimulated through CD40, they produce large amounts of IL-10 but are unable to suppress CD4+ T-cell cytokine production. Differentiated pre-naïve B cells are autoreactive, thus, they produce IgM autoantibodies with reactivity to single-stranded deoxyribonucleic acid. In SLE, pre-naïve B cells have increased expression of costimulatory molecules but reduced ability of producing IL-10, resulting in increased CD4+ T-cell proliferation and the development of autoimmunity [21].

IL-6-producing B Cells and Autoimmunity

Activated B cells are a source of IL-6 production, promoting by that Tfh cell differentiation. The lack of IL-6-producing B cells was shown to decrease spontaneous GC formation in a mouse model of SLE, thus, inhibiting the development of autoimmunity and the formation of switched autoantibodies. This finding suggests that IL-6-producing B cells contribute to autoimmunity through local IL-6 production, inducing by that Tfh differentiation and autoimmune GC formation [22]. IL-6 drives terminal B-cell differentiation and secretion of immunoglobulins. In one study, SLE-like disease parameters were studied in IL-6-deficient BXSB mice. Survival of IL-6-deficient mice was significantly prolonged in association with reduced autoimmune manifestations. B cells costimulated with TLR7 and BCR produced high levels of IL-6 which was further enhanced by IFN-1 stimulation. This suggests that high production of IL-6 by B cells increased by IFN-1 and TLR7 accelerates autoimmunity and the progression of SLE-like disease [23]. In a recent study, high sensitive C-reactive proteins (hs-CRP) and IL-6 levels were analyzed in SLE in relation with SLE disease activity. Mean hs-CRP levels were significantly higher in SLE than in controls. Similarly, IL-6 levels were significantly higher in active SLE as compared with inactive SLE. This study confirms a good correlation between IL-6 and disease activity indicating its direct involvement in SLE-related inflammation [24]. The distribution of transitional B-cell subsets in patients with systemic sclerosis was found to be altered in association with increased IL-6 production and altered self-tolerance. Defects in B-lymphocyte tolerance exist in parallel with altered apoptosis following BCR signaling and the failure to suppress autoreactive B cells, namely, the failure in regulating Scl-70 production. These data emphasize the role of autoreactive IL-6-producing transitional B cells in the pathogenesis of systemic sclerosis [25]. In a most recent study, anti-IL-6 therapy restored abnormal B-cell functions, namely, cytokine-mediated inflammation and autoreactivity. Rheumatoid arthritis B cells produce higher amounts of proinflammatory cytokines such as IL-8, IL-6, and others. Being continuously hyperactive, they become defective in their ability to maintain protective functions. Anti-IL-6 therapy reversed B-cell abnormalities including increased cytokine levels and loss of tolerance, indicating that abnormal IL-6 signaling is responsible for most humoral defects in RA [26].

IFNs and B Cells in Autoimmunity

When B cells are stimulated by the TLR9 agonists-CpGs they proliferate and they secrete antibodies and many cytokines including IL-6. Toll-like receptor 9 agonists are also used in many adjuvants to boost both innate and adaptive immunity. In response to these adjuvants, B cells secrete proinflammatory cytokines such as type 1 IFNs pointing to the different pathways of stimulation by which they play role in different immune responses [27]. The mechanisms by which autoreactive B cells generate somatically mutated and class-switched pathogenic autoantibodies within developed GCs are continuously investigated. A possible mechanism in this respect is that B-cell-intrinsic IFN-γ receptor and STAT1 signaling are required for GC and Tfh cell formation. B-cell-specific IFN-γ receptor deficiency in autoimmune mice models resulted in reduced Tfh responses and altered titers of autoantibodies. IFN-γ deficiency did not affect GC, Tfh cell, or antibody responses against T-cell-dependent foreign antigens, suggesting that IFN-γ receptor signaling is uniquely important for autoantibody responses, but not for polyclonal antibody production. This suggests that IFN-γ signaling is central for the development of autoimmunity and therefore can be a potential target for a better beneficial treatment of SLE [28].

IN SUMMARY

The role of B cells in healthy and disease immune responses is increasingly studied. Long-lived plasma cells are important in maintaining antibody secretion against foreign antigens and following vaccinations. In autoimmunity, autoreactive B cells are the source of specific autoantibodies but also of proinflammatory cytokines. Many signaling pathways are recently reported, aiming to identify their complexity. Some of these are summarized in this chapter.

REFERENCES

[1] Adler LN, Jiang W, Bhamidipati K, Millican M, Macaubas C, Hung SC, Mellins ED. The other function: class II-restricted antigen presentation by B cells. Front Immunnol 2017;8:319.

[2] Choi SC, Morel L. B cell contribution of the CD4+ T cell inflammatory phenotypes in systemic lupus erythematosus. Autoimmunity 2017;50:37–41.

[3] Chan O, Shlomchik MJ. A new role for B cells in systemic autoimmunity: B cells promote spontaneous T cell activation in MRL-lpr/lpr mice. J Immunol 1998;160:51–9.

[4] Falcone M, Lee J, Patstone G, Yeung B, Sarvetnick N. B lymphocytes are crucial antigen-presenting cells in the pathogenic autoimmune response to GAD65 antigen in nonobese diabetic mice. J Immunol 1998;161:1163–8.

[5] Barnett LG, Simkins HM, Barnett BE, Korn LL, Johnson AL, Wherry EJ, et al. B cell antigen presentation in the initiation of follicular helper T cell and germinal center differentiation. J Immunol 2014;192:3607–17.

[6] Zaretsky I, Atrakchi O, Mazor RD, Stoler-Barak L, Biram A, Feigelson SW, et al. ICAMs support B cell interactions with T follicular helper cells and promote clonal selection. J Exp Med 2017;214:3435–48.

[7] Liu J, Brutkiewicz RR. The toll-like receptor 9 signaling pathway regulates MRI-mediated bacterial antigen presentation in B cells. Immunology 2017;152:232–42.

[8] Kuklina EM, Smirnova EN, Nekrasova IV, Balashova TS. Role of B cells in presentation of autoantigens to CD4+ T cells in patients with autoimmune thyroiditis. Dokl Biol Sci 2015;464:263–6.

[9] Engeroff P, Fellmann M, Yerly D, Bachmann MF, Vogel M. A novel recycling mechanism of native IgE-antigen complexes in human B cells facilitates transfer of antigen to dendritic cells for antigen presentation. J Allergy Clin Immunol 2018;142:557–685.

[10] Huck S, Jamin C, Younou P, Zouali M. High density expression of CD95 on B cells and underrepresentation of the B-1 cell subset in human lupus. J Autoimmun 1998;11:449–55.

[11] Fleischer SJ, Giesecke C, Mei HE, Lipsky PE, Daridon C, Dorner T. Increased frequency of unique spleen tyrosine kinase bright memory B cell population in systemic lupus erythematosus. Arthritis Rheumatol 2014;66:3424–35.

[12] Simon D, Balogh P, Bognar A, Kellermayer Z, Engelmann P, Nemeth P, et al. Reduced non-switched memory B cell subsets cause imbalance in B cell repertoire in systemic sclerosis. Clin Exp Rheumatol 2016;34(100):30–6.

[13] Torigoe M, Iwata S, Nakayamada S, Sakata K, Zhang M, Hajime M, et al. Metabolic reprogramming commits differentiation of human CD27+IgD+ B cells to plasmablasts or CD27-IgD- cells. J Immunol 2017;199:425–34.

[14] Inui M, Hirota S, Hirano K, Fujii H, Sugahara-Tobinai A, et al. Human CD43+ B cells are closely related not only to memory B cells phenotypically but also to plasmablasts developmentally in healthy in heathy individuals. Int Immunol 2015;27:346–55.

[15] Molnarfi N, Bjarnadottir K, Benkhoucha M, Juillard C, Lalive PH. Activation of human B cells negatively regulates TGF-β production. J NeuroInflamm 2017;14:13.

[16] Sellam J, Miceli-Richard C, Gottenberg JE, Ittah M, Lavie F, Lacabaratz C, et al. Decreased B cell activating factor receptor expression on peripheral lymphocytes associated with increased disease activity in primary Sjogren's syndrome and systemic lupus erythematosus. Ann Rheum Dis 2007;66:790–7.

[17] Zhao LD, Li Y, Smith Jr MF, Wang JS, Zhang W, Tang FL, et al. Expression of BAFF/BAFF receptors and their correlation with disease activity in Chinese SLE patients. Lupus 2010;19:1534–49.

[18] Lepse N, Land J, Rutgers A, Kallenberg CG, Stegeman CA, Abdulahad WH, Heeringa P. Toll-like receptor 9 activation enhances B cell activating factor and interleukin-21 induced anti-proteinase 3 autoantibody production in vitro. Rheumatology (Oxf) 2016;55:162–72.

[19] Peng H, Wang W, Zhou M, Li R, Pan HF, Ye DQ. Role of interleukin-10 and interleukin-10 receptor in systemic lupus erythematosus. Clin Rheumatol 2013;32:1255–66.

[20] van der Geest KS, Lorencetti PG, Abdulahad WH, Horst G, Huitema M, Roozendaal C, et al. Aging-dependent decline of IL-10 producing B cells coincides with production of antinuclear antibodies but not rheumatoid factors. Exp Gerontol 2016;75:24–9.

[21] Sim JH, Kim HR, Chang SH, Kim IJ, Lipsky PE, Lee J. Autoregulatory function of interleukin-10-producing pre-naïve B cells is defective in systemic lupus erythematosus. Arthritis Res Ther 2015;17:190.

[22] Arkatkar T, Du SW, Jacobs HM, Dam EM, Hou B, Buckner JH, et al. B cell derived IL-6 initiates spontaneous germinal center formation during systemic autoimmunity. J Exp Med 2017;214:3207–17.

[23] Jain S, Park G, Sproule TJ, Christianson GJ, Leeth CM, Wang H, et al. Interleukin 6 accelerates mortality by promoting the progression of the systemic lupus erythematosus-like disease of BXSB.Yaa mice. PLoS One 2016;11:e0153059.

[24] Umare V, Nadkarni A, Nadker M, Rajadhyksha A, Khadilkar P, Ghosh K, Pradhan VD. Do high sensitivity C-reactive protein and serum IL-6 levels correlate with disease activity in systemic lupus erythematosus patients? J Postgrad Med 2017;63:92–5.

[25] Taher TE, Ong VH, Bystrom J, Hillion S, Simon Q, Denton CP, et al. Defective regulation of autoreactive IL-6-producing transitional B lymphocytes is associated with disease in patients with systemic sclerosis. Arthritis Rheumatol 2018;70:450–61.

[26] Fleischer S, Ries S, Shen P, Lheritier A, Cazals F, Burmester GR, et al. Anti-interleukin-6 signaling therapy rebalances the disrupted cytokine production of B cells from patients with active rheumatoid arthritis. Eur J Immunol 2018;48:194–203.

[27] Akkaya M, Akkaya B, Miozzo P, Rawat M, Pena M, Sheehan PW, et al. B cells produce type 1 IFNs in response to the TLR9 agonists CpGs conjugated to cationic lipids. J Immunol 2017;199:931–40.

[28] Domeier PP, Chodisetti SB, Soni C, Schell SL, Elias MJ, Wong EB, et al. IFN-γ receptor and STAT1 signaling in B cells are central to spontaneous germinal center formation and autoimmunity. J Exp Med 2016;213:715–32.

Chapter 4

B Regulatory Cells in Autoimmunity

Zahava Vadasz[1], Elias Toubi[2]
[1]The Division of Allergy and Clinical Immunology, Bnai-Zion Medical Center, Faculty of Medicine, Technion, Haifa-Israel; [2]Bnai-Zion Medical Center, Faculty of Medicine, Haifa, Israel

INTRODUCTION

Traditionally, the main role of B cells was considered to be the source of antibody production. Normally, they produce antibodies against bacterial or viral invaders, but they also produce low affinity and low titers of autoantibodies. B cells are also antigen-presenting cells (APC) and as such, they activate Th1 and Th2 effector cells and induce relevant proinflammatory cytokines. When autoreactive B cells are continuously triggered by autoantigens or immune complexes, plasma cells are switched and become IgG autoantibody producers. Many factors such as B lymphocyte factor and IL-6 are responsible for the breakdown of self-tolerance and the development of autoimmune diseases such as systemic lupus erythematosus (SLE) [1,2]. The identification of a subset of B cells as producers of inhibitory cytokines such as IL-10 and later TGF-β, IL-35, and IgG4 established the issue of B regulatory (Breg) cells being highly important in regulating immune-mediated inflammation. The understanding that this subset of cells has many faces and that the continuous reporting on Breg cells is a big family requires a better identification and characterization of this important subset of cells.

IL-10–PRODUCING B REGULATORY CELLS

The role of IL-10–producing Breg cells was recognized many years ago. In one of the earliest studies, they were characterized being able to suppress the progression of intestinal inflammation in a murine model. They were shown to downregulate inflammation by decreasing IL-1–mediated responses and STAT3 activation rather than by altering polarized T effector cell responses [3]. Subsequently, IL-10 production by a subset of B cells was shown to be increased when arthritogenic splenocytes were activated using anti-CD40. The transfer of these Bregs into a mice model of collagen-induced arthritis (CIA) inhibited T helper cell differentiation and prevented the development of arthritis. The failure of B cells, isolated from IL-10 knockout mice, to induce this regulatory function alluded to the fact that this protective function of B cells is IL-10 dependent [4]. The next step was to study several membrane markers for a better characterization of this subset of B cells. One of these early reports was the one showing that CD25highCD1dhigh B cells are of immune regulatory property in patients suffering from rheumatoid arthritis (RA). They were shown to be CD27high (memory B cells) and IL-10 producing [5]. The presence of higher amounts of CD25highCD1dhigh B cells was reported to be in association with inactive antineutrophil cytoplasmic antibody–related vasculitis. However, lower amounts of these Breg cells were found to be in association with active disease [6]. In this respect, our group reported Breg cells as being CD25highCD86highCD1d high. The incubation of these cells with autologous Treg cells induced their increased FoxP3 and IL-10 expression, but most importantly, they also increased their suppressive functional property [7]. The other subgroup of IL-10–producing Breg cells is CD38highCD1dhighCD424high cells. These were shown to suppress TNF-α and IFN-γ secretion from activated effector T cells in normal individuals. However, when these Breg cells were evaluated in SLE patients, they failed to achieve a proper regulatory effect, thereby suggesting they play an important role in the pathogenesis of SLE [8].

CD5HIGHIL-10HIGH B REGULATORY CELLS

During the same period as the above-identified Breg cells, many reported about CD5+ B cells being IL-10 producing and of regulatory properties in many immune-mediated responses. In one of the early studies, the trigger of toll-like receptor (TLR) 9 was found to induce the secretion of high amounts of IL-10 from CD5+ B cells but not from CD5− B cells. The secretion of IL-10 by CD5+ B cells prevented optimal IL-12 secretion by immature DCs, thus inhibiting Th1 priming. This suggested that CD5+ B cells could be identified as CD5highIL-10high Breg cells [9]. In another study, T cell–mediated inflammation was enhanced when assessed in CD19-deficient mice. This inflammation was negatively regulated by a subset of Breg cells that were identified as CD5highCD1dhigh. Adoptive transfer of these Breg cells suppressed T cell–mediated inflammation in an IL-10–dependent manner, thereby establishing CD5highIL-10high as a unique subset of potent regulatory cells [10]. In a mice model of experimental autoimmune encephalomyelitis (EAE), the progression of disease symptoms was noticed following the depletion of IL-10–producing CD5highCD1dhigh B cells. In this case, the adoptive transfer of these cells in B cell–depleted mice, before EAE induction, delayed EAE progression. However, the transfer of Breg cells during disease progression was of no beneficial effect, suggesting that the timing of Breg initiation is crucial [11]. The lack or loss of CD5high Breg cells has been demonstrated by exacerbated symptoms in EAE, chronic colitis, contact hypersensitivity, CIA, and nonobese diabetic mouse models. Here again, it is demonstrated that Breg cell function is mediated by the production of IL-10 by either B-1, marginal zone (MZ), or transitional 2-MZ precursor B cell subsets [12]. The presence of CD5high B lymphocytes was looked in human spondyloarthritis (SpA). Peripheral blood B cells from patients with SpA, RA, and healthy individuals were studied by flow cytometry. Sorted CD5+ and CD5– B cells were analyzed for the expression of co-stimulatory molecules and cytokine production. CD5+ B cells from patients with SpA expressed increased levels of human-leucocyte -antigen- DR (HLA-DR) but low levels of CD80 and CD86. In vitro activation of Breg cells failed to induce an increased expression of CD86 but induced significant amounts of IL-10 and IL-6. The expansion of CD5high B cells in SpA is speculated to be the result of continuous compensatory responses in an attempt to attenuate inflammatory responses [13]. The role of CD5high Breg cells was additionally evaluated in a mouse model of CIA. In this case, decreased numbers of IL-10–producing Breg cells were found to be in association with increased IL-17–producing CD4+ T (Th17) cells in both spleen and draining lymph nodes of mice during the active stage of disease. When CD5highIL-10high Breg cells were transferred to these mice, one could notice a marked delay of arthritis and altered severity of joint damage. These findings suggest that the regulatory role of CD5high Breg cells in CIA is mediated via the suppression of Th-17 cell generation [14]. The issue of how to efficiently increase the number of CD5+ B cells and how to improve their IL-10 production was also assessed. The incubation of B cells with anti-CD40 and IL-4 increased the ability of CD5+ B cells to secrete IL-10. Further incubation of these cells with IL-21 resulted in CD5+ B cell expansion and increased IL-10 secretion. This suggested that regulatory B cells control T cell autoimmunity through IL-21–dependent cognate interactions [15]. While sharing similar regulatory mechanisms, such as IL-10 dependency, Breg cells differ in exhibiting their suppressive effects by expressing other inhibitory molecules such as TGF-β, PDL-1, FoxP3, and Fas-ligand (FasL). In a recent study, our group was able to show that both IL-10 and FoxP3 expressions were found to be significantly increased in activated CD19+CD25high B cells of active SLE patients when compared to these of the normal controls. At this point, CD25highFoxP3high cells were also found to be IL-10–producing B cells. The expansion of this subgroup of cells was found to be in positive correlation with increased systemic lupus erythematous disease activity index (Score) (SLEDAI) and in association with lupus nephritis [16]. In agreement with these findings, CD19+CD25highFoxP3high Breg cells were found to be increased in the cerebrospinal fluid of active patients with relapsing-remitting multiple sclerosis when analyzed in patients in remission. The expansion of these cells suggests that an increased number of Breg cells is required to suppress (though not efficiently) immune-mediated responses and to prevent further inflammatory responses [17]. Contrary to the above findings, decreased amounts of CD19+FoxP3high B cells were reported in patients suffering from RA, in negative association with disease severity scores and in negative correlation with erythrocyte sedimentation rate and C-reactive protein levels [18]. In a recent study, the adoptive transfer of FoxP3-expressing Breg cells into a mouse model resulted in the amelioration of autoimmune arthritis in association with increased Treg/Th17 balance [19]. Although described in CD19+CD25high (as mentioned above), most reports suggest that FoxP3-expressing B cells are mostly found in CD5high B cells. They are reported to comprise 8.5% of all CD19+CD5+ B cells and are considered a unique subset of regulatory B cells [20]. CD19+CD5highFoxP3high Breg cells were reported to be involved in non–IgE-mediated food allergies, namely, playing a role in maintaining tolerance to milk allergies [21]. The reporting on FoxP3 expression in Breg cells is still controversial and should be carefully evaluated by excluding many potential options of artificial contamination. Recently, attention has been directed to a new subset of Breg cells characterized as CD5highFas-ligand (FasLhigh) and hence they have been dubbed "killer" B cells. Increased FasL expression on B cells was first reported in infectious diseases such as in schistosomal infection where by inducing increased apoptosis of cytotoxic T cells they prevented efficient antiviral immune responses and enabled the persistence of this infection. A culture of purified B cells with recombinant IL-4, IL-10, and soluble egg antigens led to the increased expression of FasL on these B cells [21]. In line with this, killer Breg cells were reported to prevent efficient antitumor immune responses allowing the spread of many malignancies [22]. In a study by our group (unpublished), we assessed the role of these cells in the chronic hepatitis C virus (HCV) infection and asked if they contribute to the increased viral load and persistence of HCV and its related autoimmunity. Here also, CD19+CD5highFasLhigh cells were found to increase significantly in HCV patients when compared with those in healthy individuals. The incubation of these cells, purified from HCV patients, with autologous CD8+ T cells enhanced their apoptosis and was shown to be IL-10 dependent. Finally, the expansion of killer Breg cells in HCV was in positive correlation with an increased viral load and with the presence of

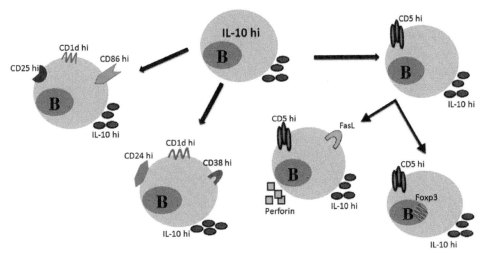

FIGURE 4.1 B regulatory cells are identified as IL-10–producing cells but with many different phenotypic faces: (1) They are CD25highCD86high. (2) They are CD38highCD24high. Recently, CD5high B cells are appreciated as a main subset of B regulatory cells, some of which are Fas-ligand expressing and some identified to be FoxP3 expressing.

autoantibodies such as anticardiolipin and rheumatoid factor. In recent years, many studies have focused on the role of killer B cells in autoimmunity. In this respect, FasL-expressing B cells were assessed in a mouse model of CIA in which all CD4+ T cells recognize a single peptide of type II collagen. Increased arthritis severity was found to be associated with altered numbers of CD5+ B cells. FasL was highly expressed on CD5high but not on CD5low B cells, and when CD5highFasLhigh B cells were cocultured with antigen-dependent T cells, they resulted in their increased apoptosis. In addition, reduced production of IL-17 was noted when antigen-driven T cells were cocultured with these Breg cells. The direct killing effect of FasL-expressing B cells was confirmed by using an antigen-specific T cell hybridoma line. Reduced numbers of these killer Breg cells and therefore reduced antigen-driven T cell apoptosis are associated with disease severity [23]. See Fig. 4.1.

OTHER REGULATORY MOLECULES/CYTOKINES

B Regulatory Cells and IgG4

During the process of successful immunotherapy for allergic diseases, we usually see a decrease of specific IgE and a gradual increase of allergen-specific IgG4 antibodies. The clinical improvement of allergic symptoms correlates with a 10- to 100-fold decrease of allergen-specific IgE/IgG4 ratio. IgG4 is well-appreciated for its antiinflammatory properties; e.g., their low affinity of activating FcERI receptors and their low ability of complement activation [24]. The differentiation and isotype switching of human B cells is partly IL-10 dependent. It inhibits IL-4–induced IgE class switch recombination on one side but promotes IgG4 production by B cells on the other side. The issue of whether all IL-10–producing B cells are IgG4 producers or IgG4-producing B cells is a subset of these cells being expanded under specific allergen/antigen stimulation is not clear enough. In this respect, it was shown that IgG4 is produced more than 15-fold from purified IL-10BRI cells than from general B cells, whereas other immunoglobulin isotypes were produced at equal rates [25–29]. When B cells, specific to the major bee venom allergen, were isolated and analyzed from healthy beekeepers, they were found to express increased levels of IL-10 and mature IgG4mRNA [30]. The clinical significance of IgG4-expressing B cells in beekeepers was evaluated. First, it was shown that phospholipase A2–specific (bee venom) B cells from beekeepers are mainly IL-10 and IgG4-producing B cells. Furthermore, these B cells were evaluated in allergic individuals to bee venom after successful immunotherapy. In this case, IL-10 and IgG4-producing B cells were significantly increased to almost the same levels seen in healthy beekeepers, postulating that successful allergen immunotherapy is linked to increased serum IgG4 and IL-10 [29,31]. In parasite infections, such as the Schistosoma mansoni infection in children, it was found that a correlation exists between increased IL-10 production in response to parasitic antigens and the decreased incidence of atopy. In line with this finding, the protective role of high levels of IgG4 antibodies in helminth-infected subjects was reported and discussed in other studies [32]. IL-10–producing in general and IgG4-producing Breg cells in specific diseases seem to perform as two important arms in maintaining immune tolerance, namely, preventing proinflammatory immune responses to allergens [29].

B Regulatory Cells and IL-35

B cells have been shown to mediate the regulatory effects independent of IL-10 secretion. Thus, many attempts were made to find\demonstrate other suppressive mediators that could account for their broader biological functions in immune regulation. Several studies have focused on elucidating the potential of enhancing Breg functions, e.g., drive IL-10 secretion, or act independently or synergistically with IL-10 to elicit maximal regulatory functions. In transcriptome analysis of activated B cells (with TLR4 and CD40 co-stimulation) Ebi3, the beta chain of the inhibitory cytokine, IL-35, emerged as one of the differentially regulated genes [33]. In this study, it was also found that B cells constitutively express the IL-35 alpha chain, p35, but do not express p40. Therefore, following B cell stimulation, there is increased Ebi3 and p35 transcription and IL-35 secretion, identifying B cells as a novel source of IL-35. In an in vivo model of B cell–restricted IL-35–deficient mice, it was found that these mice developed exacerbated EAE but were protected from *S. typhimurium* (Salmonella)–induced sepsis relative to the controls [33]. These responses were the result of the enhanced antigen-presenting potential of IL-35–deficient B cells (as was demonstrated by higher expression of major histocompatibility complex (MHC) class II, CD80, CD86), thereby stimulating CD4+ T cells to secrete proinflammatory cytokines and induce a higher proliferation rate. Thus, it seems that the suppressive effects of B cells–derived IL-35 are mainly because of their ability to regulate APC function of B cells and thereby limiting autoimmunity or mediating pathogen clearance. In another study, it was shown that the addition of recombinant IL-35 induced IL-10- and IL-35 secreting Bregs (IL-10+\IL-35+ Breg cells) that efficiently suppressed proliferation of CD19 + B cells [34]. IL-35+ Breg cells efficiently inhibited the progression of the initial and established stages of experimental autoimmune uveitis (EAU). This inhibition was mediated by the expansion of endogenous Bregs and Tregs and inhibition of pathogenic Th1 and Th17 effector cells. To emphasize the relationships between IL-10 and IL-35 to the suppressive ability of Breg cells, B cells deficient in IL-12a, IL-12Rb2, and IL-10 were cultured in the presence of rIL-35 and evaluated for their capacity to decrease EAU. In this study it was found that the loss of IL-10 completely abrogated the suppressive effects of IL-35; thus, it seems that IL-10 is the final mediator in the suppressive ability of IL-35+ Bregs [34]. In conjunction with this, it was demonstrated that the addition of the neutralizing IL-10 antibody abrogated the suppressive effects of rIL-35. Thus, the finding that the addition of rIL-35 to human B cells induces IL-10 expression and thereby inhibiting B cell proliferation and proinflammatory activation suggests that IL-35 may hold a promise for autologous Breg induction [35].

B Regulatory Cells and CD72

The activation and proliferation of B cells is usually balanced/regulated by many B cell receptors and co-receptors such as FcγRIIb, CD22, PIR-B, and CD72 among others. When B cells are overactivated or when autoreactive B cells are expanded, a regulation of their activation threshold is required to maintain their balanced immune response. Co-receptors such as CD72 are one of these regulators, the role of which is recently appreciated in the maintenance of self-tolerance [36]. CD72 (a 45kDa type II transmembrane glycoprotein) is a B cell co-receptor, the extracellular domain of which contains C-type lectin-like domain, and its intracellular N-terminal region has an immune-receptor tyrosine-based inhibition motif (ITIM). CD72 is expressed as a homodimer on all B cell lineages except plasma cells and functions as inhibitory co-receptor, which negatively regulates B cell receptor (BCR) signaling [37]. By signaling CD72, cytoplasmic ITIMs are recruited and phosphorylated to induce the activation of phosphatases such as SH2 domain-containing protein tyrosine phosphatases, followed by the inhibition of BCR signaling. BCR-mediated signals are therefore enhanced in CD72-deficient cells or when CD72 expression on B cells is neutralized by blocking Monoclonal antibodies (mAbs) [38]. In addition, decreased CD72 expression on B cells blocks BCR-mediated cell death, promotes B cells survival and proliferation, and increases the expression of MHC class II [39]. The suppressive role of CD72 attracted attention because of its importance in autoimmune diseases mainly in preventing SLE. SLE is a systemic autoimmune disease characterized by the loss of B cell tolerance and the increased population and activity of autoreactive B cells against various nuclear antigens. Studies regarding the pathophysiology of SLE have emphasized the pivotal role of B cells in this disease, not only as a producer of autoantibodies and proinflammatory cytokines but also as a regulator of autoantigen reactive T cells. CD72 has an important role in the development of an SLE-like disease in animal models. CD72-deficient mice spontaneously produce hyperproliferative and hyperactive B cells with increased production of antinuclear autoantibodies [40]. Moreover, polymorphism in the extracellular domain of CD72 was reported to be associated with SLE in mice. In mice, the CD72^c allele is a crucial modifier gene that promotes lupus [16]; however, the replacement of CD72^c with the CD72^b allele reduces SLE disease severity [41]. In humans, several CD72 polymorphisms were identified in the upstream coding region and introns. One study defined the point mutation FCGR2B-Ile232Thr in the FcγRIIb inhibitory receptor as a risk factor for SLE in individuals who carry the CD72*1 haplotype and as a resistance factor for the CD72*2 haplotype [25]. Another polymorphism is defined as one or two repeats of 13 nucleotides in intron 8, leading to the skipping of exon 8 coding and to the alternative splicing of exon 9-CD72Δex8 isoform [42]. At a later date, the same group tried to understand the biological advance of CD72Δex8 compared with CD72 full length. This study revealed that CD72Δex8 does not regulate BCR signaling but actually accumulates in the endoplasmic reticulum and therefore can regulate antibody production [43]. The importance of CD72 expression on immune cells has been assessed in many studies. In one of these, the expression of CD72 protein and mRNA in peripheral blood mononuclear cells from adolescent patients with SLE was significantly decreased when compared with that on B cells of controls [44]. In another study, the decreased expression of CD72 and increased IgG class switching were documented on B cells from patients with lupus nephritis [45]. In this respect, we reported on CD72 expression on activated B cells being significantly lower in SLE patients, in correlation with SLE disease activity, namely the SLEDI score. In addition, we were able to demonstrate that semaphorin3A (sema3A) could reconstruct the regulatory function of B cells by upregulating CD72 expression on B cells [22]. In another study published by our group, we looked at the soluble form of CD72 (sCD72) in SLE patients' serum as compared with the normal controls. Here, we revealed higher levels of sCD72 in SLE patients' serum when compared with RA patients (disease control) and healthy controls. These higher levels were found in correlation with disease severity, namely, with lupus nephritis and increased titers of relevant autoantibodies [46]. A more recent study showed that CD72 binds to a lupus-related self-antigen Sm/RNP antigen and by doing so can specifically inhibit B cell response to the endogenous TLR7 ligand [27]. Taken all the above-mentioned data, it is convincing that CD72 is an important B cell regulator that has an important role in SLE pathogenesis and in maintaining self-tolerance.

B Regulatory Cells and Semaphorin3A

Semaphorins are a large family of membrane-bound and secreted proteins that were found as axonal guidance molecules during neurodevelopment. Semaphorins are continuously reported as being important regulators of immune-mediated responses, and thus, they are also called "immune semaphorins." They are expressed on most immune cells such as T, B, and macrophages and were shown to be involved in all phases of both normal and pathological immune responses [47–49]. In the last decade, sema3A was recognized as one of the most active semaphorins in the modulation of inflammatory conditions thereby receiving special attention. The expression of sema3A and its receptors, neuropilin-1 (NP-1), NP-2, and plexins, was found to be increased on differentiating macrophages and activated T cells, suggesting that they may be frontline players in immune-mediated diseases [49,50]. In several publications, sema3A was found to decrease T cells proliferation and proinflammatory cytokines' production. Similarly, sema3A was also found to be involved in the regulation of human thymocyte migration and proven to inhibit triggered chemotaxis by CXCL12 [51,52]. Our research group published several reports in which the relationship between sema3A and SLE was assessed. Sema3A serum levels were found to be significantly lower in SLE patients than that in RA patients (55.04 ± 16.30 ng/mL vs. 65.54 ± 14.82 ng/mL, $P = .018$) and much lower in normal individuals (55.04 ± 16.30 ng/mL vs. 74.41 ± 17.60 ng/mL, $P < .0001$). Lower serum sema3A levels in SLE patients were found to be in negative correlation with SLE disease activity, renal damage, and the presence of relevant autoantibodies ($R = -0.89$, $P < .0001$) [53]. Being the source of autoantibodies and proinflammatory cytokines, the regulatory status of B cells in respect with sema3a was also evaluated. The expression of sema3A on Breg cells, namely CD19+CD25high and NP-1+, was analyzed. As expected, sema3A expression on these cells was significantly lower in SLE patients when compared with the B cells from normal individuals, suggesting this to be partially responsible for B cell autoreactivity in SLE. Our other finding was the downregulation of NP-1 expression on B cells from SLE patients, suggesting that both sema3A and NP-1 are essential in the process of regulating autoimmunity in SLE [53]. Autoreactive B cells in SLE are characterized by the overexpression of TLR9 and increased production of IL-6 and IFN-γ. This increased expression was found to be in positive association with SLE disease severity and with anti-dsDNA antibody production. Considering sema3A to be an important regulator in autoimmune diseases, we analyzed the possibility of lowering TLR9 expression on B cells by co-culturing them with sema3A. We found that the addition of recombinant human sema3A to activated B cells of SLE patients decreased the expression of TLR9, thereby strengthening the idea of using sema3A as a therapeutic agent for SLE [13]. Being a marker of both Treg and Breg cells, we assessed the soluble and membrane-bound sema3A in 17 patients with familial Mediterranean fever (FMF) during attacks and when in remission. Eight patients with smoldering disease and 12 healthy controls were included. The serum level of sema3A was recorded as much lower in FMF patients during attacks or remission compared to serum levels in healthy controls (242 ± 9.8 ng/mL vs. 232 ± 22.7 ng/mL vs. 323 ± 160 ng/mL respectively, $P < .05$). In addition, the expression of sema3A on Breg cells ($69.5\% \pm 9$ during attack vs. $83.4\% \pm 5.8$ in remission vs. $82.6 \pm 6.4\%$ normal controls, $P < .05$) and also on Treg cells was significantly lower in FMF patients during attacks but was normalized when in remission. Therefore, it is possible that healthy Treg and Breg cells, namely the proper expression of sema3A, are required to end FMF attacks [54]. Due to the above finding, sema3A should be considered a promising therapeutic tool that should be applied in a broad spectrum of immune-mediated diseases. See Fig. 4.2.

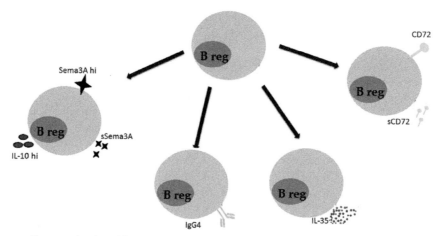

FIGURE 4.2 B regulatory cells express/produce different regulatory molecules. Of these important roles in maintaining self-tolerance are sema3A (both membrane bound and soluble); IgG4-producing B cells; IL-35–producing B cells; and CD72 (both membrane bound and soluble).

CONCLUSION

The evolving complexity of regulatory cells/molecules in maintaining normal immune responses is only the first step toward an understanding of how Breg cells are important in preventing autoimmunity and in decreasing the production of proinflammatory cytokines. Further studies are required to establish whether naïve Breg cells are one subset of B cells that by stimulating them accordingly, they are induced to develop into different faces and types of Breg cells with different functions. The next issue requiring our attention is to determine the specificity of all Breg faces and to learn if they are indeed antigen specific, namely, how to apply this specificity in different autoimmune diseases.

REFERENCES

[1] Steri M, Orru V, Idda ML, Pitzalis M, Pala M,Zara I, et al. Overexpression of the cytokine BAFF and autoimmunity risk. N Engl J Med 2017;376:1615–26.

[2] Cimaz R. Systemic-onset Juvenile idiopathic arthritis. Autoimmun Rev 2016;15:931–4.

[3] Mizoguchi A, Mizoguchi E, Takedatsu II, Blumberg RS, Bhan AK. Chronic intestinal inflammatory condition generates IL-10-producing regulatory B cell subset characterized by CD1d up regulation. Immunity 2002;16:219–30.

[4] Mauri C, Gray D, Mushtaq N, Londel M. Prevention of arthritis by interleukin 10-producing B cells. J Exp Med 2003;197:489–501.

[5] Amu S, Tarkowski A, Dorner T, Bokarewa M, Briilert M. The human immunomodulatory CD25+ B cell population belongs to the memory B cell pool. Scand J Immunol 2007;66:77–86.

[6] Dumoitier N, Terrier B, London J, Lofek S, Mouton L. Implication of B lymphocytes in the pathogenesis of ANCA-associated vasculitides. Autoimmun Rev 2015;14:996–1004.

[7] Kessel A, Haj T, Peri R, Snir A, Melamed D, Sabo E, Toubi E. Human CD19+CD25 high B regulatory cells suppress proliferation of CD4+ T cells and enhance Foxp3 and CTLA-4 expression in T-regulatory cells. Autoimmun Rev 2012;11:670–7.

[8] Blair PA, Norena LY, Flores-Borja F, Rawlings DJ, Isenberg DA, Ehrenstein MR, Mauri C. CD19+CD24highCD38high B cells exhibit regulatory capacity in healthy individuals but are functionally impaired in systemic lupus erythematosus. Immunity 2010;32:129–40.

[9] Sun CM, Deriaud E, Leclerc C, Lo-Man R. Upon TLR9 signaling, CD5+ B cells control the IL-21-dependent Th1 priming capacity of neonatal DCs. Immunity 2005;22:467–77.

[10] Yanaba K, Bouaziz JD, Haas KM, Foe JC, Fujimoto M, Tedder TF. A regulatory B cell subset with a unique CD1dCD5+ phenotype controls T cell-dependent inflammatory responses. Immunity 2008;28:639–59.

[11] Matsushita T, Ynaba K, Bouaziz JD, Fujimoto M, Tedder TF. Regulatory B cells inhibit EAE initiation in mice while other B cells promote disease progression. J Clin Investig 2008;118:3420–30.

[12] Bouaziz JD, Yanaba K, Tedder TF. Regulatory B cells as inhibitors of immune responses and inflammation. Immunol Rev 2008;224:201–14.

[13] Cantaert T, Doorenspleet ME, Francosalinas G, Paramarta JE, Klarenbeek PL, Tiersma Y, et al. Increased numbers of CD5+ B lymphocytes with a regulatory phenotype in spondyloarthritis. Arthritis Rheum 2012;64:1859–68.

[14] Yang M, Deng J, Liu Y, Ko KH, Wang X, Jiao Z, et al. IL-10-producing regulatory B10 cells ameliorate collagen-induced arthritis via suppressing Th17 cell generation. Am J Pathol 2012;180:2375–85.

[15] Yoshizaki A, Miyagaki T, Dilillo DJ, Matsushita T, Horikawa M, Kountikov EI, et al. Regulatory B cells control T-cell autoimmunity through IL-21 dependent cognate interactions. Nature 2012;491:264–8.

[16] Vadasz Z, Peri R, Eiza N, Slobodin G, Balbir-Gurman A, Toubi E. The expansion of CD25highIL-10highFoxP3high B regulatory cells is in association with SLE disease activity. J Immunol Res 2015:1–6.

[17] de Andres C, Tejera-Alhambra M, Alonso B, Valor L, Teijeiro R, Ramos-Medina R, et al. New regulatory CD19+CD25+ B-cell subset in clinically isolated syndrome and multiple sclerosis relapse, Changes after glucocorticoids. J Neuroimmunol 2014;270:37–44.

[18] Guo Y, Zhang M, Qin X, Wang X. Changes in peripheral CD19+Foxp3+ and CD19+TGF-β+ regulatory B cell populations in rheumatoid arthritis patients with interstitial lung disease. J Thorac Dis 2015;7:471–7.

[19] Park MK, Jung YO, Lee SY, Lee SH, Heo YJ, Kim EK, et al. Amelioration of autoimmune arthritis by adoptive transfer of FoxP3-expressing regulatory B cells is associated with Treg/Th17 cell balance. J Transl Med 2016;14:191.

[20] Noh J, Choi WS, Noh G, Lee JH. Presence of FoxP3-expressing CD19+CD5+ B cells in human peripheral blood mononuclear cells: human CD19+CD5+FoxP3+ regulatory B cells. Immune Netw 2010;10:247–9.

[21] Noh J, Noh G. Allergen specific responses of CD19high and CD19low B cells in non-IgE mediated food allergy of late eczematous reactions in atopic dermatitis: presence of IL-17 and IL-32 producing regulatory B cells (Br17 & Br32). Inflamm Allergy Drug Targets 2012;11:320–9.

[22] Lundy SK, Boros DL. Fas ligand-expressing B-1a lymphocytes mediate CD4+ T-cell apoptosis during schistosomal infection: induction by interleukin 4 (IL-4) and IL-10. Infect Immun 2002;70:812–9.

[23] Tao H, Lu L, Xia Y, Dai F, Wang Y, Bao Y, et al. Anti-tumor effector B cells directly kill tumor cells via Fas/FasL pathway and are regulated by IL-10. Eur J Immunol 2015;45:999–1009.

[24] van der Neut Kolfschoten M, Schuurman J, Losen M, Bleeker WK, Martinez P, Vermeulen E, et al. Anti-inflammatory activity of human IgG4 antibodies by dynamic Fab arm exchange. Science 2007;317:1554–7.

[25] Jiménez-Saiz R, Patil SU. The Multifaceted B cell Response in Allergen Immunotherapy. Curr Allergy Asthma Rep 2018;18(12):66.

[26] Moore KW, de Waal Malefyt R, Coffman RL, O'Garra A. Interleukin-10 and the interleukin-10 receptor. Annu Rev Immunol 2001;19:683–765.

[27] Akdis CA, Blesken T, Akdis M, Wuthrich B, Blaser K. Role of interleukin 10 in specific immunotherapy. J Clin Investig 1998;102:98–106.

[28] Jeannin P, Lecoanet S, Delneste Y, Gauchat JF, Bonnefoy JY. IgE versus IgG4 production can be differentially regulated by IL-10. J Immunol 1998;160:3555–61.

[29] van de Veen W, Barbara Stanic B, Yaman G, Wawrzyniak M, Sollner S, Akdis DG, et al. IgG4 production is confined to human IL-10–producing regulatory B cells that suppress antigen-specific immune responses. J Allergy Clin Immunol 2013;131:1204–12.

[30] van de Veen W, Stanic B, Wirz OF, Jansen K. Anna Globinska A, Akdis M. Role of regulatory B cells in immune tolerance to allergens and beyond. J Allergy Clin Immunol 2016;138:654–65.

[31] Akdis CA, Akdis M. Mechanisms of allergen-specific immunotherapy. J Allergy Clin Immunol 2011;127:18–29.

[32] van den Biggelaar AH, van Ree R, Rodrigues LC, Lell B, Deelder AM, Kremsner PG, et al. Decreased atopy in children infected with Schistosoma haematobium: a role for parasite-induced interleukin-10. Lancet 2000;356:1723–7.

[33] Shen P, Roch T, Lampropoulou V, O'Connor RA, Stervbo U, Hilgenberg E, Ries S, et al. IL-35-producing B cells are critical regulators of immunity during autoimmune and infectious diseases. Nature 2014;507(7492):366–70. 20.

[34] Wang RX, Yu CR, Dambuza IM, Mahdi RM, Dolinska MB, Sergeev V, Wingfield PT, Kim SH, Egwuagu CE. Interleukin-35 induces regulatory B cells that suppress autoimmune disease. Nat Med 2014;20(6):633–41.

[35] Sawant DV, Hamilton K, Vignal DAA. Interleukin-35: expanding its job profile. J Interferon Cytokine Res 2015;35(7):499–512.

[36] Sabo MC, Luca VC, Prentoe J, Hopcraft KJ, Blight K, Yi M, Lemon JK, Bukh BJ, Evans MJ, Fremont DH, Diamond MS. Neutralizing monoclonal antibodies against hepatitis C virus E2 protein bind discontinuous epitopes and inhibit infection at a postattachment step. J Virol 2011;85:7005–19.

[37] Vivier E, Raulet DH, Moretta A, Caligiuri MA, Zitvogel L, Lanier LL, Yokoyama WM, Ugolini S. Innate or adaptive immunity? The example of natural killer cells. Science 2011;331:44–9.

[38] Piazzolla G, Tortorella C, Schiraldi O, Antonaci S. Relationship between interferon-gamma, interleukin-10, and interleukin-12 production in chronic hepatitis C and in vitro effects of interferon-alpha. J Clin Immunol 2000;20:54–61.

[39] Ray RB, Lagging LM, Meyer K, Steele R, Ray R. Transcriptional regulation of cellular and viral promoters by the hepatitis C virus core protein. Virus Res 1995;37:209–20.

[40] Toubi E, Kessel A, Goldstein L, Slobodin G, Sabo E, Shmuel Z, Zuckerman E. Enhanced peripheral T-cell apoptosis in chronic hepatitis C virus infection: association with liver disease severity. J Hepatol 2001;35:774–80.

[41] Lee JH, Noh J, Noh G, Choi WS, Lee SS. IL-10 is predominantly produced by CD19(low)CD5(+) regulatory B Cell subpopulation: characterisation of CD19 (high) and CD19(low) subpopulations of CD5(+) B cells. Yonsei Med J 2011;52:851–5.

[42] Mariani SM, Krammer PH. Differential regulation of TRAIL and CD95 ligand in transformed cells of the T and B lymphocyte lineage. Eur J Immunol 1998;28:973–82.

[43] Bonardelle D, Benihoud K, Kiger N, Bobe P. B lymphocytes mediate Fas-dependent cytotoxicity in MRL/lpr mice. J Leukoc Biol 2005;2005(78):1052–9.

[44] Lundy SK, Fox DA. Reduced Fas ligand-expressing splenic CD5+ B lymphocytes in severe collagen-induced arthritis. Arthritis Res Ther 2009;11:R128.

[45] Noh J, Lee JH, Noh G, Bang SY, Kim HS, Choi WS, Cho S, Lee SS. Characterisation of allergen-specific responses of IL-10-producing regulatory B cells (Br1) in cow milk allergy. Cell Immunol 2010;264:143–9.

[46] Velupillai P, Harn DA. Oligosaccharide-specific induction of interleukin 10 production by B220+ cells from schistosome-infected mice: a mechanism for regulation of CD4+ T-cell subsets. Proc Natl Acad Sci USA 1994;91:18–22.

[47] Gherardi E, Love CA, Esnouf RM, Jones EY. The sema domain. Curr Opin Struct Biol 2004;14:669–78.

[48] Tamagnone L, Comoglio PM. Signaling by semaphorin receptors: cell guidance and beyond. Trends Cell Biol 2000;10:377–83.

[49] Mendes-da-Cruz DA, Lepelletier Y, Brignier AC, Smaniotto S, Renand A, Milpied P, et al. Neuropilins, semaphorins, and their role in thymocyte development. Ann NY Acad Sci 2009;1153:20–8.

[50] Vadasz Z, Toubi E. Semaphorins: their dual role in regulating immune-mediated diseases. CRAI 2014;47(1):17–25.

[51] Lepelletier Y, Smaniotto S, Hadj-Slimane R, Villa-Verde DM, Nogueira AC, Dardenne M, Hermine O, Savino W. Control of human thymocyte migration by Neuropilin-1/Semaphorin-3A-mediated interactions. Proc Natl Acad Sci USA 2007;104(13):5545–50. 27.

[52] Garcia F, Lepelletier Y, Smaniotto S, Hadj-Slimane R, Dardenne M, Hermine O, Savino W. Inhibitory effect of semaphorin-3A, a known axon guidance molecule, in the human thymocyte migration induced by CXCL12. J Leukoc Biol 2012;91(1):7–13.

[53] Vadasz Z, Haj T, Halasz K, Rosner I, Slobodin G, Attias D, Kessel A, Kessler O, Neufeld G, Toubi E. Semaphorin 3A is a marker for disease activity and a potential immunoregulator in systemic lupus erythematosus. Arthritis Res Ther 2012;14(3):R146.

[54] Rimar D, Rosner I, Slobodin G, Rozenbaum M, Halasz K, Jiries N, et al. Semaphorin3A, a potential immune regulator in familial Mediterranean fever. Clin Exp Rheumatol 2016;34:S52–5.

FURTHER READING

[1] Hagan P, Blumenthal UJ, Dunn D, Simpson AJ, Wilkins HA. Human IgE, IgG4 and resistance to reinfection with schistosoma haematobium. Nature 1991;349:243–5. 45.

[2] Rihet P, Demeure CE, Dessein AJ, Bourgois A. Strong serum inhibition of specific IgE correlated to competing IgG4, revealed by a new methodology in subjects from a S. mansoni endemic area. Eur J Immunol 1992;22:2063–70.

[3] Kurniawan A, Yazdanbakhsh M, van Ree R, Aalberse R, Selkirk ME, Partono F, et al. Differential expression of IgE and IgG4 specific antibody responses in asymptomatic and chronic human filariasis. J Immunol 1993;150:3941–50.

Chapter 5

T Cells in Autoimmune Diseases

Amir Sharabi[1,2], George C. Tsokos[1]

[1]*Division of Rheumatology, Beth Israel Deaconess Medical Center, Harvard Medical School, Boston, MA, United States;* [2]*Department of Clinical Microbiology and Immunology, Sackler School of Medicine, Tel Aviv University, Tel Aviv, Israel*

INTRODUCTION

T cells develop in the thymus from bone marrow–derived hematopoietic cell precursor, and during their development they acquire their T cell receptor (TCR) that is educated not to recognize self-antigens. During this selection process, the T cells gain and lose the expression of CD4 and CD8 co-receptors that eventually result in the generation of conventional T cells and T regulatory (Treg) cells that can be sent out to the periphery [1]. However, some autoreactive T cells do leak into the periphery as T cell selection in the thymus is not protected totally from mistakes. Furthermore, in circumstances of deletion of genes that are critical for T cell development in the thymus, such as phosphatase and tensin homolog (PTEN), a potent negative regulator of PI3K signaling [2], and zeta-chain-associated protein kinase 70 (ZAP-70) that is critical for the depletion of autoreactive T cells [3], autoimmune diseases will ultimately develop. The thymic autoreactive T cells, which escape to the periphery, will be later controlled by peripheral tolerance mechanisms able to prevent autoreactive T cells from inducing pathogenic immune responses in target organs. The breakdown of peripheral T cell tolerance to self-antigens enables autoreactive T cells to become active and mediate the effector immune responses through inflammation and support to autoantibody-producing B cells.

GENETIC PREDISPOSITION AND T CELL GENETIC VARIANTS IN AUTOIMMUNE DISEASES

Genome-wide association studies have shown that the susceptibility for developing autoimmune diseases is rather polygenic with multiple genetic variants [4]. The highest genetic risk derives from *MHC loci*, which indicates a key role for antigen recognition by T cells for them to become pathogenic. Additional genetic variants include CD25 (IL-2 receptor, α chain), IL-2, CTLA-4, serine/threonine protein phosphatase 2A (PP2A), and tyrosine protein phosphatase [5,6]. Alternative splicing of T cell genes gives rise to several splice gene variants that are pathogenic. Alternative splicing of the CD3 zeta mRNA in systemic lupus erythematosus (SLE) T cells results in an unstable variant, which contributes to abnormalities with TCR signaling [7]. Furthermore, *CD44v3* and *CD44v6* are common splice isoforms of the *CD44* gene in SLE T cells, which have been shown to correlate with the extent of disease activity, the presence of lupus nephritis, and with positivity for anti-dsDNA antibodies [8]. CD44 variant isoforms are important for the homing capacity of T cells to target organs. In addition, the products of alternative spliced *CREM* gene, cAMP responsive element modulator alpha (*CREMα*) and cAMP early repressor I (*ICER*), represent transcriptional repressors of certain functional repressions. Lupus-prone B6.lpr mice deficient of *ICER/CREM* are protected from systemic and organ specific autoimmunity [9].

T CELLS IN THE PATHOGENESIS OF AUTOIMMUNE DISEASES

There are different subsets of T cells that are defined by their TCR composition (e.g., αβ chains or γδ chains), the expression of co-receptors, namely CD4 for T helper (Th) cells and CD8 for T cytotoxic (Tc) cells, and the expression of master genes, transcription factors, and cytokines. Most of T cell subsets have a role in the pathogenesis of autoimmune diseases (Fig. 5.1), either because of the expression and production of pathogenic cytokines or because of impaired or excessive function.

Th17 Cells

CD4 T cells that express the transcription factor ROR-γt produce on stimulation the proinflammatory cytokines IL-17, IL-21, IL-22, IFN-γ, and Granulocyte-monocyte colony-stimulating factor (GM-CSF), all of which promote the development of autoimmune diseases in mice and humans [10,11]. In target organs they generate ectopic lymphoid follicles [12], wherein B cells are activated and become autoreactive [13,14].

Mosaic of Autoimmunity. https://doi.org/10.1016/B978-0-12-814307-0.00005-0

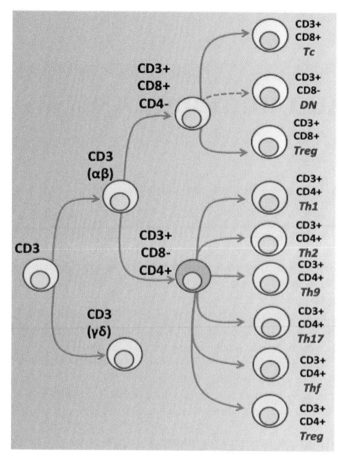

FIGURE 5.1 T cell subsets playing role in autoimmune disease.

Double-Negative T Cells

These cells are αβ TCR T cells that do not express CD4 and CD8. Their origin is not clear; however, because they share genes with those of CD8 T cells, it is suggested that at least some of them originate from autoreactive CD8+ T cells that were stimulated continuously [15–17]. In mice, the repression of *CD8 locus* is triggered by engagement of these cells with autoantigens [18]. In patients with SLE, CREMα mediates CD8 repression through binding to the *CD8 locus* and the recruitment of HDAC1 and DNMT1, which turn the chromatin inaccessible [19]. In several autoimmune diseases, double-negative (DN) T cells are expanded and may comprise 1%–5% of peripheral T cells. They produce IL-17 and can help B cells to produce autoantibody. IL-17–producing DN T cells accumulate in the kidney and probably other tissues [20–23].

γδ T Cells

These cells represent a minor T cell population that has adaptive and innate-like characteristics important for mucosal immunity [24]. They can present antigen, secrete inflammatory cytokines, promote antibody production, and inhibit Treg cells, thereby playing a pathogenic role in autoimmune diseases [25]. Stress molecules such as those of the HSP60 family augment γδ T cell activity. γδ T cells affect dendritic cells to produce IL-17 resulting in inflammatory cell infiltration in the kidney, and depletion of γδ T cells can diminish this infiltration [26–28].

T Follicular Helper Cells

These are CD4 T cells that express the transcription factor Bcl6 and the chemokine receptor CXCR5, which enable them to migrate into germinal centers. Within the germinal centers of lymph nodes and kidneys, T follicular helper (Tfh) cells help the activation of B cells and lead to differentiation of long-lived plasma cells. This process yields the production of high-affinity autoantibodies as it leads to immunoglobulin class switching [29–32]. Tfh cells are frequent in autoimmune diseases, and their pathogenic role in SLE has been demonstrated in murine models [31]. In patients with SLE, the number of Tfh cells correlates with both the numbers of plasmablasts and the titers of anti-dsDNA autoantibodies. Interestingly, a subset of Tfh cells in SLE patients was shown to secrete IL-17 and promote B cell activation in the kidney leading to the development of nephritis [29].

Th1 Cells

These are CD4 T cells that express the αβ TCR and IFN-γ as their signature cytokine. These are the pathogenic cells that mediate the development of diffuse proliferative lupus nephritis and crescentic glomerulonephritis, anti–GBM-induced glomerulonephritis, and antineutrophil cytoplasmic antibody (ANCA)–associated vasculitis [33–35].

Th2 Cells

These are CD4 T cells that express the αβ TCR and produce IL-4 as their signature cytokine. IL-4 activates signal transducer and activator of transcription 6 (STAT6) and leads to the expression of their principle transcription factor, GATA. They also secrete IL-5, IL-6, IL-9, IL-13, and IL-17E that support the humoral response. Th2 cells mediate the development of membranous lupus nephritis in MRL/lpr mice whose Th1 response is genetically deleted [37]. It is noteworthy that in addition to the effects of Th cells on B cells, BAFF and APRIL are B cell survival and growth factors that contribute to the pathogenicity of B cells, and patients with autoimmune diseases produce high levels of these factors [36].

Th9 Cells

Th9 cells secrete IL-9 and require TGF-β and IL-4 for their induction [38,39]. They express Foxp3 and IL-4 but at much lower levels than Tregs and Th2 cells, respectively. TGF-β promotes the development of Th9 cells in both mice and humans through the induction of the ETS-transcription factor PU.1 [40,41]. PU.1 binds to the IL-9 promoter and promotes Th9 subset polarization. IL-4 activates STAT6, which stimulates an increase of IL-9 in Th9 cells. MRL/lpr mice with established lupus have expanded Th9 cells in their spleens and kidneys, which correlate with the production of anti-dsDNA antibodies [42]. In addition, experimental autoimmune encephalomyelitis (EAE) could be induced by Th9 cells and IL-9, and the inflammation in the central nervous system was shown to be independent of Th1 and Th17 cells [43].

CD8 T Cells

In addition to their cytotoxic role they have against intracellular pathogens and tumors, CD8 T cells are known for their ability to regulate autoimmune and allergic diseases [44]. In experimental autoimmune glomerulonephritis, depletion of CD8+ T cells reduced the severity of disease [45]. Furthermore, in SLE and ANCA-associated vasculitis, an altered gene expression profile in CD8+ T cells was shown to correlate with a negative disease outcome [46]. Also, patients with ANCA-associated nephritis and lupus nephritis have a higher urinary CD8 to CD4 T cell ratio [47].

CD4 Treg Cells

Among the CD4 and CD8 T cells, the most studied Treg cell population resides within the CD4 T cells that express the αβ TCR and the master gene Foxp3. Those CD4 Treg cells develop in the thymus and have typical characteristics that enable them to suppress the immune response [48]. CD4 Treg cells also play a role in tissue repair [49,50]. Defects in several signaling molecules and pathways were shown to hamper Treg cell function, including PP2A, mechanistic target of rapamycin (mTOR) C1, PI3 phosphatase, PTEN, and calcium/calmodulin-dependent protein kinase IV (CaMKIV) [49]. In autoimmune diseases, both decreased numbers and compromised function have been implicated [51,52].

CD8 Treg Cells

These are CD8 T cells of multiple subsets that have suppressive capabilities. Their number, function, or both are impaired in patients with autoimmune diseases and in murine models of autoimmunity [53]. Frequent subsets of CD8 Treg cells express low levels of CD28. CD8 knockout mice that were induced with EAE improved their outcome following the adoptive transfer of CD8+CD28low T cells from wild-type animals [54]. Furthermore, in murine SLE, treatment with tolerogenic peptides ameliorated the disease manifestations through the induction of CD8 and CD4 Treg cells [55,56], and CD8 Treg cells were essential for the optimal function of CD4 Treg cells [56,57], suggesting a cross talk between CD8 and CD4 Treg cells.

MOLECULAR PATHWAYS IN PATHOGENIC AUTOREACTIVE T CELLS

Central pathways in T cell development in the thymus, which result in the development of autoimmune diseases, are beyond the scope of this manuscript, but mostly related to interference with the process of educating the TCR recognition of self-antigens and the deletion of autoreactive T cells [1–3]. The main molecular pathways in the periphery that participate in the induction and activation of autoreactive T cells are described here (Fig. 5.2).

CD3 Zeta

This T cell surface molecule is part of the CD3 complex, which transduces the signaling from TCR following antigen recognition. Single-nucleotide polymorphisms in the *CD3 zeta locus* affect its expression, and it is downregulated in several autoimmune diseases [58–60]. Consequently, decreased expression of *CD3 zeta* can lead to the migration and accumulation of peripheral T cells in tissues where they produce IFN-γ and IL-17 and trigger inflammation [61–63]. T cells with decreased CD3 *zeta* expression have a higher capacity to infiltrate tissues partly because they overexpress the adhesion molecule CD44 [64]. T cells from patients with SLE also express elevated levels of CD44 and specifically *v6* variant of CD44, which has been associated with lupus nephritis [8].

Rho-Associated Protein Kinase

This is a serine/threonine kinase that phosphorylates ezrin/radixin/moesin (ERM) protein complex for the regulation of cell migration [65], and the CD44–Rho-associated protein kinase (ROCK)–ERM axis is activated in patients with autoimmune diseases, including SLE [66–68]. Inflammatory conditions for mesangial cells and podocytes also result in ROCK activation [69]. Rock activation can also result in the development of Th17 cells [68].

Protein Phosphatase 2A

This is a serine/threonine phosphatase composed of three subunits (each with different isoforms), which is involved in pivotal cellular reactions and responses, including transcription, and cell migration and survival [70]. PP2A-beta subunit plays a role in the survival of autoreactive T cells as it controls T cell apoptosis following IL-2 deprivation, and T cells from patients with SLE have decreased levels of PP2A-beta subunit [71]. In Treg cells, however, it is required for their development through the suppression of mTORC1 [72]. Interestingly, mice whose T cells overexpress PP2A do not develop autoimmune syndrome spontaneously, yet on challenge with anti-GBM antibody, they develop glomerulonephritis that is responsive to treatment with anti–IL-17 antibody [73].

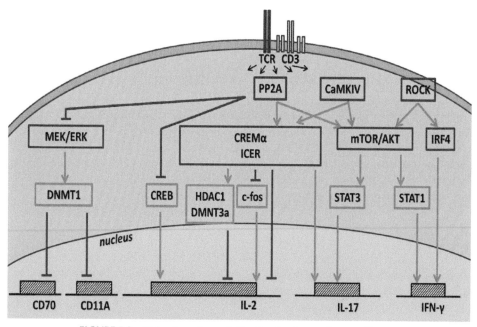

FIGURE 5.2   Molecular pathways in T cells related to autoimmune disease.

CREM

This is a family of transcription factors that become activated following intracellular increase in cAMP. Two isoforms, CREMα and ICER, play a role in T cell differentiation, epigenetic-regulated suppression of IL-2, and regulation of CD8 expression by CREMα [9,19,74–78]. CREMα is increased in SLE T cells and represses IL-2 transcription through at least three pathways: (1) binding to CREB-binding site to withhold the transcription initiation machinery, (2) the recruitment of HDAC1 and DNMT-3a to impose epigenetic closure of the IL-2 locus, and (3) binding and repressing c-fos to reduce AP-1 formation required for IL-2 transcription [74,75]. CREMα together with ICER result in demethylation and acetylation of the IL-17 promoter, processes that upregulate IL-17 transcription [9,74,75].

Calcium/Calmodulin-Dependent Protein Kinase IV

This is a serine/threonine kinase that regulates gene expression through transcription factors associated with activation and development of T cell subsets. In SLE patients and lupus-prone mice, the expression of CaMKIV is increased in T cells following their activation [77,78]. This results in decreased IL-2 production and compromised Treg cell function [77]. Specifically, in SLE T cells, CaMKIV enhances the binding of CREMα to the IL-2 promoter and reduces its activity [78]. Depletion of CaMKIV in T cells from both mice and human with SLE recovers IL-2 production and Treg cell differentiation [77]. CaMKIV also promotes Th17 cell differentiation through the Akt/mTOR pathway [79] and the recruitment of these cells into tissues, including the kidneys [80], where it affects the function of mesangial cells [81] and podocytes [82].

Mechanistic Target of Rapamycin Pathway

mTOR is a serine/threonine kinase that regulates T cell activation, proliferation, and survival, and it is frequently activated in autoimmune diseases [83]. There are two major mTOR complexes, namely mTORC1 and mTORC2, and the former plays a role in Th1 and Th17 cell differentiation, whereas the latter is essential for Th2 differentiation [84]. In SLE, the mTORC1 is activated by PI3K/Akt pathway, CaMKIV, and ROCK [68,79,85], which impairs Treg cells and increases the development and tissue recruitment of Th1 and Th17 cells to target organs [86].

Signal Transducer and Activator of Transcription

This is a family of signaling molecules downstream the cytokine receptors that dictate the differentiation and function of immune cells, including T cells. Following the engagement of a cytokine receptor, STAT molecules are phosphorylated by janus kinases and become activated. For instance, STAT4 promotes Th1 cell differentiation in response to IL-12; STAT6 promotes Th2 cell differentiation in response to IL-4; STAT3 promotes Th17 or Tfh cells in response to IL-6, IL-21, IL-23, and TGF-β; and STAT5 promotes Treg cells in response to IL-2 and TGF-β. These differentiation events of T cells are regulated by mTOR pathway [87]. SLE T cells express high levels of STAT3 [88], and STAT3-induced IL-17 production and Tfh cell differentiation are required for infiltration and accumulation of immune complexes in murine lupus nephritis [89,90].

EPIGENETICS AND AUTOIMMUNITY

Epigenetic pathways enable cells to make functional adjustments through the expression or repression of genes in response to a variety of stimuli ranging from cell surface molecules to signaling molecules. Methylation of DNA CpGs and histone modifications are common epigenetic mechanisms, and gene expression is increased when DNA is hypomethylated [91]. In SLE, genes that are hypomethylated and play a pathogenic role include CD70, CD11A, CD40L, IL-4, IL-10, IL-13, and IL-17 [91,92]. Furthermore, *PP2A* gene is hypomethylated in SLE T cells [93], and increased activity of PP2A results in ERK/MEK dephosphorylation and decreased DNMT1 activity with a resultant hypomethylation of the pathogenic molecules, CD70 and CD11a [94].

CONCLUDING REMARKS

The study of T cells in patients with systemic autoimmunity and lupus-prone mice has generated novel insights into the pathogenesis of the disease and more importantly in the expression of organ damage. Study of T cell subsets has demonstrated the poor function of Treg cells and the poor control of the autoimmune and the inflammatory responses. Recognition of the expansion of DN T cells has provided insight into their ability to help B cells to produce anti-dsDNA antibodies and to produce the proinflammatory cytokine IL-17 in the periphery and when they infiltrate the kidney. Study of the CD8 cell subset and their poor cytotoxic function has provided a better understanding of the inability of SLE patients to fend off infections. More importantly, detailed studies of the biochemistry of T cell signaling events and gene transcription processes have unveiled a number of plausible treatment targets and biomarkers of disease activity. For example, a ROCK inhibitor is in Phase II trial, and mTOR inhibitors have been considered enthusiastically along with Syk and CaMKIV inhibitors. Low-dose IL-2 has been extolled in uncontrolled reports, whereas an anti-p40 (IL-23) monoclonal antibody has completed a successful Phase II trial. In parallel, a number of surface molecules (CD44v3 or C6) or gene expression profiles have been shown to have biomarker value. Yet, T cells in patients with SLE and other autoimmune diseases present enormous complexity, and continuous intense studies will reveal not only novel targets and biomarkers but also potential to develop tools toward personalized medicine.

REFERENCES

[1] Klein L, Kyewski B, Allen PM, Hogquist KA. Positive and negative selection of the T cell repertoire: what thymocytes see (and don't see). Nat Rev Immunol 2014;14:377–91.

[2] Liu X, Karnell JL, Yin B, Zhang R, Zhang J, Li P, Choi Y, Maltzman JS, Pear WS, Bassing CH, Turka LA. Distinct roles for PTEN in prevention of T cell lymphoma and autoimmunity in mice. J Clin Investig 2010;120:2497–507.

[3] Negishi I, Motoyama N, Nakayama K, Nakayama K, Senju S, Hatakeyama S, Zhang Q, Chan AC, Loh DY. Essential role for ZAP-70 in both positive and negative selection of thymocytes. Nature 1995;376:435–8.

[4] Cotsapas C, Hafler DA. Immune-mediated disease genetics: the shared basis of pathogenesis. Trends Immunol 2013;34:22–6.

[5] Wellcome Trust Case Control Consortium. Genome-wide association study of 14,000 cases of seven common diseases and 3,000 shared controls. Nature 2007;447:661–78.

[6] Tan W, Sunahori K, Zhao J, Deng Y, Kaufman KM, Kelly JA, Langefeld CD, Williams AH, Comeau ME, Ziegler JT, et al. BIOLUPUS Network; GENLES Network. Association of PPP2CA polymorphisms with systemic lupus erythematosus susceptibility in multiple ethnic groups. Arthritis Rheum 2011;63:2755–63.

[7] Nambiar MP, et al. T cell signaling abnormalities in systemic lupus erythematosus are associated with increased mutations/polymorphisms and splice variants of T cell receptor zeta chain messenger RNA. Arthritis Rheum 2001;44:1336–50.

[8] Crispin JC, et al. Expression of CD44 variant isoforms CD44v3 and CD44v6 is increased on T cells from patients with systemic lupus erythematosus and is correlated with disease activity. Arthritis Rheum 2010;62:1431–7.

[9] Yoshida N, et al. ICER is requisite for Th17 differentiation. Nat Commun 2016;7:12993.

[10] Miossec P, Korn T, Kuchroo VK. Interleukin-17 and type 17 helper T cells. N Engl J Med 2009;361:888–98.

[11] Gaffen SL, Jain R, Garg AV, Cua DJ. The IL-23-IL-17 immune axis: from mechanisms to therapeutic testing. Nat Rev Immunol 2014;14:585–600.

[12] Deteix C, et al. Intragraft Th17 infiltrate promotes lymphoid neogenesis and hastens clinical chronic rejection. J Immunol 2010;184:5344–51.

[13] Mitsdoerffer M, et al. Proinflammatory T helper type 17 cells are effective B-cell helpers. Proc Natl Acad Sci USA 2010;107:14292–7.

[14] Schaffert H, et al. IL-17-producing CD4+ T cells contribute to the loss of B-cell tolerance in experimental autoimmune myasthenia gravis. Eur J Immunol 2015;45:1339 47.

[15] Thomson CW, Lee PL, Zhang L. Double negative regulatory T cells. non-conventional regulators. Immunol Res 2006;35:163–78.

[16] Rodríguez-Rodríguez N, et al. Programmed cell death 1 and Helios distinguish TCR-αβ+ double-negative (CD4-CD8-) T cells that derive from self-reactive CD8 T cells. J Immunol 2015;194:4207–14.

[17] Crispín JC, Tsokos GC. Human TCR-alpha beta+ CD4- CD8- T cells can derive from CD8+ T cells and display an inflammatory effector phenotype. J Immunol 2009;183:4675–81.

[18] Rodríguez-Rodríguez N, et al. Pro-inflammatory self-reactive T cells are found within murine TCR-αβ+ CD4– CD8– PD-1+ cells. Eur J Immunol 2016;46:1383–91.

[19] Hedrich CM, Crispín JC, Rauen T, Ioannidis C, Koga T, Rodriguez Rodriguez N, Apostolidis SA, Kyttaris VC, Tsokos GC. cAMP responsive element modulator (CREM) α mediates chromatin remodeling of CD8 during the generation of CD3+ CD4- CD8- T cells. J Biol Chem 2014;289:2361–70.

[20] Crispín JC, et al. Expanded double negative T cells in patients with systemic lupus erythematosus produce IL-17 and infiltrate the kidneys. J Immunol 2008;181:8761–6.

[21] Oliveira JB, et al. Revised diagnostic criteria and classification for the autoimmune lymphoproliferative syndrome (ALPS): report from the 2009 NIH International Workshop. Blood 2010;116:e35–40.

[22] Alunno A, et al. CD4–CD8– T-cells in primary Sjögren's syndrome: association with the extent of glandular involvement. J Autoimmun 2014;51:38–43.

[23] Tarbox JA, et al. Elevated double negative T cells in pediatric autoimmunity. J Clin Immunol 2014;34:594–9.

[24] Lalor SJ, McLoughlin RM. Memory γδ T cells-newly appreciated protagonists in infection and immunity. Trends Immunol 2016;37:690–702.

[25] Paul S, et al. Role of gamma-delta (γδ) T cells in autoimmunity. J Leukoc Biol 2015;97:259–71.

[26] Turner JE, et al. IL-17A production by renal γδ T cells promotes kidney injury in crescentic GN. J Am Soc Nephrol 2012;23:1486–95.

[27] Peng X, et al. IL-17A produced by both γδ T and Th17 cells promotes renal fibrosis via RANTES-mediated leukocyte infiltration after renal obstruction. J Pathol 2015;235:79–89.

[28] Yin S, et al. Hyperactivation and in situ recruitment of inflammatory Vδ2 T cells contributes to disease pathogenesis in systemic lupus erythematosus. Sci Rep 2014;5:14432.

[29] Liarski VM, Kaverina N, Chang A, Brandt D, Yanez D, Talasnik L, Carlesso G, Herbst R, Utset TO, Labno C, Peng Y, Jiang Y, Giger ML, Clark MR. Cell distance mapping identifies functional T follicular helper cells in inflamed human renal tissue. Sci Transl Med 2014;6:230ra46.

[30] Craft JE. Follicular helper T cells in immunity and systemic autoimmunity. Nat Rev Rheumatol 2012;8:337–47.

[31] Ueno H. T follicular helper cells in human autoimmunity. Curr Opin Immunol 2016;43:24–31.

[32] Morita R, et al. Human blood CXCR5+CD4+ T cells are counterparts of T follicular cells and contain specific subsets that differentially support antibody secretion. Immunity 2011;34:108–21.

[33] Hünemörder S, et al. TH1 and TH17 cells promote crescent formation in experimental autoimmune glomerulonephritis. J Pathol 2015;237:62–71.

[34] Steinmetz OM, et al. CXCR3 mediates renal Th1 and Th17 immune response in murine lupus nephritis. J Immunol 2009;183:4693–704.

[35] Paust HJ, et al. CXCR3+ regulatory T cells control TH1 responses in crescentic GN. J Am Soc Nephrol 2016;27:1933–42.

[36] Shimizu S, et al. Membranous glomerulonephritis development with Th2-type immune deviations in MRL/lpr mice deficient for IL-27 receptor (WSX-1). J Immunol 2005;175:7185–92.

[37] Hiepe F, Radbruch A. Plasma cells as an innovative target in autoimmune disease with renal manifestations. Nat Rev Nephrol 2016;12:232–40.

[38] Veldhoen M, Uyttenhove C, van Snick J, Helmby H, Westendorf A, Buer J, Martin B, Wilhelm C, Stockinger B. Transforming growth factor-beta 'reprograms' the differentiation of T helper 2 cells and promotes an interleukin 9-producing subset. Nat Immunol 2008;9:1341–6.

[39] Dardalhon V, Awasthi A, Kwon H, Galileos G, Gao W, Sobel RA, Mitsdoerffer M, Strom TB, Elyaman W, Ho IC, Khoury S, Oukka M, Kuchroo VK. IL-4 inhibits TGF-beta-induced Foxp3+ T cells and, together with TGF-beta, generates IL-9+IL-10+ Foxp3(-) effector T cells. Nat Immunol 2008;9:1347–55.

[40] Chang HC, Sehra S, Goswami R, Yao W, Yu Q, Stritesky GL, Jabeen R, McKinley C, Ahyi AN, Han L, Nguyen ET, Robertson MJ, Perumal NB, Tepper RS, Nutt SL, Kaplan MH. The transcription factor PU.1 is required for the development of IL-9-producing T cells and allergic inflammation. Nat Immunol 2010;11:527–34.

[41] Jabeen R, Kaplan MH. The symphony of the ninth: the development and function of Th9 cells. Curr Opin Immunol 2012;24:303–7.

[42] Yang J, Li Q, Yang X, Li M. Interleukin-9 is associated with elevated anti-double-stranded DNA antibodies in lupus-prone mice. Mol Med 2015;21:364–70.

[43] Jäger A, Dardalhon V, Sobel RA, Bettelli E, Kuchroo VK. Th1, Th17, and Th9 effector cells induce experimental autoimmune encephalomyelitis with different pathological phenotypes. J Immunol 2009;183:7169–77.

[44] Kim HJ, Cantor H. Regulation of self-tolerance by Qa-1-restricted CD8(+) regulatory T cells. Semin Immunol 2011;23:446–52.

[45] Reynolds J, Norgan VA, Bhambra U, Smith J, Cook HT, Pusey CD. Anti-CD8 monoclonal antibody therapy is effective in the prevention and treatment of experimental autoimmune glomerulonephritis. J Am Soc Nephrol 2002;13:359–69.

[46] McKinney EF, Lyons PA, Carr EJ, Hollis JL, Jayne DR, Willcocks LC, Koukoulaki M, Brazma A, Jovanovic V, Kemeny DM, Pollard AJ, Macary PA, Chaudhry AN, Smith KG. A CD8+ T cell transcription signature predicts prognosis in autoimmune disease. Nat Med 2010;16:586–91.

[47] Kopetschke K, et al. The cellular signature of urinary immune cells in Lupus nephritis: new insights into potential biomarkers. Arthritis Res Ther 2015;17:94.

[48] Josefowicz SZ, Lu LF, Rudensky AY. Regulatory T cells: mechanisms of differentiation and function. Annu Rev Immunol 2012;30:531–64.

[49] Kasper IR, Apostolidis SA, Sharabi A, Tsokos GC. Empowering regulatory T cells in autoimmunity. Trends Mol Med 2016;22:784–97.

[50] Arpaia N, et al. A distinct function of regulatory T cells in tissue protection. Cell 2015;162:1078–89.

[51] Ferretti C, La Cava A. Adaptive immune regulation in autoimmune diabetes. Autoimmun Rev 2016;15:236–41.

[52] Ghali JR, Wang YM, Holdsworth SR, Kitching AR. Regulatory T cells in immune-mediated renal disease. Nephrology (Carlton) 2016;21:86–96.

[53] Costantino CM, Baecher-Allan CM, Hafler DA. Human regulatory T cells and autoimmunity. Eur J Immunol 2008;38:921–4.

[54] Najafian N, Chitnis T, Salama AD, Zhu B, Benou C, Yuan X, Clarkson MR, Sayegh MH, Khoury SJ. Regulatory functions of CD8+CD28- T cells in an autoimmune disease model. J Clin Investig 2003;112:1037–48.

[55] Hahn BH, Singh RP, La Cava A, Ebling FM. Tolerogenic treatment of lupus mice with consensus peptide induces Foxp3-expressing, apoptosis-resistant, TGFbeta-secreting CD8+ T cell suppressors. J Immunol 2005;175:7728–37.

[56] Sharabi A, Mozes E. The suppression of murine lupus by a tolerogenic peptide involves foxp3-expressing CD8 cells that are required for the optimal induction and function of foxp3-expressing CD4 cells. J Immunol September 1, 2008;181(5):3243–51.

[57] Arazi A, Sharabi A, Zinger H, Mozes E, Neumann AU. In vivo dynamical interactions between CD4 Tregs, CD8 Tregs and CD4+ CD25- cells in mice. PLoS One 2009;4:e8447.

[58] Moulton VR, Tsokos GC. T cell signaling abnormalities contribute to aberrant immune cell function and autoimmunity. J Clin Investig 2015;125:2220–7.

[59] Li P, et al. TCR-CD3ζ gene polymorphisms and expression profile in rheumatoid arthritis. Autoimmunity 2016;49:466–71.

[60] Zayed H. Genetic epidemiology of type 1 diabetes in the 22 Arab countries. Curr Diab Rep 2016;16:37.

[61] Zhang Z, et al. TCRzetadim lymphocytes define populations of circulating effector cells that migrate to inflamed tissues. Blood 2007;109:4328–35.

[62] Yoshimoto K, Setoyama Y, Tsuzaka K, Abe T, Takeuchi T. Reduced expression of TCR zeta is involved in the abnormal production of cytokines by peripheral T cells of patients with systemic lupus erythematosus. J Biomed Biotechnol 2010;2010:509021.

[63] Ferraccioli G, Zizzo G. The potential role of Th17 in mediating the transition from acute to chronic autoimmune inflammation: rheumatoid arthritis as a model. Discov Med 2011;11:413–24.

[64] Deng GM, Beltran J, Chen C, Terhorst C, Tsokos GC. T Cell CD3ζ deficiency enables multiorgan tissue inflammation. J Immunol 2013;191:3563–7.

[65] Loirand G. Rho kinases in health and disease: from basic science to translational research. Pharmacol Rev 2015;67:1074–95.

[66] Nishikimi T, Matsuoka H. Molecular mechanisms and therapeutic strategies of chronic renal injury: renoprotective effect of rho-kinase inhibitor in hypertensive glomerulosclerosis. J Pharmacol Sci 2006;100:22–8.

[67] Komers R. Rho kinase inhibition in diabetic kidney disease. Br J Clin Pharmacol 2013;76:551–9.

[68] Isgro J, et al. Enhanced rho-associated protein kinase activation in patients with systemic lupus erythematosus. Arthritis Rheum 2013;65:1592–602.

[69] Hayashi K, et al. Molecular mechanisms and therapeutic strategies of chronic renal injury: role of rho-kinase in the development of renal injury. J Pharmacol Sci 2006;100:29–33.

[70] Sharabi A, Kasper IR, Tsokos GC. The serine/threonine protein phosphatase 2A controls autoimmunity. Clin Immunol 2017;17:S1521–6616.

[71] Crispín JC, Apostolidis SA, Finnell MI, Tsokos GC. Induction of PP2A Bβ, a regulator of IL-2 deprivation-induced T-cell apoptosis, is deficient in systemic lupus erythematosus. Proc Natl Acad Sci USA 2011;108:12443–8.

[72] Apostolidis SA, et al. Phosphatase PP2A is requisite for the function of regulatory T cells. Nat Immunol 2016;17:556–64.

[73] Crispín JC, et al. Cutting edge: protein phosphatase 2A confers susceptibility to autoimmune disease through an IL-17-dependent mechanism. J Immunol 2012;188:3567–71.

[74] Rauen T, Hedrich CM, Tenbrock K, Tsokos GC. cAMP responsive element modulator: a critical regulator of cytokine production. Trends Mol Med 2013;19:262–9.

[75] Hedrich CM, et al. cAMP response element modulator α controls IL2 and IL17A expression during CD4 lineage commitment and subset distribution in lupus. Proc Natl Acad Sci USA 2012;109:16606–11.

[76] Hedrich CM, et al. cAMP-responsive element modulator α (CREMα) trans-represses the transmembrane glycoprotein CD8 and contributes to the generation of CD3+CD4-CD8- T cells in health and disease. J Biol Chem 2013;288:31880–7.

[77] Koga T, Ichinose K, Mizui M, Crispín JC, Tsokos GC. Calcium/calmodulin-dependent protein kinase IV suppresses IL-2 production and regulatory T cell activity in lupus. J Immunol 2012;189:3490–6.

[78] Juang YT, Wang Y, Solomou EE, Li Y, Mawrin C, Tenbrock K, Kyttaris VC, Tsokos GC. Systemic lupus erythematosus serum IgG increases CREM binding to the IL-2 promoter and suppresses IL-2 production through CaMKIV. J Clin Investig 2005;115:996–1005.

[79] Koga T, et al. CaMK4-dependent activation of AKT/mTOR and CREM-α underlies autoimmunity-associated Th17 imbalance. J Clin Investig 2014;124:2234–45.

[80] Koga T, et al. CaMK4 facilitates the recruitment of IL-17-producing cells to target organs through the CCR6/CCL20 axis in Th17-driven inflammatory diseases. Arthritis Rheumatol 2016;68:1981–8.

[81] Ichinose K, Rauen T, Juang YT, Kis-Toth K, Mizui M, Koga T, Tsokos GC. Cutting edge: calcium/Calmodulin-dependent protein kinase type IV is essential for mesangial cell proliferation and lupus nephritis. J Immunol 2011;187:5500–4.

[82] Ichinose K, Ushigusa T, Nishino A, Nakashima Y, Suzuki T, Horai Y, Koga T, Kawashiri SY, Iwamoto N, Tamai M, Arima K, Nakamura H, Obata Y, Yamamoto K, Origuchi T, Nishino T, Kawakami A, Tsokos GC. Lupus nephritis IgG induction of calcium/calmodulin-dependent protein kinase IV expression in podocytes and alteration of their function. Arthritis Rheumatol 2016;68:944–52.

[83] Perl A. Activation of mTOR (mechanistic target of rapamycin) in rheumatic diseases. Nat Rev Rheumatol 2016;12:169–82.

[84] Delgoffe GM, Pollizzi KN, Waickman AT, Heikamp E, Meyers DJ, Horton MR, Xiao B, Worley PF, Powell JD. The kinase mTOR regulates the differentiation of helper T cells through the selective activation of signaling by mTORC1 and mTORC2. Nat Immunol 2011;12:295–303.

[85] Suárez-Fueyo A, Barber DF, Martínez-Ara J, Zea-Mendoza AC, Carrera AC. Enhanced phosphoinositide 3-kinase δ activity is a frequent event in systemic lupus erythematosus that confers resistance to activation-induced T cell death. J Immunol 2011;187:2376–85.

[86] Kshirsagar S, et al. Akt-dependent enhanced migratory capacity of Th17 cells from children with lupus nephritis. J Immunol 2014;193:4895–903.

[87] Saleiro D, Platanias LC. Intersection of mTOR and STAT signaling in immunity. Trends Immunol 2015;36:21–9.

[88] Harada T, et al. Increased expression of STAT3 in SLE T cells contributes to enhanced chemokine-mediated cell migration. Autoimmunity 2007;40:1–8.

[89] Amarilyo G, Lourenço EV, Shi FD, La Cava A. IL-17 promotes murine lupus. J Immunol 2014;193:540–3.

[90] Yiu G, et al. Development of Th17-associated interstitial kidney inflammation in lupus-prone mice lacking the gene encoding STAT-1. Arthritis Rheumatol 2016;68:1233–44.

[91] Hedrich CM, Crispin JC, Tsokos GC. Epigenetic regulation of cytokine expression in systemic lupus erythematosus with special focus on T cells. Autoimmunity 2014;47:234–41.

[92] Patel DR, Richardson BC. Dissecting complex epigenetic alterations in human lupus. Arthritis Res Ther 2013;15:201.

[93] Sunahori K, Juang YT, Tsokos GC. Methylation status of CpG islands flanking a cAMP response element motif on the protein phosphatase 2Ac alpha promoter determines CREB binding and activity. J Immunol 2009;182:1500–8.

[94] Sunahori K, Nagpal K, Hedrich CM, Mizui M, Fitzgerald LM, Tsokos GC. The catalytic subunit of protein phosphatase 2A (PP2Ac) promotes DNA hypomethylation by suppressing the phosphorylated mitogen-activated protein kinase/extracellular signal-regulated kinase (ERK) kinase (MEK)/phosphorylated ERK/DNMT1 protein pathway in T-cells from controls and systemic lupus erythematosus patients. J Biol Chem 2013;288:21936–44.

Chapter 6

Th17 Cells

Alessia Alunno, Elena Bartoloni, Roberto Gerli
Rheumatology Unit, Department of Medicine, University of Perugia, Perugia, Italy

HISTORICAL ASPECTS

Following the seminal work by Mosmann et al. in 1986, in mice [1], Romagnani et al. confirmed 5 years later that human CD4+ T helper (Th) cells can also be classified into two major functionally different subsets on the basis of the different cytokines they produce [2]. Th1 cells produce interferon (IFN) γ and lymphotoxin (LT) α, whereas Th2 cells produce IL-4, IL-5, and IL-13 [3]. IL-17 was identified in 1993 in rodents, with the name of cytotoxic T lymphocyte–associated antigen 8, and in 1995 in humans [4,5]. Subsequently, it was found that IL-17 family consists of six members, from A to F, and the term IL-17 usually refers to IL-17A. IL-17 receptor (IL-17R), identified in 1995, is present on the surface of many immune and nonimmune cells, thereby explaining the multifaceted effects mediated by this cytokine. The IL-17R family includes five subunits, from IL-17RA to IL-17RE, although IL-17A binds to a complex of two IL-17A and one IL-17C subunits. The downstream signal is transduced via a tumor necrosis factor (TNF) receptor–associated factor (TRAF) 6–dependent and a TRAF6-independent pathways. The TRAF6-dependent pathway culminates with the activation of NF-κB and the transcription of proinflammatory genes. Although initially defined as a T cell–related cytokine, the peculiar T cell subset able to secrete IL-17 was identified only in 2005 in mice and in 2007 in humans and was named Th17 [6–8].

TH17 CELL DEVELOPMENT AND PLASTICITY

The polarization of naïve T cells toward a Th17 cell is a multistep process. The upregulation of the retinoic acid orphan receptor (ROR) γt transcription, the expression of IL-17, and the stabilization of the Th17 phenotype require a peculiar cytokine milieu that includes IL-6, TGF-β, IL-21, IL-1β, and IL-23 [6,9]. In detail, IL-6, TGF-β, and IL-21 initiate this process by inducing the expression of RORγt in naïve T cells. Subsequently, IL-6 and IL-1β generate a positive loop to enhance this polarization and finally IL-23 promotes the expansion and stabilization of the Th17 phenotype [6,10–13]. In addition, Th17 cells are able to secrete IL-21 and IL-22, the former acting as paracrine stimulus to further boost Th17 cells. An intriguing aspect of Th17 physiology is the developmental plasticity with the regulatory counterpart of the immune system, the Treg cells. It has been widely demonstrated that TGF-β is a common triggering stimulus for both cell subsets and a naïve T cell can be transformed in either a Th17 or a Treg cell according to the concurrent presence or absence of IL-6 and IL-23 [14,15]. Furthermore, the evaluation of a forkhead box protein (Foxp3) reporter mouse to tag the specific transcription factor of Treg cells revealed that fully committed Treg cells can be turned into a Th17 cell and vice versa in an IL-6–dependent manner [16]. Finally, the direct investigation of Th17 cell fate allowed to clarify additional aspects of Th17 cell plasticity. This dynamic process occurs in physiological conditions and in pathological settings such as chronic inflammatory diseases [17]. Fully differentiated Th17 cells can deviate toward a Th1 phenotype, hence acquiring the ability to secrete IFN-γ, which is useful for host defense against infections, but can be detrimental synergizing the action of Th1 lymphocytes in the development of chronic inflammatory diseases [18–21]. Another interesting aspect is represented by the conversion of Th17 cells into follicular helper T cells (Tfh) in Peyer's patches orchestrating B cell help and eventually IgA production [22].

TH17 CELLS AND HEALTH

IL-17 is a pleiotropic cytokine involved in several physiological processes. In normal conditions, Th17 cells represent a leading player in the scenario of host defense against pathogens [23]. Owing to its capability to induce the secretion of many proinflammatory cytokines, chemokines, and other mediators, such as matrix metalloproteinases and prostaglandins, IL-17 is a keystone in cellular and humoral immune response. With regard to the first level of defense, namely epithelial barriers, IL-17 is able to increase the release of antimicrobial proteins, such as beta-defensin-2, mucins (MUC5AC and MUC5B), and S100 proteins (S100A7, S100A8, and S100A9) [24,25], as well as of IgA [26]. If the barrier integrity is lost and proinflammatory cytokines such as IL-6 and IL-1β are released, a peculiar IL-17–producing cell subset, the so-called "innate-like lymphocytes," is recruited. γδ T cells and innate lymphoid cells (ILCs) further contribute to the local IL-17 balance and following the synergistic action of IL-17, TNF-α, and chemokines, macrophages and neutrophils are recruited at the site of injury [27,28].

The ability to induce neutrophil recruitment makes Th17 cells particularly relevant in the context of immune responses against extracellular pathogens [29]. In fact, this feature is important for host defense against Gram-negative bacteria such as Klebsiella pneumoniae and *Pseudomonas aeruginosa*, as well as accounts for the prominent antifungal activity of IL-17 [30]. Congenital or acquired defects of the Th17 immune response have been associated with chronic mucocutaneous candidiasis [31,32], and specific genetic defects of Th17 cells are associated with recurrent infections of other etiology [33,34]. With regard to intracellular pathogens, although IL-17–producing cells are not as important as IFN-γ–producing cells, their role in inducing neutrophils is still important in this scenario [35]. Furthermore, it is intriguing the observation of a plasticity of Th17 and ILC3 cells that, under specific circumstances, can divert toward a type 1 response and synergize with Th1 cells [17]. Finally, in the case of Mycobacterium tuberculosis infection, Th17 cells are crucial for the development of an effective memory T cell response [36,37].

TH17 CELLS AND SYSTEMIC AUTOIMMUNE DISEASES

The evidence that IL-17 knockout (KO) mice are less prone to develop autoimmune diseases such as type 1 diabetes, collagen-induced arthritis, experimental autoimmune encephalomyelitis, and Sjögren's syndrome (SS) prompted intense investigation in this field [38–40]. As summarized in Table 6.1, the assessment of IL-17 and related cytokines in sera, other biologic fluids, and target tissues from patients with rheumatoid arthritis (RA), systemic lupus erythematosus (SLE), and primary (p) SS, as well as phenotypic and functional analysis performed in peripheral blood mononuclear cells, revealed many facets of IL-17 axis in systemic autoimmune diseases and provided the rationale to pursue possible targeting of such system for therapeutic purposes [93–97].

Rheumatoid Arthritis

In the context of RA pathogenesis, data from experimental models of the disease support the role of IL-17 in pannus growth, synovial neoangiogenesis, and development of bone erosions [98–103,123]. In humans, in vitro studies revealed that recombinant IL-17 is able to potentiate the expression of proinflammatory cytokines such as TNF-α and prostaglandin E2 and synergize their effects in synovial tissue cells, confirming its role in inducing pannus growth and osteoclastogenesis in vivo [41,42,99]. Interestingly, such synergistic effects seem to change from patient to patient as the blockade of either or both cytokine results in different inhibition of bone resorption [104,105]. Furthermore, the proangiogenic potential of IL-17 is also confirmed by the evidence that its recombinant form enhances the production of vascular endothelial growth factor A in RA synovial fibroblasts [66]. To date, a consistent body of evidence is available with regard to IL-17 and Th17 cells in RA [106]. The first studies aimed at measuring IL-17 in RA serum and synovial fluid date back in early 2000s. In most cohorts, IL-17 was increased in both kind of samples compared with normal or osteoarthritis (OA) controls [41–52]. In the majority of cases, also the proportion of circulating Th17 cells was higher compared with controls and paralleled the serum concentration of IL-17 [52,57–65]. IL-17 expression was also increased in RA synovial tissue compared with OA controls [41,42,47,49,53–56]. It is interesting to note that according to the aforementioned plasticity of Th17 cells, FoxP3+Th17 cells have been demonstrated in rheumatoid synovial membrane and they show a more pathogenic behavior compared with Th17 cells originating from naïve T cells [15]. Finally, it has been speculated that Th17 cells and IL-17 may act as biomarker of higher disease activity or more severe disease. In fact, most studies agree that serum IL-17 concentration [46,50,56], circulating Th17 cell percentage [57,61,65], and IL-17 synovial tissue expression [55,66] positively correlate with the disease activity score on 28 joints. Serum IL-17 levels appear to be directly correlated with both erythrocyte sedimentation rate and C-reactive protein [50,67]. Synovial fluid Th17-cell percentage is directly correlated with the degree of synovial intimal lining layer hyperplasia [56] and with the ultrasound power Doppler signal in the corresponding joint [66].

Systemic Lupus Erythematosus

Owing to its multifaceted functional activity, IL-17 can participate in several aspects of SLE pathogenesis. The induction of inflammatory mediators, the interplay with autoreactive B lymphocytes, and the fostering of T lymphocyte migration to

TABLE 6.1 Indicators of Th17 Cells and IL-17 Involvement in the Pathogenesis of Rheumatoid Arthritis, Systemic Lupus Erythematosus, and Primary Sjögren's Syndrome

Disease	Findings	References
Rheumatoid arthritis	• ↑ PB IL-17 versus HD or OA	[41–52]
	• ↑ SF IL-17 versus OA	[41–52]
	• ↑ SM IL-17 compared to OA	[41,42,47,49,53–56]
	• ↑ PB Th17 cells compared to HD	[52,57–65]
	• ↑ SM Th17 cells compared to OA	[41,42,47,49,53–56]
	• Association of PB IL-17 with DAS28	[46,50,56]
	• Association of PB Th17 cells with DAS28	[57,61,65]
	• Association of SM IL-17 with DAS28	[55,66]
	• Association of PB IL-17 with ESR and CRP	[50,67]
	• Association of SF Th17 cells with degree of SM hyperplasia	[56]
	• Association of SF Th17 cells with US PD	[66]
Systemic lupus erythematosus	• ↑ PB IL-17 versus HD	[68–77]
	• ↑ Renal IL-17 in lupus nephritis	[78]
	• ↑ Cutaneous IL-17 in lesional areas	[79]
	• ↑ CSF IL-17 in CNS lupus	[80]
	• Association of PB IL-17 with SLEDAI	[78]
	• No association of PB IL-17 with SLEDAI	[75,76]
	• Predictive value of PB IL-17 levels for nephritis evolution	[78]
	• Association of glomerular IL-17 with extent of histologically proven damage, proteinuria, hematuria, and blood urea nitrogen	[81,82]
Primary Sjögren's syndrome	• ↑ PB IL-17 in a small patient subgroup	[83–86]
	• ↑ IL-17 in MSGs	[83,84,87]
	• Association of PB IL-17 with longer disease duration	[86]
	• Association of PB IL-17 with presence of GCs in MSGs	[86]
	• Association of MSG IL-17 with glandular inflammation extent	[83,84,87]
	• ↑ IL-17 in saliva versus xerostomia of other etiology	[88]
	• ↑ IL-17 in tears versus dry eye of other etiology	[89–92]
	• No association of salivary IL-17 with glandular damage	[88]

CNS, central nervous system; *CRP*, C-reactive protein; *CSF*, cerebrospinal fluid; *DAS28*, disease activity score on 28 joints; *ESR*, erythrocyte sedimentation rate; *GCs*, germinal center–like structures; *HD*, healthy donors; *MSGs*, minor salivary glands; *OA*, osteoarthritis; *PB*, peripheral blood; *SF*, synovial fluid; *SM*, synovial membrane.

target tissues explain why IL-17 is a leading actor in this scenario [107]. However, it is interesting to note that data from different animal models about the role of Th17 cells in lupus nephritis are conflicting. In IL-17 KO MRL/*lpr* mice, the natural history of lupus nephritis is not affected [108], whereas B6 KO mice are resistant to the induction of concanavalin A–activated lymphocyte-derived DNA (ALD-DNA) lupus nephritis, even when higher doses compared with those effective in wild-type (WT) mice are employed [109], and B6.lpr IL-17R KO mice are protected from poly I:C–induced glomerulo-nephritis [110]. On the other hand, following the induction of ALD-DNA lupus nephritis in the WT BALB/c mice, IL-17 serum levels are strongly correlated with pathology score of kidney, serum levels of anti-dsDNA, and levels of proteinuria. In addition, the overexpression of IL-17 by an adenovirus construct that expresses murine IL-17 before the immunization with ALD-DNA leads to worse kidney damage compared with mice injected with the control adenovirus. Finally, IL-17 blockade significantly ameliorates ALD-DNA–induced lupus nephritis [109]. Likewise, IL-17 blockade in NZB/NZW mice leads to an improvement of lupus nephritis [108]. With regard to the human counterpart, the majority of studies agree that serum levels of IL-17 and circulating Th17 cells are increased in SLE [68–77]. Serum IL-17 levels strongly correlate with disease activity and are particularly elevated in particular subgroups of patients with glomerulonephritis [74,111–113], neurological manifestations [75,76], and pulmonary manifestations [114]. In this regard, IL-17 serum levels have also been suggested as biomarkers to monitor patients with specific manifestations, but currently available data are conflicting [75,76,78]. Increased levels of IL-17 have been also observed in target organs of the disease including kidney [78], skin [79], and central nervous system [80]. With regard to renal disease, glomerular IL-17 levels correlate with the extent of histologically proven damage, proteinuria, hematuria, and blood urea nitrogen level [81,82]. IL-17 has also been detected at mRNA level in urine sediment of patients with lupus nephritis [115]. In this scenario, besides conventional CD4+ Th17 cells, a peculiar T lymphocyte subsets lacking CD4 and CD8 on cell surface (double negative, DN) is crucial for the local IL-17 balance in kidneys [116].

Primary Sjögren's Syndrome

The first evidence that the overexpression of IL-17 in salivary glands of nonsusceptible mice was able to trigger an SS-like condition dates back in 2008 and was followed by the demonstration that IL-17 KO mice do not develop salivary gland inflammation despite being immunized with salivary gland peptides [40,124]. In the latter model, the adoptive transfer of Th17 cells was able to induce a focal sialadenitis similar to that of WT mice [40]. It became therefore clear that this cytokine and, in consequence, Th17 cells play a key role in the induction of pSS [94,117]. Besides conventional CD4+ Th17 cells, there is evidence that also CD8+ T cells, DN T cells, and mast cells contribute to IL-17 balance in pSS [118–122]. Unlike RA, the body of evidence regarding IL-17 in pSS serum is rather scarce. However, the few available studies agree that only a subgroup of pSS display detectable serum levels of IL-17 [83–86]. Of interest, this subset of IL-17+ pSS patients has longer disease duration, less prevalence of parotid gland swelling, and ectopic lymphoid, germinal center–like structures in minor salivary glands (MSGs) [86]. These findings fit with the evidence that although an overall increase of circulating CD4+ Th17 and DN T cells can be detected in pSS, there are differences in their proportion according to the phase of the disease. In fact, while in early pSS CD4+ Th17 cells are expanded and DN T cells are comparable with those of normal subjects, in patients with established disease, DN T cells are expanded and CD4+ Th17 cells are comparable with those of normal subjects [84,119–121]. Furthermore, pSS MSGs always express IL-17 and such expression parallels the severity of the inflammatory infiltrate [83,84,87]. In addition, DN, but not CD4+ Th17, cells have been associated with the same parameter and also with the development of ectopic lymphoid structures [121]. Finally, the few studies assessing IL-17 in saliva and tears of pSS patients revealed increased levels of this cytokine compared with subjects with dry mouth or dry eye of other etiology, but no association with MSG inflammation or other clinical and serological features was observed [88–92].

CONCLUDING REMARKS

Th17 cells are a pleiotropic T cell subset involved in several physiological and pathological processes but, although several aspects of their function have been unmasked, many others need to be fully elucidated. From their crucial role in host defense to their capability to orchestrate tissue damage in inflammatory diseases, Th17 cells have attracted a lot of attention in different fields over the last decades, and the possible therapeutic targeting of the IL-17 axis in autoimmune diseases is under intense investigation.

REFERENCES

[1] Mosmann TR, Cherwinski H, Bond MW, Giedlin MA, Coffman RL. Two types of murine helper T cell clone. I. Definition according to profiles of lymphokine activities and secreted proteins. J Immunol 1986;175:5–14.

[2] Romagnani S. Human TH1 and TH2 subsets: doubt no more. Immunol Today 1991;12:256–7.

[3] Romagnani S. Lymphokine production by human T cells in human disease states. Annu Rev Immunol 1994;12:227–57.

[4] Rouvier E, Luciani MF, Mattei MG, Denizot F, Golstein P. CTLA-8, cloned from an activated T cell, bearing AU-rich messenger RNA instability sequences, and homologous to a herpesvirus saimiri gene. J Immunol 1993;150:5445–56.

[5] Yao Z, Painter SL, Fanslow WC, Ulrich D, Macduff BM, Spriggs MK, Armitage RJ, Human IL. 17: a novel cytokine derived from T cells. J Immunol 1995;155:5483–6.

[6] Harrington LE, Hatton PR, Mangan H, Turner TL, Murphy TL, Murphy KM, Weaver CT. Interleukin17-producing CD41 effector T cells develop via lineage distinct from the T helper type 1 and 2 lineages. Nat Immunol 2005;6:1123–32.

[7] Acosta-Rodriguez EV, Rivino L, Geginat J, Jarrossay D, Gattorno M, Lanzavecchia A, Sallusto F, Napolitani G. Surface phenotype and antigen specificity of human interleukin 17-producing T helper memory cells. Nat Immunol 2007;8:639–46.

[8] Annunziato F, Cosmi L, Santarlasci V, Maggi L, Liotta F, Mazzinghi B, Parente E, Filì L, Ferri S, Frosali F, Giudici F, Romagnani P, Parronchi P, Tonelli F, Maggi E, Romagnani S. Phenotypic and functional features of human Th17 cells. J Exp Med 2007;204:1849–61.

[9] O'Shea JJ, Paul WE. Mechanisms underlying lineage commitment and plasticity of helper CD4+ T cells. Science 2010;327(5969):1098–102.

[10] Kolls JK, Linden A. Interleukin-17 family members and inflammation. Immunity 2004;21:467–76.

[11] Aggarwal S, Ghilardi N, Xie M, de Sauvage FJ, Gurney AL. Interleukin 23 promotes a distinct CD4 T cell activation state characterized by the production of interleukin 17. J Biol Chem 2003;278(3):1910–4.

[12] Noack M, Miossec P. Th17 and regulatory T cell balance in autoimmune and inflammatory diseases. Autoimmun Rev 2014;13(6):668–77.

[13] Weaver CT, Hatton RD, Mangan PR, Harrington LE. IL-17 family cytokines and the expanding diversity of effector T cell lineages. Annu Rev Immunol 2007;25:821–52.

[14] Lee YK, Mukasa R, Hatton RD, Weaver CT. Developmental plasticity of Th17 and Treg cells. Curr Opin Immunol 2009;21:274–80.

[15] Komatsu N, Okamoto K, Sawa S, Nakashima T, Oh-Hora M, Kodama T, Tanaka S, Bluestone JA, Takayanagi H. Pathogenic conversion of Foxp3(+) T cells into TH17 cells in autoimmune arthritis. Nat Med January 2014;20(1):62–8.

[16] Sharma MD, Hou DY, Liu Y, Koni PA, Metz R, Chandler P, Mellor AL, He Y, Munn DH. Indoleamine 2,3-dioxygenase controls conversion of Foxp3+ Tregs to TH17-like cells in tumor draining lymph nodes. Blood 2009;113:6102–11.

[17] Hirota K, Duarte JH, Veldhoen M, Hornsby E, Li Y, Cua DJ, Ahlfors H, Wilhelm C, Tolaini M, Menzel U, Garefalaki A, Potocnik AJ, Stockinger B. Fate mapping of IL-17-producing T cells in inflammatory responses. Nat Immunol 2011;12:255–63.

[18] Harbour SN, Maynard CL, Zindl CL, Schoeb TR, Weaver CT. Th17 cells give rise to Th1 cells that are required for the pathogenesis of colitis. Proc Natl Acad Sci USA 2015;112(22):7061–6.

[19] Morrison PJ, Bending D, Fouser LA, Wright JF, Stockinger B, Cooke A, Kullberg MC. Th17-cell plasticity in Helicobacter hepaticus-induced intestinal inflammation. Mucosal Immunol 2013;6:1143–56.

[20] Ahlfors H, Morrison PJ, Duarte JH, Li Y, Biro J, Tolaini M, Di Meglio P, Potocnik AJ, Stockinger B. IL-22 fate reporter reveals origin and control of IL-22 production in homeostasis and infection. J Immunol 2014;193:4602–13.

[21] Jostins L, Ripke S, Weersma RK, Duerr RH, McGovern DP, Hui KY, Lee JC, Schumm LP, Sharma Y, Anderson CA, Essers J, Mitrovic M, Ning K, Cleynen I, Theatre E, Spain SL, Raychaudhuri S, Goyette P, Wei Z, Abraham C, Achkar JP, Ahmad T, Amininejad L, Ananthakrishnan AN, Andersen V, Andrews JM, Baidoo L, Balschun T, Bampton PA, Bitton A, Boucher G, Brand S, Büning C, Cohain A, Cichon S, D'Amato M, De Jong D, Devaney KL, Dubinsky M, Edwards C, Ellinghaus D, Ferguson LR, Franchimont D, Fransen K, Gearry R, Georges M, Gieger C, Glas J, Haritunians T, Hart A, Hawkey C, Hedl M, Hu X, Karlsen TH, Kupcinskas L, Kugathasan S, Latiano A, Laukens D, Lawrance IC, Lees CW, Louis E, Mahy G, Mansfield J, Morgan AR, Mowat C, Newman W, Palmieri O, Ponsioen CY, Potocnik U, Prescott NJ, Regueiro M, Rotter JI, Russell RK, Sanderson JD, Sans M, Satsangi J, Schreiber S, Simms LA, Sventoraityte J, Targan SR, Taylor KD, Tremelling M, Verspaget HW, De Vos M, Wijmenga C, Wilson DC, Winkelmann J, Xavier RJ, Zeissig S, Zhang B, Zhang CK, Zhao H, International IBD Genetics Consortium (IIBDGC), Silverberg MS, Annese V, Hakonarson H, Brant SR, Radford-Smith G, Mathew CG, Rioux JD, Schadt EE, Daly MJ, Franke A, Parkes M, Vermeire S, Barrett JC, Cho JH. Host-microbe interactions have shaped the genetic architecture of inflammatory bowel disease. Nature 2012;491:119–24.

[22] Hirota K, Turner JE, Villa M, Duarte JH, Demengeot J, Steinmetz OM, Stockinger B. Plasticity of Th17 cells in Peyer's patches is responsible for the induction of T cell dependent IgA responses. Nat Immunol 2013;14:372–9.

[23] Veldhoen M. Interleukin 17 is a chief orchestrator of immunity. Nat Immunol 2017;18(6):612–21.

[24] Pennino D, Eyerich K, Scarponi C, Carbone T, Eyerich S, Nasorri F, Garcovich S, Traidl-Hoffmann C, Albanesi C, Cavani A. IL-17 amplifies human contact hypersensitivity by licensing hapten nonspecific Th1 cells to kill autologous keratinocytes. J Immunol 2010;184:4880–8.

[25] Chiricozzi A, Nograles KE, Johnson-Huang LM, Fuentes-Duculan J, Cardinale I, Bonifacio KM, Gulati N, Mitsui H, Guttman-Yassky E, Suárez-Fariñas M, Krueger JG. IL-17 induces an expanded range of downstream genes in reconstituted human epidermis model. PLoS One 2014;9:e90284.

[26] Liévin-Le Moal V, Servin AL. The front line of enteric host defense against unwelcome intrusion of harmful microorganisms: mucins, antimicrobial peptides, and microbiota. Clin Microbiol Rev 2006;19:315–37.

[27] Martin B, Hirota K, Cua DJ, Stockinger B, Veldhoen M. Interleukin-17-producing γδ T cells selectively expand in response to pathogen products and environmental signals. Immunity 2009;31:321–30.

[28] Satoh-Takayama N, Vosshenrich CA, Lesjean-Pottier S, Sawa S, Lochner M, Rattis F, Mention JJ, Thiam K, Cerf-Bensussan N, Mandelboim O, Eberl G, Di Santo JP. Microbial flora drives interleukin 22 production in intestinal NKp46+ cells that provide innate mucosal immune defense. Immunity 2008;29:958–70.

[29] McKenzie BS, Kastelein RA, Cua DJ. Understanding the IL-23-IL-17 immune pathway. Trends Immunol 2006;27.17–23.

[30] Huang W, Na L, Fidel PL, Schwarzenberger P. Requirement of interleukin-17A for systemic anti-Candida albicans host defence in mice. J Infect Dis 2004;190:624–31.

[31] Eyerich K, Foerster S, Rombold S, Seidl H-P, Behrendt H, Hofmann H, Ring J, Traidl-Hoffmann C. Patients with chronic mucocutaneous candidiasis exhibit reduced production of Th17- associated cytokines IL-17 and IL-22. J Investig Dermatol 2008;128:2640–5.

[32] Puel A, Cypowyj S, Bustamante J, Wright JF, Liu L, Lim HK, Migaud M, Israel L, Chrabieh M, Audry M, Gumbleton M, Toulon A, Bodemer C, El-Baghdadi J, Whitters M, Paradis T, Brooks J, Collins M, Wolfman NM, Al-Muhsen S, Galicchio M, Abel L, Picard C, Casanova JL. Chronic mucocutaneous candidiasis in humans with inborn errors of interleukin-17 immunity. Science 2011;332:65–8.

[33] Milner JD, Brenchley JM, Laurence A, Freeman AF, Hill BJ, Elias KM, Kanno Y, Spalding C, Elloumi HZ, Paulson ML, Davis J, Hsu A, Asher AI, O'Shea J, Holland SM, Paul WE, Douek DC. Impaired T(H)17 cell differentiation in subjects with autosomal dominant hyper-IgE syndrome. Nature 2008;452:773–6.

[34] Ma CS, Chew GY, Simpson N, Priyadarshi A, Wong M, Grimbacher B, Fulcher DA, Tangye SG, Cook MC. Deficiency of Th17 cells in hyper IgE syndrome due to mutations in STAT3. J Exp Med 2008;205:1551–7.

[35] Zhang Y, Wang H, Ren J, Tang X, Jing Y, Xing D, Zhao G, Yao Z, Yang X, Bai H. IL-17A synergizes with IFN-γ to upregulate iNOS and NO production and inhibit chlamydial growth. PLoS One 2012;7:e39214.

[36] Khader SA, Bell GK, Pearl JE, Fountain JJ, Rangel-Moreno J, Cilley GE, Shen F, Eaton SM, Gaffen SL, Swain SL, Locksley RM, Haynes L, Randall TD, Cooper AM. IL-23 and IL-17 in the establishment of protective pulmonary CD4+ T cell responses after vaccination and during Mycobacterium tuberculosis challenge. Nat Immunol 2007;8:369–77.

[37] Trentini MM, de Oliveira FM, Kipnis A, Junqueira-Kipnis AP. The role of neutrophils in the induction of specific Th1 and Th17 during vaccination against tuberculosis. Front Microbiol 2016;7:898.

[38] Hsu HC, Yang P, Wang J, Wu Q, Myers R, Chen J, Yi J, Guentert T, Tousson A, Stanus AL, Le TV, Lorenz RG, Xu H, Kolls JK, Carter RH, Chaplin DD, Williams RW, Mountz JD. Interleukin 17–producing T helper cells and interleukin 17 orchestrate autoreactive germinal center development in autoimmune BXD2 mice. Nat Immunol 2008;9:166–75.

[39] Kuriya G, Uchida T, Akazawa S, Kobayashi M, Nakamura K, Satoh T, Horie I, Kawasaki E, Yamasaki H, Yu L, Iwakura Y, Sasaki H, Nagayama Y, Kawakami A, Abiru N. Double deficiency in IL-17 and IFN-γ signalling significantly suppresses the development of diabetes in the NOD mouse. Diabetologia 2013;56:1773–80.

[40] Lin X, Rui K, Deng J, Tian J, Wang X, Wang S, Ko KH, Jiao Z, Chan VS, Lau CS, Cao X, Lu L. Th17 cells play a critical role in the development of experimental Sjögren's syndrome. Ann Rheum Dis 2015;74(6):1302–10.

[41] Kotake S, Udagawa N, Takahashi N, Matsuzaki K, Itoh K, Ishiyama S, Saito S, Inoue K, Kamatani N, Gillespie MT, Martin TJ, Suda T. IL-17 in synovial fluids from patients with rheumatoid arthritis is a potent stimulator of osteoclastogenesis. J Clin Investig 1999;103(9):1345–52.

[42] Moran EM, Mullan R, McCormick J, Connolly M, Sullivan O, Fitzgerald O, Bresnihan B, Veale DJ, Fearon UE. Human rheumatoid arthritis tissue production of IL-17A drives matrix and cartilage degradation: synergy with tumour necrosis factor-α, Oncostatin M and response to biologic therapies. Arthritis Res Ther 2009;11(4):R113.

[43] Ziolkowska M, Koc A, Luszczykiewicz G, Ksiezopolska-Pietrzak K, Klimczak E, Chwalinska-Sadowska H, Maslinski W. High levels of IL-17 in rheumatoid arthritis patients: IL-15 triggers in vitro IL-17 production via cyclosporin A-sensitive mechanism. J Immunol 2000;164(5):2832–8.

[44] Kageyama Y, Ichikawa T, Nagafusa T, Torikai E, Shimazu M, Nagano AM. Etanercept reduces the serum levels of interleukin-23 and macrophage inflammatory protein-3 alpha in patients with rheumatoid arthritis. Rheumatol Int 2007;28(2):137–43.

[45] Chen DY, Chen YM, Chen HH, Hsieh CW, Lin CC, Lan JL. Increasing levels of circulating Th17 cells and interleukin-17 in rheumatoid arthritis patients with an inadequate response to anti-TNF-α therapy. Arthritis Res Ther 2011;13(4):R126.

[46] Metawi SA, Abbas D, Kamal MM, Ibrahim MK. Serum and synovial fluid levels of interleukin-17 in correlation with disease activity in patients with RA. Clin Rheumatol 2011;30(9):1201–7.

[47] Kenna TJ, Brown MA. The role of IL-17-secreting mast cells in inflammatory joint disease. Nat Rev Rheumatol 2013;9(6):375–9.

[48] Arroyo-Villa I, Bautista-Caro MB, Balsa A, Aguado-Acín P, Nuño L, Bonilla-Hernán MG, Puig-Kröger A, Martín-Mola E, Miranda-Carús ME. Frequency of Th17 CD4+ T cells in early rheumatoid arthritis: a marker of anti-CCP seropositivity. PLoS One 2012;7(8):e42189.

[49] van Baarsen LG, Lebre MC, van der Coelen D, Aarrass S, Tang MW, Ramwadhdoebe TH, Gerlag DM, Tak PP. Heterogeneous expression pattern of interleukin-17A (IL-17A), IL-17F and their receptors in synovium of rheumatoid arthritis, psoriatic arthritis and osteoarthritis: possible explanation for non-response to anti-IL-17 therapy. Arthritis Res Ther 2014;16(4):426.

[50] Kim J, Kang S, Kim J, Kwon G, Koo S. Elevated levels of T helper 17 cells are associated with disease activity in patients with rheumatoid arthritis. Ann Lab Med 2013;33(1):52–9.

[51] Shen H, Goodall JC, Hill Gaston JS. Frequency and phenotype of peripheral blood Th17 cells in ankylosing spondylitis and rheumatoid arthritis. Arthritis Rheum 2009;60(6):1647–56.

[52] Fazaa A, Ben Abdelghani K, Abdeladhim M, Laatar A, Ben Ahmed M, Zakraoui L. The level of interleukin-17 in serum is linked to synovial hypervascularisation in rheumatoid arthritis. Joint Bone Spine 2014;81:550–1.

[53] Shahrara S, Huang Q, Mandelin 2nd AM, Pope RM. TH-17 cells in rheumatoid arthritis. Arthritis Res Ther 2008;10(4):R93.

[54] Hueber AJ, Asquith DL, Miller AM, Reilly J, Kerr S, Leipe J, Melendez AJ, McInnes IB. Mast cells express IL-17A in rheumatoid arthritis synovium. J Immunol 2010;184(7):3336–40.

[55] Li N, Wang JC, Liang TH, Zhu MH, Wang JY, Fu XL, Zhou JR, Zheng SG, Chan P, Han J. Pathologic finding of increased expression of interleukin-17 in the synovial tissue of rheumatoid arthritis patients. Int J Clin Exp Pathol 2013;6(7):1375–9.

[56] Melis L, Vandooren B, Kruithof E, Jacques P, De Vos M, Mielants H, Verbruggen G, De Keyser F, Elewaut D. Systemic levels of IL-23 are strongly associated with disease activity in rheumatoid arthritis but not spondyloarthritis. Ann Rheum Dis 2010;69(3):618–23.

[57] Niu Q, Cai B, Huang ZC, Shi YY, Wang LL. Disturbed Th17/Treg balance in patients with rheumatoid arthritis. Rheumatol Int 2012;32(9):2731–6.

[58] Samson M, Audia S, Janikashvili N, Ciudad M, Trad M, Fraszczak J, Ornetti P, Maillefert JF, Miossec P, Bonnotte B. Brief report: inhibition of interleukin-6 function corrects Th17/Treg cell imbalance in patients with rheumatoid arthritis. Arthritis Rheum 2012;64(8):2499–503.

[59] Lina C, Conghua W, Nan L, Ping Z. Combined treatment of etanercept and MTX reverses Th1/Th2, Th17/Treg imbalance in patients with rheumatoid arthritis. J Clin Immunol 2011;31(4):596–605.

[60] Guggino G, Giardina A, Ferrante A, Giardina G, Schinocca C, Sireci G, Dieli F, Ciccia F, Triolo G. The in vitro addition of methotrexate and/or methylprednisolone determines peripheral reduction in Th17 and expansion of conventional Treg and of IL-10 producing Th17 lymphocytes in patients with early rheumatoid arthritis. Rheumatol Int 2015;35(1):171–5.

[61] Zhang L, Li YG, Li YH, Qi L, Liu XG, Yuan CZ, Hu NW, Ma DX, Li ZF, Yang Q, Li W, Li JM. Increased frequencies of th22 cells as well as th17 cells in the peripheral blood of patients with ankylosing spondylitis and rheumatoid arthritis. PLoS One 2012;7(4):e31000.

[62] van Hamburg JP, Corneth OB, Paulissen SM, Davelaar N, Asmawidjaja PS, Mus AM, Lubberts E. IL-17/Th17 mediated synovial inflammation is IL-22 independent. Ann Rheum Dis 2013;72(10):1700–7.

[63] Henriques A, Gomes V, Duarte C, Pedreiro S, Carvalheiro T, Areias M, Caseiro A, Gabriel AJ, Laranjeira P, Pais ML, da Silva JA, Paiva A. Distribution and functional plasticity of peripheral blood Th(c)17 and Th(c)1 in rheumatoid arthritis. Rheumatol Int 2013;33(8):2093–9.

[64] Sarkar S, Fox DA. Targeting Il-17 and th17 cells in rheumatoid arthritis. Rheum Dis Clin N Am 2010;36(2):345–66.

[65] Miao J, Zhang K, Lv M, Li Q, Zheng Z, Han Q, Guo N, Fan C, Zhu P. Circulating Th17 and Th1 cells expressing CD161 are associated with disease activity in rheumatoid arthritis. Scand J Rheumatol 2014;43(3):194–201.

[66] Gullick NJ, Evans HG, Church LD, Jayaraj DM, Filer A, Kirkham BW, Taams LS. Linking power Doppler ultrasound to the presence of Th17 cells in the rheumatoid arthritis joint. PLoS One September 1, 2010;5(9).

[67] Shen H, Xia L, Lu J, Xiao W. Infliximab reduces the frequency of interleukin 17-producing cells and the amounts of interleukin 17 in patients with rheumatoid arthritis. J Investig Med 2010;58(7):905–8.

[68] Yu B, Guan M, Peng Y, Shao Y, Zhang C, Yue X, Zhang J, Yang H, Zou H, Ye W, Wan J, Zhang W. Copy number variations of interleukin-17F, interleukin-21, and interleukin-22 are associated with systemic lupus erythematosus. Arthritis Rheum 2011;63:3487–92.

[69] Bălănescu P, Bălănescu E, Tănăsescu C, Nicolau A, Tănăsescu R, Grancea C, Vagu C, Ruță S, Bleoțu C. T helper 17 cell population in lupus erythematosus. Rom J Intern Med 2010;48(3):255–9.

[70] Rana A, Minz RW, Aggarwal R, Anand S, Pasricha N, Singh S. Gene expression of cytokines (TNF-alpha, IFN-gamma), serum profiles of IL-17 and IL-23 in paediatric systemic lupus erythematosus. Lupus 2012;21(10):1105–12.

[71] Torricelli M, Bellisai F, Novembri R, Galeazzi LR, Iuliano A, Voltolini C, Spreafico A, Galeazzi M, Petraglia F. High levels of maternal serum IL-17 and activin A in pregnant women affected by systemic lupus erythematosus. Am J Reprod Immunol 2011;66(2):84–9.

[72] Chen XQ, Yu YC, Deng HH, Sun JZ, Dai Z, Wu YW, Yang M. Plasma IL-17A is increased in new-onset SLE patients and associated with disease activity. J Clin Immunol 2010;30(2):221–5.

[73] Ballantine LE, Ong J, Midgley A, Watson L, Flanagan BF, Beresford MW. The proinflammatory potential of T cells in juvenile-onset systemic lupus erythematosus. Pediatr Rheumatol Online J 2014;12:4.

[74] Rastin M, Soltani S, Nazemian F, Sahebari M, Mirfeizi SZ, Tabasi N, Mahmoudi M. Expression of T Helper 17 and regulatory T cell cytokines and molecules in glomerulonephritis class IV systemic lupus erythematosus. Iran J Kidney Dis 2016;10(3):113–8.

[75] Vincent FB, Northcott M, Hoi A, Mackay F, Morand EF. Clinical associations of serum interleukin-17 in systemic lupus erythematosus. Arthritis Res Ther 2013;15:R97.

[76] Mok MY, Wu HJ, Lo Y, Lau CS. The relation of interleukin 17 (IL-17) and IL-23 to Th1/Th2 cytokines and disease activity in systemic lupus erythematosus. J Rheumatol 2010;37:2046–52.

[77] Zhao XF, Pan HF, Yuan H, Zhang WH, Li XP, Wang GH, Wu GC, Su H, Pan FM, Li WX, Li LH, Chen GP, Ye DQ. Increased serum interleukin 17 in patients with systemic lupus erythematosus. Mol Biol Rep 2010;37(1):81–5.

[78] Abdel Galil SM, Ezzeldin N, El-Boshy ME. The role of serum IL-17 and IL-6 as biomarkers of disease activity and predictors of remission in patients with lupus nephritis. Cytokine 2015;76(2):280–7.

[79] Tanasescu C, Balanescu E, Balanescu P, Olteanu R, Badea C, Grancea C, Vagu C, Bleotu C, Ardeleanu C, Georgescu A. IL-17 in cutaneous lupus erythematosus. Eur J Intern Med 2010;21:202–7.

[80] Lu XY, Zhu CQ, Qian J, Chen XX, Ye S, Gu YY. Intrathecal cytokine and chemokine profiling in neuropsychiatric lupus or lupus complicated with central nervous system infection. Lupus 2010;19:689–95.

[81] Chen DY, Chen YM, Wen MC, Hsieh TY, Hung WT, Lan JL. The potential role of Th17 cells and Th17-related cytokines in the pathogenesis of lupus nephritis. Lupus 2012;21:1385–96.

[82] Wang Y, Ito S, Chino Y, Goto D, Matsumoto I, Murata H, Tsutsumi A, Hayashi T, Uchida K, Usui J, Yamagata K, Sumida T. Laser microdissection-based analysis of cytokine balance in the kidneys of patients with lupus nephritis. Clin Exp Immunol 2010;159:1–10.

[83] Nguyen CQ, Hu MH, Li Y, Stewart C, Peck AB. Salivary gland tissue expression of interleukin-23 and interleukin-17 in Sjögren's syndrome: findings in humans and mice. Arthritis Rheum 2008;58(3):734–43.

[84] Fei Y, Zhang W, Lin D, Wu C, Li M, Zhao Y, Zeng X, Zhang F. Clinical parameter and Th17 related to lymphocytes infiltrating degree of labial salivary gland in primary Sjögren's syndrome. Clin Rheumatol 2014;33(4):523–9.

[85] Reksten TR, Jonsson MV, Szyszko EA, Brun JG, Jonsson R, Brokstad KA. Cytokine and autoantibody profiling related to histopathological features in primary Sjögren's syndrome. Rheumatology (Oxford) 2009;48(9):1102–6.

[86] Alunno A, Bistoni O, Caterbi S, Bartoloni E, Cafaro G, Gerli R. Serum interleukin-17 in primary Sjögren's syndrome: association with disease duration and parotid gland swelling. Clin Exp Rheumatol 2015;33(1):129.

[87] Katsifis GE, Rekka S, Moutsopoulos NM, Pillemer S, Wahl SM. Systemic and local interleukin-17 and linked cytokines associated with Sjögren's syndrome immunopathogenesis. Am J Pathol 2009;175(3):1167–77.

[88] Ohyama K, Moriyama M, Hayashida JN, Tanaka A, Maehara T, Ieda S, Furukawa S, Ohta M, Imabayashi Y, Nakamura S. Saliva as a potential tool for diagnosis of dry mouth including Sjögren's syndrome. Oral Dis 2015;21(2):224–31.

[89] Kang MH, Kim MK, Lee HJ, Lee HI, Wee WR, Lee JH. Interleukin-17 in various ocular surface inflammatory diseases. J Korean Med Sci 2011;26(7):938–44.

[90] Lee SY, Han SJ, Nam SM, Yoon SC, Ahn JM, Kim TI, Kim EK, Seo KY. Analysis of tear cytokines and clinical correlations in Sjögren's syndrome dry eye patients and non- Sjögren's syndrome dry eye patients. Am J Ophthalmol 2013;156(2). 247–253.e1.

[91] Tan X, Sun S, Liu Y, Zhu T, Wang K, Ren T, Wu Z, Xu H, Zhu L. Analysis of Th17-associated cytokines in tears of patients with dry eye syndrome. Eye (Lond) 2014;28(5):608–13.

[92] Chung JK, Kim MK, Wee WR. Prognostic factors for the clinical severity of keratoconjunctivitis sicca in patients with Sjögren's syndrome. Br J Ophthalmol 2012;96(2):240–5.

[93] Alunno A, Manetti M, Caterbi S, Ibba-Manneschi L, Bistoni O, Bartoloni E, Valentini V, Terenzi R, Gerli R. Altered immunoregulation in rheumatoid arthritis: the role of regulatory T cells and proinflammatory Th17 cells and therapeutic implications. Mediators Inflamm 2015;2015:751793.

[94] Alunno A, Carubbi F, Bartoloni E, Bistoni O, Caterbi S, Cipriani P, Giacomelli R, Gerli R. Unmasking the pathogenic role of IL-17 axis in primary Sjögren's syndrome: a new era for therapeutic targeting? Autoimmun Rev 2014;13(12):1167–73.

[95] Alunno A, Carubbi F, Bistoni O, Bartoloni E, Valentini V, Gerli R. Novel therapeutic strategies in primary Sjögren's syndrome. Isr Med Assoc J 2017;19(9):576–80.

[96] Montanucci P, Alunno A, Basta G, Bistoni O, Pescara T, Caterbi S, Pennoni I, Bini V, Gerli R, Calafiore R. Restoration of t cell substes of patients with type 1 diabetes mellitus by microencapsulated human umbilical cord Wharton jelly-derived mesenchymal stem cells: an in vitro study. Clin Immunol 2016;163:34–41.

[97] Paley MA, Strand V, Kim AH. From mechanism to therapies in systemic lupus erythematosus. Curr Opin Rheumatol 2017;29(2):178–86.

[98] Sato K, Suematsu A, Okamoto K, Yamaguchi A, Morishita Y, Kadono Y, Tanaka S, Kodama T, Akira S, Iwakura Y, Cua DJ, Takayanagi H. Th17 functions as an osteoclastogenic helper T cell subset that links T cell activation and bone destruction. J Exp Med 2006;203(12):2673–82.

[99] Ito H, Yamada H, Shibata TN, Mitomi H, Nomoto S, Ozaki SH. Dual role of interleukin-17 in pannus growth and osteoclastogenesis in rheumatoid arthritis. Arthritis Res Ther 2011;13(1):R14.

[100] Moon YM, Yoon BY, Her YM, Oh HJ, Lee JS, Kim KW, Lee SY, Woo YJ, Park KS, Park SH, Kim HY, Cho ML. IL-32 and IL-17 interact and have the potential to aggravate osteoclastogenesis in rheumatoid arthritis. Arthritis Res Ther 2012;14(6):R246.

[101] SJ1 K, Chen Z, Chamberlain ND, Volin MV, Swedler W, Volkov S, Sweiss N, Shahrara S. Angiogenesis in rheumatoid arthritis is fostered directly by toll-like receptor 5 ligation and indirectly through interleukin-17 induction. Arthritis Rheum 2013;65(8):2024–36.

[102] Pickens SR, Volin MV, Mandelin 2nd AM, Kolls JK, Pope RM, Shahrara S. IL-17 contributes to angiogenesis in rheumatoid arthritis. J Immunol 2010;184(6):3233–41.

[103] Miossec P. Update on interleukin-17: a role in the pathogenesis of inflammatory arthritis and implication for clinical practice. RMD Open 2017;3(1):e000284.

[104] Chabaud M, Lubberts E, Joosten L, van Den Berg W, Miossec P. IL-17 derived from juxta-articular bone and synovium contributes to joint degradation in rheumatoid arthritis. Arthritis Res 2001;3:168–77.

[105] Chabaud M, Miossec P. The combination of tumor necrosis factor alpha blockade with interleukin-1 and interleukin-17 blockade is more effective for controlling synovial inflammation and bone resorption in an ex vivo model. Arthritis Rheum 2001;44:1293–303.

[106] Benedetti G, Miossec P. Interleukin 17 contributes to the chronicity of inflammatory diseases such as rheumatoid arthritis. Eur J Immunol 2014;44(2):339–47.

[107] Li D, Guo B, Wu H, Tan L, Chang C, Lu Q. Interleukin-17 in systemic lupus erythematosus: a comprehensive review. Autoimmunity 2015;48(6):353–61.

[108] Schmidt T, Paust HJ, Krebs CF, Turner JE, Kaffke A, Bennstein SB, Koyro T, Peters A, Velden J, Hünemörder S, Haag F, Steinmetz OM, Mittrücker HW, Stahl RA, Panzer U. Function of the Th17/interleukin-17A immune response in murine lupus nephritis. Arthritis Rheumatol 2015;67(2):475–87.

[109] Wen Z, Xu L, Xu W, Yin Z, Gao X, Xiong S. Interleukin-17 expression positively correlates with disease severity of lupus nephritis by increasing anti-double-stranded DNA antibody production in a lupus model induced by activated lymphocyte derived DNA. PLoS One 2013;8(3):e58161.

[110] Ramani K, Biswas PS. Interleukin 17 signaling drives Type I Interferon induced proliferative crescentic glomerulonephritis in lupus-prone mice. Clin Immunol 2016;162:31–6.

[111] Biswas PS, Aggarwal R, Levesque MC, Maers K, Ramani K. Type I interferon and T helper 17 cells co-exist and co-regulate disease pathogenesis in lupus patients. Int J Rheum Dis 2015;18(6):646–53.

[112] AlFadhli S, AlFailakawi A, Ghanem AA. Th-17 related regulatory network in the pathogenesis of patients with systemic lupus erythematosus and lupus nephritis. Int J Rheum Dis 2016;19(5):512–20.

[113] Xing Q, Wang B, Su H, Cui J, Li J. Elevated Th17 cells are accompanied by FoxP3+ Treg cells decrease in patients with lupus nephritis. Rheumatol Int 2012;32(4):949–58.

[114] Hammad A, Osman E, Mosaad Y, Wahba M. Serum interleukin-17 in Egyptian children with systemic lupus erythematosus: is it related to pulmonary affection? Lupus 2017;26(4):388–95.

[115] Kwan BC, Tam LS, Lai KB, Lai FM, Li EK, Wang G, Chow KM, Li PK, Szeto CC. The gene expression of type 17 T-helper cell-related cytokines in the urinary sediment of patients with systemic lupus erythematosus. Rheumatology (Oxford) 2009;48:1491–7.

[116] Crispín JC, Oukka M, Bayliss G, Cohen RA, Van Beek CA, Stillman IE, Kyttaris VC, Juang YT, Tsokos GC. Expanded double negative T cells in patients with systemic lupus erythematosus produce IL-17 and infiltrate the kidneys. J Immunol 2008;181(12):8761–6.

[117] Alunno A, Carubbi F, Bistoni O, Caterbi S, Bartoloni E, Mirabelli G, Cannarile F, Cipriani P, Giacomelli R, Gerli R. T regulatory and T helper 17 cells in primary Sjögren's syndrome: facts and perspectives. Mediators Inflamm 2015;2015:243723.

[118] Sakai A, Sugawara Y, Kuroishi T, Sasano T, Sugawara S. Identification of IL-18 and Th17 cells in salivary glands of patients with Sjögren's syndrome, and amplification of IL-17-mediated secretion of inflammatory cytokines from salivary gland cells by IL-18. J Immunol 2008;181(4):2898–906.

[119] Kwok SK, Cho ML, Her YM, Oh HJ, Park MK, Lee SY, Woo YJ, Ju JH, Park KS, Kim HY, Park SH. TLR2 ligation induces the production of IL-23/IL-17 via IL-6, STAT3 and NF-κB pathway in patients with primary Sjögren's syndrome. Arthritis Res Ther 2012;14(2):R64.

[120] Alunno A, Bistoni O, Bartoloni E, Caterbi S, Bigerna B, Tabarrini A, Mannucci R, Falini B, Gerli R. IL-17-producing CD4−CD8− T cells are expanded in the peripheral blood, infiltrate salivary glands and are resistant to corticosteroids in patients with primary Sjögren's syndrome. Ann Rheum Dis 2013;72(2):286–92.

[121] Alunno A, Carubbi F, Bistoni O, Caterbi S, Bartoloni E, Bigerna B, Pacini R, Beghelli D, Cipriani P, Giacomelli R, Gerli R. CD4-CD8- T-cells in primary Sjögren's syndrome: association with the extent of glandular involvement. J Autoimmun 2014;51:38–43.

[122] Ciccia F, Guggino G, Rizzo A, Alessandro R, Carubbi F, Giardina A, Cipriani P, Ferrante A, Cannizzaro A, Giacomelli R, Triolo G. Rituximab modulates IL-17 expression in the salivary glands of patients with primary Sjögren's syndrome. Rheumatology (Oxford) 2014;53(7):1313–20.

[123] Chabaud M, Durand JM, Buchs N, Fossiez F, Page G, Frappart L, Miossec P. Human interleukin-17: a T cell-derived proinflammatory cytokine produced by the rheumatoid synovium. Arthritis Rheum 1999;42(5):963–70.

[124] Nguyen CQ, Yin H, Lee BH, Carcamo WC, Chiorini JA, Peck AB. Pathogenic effect of interleukin-17A in induction of Sjögren's syndrome-like disease using adenovirus mediated gene transfer. Arthritis Res Ther 2010;12(6):R220.

Chapter 7

Natural Killer Cells in Autoimmunity

Maria Sole Chimenti, Paola Conigliaro, Giulia Lavinia Fonti, Roberto Perricone
Rheumatology, Allergy and Clinical Immunology – University of Rome "Tor Vergata", Rome, Italy

NATURAL KILLER CELLS

Cantor, Wigzell, Playfair, and other authors described between 1974 and 1977 a novel lymphocyte effector function mediated by cells that were large granulocytic lymphocytes yet were considered neither T cells nor B cells and did not use related families of antigen receptors [1]. These cells, called large granular lymphocytes or better known as natural killer (NK) cells, are part of the innate immune system and respond rapidly to a variety of insults via cytokine secretion and cytolytic activity [2–5]. Their main role is antiviral immune response and the effector function is perceived to be an important first line of innate immunity across viral, bacterial, and parasitic infections [6]. NK cells, which are thymus-independent and do not require preimmunization [7], thus reflecting their innate character, express the activation markers CD6, CD56, and CD57, the inhibitory marker CD158a, and CD94, which can be either inhibitory or activatory.

Human NK cells can be classified into two subsets, depending on their immunophenotype and function: $CD56^{dim}$ and $CD56^{bright}$. $CD56^{dim}$ constitutes 90% of the total NK cell population in peripheral blood and these express a low-affinity receptor for the constant region of immunoglobulin G (IgG), FcγRIIIa (CD16). Functionally, these have high cytotoxic activity. Approximately 10% of NK cells belong to the $CD56^{bright}$ subset and they are mostly involved in the production of cytokines. Table 7.1 summarizes the most relevant cellular receptors discovered on NK surface [8].

NK cell functioning is controlled by many inhibitory or activating receptors. The family of inhibitory receptors consists of the killer immunoglobulin-like receptors (KIR) or Ig-like receptors (CD158), the C-type lectin receptors (CD94-NKG2A), and leukocyte inhibitory receptors (LIR1, LAIR-1). Activating receptors are the natural cytotoxicity receptors (NKp46, NKp44), C-type lectin receptors (NKG2D, CD94-NKG2C), and Ig-like receptors (2B4). As different NK cells express different combinations of inhibitory or activating receptors, there is sizeable heterogeneity within the NK cell population. A particular NK cell typically expresses two to four inhibitory receptors in addition to an array of activation receptors. Indeed, they have a very sophisticated program for control of activation and killing, which is now understood to be a highly complex system of diverse, inhibitory, and activatory receptor-ligand interactions, sensing changes in MHC (major histocompatibility complex) expression. Recent data have shown that NK cells in addition to direct cytotoxic and antiviral functions are not solely killers but can also act as regulators of adaptive immunity, for example, by interacting and providing stimulatory signals for the components of the adaptive immune system, including T cells and DCs (dendritic cells). This interaction implies a broad role in immunity and potential involvement in a wide range of diseases, including infections, cancers, and especially autoimmune disorders. NK cells involvement in the regulation of inflammatory and autoimmune responses (loss of self-tolerance at multiple steps) is well established, and the paradigm that innate immunity plays an instructive role in the adaptive immune response is well established as well [9,10]. Recent studies suggest that NK cells may play distinct roles during different forms and at different stages of autoimmune response. There has been growing interest to clarify and understand the biological functions of NK cells particularly concerning their role in inflammatory and autoimmune response, both in animal models and humans [11,12]. However, mechanisms underlying NK cells involvement in autoimmune diseases remain foggy and may often bring to a dichotomy. Thus, it has been suggested that NK cells may either prevent/limit autoimmune responses [13–16] or may have a permissive role in autoimmunity.

There is clear evidence that KIR is implicated in human autoimmune disorders. A number of associations have been identified between risk of autoimmune disease and proposed activating KIR or KIR/human leukocyte antigen (HLA) genotypes accompanied by a lack of inhibition. Indeed, in humans, one of the key receptor families contributing to the NK cell receptor repertoire is the KIR family. Similar to many NK cell receptors, KIRs are expressed on T cells in addition to NK cells, affirming their role in adaptive immunity [17]. They are distinct from many other NK cell receptors, however, in that they are both diverse and rapidly evolving. It could be expected that the existence of KIR/HLA genotypes that tune NK cells in favor of active interactions may be beneficial in some contexts of

Mosaic of Autoimmunity. https://doi.org/10.1016/B978-0-12-814307-0.00007-4

TABLE 7.1 Immune Characteristics of Natural Killer Receptors Based on Their Immunophenotype and Function

Receptor	Ligand	Function
KIR or Ig-like receptors CD158	I Class HLA	Inhibitory
CD94-NKG2A	HLA-E	Inhibitory
LIR1, LAIR-1	Collagen	Inhibitory
SIGLEC-3/7/9 (CD33)	Sialic acid	Inhibitory
KLRG1	Cadherins	Inhibitory
NKR-P1A KLRB1	CLEC2D LLTI	Inhibitory
LIR1 (ILT2, LILRB1)	I Class HLA	Inhibitory
KIR2DL1, KIR2DL2, KIR2DL3	HLA-C	Inhibitory
KIR3DL1 KIR3DL2	HLA-A or B	Inhibitory
KIR2DS1	HLA-C	Activating
DAP10 (HCS1)	MICA, MICB, ULBP1	Activating
CD160	HLA-C	Activating
NKG2D, CD94-NKG2C	HLA-E	Activating
Ig-like receptors (2B4)	CD48	Activating
CD16 (FCgRIIIA)	IgG	Activating
NKp30	B7-H6, CMV pp65, BAT-3	Activating
DNAM1(CD226)	Nectin 2(CD112, PVRL2)	Activating
CD27	CD70	Activating
PSGL1	L-Selectin (CD62L)	Activating
NKp46, NKp44	Viral HA	Activating

BAT-3, HLA-B–associated transcript 3; *CD94-NKG2A*, C-type lectin receptors; *CMV pp65*, cytomegalovirus; *DNAM1*, DNAX accessory molecule 1; *HA*, hemagglutinin; *HLA*, human leukocyte antigen; *KIR*, killer immunoglobulin-like receptor; *KLRG1*, killer cell lectin-like receptor G1; *LAIR-1*, leukocyte-associated immunoglobulin-like receptor 1; *LILR*, leukocyte immunoglobulin-like receptor; *LIR1*, leukocyte inhibitory receptors; *MICA*, MHC class I polypeptide-related sequence A; *NCR*, natural cytotoxicity receptor; *NK*, natural killer; *NKG2D, CD94-NKG2C*, C-type lectin receptors; *PSGL1*, P-selectin glycoprotein ligand-1.

infectious disease and in some cases this mechanism may predispose to autoimmunity. For example, in rheumatoid vasculitis enhanced disease risk seems to be associated with presence of the KIR2DS2 gene. H. Segharfid et al. demonstrated that expression of activating KIR, in the absence of an inhibitory receptor for self–MHC-I, may contribute to autoimmune disorders. In this case, the activating KIR expressed in effector T cells may synergize with the signals transduced by T cell receptor (TCR), otherwise insufficient for an autoantigen alone, to elicit an autoimmune response [18]. A related condition appears in type 1 diabetes, where the disease was associated with an increase in KIR2DS2/HLA ligand pairs in the presence of diminished inhibitory interactions. Finally, the spondyloarthritis show a strong association with HLAB27, making it of interest to determine whether this may involve the interaction with KIR3DL2.

The only identified gene with polymorphisms associated with systemic lupus erythematosus (SLE) that appears relevant to NK cells is the one encoding for the CD16 or FCγRIIIA. This receptor is present on the surface of NK cells, and the associated variant is of low binding capacity, thus resulting in altered (diminished) NK cells adhesion and function that may have important consequences in SLE pathogenesis. SLAM family receptors are important immunomodulatory receptors involved in the cross talk between a number of immune cells [19]. SLAM locus is genetically associated with SLE [20–24], and recent data suggest involvement of SLAM receptors in SLE pathogenesis. The expression of the SLAM family receptors CD319 and CD229 was dynamically regulated on pDCs (plasmacytoid dendritic cells) and CD56^{dim} NK cells by RNA-ImmunoComplexes (RNA-ICs) typically found in lupus. Moreover, the expression of the SLAM molecules on pDCs and NK cells from patients with SLE was decreased: patients with SLE had decreased expression of CD84 and CD319 on circulating pDCs. The exact consequence of the altered expression of SLAM molecules in SLE NK cells is unknown, but it might reflect several previous observations. For instance, the lower expression of CD229 on CD56^{dim} cells may contribute to the decreased cytotoxicity of SLE NK cells. In contrast, the increased expression of SLAM molecules on CD56^{bright} NK cells may play a role in the increased proinflammatory cytokine production in SLE. SLAM family of receptors is implicated in autoimmune disease processes and they may have the role of biomarkers and therapeutic targets in SLE [25]. It is relevant to underline that autoimmune diseases are multifactorial diseases, in which there is a high number of genes involved. However, from the previous studies, it is clear how genes modulating NK cells number and response may be deeply implicated in the pathogenesis of autoimmunity and further studies are needed to clarify this issue. Recently, it has been individuated as another pool of cells, called natural killer T (NKT) cells, which act as a link between innate and adaptive immunity. They are a subset of T lymphocytes characterized by a restricted expression of TCR and they recognize glycolipid antigens, such as α-galactosylceramide (α-GalCer), presented by MHC I–like molecule CD1d. They are able to activate a variety of immune cells, such as monocytes, DCs, NK cells, T cells, and B cells, by rapidly producing Th1 and Th2 cytokines, such as IFN-γ and IL-4. Thus, NKT cells act as regulatory and/or effector cells. Due to their characteristics, they are implicated in a broad range of diseases, including autoimmune diseases such as rheumatoid arthritis (RA) and SLE [26].

NATURAL KILLER CELLS AND AUTOIMMUNITY

Several studies regarding NK cells and autoimmunity mainly focused on the number or status of the NK cells at different levels within patients affected by inflammatory/autoimmune diseases that share inflammatory/autoimmune features usually compared with healthy controls. Previous reports showed that number of circulating NK cells can be frequently altered depending on the disease taken into consideration. These include multiple sclerosis (MS), RA, type 1 diabetes mellitus, Sjögren's syndrome, and miastenia gravis [23–27], diseases that are characterized by a predominant Th1 cytokine expression in the target tissue. It has been proposed that NK cells play a regulatory role in autoimmunity in these conditions. Indeed, it has been hypothesized that NK cells may act as a source of Th2 cytokines, which, when reduced, allows an overabundance of Th1 cytokines and resultant autoimmune activity [28].

Roles attributed to NK cells in various clinical and experimental autoimmune diseases include a pathogenic function through inappropriate activation, on one hand, and suppressive functions through lysis of DCs or activated T cells on the other hand. A protective role for NK cells in murine diabetes was reported recently as it was suggested in patients with MS. These evidences were confirmed in mouse myelin oligodendrocyte glycoprotein–induced experimental autoimmune encephalomyelitis [29,30].

Questions arise whether the altered number of NK cells is a consequence of the pathological status or a primary condition that leads into the disease, if NK cells play a protective (and physiological) role or if they can be considered pathological under certain conditions.

Although NK cells were initially described primarily in the context of tumor surveillance and viral immunity, there have been a number of observations made about possible contributions to autoimmunity [17,19]. The new knowledge on NK cell biology implicates NK cells as possible players in all the phases of autoimmune response and interesting results have emerged. In this context, NK cells have been identified in target organs of patients suffering from diverse autoimmune diseases such as RA (localized in the synovial tissue) or MS (localized in the brain lesions).

Given their capacity to kill other cells and to produce IFN-γ, which is recognized as a damage mediator, it seems that NK cells may rather have a disease-promoting role in autoimmunity than a protective role. The interaction with the adaptive immune system could facilitate both the priming phase and the effector phase of the immune response with NK cells. However, to promote disease, it has been suggested that NK cells must produce IFN-γ. IL-21 also might act by stimulating NK cells to become disease-promoting, possibly by stimulating their IFN-γ secretion. It has also been suggested that NK cells may play a pathogenic role during late stages of autoimmunity in a virally induced model of autoimmune diabetes [31]. Even aggressive insulitis and the presence of NK cells in the infiltrate may be associated and, in-line with this finding, diabetes incidence is decreased when NK cells are depleted in other two induced models of diabetes, suggesting a role for NK cells in the late stages of disease also in these diabetes models.

It is evident that NK cells may be both protective and pathogenic in different disease models and sometimes even in the same disease. Functional differences between NK cells at different anatomical localizations and the adaptability, or flexibility, of effector responses in NK cells may also explain differences in such responses [32].

NK cells that usually represent the 10%–15% of peripheral blood lymphocytes and the 5% of all mononuclear cells in peripheral lymph nodes have the capability of migrating into peripheral tissue and in the target organs of autoimmunity. As previously evidenced, localization of NK cells might have a crucial role in determining which effect they could have on autoimmune diseases as it may happen in the decidua of recurrent spontaneous aborters. Cytokine milieu and other stimuli acting on different cell surface receptors such as KIR, present in the target organ, may differently trigger NK cells response and influence the role played in different autoimmune diseases [33]. Moreover, the microenvironment in which they mature triggers differential effector responses in NK cells, as different molecules have unique effects on NK cell effector functions, as clearly demonstrated by diverse effects exerted by IL-5, IL-6, IL-15, TNF-α, βhCG, progesterone, and prolactin during pregnancy.

NATURAL KILLER IN AUTOIMMUNE DISEASES
Rheumatoid Arthritis

NK cells comprised a significant fraction of the lymphocytes (8%–25%) in the synovial fluid of RA patients and could be detected in the joint early during the disease course. Similar to the observations in the cerebrospinal fluid of MS patients, the majority of the NK cells in the synovial fluid of RA patients were CD56^{bright} (~60% of NK cells) with elevated expression of CD94/NKG2A and decreased expression of KIRs and CD16. The CD56^{bright} subpopulation of NK cells was also found in the blood of RA patients (and normal controls) but at much lower frequencies (~10% of NK cells) [34]. NK cells within the synovium also showed upregulated expression of several chemokine receptors and adhesion molecules that may participate in preferential recruitment into the synovium. Synovial CD56^{bright} NK cells expressed higher levels of activation markers (CD69 and NKp44) and produced more TNF-α and IFN-γ than CD56^{bright} NK cells from the peripheral blood of the same patients. Synovial NK cells could induce monocytes to differentiate into DCs and have also been shown to produce IL-22, a cytokine that induces proliferation of synovial fibroblasts. Aberrant expression of MHC class I polypeptide-related sequence A in the inflamed synovium may augment CD56^{bright} NK cell activation, resulting in dysregulated production of proinflammatory cytokines rather than in immunoregulation [18]. Taken together, these findings suggest that the enrichment of CD56^{bright} NK cells may contribute to the initiation and/or perpetuation of dysregulated production of proinflammatory cytokines in the synovium of RA patients. In contrast to the accumulation of activated CD56^{bright} NK cells in the synovium, patients with RA have decreased circulating NK cells in their peripheral blood. In addition to the numeric deficit, peripheral blood NK cells in RA patients have decreased cytotoxicity on a per cell basis. These observations in conjunction with the genetic associations between inflammatory arthritis and KIR haplotypes support the hypothesis that dysregulation of cytokine production by CD56^{bright} NK cells in the synovium and/or decreased cytotoxicity by peripheral CD56^{dim} NK cells may contribute to pathogenesis of RA. This hypothesis is further corroborated by findings in several distinct murine models of inflammatory arthritis (for example, collagen-induced arthritis and *Staphylococcus aureus*–associated arthritis), which have demonstrated that NK cell depletion results in earlier onset of arthritis, more severe disease, and increased autoantibody and IL-17 production [35]. Interestingly, reduced peripheral NK cell numbers and decreased cytotoxicity were also observed in the collagen-induced arthritis model. NK cell–generated IFN-γ was shown to suppress the generation of IL-17 cells (collagen-induced arthritis model) and neutrophil recruitment to the affected joints (K/BxN model, an autoantibody model of arthritis) [34]. In RA, NK cells are also implicated in dysregulated osteoclastogenesis. They secrete a variety of cytokines that could have a disease-promoting or a disease-controlling role in RA. Numerous cytokines have been individuated as principal factors of the processes that contribute to the joint disease progression. One of the most potent osteoclastogenic cytokines which is pivotal in the pathogenesis of RA is TNF-α. It has been demonstrated that TNF-α works in synergism with IL-15 in patient affected by RA to induce receptor acquisition by NK cells and to activate NF-κB. NF-κB signaling pathways can mediate crucial events in the inflammatory response by chondrocytes, leading to extracellular matrix damage and cartilage destruction. IL-15 may stimulate the expression of PLD1-induced RANKL in rheumatoid synovial fibroblasts and, in collaboration with IL-2, may stimulate T cells activation, resulting in enhanced TNF-α production, NK cell proliferation and activation, and IFN-γ production. These data may explain why levels of IL-15 are increased with RA disease duration in the serum and synovial membrane of patient affected by this disease. In a recent work, Hye-Mi Jin and collaborators investigated the role played by NKT cells in osteoclastogenesis and their effects on inflammatory bone destruction. In healthy population, α-GalCer, presented by MHC class I–like molecule CD1d, stimulating NKT cells, have a regulatory effect on osteoclastogenesis. They demonstrated that patients affected by RA have an NKT cell dysfunction, but the administration of α-GalCer ameliorates arthritis and has a protective effect against inflammatory bone destruction via IFN-γ induction. Indeed, NKT cells inhibit in vitro osteoclastogenesis in a cell contact–independent manner (i.e., by antiresorptive cytokine secretion), inducing an increment of bone volumes, percent bone volumes, and trabecular thicknesses [26].

Systemic Lupus Erythematosus

NK cells are reduced within SLE patients. Indications of a relevant role of NK cells in SLE were derived from their analysis in SLE-affected organs. In particular, NK cells contribute directly to renal injury by killing tubular epithelial cells during renal ischemia-reperfusion injury and that NK cells are involved in mediating damage in long-term kidney transplants. Spada and collaborators have investigated the expression of MICA in lupus nephritis patients. In three murine models of SLE, they found increased NKG2D ligand levels in glomeruli, even at the predisease stage, which indicates that local NKG2D ligand expression might promote NK cell activity and drive kidney injury. They also suggest the role of a chemoat-tractant chemokine, the CX3CL1, in an early stage of disease, as an NK cells recruiter in kidney damage [36]. Huang et al. demonstrated that NK cells implicated in kidney damage produce high levels of cytotoxic granules (perforin and granzyme B) and IFN-γ, responsible for promoting and sustaining inflammation in nephritic lupus kidney. They also reported that the majority of NK cells that infiltrate kidney in mice with active disease express CD226, another important NK-activating receptor [37].

Despite the large amount of studies conducted on reduced NK cell numbers in SLE, this phenomenon still remains unexplained. Probably, NK cells in peripheral blood mononuclear cells are depleted as a result of death or NK cell migra-tion to target organs in SLE because of the expression of CXCR3. More researches are required to better understand the real mechanism under this process.

Moreover, in a recent study conducted by Green and collaborators, it has been demonstrated as a role of NKT cells in regulation of plasma IgG levels in patients with SLE. Actually, high levels of plasma IgG in patients with SLE and their first-degree relatives and high levels of IgG anti-dsDNA antibodies in patients were observed to be associated with a low frequency of NKT cells. The real mechanism of this process is still unknown [38].

Psoriasis and Psoriatic Arthritis

NK cell number and activity may also be reduced in patients with psoriasis or psoriatic arthritis (PsA) when compared with normal controls. However, cells expressing NK cell antigens are present in plaques of psoriasis and it is thought that these cells may play a key role in the pathogenesis of psoriasis. But how are NK cell levels determined? A key role is attributed to a strong involvement of genetic factors. Also in patients affected by SLE, alleles for susceptibil-ity have been described in the MICA, and the activating receptor NKG2D can modulate NK cells in the same way. Fangming Tang et al. demonstrated that NKG2D expression is considerably high on NK cells isolated from the joints compared with those isolated from the blood of PsA patients, suggesting that the microenvironment of the inflamed joint was capable of driving upregulation of NKG2D. These data, related to the high expression of MICA in PsA patient synovial tissue, underline the relevance of the joint microenvironment in influencing immune responses. In addition, NK cells–dependent joint inflammation may be activated by IL 15 by arming the cytolytic NKG2D pathway in NK cells: they recruit granulocytes and mast cells, two cell types which participate in the aberrant inflammatory responses of PsA, responsible of directly killing MIC expressing synovial cells and releasing arachidonic acid; this mechanism can be improved by cPLA2 upregulation [39].

Concerning therapy, a significant correlation between peripheral blood value of NK cells, TNF-α pathway, and clinical response to treatment with TNF-α inhibitors was demonstrated. An early and permanent increase up to normalization of NK in PsA patients treated with etanercept was observed: the increase of NK cell number occurred only in those patients who achieved a good–moderate clinical response, suggesting a relationship between peripheral blood cells levels and clinical outcome [40].

NATURAL KILLER CELLS, THE PARADIGM OF PREGNANCY AND AUTOIMMUNITY

A deeper insight into apparently unexplained recurrent spontaneous abortion (RSA) shows increasing evidences support-ing a role for NK cells [41]. NK cells constitute the predominant leukocyte population present in the endometrium at the time of implantation and in early pregnancy [42]. Uterine NK (uNK) cells differ from NK cells in other sites of the body. Mature uNK cells contain numerous granules (rich in perforin, granzymes, granulysin), but, unlike peripheral blood NK cells, uNK cells are only weakly cytotoxic in vitro and do not kill trophoblasts in vivo. They not only seem to both differ-entiate and proliferate in the uterus but also migrate from the periphery. uNK cells express NKp46, NKp44, and NKp30 [43]. Despite NK cells playing a fundamental role for successful pregnancies, increased number and killing activity of NK cells in the peripheral blood in RSA can predict the likelihood of another miscarriage and they are considered as prognostic factor for sterility, infertility and miscarriage. In fact, high concentrations of NK cells of the conventional

TABLE 7.2 Possible Roles of Natural Killer Cells in Pregnancy [6]

1. Physiologic
   a. Immunosurveillance
   b. Angiogenesis
   c. Remodeling of the spiral arteries to uteroplacental arteries
   d. Supporting proper trophoblast and placental growth
   e. Vascularization of the deciduas
   f. Production of immunomodulatory molecules
2. Pathologic
   a. Killing cytolytic activity
   b. Inhibiting placental human chorionic gonadotrophin secretion
   c. Complement activation
   d. Cytokine imbalance
   e. Failure in the generation of Th2-type responses
   f. Activate antigen-presenting cells leading to the development of Th1 responses

CD56 + 16–type have been found in the blood, uterus, and placental biopsies of women who have abortions suggesting that the cytotoxic activity is probably present also at the implantation site. Available data support that during the early stages of normal pregnancy, uNK cells proliferate significantly in situ, under the influence of IL-15 and prolactin. The expanded uNK population then plays an important role through cytokine production in mediating the angiogenesis necessary for continuation of the pregnancy [44–46]. Decidual NK (dNK) cells maintain immune tolerance by antagonizing T_H17 cells. IFN-γ is closely involved in this effect, and the main source of IFN-γ is confined to the CD56^{bright}CD27$^+$ dNK subset. Evidence emerged concerning that the regulatory process is critical for successful pregnancy and that NK cells play a key role in the control of local inflammation to ensure optimal fetal development at the maternal–fetal interface. One of the functions of NK cells at the maternal–fetal interface is to inhibit local inflammation and maintain immune balance. During normal pregnancy, dNK cells act as sentinel cells to control local inflammation, which is critical for maintaining tolerance at the fetal–maternal interface. However, this regulatory mechanism has limits because NK cells can become altered by the inflammatory environment in that the non-NK cells in the decidua secrete high levels of IL-1β and IL-6, which promote the expansion and recruitment of Th17 cells. In RSA, creation of an imbalance in Th1–Th2 response, resulting in a prevalent Th1 cytokine environment in the periphery, may lead into NK cell activation and proliferation, which could result in migration of cytotoxic NK cells into the uterus and in turn contribute to mechanisms involved in miscarriage. Alternatively, the local endometrial immune assessment may be disrupted at a variety of levels, causing defects in homing of the proper NK population to the uterus, local production of cytokines and hormones such as IL-15 and prolactin, and impairment of more downstream events such as production of immunoregulatory factors by uNK cells (Table 7.2). It has been demonstrated as a decreased expression of NKp46 in peripheral blood in women with previous reproductive failures in peritoneal fluid in women with pelvic endometriosis, as well as in peripheral blood in pregnant women with gestational diabetes mellitus. These studies suggest that regulation of NKp46 expression in various types of NK cells may be one of the key factors in reproductive failure. Additionally, analysis of NKp46 expression may be a useful tool to investigate and diagnose reproductive failures [43]. An important evidence of as to how NK cells may behave as pathogenic effectors in RSA comes from a recent study that showed NK cells possibly playing a role in the pathogenesis of abortive events in a subpopulation of antiphospholipid syndrome (APS)-RSA patients, which previously has been explained in terms of autoimmune specific reactions (antiphospholipid, aPL-mediated) [47]. NK cells were found elevated both in absolute number and in percentage in a subpopulation of APS-RSA patients, which show specific features in terms of high NK cells levels (>15%) and early abortion (within the gestational week, GW). Interestingly, NK cell levels were elevated not only when compared with normal healthy controls but also when compared with other RSA populations (except idiopathic) or with another APS population not presenting RSA and overall they were higher than the APS-RSA subpopulation showing late abortions (after the 10th GW). These evidences support the hypothesis that a high number of circulating NK cells could be a not specific but important peculiarity of tendency to miscarriage: in these patients, the high NK value may not be linked to the condition of being pregnant, but present yet before, as a distinctive mark of their immunity system and may cause damage perhaps because of their ability to provide an early source of cytokines and to activate Antigen Presenting Cells (APCs) leading to the development of pathogenic Th1 responses. Whether is the clue of NK cells in pregnancy, it is an evidence that under certain conditions they may switch from their natural protective role and become aggressive and damaging even leading into (early) abortion.

REFERENCES

[1] Perricone R, Perricone C, De Carolis C, Shoenfield Y. NK cells in autoimmunity: a two-edged weapon of the immune system. Autoimmun Rev 2008;7:384–90.

[2] Ljunggren HG, Karre K. In search of the 'missing self': MHC molecules and NK cell recognition. Immunol Today 1990;11:237–44.

[3] Lanier LL. Natural killer cell receptor signaling. Curr Opin Immunol 2003;15:308–14.

[4] Lanier LL. The origin and functions of natural killer cells. Clin Immunol 2000;95:14–8.

[5] Seaman WE. Natural killer and natural killer T cells. Arthritis Rheum 2000;43:1204–17.

[6] Biron CA, Nguyen KB, Pien GC, Cousens LP, Salazar-Mather TP. Natural killer cells in antiviral defense: function and regulation by innate cytokines. Annu Rev Immunol 1999;17:189–220.

[7] Yokoyama WM, Kim S, French AR. The dynamic life of natural killer cells. Annu Rev Immunol 2004;22:405–29.

[8] Mandal A, Viswanathan C. Natural killer cells: in health and disease. Hematol Oncol Stem Cell Ther 2015;8:47–55.

[9] Raulet DH. Interplay of natural killer cells and their receptors with the adaptive immune response. Nat Immunol 2004;5:996–1002.

[10] Shi F, Ljunggren HG, Sarvetnick N. Innate immunity and autoimmunity: from self protection to self-destruction. Trends Immunol 2001;22:97–101.

[11] Zimmer J, Bausinger H, De La Salle H. Autoimmunity mediated by innate immune effector cells. Trends Immunol 2001;22:300–1.

[12] French AR, Yokoyama WM. Natural killer cells and autoimmunity. Arthritis Res Ther 2004;6:8–14.

[13] Smeltz RB, Wolf NA, Swanborg RH. Inhibition of autoimmune T cell responses in the DA rat by bone marrow-derived NK cells in vitro: implications for autoimmunity. J Immunol 1999;163:1390–7.

[14] Matsumoto Y, Kohyama K, Aikawa Y, Shin T, Kawazoe Y, Suzuki Y, Tanuma N. Role of natural killer cells and TCRγδ T cells in acute autoimmune encephalomyelitis. Eur J Immunol 1998;28:1681–8.

[15] Zhang B, Yamamura T, Kondo T, Fujiwara M, Tabira T. Regulation of experimental autoimmune encephalomyelitis by natural killer (NK) cells. J Exp Med 1997;186:1677–87.

[16] Fort MM, Leach MW, Rennick DM. A role for NK cells as regulators of CD4+ T cells in a transfer model of colitis. J Immunol 1998;161:3256–61.

[17] Khakoo SI, Carrington M. KIR and disease: a model system or system of models. Immunol Rev 2006;214:186–201.

[18] Shegarfi H, Naddafi F, Mirshafiey A. Natural killer cells, T. role in rheumatoid arthritis: friend or foe? Sci World J 2012;2012:491974.

[19] Jie HB, Sarvetnick N. The role of NK cells and NK cell receptors in autoimmune disease. Autoimmunity 2004;37:147–53.

[20] Erkeller-Yüsel F, Hulstaart F, Hannet I, Isenberg D, Lydyard P. Lymphocyte subsets in a large cohort of patients with systemic lupus erythematosus. Lupus 1993;2:227–31.

[21] Majewski S, Wasik M, Jabłońska S, Kamiński M, Fraczykowska M. Defective natural-killer- and killer-cell activity associated with increased polymorphonuclear leukocyte adherence in psoriasis. Arch Dermatol Res 1986;278:264–9.

[22] Jones CD, Guckian M, el-Ghorr AA, Gibbs NK, Norval M. Effects of phototherapy on the production of cytokines by peripheral blood mononuclear cells and on systemic antibody responses in patients with psoriasis. Photodermatol Photoimmunol Photomed 1996;12:204–10.

[23] Kastrukoff LF, Morgan NG, Zecchini D, White R, Petkau AJ, Satoh J, Paty DW. A role for natural killer cells in the immunopathogenesis of multiple sclerosis. J Neuroimmunol 1998;86:123–33.

[24] Negishi K, Waldeck N, Chandy G, Buckingham B, Kershnar A, Fisher L, Gupta S, Charles MA. Natural killer cell and islet cell activities in type I (insulin dependent) diabetes. Diabetologica 1986;29:352–7.

[25] Hagberg N, Theorell J, Schlums H, Eloranta ML, Bryceson YT, Rönnblom L. Systemic lupus erythematosus immune complexes increase the expression of SLAM family members CD319 (CRACC) and CD229 (LY-9) on plasmacytoid dendritic cells and CD319 on CD56dim NK cells. J Immunol 2013;191:2989–98.

[26] Jin HM, Kee SJ, Cho YN, Kang JH, Kim MJ, Jung HJ, Park KJ, Kim TJ, Lee SI, Choi H, Koh JT, Kim N, Park YW. Dysregulated osteoclastogenesis is related to natural killer T cell dysfunction in rheumatoid arthritis. Arthritis Rheumatol 2015;67:2639–50.

[27] Sibbitt Jr WL, Bankhurst AD. Natural killer cells in connective tissue disorders. Clin Rheum Dis 1985;11:507–21.

[28] Colucci F, Di Santo JP, Leibson PJ. Natural killer cell activation in mice and men: different triggers for similar weapons? Nat Immunol 2002;3:807–13.

[29] Takahashi K, Aranami T, Endoh M, Miyake S, Yamamura T. The regulatory role of natural killer cells in multiple sclerosis. Brain 2004;127:1917–27.

[30] Lee IF, Qin H, Trudeau J, Dutz J, Tan R. Regulation of autoimmune diabetes by complete Freund's adjuvant is mediated by NK cells. J Immunol 2004;172:937–42.

[31] Baxter AG, Smyth MJ. The role of NK cells in autoimmune disease. Autoimmunity 2002;35:1–14.

[32] Johansson S, Berg L, Hall H, Höglund P. NK cells: elusive players in autoimmunity. Trends Immunol 2005;26:613–8.

[33] Perussia B, Chen Y, Loza MJ. Peripheral NK cell phenotypes: multiple changing of faces of an adapting, developing cell. Mol Immunol 2005;42:385–95.

[34] Fogel LA, Yokoyama WM, French AR. Natural killer cells in human autoimmune disorders. Arthritis Res Ther 2013;15:216.

[35] Conigliaro P, Scrivo R, Valesini G, Perricone R. Emerging role for NK cells in the pathogenesis of inflammatory arthropathies. Autoimmun Rev 2011;10:577–81.

[36] Spada R, Rojas JM, Barber DF. Recent findings on the role of natural killer cells in the pathogenesis of systemic lupus erythematosus. J Leukoc Biol 2015;98:479–87.

[37] Huang Z, Fu B, Zheng SG, Li X, Sun R, Tian Z, Wei H. Involvement of CD226+ NK cells in immunopathogenesis of systemic lupus erythematosus. J Immunol 2011;186:3421–31.

[38] Green MR, Kennell AS, Larche MJ, Seifert MH, Isenberg DA, Salaman MR. Natural killer T cells in families of patients with systemic lupus erythematosus their possible role in regulation of IgG production. Arthritis Rheum 2007;56:303–10.

[39] Tang F, Sally B, Ciszewski C, Abadie V, Curran SA, Groh V, Fitzgerald O, Winchester RJ, Jabri B. Interleukin 15 primes natural killer cells to kill via NKG2D and cPLA2 and this pathway is active in psoriatic arthritis. PLoS One 2013;8:e76292.

[40] Conigliaro P, Triggianese P, Perricone C, Chimenti MS, Di Muzio G, Ballanti E, Guarino MD, Kroegler B, Gigliucci G, Grelli S, Perricone R. Restoration of peripheral blood natural killer and B cell levels in patients affected by rheumatoid and psoriatic arthritis during etanercept treatment. Clin Exp Immunol 2014;177:234–43.

[41] Tincani A, Rebaioli CB, Frassi M, Taglietti M, Gorla R, Cavazzana I, Faden D, Taddei F, Lojacono A, Motta M, Trepidi L, Meroni P, Cimaz R, Ghirardello A, Doria A, Pisoni MP, Muscarà M, Brucato A. Pregnancy Study Group of Italian Society of Rheumatology. Pregnancy and autoimmunity: maternal treatment and maternal disease influence on pregnancy outcome. Autoimmun Rev 2005;4:423–8.

[42] De Carolis C, Perricone C, Perricone R. War and peace at the feto-placental front line: recurrent spontaneous abortion. Isr Med Assoc J 2014;16:667–8.

[43] Fukui A, Funamizu A, Fukuhara R, Shibahara H. Expression of natural cytotoxicity receptors and cytokine production on endometrial natural killer cells in women with recurrent pregnancy loss or implantation failure, and the expression of natural cytotoxicity receptors on peripheral blood natural killer cells in pregnant women with a history of recurrent pregnancy loss. J Obstet Gynaecol Res 2017;43:1678–86.

[44] Balasch J. Antiphospholipid antibodies: a major advance in the management of recurrent abortion. Autoimmun Rev 2004;3:228–33.

[45] Asherson RA, Cervera R. The antiphospholipid syndrome: multiple faces beyond the classical presentation. Autoimmun Rev 2003;2:140–51.

[46] Hanna J, Goldman-Wohl D, Hamani Y, Avraham I, Greenfield C, Natanson-Yaron S, Prus D, Cohen-Daniel L, Arnon TI, Manaster I, Gazit R, Yutkin V, Benharroch D, Porgador A, Keshet E, Yagel S, Mandelboim O. Decidual NK cells regulate key developmental processes at the human fetal-maternal interface. Nat Med 2006;12:1065–74.

[47] Perricone C, De Carolis C, Giacomelli R, Zaccari G, Cipriani P, Bizzi E, Perricone R. High levels of NK cells in the peripheral blood of patients affected with anti-phospholipid syndrome and recurrent spontaneous abortion: a potential new hypothesis. Rheumatology (Oxford) 2007;46:1574–8.

Chapter 8

Dendritic Cells: The Orchestrators of the Inflammatory Response in Autoimmune Diseases

Jiram Torres-Ruiz[1,2], Yehuda Shoenfeld[2,3]

[1]Department of Immunology and Rheumatology, Instituto Nacional de Ciencias Médicas y Nutrición Salvador Zubirán, Mexico City, Mexico;

[2]Zabludowicz Center for Autoimmune Diseases, Sheba Medical Center, affiliated to Sackler Faculty of Medicine, Tel Aviv University, Tel Aviv, Israel;

[3]Laboratory of the Mosaics of Autoimmunity, Saint-Petersburg University, Saint-Petersburg, Russian Federation

INTRODUCTION

Dendritic cells (DCs) are stellar-shaped leukocytes derived from the bone marrow that reside in the tissues and are responsible for capturing antigens from the local environment [1]. As professional antigen-presenting cells, in the steady state they favor central tolerance by the generation of regulatory T cells (Tregs) centrally in the thymus [2] and peripherally as they migrate in a small amount to the lymph nodes and present antigens to lymphocytes to favor a state of anergy in effector cells by expressing inhibitory molecules such as programmed death 1 (PD1) and cytotoxic T lymphocyte antigen 4 in T cells [2], as well as through the induction of Tregs through the secretion of transforming growth factor (TGF-β) and retinoic acid [2].

Although there are several DC subtypes distributed in almost all organs, skin, mucosa, and lymphoid tissue [3], globally, conventional dendritic cells (cDCs), those derived from monocytes and plasmacytoid dendritic cells (pDCs) have been linked to autoimmunity in several studies. pDCs are considered to be professional producers of IFN-α, but they also secrete TNF-α and IL-6 [4]. Type I IFNs are key cytokines in autoimmunity because they induce the maturation of cDC, promote antibodies secretion, and are able to promote the Th1 and CD8+ response [5].

DCs have a finger-like projection morphology and carry several pattern recognition receptors (PRRs) such as toll-like receptors (TLRs) [2], C-type lectin receptors, and intracytoplasmic nucleotide-binding oligomerization domain (NOD)-type receptors [6]. Multiple agents activate DCs, including microorganisms, dead cells (through alarmins such as heat shock proteins, high mobility group box 1 protein [HMGB-1], β-defensins, uric acid [UA]), cells of the innate and adaptive immune system, and pathogen-associated molecular patterns (PAMPs) [6]. Stimuli that induce DCs maturation include lipopolysaccharide (LPS), DNA, RNA, TNF-α, IL-1, IL-6, tissue factors, heat shock proteins, and CD154 from T lymphocytes [7]. In contrast, the low-affinity signal in T lymphocytes, IL-10, TGF-β, prostaglandins, and corticosteroids tend to modify the maturation of DCs and to divert the immune response toward Th2 [7].

When there is tissue damage or an infectious event, DCs migrate to the lymph nodes where they mature and increase the expression of peptides of the major histocompatibility complex (MHC), co-stimulatory molecules, chemokine receptors, and the production of key cytokines for the differentiation of effector T cells [1]. Thereafter, the cDC can polarize the response of helper T cells. The increased expression of TLR3 by CD141+DCs and their ability to produce IFN-β, CXCL-10, and IL-12p70 favor Th1. Nonlymphoid tissue residents cDCs induce Th1 and Th2 equally while Langerhans cells preferably induce a Th2 response [8]. On the other hand, CD1c+DCs induce a Th1 and Th17 response after stimulation of TLR7 combined with TLR4, TLR3, RIG-I, and MDA-5 [9].

The relationship between systemic autoimmunity and DCs has been demonstrated in several animal models including those deficient in IL-2, where the expansion of cDCs and pDCs entails an increased production of IL-12, IFN-γ leading to Th1 expansion and the death of BALB/C mice in 3–5 weeks secondary to autoimmune hemolytic anemia [10]. On the other hand, a higher expression of type I IFN-regulated genes (IFN signature) has been found in diverse autoimmune diseases and pDCs are the main source of IFN-α [11]. When peripheral blood monocytes are

Mosaic of Autoimmunity. https://doi.org/10.1016/B978-0-12-814307-0.00008-6

cultured with Granulocyte Macrophage Colony Stimulating Factor (GM-CSF) and IFN-α, they acquire the morphology of DCs with intense expression of TLR7 and increased secretion of IL-18 [11]. In addition, these cells produced higher amounts of IL-1β, IL-6, IL-10, and TNF-α, are capable of inducing a Th1 phenotype even in the absence of IL-12p70, and, by their increased expression of MHC-I, stimulate antigen-specific CD8+ T lymphocytes [11], which indicates that IFN-α is a key cytokine in the pathogenic autoimmune response and persistent inflammation in autoimmune diseases.

EVIDENCE OF THE PARTICIPATION OF DCS IN THE PATHOPHYSIOLOGY OF VARIOUS AUTOIMMUNE DISEASES

In Table 8.1, we summarize the main studies involving abnormalities in DCs in a diversity of tissues and/or animal models of autoimmune diseases.

Dendritic Cells in Systemic Lupus Erythematosus

Systemic lupus erythematosus (SLE) is the prototype of systemic autoimmune disease and is characterized by loss of tolerance to intracellular antigens, especially chromatin antigens and ribonucleoproteins that promote damage by immune complexes deposition in virtually any organ. Virtually all leukocytes from patients with SLE are more predisposed to die and apoptotic blebs are a source of autoantigens [12]. In addition to this, it is known that patients with SLE have defects in phagocytosis, which promotes that the autoantigens persist in the environment making them accessible to the immune system [12]. In SLE patients, apoptotic blebs are accompanied by damage-associated molecular patterns (DAMPs) such as HMGB-1, which is a ligand for TLR2, TLR4, and the receptor for advanced glycation end products [12]. The activation of these PRRs promotes the expression of CD83, CD86, and MHC-II in myeloid dendritic cells (mDCs) in vitro [12]. In this way, activated DCs can stimulate CD4+ T lymphocytes to promote the production of cytokines and stimulate the secretion of autoantibodies.

Another potential source of autoantigens in SLE is NETosis, which is a new mechanism of cell death where neutrophils extrude their decondensed chromatin as a network decorated with nuclear and cytoplasmic protein components named neutrophil extracellular traps (NETs) [13]. The NETs are a source of chromatin antigens including dsDNA, histones and nucleosomes, but patients with SLE have neutrophils with greater predisposition to carry out NETosis, and within the components of the NETs there have been found alarmins and antimicrobial peptides such as HMGB-1 and LL-37 [13]. The combination of LL-37 with anti-RNP has been shown to enhance the production IFN-α pDCs [13].

Type I IFNs play a key role in the pathogenesis of SLE [2]. The pDCs endocyte the immunoglobulin-DNA, RNA, and nucleoprotein complexes through the IgG FcγRIIa (CD32) low-affinity receptor, and the nucleic acids activate TLR7 and TLR9 in the endosomes promoting the synthesis of type I IFN, which increases the production of IL-6, TNF-α, and costimulatory molecules in DCs [12]. In addition, type I IFNs favor the CD4+ differentiation toward Th1 and augment the T cytotoxic response and the production of immunoglobulins by B lymphocytes [14]. The DCs in lupus not only present antigens and orchestrate autoimmunity but also present a source of IFN-α that perpetuates the pathogenic inflammatory response. The abnormal mechanisms of cell death in lupus are a key source of self-antigens that activate DCs to initiate the disease.

Dendritic Cells in Primary Sjögren's Syndrome

Primary Sjögren's syndrome (pSS) is an autoimmune epithelitis characterized by keratoconjunctivitis sicca and a variable occurrence of systemic manifestations [15]. The participation of DCs in pSS-like autoimmunity is observed in Dcir-deficient animal models. Dcir is a C-type lectin immune receptor expressed mainly in DCs [16]. The deficiency of this receptor causes arthritis, enthesitis, sialadenitis, antinuclear antibodies, anti-Ro, anti-La antibodies, and rheumatoid factor in mice [16]. Because patients with pSS have type I IFN signature in approximately 50% of cases, it is possible that pDCs may be involved in the pathophysiology of the disease [15]. In addition, DCs have been shown to be an important source of IL-7, a key cytokine in the pathogenesis of pSS [17].

In the normal salivary gland, DCs are found between the epithelial cells in acini and ducts with extensions that extend basally and apically to the ducts lumen, as well as in the interstitial tissue [15]. Most studies that have evaluated DCs in patients with pSS have shown that they decrease in peripheral blood during the disease, which could

TABLE 8.1 Main Studies Demonstrating Quantitative and Qualitative Alterations in Dendritic Cells (DCs) of Patients With Autoimmune Diseases

Disease	Model/Type of DC/Tissue	Principal Finding	References
Systemic lupus erythematosus	Myeloid dendritic cells (mDCs) ↓ Lin⁻HLA-DR⁺CD4⁺ DCs ↓ CD11c⁺ mDC frequency	↓ T cell stimulation capacity	[57–60]
	Normal basal and lipopolysaccharide (LPS)–induced CD80, CD83, CD86 ↓ HLA-DR induction	No difference in TNF-α, IL-1β, IL-6, IL-12 on LPS and IFN-γ stimulation ↑ IL-6 in CD86 high expressing DCs	[61,62]
	Normal mDC frequency CD80 and CD40 either ↑ or normal in mDCs ↑ CD86 ↑ BLyS ↓ CD83	↑ IL-8 secretion ↑ T cell proliferation and activation capacity	[63–66]
	Plasmacytoid dendritic cells (pDCs)	↓ pDCs frequency	[58,59,61]
	↑ pDCs in active versus active LN patients Presence of pDCs in LN kidney ↑ pDCs frequency Normal CD40, CD80, CD86 expression	↑ Allogeneic T cell proliferation, ↓ FoxP3 expression in co-cultured CD4⁺ T cells Persistent IL-10 mRNA expression and lack toll-like receptor (TLR9) induction on apoptotic cells stimulation	[63,67]
	Normal pDC frequency ↓ ChemR23 expression in pDCs	↓ IFN-α production per pDC on CpG stimulation	[62,68]
	Normal CD40 and CD80 expression	↑ Basal and CCL19-induced migration in pDCs	[66]
Primary Sjögren's syndrome	Human minor salivary gland biopsy	Upregulation of type I and II IFN genes Increased expression of TLR8 and TLR9 ↑ pDCs in salivary glands	[69]
	pDC	No difference in peripheral blood vs. healthy controls Lower percentage and decreased numbers during active disease Present in salivary glands	[69–74]
	Conventional dendritic cells (cDCs)	Lower percentage, no functional differences vs. healthy controls Present in salivary glands	
Multiple sclerosis (MS)	Cladribine treatment	pDC increased during treatment Clinical improvement	[75]
	IFN-β	cDC decreased during treatment pDC increased during treatment	
	pDCs	Located in white matter, leptomeninges, and cerebrospinal fluid (CSF), specially during exacerbations	[14]
		↓ CD40 in primary-progressive vs. secondary-progressive MS ↓ CD40 upregulation in relapsing-remitting MS	[76,77]
		↓ CD86 in relapsing-remitting MS	
		↓ CD123 in primary-progressive vs. secondary-progressive MS	
		↓ IFN-α in relapsing-remitting MS	[77–80]
		↑ IFN-α, IL-6, TNF-α in relapsing-remitting MS	
		↓ IFN-γ in relapsing-remitting MS	
		Impaired Treg induction MS	
		↑ IL-17 MS	[81]

Continued

TABLE 8.1 Main Studies Demonstrating Quantitative and Qualitative Alterations in Dendritic Cells (DCs) of Patients With Autoimmune Diseases—cont'd

Disease	Model/Type of DC/Tissue	Principal Finding	References
	cDC	↑ CD40 on CSF and on relapsing-remitting vs. blood and secondary-progressive MS	[76,82,83]
		↑ CD80 on CSF and in secondary-progressive vs. blood and relapsing-remitting MS	
		↓ CD80 In primary-progressive MS	
		↑ CD86, HLA-DR in CSF vs. peripheral blood	
		↓ CD86 in primary-progressive vs. relapsing-remitting MS	
		↓ PDL-1 In secondary-progressive vs. relapsing-remitting MS	
		↑ IL-12p70 in secondary-progressive MS	[83]
		↑ IL-23p19 in relapsing-remitting MS	
		↑ TNF-α in secondary-progressive vs. relapsing-remitting MS	
		↑ IFN-γ/IL-4/IL-13 in relapsing-remitting vs. secondary-progressive MS	
Rheumatoid arthritis	Synovial tissue	cDCs and pDC sin perivascular regions	[84]
	Peripheral blood	Same percentage of pDCs in comparison to healthy controls	
	Synovial fluid	Higher proportion of CD11c+DC vs. CD123+DC	
Type 1 diabetes mellitus	pDCs	Expanded in peripheral blood	[5,85]
		Lower frequency in peripheral blood	[86]
	cDC and pDC	Lower absolute numbers in peripheral blood	[87]
Idiopathic inflammatory myopathies	Muscle biopsy of DM and PM patients	Higher fascin+DC, lower langerin+DC	[88]
	Muscle biopsy of PM patients	mDC invading nonnecrotic myober regions	[89]
	Skin biopsy of DM patients	Higher frequency of pDCs	[90]
Inflammatory bowel disease	Colon biopsy	Higher frequency of langerin+immature dendritic cells	[91]
	Colon biopsy	Higher DC-SIGN+DCs expressing CD80 and producing IL-12 and IL-18 in comparison to healthy controls	[92]

indicate that they migrate to the tissues to cause damage and perpetuate the autoimmune response [15]. In fact, in severe salivary gland lesions of patients with pSS, there are fascin(+) DCs that form networks with B and T lymphocytes and germinal centers [15].

At the same time, epithelial cells of patients with pSS express CD40 and produce chemokines such as BCA-1 (CXCL13), TARC (CCL17), ELC (CCL19), SLC (CCL21), and MDC (CCL22) that attract DCs [15]. Apparently, salivary acinar cells attract and activate DCs in response to environmental stimuli or viral infections. Once in the glandular tissue, DCs favor the formation of germinal centers with the consequent sialadenitis.

Dendritic Cells in Systemic Sclerosis

Systemic sclerosis (SSc) is an autoimmune disease characterized by vasculopathy, autoantibodies, and diffuse deposition of collagen in skin and internal organs secondary to overactivation of fibroblasts [18]. Despite the difficulty of studying DCs in patients with SSc, it is known that fibroblasts appear to recruit DCs in the skin and in the inflamed lung, as demonstrated by the co-localization between fibroblasts and CD1a DCs in skin lesions [18]. In addition, the secretion of TGF-β1 IL-4, IL-5, and IL-13 by DCs could favor fibrogenesis in SSc patients [18].

Dendritic Cells in Multiple Sclerosis

Multiple sclerosis (MS) is a demyelinating disease of the central nervous system [14]. Apparently, the triggering event involves the activation of peripheral cDCs and CD4+ T lymphocytes that penetrate the blood–brain barrier and cause neuronal damage [14]. Both MS and its animal model, the experimental autoimmune encephalomyelitis (EAE), are autoimmune diseases mediated by the cooperating subpopulations Th1 and Th17 [19]. The DCs of patients with MS are able to induce the production of IFN-γ in mononuclear cells [20], favoring a Th1 phenotype, whereas in EAE the mature DCs secrete IL-6 and TGF-β1 with the consequent decrease in Tregs and increase in Th17 [21]. The DCs polarize the T lymphocytes to Th17 expressing IL-6 in the cytoplasmic membrane (IL-6 trans-presentation) [22]. This kind of IL-6 signal transduction is important because it forms clusters of activated T cells, and the elimination of IL-6 trans-presenting DCs induces the production of IFN-γ, decreases the secretion of IL-17, and suppresses the development of EAE [22]. In this regard, IFN-β is essential because in EAE, IFN-β-deficient mice have an increased Th17 [19]. In MS, DCs derived from TNF-α and iNOS secreting monocytes can activate CD8+ T cells and favor the secretion of IFN-γ and IL-17, which contributes to the recruitment of other leukocytes and neuronal damage [14].

Regarding other types of DCs, the kinetics of appearance of pDCs in EAE is fundamental. Depletion of pDCs before the disease onset gives protection reducing Th17 differentiation and augmenting the Th1 response and the expression of FoxP3 in splenocytes. If pDCs are absent 1 week after the disease onset, the symptoms are exacerbated [23]. In MS, DCs activate CD4+ in the periphery and orchestrate the pathogenic immune response to induce a Th1 and Th17 response once these cells migrate to neuronal tissue.

Dendritic Cells in Type 1 Diabetes Mellitus

Type 1 diabetes mellitus (T1DM) is an autoimmune disease characterized by the infiltration of autoreactive T cells into the pancreas leading to destruction of beta cells and impediment of insulin production [24]. DCs are able to capture pancreatic antigens and present them to CD4+ and CD8+ T cells [24]. In animal models of T1DM, it has been shown that most DCs that infiltrate islets are CD11c+ and have a monocytic origin [25]. The release of DNA into the extracellular space after tissue damage (for example, after a viral infection) is able to activate TLR9 in pDCs, favoring the synthesis of IFN-α and the triggering of DM1, probably through the maturation of mDCs [26]. CD11c+CD11b+CD8α DCs activate T lymphocytes for the onset of insulitis [27]. In addition, DM1 is strongly associated with HLA-DR3/DQ2 and HLA-DR4/DQ8, and it has been shown that DCs from T1DM patients present three immunogenic peptides (preproinsulin, islet tyrosine phosphatase insulinoma associated Ag-2, and glutamic acid decarboxylase 65) through these risk HLA [28]. It is possible that in the face of tissue damage secondary to viral infections, there will be release of antigens that are captured by DCs and subsequently presented to CD4+ to promote insulitis and the development of T1DM in a genetically predisposed individual.

Dendritic Cells in Psoriasis

Psoriasis is a chronic inflammatory skin disease characterized by erythematous squamous plaques that affect 2%–3% of the population [29]. In psoriasis, DCs are fundamental in the polarization of Th cells to a Th17 and Th1 phenotype by the production of IL-23 and IL-12 [30,31]. Thereafter, T cells produce IL-17, IFN-γ, TNF-α, and IL-22 that amplify inflammation and promote keratinocyte hyperplasia [31]. Apparently keratinocytes initiate the immune response after tissue damage. Psoriasis lesions can be triggered after a trauma (Koebner's phenomenon), infections, or medication use, where the damage to keratinocytes releases the antimicrobial peptide LL-37 that forms complexes with RNA and DNA and activates the mDCs and pDCs through to TLR8 and TLR9, respectively, to induce inflammation and favor the secretion of type I IFN [29].

Dendritic Cells in Inflammatory Bowel Disease

Inflammatory bowel disease (IBD) is a chronic relapsing inflammatory condition of the gastrointestinal tract that mainly encompasses ulcerative colitis (UC) and Crohn's disease (CD) [32]. One hundred trillion of bacteria, viruses, fungi, and protozoans habitat the human gastrointestinal mucosa [32]. The imbalance in the microbial system that leads to intestinal disorders (dysbiosis) is a key feature of the pathophysiology of IBD [32]. In the steady state and when intestinal homeostasis is present, the sampling of certain bacterial components such as polysaccharide A from *Bacteroides fragilis* by DCs leads to the induction of Tregs and the consequent secretion of IL-10 [32]. In IBD on the other hand, certain genetic and environmental factors lead to dysbiosis, which lead to uncontrolled inflammation, hyperactivation of Th1 and Th17 cells, and decreased differentiation of Tregs [32].

DCs seem to play an important role in the pathophysiology of IBD because animal models have shown that they are capable of priming T cells to develop a pathogenic autoimmune response, and because of their secretion of proinflammatory cytokines, they perpetuate the pathogenic autoimmunity [33]. A local inflammatory environment promotes the maturation of local DCs, which can pick up local antigens, migrate to lymphoid tissues, and expand the pathogenic autoimmune response [33]. In UC it has been shown that DCs release macrophage-inhibiting factor, a cytokine able to enhance their capability to activate T lymphocytes [34].

Nevertheless, DCs studies in patients with IBD have been contradictory, as some have shown a predominance of immature DCs while others have demonstrated raised CD40, CD80, CD83, and CD80 expression in DCs from patients with IBD compared to controls [35,36]; however, the role of DCs as orchestrators of the pathogenic autoimmune response in IBD is frank because they are distributed throughout the intestinal mucosa and polarize the immune response to a Th1 and Th17 phenotype when they are activated by the microbiota PAMPs in the context of dysbiosis.

Dendritic Cells in Rheumatoid Arthritis

Rheumatoid arthritis (RA) is a systemic autoimmune disease characterized mainly by the presence of chronic polyarthritis with the variable occurrence of extra-articular manifestations [37]. DCs in RA show an activated phenotype and produce chemokines such as IL-12 and IL-23 that promote differentiation toward Th1 and Th17 [38]. The presence of antigens with posttranslational modifications such as citrullination is important in the pathogenesis of RA because they may lead to an enhanced immune response. In this regard, DCs in the synovium may uptake these antigens [7] and present them more efficiently than DCs of control subjects [39] The pDCs contribute to inflammation through the production of IFN-α, IFN-β, IL-18, IL-23, and BAFF [38]. Finally, DCs derived from monocytes in RA are able to produce TNF, IL-6, and IL-1β, which in turn bias the T cell response toward Th17 [7]. Probably, pDCs of patients with RA favor the B cells survival and the maturation of DCs, which uptake immunogenic citrullinated antigens and present them to T lymphocytes, leading to synovitis and joint destruction.

Dendritic Cells in Idiopathic Inflammatory Myopathies

Idiopathic inflammatory myopathies (IIM) are a heterogeneous group of diseases characterized by proximal muscle weakness, increased Creatine kinase (CK), myopathic findings in electromyography, and inflammatory infiltrate in muscle biopsy [40]. Included in the spectrum of IIM are dermatomyositis (DM), polymyositis (PM), necrotizing myopathy, and antisynthetase syndrome (AS) [40]. The first evidence of the participation of DCs in IIM is the presence of immature DCs infiltrating the muscle in these diseases [41]. On the other hand, anti–histidyl synthetase (HisRS) antibodies are the most frequent type of antisynthetase antibodies and previous works have demonstrated that the NH_2-terminal domain of HisRS is chemotactic for immature DCs [42]. In muscle biopsies of DM and juvenile DM patients, DCs are located mainly in the perivascular space, whereas in PM they penetrate deep into the muscle [43]. The recruitment of DCs can be facilitated in muscle by the secretion of CXCR4 CCL19 CCL21 by mononuclear cells [43].

DCs in IIM also produce IL-18, which favors the proliferation and differentiation of naïve T cells [44], and pCDs are involved in the type IFN signature found in patients with DM because it is known that they are present in the perimysial, fascial, and endomysial inflammatory infiltrate [45].

Dendritic Cells in the Autoimmune/Autoinflammatory Syndrome Induced by Adjuvants

Due to the abundance in the expression of PRRs, DCs are fundamental in the autoimmune reactions induced by adjuvants. The prototypes of these reactions are macrophagic myofasciitis and adverse reactions after vaccines. In macrophagic myofasciitis, aluminum hydroxide (Al (OH)$_3$) persists for years after the administration of a vaccine [46]. The adjuvant is found at injection sites and in the body of patients with the disease, which is characterized by myalgias, arthralgias, chronic fatigue, and an inflammatory infiltrate of PAS(+) macrophages that express MHC-I and that show aluminum in their cytoplasm by electron microscopy [46]. At the same time, there are CD8+ T cells and damaged muscle fibers in the muscle biopsy [46].

Aluminum hydroxide (Al (OH)$_3$) favors tissue damage with the consequent release of UA and activation of the NALP3 inflammasome on DCs, with the consequent chemotaxis of neutrophils, eosinophils, and mononuclear cells to the injection site [46]. After that, there is activation of the immune system and the bias of the immune response toward a Th2 phenotype [46,47]. When UA is released into the extracellular space, it is recognized as DAMP, promoting the capture of antigens by inflammatory monocytes at the site of injury [46]. Posteriorly, those monocytes migrate to the lymph nodes where they mature to DCs and activate CD4+ T cells [46].

Aluminum also directly activates the NALP3 inflammasome on DCs with the consequent release of IL-1β [46,47]. Aluminum enhances the normal function of DCs, but in a subject genetically predisposed (for example, a carrier of HLA-DRB1*01), it can promote the development of chronic inflammation with systemic manifestations as in macrophage myofasciitis.

TOLEROGENIC DENDRITIC CELLS

Immature DCs and pDCs are considered to be naturally tolerogenic because of their low expression of MHC and co-stimulatory molecules. For example, immature DCs are able to induce tolerance in an EAE model when they are administered intravenously by increasing the production of IL-10 and Tregs [48]. However, tolerogenic dendritic cells (tolDCs) derived from peripheral blood have been generated in multiple in vitro models by cytokines such as IL-10, TGF-β, or with immunosuppressive drugs such as cyclosporine, rapamycin, mycophenolate mofetil, vitamin D3, dexamethasone, or other agents such as N-acetyl-cysteine, glucosamine, HLA-G, cAMP, or PGE2 [49].

TolDCs can be conventional or plasmacytoid and maintain peripheral tolerance through anergy and apoptosis of autoreactive T cells and through the induction of Tregs [50]. TolDCs can also exert their action by the expression of indoleamine 2,3-dioxygenase or programmed death ligand 1 (PDL-1) [49]. Its objective is to reestablish antigen-specific tolerance without promoting general immunosuppression [50]. The tolDCs do not change their phenotype in vitro, that is, even after being stimulated they do not favor the activation of self-reactive cells [50].

TolDCs have been tested mainly in animal models of MS and RA. For example, the use of tolDCs transfected with lentiviruses that inhibit the production of CD40 and IL-23 decreases the phenotype of EAE by inhibiting differentiation toward Th17 and increasing the production of IL-10 [51]. It is possible that the manipulation of transcription factors in DCs is able to modulate the immune response, for example; the increase in the expression of SOCS3 in DCs polarizes the immune response toward Th2 and decreases the symptomatology of EAE [52]. Other molecules such as LPS decrease the phenotype of EAE by creating tolDCs that reduce ROR-γt and IFN-γ in T cells prestimulated with myelin oligodendrocyte glycoprotein (MOG) [53]. The use of DCs expressing TRAIL (a member of the superfamily of TNF receptors) or PDL-1 together with MOG favors the formation of Tregs and the apoptosis of effector T cells in a murine model of EAE [54,55].

In animal models of collagen-induced arthritis, the IL-10 and TGF-β induced tolDCs have been shown to decrease the severity of the disease by increasing Tregs [38,56]. Despite the technical difficulties involved in the development and administration of tolDCs in humans, their efficacy in animal models offer hope for a personalized treatment of autoimmune diseases without the need for global immunosuppression.

CONCLUSIONS

In a genetically predisposed individual, infections and tissue damage induced favor the activation of DCs. When there are alterations in central or peripheral tolerance, the antigenic presentation and production of cytokines by DCs promotes the polarization of helper cells toward Th1 and Th17, which in turn promote tissue damage through a pathogenic autoimmune response. In Fig. 8.1, we propose a general model to explain the participation of DCs as triggers and perpetuating agents in autoimmune diseases.

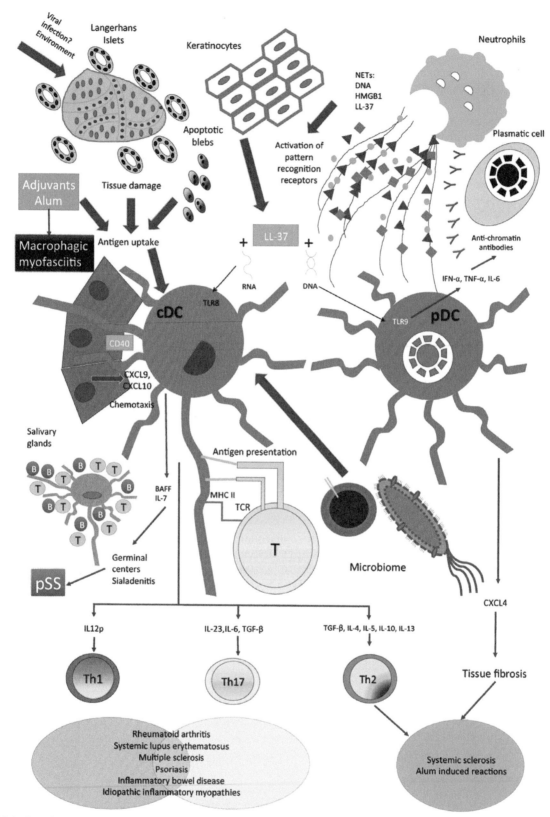

FIGURE 8.1 In patients with autoimmune diseases, epithelial and connective tissue cells secrete various chemokines that attract dendritic cells (DCs). In response to environmental stimuli including tissue damage, NETosis, infections, or the use of adjuvants such as alum, there is activation of the transmembrane and cytoplasmic pattern recognition receptors (PRRs) in DCs leading to the secretion of proinflammatory cytokines. As a result, there is a polarization of the Th response toward Th1 and Th17, which are known to be involved in the pathophysiology of many autoimmune diseases. DCs are also professional antigen-presenting cells, especially of those antigens containing posttranslational modifications and as professional type I producers, pDC induce the maturation of myeloid dendritic cells and the secretion of autoantibodies by B cells, expanding the inflammatory response. Finally, the secretion of TFG-β and IL-13 may relate dendritic cells with fibrosis in patients with systemic sclerosis.

REFERENCES

[1] Wu L, Dakic A. Development of dendritic cell system. Cell Mol Immunol 2004;1(2):112–8.

[2] Kim JM, Park SH, Kim HY. Kwok SKA plasmacytoid dendritic cells-type I interferon Axis is critically implicated in the pathogenesis of systemic lupus erythematosus. Int J Mol Sci 2015;16(6):14158–70.

[3] Chen K, Wang JM, Yuan R, et al. Tissue-resident dendritic cells and diseases involving dendritic cell malfunction. Int Immunopharmacol 2016;34:1–15.

[4] Xie ZX, Zhang HL, Wu XJ, Zhu J, Ma DH, Jin T. Role of the immunogenic and tolerogenic subsets of dendritic cells in multiple sclerosis. Mediators Inflamm 2015;2015:513295.

[5] Xia CQ, Peng R, Chernatynskaya AV, et al. Increased IFN-alpha-producing plasmacytoid dendritic cells (pDCs) in human Th1-mediated type 1 diabetes: pDCs augment Th1 responses through IFN-alpha production. J Immunol 2014;193(3):1024–34.

[6] Blanco P, Palucka AK, Pascual V, Banchereau J. Dendritic cells and cytokines in human inflammatory and autoimmune diseases. Cytokine Growth Factor Rev 2008;19(1):41–52.

[7] Lutzky V, Hannawi S, Thomas R. Cells of the synovium in rheumatoid arthritis. Dendritic cells. Arthritis Res Ther 2007;9(4):219.

[8] Boltjes A, Van Wijk F. Human dendritic cell functional specialization in steady-state and inflammation. Front Immunol 2014;5:131.

[9] Leal Rojas IM, Mok WH, Pearson FE, Minoda Y, Kenna TJ, Barnard RT, Radford KJ. Human blood CD1c+ dendritic cells promote Th1 and Th17 effector function in memory CD4+ T cells. Front Immunol 2017;8:971.

[10] Isakson SH, Katzman SD, Hoyer KK. Spontaneous autoimmunity in the absence of IL-2 is driven by uncontrolled dendritic cells. J Immunol 2012;189(4):1585–93.

[11] Mohty M, Vialle-Castellano A, Nunes JA, Isnardon D, Olive D, Gaugler B. IFN- Skews monocyte differentiation into toll-like receptor 7-expressing dendritic cells with potent functional activities. J Immunol 2003;171(7):3385–93.

[12] Chan VS, Nie YJ, Shen N, Yan S, Mok MY, Lau CS. Distinct roles of myeloid and plasmacytoid dendritic cells in systemic lupus erythematosus. Autoimmun Rev 2012;11(12):890–7.

[13] Garcia-Romo GS, Caielli S, Vega B, et al. Netting neutrophils are major inducers of type I IFN production in pediatric systemic lupus erythematosus. Sci Transl Med 2011;3(73):73ra20.

[14] Galicia G, Gommerman JL. Plasmacytoid dendritic cells and autoimmune inflammation. Biol Chem 2014;395(3):335–46.

[15] Hillen MR, Ververs FA, Kruize AA, Van Roon JA. Dendritic cells, T-cells and epithelial cells: a crucial interplay in immunopathology of primary Sjögren's syndrome. Expert Rev Clin Immunol 2014;10(4):521–31.

[16] Fujikado N, Saijo S, Yonezawa T, et al. Dcir deficiency causes development of autoimmune diseases in mice due to excess expansion of dendritic cells. Nat Med 2008;14(2):176–80.

[17] Van Roon JA, Kruize AA, Radstake TR. Editorial: interleukin-7 and its receptor: the axis of evil to target in Sjogren's syndrome? Arthritis Rheum 2013;65(8):1980–4.

[18] Lu TT. Dendritic cells: novel players in fibrosis and scleroderma. Curr Rheumatol Rep 2012;14(1):30–8.

[19] Pennell LM, Fish EN. Interferon-beta regulates dendritic cell activation and migration in experimental autoimmune encephalomyelitis. Immunology 2017;152(3):439–50.

[20] Huang YM, Stoyanova N, Jin YP, Teleshova N, Hussien Y, Xiao BG, Fredrikson S, Link H. Altered phenotype and function of blood dendritic cells in multiple sclerosis are modulated by IFN-beta and IL-10. Clin Exp Immunol 2001,124(2):306 14.

[21] Lu P, Cao Y, Wang M, et al. Mature dendritic cells cause Th17/Treg imbalance by secreting TGF-beta1 and IL-6 in the pathogenesis of experimental autoimmune encephalomyelitis. Cent Eur J Immunol 2016;41(2):143–52.

[22] Heink S, Yogev N, Garbers C, et al. Trans-presentation of IL-6 by dendritic cells is required for the priming of pathogenic TH17 cells. Nat Immunol 2017;18(1):74–85.

[23] Isaksson M, Ardesjo B, Ronnblom L, et al. Plasmacytoid DC promote priming of autoimmune Th17 cells and EAE. Eur J Immunol 2009;39(10):2925–35.

[24] Da Silva RC, Cunha Tavares Nde A, Moura R, et al. DC-SIGN polymorphisms are associated to type 1 diabetes mellitus. Immunobiology 2014;219(11):859–65.

[25] Klementowicz JE, Mahne AE, Spence A, et al. Cutting edge: origins, recruitment, and regulation of CD11c+ cells in inflamed islets of autoimmune diabetes mice. J Immunol 2017;199(1):27–32.

[26] Guerder S, Joncker N, Mahiddine K, Serre L. Dendritic cells in tolerance and autoimmune diabetes. Curr Opin Immunol 2013;25(6):670–5.

[27] Abram DM, Fernandes LGR, Ramos Filho ACS, Simioni PU. The modulation of enzyme indoleamine 2,3-dioxygenase from dendritic cells for the treatment of type 1 diabetes mellitus. Drug Des Dev Ther 2017;11:2171–8.

[28] Van Lummel M, Van Veelen PA, De Ru AH, et al. Dendritic cells guide islet autoimmunity through a restricted and uniquely processed peptidome presented by high-risk HLA-DR. J Immunol 2016;196(8):3253–63.

[29] Lowes MA, Suarez-Farinas M, Krueger JG. Immunology of psoriasis. Annu Rev Immunol 2014;32:227–55.

[30] Harden JL, Krueger JG, Bowcock AM. The immunogenetics of Psoriasis: a comprehensive review. J Autoimmun 2015;64:66–73.

[31] Kim J, Krueger JG. The immunopathogenesis of psoriasis. Dermatol Clin 2015;33(1):13–23.

[32] Zhang M, Sun K, Wu Y, Yang Y, Tso P, Wu Z. Interactions between intestinal microbiota and host immune response in inflammatory bowel disease. Front Immunol 2017;8:942.

[33] Leon F, Smythies LE, Smith PD, Kelsall BL. Involvement of dendritic cells in the pathogenesis of inflammatory bowel disease. Adv Exp Med Biol 2006;579:117–32.

[34] Murakami H, Akbar SM, Matsui H, Horiike N, Onji M. Macrophage migration inhibitory factor activates antigen-presenting dendritic cells and induces inflammatory cytokines in ulcerative colitis. Clin Exp Immunol 2002;128(3):504–10.

[35] Stagg AJ, Hart AL, Knight SC, Kamm MA. The dendritic cell: its role in intestinal inflammation and relationship with gut bacteria. Gut 2003;52(10):1522–9.

[36] Vuckovic S, Florin TH, Khalil D, et al. CD40 and CD86 upregulation with divergent CMRF44 expression on blood dendritic cells in inflammatory bowel diseases. Am J Gastroenterol 2001;96(10):2946–56.

[37] Angelotti F, Parma A, Cafaro G, Capecchi R, Alunno A, Puxeddu I. One year in review 2017: pathogenesis of rheumatoid arthritis. Clin Exp Rheumatol 2017;35(3):368–78.

[38] Schinnerling K, Soto L, Garcia-Gonzalez P, Catalan D, Aguillon JC. Skewing dendritic cell differentiation towards a tolerogenic state for recovery of tolerance in rheumatoid arthritis. Autoimmun Rev 2015;14(6):517–27.

[39] Waalen K, Førre O, Teigland J, Natvig JB. Human rheumatoid synovial and normal blood dendritic cells as antigen presenting cell–comparison with autologous monocytes. Clin Exp Immunol 1987;70(1):1–9.

[40] Milone M. Diagnosis and management of immune-mediated myopathies. Mayo Clin Proc 2017;92(5):826–37.

[41] Chevrel G, Page G, Miossec P. Novel aspects on the contribution of T cells and dendritic cells in the pathogenesis of myositis. Autoimmunity 2006;39(3):171–6.

[42] Howard OM, Zack, Dong HF, Yang De, et al. Histidyl–tRNA synthetase and asparaginyl–tRNA synthetase, autoantigens in myositis, activate chemokine receptors on T Lymphocytes and immature dendritic cells. J Exp Med 2002;196(6):781–91.

[43] De Padilla CM, Reed AM. Dendritic cells and the immunopathogenesis of idiopathic inflammatory myopathies. Curr Opin Rheumatol 2008;20(6):669–74.

[44] Tucci M, Quatraro C, Dammacco F, Silvestris F. Increased IL-18 production by dendritic cells in active inflammatory myopathies. Ann N Y Acad Sci 2007;1107:184–92.

[45] Li L, Dai T, Lv J, et al. Role of Toll-like receptors and retinoic acid inducible gene I in endogenous production of type I interferon in dermatomyositis. J Neuroimmunol 2015;285:161–8.

[46] Israeli E, Agmon-Levin N, Blank M, Shoenfeld Y. Macrophagic myofaciitis a vaccine (alum) autoimmune-related disease. Clin Rev Allergy Immunol 2011;41(2):163–8.

[47] Kool M, Petrilli V, De Smedt T, et al. Cutting edge: alum adjuvant stimulates inflammatory dendritic cells through activation of the NALP3 inflammasome. J Immunol 2008;181(6):3755–9.

[48] Zhou F, Ciric B, Zhang GX, Rostami A. Immune tolerance induced by intravenous transfer of immature dendritic cells via up-regulating numbers of suppressive IL-10(+) IFN-gamma(+)-producing CD4(+) T cells. Immunol Res 2013;56(1):1–8.

[49] Mok M. Tolerogenic dendritic cells: role and therapeutic implications in systemic lupus erythematosus. Int J Rheum Dis 2015;18(2):250–9.

[50] Gross CC, Jonuleit H, Wiendl H. Fulfilling the dream: tolerogenic dendritic cells to treat multiple sclerosis. Eur J Immunol 2012;42(3):569–72.

[51] Kalantari T, Karimi MH, Ciric B, Yan Y, Rostami A, Kamali-Sarvestani E. Tolerogenic dendritic cells produced by lentiviral-mediated CD40- and interleukin-23p19-specific shRNA can ameliorate experimental autoimmune encephalomyelitis by suppressing T helper type 17 cells. Clin Exp Immunol 2014;176(2):180–9.

[52] Li Y, Chu N, Rostami A, Zhang GX. Dendritic cells transduced with SOCS-3 exhibit a tolerogenic/DC2 phenotype that Directs type 2 Th cell differentiation in vitro and in vivo. J Immunol 2006;177(3):1679–88.

[53] Zhou F, Ciric B, Zhang GX, Rostami A. Immunotherapy using lipopolysaccharide-stimulated bone marrow-derived dendritic cells to treat experimental autoimmune encephalomyelitis. Clin Exp Immunol 2014;178(3):447–58.

[54] Hirata S, Matsuyoshi H, Fukuma D, et al. Involvement of regulatory T cells in the experimental autoimmune encephalomyelitis-preventive effect of dendritic cells expressing myelin oligodendrocyte glycoprotein plus TRAIL. J Immunol 2007;178(2):918–25.

[55] Hirata S, Senju S, Matsuyoshi H, Fukuma D, Uemura Y, Nishimura Y. Prevention of experimental autoimmune encephalomyelitis by transfer of embryonic stem cell-derived dendritic cells expressing myelin oligodendrocyte glycoprotein peptide along with TRAIL or programmed Death-1 ligand. J Immunol 2005;174(4):1888–97.

[56] Ning B, Wei J, Zhang A, et al. Antigen-specific tolerogenic dendritic cells ameliorate the severity of murine collagen-induced arthritis. PLoS One 2015;10(6):e0131152.

[57] Scheinecker C, Zwolfer B, Koller M, Manner G, Smolen JS. Alterations of dendritic cells in systemic lupus erythematosus: phenotypic and functional deficiencies. Arthritis Rheum 2001;44(4):856–65.

[58] Migita K, Miyashita T, Maeda Y, et al. Reduced blood BDCA-2+ (lymphoid) and CD11c+ (myeloid) dendritic cells in systemic lupus erythematosus. Clin Exp Immunol 2005;142(1):84–91.

[59] Fiore N, Castellano G, Blasi A, et al. Immature myeloid and plasmacytoid dendritic cells infiltrate renal tubulointerstitium in patients with lupus nephritis. Mol Immunol 2008;45(1):259–65.

[60] Koller M, Zwolfer B, Steiner G, Smolen JS, Scheinecker C. Phenotypic and functional deficiencies of monocyte-derived dendritic cells in systemic lupus erythematosus (SLE) patients. Int Immunol 2004;16(11):1595–604.

[61] Tucci M, Quatraro C, Lombardi L, Pellegrino C, Dammacco F, Silvestris F. Glomerular accumulation of plasmacytoid dendritic cells in active lupus nephritis: role of interleukin-18. Arthritis Rheum 2008;58(1):251–62.

[62] Henriques A, Ines L, Carvalheiro T, et al. Functional characterization of peripheral blood dendritic cells and monocytes in systemic lupus erythematosus. Rheumatol Int 2012;32(4):863–9.

[63] Jin O, Kavikondala S, Sun L, et al. Systemic lupus erythematosus patients have increased number of circulating plasmacytoid dendritic cells, but decreased myeloid dendritic cells with deficient CD83 expression. Lupus 2008;17(7):654–62.

[64] Decker P, Kotter I, Klein R, Berner B, Rammensee HG. Monocyte-derived dendritic cells over-express CD86 in patients with systemic lupus erythematosus. Rheumatology (Oxford) 2006;45(9):1087–95.

[65] Ding D, Mehta H, Mccune WJ, Kaplan MJ. Aberrant phenotype and function of myeloid dendritic cells in systemic lupus erythematosus. J Immunol 2006;177(9):5878–89.

[66] Gerl V, Lischka A, Panne D, et al. Blood dendritic cells in systemic lupus erythematosus exhibit altered activation state and chemokine receptor function. Ann Rheum Dis 2010;69(7):1370–7.

[67] Jin O, Kavikondala S, Mok MY, et al. Abnormalities in circulating plasmacytoid dendritic cells in patients with systemic lupus erythematosus. Arthritis Res Ther 2010;12(4):R137.

[68] Kwok SK, Lee JY, Park SH, et al. Dysfunctional interferon-alpha production by peripheral plasmacytoid dendritic cells upon Toll-like receptor-9 stimulation in patients with systemic lupus erythematosus. Arthritis Res Ther 2008;10(2):R29.

[69] Gottenberg JE, Cagnard N, Lucchesi C, et al. Activation of IFN pathways and plasmacytoid dendritic cell recruitment in target organs of primary Sjögren's syndrome. Proc Natl Acad Sci U S A 2006;103(8):2770–5.

[70] Ozaki Y, Ito T, Son Y, et al. Decrease of blood dendritic cells and increase of tissue-infiltrating dendritic cells are involved in the induction of Sjogren's syndrome but not in the maintenance. Clin Exp Immunol 2010;159(3):315–26.

[71] Wildenberg ME, Van Helden-Meeuwsen CG, Van De Merwe JP, Drexhage HA, Versnel MA. Systemic increase in type I interferon activity in Sjögren's syndrome: a putative role for plasmacytoid dendritic cells. Eur J Immunol 2008;38(7):2024–33.

[72] Ozaki Y, Amakawa R, Ito T, et al. Alteration of peripheral blood dendritic cells in patients with primary Sjogren's syndrome. Arthritis Rheum 2001;44(2):419–31.

[73] Vogelsang P, Brun JG, Oijordsbakken G, Skarstein K, Jonsson R, Appel S. Levels of plasmacytoid dendritic cells and type-2 myeloid dendritic cells are reduced in peripheral blood of patients with primary Sjogren's syndrome. Ann Rheum Dis 2010;69(6):1235–8.

[74] Thewissen K, Nuyts AH, Deckx N, et al. Circulating dendritic cells of multiple sclerosis patients are proinflammatory and their frequency is correlated with MS-associated genetic risk factors. Mult Scler 2014;20(5):548–57.

[75] Mitosek-Szewczyk K, Tabarkiewicz J, Wilczynska B, et al. Impact of cladribine therapy on changes in circulating dendritic cell subsets, T cells and B cells in patients with multiple sclerosis. J Neurol Sci 2013;332(1–2):35–40.

[76] Lopez C, Comabella M, Al-Zayat H, Tintore M, Montalban X. Altered maturation of circulating dendritic cells in primary progressive MS patients. J Neuroimmunol 2006;175(1–2):183–91.

[77] Stasiolek M, Bayas A, Kruse N, et al. Impaired maturation and altered regulatory function of plasmacytoid dendritic cells in multiple sclerosis. Brain 2006;129(Pt 5):1293–305.

[78] Bayas A, Stasiolek M, Kruse N, Toyka KV, Selmaj K, Gold R. Altered innate immune response of plasmacytoid dendritic cells in multiple sclerosis. Clin Exp Immunol 2009;157(3):332–42.

[79] Hirotani M, Niino M, Fukazawa T, et al. Decreased interferon-alpha production in response to CpG DNA dysregulates cytokine responses in patients with multiple sclerosis. Clin Immunol 2012;143(2):145–51.

[80] Balashov KE, Aung LL, Vaknin-Dembinsky A, Dhib-Jalbut S, Weiner HL. Interferon-beta inhibits toll-like receptor 9 processing in multiple sclerosis. Ann Neurol 2010;68(6):899–906.

[81] Schwab N, Zozulya AL, Kieseier BC, Toyka KV, Wiendl H. An imbalance of two functionally and phenotypically different subsets of plasmacytoid dendritic cells characterizes the dysfunctional immune regulation in multiple sclerosis. J Immunol 2010;184(9):5368–74.

[82] Pashenkov M, Huang YM, Kostulas V, Haglund M, Soderstrom M, Link H. Two subsets of dendritic cells are present in human cerebrospinal fluid. Brain 2001;124(Pt 3):480–92.

[83] Karni A, Abraham M, Monsonego A, et al. Innate immunity in multiple sclerosis: myeloid dendritic cells in secondary progressive multiple sclerosis are activated and drive a proinflammatory immune response. J Immunol 2006;177(6):4196–202.

[84] Cavanagh L, Boyce A, Smith L, Padmanabha J, Filgueira L, Pietschmann P, Thomas R. Rheumatoid arthritis synovium contains plasmacytoid dendritic cells. Arthritis Res Ther 2005;7(2):R230–40.

[85] Allen JS, Pang K, Skowera A, et al. Plasmacytoid dendritic cells are proportionally expanded at diagnosis of type 1 diabetes and enhance islet autoantigen presentation to T-cells through immune complex capture. Diabetes 2009;58(1):138–45.

[86] Chen X, Makala LH, Jin Y, et al. Type 1 diabetes patients have significantly lower frequency of plasmacytoid dendritic cells in the peripheral blood. Clin Immunol 2008;129(3):413–8.

[87] Vuckovic S, Withers G, Harris M, et al. Decreased blood dendritic cell counts in type 1 diabetic children. Clin Immunol 2007;123(3):281–8.

[88] Gendek-Kubiak H, Gendek EG. Fascin-expressing dendritic cells dominate in polymyositis and dermatomyositis. J Rheumatol 2013;40(2):186–91.

[89] Greenberg SA, Pinkus GS, Amato AA, Pinkus JL. Myeloid dendritic cells in inclusion-body myositis and polymyositis. Muscle Nerve 2007;35(1):17–23.

[90] Wenzel J, Schmidt R, Proelss J, Zahn S, Bieber T, Tuting T. Type I interferon-associated skin recruitment of CXCR3+ lymphocytes in dermatomyositis. Clin Exp Dermatol 2006;31(4):576–82.

[91] Kaser A, Ludwiczek O, Holzmann S, et al. Increased expression of CCL20 in human inflammatory bowel disease. J Clin Immunol 2004;24(1):74–85.

[92] Te Velde AA, Van Kooyk Y, Braat H, et al. Increased expression of DC-SIGN+IL-12+IL-18+ and CD83+IL-12-IL-18- dendritic cell populations in the colonic mucosa of patients with Crohn's disease. Eur J Immunol 2003;33(1):143–51.

Chapter 9

The Complement System

Elisabetta Greco, Maria Domenica Guarino, Eleonora Ballanti, Roberto Perricone
Rheumatology, Allergy and Clinical Immunology – University of Rome "Tor Vergata", Rome, Italy

INTRODUCTION

The complement system is a component of the innate immune system, which consists of physical, cellular, and chemical elements. Traditionally, the main function of the complement system was believed to be limited to the recognition and elimination of pathogens through direct killing and/or stimulation of phagocytosis (innate responses) [1,2]. In recent years, the immunoregulatory functions of the complement system were demonstrated and it was determined that the complement proteins play an important role in modulating adaptive immunity and in bridging innate and adaptive responses [3]. The contribution of complement to the development of humoral immunity has been confirmed through a series of elegant studies and a body of data has accumulated demonstrating that the activation of the complement system is also critical to the development of T cell immunity [4].

The complement system comprises more than 30 plasma and membrane-bound proteins [3,5]. The activation of these proteins occurs through three possible pathways: the classical, the alternative, and the lectin pathway. All three pathways are activated according to a cascade system, with activation of one factor leading to the activation of the next.

PATHWAYS OF COMPLEMENT SYSTEM ACTIVATION

The pathways of complement system activation constitute enzyme cascades, analogous to the coagulation, fibrinolysis, and kinin pathways. Several complement proteins are cleaved during activation of the system, and the fragments are generally designated with suffixes "a" and "b." All three pathways lead to the cleavage of C3 and finally converge at the activation of C5 (Fig. 9.1). The activation of the classical pathway is dependent on immunoglobulins IgM or IgG, present in immune complexes (IC) and binding to the C1 complex [6]. The binding of C1q to antibody leads to activation of C4 and C2 inducing the formation of the C4bC2a complex, also known as classical pathway's C3 convertase [7]. If the activation occurs through the alternative pathway, factor D, a serine protease, cleaves factor B, which is complexed with spontaneously hydrolyzed iC3b, leading to formation of Ba and Bb. Bb and C3b generate the C3 convertase of the alternative pathway, C3bBb. Properdin increases the stability of this enzyme [8]. The lectin pathway becomes activated, when either mannose-binding lectin (MBL) or ficolins recognize carbohydrate patterns on microbes and activate C2 and C4 through MBL-associated serine proteases (MASP), with the formation of the same C3 convertase as the classical pathway, C4bC2a [7]. Likewise, the classical and lectin pathways generate the same C5 convertase (C3bC4bC2a), whereas the alternative pathway generates a different C5 convertase (C3bBbC3b). The activation of C5 produces C5a (a potent chemoattractant) and C5b, which forms the membrane attack complex (MAC) C5b-9, able to cause cell lysis. In addition to cell lysis, effects of complement activation include activation of granulocytes and endothelia by sublytic quantities of MAC; deposition of C3 fragments (e.g., C3b, iC3b) on membranes and/or particles leading to opsonization and enhanced phagocytosis; IC clearance; clearance of apoptotic bodies; alterations in immune cell signal transduction, adhesion activation, and cytokine production; anaphylatoxin-mediated effects [4] (Fig. 9.2).

REGULATION OF THE COMPLEMENT SYSTEM

To avoid excessive complement activation and thus protect the host, the complement system is tightly controlled by proteins present in the fluid phase and on cell membranes [9]. Interestingly, evidence shows that many pathogenic microorganisms interact with these complement regulators to elude the immune system [10].

Several proteins regulating the complement system decrease the activity of C3 convertases in the classical and alternative pathways, enzymes that catalyze key reactions during the activation of the complement system. Moreover, important

Mosaic of Autoimmunity. https://doi.org/10.1016/B978-0-12-814307-0.00009-8

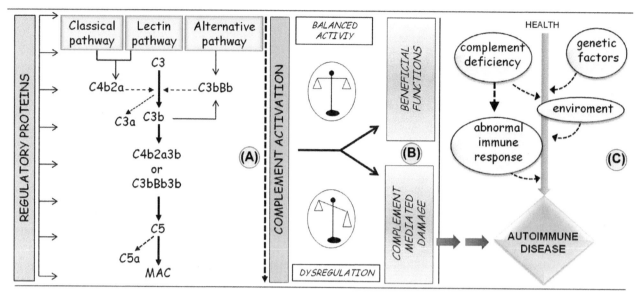

FIGURE 9.1 Activation of the complement system occurs through three possible pathways: the classical, the alternative, and the lectin pathway (A). All the pathways lead to the cleavage of C3 and finally converge at the activation of C5, with possible formation of the membrane attack complex (A). To avoid excess complement activation, the complement system is tightly controlled by several regulatory proteins, which act at different points of complement cascade (A). When the mechanisms that regulate this delicate balance do not work correctly, complement (that usually mediates beneficial functions) may cause damage by induction and augmentation of inflammation (B). Its intervention has been implicated in the pathogenesis of several autoimmune diseases (C).

control proteins are involved in the regulation of C1 activity and of the MAC [9]. When the mechanisms that regulate this delicate balance do not work properly or there is an overactivation of the complement system exceeding the capacity of the regulatory mechanisms, the complement system may cause damage by induction and amplification of inflammation [3] (Fig. 9.1).

The importance of the regulatory mechanisms is evident in hereditary angioedema (HAE). In this disease the deficiency of C1 inhibitor (C1INH), a multifunctional serine protease inhibitor, causes inappropriate activation of the complement system and of the other plasma enzymatic systems (contact system, coagulation system) that result in recurrent episodes of angioedema involving the skin and the mucosa [11].

Paroxysmal nocturnal hemoglobinuria is another example of the consequences of the failure to regulate the complement system. In such disease, a somatic mutation in the phosphatidylinositol glycan class A gene causes a deficiency of a protein required for the synthesis of glycosylphosphatidylinositol, the lipid that anchors several proteins to cell membranes [12]. As a result, two molecules anchored by glycosylphosphatidylinositol, decay-accelerating factor or CD55 (which regulates the formation of C3 convertase) and CD59 (which inhibits the formation of the MAC), are lacking on cell membrane, thus increasing susceptibility of erythrocytes to complement and leading to intravascular hemolysis [12].

COMPLEMENT SYSTEM AS MEDIATOR OF TISSUE DAMAGE

Several studies demonstrated that the complement system is involved in inflammatory tissue damage. The activation of the complement system in the tissues occurs through IC, which trigger the classical complement pathway [5] (Fig. 9.2). Moreover, in ischemic tissues, phospholipids and mitochondrial proteins, normally sequestrated in the cells, are exposed and are able to activate the complement system either directly by binding C1q or MBL or indirectly by binding natural antibodies or C-reactive protein (CRP) [5]. CRP can activate the classical pathway by binding C1q. Furthermore, necrotic cells and tissues lack the regulatory molecules that normally prevent the binding of complement proteins [5].

C1q has long been considered an innate immune molecule. Its complement-independent functions on immune and nonimmune cells serve to highlight a critical role in maintaining homeostasis. C1q's interaction with novel receptors linked to immune tolerance and prevention of autoimmunity and neuronal inflammation are fascinating areas for further investigation [13].

Inappropriate activation of the complement system causes the release of several proinflammatory mediators, such as anaphylatoxins C3a and C5a, which, in turn, are able to stimulate the synthesis of other proinflammatory mediators [14]. C5a is also a potent chemoattractant for neutrophils, monocytes, and eosinophils [14]. In addition, the MAC can contribute

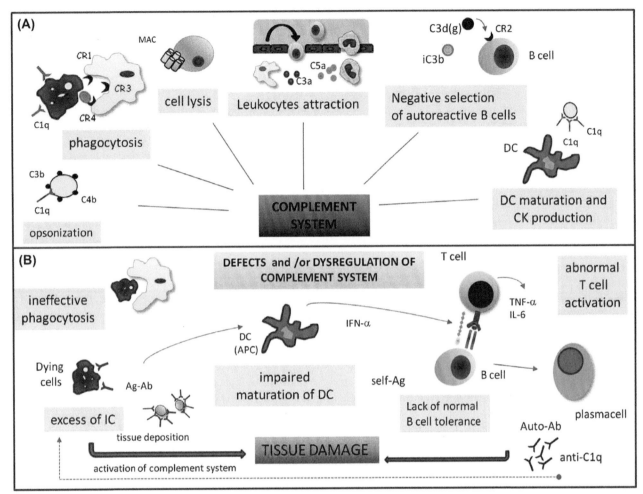

FIGURE 9.2 Complement involvement in physiological conditions and autoimmune diseases. (A) Complement proteins play an important role in modulating innate and adaptive responses of immune system. Opsonization, phagocytosis, cell lysis, leukocytes attraction, and activation are important mechanisms for pathogens and cellular debris elimination. (B) Both defects and dysregulation of complement proteins have been involved in autoimmune diseases pathogenesis. In patients with complement proteins' defects poor clearance of IC and dying cells is observed with inflammatory tissue damage and release of autoantigens. Lack of normal B cell tolerance causes production of autoantibodies, including antibodies against complement proteins. A central role is played by DCs, whose polarization is deeply influenced by complement proteins. C1q interacting with APC results in diminished proinflammatory T subsets. Conversely, defects of C1q or neutralization by anti-C1q causes proinflammatory T cell activation. *Ab*, antibodies; *Ag*, antigen; *APC*, antigen-presenting cell; *CK*, cytokines; *DC*, dendritic cells; *IC*, immune complexes.

to inflammation and tissue damage. Formation of the terminal complement complex C5b-9 can lead to cell death by necrosis or apoptosis [14].

The contribution of the complement system to tissue damage is exemplified by necrosis following ischemia. In fact, the activation of the complement system has been demonstrated in areas of myocardial infarction and cerebral stroke [5,15].

COMPLEMENT SYSTEM AND AUTOIMMUNITY

The relation between the complement system and autoimmunity is apparently paradoxical. If on one hand the complement system is activated and contributes to tissue damage in autoimmune diseases, on the other hand, deficiency of the complement proteins leads to autoimmunity and it is challenging reconciling these two aspects.

The complement system is involved in the pathogenesis and contributes to the clinical manifestations of several autoimmune diseases (Fig. 9.1), such as systemic lupus erythematosus (SLE), anti–glomerular basement membrane disease, vasculitides, Sjögren's syndrome (SS), antiphospholipid antibody syndrome (APS), systemic sclerosis (SSc), dermatomyositis (DM), and rheumatoid arthritis (RA) [16].

Paradoxically, complement system deficiencies are also associated with autoimmune diseases. The prevalence of complement system's deficiencies in the population is difficult to assess. Most heterozygotic complement-deficient individuals are clinically normal. Generally, only C1-INH (autosomal dominant), properdin (X-linked recessive), and homozygotic complement-deficient individuals present with clinical diseases. Deficiencies of components of the complement system may result in a wide variety of clinical presentations, including recurrent bacterial infections, HAE, rheumatic disorders, leukocyte adhesion deficiency, and hemolytic-uremic syndrome (HUS) [17].

Autoimmune disorders, mainly SLE, can be the common clinical manifestation of genetically determined disorders of the complement system, and they are most frequently observed in patients with deficiencies of the early components of the classical pathway. While over 30% of patients with C2 deficiency and nearly 80% of patients with either C3 or C4 deficiency present autoimmune manifestations, less than 10% of the patients with deficiencies of C5–9 develop similar clinical evidences. The most common presentation is SLE, but discoid lupus, DM, scleroderma, and glomerulonephritis were also reported [18].

Several theories have been proposed to explain the association between deficiencies of components of the complement system and autoimmune diseases. The majority of these focus on the inadequate clearance of IC in presence of reduced levels of complement system's components [19]. An excess of IC may deposit in the tissues, resulting in inflammatory damage and release of autoantigens that trigger an autoimmune response (Fig. 9.2). Alternatively, the presence of high concentration of apoptotic cells (AC) due to poor clearance may be sufficient to elicit an autoimmune response [20] (Fig. 9.2).

In particular, among complement proteins, a primary role in clearance activity is attributed to the first component of the complement C1q. This can directly and indirectly opsonize AC for phagocytosis by macrophages. It can directly bind AC and mediate AC phagocytosis through CD91 or LRP-1 (low-density lipoprotein receptor-related protein 1) on macrophages. It can also bind indirectly, through CRP and IgM, to cause complement activation and C3 deposition [21,22].

A third hypothesis suggests that the complement system favors the development of tolerance against self [23].

The complement system is needed for the elimination of self-reactive lymphocytes during maturation of the immune system. Hence, deficiencies of the complement system result in lack of normal B cell tolerance and production of autoantibodies [24,25] (Fig. 9.2).

Moreover, recent data seem to demonstrate that complement system's proteins, in particular C1q, act as a strong signal for dendritic cells (DCs) [26]. Mature DCs are the most powerful antigen-presenting cells (APCs) able to induce and direct the differentiation of naive T cells. Depending on the maturation signal and the cytokine environment, DCs may stimulate CD4+ helper, CD8+ cytotoxic, or regulatory T cells, inducing tolerance (Fig. 9.2). C1q plays an important role in the initiation of DCs maturation and induction of cytokine production, suggesting that, in the absence of this complement system's protein, DC functions might be impaired. Therefore, C1q-containing IC and C1q opsonized AC and pathogens most probably play a role in both the induction and regulation of immunity and autoimmunity [26]. Benoit et al. have recently identified specific molecular pathways induced by C1q. They demonstrated that C1q bounds to autologous apoptotic lymphocytes modulating the expression of genes associated with JAK/STAT signaling, chemotaxis, immunoregulation, and NLRP3 inflammasome activation in LPS-stimulated human monocyte-derived macrophages. These results underline the role of C1q in suppressing macrophage-induced inflammation and providing potential therapeutic targets to control macrophage polarization and thus inflammation and autoimmune reactions [27]. The protective role of the complement system from autoimmune conditions is also expressed by the role of complement receptors 1 (CR1) and 2 (CR2), the defect of which has been associated with increased susceptibility to autoimmune diseases [18]. These receptors, found on erythrocytes, hematopoietic cells, follicular DCs, and B cells, are capable of binding C3 activation fragments. CR2 binds C3d and iC3b. It has been demonstrated that CR2 is able to amplify antigen-induced B cell activation through surface IgM (sIgM), to rescue peripheral B cells from sIgM-mediated apoptosis, to promote antigen processing and presentation of C3d-bound targets, to modulate the expression of co-stimulatory molecules, to stabilize the B cell receptor in lipid rafts, and to target IC to germinal centers in secondary lymphoid organs [19]. Many of these functions may occur via interactions of CR2 with CD19 and CD81 on the B cell surface, where these receptors form a multimolecular signal transduction complex.

While the role as an activating receptor of CR2 is better defined, the exact function of CR1 on B cells is yet to be determined [28]. CR1 binds the C3b and with lower affinity, iC3b and C4b, and it is capable of transmitting both activating and inhibitory signals to human B cells.

Expression of CR2 and CR1 on human B cells has been studied in some human autoimmune diseases. It was observed that patients with SLE had abnormalities in the expression of both CR2 and CR1 on B lymphocytes. Peripheral B cells showed a marked decrease in both CR2 and CR1 density as compared with control subjects [29,30]. RA patients also had fewer CR1 and CR2 positive B cells and decreased receptor expression compared with healthy subjects [31].

COMPLEMENT SYSTEM AND AUTOIMMUNE DISEASES

Systemic Lupus Erythematosus

SLE is the prototype of a multiorgan autoimmune disease. As found in several other autoimmune disorders, SLE pathogenesis is multifactorial lying on genetic and environmental factors and on abnormalities of both the innate and the adaptive immune system. The role of the complement system in the pathogenesis of SLE is apparently paradoxical; while complement activation contributes to SLE-associated inflammation, complement deficiency is also a risk factor for SLE development. Genetic deficiency of several components of the classical pathway (including C1q, C1r, C1s, C4, and C2) is associated with the development of SLE [32].

The hypothesis invoked to explain the involvement of the complement system in the pathogenesis of SLE is known as the "waste-disposal" hypothesis [33]. According to this hypothesis, complement system's proteins play a role in clearing IC and AC from both tissues and circulation. Failing this activity of the complement system, waste material—consisting of partially degraded components of the cytoplasm and nucleus—could accumulate and elicit an autoimmune response (Fig. 9.2). The "waste-disposal" hypothesis envisages the following steps. The first step is the failure to clear autoantigens [5]. The second step is the uptake of autoantigen by immature DCs in the presence of inflammatory cytokines, which causes these cells to mature into APCs, allowing the presentation of autoantigens to T cells [5]. The third step is the provision of help by T cells to autoreactive B cells, which have taken up autoantigen by means of their immunoglobulin receptors. Such B cells mature into plasma cells that secrete autoantibodies [2].

SLE-like disease associated with complement system's deficiencies clinically differs from SLE disease without complement system's deficiencies. In patients with SLE-like disease and complement system's deficiency, the onset is at a younger age; renal, pulmonary, and pericardial involvement are less conspicuous, but annular photosensitive skin rashes are more prominent. Fulminant glomerulonephritis, progressive nephritis, and renal failure are also far less common in patients with SLE-like disease and complement system's deficiency. Antinuclear antibodies, anti-DNA antibodies, are usually relatively low or absent in patients with SLE-like disease, whereas anti-Ro antibodies are often elevated [17].

The severity of SLE-like disease varies according to the position of the missing component within the classical pathway of activation (C1>C4>C2) [34]. Inherited deficiencies of C1q and C4 are invariably associated with the development of a severe SLE-like disease early in life, whereas C2 deficiency is only weakly associated with a milder form of SLE [34].

In the case of C3 deficiency, the clinical picture is rather different [5]. It is characterized by recurrent pyogenic infections, membranoproliferative glomerulonephritis, and rashes and it is rarely associated with SLE.

The initial cause of complement activation in SLE is thought to be the formation of high levels of IC that activate complement via the classical pathway [33]. Key mediators of tissue damage induced by the complement system are the anaphylatoxins (C3a and C5a) and MAC. Histologic data indicate that the activation of the complement system substantially contributes to tissues damages in patients with SLE. Deposits of C3, C4, and associated complement fragments are easily detected in biopsies of inflamed tissues from patients with SLE [35]. In these patients, the MAC is localized in the basement membrane zone of cutaneous lesions and, compared with clinically normal tissues, more prominent MAC deposits have been observed in inflamed tissues [36].

Immunofluorescence studies in SLE patients have shown deposits of immunoglobulins and complement in renal glomeruli and vessels in spleen, heart, skin, and liver. There is evidence that in SLE nephritis, the activation of the complement system is triggered by the deposition of IC in the glomerulus, either through the blood flow or by in situ formation [37,38].

In patients with active SLE, low complement concentrations and activation of the complement system are characteristic findings and are routinely evaluated for diagnostic and disease monitoring purposes. Moreover, clinically inactive SLE patients with low levels of C3, who are often classified as serologically active clinically quiescent, have a higher risk of lupus flares than inactive SLE patients with normal complement C3 levels [39].

In vivo complement activation can be demonstrated by tests for complexes or split products formed during the activation of the complement system. Several studies have shown that such measurements are more sensitive than regular measurement of CH50 or complement native components, such as C1q, C4, and C3, to verify complement activation and disease activity [39].

In addition to the previously mentioned reduced expression of complement receptors on B cells in SLE patients [40,41], these are also reduced on erythrocytes. On red blood cells, CR1 acts as a binding molecule for particles carrying C3b clusters (for example, parasites and bacteria) further transporting them to the fixed mononuclear phagocytic system in the liver, spleen, and bone marrow [40]. There is evidence that reduction of CR1 levels on erythrocytes correlates with disease activity in SLE [41].

Approximately one-third of patients with SLE show elevated levels of anti-C1q antibodies. Experimental models seem to demonstrate that they are directed against a neoepitope of C1q not expressed in the intact C1q complex. Moreover, anti-C1q autoantibodies are thought to have a pathogenic role by amplifying local complement activation: IC containing anti-C1q antibodies are more potent at activating complement than IC alone [42]. These autoantibodies are associated with severe disease, with occurrence of glomerulonephritis and with intense activation of classical pathway [40].

Rheumatoid Arthritis

To date, the pathogenesis of RA is not fully understood but there is increasing evidence of the role played by components of the complement system's cascade [43]. Animal models suggest that the immunization with type II collagen (CII), the major constituent protein of cartilage in diarthrodial joints, induces autoimmune arthritis resembling RA (collagen-induced arthritis) [44–47]. C3 or factor B–deficient mice immunized with bovine CII showed reduction or complete remission of clinical or histologic signs of arthritis [48]. Moreover, the systemic administration of anti-C5 monoclonal antibody (mAb) prevented the onset of arthritis and improved established disease [49].

Although increased complement system activation is plausibly related to the onset and/or augmentation of inflammation in RA, complement system's deficiencies may also induce RA. In particular, C1q and C2 deficiencies are correlated to the development of RA [50,51].

Tes

Plasma levels of most of the complement system's components are maintained by hepatic synthesis. We evaluated plasma levels of complement system's components in 114 patients with active RA. Mean C3 and C4 plasma levels observed in patients with active RA were significantly higher than in controls. This finding is consistent with the presence of an underlining inflammatory process [52] and confirms that complement system's proteins may act as acute phase proteins, with increased hepatocyte synthesis occurring in response to inflammatory cytokines [53–56].

However, it has to be noted that the synthesis of complement system's components also occurs in extrahepatic sites and in chronically inflamed tissues such as the rheumatoid joint [57–60]. Synovial membrane cells, which seem to be responsible for the synthesis of complement system's components, include lining cells, fibroblasts, mononuclear phagocytes, and endothelial cells [61].

Evidence of complement system activation in the synovial fluid is abundant. Levels of complement proteins are generally depressed in the synovial fluid of patients with RA, reflecting consumption of complement. Moreover, elevated levels of several complement cleavage products, such as C3a, C3c, C5a, sC5b-9, Bb, C1-C1INH complexes, have been observed in the synovial fluid [62–65]. Some studies demonstrated low levels of MAC inhibitors in synovial fluid and tissue of RA patients. This observation might justify lytic or sublytic attacks on local cells [64,66].

Several mechanisms of complement system activation have been proposed in RA patients. RA patients have increased levels of circulating IC [67,68], also including rheumatoid factors (RFs), and they can activate the classical pathway of the complement system [69–72]. Although the activation of the classical pathway is predominant [73], the alternative pathway is also activated in RA synovium as demonstrated by decreased levels of factor B and properdin and increased levels of Ba in the synovial fluid [74]. Increased complement activation via the lectin pathway could also play a role in RA. Changes in IgG glycosylation cause an increase in binding of MBL resulting in increased complement activation [75].

Trouw et al. suggested that another trigger for complement activation could be IC containing RA-associated antibodies, in particular anticitrullinated protein antibodies (ACPAs) and/or RF [76]; ACPA from RA patients may activate complement via both the classical and the alternative pathways [77].

Molecules released from the extracellular matrix of cartilage, including osteomodulin, chondroadherin, fibromodulin, the G3 domain of aggrecan, and cartilage oligomeric matrix protein (COMP), are also potent triggers for complement activation [78–81]. Moreover, local complement activation within affected joints could additionally be triggered by dead cells [82], extracellular DNA [83], and CRP [84].

Several studies failed to demonstrate a correlation between local and systemic activation of the complement system in RA and reported higher levels of complement cleavage products in synovial fluid than in plasma. These findings are consistent with a prevalent local activation of the complement system's cascade. The possible association between the activation of the complement system and disease activity has to be noted. Some authors reported a correlation between levels of complement system's cleavage products and disease activity in RA patients [62,85].

Other Inflammatory Arthritides

There is limited availability of data in literature about role of complement system's proteins in other inflammatory arthritides.

Studies conducted in psoriatic patients have shown increased plasma concentrations of iC3b, C4d, and Bb fragments, especially in patients with erythrodermic pustular psoriasis and psoriatic arthritis (PsA) [86]. Partsch et al. have reported relatively low levels of the C3c cleavage product in synovial fluid from PsA patients, similar to that observed in patients with osteoarthritis (OA) [87].

A possible implication of complement activation in the pathogenesis of PsA is supported by the finding of impaired expression of complement regulators in these patients. Triolo et al. reported low expression of erythrocyte membrane-anchored CD59, an important membrane inhibitor of MAC. In keeping with this observation, increased SC5b-9 plasma levels were detected in patients with active disease and an inverse correlation was also found between SC5b-9 plasma levels and CD59 expression levels [88]. Rivas et al. found a statistically significant decrease of CR1 density on erythrocyte membranes in PsA patients with polyarthritis compared with controls. An inverse correlation between CRl concentration and the articular index of PsA patients has been reported and this finding is suggestive of a correlation between CRl levels and disease severity in PsA patients [89].

Our group has recently conducted a study evaluating the complement system in PsA treated with antitumor necrosis factor agents, which demonstrated that moderate to severe PsA disease is associated with higher C3 and C4 plasma levels with respect to healthy subjects [90]. Moreover, Torres et al., in 2014 [91], hypothesized that C3 may be a better marker of cardiometabolic risk than CRP; in fact within psoriasis patients, C3 levels were independently associated with abdominal visceral fat, insulin resistance, metabolic syndrome, and oxidized LDL-cholesterol, while CRP did not.

Low-grade inflammation is thought to be an important factor also in the development of OA, and several studies have found evidence of complement activation in the synovium or synovial fluid of patients with OA. Struglics et al. found that complement activation fragments C4d, CebBbP, and soluble MAC were increased in OA synovial fluid relative to the synovial fluid of healthy knee joints [92].

Systemic Sclerosis

SSc is a complex autoimmune disorder characterized by microvascular damage and progressive fibrosis of the skin and visceral organs, especially the lungs, heart, and kidneys. The pathogenesis of SSc remains poorly understood, but a growing body of evidence suggests that activation of the complement system may be involved in the disease.

Reduced complement levels in SSc patients were first observed in 1967 [93]. Senaldi et al. subsequently demonstrated higher level of complement fragments in patients with SSc, in particular those with diffuse cutaneous SSc, with respect to controls. They postulated a direct correlation between the complement system activation and clinical severity [94]. In the light of these findings, low C3 levels were identified as candidate parameter for inclusion in the American College of Rheumatology classification criteria for SSc [95]. In 2001, hypocomplementemia was included among the parameters used to assess the disease activity score by the European Scleroderma Study Group [96].

Hudson et al. studied a cohort of 321 patients with SSc. It was observed that there were no differences in the clinical presentation of the disease between patients with normal or low complement levels; however, hypocomplementemia was associated with features of overlap disease. In particular, inflammatory myositis and vasculitis were more frequent in patients with low levels of complement system's proteins compared with patients with normal values [97].

Furthermore, in 2010 a study of SSc patients showed increased levels of factor H, a complement regulator, which had impaired function [98]. The development of a mini factor H has been shown to reduce abnormal C3 deposition in a factor H deficient mouse model [99]. In 2014, it was shown that while the lectin pathway of complement system was not a cause of SSc, it contributes to exacerbate symptoms following ischemia and reperfusion [100].

Antiphospholipid Antibodies Syndrome

APS is classified as the association of arterial and/or venous thromboses and/or obstetric morbidity in patients who test positive for antiphospholipid antibodies (aPL) on two occasions at least 12 weeks apart.

The pathogenic mechanisms underlying aPL antibodies induced thrombosis are not completely understood. It is well established that activated complement fragments themselves have the capacity to bind and activate inflammatory and endothelial cells, as well as to induce a prothrombotic phenotype, either through the MAC directly or through C5a receptor (CD88)–mediated effects [101,102].

An important role of complement activation in APS was demonstrated in several murine models of aPL-related pregnancy loss [103]. Complement products C3a and C5a were assumed to cause placental inflammation, and mice deficient in C3, C4, C5, or C5a receptors was protected from fetal loss induced by aPL-IgG [104]. Afterward, it has been described that complement activation contributes to aPL-mediated thrombosis in mice as demonstrated by the ability of C5 inhibitors to prevent thrombosis in animals receiving passive transfer of human aPL-IgG antibodies [105,106]. Complement activation by aPL leads to generation of the anaphylatoxin C5a, which recruits neutrophils and monocytes, activates endothelial cells and platelets, and induces expression of tissue factor [107,108].

Moreover complement can be activated by the binding of C3 fragment to the Fc receptor of aPL antibodies or by the formation of autoantibodies against C1q, which are frequently detected in patients with APS [109]. However, while increased levels of complement activation products have been detected in patients with APS, these have not been demonstrated to correlate with thrombosis [110]. Complement factor H, a homologue of β2GPI, also binds to anionic phospholipids and a recent report showed that autoantibodies against factor H are prevalent in patients with APS and are related to recurrent venous thrombosis [111]. In addition, there is evidence supporting activation of the classical and alternative complement pathways in patients with catastrophic APS (CAPS) [112], and eculizumab (humanized anti-C5a monoclonal antibody) has been successfully used in CAPS and APS thrombotic microangiopathy [112–116].

Inflammatory Myopathies

Inflammatory myopathies can be differentiated into DM, polymyositis (PM), necrotizing autoimmune myopathy, and sporadic inclusion body myositis.

There is increasing evidence that complement-mediated microangiopathy plays a pathogenic role in DM.

The primary antigenic target in DM is the endothelium of the endomysial capillaries. Putative antibodies directed against endothelial cells activate C3. In its turn, activated C3 leads to formation of C3b and C4b fragments and MAC, which can be detected early in the course of the disease both in serum and in the capillaries before inflammatory or structural changes are observed in the muscular tissue [117]. Immunohistochemically, the deposition of MAC C5b-9 on perifascicular endomysial capillaries is regarded as a diagnostic hallmark of DM and the extent of C5b-9 deposits seems to be associated with the clinical course of the disease. Capillary complement deposits induce swollen endothelial cells, vacuolization, capillary necrosis, perivascular inflammation, ischemia, and destruction of muscle fibers [118]. Furthermore, nerve pathology during DM, demonstrating deposition of C5b-9 around small blood vessels and capillaries in the endoneurium, supports the possibility that complement-mediated damage could be a unifying pathogenic mechanism of muscle and nerve injury due to DM [119].

Moreover, the deposition of MAC was found in a high proportion of biopsies from skin lesions of DM patients and was absent in unaffected skin, suggesting that the complement system is also involved in the pathogenesis of skin lesions [120, 121].

Sjogren Syndrome

Primary SS is a chronic autoimmune disorder characterized by lymphocytic infiltration of the exocrine glands, predominantly the salivary and lacrimal glands, which leads to their gradual destruction and consequent oral and ocular dryness. Approximately one in three patients will unquestionably develop severe systemic manifestations; among those manifestations that severely complicate the disease and result in an increased risk of death, non-Hodgkin's lymphoma (NHL) is the most deleterious [122].

In patients with primary SS, there is growing interest in determining the negative prognostic significance of low complement levels. The prevalence of hypocomplementemia in SS patients has been evaluated in several studies. Skopouli et al. reported that low serum C4 complement levels, mixed monoclonal cryoglobulinemia (MMC), and purpura at primary SS diagnosis were strong predictors for NHL development. Low C4 levels and MMC were the most important predictors and correlated with each other [123]. Several other authors have also recognized decreased complement levels as a predictive marker for lymphoma development. In the prognostic model proposed by Ioannidis et al., low C4 levels along with palpable purpura could identify the few patients at risk of dying from lymphoma [124], while Baimpa et al. showed that among other clinical and laboratory parameters, MMC and low C4 levels were strong lymphoma predictors [125].

Brito-Zeron et al. found a higher risk of mucosa-associated lymphoid tissue (MALT) lymphoma in patients presenting with systemic activity, positive cryoglobulins (CG), and low C3 levels at primary SS diagnosis and a high risk of non-MALT lymphomas in those patients with monoclonal gammopathy and low C4 levels [126].

Low complement levels seem to be associated with systemic SS features, including extraglandular features (fever, articular and cutaneous involvement, vasculitis, and peripheral neuropathy) and immunological markers (cryoglobulinemia, RF) [127]. These results support the inclusion of complement level determination as a predictor of SS outcome both at diagnosis and routinely during the clinical follow-up.

Vasculitides

Vasculitides are defined by the presence of leukocytes in the vessel wall with reactive damage. Depending on the specific vasculitic disorder, affected vessels vary in size, type, and location. Many vasculitic disorders are caused by IC and the activation of the complement system is involved in their pathogenesis.

In particular, complement involvement was demonstrated in small-vessel vasculitides, as described in the next paragraphs.

Antineutrophil Cytoplasmic Antibody-Associated Vasculitides

Antineutrophil cytoplasmic antibody (ANCA)–associated vasculitides (AAV) are a group of primary small-vessel vasculitis with three distinct clinical entities, including granulomatosis with polyangiitis (formerly Wegener's granulomatosis), microscopic polyangiitis (MPA), and eosinophilic granulomatosis with polyangiitis (formerly Churg–Strauss syndrome). Kidneys and lungs are the most commonly involved organs and ANCA, directed against proteinase 3 (PR3) or to myeloperoxidase (MPO), is the serological marker of AAV [128,129]. These small-vessel vasculitides are characterized by necrotizing inflammation of the vessel wall, particularly of small arteries, arterioles, capillaries, and venules.

In AAV, the adaptive immune response, expressed by the ANCAs, interacts with innate immunity, in particular with neutrophils and the complement system. Together they target the endothelium, resulting in necrotizing vasculitis [130].

In vitro data demonstrate that in AAV the complement system constitutes an amplification loop for ANCA-induced neutrophil activation. Schreiber et al. showed that supernatants from ANCA-activated neutrophils activate the complement system via the alternative pathway, resulting in the production, among others, of C5a [131]. C5a was able to prime neutrophils for ANCA-induced activation, and blocking of the C5a receptor on neutrophils abrogated this process.

The first evidence of the role of complement activation in the pathogenesis of AAV was provided by the mouse model of MPO-ANCA vasculitis by Xiao et al. C5-deficient mice or wild-type mice pretreated with cobra venom factor to deplete complement failed to develop glomerulonephritis and vasculitis [132].

Although little immunoglobulin and complement deposition is found in the glomerular capillary walls of patients with AAV, several studies have found a certain degree of IC and complement C3c deposition in renal samples from these patients, which was associated with heavier proteinuria and poorer renal function [133,134]. According to these findings, compounds interfering with the complement cascade should be explored as therapeutic options for AAV.

Cryoglobulinemia

CG are an abnormal group of serum proteins that share the common property of reversible precipitation at low temperatures. It is widely accepted that the majority of CG are either intact monoclonal immunoglobulins or IC in which one component, usually IgM, exhibits antibody activity to IgG. The latter are known as mixed CG [135].

Monoclonal CG are usually associated with hematological disorders, whereas mixed CG are found in many infectious and systemic disorders. Essential mixed cryoglobulinemia shows a striking association with hepatitis C virus infection (>90%). It is a systemic vasculitis (leukocytoclastic vasculitis) affecting cutaneous vessels and multiple visceral organs [136]. The classical pathway of the complement system is usually activated in both essential and secondary cryoglobulinemia. Decreased C4 and C2 levels are observed together with slightly altered C3 levels. Late complement components are also insignificantly affected, although modest elevations have been reported. Diminished serum levels of complement components may reflect ongoing consumption by CG-containing IC [137,138].

Henoch-Schönlein Purpura/IgA Nephropathy

Henoch-Schönlein purpura nephritis (HSPN) and IgA nephropathy (IgAN) are currently considered related diseases. Both diseases display similar histologic features and IgA abnormalities. The common clinical pattern of IgAN is an indolent progressive disease with slowly increasing proteinuria and loss of the renal function associated with episodes of macroscopic hematuria in half of the patients. In the majority of patients, HSPN is characterized by acute onset followed by full recovery [139]. The activation of the complement pathway is likely to be involved in the pathophysiology of glomerular lesions. Glomerular depositions of MBL, L-ficolin, MASP, and C4d are reported in the vast majority of patients with HSPN and IgAN. These findings, together with the absence C1q, are supportive of the predominant activation of the lectin pathways of the complement system as pathophysiological mechanism [140]. The deposition of complement fragments, derived from the activation of the lectin pathway, has been shown to be associated with a higher degree of proteinuria and hematuria, as well as with more severe histological lesions in both HSPN and IgAN patients [140–142]. These findings emphasize the need for further studies to assess the potential significance of the measurement of blood, and urinary complement splits products and MAC to evaluate the disease activity.

COMPLEMENT-TARGETED THERAPY

The complement system is increasingly recognized to have a causal link with tissue damage during ischemic, inflammatory, and autoimmune diseases. This makes the complement system an attractive target for the treatment of a wide range of diseases. Any of the three complement activation pathways, as well as the common final effector pathway, can be therapeutically targeted, providing wide opportunities for inhibition of the complement system.

Several compounds interfering with complement system cascade have been studied in experimental models for autoimmune diseases. The main therapeutic strategies are inhibition of complement activation components, inhibition of complement receptors, and inhibition of MAC [143]. Different molecules believed to have complement modulation properties have been studied in several animal models for arthritis. These include soluble CR1 [144] (which suppresses complement system activation at the main gathering point C3), C3a [145] and C5a [146] receptor antagonists (which can be used to control the anaphylatoxins C3a and C5a), and recombinant CD59 [147] (which inhibits the formation of MAC). Although PMX53, a C5a mimetic compound that binds the C5a receptor, had shown encouraging results in rats, where a significant improvement of arthritis was observed with no side effect [146], its use in RA patients did not match the expectation [148].

Only two complement modulators have been approved for use in human. Eculizumab binds to the complement protein C5 inhibiting its cleavage and is indicated for the treatment of paroxysmal nocturnal hemoglobinuria and HUS [149,150]. C1INH and recombinant C1INH plasma-derived C1 esterase inhibitor are indicated for the treatment of HAE [151].

Eculizumab has been reported to lack efficacy in patients with RA [148], although it appears to be an effective therapy for HUS in the context of SLE [152]; whether or not eculizumab is effective in treating nonthrombotic lupus nephritis requires further investigation. As already mentioned in the previous paragraph, eculizumab has also shown to be effective in the treatment of a patient with CAPS [113–116]. In AAV, a phase III trial of a C5aR antagonist, CCX168, is currently underway and will evaluate the proportion of patients achieving remission at 26 and 52 weeks [153], while Jayne et al. already demonstrated that CCX168 could substitute high-dose steroids in patients with AAV [154].

An additional strategy to be considered is the replacement of missing complement system's proteins to reverse the effects of complement deficiencies. However, this approach presents several potential drawbacks. Firstly, purified or engineered complement proteins are not available for treatment purposes and whole plasma preparations would have to be used, with obvious complications of plasma treatment. Secondly, the replacement of a missing complement protein may be followed by complement activation and tissue damage. Finally, exposure to a protein that is genetically deficient may cause development of antibodies. At present, only anecdotal observations have been reported [41].

The modulation of the complement system is one of the benefits associated with the use of high-dose intravenous immunoglobulins (IVIg) in autoimmune conditions. The complement systems modulating effect exhibited by IVIg can be explained by several mechanisms. First, activated C3 and C4 may bind to immunoglobulin molecules, which then serve as scavengers, hence avoiding in situ deposition of these fragments. Second, C1q may bind to immunoglobulin leading to a deviation of C1 binding from its target to the IVIg [155]. Third, IVIg may enhance the inactivation of C3 in complex with immunoglobulins and thus downregulate the C3 convertase activity [156]. Finally IVIg are able to cause a mild and controlled activation of the complement system. This is not harmful per se and it may reduce a pathological activation observed in the pathogenesis of autoimmune disease [155]. A broadly applicable anti-C therapeutic agent, useful in acute and chronic conditions, should be inexpensive, highly specific, either have a very long plasma half-life or be active orally, and be able to block the pathological activation of the complement system while causing minimal disruption of the systemic complement function [157]. None of the currently available agents satisfy these requirements, but data derived from preclinical studies and initial clinical trials suggest that complement modulation could become an important therapeutic strategy in autoimmune conditions in the next decades.

REFERENCES

[1] Ballanti E, Perricone C, Greco E, Ballanti M, Di Muzio G, Chimenti MS, Perricone R. Complement and autoimmunity. Immunol Res 2013;56(2–3):477–91.

[2] Morgan BP, Marchbank KJ, Longhi MP, Harris CL, Gallimore AM. Complement: central to innate immunity and bridging to adaptive responses. Immunol Lett 2005;97:171–9.

[3] Walport MJ. Complement. First of two parts. N Engl J Med 2001;344:1058–66.

[4] Hawlisch H, Köhl J. Complement and Toll-like receptors: key regulators of adaptive immune responses. Mol Immunol 2006;43:13–21.

[5] Walport MJ. Complement. Second of two parts. N Engl J Med 2001;344:1140–4.

[6] Nauta AJ, Castellano G, Xu W, Woltman AM, Borrias MC, Daha MR, et al. Opsonization with C1q and mannose-binding lectin targets apoptotic cells to dendritic cells. J Immunol 2004;173:3044–50.

[7] Gál P, Dobó J, Závodszky P, Sim RB. Early complement proteases: C1r, C1s and MASPs. A structural insight into activation and functions. Mol Immunol 2009;46:2745–52.

[8] Rus H, Cudrici C, Niculescu F. The role of the complement system in innate immunity. Immunol Res 2005;33:103–12.

[9] Liszewski MK, Farries TC, Lublin DM, Rooney IA, Atkinson JP. Control of the complement system. Adv Immunol 1996;61:201–83.

[10] Lindahl G, Sjöbring U, Johnsson E. Human complement regulators: a major target for pathogenic microorganisms. Curr Opin Immunol 2000;12:44–51.

[11] Davis AE. The pathophysiology of hereditary angioedema. Clin Immunol 2005;114:3–9.

[12] Boccuni P, Del Vecchio L, Di Noto R, Rotoli B. Glycosyl phosphatidylinositol (GPI)-anchored molecules and the pathogenesis of paroxysmal nocturnal hemoglobinuria. Crit Rev Oncol Hematol 2000;33:25–43.

[13] Son M, Diamond B, Santiago-Schwarz F. Fundamental role of C1q in autoimmunity and inflammation. Immunol Res 2015;63:101–6.

[14] Nauta AJ, Roos A, Daha MR. A regulatory role for complement in innate immunity and autoimmunity. Int Arch Allergy Immunol 2004;134:310–23.

[15] Théroux P, Martel C. Complement activity and pharmacological inhibition in cardiovascular disease. Can J Cardiol 2006;22(Suppl. B):18B–24B.

[16] Chen M, Daha MR, Kallenberg CG. The complement system in systemic autoimmune disease. J Autoimmun 2010;34:276–86.

[17] Pettigrew HD, Teuber SS, Gershwin ME. Clinical significance of complement deficiencies. Ann NY Acad Sci 2009;1173:108–23.

[18] Etzioni A. Immune deficiency and autoimmunity. Autoimmun Rev 2003;2:364–9.

[19] Boackle SA. Complement and autoimmunity. Biomed Pharmacother 2003;57:269–73.

[20] Bussone G, Mouthon L. Autoimmune manifestations in primary immune deficiencies. Autoimmun Rev 2009;8:332–6.

[21] Pittoni V, Valesini G. The clearance of apoptotic cells: implications for autoimmunity. Autoimmun Rev 2002;1:154–61.

[22] Lu JH, Teh BK, Wang L, Wang YN, Tan YS, Lai MC, et al. The classical and regulatory functions of C1q in immunity and autoimmunity. Cell Mol Immunol 2008;5:9–21.

[23] Carroll MC. The role of complement in B cell activation and tolerance. Adv Immunol 2000;74:61–88.

[24] Truedsson L, Bengtsson AA, Sturfelt G. Complement deficiencies and systemic lupus erythematosus. Autoimmunity 2007;40:560–6.

[25] Muñoz LE, Janko C, Schulze C, Schorn C, Sarter K, Schett G, et al. Autoimmunity and chronic inflammation - two clearance-related steps in the etiopathogenesis of SLE. Autoimmun Rev 2010;10:38–42.

[26] Csomor E, Bajtay Z, Sándor N, Kristóf K, Arlaud GJ, Thiel S, et al. Complement protein C1q induces maturation of human dendritic cells. Mol Immunol 2007;44:3389–97.

[27] Benoit ME, Clarke EV, Morgado P, Fraser DA, Tenner AJ. Complement protein C1q directs macrophage polarization and limits inflammasome activity during the uptake of apoptotic cells. J Immunol 2012;188:5682–93.

[28] Erdei A, Isaák A, Török K, Sándor N, Kremlitzka M, Prechl J, et al. Expression and role of CR1 and CR2 on B and T lymphocytes under physiological and autoimmune conditions. Mol Immunol 2009;46:2767–73.

[29] Marquart HV, Svendsen A, Rasmussen JM, Nielsen CH, Junker P, Svehag SE, et al. Complement receptor expression and activation of the complement cascade on B lymphocytes from patients with systemic lupus erythematosus (SLE). Clin Exp Immunol 1995;101:60–5.

[30] Wilson JG, Ratnoff WD, Schur PH, Fearon DT. Decreased expression of the C3b/C4b receptor (CR1) and the C3d receptor (CR2) on B lymphocytes and of CR1 on neutrophils of patients with systemic lupus erythematosus. Arthritis Rheum 1986;29:739–47.

[31] Prokopec KE, Rhodiner M, Matt P, Lindqvist U, Kleinau S. Down regulation of Fc and complement receptors on B cells in rheumatoid arthritis. Clin Immunol 2010;137:322–9.

[32] Macedo AC, Isaac L. Systemic lupus erythematosus and deficiencies of early components of the complement classical pathway. Front Immunol 2016;7:55.

[33] Manderson AP, Botto M, Walport MJ. The role of complement in the development of systemic lupus erythematosus. Annu Rev Immunol 2004;22:431–56.

[34] Pickering MC, Botto M, Taylor PR, Lachmann PJ, Walport MJ. Systemic lupus erythematosus, complement deficiency and apoptosis. Adv Immunol 2000;76:227–324.

[35] Biesecker G, Lavin L, Ziskind M, Koffler D. Cutaneous localization of the membrane attack complex in discoid and systemic lupus erythematosus. N Engl J Med 1982;306:264–70.

[36] Helm KF, Peters MS. Deposition of membrane attack complex in cutaneous lesions of lupus erythematosus. J Am Acad Dermatol 1993;28:687–91.

[37] Paronetto F, Koffler D. Immunofluorescent localization of immunoglobulins, complement, and fibrinogen in human diseases. I. Systemic lupus erythematosus. J Clin Investig 1965;44:1657–64.

[38] Lachmann PJ, Muller-Eberhard HJ, Kunkel HG, Paronetto F. The localization of in vivo bound complement in tissue section. J Exp Med 1962;115:63–82.

[39] Biesen R, Rose T, Hoyer BF, Hiepe F. Autoantibodies, complement and type I interferon as biomarkers for personalized medicine in SLE. Lupus 2016;25:823–9.

[40] Walport MJ. Complement and systemic lupus erythematosus. Arthritis Res 2002;4(Suppl. 3):S279–93.

[41] Ross GD, Yount WJ, Walport MJ, Winfield JB, Parker CJ, Fuller CR, Taylor RP, Myones BL, Lachmann PJ. Disease-associated loss of erythrocyte complement receptors (CR1, C3b receptors) in patients with systemic lupus erythematosus and other diseases involving autoantibodies and/or complement activation. J Immunol 1985;135:2005–14.

[42] Trouw LA, et al. Anti-C1q autoantibodies deposit in glomeruli but are only pathogenic in combination with glomerular C1q-containing immune complexes. J Clin Investig 2004;14:679–88.

[43] Ballanti E, Perricone C, Di Muzio G, Kroegler B, Chimenti MS, Graceffa D, Perricone R. Role of the complement system in rheumatoid arthritis and psoriatic arthritis: relationship with anti-TNF inhibitors. Autoimmun Rev 2011;10:617–23.

[44] Trentham DE, Townes AS, Kang AH. Autoimmunity to type II collagen an experimental model of arthritis. J Exp Med 1977;146:857–68.

[45] Courtenay JS, Dallman MJ, Dayan AD, Martin A, Mosedale B. Immunisation against heterologous type II collagen induces arthritis in mice. Nature 1980;283:666–8.

[46] Cathcart ES, Hayes KC, Gonnerman WA, Lazzari AA, Franzblau C. Experimental arthritis in a nonhuman primate. I. Induction by bovine type II collagen. Lab Investig 1986;54:26–31.

[47] Yoo TJ, Kim SY, Stuart JM, Floyd RA, Olson GA, Cremer MA, et al. Induction of arthritis in monkeys by immunization with type II collagen. J Exp Med 1988;168:777–82.

[48] Hietala MA, Jonsson IM, Tarkowski A, Kleinau S, Pekna M. Complement deficiency ameliorates collagen-induced arthritis in mice. J Immunol 2002;169:454–9.

[49] Wang Y, Rollins SA, Madri JA, Matis LA. Anti-C5 monoclonal antibody therapy prevents collagen-induced arthritis and ameliorates established disease. Proc Natl Acad Sci USA 1995;92:8955–9.

[50] Mizuno M. A review of current knowledge of the complement system and the therapeutic opportunities in inflammatory arthritis. Curr Med Chem 2006;13:1707–17.

[51] D'Cruz D, Taylor J, Ahmed T, Asherson R, Khamashta M, Hughes GR. Complement factor 2 deficiency: a clinical and serological family study. Ann Rheum Dis 1992;51:1254–6.

[52] Di Muzio G, Perricone C, Ballanti E, Kroegler B, Greco E, Novelli L, et al. Complement system and rheumatoid arthritis: relationships with auto-antibodies, serological, clinical features, and anti-TNF treatment. Int J Immunopathol Pharmacol 2011;24:357–66.

[53] Miura N, Prentice HL, Scheider PM, Perlmutter DH. Synthesis and regulation of the two human complement C4 genes in stable transfected mouse fibroblasts. J Biol Chem 1987;262:7298–305.

[54] Andus T, Heinrich PC, Bauer J, Trau-Thi TA, Decker K, Manuel D, et al. Discrimination of hepatocyte stimulating activity from human recombinant tumour necrosis factor α. Eur J Immunol 1988;17:1193–7.

[55] Anthony R, EL-Omar E, Lappin DF, MacSween RNM, Whaley K. Regulation of hepatic synthesis of C3 and C4 during acute-phase response in the rat. Eur J Immunol 1989;19:1405–12.

[56] Ramadori G, Van Daume J, Riedert H, Mayer Zum Buschenfelde KH. Interleukin-6, the third mediator of acute-phase reaction, modulates hepatic protein synthesis in human and mouse comparison as with interleukin-1β and tumour necrosis faclor-α. Eur J Immunol 1988;18:1259–64.

[57] Moffat GJ, Lappin D, Birnie GD, Whaley K. Complement biosynthesis in human synovial tissue. Clin Exp Immunol 1989;78:54–60.

[58] Ruddy S, Colten HR. Rheumatoid arthritis. Biosynthesis of complement proteins by synovial tissues. N Engl J Med 1974;290:1284–8.

[59] Neumann E, Barnum SR, Tarner IH, Echols J, Fleck M, Judex M, et al. Local production of complement proteins in rheumatoid arthritis synovium. Arthritis Rheum 2002;46:934–45.

[60] Guc D, Gulati P, Lemercier C, Lappin D, Birnie GD, Whaley K. Expression of the components and regulatory proteins of the alternative complement pathway and the membrane attack complex in normal and diseased synovium. Rheumatol Int 1993;13:139–46.

[61] Whaley K, Guc D, Gulati P, Lappin D. Synthesis of complement components by synovial membrane. Immunopharmacology 1992;24:83–9.

[62] Doherty M, Richards N, Hornby J, Powell R. Relation between synovial fluid C3 degradation products and local joint inflammation in rheumatoid arthritis, osteoarthritis, and crystal associated arthropathy. Ann Rheum Dis 1988;47:190–7.

[63] Oleesky DA, Daniels RH, Williams BD, Amos N, Morgan BP. Terminal complement complexes and C1/C1 inhibitor complexes in rheumatoid arthritis and other arthritic conditions. Clin Exp Immunol 1991;84:250–5.

[64] Konttinen YT, Ceponis A, Meri S, Vuorikoski A, Kortekangas P, Sorsa T, et al. Complement in acute and chronic arthritides: assessment of C3c, C9, and protectin (CD59) in synovial membrane. Ann Rheum Dis 1996;55:888–94.

[65] Jose PJ, Moss IK, Maini RN, Williams TJ. Measurement of the chemotactic complement fragment C5a in rheumatoid synovial fluids by radioim-munoassay: role of C5a in the acute inflammatory phase. Ann Rheum Dis 1990;49:747–52.

[66] Høgåsen K, Mollnes TE, Harboe M, Götze O, Hammer HB, Oppermann M. Terminal complement pathway activation and low lysis inhibitors in rheumatoid arthritis synovial fluid. J Rheumatol 1995;22:24–8.

[67] Zubler RH, Nydegger U, Perrin LH, Fehr K, McCormick J, Lambert PH, et al. Circulating and intra-articular immune complexes in patients with rheumatoid arthritis: correlation of 125IClq binding activity with clinical and biological features of the disease. J Clin Investig 1976;57:1308–19.

[68] Hay FC, Nineham LJ, Perumal R, Roitt IM. Intra-articular and circulating immune complexes and antiglobulins (IgG and IgM) in rheumatoid arthritis: correlation with clinical features. Ann Rheum Dis 1979;38:1–7.

[69] Robbins DL, Fiegal Jr DW, Leek JC, Shapiro R, Wiesner K. Complement activation by 19S IgM rheumatoid factor: relationship to disease activity in rheumatoid arthritis. J Rheumatol 1986;13:33–8.

[70] Sato Y, Sato R, Watanabe H, Kogure A, Watanabe K, Nishimaki T, et al. Complement activating properties of monoreactive and polyreactive IgM rheumatoid factors. Ann Rheum Dis 1993;52:795–800.

[71] Sato Y, Watanabe H, Kogure A, Miyata M, Watanabe K, Nishimaki T, et al. Complement-activating properties of IgM rheumatoid factors reacting with IgG subclasses. Clin Rheumatol 1995;14:425–8.

[72] Tanimoto K, Cooper NR, Johnson JS, Vaughan JH. Complement fixation by rheumatoid factor. J Clin Investig 1975;55:437–45.

[73] Ruddy S, Austen KF. Activation of the complement and properdin systems in rheumatoid arthritis. Ann NY Acad Sci 1975;256:96–104.

[74] El-Ghobarey A, Whaley K. Alternative pathway complement activation in rheumatoid arthritis. J Rheumatol 1980;7:453–60.

[75] Malhotra R, Wormald MR, Rudd PM, Fischer PB, Dwek RA, Sim RB. Glycosylation changes of IgG associated with rheumatoid arthritis can activate complement via the mannose-binding protein. Nat Med 1995;1:237–43.

[76] Trouw LA, Rispens T, Toes RE. Beyond citrullination: other post-translational protein modifications in rheumatoid arthritis. Nat Rev Rheumatol 2017;13:331–9.

[77] Trouw LA, Haisma EM, Levarht EW, van der Woude D, Ioan-Facsinay A, Daha MR, et al. Anti-cyclic citrullinated peptide antibodies from rheumatoid arthritis patients activate complement via both the classical and alternative pathways. Arthritis Rheum 2009;60:1923–31.

[78] Happonen KE. Regulation of complement by cartilage oligomeric matrix protein allows for a novel molecular diagnostic principle in rheumatoid arthritis. Arthritis Rheum 2010;62:3574–83.

[79] Melin Furst C, et al. The C type lectin of the aggrecan G3 domain activates complement. PLoS One 2013;8:e61407.

[80] Melin Furst C, et al. Quantitative mass spectrometry to study inflammatory cartilage degradation and resulting interactions with the complement system. J Immunol 2016;197:3415–24.

[81] Sjöberg A, Onnerfjord P, Mörgelin M, Heinegård D, Blom AM. The extracellular matrix and inflammation: fibromodulin activates the classical pathway of complement by directly binding C1q. J Biol Chem 2005;280:32301–8.

[82] Trouw LA, Blom AM, Gasque P. Role of complement and complement regulators in the removal of apoptotic cells. Mol Immunol 2008;45:1199–207.

[83] Van Schravendijk MR, Dwek RA. Interaction of C1q with DNA. Mol Immunol 1982;19:1179–87.

[84] Molenaar ET, Voskuyl AE, Familian A, van Mierlo GJ, Dijkmans BA, Hack CE. Complement activation in patients with rheumatoid arthritis mediated in part by C-reactive protein. Arthritis Rheum 2001;44:997–1002.

[85] Wouters D, Voskuyl AE, Molenaar ET, Dijkmans BA, Hack CE. Evaluation of classical complement pathway activation in rheumatoid arthritis: measurement of C1q-C4 complexes as novel activation products. Arthritis Rheum 2006;54:1143–50.

[86] Rosenberg EW, Noah PW, Wyatt RJ, Jones RM, Kolb WP. Complement activation in psoriasis. Clin Exp Dermatol 1990;15:16–20.

[87] Partsch G, Bauer K, Bröll H, Petera P, Dunky A, Merétey K. Complement C3 cleavage product in synovial fluids detected by immunofixation. Z Rheumatol 1991;50:82–5.

[88] Triolo G, Accardo-Palumbo A, Sallì L, Ciccia F, Ferrante A, Tedesco L, et al. Impaired expression of erythrocyte glycosyl-phosphatidylinositol-anchored membrane CD59 in patients with psoriatic arthritis. Relation to terminal complement pathway activation. Clin Exp Rheumatol 2003;21:225–8.

[89] Rivas D, Riestra-Noriega JL, Torre-Alonso JC, Rodriguez A, Gutiérrez C. Decrease in detectable complement receptor type 1 levels on erythrocytes from patients with psoriatic polyarthritis. Br J Rheumatol 1994;33:626–30.

[90] Chimenti MS, Perricone C, Graceffa D, Di Muzio G, Ballanti E, Guarino MD, et al. Complement system in psoriatic arthritis: a useful marker in response prediction and monitoring of anti-TNF treatment. Clin Exp Rheumatol 2012;30:23–30.

[91] Torres T, Bettencourt N, Mendonça D, Vasconcelos C, Silva BM, Selores M. Complement C3 as a marker of cardiometabolic risk in psoriasis. Arch Dermatol Res September 2014;306(7):653–60.

[92] Struglics A, Okroj M, Swärd P, Frobell R, Saxne T, Lohmander LS, Blom AM. The complement system is activated in synovial fluid from subjects with knee injury and from patients with osteoarthritis. Arthritis Res Ther 2016;18(1):223.

[93] Townes AS. Topics in clinical medicine. Complement's levels in disease. Johns Hopkins Med J 1967;120:337–9.

[94] Senaldi G, Lupoli S, Vergani D, Black CM. Activation of the complement system in systemic sclerosis. Relationship to clinical severity. Arthritis Rheum 1989;32:1262–7.

[95] Subcommittee for Scleroderma Criteria of the American Rheumatism Association Diagnostic and Therapeutic Criteria Committee. Preliminary criteria for the classification of systemic sclerosis (scleroderma). Arthritis Rheum 1980;23:581–90.

[96] Valentini G, Della Rossa A, Bombardieri S, Bencivelli W, Silman AJ, D'Angelo S, et al. European multicentre study to define disease activity criteria for systemic sclerosis. II. Identification of disease activity variables and development of preliminary activity indexes. Ann Rheum Dis 2001;60:592–8.

[97] Hudson M, Walker JG, Fritzler M, Taillefer S, Canadian Scleroderma Research Group, Baron M. Hypocomplementemia in systemic sclerosis, clinical and serological correlations. J Rheumatol 2007;34:1–6.

[98] Scambi C, Ugolini S, Jokiranta TS, De Franceschi L, Bortolami O. The local complement activation on vascular bed of patients with systemic sclerosis: a hypothesis-generating study. PLoS One 2015;10(2).

[99] Nichols EM, Barbour TD, Pappworth IY, Wong EK, Palmer JM, Sheerin NS, Pickering MC, Marchbank KJ. An extended mini-complement factor H molecule ameliorates experimental C3 glomerulopathy. Kidney Int 2015;88(6):1314–22.

[100] Osthoff M, Ngian GS, Dean MM, Nikpour M, Stevens W, Proudman S, Eisen DP, Sahhar J. Potential role of the lectin pathway of complement in the pathogenesis and disease manifestations of systemic sclerosis: a case-control and cohort study. Arthritis Res Ther 2014;16(6):480.

[101] Wetsel RA. Structure, function and cellular expression of complement anaphylatoxin receptors. Curr Opin Immunol 1995;7:48–53.

[102] Shin ML, Rus HG, Nicolescu FI. Membrane attack by complement: assembly and biology of terminal complement complexes. Biomembranes 1996;4:123–49.

[103] Girardi G, Berman J, Redecha P, Spruce L, Thurman JM, Kraus D, et al. Complement C5a receptors and neutrophils mediate fetal injury in the antiphospholipid syndrome. J Clin Investig 2003;112:1644–54.

[104] Salmon JE, Girardi G, Holers VM. Activation of complement mediates antiphospholipid antibody induced pregnancy loss. Lupus 2003;12:535–8.

[105] Pierangeli SS, Girardi G, Vega-Ostertag M, Liu X, Espinola RG, Salmon J. Requirement of activation of complement C3 and C5 for antiphospholipid antibody-mediated thrombophilia. Arthritis Rheum 2005;52:2120–4.

[106] Agostinis C, Durigutto P, Sblattero D, Borghi MO, Grossi C, Guida F, et al. A non-complement-fixing antibody to beta2 glycoprotein I as a novel therapy for antiphospholipid syndrome. Blood 2014;123:3478–87.

[107] Ritis K, Doumas M, Mastellos D, Micheli A, Giaglis S, Magotti P, et al. A novel C5a receptor-tissue factor cross-talk in neutrophils links innate immunity to coagulation pathways. J Immunol 2006;177:4794–802.

[108] Redecha P, Tilley R, Tencati M, Salmon JE, Kirchhofer D, Mackman N, et al. Tissue factor: a link between C5a and neutrophil activation in antiphospholipid antibody induced fetal injury. Blood 2007;110:2423–31.

[109] Oku K, Nakamura H, Kono M, et al. Complement and thrombosis in the antiphospholipid syndrome. Autoimmun Rev 2016;15:1001–4.

[110] Breen KA, Seed P, Parmar K, Moore GW, Stuart-Smith SE, Hunt BJ. Complement activation in patients with isolated antiphospholipid antibodies or primary antiphospholipid syndrome. Thromb Haemost 2012;107:423–9.

[111] Foltyn Zadura A, Memon AA, Stojanovich L, Perricone C, Conti F, Valesini G, et al. Factor H autoantibodies in patients with antiphospholipid syndrome and thrombosis. J Rheumatol 2015;42:1786–93.

[112] Barratt-Due A, Floisand Y, Orrem HL, Kvam AK, Holme PA, Bergseth G, et al. Complement activation is a crucial pathogenic factor in catastrophic antiphospholipid syndrome. Rheumatology 2016;55:1337–9.

[113] Zikos TA, Sokolove J, Ahuja N, Berube C. Eculizumab induces sustained remission in a patient with refractory primary catastrophic antiphospholipid syndrome. J Clin Rheumatol 2015;21:311–3.

[114] Shapira I, Andrade D, Allen SL, Salmon JE. Brief report: induction of sustained remission in recurrent catastrophic antiphospholipid syndrome via inhibition of terminal complement with eculizumab. Arthritis Rheum 2012;64:2719–23.

[115] Wig S, Chan M, Thachil J, Bruce I, Barnes T. A case of relapsing and refractory catastrophic antiphospholipid syndrome successfully managed with eculizumab, a complement 5 inhibitor. Rheumatology 2016;55:382–4.

[116] Lonze BE, Zachary AA, Magro CM, Desai NM, Orandi BJ, Dagher NN, et al. Eculizumab prevents recurrent antiphospholipid antibody syndrome and enables successful renal transplantation. Am J Transplant 2014;14:459–65.

[117] Dalakas MC, Hohlfeld R. Polymyositis and dermatomyositis. Lancet 2003;362(9388):971–82.

[118] Kissel JT, Mendell JR, Rammohan KW. Microvascular deposition of complement membrane attack complex in dermatomyositis. N Engl J Med 1986;314:329–34.

[119] Thy PN, Bangert C, Biliciler S, Athar P, Sheikh K. Dermatomyositis-associated sensory neuropathy: a unifying pathogenic hypothesis. J Clin Neuromuscul Dis 2014;16(1):7–11.

[120] Mascaró Jr JM, Hausmann G, Herrero C, Grau JM, Cid MC, Palou J, et al. Membrane attack complex deposits in cutaneous lesions of dermatomyositis. Arch Dermatol 1995;131:1386–92.

[121] Takada K, Bookbinder S, Furie R, Oddis C, Mojcik CF, Bombara M, Plotz P, Kissel J. A pilot study of eculizumab in patients with dermatomyositis. Arthritis Rheum 2002;46(9):S489.

[122] Papageorgiou A, Voulgarelis M, Tzioufas AG. Clinical picture, outcome and predictive factors of lymphoma in Sjögren syndrome. Autoimmun Rev 2015;14:641–9.

[123] Skopouli FN, Dafni U, Ioannidis JP, Moutsopoulos HM. Clinical evolution, and morbidity and mortality of primary Sjogren's syndrome. Semin Arthritis Rheum 2000;29:296–304.

[124] Ioannidis JP, Vassiliou VA, Moutsopoulos HM. Long-term risk of mortality and lymphoproliferative disease and predictive classification of primary Sjogren's syndrome. Arthritis Rheum 2002;46:741–7.

[125] Baimpa E, Dahabreh IJ, Voulgarelis M, Moutsopoulos HM. Hematologic manifestations and predictors of lymphoma development in primary Sjogren syndrome: clinical and pathophysiologic aspects. Medicine (Baltim) 2009;88:284–93.

[126] Brito-Zeron P, Belchin K, Fraile G, Caravia-Durán D, Maure B, et al. Characterization and risk estimate of cancer in patients with primary Sjögren syndrome. J Hematol Oncol 2017;10:90.

[127] Ramos-Casals M, Brito-Zeron P, Yague J, Akasbi M, Bautista R, Ruano M, et al. Hypocomplementaemia as an immunological marker of morbidity and mortality in patients with primary Sjogren's syndrome. Rheumatology (Oxf) 2005;44:89–94.

[128] Jennette JC, Falk RJ, Bacon PA, Basu N, Cid MC, Ferrario F, Flores-Suarez LF, et al. 2012 revised international chapel hill consensus conference nomenclature of vasculitides. Arthritis Rheum 2013;65:1–11.

[129] Chimenti MS, Ballanti E, Triggianese P, Perricone R. Vasculitides and the complement system: a comprehensive review. Clin Rev Allergy Immunol 2015;49(3):333–46.

[130] Kallenberg CGM. Pathophysiology of ANCA-associated small vessel vasculitis. Curr Rheumatol Rep 2010;12:399–405.

[131] Schreiber A, Xiao H, Jennette JC, Schneider W, Luft FC, Kettritz R. C5a receptor mediates neutrophil activation and ANCA-induced glomerulonephritis. J Am Soc Nephrol 2009;20:289–98.

[132] Xiao H, Heeringa P, Hu P, Liu Z, Zhao M, Aratani Y, Maeda N, et al. Antineutrophil cytoplasmic autoantibodies specific for myeloperoxidase cause glomerulonephritis and vasculitis in mice. J Clin Investig 2002;110:955–63.

[133] Haas M, Eustace JA. Immune complex deposits in ANCA-associated crescentic glomerulonephritis: a study of 126 cases. Kidney Int 2004;65:2145–52.

[134] Yu F, et al. Clinical and pathological features of renal involvement in propylthiouracil-associated ANCA positive vasculitis. Am J Kidney Dis 2007;49:607–14.

[135] Lospalluto J, Dorward B, Miller Jr W, Ziff M. Cryoglobulinemia based on interaction between a gamma macroglobulin and 7S gamma globulin. Am J Med 1962;32:142–5.

[136] Ferri C, Zignego AL, Pileri SA. Cryoglobulins. J Clin Pathol 2002;55:4–13.

[137] Monti G, Galli M, Invernizzi F, Pioltelli P, Saccardo F, Monteverde A, et al. Cryoglobulinaemias: a multi-centre study of the early clinical and laboratory manifestations of primary and secondary disease. GISC. Italian Group for the Study of Cryoglobulinaemias. QJM 1995;88:115–26.

[138] Tarantino A, Anelli A, Costantino A, De Vecchi A, Monti G, Massaro L. Serum complement pattern in essential mixed cryoglobulinaemia. Clin Exp Immunol 1978;32:77–85.

[139] Davin JC. Henoch-Schonlein purpura nephritis: pathophysiology, treatment, and future strategy. Clin J Am Soc Nephrol 2011;6:679–89.

[140] Hisano S, Matsushita M, Fujita T, Iwasaki H. Activation of the lectin complement pathway in Henoch-Schonlein purpura nephritis. Am J Kidney Dis 2005;45:295–302.

[141] Roos A, Rastaldi MP, Calvaresi N, Oortwijn BD, Schlagwein N, van Gijlswijk-Janssen DJ, et al. Glomerular activation of the lectin pathway of complement in IgA nephropathy is associated with more severe renal disease. J Am Soc Nephrol 2006;17:1724–34.

[142] Espinosa M, Ortega R, Gómez-Carrasco JM, López-Rubio F, López-Andreu M, López-Oliva MO, et al. Mesangial C4d deposition: a new prognostic factor in IgA nephropathy. Nephrol Dial Transplant 2009;24:886–91.

[143] Holers VM. The complement system as a therapeutic target in autoimmunity. Clin Immunol 2003;107:140–51.

[144] Goodfellow RM, Williams AS, Levin JL, Williams BD, Morgan BP. Soluble complement receptor one (sCR1) inhibits the development and progression of rat collagen-induced arthritis. Clin Exp Immunol 2000;119:210–6.

[145] Ames RS, Lee D, Foley JJ, Jurewicz AJ, Tornetta MA, Bautsch W, et al. Identification of a selective non peptide antagonist of the anaphylatoxin C3a receptor that demonstrates antiinflammatory activity in animal models. J Immunol 2001;166:6341–8.

[146] Woodruff TM, Strachan AJ, Dryburgh N, Shiels IA, Reid RC, Fairlie DP, et al. Antiarthritic activity of an orally active C5a receptor antagonist against antigen-induced monarticular arthritis in the rat. Arthritis Rheum 2002;46:2476–85.

[147] Fraser DA, Harris CL, Williams AS, Mizuno M, Gallagher S, Smith RA, et al. Generation of a recombinant, membrane-targeted form of the complement regulator CD59: activity in vitro and in vivo. J Biol Chem 2003;278:48921–7.

[148] Vergunst CE, Gerlag DM, Dinant H, Schulz L, Vinkenoog M, Smeets TJ, et al. Blocking the receptor for C5a in patients with rheumatoid arthritis does not reduce synovial inflammation. Rheumatology (Oxf) 2007;46:1773–8.

[149] Hillmen P, et al. The complement inhibitor eculizumab in paroxysmal nocturnal hemoglobinuria. N Engl J Med 2006;355:1233–43.

[150] Legendre CM, Licht C, Muus P, Greenbaum LA, Babu S, Bedrosian C, et al. Terminal complement inhibitor eculizumab in atypical hemolytic–uremic syndrome. N Engl J Med 2013;368:2169–81.

[151] Cancian M, ITACA Group. Diagnostic and Therapeutic management of hereditary angioedema due to C1-inhibitor deficiency: the Italian experience. Curr Opin Allergy Clin Immunol 2015;15(4):383–91.

[152] Bermea RS, Sharma N, Cohen K, Liarski VM. Use of eculizumab in atypical hemolytic uremic syndrome, complicating systemic lupus erythematosus. J Clin Rheumatol 2016;22:320–3.

[153] Trouw LA, Pickering MC, Blom AM. The complement system as a potential therapeutic target in rheumatic disease. Nat Rev Rheumatol 2017;13(9):538–47.

[154] Jayne DR, Bruchfeld AN, Harper L, Schaier M, Venning MC, Hamilton P, et al. CLEAR Study. Group Randomized trial of C5a receptor inhibitor avacopan in ANCA-associated vasculitis. J Am Soc Nephrol 2017;28(9):2756–67.

[155] Mollnes TE, Høgåsen K, De Carolis C, Vaquero E, Nielsen EW, Fontana L, et al. High-dose intravenous immunoglobulin treatment activates complement in vivo. Scand J Immunol 1998;48:312–31.

[156] Cicardi M, Zanichelli A. Replacement therapy with C1 esterase inhibitors for hereditary angioedema. Drugs Today 2010;46:867–74.

[157] Morgan BP, Harris CL. Complement therapeutics; history and current progress. Mol Immunol 2003;40:159–70.

Chapter 10

Autoantibodies in Disease Criteria for Systemic Autoimmune Diseases: Developments in the Last Decade

Jan Damoiseaux[1], Joyce van Beers[1], Pieter van Paassen[2]

[1]Central Diagnostic Laboratory, Maastricht University Medical Center, Maastricht, The Netherlands; [2]Department of Internal Medicine, Maastricht University Medical Center, Maastricht, The Netherlands

INTRODUCTION

Autoantibodies are increasingly recognized as important parameters in the diagnosis of systemic autoimmune diseases. Most evidently, they are included in classification criteria for these diseases (Table 10.1). Although classification criteria are intended to be used for appropriate patient inclusion in studies, they are also used for diagnostic purposes. The classification criteria for the systemic autoimmune diseases, however, do not fully recognize the implications of the many novel technologies for autoantibody detection that are nowadays available and the broader spectrum of clinical disciplines that request such tests. Several criteria include just the mere absence or presence of an autoantibody, whereas other criteria give some direction toward relevant clinical manifestations and optimal interpretation. For example, the new classification criteria for Sjögren's syndrome include the presence of anti-SSA/Ro antibodies but do not discriminate between SSA/Ro60 and Ro52/TRIM21 [1]. In the criteria for rheumatoid arthritis (RA), on the other hand, the scoring system is differentiating between low- and high antibody levels [2]. Furthermore, the Systemic Lupus International Collaborating Clinics (SLICC) criteria for systemic lupus erythematosus (SLE) make a distinction between assays for anti-dsDNA antibodies because results obtained by enzyme-linked immunosorbent assays (ELISA) are only considered relevant if the result is at least two times above the reference range [3]. Ideally, the criteria should refer to guidelines for requesting, detection, reporting, and interpretation, while taking into account the spectrum of immunoassays currently available in routine diagnostic laboratories.

The current chapter deals with the autoantibodies that are incorporated in the most recent criteria for systemic autoimmune diseases. Possible pitfalls in the interpretation of the autoantibody results will be elaborated upon. Newly discovered autoantibodies will only be mentioned if they may be on the edge of being included in novel criteria.

RHEUMATOID ARTHRITIS

With the inclusion of anticitrullinated protein antibodies (ACPA) in the 2010 American College of Rheumatology (ACR)/European League Against Rheumatism (EULAR) classification criteria for RA, the clinical value of these antibodies has been well appreciated [2,4]. The classification criteria are met if ≥6 points are scored and autoantibodies may represent 3 points. Seronegative RA only fulfills the criteria if at least 10 joints, including 1 small joint, are affected. These criteria also state that high antibody levels (3 points) have increased diagnostic value as compared with low antibody levels (2 points). The role of rheumatoid factor (RF) has been maintained in the criteria, and, as has been underscored by Eng Tan at the 14th IWAA in Kyoto (2016), this can be attributed to the pathogenic potential of these antibodies. As RF reacts with IgG, the enhanced immune complex formation and subsequent deposition in the joints may cause and/or increase local inflammation. Nevertheless, it is somewhat surprising that both ACPA and RF have attained the same weight in the criteria, while it is well known that ACPA, having almost similar sensitivity, have a far better specificity for RA than RF [4]. This difference in added diagnostic value is clearly illustrated in a study of Bossuyt et al., which compared the likelihood ratios for test result intervals of ACPA and RF [5]. In this study the positive likelihood ratio of low-level ACPA was 4.5 as compared with 2.9–4.8 for high-level RF. The positive likelihood ratio of high-level ACPA was 27.7. Although in this study only one single test was used for both ACPA and RF in a single RA cohort, the findings support the idea that the value of RF is overrated

TABLE 10.1 Diagnostic and Classification Criteria for Rheumatic Autoimmune Diseases

Disease	Criteria	Autoantibodies/Antigens	Guidelines for Autoantibodies
Rheumatoid arthritis	ACR/EULAR (2010) [2]	RF and ACPA	Definition of interpretation thresholds [2]
Systemic lupus erythematosus	ACR (1982 and 1997) [10,11]	ANA, dsDNA and Sm, LA, CL (IgM and IgG), and β2GPI (IgM and IgG)	ANA to be determined by IIF (1982) [10] ACR guideline for ANA testing (2002) [12] ACR guideline for anti-dsDNA antibody tests (2002) [13] ACR guideline for anti-Sm antibody tests (2004) [14]
	SLICC (2012) [3]	ANA, dsDNA and Sm, LA, CL (IgM, IgG, and IgA), and β2GPI (IgM, IgG, and IgA)	Anti-dsDNA >2 times reference range for ELISA [3]
Sjögren's syndrome	ACR/EULAR (2016) [1]	SSA/Ro	None
Systemic sclerosis	ACR/EULAR (2013) [29]	Centromere (CENP-B), topoisomerase I (Scl-70), and RNApol III	None
Mixed connective tissue disease	Sharp (1972) [36]	U1-RNP	None
	Alarcón-Segovia (1987) [37]	U1-RNP	Titer definition based on hemagglutination assay [37]
Autoimmune myositis • Overlap myositis • Dermatomyositis • Necrotizing myositis • Inclusion body myositis	Senécal [39]	Synthetases (Jo-1, PL7, PL12, HA, OJ, KS, ZO, EJ), RNP, PM-Scl, Ku MDA5, Mi-2, NXP2, SAE, TIF-1γ HMGCR, SRP cN-1A	None
Antiphospholipid syndrome	Sydney Criteria (2006) [20]	LA, CL (IgM and IgG), and β2GPI (IgM and IgG)	Reference to ISTH guideline for LA detection [45,46] Definition of interpretation thresholds [20]
ANCA-associated vasculitis	ACR (1990) [56]	ANCA not included	International Consensus on ANCA testing for AAV (2017) [56]
	CHCC (1994) [56]	ANCA not included	

ACR, American College of Rheumatology; ANA, antinuclear antibodies; ANCA, antineutrophil cytoplasmic antibodies; ACPA, anticitrullinated protein antibodies; β2GPI, β2 glycoprotein 1; CHCC, Chapel Hill Consensus Conference; CL, cardiolipin; EULAR, European League Against Rheumatism; ISTH, International Society on Thrombosis and Haemostasis; LA, lupus anticoagulans; RF, rheumatoid factor; RNP, ribonucleoprotein; SLICC, Systemic Lupus International Collaborating Clinics.

as compared to ACPA in the current classification criteria. Actually, this is also recognized in the discussion of the current criteria [2]. Moreover, it should be realized that the suggested cutoffs for appointing value to the autoantibody results, i.e., the cutoff provided by the company in combination with three times this cutoff for defining the range of low-positive results, reveal very diverse outcomes depending on the used immunoassay [60]. Although results of RF may be expressed in international units, which is not the case for ACPA, standardization of immunoassays remains a general concern in autoantibody testing. Probably, the cutoffs for the respective test result intervals can be better standardized if they are defined by preset specificities, as has been applied for autoantibodies in the small-vessel vasculitides [6]. Finally, the current classification criteria do not clearly define the relevance of the autoantibody isotype. This is only a minor issue for ACPA because most assays used in clinical practice are specific for the IgG isotype, but several immunoassays for RF do not discriminate between distinct isotypes. Nevertheless, although the criteria describe RF without specifying the isotype, the paragraph on the definition of the serological criteria specifically refers to IgM RF [2].

With respect to novel autoantibodies in RA, those recognizing posttranslational modifications other than citrullination seem promising. These include antibodies reacting with carbamylated proteins (CarP) or acetylated proteins [7,8]. The carbamylation involves modification of lysine residues to homocitrulline. These anti-CarP autoantibodies identify RA patients with a more severe disease course. Although there is overlap with APCA- and RF-positive RA patients, it is expected that anti-CarP antibodies will further close the gap of seronegative RA and enable to better identify individuals at risk of developing RA.

In conclusion, the 2010 ACR/EULAR classification criteria for RA will improve by considering differential rating for RF and ACPA and by explicitly defining the relevant isotype for RF; a possible role for anti-CarP autoantibodies remains to be established.

SYSTEMIC LUPUS ERYTHEMATOSUS

SLE is probably the autoimmune disease with the widest plethora of circulating autoantibodies. More than 100 different autoantibodies have been found in SLE patients [9]. On the other hand, only a limited number of these autoantibodies are included in the classification criteria as defined by the ACR and more recently by the SLICC initiative [3,10,11]. Both sets of criteria have included more or less the same autoantibodies, i.e., antinuclear antibodies (ANA) and the autoantibodies specific for dsDNA, Sm, and phospholipids. The ACR has published distinct evidence-based guidelines for detection of these antibodies [12–14].

The original ACR criteria defined that ANA are to be detected by indirect immunofluorescence (IIF) [10]. This was underscored by the ACR position statement that IIF remains the gold standard for ANA detection [15]. This item was not further discussed in the SLICC criteria [3], but the European Autoimmunity Standardisation Initiative (EASI)/International Union of Immunological Societies (IUIS) recommendations gave credit to alternative assays as long as in case of strong clinical suspicion and a negative test result that the request for an IIF test is awarded (Delphi score 9.7 ± 0.6) [16]. The ANA IIF test, however, reveals more information than just a negative or positive result. Indeed, staining intensity, often reported as a titer, and pattern may add value to the result. The International Consensus on ANA Patterns (ICAP) has reached consensus on the nomenclature and description of multiple ANA patterns (AC-1–AC-29) as observed on HEp-2 cells [17]. These not only include true nuclear patterns but also cytoplasmic patterns and mitotic patterns (see www.ANApatterns. org). Whether cytoplasmic and mitotic patterns are to be considered ANA positive, and thereby are part of the classification criteria, is not defined [18]. The relevance of distinct nuclear patterns for SLE may also be questioned. The specific autoantibodies reactive with dsDNA and Sm reveal a homogeneous (AC-1) or large/coarse speckled pattern (AC-5), respectively. On the other hand, the presence of the dense fine speckled pattern (AC-2), if monospecific for DFS70, has been suggested to exclude ANA-associated rheumatic diseases [19].

With respect to the anti-dsDNA antibodies, there is ample discussion about the optimal immunoassay to be used. This is best illustrated by the relatively low Delphi score and high standard deviation (8.0 ± 2.5) of the EASI/IUIS recommendation, stating that "the *Crithidia luciliae* IIF (CLIFT) and Farr-assay offer the best specificity; if alternative assays are used, the result is to be confirmed in one of the former assays" [16]. In addition, the SLICC criteria consider alternative assays, such as ELISA, inferior as these tests are only to be considered positive if the reference range is greater than twofold [3]. This cutoff item is somewhat surprising because it implies that the reference ranges for solid-phase immunoassays were not appropriately defined by the diagnostic companies and verified by the laboratories utilizing these assays. Furthermore, it seems that this conclusion is based on a single ELISA at the coordinating site of the SLICC cohort. Interestingly, the suspected differences in the immunoassays are not evident from diagnostic test characteristics provided in the evidence-based ACR guideline for anti-dsDNA antibody tests [13].

Antiphospholipid antibodies, the hallmark of the antiphospholipid syndrome (APS), are also part of the classification criteria for SLE. Although not specified in the ACR criteria [11], in clinical practice the antibody criteria for APS, i.e., the Sydney criteria [20], are applied. The SLICC criteria have extended the Sydney criteria by also including the IgA isotype for anticardiolipin (aCLA) and anti-β_2GPI antibodies [3]. The argument used for including the IgA isotype refers to a study showing that IgA anti-β_2GPI antibodies (but not IgA aCLA) are associated with clinical and laboratory manifestations of SLE [21]. Such an association, however, does not necessarily imply that these antibodies have added diagnostic value.

Finally, there are two SLE-associated autoantibodies that are considered clinically relevant. First, anti-C1q antibodies are clearly associated with lupus nephritis and their presence predicts renal involvement [22]. This association is even further enhanced in case of co-occurrence with anti-dsDNA antibodies and low complement levels. Second, the anti-RibP antibodies have been reported to be more prevalent in juvenile-onset SLE, associated with nephritis, and diffuse CNS involvement [9]. Of note, the anti-RibP antibodies reveal a cytoplasmic dense fine speckled pattern (AC-19) by IIF on HEp-2 cells [17].

In conclusion, the 1997 ACR and 2012 SLICC criteria for SLE will improve by differentiating between ANA patterns, by defining a clinically relevant cutoff for anti-dsDNA antibody assays based on a preset specificity, e.g., 98%, irrespective of the type of immunoassay, and by alignment of the antiphospholipid antibodies as defined for APS. Other autoantibodies, such as anti-C1q antibodies, may be relevant for classification of SLE subtypes.

SJÖGREN'S SYNDROME

In the last decade, two sets of classification criteria for the Sjögren's syndrome have been published. In the 2012 ACR criteria, presence of autoantibodies is one of the three features used for classification. The antibody category is defined as positive serum anti-SSA/Ro and/or anti-SSB/La or positive RF in combination with positive ANA with a titer ≥1:320 [23]. The more recent 2016 ACR/EULAR criteria utilize a scoring system based on five items; if the total score is ≥4, the patient can be classified as having the Sjögren's syndrome [1]. Presence of autoantibodies is a dominant item because it can reveal 3 points on the score. However, as compared to the 2012 ACR criteria, the new criteria have restricted the spectrum of autoantibodies to only anti-SSA/Ro antibodies. The combined presence of RF and ANA has been removed because they are evidently less specific for this disease, whereas the added value of anti-SSB/La probably is limited because these antibodies most often co-occur with anti-SSA/Ro antibodies. The absence or presence of anti-SSB/La antibodies, however, may distinguish between patients with mixed-type cryoglobulinemia [24]. This also holds for high-level IgM RF [25].

Although ANA is not included in the most recent classification criteria anymore, screening for anti-extractable nuclear antigens (ENA) antibodies often occurs with ANA IIF because according to the ACR this is considered the gold standard [15]. Detection of anti-SSA/Ro antibodies, however, appears less optimal by ANA IIF, and solid-phase immunoassays have better test characteristics for the Sjögren's syndrome [26]. This has resulted in the international EASI/IUIS recommendation that in case of high clinical suspicion for Sjögren's syndrome, a negative ANA IIF result should not preclude from testing for anti-SSA/Ro antibodies (Delphi score 9.9±0.1) [16].

Both the old and the new criteria do not discriminate between antibodies directed to SSA/Ro60 and Ro52/TRIM21, although it is well recognized that the latter are quite common in patients with other systemic autoimmune diseases [27]. In this respect, it is important to realize that several immunoassays utilize a mixture of SSA/Ro60 and Ro52/TRIM21, whereas others enable to discriminate between both entities. Based on a questionnaire, it appeared that discrimination between both entities occurs in less than half of the European laboratories, while only about half of these laboratories also report the results separately to the clinician [28].

In conclusion, the 2017 ACR/EULAR criteria for the Sjögren's syndrome will improve by differentiation between autoantibodies to SSA/Ro60 and Ro52/TRIM21. Screening for these antibodies is preferentially performed by antigen-specific immunoassays.

SYSTEMIC SCLEROSIS

Like for RA and Sjögren's syndrome, the 2013 ACR/EULAR criteria for systemic sclerosis are based on a scoring system [29]. Classification requires ≥9 points and these can be obtained by the presence of skin thickening of the fingers of both hands extending proximal to the metacarpophalangeal joints. The classification criteria can also be met by combinations of other clinical manifestations in the absence of autoantibodies. Nevertheless, presence of autoantibodies, i.e., anticentromere (CENP-B), antitopoisomerase I (Topo I/Scl-70), and anti-RNA polymerase III (RNApol III) antibodies, accounts for a maximum of 3 points and thereby significantly contributes to classification. For detection of the anticentromere antibodies, it is sufficient that the respective pattern (AC-3) is observed by ANA IIF; confirmation by an antigen-specific immunoassay is not required. Also the anti-Topo I antibodies reveal a very distinct pattern by ANA IIF [30]. These autoantibodies have recently been included in ICAP as pattern AC-29; antigen-specificity, though, is to be confirmed by an antigen-specific immunoassay. The anti-RNApol III antibodies reveal a nonspecific large/coarse speckled pattern (AC-5) that often will be mixed with a punctate nucleolar ANA pattern (AC-10) because of copresence of anti-RNApol I antibodies [17]. Because the prevalence of autoantibodies to RNApol III is relatively low, the clinical indications to request for this test should be restricted to those related to systemic sclerosis. As many laboratories use a standard testing algorithm for ANA-associated systemic autoimmune diseases, incorporation of anti-RNApol III antibody testing in this algorithm will result in increased numbers of false-positive results [31]. Therefore, it has been suggested to only test for these antibodies if anticentromere and anti-Topo I antibodies are negative, in combination with a clear clinical suspicion of systemic sclerosis, e.g., renal crisis [32].

Although not included in the latest classification criteria, two other sets of autoantibodies have been associated with systemic sclerosis. The presence of the first set of autoantibodies can be screened for by ANA IIF and often reveals a nucleolar staining (AC-8–AC-10). The antigens recognized include U3-RNP (fibrillarin), Th/To, NOR-90, PM-Scl, and Ku; the latter two are associated with the myositis-scleroderma overlap syndrome. These autoantibodies can be detected by multiplex dot and/or line immunoassays in combination with the autoantibodies mentioned in the criteria. Like anti-RNApol III antibodies, the prevalence of these antibodies is low. This seriously hampers verification of the assay characteristics for all antigen specificities [33]. The second set of autoantibodies associated with systemic sclerosis reacts with cell membrane receptors. These antibodies, reacting with the platelet-derived growth factor (PDGF) and G protein–coupled receptors (GPCR), are optimally detected by functional bioassays because the recognized epitopes are configuration dependent [34,35]. Therefore, it will not be easy to incorporate these autoantibodies in disease criteria as the respective assays will not be readily available in routine diagnostic laboratories.

In summary, inclusion of the anti-RNApol III antibodies in the 2013 ACR/EULAR criteria for systemic sclerosis has extended the autoantibody repertoire, but this test should not be included in the standard testing algorithm for systemic autoimmune diseases. In particular autoantibodies to PDGF and GPCR may be of added value; appropriate evaluation of the potential added value demands immunoassays other than functional bioassays.

MIXED CONNECTIVE TISSUE DISEASE

There consist several long-standing diagnostic and classification criteria for mixed connective tissue disease (MCTD) [36,37]. They have in common that the presence of anti-U1-RNP antibodies are a sine *qua non*. These autoantibodies reveal a nuclear large/course speckled ANA pattern (AC-5) on HEp-2 cells. This pattern, however, is not specific for anti-U1-RNP antibodies [17]. Therefore, these antibodies are to be confirmed by antigen-specific immunoassays. The only novelty with respect to autoantibodies in MCTD is perhaps the availability of novel immunoassays that enable detection of anti-U1-RNP antibodies. These assays present the antigen in several distinct configurations. U1-RNP is part of so-called small nuclear ribonucleoprotein particles (snRNP) and consists of three distinct components, i.e., RNP-A, RNP-C, and RNP-70. Furthermore, the respective snRNP also contains the Sm proteins. Consequently, immunoassays may be based on native U1-RNP complexes, either or not associated with Sm proteins, or separate, recombinant U1-RNP proteins (A, C, 70). Because most immunoassays currently used in routine clinical practice have been introduced years after the publications on the diagnostic and classification criteria for MCTD, these criteria do not define how to interpret the results obtained in these assays. For instance, it can be questioned if the criteria are met if autoantibodies are only directed to a single U1-RNP component. Moreover, the criteria defined by Alarcón-Segovia et al. require high-titer autoantibodies [37]. This is defined as a titer $\geq 1:1600$ in a hemagglutination assay, but this type of assay is probably not in use anymore in routine diagnostics. For the novel assays, the cutoffs for a high antibody level have not been defined. Nevertheless, it is recommended by the EASI/IUIS to report anti-U1-RNP antibodies quantitatively if MCTD is suspected [16]. Because anti-ENA antibodies are, in general, reported only qualitatively, it is not surprising that there was only limited consensus for this recommendation (Delphi score 8.2 ± 2.7).

In conclusion, optimal appreciation of anti-U1/RNP test results in the context of the classification criteria for MCTD requires better definition of "high level" as obtained in distinct immunoassays and of how to interpret reactivity to distinct components of the RNP complex.

AUTOIMMUNE MYOSITIS

Since the publication of the classification criteria as defined by Bohan and Peter [38], a still increasing number of myositis autoantibodies have been discovered. These autoantibodies have been included in the proposal for new classification criteria [39], and their discovery has thus revolutionized the understanding of the pathogenesis and categorization of the distinct disease entities. While the group of myopathies has long been referred to as idiopathic inflammatory myopathies, the strong evidence of an autoimmune pathogenesis strengthens the use of the more specific term autoimmune myositis (AIM) [39]. Based on clinical manifestations, histopathology, and specific autoantibody profiles, four major categories can be distinguished within the spectrum of AIM: overlap myositis (including the majority of patients that formerly were classified as having polymyositis), dermatomyositis, necrotizing myopathies, and inclusion body myositis [40]. First, overlap myositis traditionally includes AIMs with extramuscular symptoms often observed in other systemic autoimmune rheumatic diseases. This type of overlap myositis is associated with antibodies to Ku, PM-Scl, or RNP. Within the extended category of overlap myositis, the most distinguished group is the antisynthetase syndrome, a syndrome characterized by the combination of polymyositis, interstitial lung disease, Raynaud's phenomenon, mechanic's hands, and arthritis. The name of this subgroup refers to the autoantibodies observed in the antisynthetase syndrome because they react with tRNA synthetases. While Jo-1 or anti-histidyl-tRNA synthetase is the most prevalent and well-known autoantibody, at least seven other tRNA synthetases (anti-EJ, anti-Ha, anti-KS, anti-OJ, anti-PL7, anti-PL12, and anti-Zo) have been identified as autoantigen in this syndrome. Second, dermatomyositis is recognized by a combination of skin rashes and proximal skeletal muscle weakness, but no overlap features. The dermatomyositis-specific autoantibodies (anti-MDA5, anti-Mi2, anti-NXP-2, anti-SAE, and anti-TIF1γ) cover only about 50% of the cohort of dermatomyositis patients, leaving space for the further discovery of novel autoantibodies. Importantly, some of these autoantibodies, i.e., anti-NXP2 and anti-TIF1γ, are associated with malignancy. Third, the category of necrotizing myopathies presents with prominent muscle fiber necrosis with limited infiltration of inflammatory cells on regeneration. In particular autoantibodies to 3-hydroxy-3-methylglutaryl coenzyme A reductase (HMGCR) are considered as a biomarker for necrotizing myopathies [41]. Indeed, up to 50% of these patients may have these autoantibodies and this typically includes patients on treatment with statins. This association with statins is rather limited as the presence of anti-HMGCR autoantibodies is exceptional in statin users, while about one-third of the patients with anti-HMGCR autoantibodies never used statins. Interestingly, in latter group of patients, the presence of the autoantibodies is associated with malignancy [42]. Besides anti-HMGCR, anti–signal recognition particle antibodies are present in this category of AIM. The final category of AIM entails inclusion body myositis with the clinical hallmarks of slowly progressive asymmetric muscle weakness. As this condition is resistant to conventional immunosuppressive treatment, an autoimmune pathogenesis was for long held unlikely. This conclusion became debated on the recent discovery of autoantibodies to cytosolic 5′-nucleotidase 1A (cN-1A) in a subset of patients [43]. However, these antibodies are not specific as they are also prevalent in Sjögren's syndrome and SLE.

The total of about 20 AIM autoantibodies is a challenge for the diagnostic laboratory. Many of these autoantibodies, in particular the antisynthetase antibodies, are poorly recognized in the ANA IIF test. Hence, there is high consensus on the EASI/IUIS recommendation that a negative ANA result should not deter from further testing for AIM autoantibodies (Delphi score 9.9 ± 0.1) [16]. Considering the wide spectrum of AIM autoantibodies and the limitation of ANA IIF as screening test for these autoantibodies, multiplex testing seems the best alternative [44]. Also the multiplex assays, predominantly line immunoassays (LIA) or dot immunoassays (DIA), harbor several disadvantages: they do not cover the whole spectrum of AIM autoantibodies; they do not correlate perfectly with the gold standard immunoprecipitation assays; and, due to the low prevalence of the autoantibodies, verification of the assay characteristics is hard to perform for all antigen specificities. Finally, with increasing numbers of autoantigens in the test, the chance of a false-positive result will increase accordingly. These shortcomings can be partially overcome by restricted use of the tests, i.e., guided by predefined disease manifestations and in specialized laboratories only.

In conclusion, the novel proposal for classification of AIM has incorporated the whole spectrum of autoantibodies identified. This has underscored the autoimmune component in these diseases and, in addition, has enabled to further support distinct disease entities. As ANA IIF is not the optimal screening strategy for AIM, multiplex immunoassays are to be preferred when restricted to patients with the relevant clinical manifestations.

ANTIPHOSPHOLIPID SYNDROME

The 2006 classification criteria for the APS have further extended the important role of autoantibodies in this disease. These antibodies include lupus anticoagulant (LA), aCLA, and anti-β_2GPI antibodies [20]. A novel positive phospholipid autoantibody finding should be confirmed after 12 weeks to further improve the specificity. Detection of LA is to be performed according to the International Society on Haemostasis and Thrombosis (ISTH) guidelines [45,46]. In short, this guideline prescribes screening with a combination of dRVVT and aPTT, mixing with normal plasma to exclude coagulation factor deficiencies, and confirming phospholipid dependence by adding a surplus of phospholipids. The overall result, i.e., LA negative or positive, is to be reported to the clinician.

In the last decade, some alternative guidelines have been published. These include guidelines from the British Committee for Standards in Haematology (BCSH) and the Clinical and Laboratory Standards Institute (CLSI) [47]. Major differences with the ISTH guideline include (1) the acceptance of alternative screening assays, (2) the switch between mixing and confirming steps (CLSI), (3) application of a 97.5 percentile cutoff for screening instead of the 99 percentile of the ISTH guideline, and (4) the advice toward testing patients on vitamin K antagonists [47]. With respect to the reduced cutoff for the screening assay, it is evident that for screening assays, sensitivity is more important than specificity. Because such screening test is followed by mixing and confirming steps, the risk of reporting a false-positive result to the clinician is not at stake. Interestingly, Moore remarked that the ISTH recommendation to verify the 99 percentile cutoff locally by analyzing 40 donors is statistically incorrect because this requires more analyses. Finally, with respect to appropriate detection of LA, it is to be mentioned that treatment with the new oral anticoagulants, such as anti-factor Xa and anti-factor IIa, interferes with the LA screening assays revealing false-positive results [48].

The APS classification criteria also give rise to some discussion with respect to the cutoff for the aCLA and anti-β_2GPI antibody assays. For aCLA, antibody levels above 40 U/mL or above the 99th percentile are considered clinically relevant. The value of 40 U/mL should be traceable to the Harris Standard and is then expressed as IgG antiphospholipid units (GPL) or IgM antiphospholipid units (MPL) for IgG and IgM aCLA, respectively [49]. For most immunoassays used in routine clinical practice, the cutoff defined by the 99th percentile significantly differs from the level of 40 GPL/MPL. Moreover, due to the introduction of novel immunoassays, such as chemiluminescent immunoassays, addressable laser bead immunoassays, and LIA/DIA, standardization of the clinically relevant cutoff value has become even more complicated.

For the anti-β_2GPI antibody assays, only the 99th percentile is mentioned in the criteria. Recently, international standards for IgG and IgM anti-β_2GPI antibodies have become available, but they are not incorporated yet in commercially available assays [50,51]. Thus far, the APS classification criteria for autoantibodies are restricted to the IgG and IgM isotypes. As mentioned already, the SLICC criteria for SLE [3] have also included the IgA isotype. However, the diagnostic value of IgA antibodies in APS is still a matter of debate [52].

Because the autoantibodies currently included in the classification criteria are far from optimal as diagnostic markers, on the one hand there is a continuous search for novel markers, and on the other hand the APS antibodies might be better regarded as risk factors for occurrence of clinical manifestations. Interesting novel immunoassays include detection of antibodies directed to domain I of β2GPI [53], as well as antibodies to phosphatidylserine–prothrombin (PS/PT) complexes [54]. As the results of the accuracy of these novel autoantibodies for diagnosing APS are conflicting, introduction of these assays in routine clinical practice awaits further verification [52]. Nevertheless, the anti-PS/PT antibodies have been included in a risk stratification system, the Global Antiphospholipid Syndrome Score (GAPSS), which enables prediction of thrombosis or pregnancy loss in SLE patients [55]. Surprisingly, while in general triple positivity, LA, IgG, and high-level autoantibodies are considered the most important risk factors, GAPSS appoints most value to aCLA and does not differentiate between IgM and IgG isotypes. This might be because of the fact that GAPSS has been based on a relatively small (developmental and validation) cohort of only SLE patients.

In conclusion, the 2006 Sydney classification criteria for APS not only include a number of autoantibodies but also give information about the type of immunoassay to be performed and about the way results are to be interpreted. Alignment of the distinct guidelines for detection of LA and of the clinically relevant cutoff may further improve these criteria. In the end, the antiphospholipid antibodies may be better regarded as risk factors instead of diagnostic markers for APS.

ANCA-ASSOCIATED VASCULITIS

Although the test results for antineutrophil cytoplasmic antibodies (ANCA) are not included in the classification criteria for ANCA-associated vasculitis (AAV), they are part of the 2012 Chapel Hill Nomenclature consensus [56]. In addition, there are international consensus reports on how to test for ANCA in AAV. The first 1999 international consensus on ANCA testing prescribed screening with IIF on ethanol-fixed neutrophils, and if positive, reflex testing for both MPO- and PR3-ANCA [57]. Due to new developments and technical improvements, the test characteristics of the currently available immunoassays outperform IIF tests, even if these IIF tests combine ethanol with formalin-fixed neutrophils and ANA on HEp-2 cells [58]. These data have resulted in a revised 2017 international consensus stating that high-quality immunoassays can be used as the primary screening method for patients suspected of having AAV, without the categorical need for IIF [56]. If results are negative for both MPO- and PR3-ANCA, and there is high suspicion of small-vessel vasculitis, the use of another immunoassay is recommended to increase the sensitivity. On the other hand, if low-positive results are obtained, it is advised to perform a second test to increase the specificity.

Like for other autoantibody assays, also for ANCA detection, there is a lack of standardization. Introduction of standard preparations is considered promising, but there is still a long way to go. An alternative approach, i.e., harmonization of interpretation based on likelihood ratios for test result intervals, seems more feasible. When test result intervals are defined by preset thresholds for specificity, the associated likelihood ratios are very similar for distinct immunoassays [5]. Moreover, the percentage of AAV patients within each test result interval is also very similar. Representation of these results in a graph of pretest probability versus posttest probability will greatly facilitate the interpretation of the ANCA results [5,56].

In conclusion, the current ACR and Chapel Hill criteria for the distinct entities of ANCA-associated vasculitis will benefit from including the ANCA test results. Ideally, test results are presented as likelihood ratios for test result intervals to further improve the added value in the clinical context of the patient.

CONCLUSION

Keeping in mind that classification criteria are not designed for diagnostic purposes, it is evident from the current classification criteria for systemic autoimmune diseases that autoantibodies are well recognized for their added value in defining the distinct disease types. The diagnostic value of an autoantibody test result, however, is determined by several items (Fig. 10.1). First, requesting for a specific test should be restricted to those patients who have a sufficiently high pretest probability based on clinical manifestations. Gating strategies, as applied for AAV [56], may significantly reduce the number of false-positive results without affecting the identification of patients with the respective disease. Second, the type of assay performed will influence the quality of the result. Critical parameters include the exposition of clinically relevant epitopes and the recognition of the autoantibody isotype/subclass by the secondary antibodies. Third, reporting of results may be

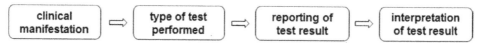

FIGURE 10.1 Critical items that determine the added value of a test result for autoantibodies.

limited to negative/positive or extended to (semi)quantitative results or even to likelihood ratios for test result intervals [59]. Also additional information, e.g., the type of assay or the IIF pattern, will enable better interpretation of the reported results. Finally, the test results are to be interpreted in the context of the clinical manifestations. Critical appraisal of these issues, therefore, warrants the highest diagnostic value of a test result but may also improve the quality of classification criteria.

REFERENCES

[1] Shiboski CH, Shiboski SC, Seror R, et al. 2016 American College of Rheumatology/European League against Rheumatism classification criteria for primary Sjögren's syndrome: a consensus and data-driven methodology involving three international patient cohorts. Ann Rheum Dis 2017;76:9–16.

[2] Aletaha D, Neogi T, Silman AJ, et al. 2010 Rheumatoid arthritis classification criteria: an American College of Rheumatol-ogy/European League against Rheumatism collaborative initiative. Ann Rheum Dis 2010;69:1580–8.

[3] Petri M, Orbai AM, Alarcón GS, et al. Derivation and validation of systemic lupus international collaborating clinics classification criteria for systemic lupus erythematosus. Arthritis Rheum 2012;64:2677–86.

[4] Van Venrooij W, Van Beers JJBC, Pruijn GJM. Anti-CCP antibodies: the past, the present and the future. Nat Rev Rheumatol 2011;7:391–8.

[5] Bossuyt X, Coenen D, Fieuws S, et al. Likelihood ratios as a function of antibody concentration for anti-cyclic citrullinated peptide antibodies and rheumatoid factor. Ann Rheum Dis 2009;68:287–9.

[6] Bossuyt X, Rasmussen N, van Paassen, et al. A multicentre study to improve clinical interpretation of proteinase-3 and myeloperoxidase anti-neutrophil cytoplasmic antibodies. Rheumatology (Oxford) 2017;56:1533–41.

[7] Trouw LA, Huizinga TW, Toes RE. Autoimmunity in rheumatoid arthritis: different antigens–common principles. Ann Rheum Dis 2013;72(Suppl. 2):ii132-6.

[8] Juarez M, Bang H, Hammar F, et al. Identification of novel antiacetylated vimentin antibodies in patients with early inflammatory arthritis. Ann Rheum Dis 2016;75:1099–107.

[9] Sherer Y, Gorstein A, Fritzler MJ, et al. Autoantibody explosion in systemic lupus erythematosus: more than 100 different antibodies found in SLE patients. Semin Arthritis Rheum 2004;34:501–37.

[10] Tan EM, Cohen AS, Fries JF, et al. The 1982 revised criteria for the classification of systemic lupus erythematosus. Arthritis Rheum 1982;25:1271–7.

[11] Hochberg MC. Updating the American College of Rheumatology revised criteria for the classification of systemic lupus erythematosus. Arthritis Rheum 1997;40:1725.

[12] Solomon DH, Kavanaugh AJ, Schur PH, et al. Evidence-based guidelines for the use of immunologic tests: antinuclear antibody testing. Arthritis Rheum 2002;47:434–44.

[13] Kavanaugh AF, Solomon DH. Guidelines for immunologic laboratory testing in the rheumatic diseases: anti-DNA antibody tests. Arthritis Rheum 2002;47:546–555.

[14] Benito-Garcia E, Schur PH, Lahita R, et al. Guidelines for immunologic laboratory testing in the rheumatic diseases: anti-Sm and anti-RNP antibody tests. Arthritis Rheum 2004;51:1030–44.

[15] Meroni PL, Schur PH. ANA screening: an old test with new recommendations. Ann Rheum Dis 2010;69:1420–2.

[16] Agmon-Levin N, Damoiseaux J, Kallenberg C, et al. International recommendations for the assessment of autoantibodies to cellular antigens referred to as anti-nuclear antibodies. Ann Rheum Dis 2014;73:17–23.

[17] Chan EK, Damoiseaux J, Carballo OG, et al. Report of the first international consensus on standardized nomenclature of antinuclear antibody HEp-2 cell patterns 2014-2015. Front Immunol 2015;6:412.

[18] Damoiseaux J, von Mühlen CA, Garcia-De La Torre I, et al. International consensus on ANA patterns (ICAP): the bumpy road towards a consensus on reporting ANA results. Auto Immun Highlights 2016;7:1.

[19] Mahler M, Meroni PL, Bossuyt X, et al. Current concepts and future directions for the assessment of autoantibodies to cellular antigens referred to as anti-nuclear antibodies. J Immunol Res 2014;2014:315179.

[20] Miyakis S, Lockshin MD, Atsumi T, et al. International consensus statement on an update of the classification criteria for definite antiphospholipid syndrome (APS). J Thromb Haemost 2006;4:295–306.

[21] Mehrani T, Petri M. Association of IgA Anti-beta2 glycoprotein I with clinical and laboratory manifestations of systemic lupus erythematosus. J Rheumatol 2011;38:64–8.

[22] Orbai AM, Truedsson L, Sturfelt G, et al. Anti-C1q antibodies in systemic lupus erythematosus. Lupus 2015;24:42–9.

[23] Shiboski SC, Shiboski CH, Criswell LA, et al. American College of Rheumatology classification criteria for Sjögren's syndrome: a data-driven, expert consensus approach in the Sjögren's International Collaborative Clinical Alliance cohort. Arthritis Care Res (Hoboken) 2012;64:475–87.

[24] Quartuccio L, Baldini C, Priori R, et al. Cryoglobulinemia in Sjögren syndrome: a disease subset that links higher systemic disease activity, autoimmunity, and local B cell proliferation in mucosa-associated lymphoid tissue. J Rheumatol 2017;44:1179–83.

[25] Damoiseaux J, Cohen Tervaert JW. Diagnostics and treatment of cryoglobulinaemia: it takes two to tango. Clin Rev Allergy Immunol 2014;47:299–310.

[26] Op De Beeck K, Vermeersch P, Verschueren P, et al. Detection of antinuclear antibodies by indirect immunofluorescence and by solid phase assay. Autoimmun Rev 2011;10:801–8.

[27] Ghillani P, André C, Toly C, et al. Clinical significance of anti-Ro52 (TRIM21) antibodies non-associated with anti-SSA 60kDa antibodies: results of a multicentric study. Autoimmun Rev 2011;10:509–13.

[28] Damoiseaux J, Agmon-Levin N, Van Blerk M, et al. From ANA-screening to antigen-specificity: an EASI-survey on the daily practice in European countries. Clin Exp Rheumatol 2014;32:539–46.

[29] van den Hoogen F, Khanna D, Fransen J, et al. 2013 classification criteria for systemic sclerosis: an American College of Rheumatology/European League against Rheumatism collaborative initiative. Arthritis Rheum 2013;65:2737–47.

[30] Dellavance A, Gallindo C, Soares MG, et al. Redefining the Scl-70 indirect immunofluorescence pattern: autoantibodies to DNA topoisomerase I yield a specific compound immunofluorescence pattern. Rheumatology (Oxford) 2009;48:632–7.

[31] Damoiseaux J. Are autoantibodies to RNA-polymerase III to be incorporated in routine diagnostic laboratory algorithms for systemic autoimmune rheumatic diseases? Ann Rheum Dis 2014;73:e29.

[32] Bonroy C, Smith V, Van Steendam K, et al. The integration of the detection of systemic sclerosis-associated antibodies in a routine laboratory setting: comparison of different strategies. Clin Chem Lab Med 2013;51:2151–60.

[33] Bonroy C, Van Praet J, Smith V, et al. Optim ization and diagnostic performance of a single multiparameter lineblot in the serological workup of systemic sclerosis. J Immunol Methods 2012;379:53–60.

[34] Baroni SS, Santillo M, Bevilacqua F, et al. Stimulatory autoantibodies to the PDGF receptor in systemic sclerosis. N Engl J Med 2006;354:2667–76.

[35] Cabral-Marques O, Riemekasten G. Functional autoantibodies targeting G protein-coupled receptors in rheumatic diseases. Nat Rev Rheumatol 2017;13:648–56.

[36] Sharp GC, Irvin WS, Tan EM, et al. Mixed connective tissue disease—an apparently distinct rheumatic disease syndrome associated with a specific antibody to an extractable nuclear antigen (ENA). Am J Med 1972;52:148–59.

[37] Alarcon-Segovia D, Cardiel MH. Comparison between 3 diagnostic criteria for mixed connective tissue disease. Study of 593 patients. J Rheumatol 1989;16:328–34.

[38] Bohan A, Peter JB. Polymyositis and dermatomyositis (first of two parts). N Engl J Med 1975;292:344–7.

[39] Senécal JL, Raynauld JP, Troyanov Y. Editorial: a new classification of adult autoimmune myositis. Arthritis Rheum 2017;69:878–84.

[40] Benveniste O, Stenzel W, Allenbach Y. Advances in serological diagnostics of inflammatory myopathies. Curr Opin Neurol 2016;29:662–73.

[41] Musset L, Allenbach Y, Benveniste O, et al. Anti-HMGCR antibodies as a biomarker for immune-mediated necrotizing myopathies: a history of statins and experience from a large international multi-center study. Autoimmun Rev 2016;15:983–93.

[42] Mammen AL. Statin-associated autoimmune myopathy. N Engl J Med 2016;374:664–9.

[43] Herbert MK, Stammen-Vogelzangs J, Verbeek MM, et al. Disease specificity of autoantibodies to cytosolic 5'-nucleotidase 1A in sporadic inclusion body myositis versus known autoimmune diseases. Ann Rheum Dis 2016;75:696–701.

[44] Damoiseaux J. Multiparametric autoimmune diagnostics: recent advances. Pathol Lab Med Int 2016;8:15–25.

[45] Pengo V, Tripodi G, Reber G, et al. Update of the guidelines for lupus anticoagulant detection. J Thromb Haemost 2009;7:1737–40.

[46] Pengo V. ISTH guidelines on lupus anticoagulant testing. Thromb Res 2012;130:S76–7.

[47] Moore GW. Recent guidelines and recommendations for laboratory detection of lupus anticoagulants. Semin Thromb Hemost 2014;40:163–71.

[48] Hoxha A, Banzato A, Ruffatti A, et al. Detection of lupus anticoagulant in the era of direct oral anticoagulants. Autoimmun Rev 2017;16:173–8.

[49] Harris EN. The second international anticardiolipin standardization workshop: the Kingston Anticardiolipin Antibody Study (KAPS) group. Am J Clin Pathol 1990;101:616–24.

[50] Willis R, Grossi C, Orietta Borghi M, et al. International standards for IgG and IgM anti-β2glycoprotein antibody measurement. Lupus 2014;23:1317–9.

[51] Willis R, Pierangeli SS, Jaskowski TD, et al. Performance characteristics of commercial immunoassays for the detection of IgG and IgM antibodies to β2 glycoprotein I and an initial assessment of newly developed reference materials for assay calibration. Am J Clin Pathol 2016;145:796–805.

[52] Sciascia S, Amigo MC, Roccatello D, et al. Diagnosing antiphospholipid syndrome: 'extra-criteria' manifestations and technical advances. Nat Rev Rheumatol 2017;13:548–60.

[53] Mahler M, Norman GL, Meroni PL, et al. Autoantibodies to domain 1 of beta 2 glycoprotein 1: a promising candidate biomarker for risk management in antiphospholipid syndrome. Autoimmun Rev 2012;12:313–7.

[54] Sciascia S, Sanna G, Murru V, et al. Anti-prothrombin (aPT) and anti-phosphatidylserine/prothrombin (aPS/PT) antibodies and the risk of thrombosis in the antiphospholipid syndrome. A systematic review. Thromb Haemost 2014;111:354–64.

[55] Sciascia A, Sanna G, Murru V, et al. GAPSS: the global anti-phospholipid syndrome score. Rheumatology (Oxford) 2013;52:1397–403.

[56] Bossuyt X, Cohen Tervaert JW, Arimura Y, et al. Position paper: revised 2017 international consensus on testing of ANCAs in granulomatosis with polyangiitis and microscopic polyangiitis. Nat Rev Rheumatol 2017;13:683–92.

[57] Savige J, Gillis D, Benson E, et al. International consensus statement on testing and reporting of antineutrophil cytoplasmic antibodies (ANCA). Am J Clin Pathol 1999;111:507–13.

[58] Damoiseaux J, Csernok E, Rasmussen N, et al. Detection of antineutrophil cytoplasmic antibodies (ANCAs): a multicentre European Vasculitis Study Group (EUVAS) evaluation of the value of indirect immunofluorescence (IIF) versus antigen-specific immunoassays. Ann Rheum Dis 2017;76:647–53.

[59] Bossuyt X. Clinical performance characteristics of a laboratory test. A practical approach in the autoimmune laboratory. Autoimmun Rev 2009;8:543–548.

[60] Van Hoovels L, Jacobs J, Vander Cruyssen B, et al. Performance characteristics of rheumatoid factor and anti-cyclic citrullinated peptide antibody assays may impact ACR/EULAR classification of rheumatoid arthritis. Ann Rheum Dis 2018;77:667–77.

Chapter 11

Anti-DFS70 Antibodies: A New Protective Autoantibodies?

Dolores Pérez

Zabludowitz Center for Autoimmune Diseases, Sheba Medical Center, Tel-Hashomer, Israel

Antibodies producing a dense fine speckled (DFS) pattern on the antinuclear antibodies indirect immunofluorescence (IIF) assay on HEp-2 cells, which also recognized the dense fine speckled autoantigen of 70 kD (DFS70). The nuclear DFS-IIF staining pattern is recognized as a unique speckled pattern distributed throughout interphase nuclei and metaphase chromatin [1].

The DFS pattern is highly subjective and vulnerable to suffer variations according to the manufacturer of HEp-2 cells. Consequently, the recognition of the DFS pattern is challenging and the anti-DFS70 antibodies require the confirmation with specific immunoassays. The anti-DFS70 autoantibodies can be detected by different solid phase assays with high specificity such as ELISA, line immunoblot, or chemiluminescence assay. However, the development of two specific assays for the detection of anti-DFS70 antibodies has improved the specificity of the IIF for the detection of these autoantibodies. These assays are the immunoabsorption test and the use of HEp-2 cells knock-out for the DFS70 protein [2,3].

The autoantigen was initially termed DFS70 according to the IIF pattern but was later identified as the lens epithelium grown factor of 75 kD (LEDGF/p75), a DNA binding transcription coactivator, which plays an important role in promoting resistance to stress-induced cell death in inflammation, autoimmune conditions, and cancer. DFS70 is upregulated in a variety of cells and tissues in response to environmental stressors (viral infections, cytotoxic drugs, ultraviolet B, hyperthermia) and promotes cell survival by engaging in multiple complexes in the chromatin and transcriptionally activating stress-protective, antioxidant, and inflammatory-related genes. In addition, this protein is involved in the mechanism of human immunodeficiency virus 1 (HIV-1), a new prointegration on the host cells by direct interaction with HIV-integrate (HIV-IN) [4,5].

The anti-DFS70 antibodies are preferably detected in apparently healthy individuals with prevalence around 10%. The prevalence in patients with SARD ranges between 0.5% and 3% [6]. Anti DFS70 antibodies are rarely found in SARD patients and when present, they are usually accompanied by the presence of additional SARD-related autoantigens. The anti-DFS70 antibodies are more frequent in people younger than 30–35 years old. The autoantibodies are typically immunoglobulin G and can circulate in high titer in apparently healthy individuals who stay healthy after years of follow-up. Consequently, the presence of isolated anti-DFS70 antibodies has been proposed as a valuable biomarker that helps to role out a diagnosis of SARD, including systemic lupus erythematosus, systemic sclerosis, Sjögren syndrome, idiopathic inflammatory myopathies, and mixed connective tissue disease [7,8].

These autoantibodies can be found in patients with diverse inflammatory conditions such as autoantibodies related to chronic inflammatory conditions, autoimmune thyroiditis, in Vogt–Koyanagi–Harada syndrome, atopic dermatitis, in prostate cancer, and eye diseases. However, the clinical relevance of these antibodies in the diseases remains largely unclear. None of the associations were verified unambiguously and became part of routine diagnosis so far [9].

The clinical and biological significance of the anti-DFS70 antibodies is still unclear. Depending on the context, they could play various roles. Because of his high prevalence in healthy subjects, it has been suggested that the anti-DFS70 antibodies are natural autoantibodies. The anti-DFS70 antibodies may serve a protective role by removing the DFS70 protein and its cleavage fragments from cellular debris generation during noninflammatory apoptotic cell death. The anti-DFS70 antibodies could confer a protective advantage to patients due to blockade of its HIV-IN binding functions [5]. They could also play a pathogenic role by binding to extracellular released DFS70 autoantigens and by preventing it from entering cells where it could activate a stress survival pathway. The antibodies could be indicative of an undetected chronic inflammatory response because they are associated with increased oxidative stress and aberrant expression or functions of the DFS70 antigen that alters its immunogenicity [10]. The clinical significance of the anti-DFS70 antibodies in health and disease is still unclear.

Mosaic of Autoimmunity. https://doi.org/10.1016/B978-0-12-814307-0.00011-6

REFERENCES

[1] Bentow C, Fritzler MJ, Mummert E, Mahler M. Recognition of the dense fine speckled (DFS) pattern remains challenging: results from an international internet-based survey. Auto Immun Highlights December 2016;7(1):8.

[2] Bizzaro N, Pesente F, Cucchiaro F, Infantino M, Tampoia M, Villalta D, et al. Anti-DFS70 antibodies detected by immunoblot methods: a reliable tool to confirm the dense fine speckles ANA pattern. J Immunol Methods September 2016;436:50–3.

[3] Bentow C, Rosenblum R, Correia P, Karayev E, Karayev D, Williams D, et al. Development and multi-center evaluation of a novel immunoadsorption method for anti-DFS70 antibodies. Lupus July 2016;25(8):897–904.

[4] Perez D, Azoulay D. Anti-DFS70 autoantibodies in HIV-1-positive individuals. Curr Opin Rheumatol July 2018;30(4):361–4.

[5] Basu A, Sanchez TW, Casiano CA. DFS70/LEDGFp75: an enigmatic autoantigen at the interface between autoimmunity, AIDS, and cancer. Front Immunol 2015;6:116.

[6] Shovman O, Gilburd B, Chayat C, Amital H, Langevitz P, Watad A, et al. Prevalence of anti-DFS70 antibodies in patients with and without systemic autoimmune rheumatic diseases. Clin Exp Rheumatol July 27, 2017.

[7] Seelig CA, Bauer O, Seelig HP. Autoantibodies against DFS70/LEDGF exclusion markers for systemic autoimmune rheumatic diseases (SARD). Clin Lab 2016;62(4):499–517.

[8] Mahler M, Parker T, Peebles CL, Andrade LE, Swart A, Carbone Y, et al. Anti-DFS70/LEDGF antibodies are more prevalent in healthy individuals compared to patients with systemic autoimmune rheumatic diseases. J Rheumatol November 2012;39(11):2104–10.

[9] Conrad K, Rober N, Andrade LE, Mahler M. The clinical relevance of anti-DFS70 autoantibodies. Clin Rev Allergy Immunol April 2017;52(2):202–16.

[10] Mahler M, Meroni PL, Andrade LE, Khamashta M, Bizzaro N, Casiano CA, et al. Towards a better understanding of the clinical association of anti-DFS70 autoantibodies. Autoimmun Rev February 2016;15(2):198–201.

Chapter 12

Genetics and Autoimmunity: Recent News

Carlo Perricone[1], Cinzia Ciccacci[2], Fulvia Ceccarelli[1], Enrica Cipriano[1], Andrea Latini[2], Giuseppe Novelli[2], Paola Borgiani[2], Fabrizio Conti[1]

[1]Rheumatology, Department of Internal Medicine, Sapienza University of Rome, Rome, Italy; [2]Department of Biomedicine and Prevention, Section of Genetics, School of Medicine, University of Rome Tor Vergata, Rome, Italy

INTRODUCTION

Autoimmune diseases (ADs) have a complex pathogenesis in which an interaction between individual genetic predisposition and environmental, hormonal and immunological factors lead to protean clinical forms with specific features [1]. The genes involved in autoimmunity confer susceptibility or resistance to infections, increase the risk of developing an allergic or autoimmune reaction and often codify for antibodies, cytokines, and surface antigens active in cell recognition. Variations in these genes cause dysfunctions in the immune system and underlie immunodeficiencies, ADs, allergies, and cancer [1].

Several studies suggest the need of a genetic predisposition in the pathogenesis of ADs [2]. For instance, when considering systemic lupus erythematosus (SLE), a higher frequency of the disease has been demonstrated in identical twins compared with dizygotic twins, with a concordance rate of 24%–57% compared to 6.2% in dizygotic twins [2]. In addition, family members of patients with SLE have a higher risk of developing the disease ranging from 5% to 12% [3]. Moreover, the disease has a greater frequency in some ethnic groups as in Asian populations, Afro-American and Afro-Caribbean [4].

Moreover, ADs, such as SLE, can be rarely monogenic and more frequently polygenic. For instance, SLE can result from a deficiency of a single genetic factor (for example, the components of complement C1q and C4), but more frequently from the combined effect of variations in a large number of genes [4].

The genetic contribution of ADs has been mainly evaluated by means of two approaches: the linkage studies in the past decades and, more recently, the association studies [5]. Regarding the linkage studies, genome scans use polymorphisms to identify susceptibility loci in multiplex families. They rely on either multiallelic markers (polymorphic microsatellites) spaced at regular intervals on the genome or the far more numerous biallelic markers. Genetic material from at least two affected siblings (affected sib pairs, ASPs) must be available. Linkage manifests as greater locus similarity in ASPs than predicted by Mendelian laws. Chromosomal regions exhibiting increased alleles sharing are likely to contain susceptibility genes. A huge advantage of this approach is that no preliminary hypothesis (e.g., regarding the position of loci) is required. On the contrary, the association studies can be used to test candidate susceptibility genes. A gene may be a likely candidate either because of its function or the potential pathophysiological impact of its allelic variants or because of its location within a region of interest identified by genome screening. In the case–control approach, unrelated patients are compared to unrelated matched healthy controls of identical ethnicity, so that presence of the disease is ideally the only difference between the two groups. This study is easy to conduct, but bias related to differences between cases and controls is difficult to eliminate (stratification bias) and it may lead to false-positive findings due to random differences in genotype distribution between the two groups [5].

In last decades, the improving of genomic technology has seen the advent of genome-wide association (GWA) studies that allowed to investigate hundreds of thousands of SNPs contemporary without an a priori hypothesis [6].

In recent years, the study of genetic of ADs received a big impulse by the use of large-scale genotyping studies and by comprehensive gene expression analysis that allowed to identify key molecular pathways, but also by epigenetic studies, as epigenetic signatures have been found to be involved in various disease etiologies. Nowadays, new genome-based applications have made their appearance into modern clinical practice with next-generation sequencing opening a new door on the road to the full determination of the genetic mechanisms of ADs [7].

Mosaic of Autoimmunity. https://doi.org/10.1016/B978-0-12-814307-0.00012-8

THE HUMAN LEUKOCYTE ANTIGEN SYSTEM

The major histocompatibility complex (MHC) system is the most polymorphic gene cluster of the mammal genome. In humans, this is a genomic locus extended to approximately 3.6 Mb located on the short arm of chromosome 6 (6p21.3), and it is known as the human leukocyte antigen (HLA) system. The concept of the extended MHC, spanning about 7.6 Mb of the genome, has been recently established by the finding that linkage disequilibrium (LD) and MHC-related genes exist outside the classically defined locus [8]. The fact that there are genes inherited in close association with HLA alleles contributes to reinforce the idea that many genes are involved in the development of ADs and explains how the positivity of a single polymorphism is not enough to develop the disease.

HUMAN LEUKOCYTE ANTIGEN GENES AND AUTOIMMUNE DISEASES

The molecular mechanism underlying the associations between MHC (HLA) and autoimmune diseases has not yet been fully clarified. In many cases it reflects LD phenomena between HLA alleles and the physically mapped gene disease in the MHC region. In other cases, however, the association found reflects the amino acid structure of the HLA molecule. In fact, the primary function of HLA class II antigens is to bind the peptide antigens and to present them to CD4+ and CD8+ cells. Therefore, it is possible that some antigenic structures may be presented as autoantigens to the competent cells. Other proposed mechanisms concern the ability to influence the clonal selection of T cells, at thymic level, by some HLA alleles, or the stimulation of different cytokines.

The HLA encodes mostly immune-associated genes distributed in three regions: class I, class II, and class III, which are related by the structure and function of the proteins that they encode [9]. The main function of HLA gene products is the presentation of antigens to the immune cells. For instance, class I gene products (HLA-A, B, and C) are in charge of presenting endogenous peptides, which are usually related to viral infections. In contrast, the class II coded molecules (HLA-DR, DP, and DQ) present exogenous peptides such as bacterial antigens. Finally, the class III region codifies immune regulatory molecules, e.g., tumor necrosis factor (TNF), C3, C4, and C5 of complement and heat shock proteins [10].

From the evolutionary point of view, the HLA system is highly conserved as its proper function is crucial for the immune response against pathogens. The proteins codified in this region regulate and interact with other proteins, which can be codified within the same region or not. This system must ensure the correct recognition and presentation of a tremendous diversity of pathogens and potentially harmer factors. Therefore, even if these proteins are highly conserved, their genes are also the most polymorphic; in particular those codifying for HLA class I and II. This variability is represented in a huge number of alleles, which cause slight variations in the structure of the proteins giving to a single individual the capability to react against different pathogens conserving the essential structure and the function [11,12]. For instance, at September 2018, the number of alleles reported for human HLA I and II is 18,771 (http://hla.alleles.org/nomenclature/stats.html). Indeed, the number of different alleles in HLA class I is 13,680, whereas for class II is 5091. The comparison between the genomic sequences of class I and class II alleles shows that variations, in particular, nucleotide substitutions, are concentrated in the exons that encode areas that directly interact with the pathogen molecules and with the T cell receptor [13].

Polymorphisms in HLA class II genes and haplotypes have been associated with multiple ADs. HLA class II molecules (HLADR, HLADQ, and HLADP) are exclusively expressed in immunocompetent or antigen-presenting cells (i.e., macrophages) to present peptides to T helper cells. HLA-DR is αβ heterodimer composed by two different subunits codified by the HLA-DRA locus for the DR-α chain, and by four loci, of which no more than three are functional and no more than two on a single chromosome, for the DR-β chain. HLA-DP and DQ have also two subunits encoded by two loci, DPA1 and DPB1 and DQA and DQB, respectively. The interaction of both molecules forms a groove between the alfa 1 and the beta 1 domains where peptides from exogenous origin can bind [14]. There is strong LD within this region; for instance, the HLA-DRB1 is strongly linked to the HLA-DQB1.

The HLA-DRB1 gene codifies for the beta chain of one of the HLA-II being the most polymorphic gene within the HLA II region, followed by HLA-DPB1 and HLA-DQB1. The distribution of single nucleotide polymorphisms within the HLA region is higher in the Beta1 domain, which is the region in contact with the foreign peptides that will be presented to the immune system. This fact gives to all individuals a better chance to respond to a more widely range of infections [15]. Because of such high variability, genetic studies have shown the strong association between HLA-DRB1 polymorphisms and different diseases, in particular those with an autoimmune fingerprint (Table 12.1).

The mechanisms relating HLA polymorphisms and ADs are not clearly understood. One long-held view suggests a breakdown in immunological tolerance to self-antigens through aberrant class II presentation of self or foreign peptides to autoreactive T lymphocytes [16]. It seems likely that specific MHC-II alleles determine the targeting of particular autoantigens resulting in disease-specific associations. Interestingly, a metaanalysis performed in Latin American populations

TABLE 12.1 *HLA-DRB1* Risk Polymorphisms in Several Autoimmune Diseases

Disease	HLA Allele	Population
Diabetes mellitus type 1	DRB1*03,*04,*04:01,*04:02,*04:05	Latin American, Caucasians
Multiple sclerosis	DRB1*15:01,*15:03	Latin American, Caucasians
Rheumatoid arthritis	HLA-DRB1*01:01,*01:02,*04:01, *04:04,*04:05,*04:05,*04:08	Caucasians, Israeli, Latin Americans, Japanese
Autoimmune hepatitis	DRB1*13:01	
Antiphospholipid syndrome		
Celiac disease	Non-DRB1	
Systemic lupus erythematous	DRB1*03:01,*15:01,*08:01	Latin American, Caucasians
Sjögren's syndrome	DRB1*03:01,*11:01,*11:04	Latin American, Caucasians, Israelis
Ankylosing spondylitis	Non-DRB1	
Psoriatic arthritis	Non-DRB1	
Myasthenia gravis	DRB1*15:01	Caucasians
Primary biliary cirrhosis	DRB1*08,*14	Caucasians
Pemphigus vulgaris	DRB1*14	Caucasians
Autoimmune thrombotic thrombocytopenic purpura	DRB1*11	Caucasians
Giant cell arteritis	DRB1*04	Caucasians
Macrophagic myofasciitis	DRB1*01	Caucasians

of six different ADs showed that specific polymorphisms in the HLA-DRB1 are shared between more than one AD. To be precise, the allele DRB1*04·01 is a risk factor for Type 1 diabetes (T1D) and rheumatoid arthritis (RA); DRB1*03:01 is associated with T1D, SLE, and SS; and, finally, the DRB1*04:05 is associated with T1D, RA, and autoimmune hepatitis [17]. In SLE in the last years, the major susceptibility genes observed through candidate gene studies were HLA-DRB1, FcγR2A, PTPN22, and STAT4. In recent times, the more extensive usage of the GWA studies allowed the discovery of novel loci associated with the disease [18,19]. These findings have made possible to classify the manifestations of SLE in different categories: those influenced by the cumulative effects of multiple genes, those influenced by a single gene locus, and those that to date does not appear to correlate with a particular genetic predisposition. The most significant reported association is with the HLA class II, although a number of factors, including long-range LD across disease-associated haplotypes, have hampered investigations and association. The most consistent HLA II association with SLE resides with HLA-DRB1*0301 (DR3) and HLA-DRB1*1501 (DR2) and their respective haplotypes in Caucasian populations [20]. In 2002, a family-based association study identified three microsatellite-inferred risk haplotypes in European lupus families: DRB1*1501/DQB1*0602, DRB1*0301/DQB1*0201, and DRB1*0801/DQB1*0402 [21]. Studies have demonstrated the role of these alleles not only in the onset of the disease but also in modulating the presence of specific clinical and laboratory manifestations. In particular HLADRB1*1501 (DR2) has been associated with positivity for anti-dsDNA and an increased risk of developing renal involvement [21]. Bang et al. have investigated the association of HLA-DRB1 alleles with SLE susceptibility and clinical features in a Korean population. They identified four HLA-DRB1 alleles associated with increased susceptibility to SLE (two previously detected alleles, *15:01 and *09:01; two novel alleles, *08:03 and *07:01). In addition, protective effects on the development of SLE were observed for two novel alleles (HLA-DRB1*12:02, *11:01). The SLE-risk alleles promoted the production of autoantibodies including anti-Sm and diverse clinical manifestations [22]. A recent metaanalysis concluded that the HLA-DR4, DR11, DR14 alleles might be protective factors for SLE, and HLA-DR3, DR9, DR15 were shown to be strong risk factors. In addition, HLA-DR4 and DR11 alleles might be protective factors for lupus nephritis and DR3 and DR15 suggest a risk role [23].

GENETIC BASES OF RHEUMATOID ARTHRITIS

RA (OMIM # 180300) is a chronic, autoimmune, systemic, inflammatory disease that mainly affects the joints. This multifactorial disease leads to the progressive destruction of the joints. Environmental and genetic factors seem to be responsible for susceptibility and disease phenotype. The prevalence of RA ranges from 2% to 12% in patients' first-degree relatives and rises to 12%–30% in dyzygotic twins and 5%–10% in monozygotic twins, compared to a prevalence in the general population of 0.2%–1% in most ethnic groups. Surprisingly, some Native American groups show a relatively higher prevalence (>2%), while it is low in African populations and in Southeast Asia (<0.3%) [24,25]. There are at least 30 genetic regions found associated with RA [26].

The region with the most significant association is once again the HLA. Several studies have shown an association with the HLA-DR region, which represents a highly polymorphic group, and mostly with alleles of the HLA-DRB1 gene [27], particularly in patients with antibodies directed against citrullinated proteins and peptides (ACPA). This region is called the shared epitope because several alleles share a common tract of amino acid residues. It is currently believed that all HLA-DRB1 alleles of the shared epitope region are able to provide antigens that increase susceptibility to RA, as well as the likelihood of developing a more aggressive, more erosive, and rapidly progressive disease phenotype. In a Korean population, patients heterozygous for HLA-DRB1*0405 or *0901 have an increased risk (up to 60 times) of developing RA.

An environmental factor that seems to interact with HLA-DRB1 alleles is cigarette smoking (see relative chapter), and a synergistic gene–environment effect, among HLA-DRB1, PTPN22, and cigarette smoking, and the development of a seropositive disease phenotype has been demonstrated [28].

Recently, GWA studies have permitted that numerous genes have been identified outside the HLA region in association not only with predisposition to disease but also to the clinical phenotypes and response to therapies.

Among these, Peptidylarginine deiminases citrullinating enzyme 4 (PADI4), protein tyrosine phosphatase, nonreceptor type 22 (PTPN22), tumor necrosis factor receptor-associated factor 1, complement component 5 (TRAF1-C5), signal transducer and activator of transcription 4 (STAT4), and Fcγ receptors (FCGR) seem to show the most significant associations.

The genetic association with PTPN22, an intracellular tyrosine phosphatase that encodes for LYP, a potent T cell activation inhibitor, is of interest for several reasons. It shows the strongest association among non-HLA genes on Caucasian populations. The nonsynonymous polymorphism (rs2476601) at position 620 involves the mutation from arginine (R) to tryptophan (W). Although it has been shown that the 620W variant reduces the binding of PTPN22 to the Csk intracellular kinase, it is unclear exactly how this variant is able to influence the risk of disease. The presence of a single copy of the 620W allele almost doubles the risk of developing RA, while with two copies of the 620W, the risk is three times higher. It has been hypothesized that a less-effective downregulation of T cells can occur, leading to an increased risk of developing autoimmunity [29,30].

Some genes moreover seem to have the ability to influence the course of the disease. For instance, in a study of our group, not only we confirmed an association with rs7574865 in the STAT4 gene, and a protective effect of rs1800872 in the IL10 gene, but we also described associations with clinical phenotypes [31]. The presence of rheumatoid factor was associated with rs1800872 variant in IL10, whereas rs2910164 in MIR146A showed a protective effect. ACPA were associated significantly with rs7574865 in STAT4. The SNP rs2233945 in the PSORS1C1 gene was protective regarding the presence of bone erosions, whereas rs2542151 in PTPN2 gene was associated with joint damage [31]. In another study, we found that polymorphisms in STAT4, PTPN2, PSORS1C1, and TRAF3IP2 are associated with response to TNF-i treatment in RA patients, suggesting that genes may be used in the future as predictors of response to biological therapies [32].

GENETICS OF SYSTEMIC LUPUS ERYTHEMATOSUS

SLE and other ADs share many of the risk loci identified, suggesting the involvement of common pathways in ADs. Moreover, the existence of common genetic susceptibility was already suggested by the clustering of multiple ADs within families, including families with SLE. This genetic overlap is exemplified by the well-known associations of certain HLA loci with multiple AD as well as non-HLA risk loci in different pathways such as STAT4 and IL-10. In this context, Th17 and B cell-mediated pathways seem to play a major role in disease pathogenesis [2].

Moreover, type I interferon (IFN) has an important pathogenic role in SLE. Some variants of the IFN regulatory factor 5 (IRF5) gene are associated with an increased risk of SLE. IRF5 encodes for a transcription factor responsible for the innate immune response during viral infections. The IFN regulatory factors are a family of transcriptional regulators that have a DNA-binding domain [33,34]. IRF5 is expressed by B cells and dendritic cells and activates genes of encoding for inflammatory cytokines, including TNF, IL-12, IL-6, and IFN [35]. In fact, a large GWA, subsequently replicated, showed a strong association between polymorphisms of IRF5 and SLE. This association was firstly found in Scandinavian populations and later confirmed in other populations [36]. Yet, little is known about the functional significance of IRF5 SNPs. Feng et al. recently evaluated the contribution of four risk alleles (CGGGG ins/del, r22004640, rs10954213, and rs10488631) in IRF5 gene in modifying transcription and expression of IRF5 protein in SLE [37]. In their study, the authors suggested that patients with SLE have a higher expression of IRF5. Similarly, the expression of the IRF5 protein has been associated with the risk haplotype H2, and the expression of IRF5 was upregulated in 25% of monocytes and myeloid dendritic cells of patients carrying homozygous H2 haplotype. These results suggest that the high levels of IFN observed in SLE patients could be due to genetic variants associated with aberrant expression of IRF5 [37].

The polymorphisms of some genes associated with SLE are involved in T mediated pathways (CD3-ζ9 and PP2Ac10). A recent study identified TNIP1, PRDM1, JAZF1, UHRF1BP1, and IL10 as risk loci for SLE [38]. An alteration in the number of copies of certain genes such as C4, FCGR3B, and TLR7, has been linked to SLE susceptibility [39]. A locus on the long arm of chromosome 1 (1q23-24) in which the genes encoding for the C-reactive protein are located—the so-called pentraxin locus—was associated with susceptibility to SLE in several populations [40,41].

TREX1 is a gene that encodes a protein acting as an intracellular DNase in mammals. Some polymorphisms of TREX1 showed a correlation with the presence of anti-SSA/Ro and anti-dsDNA antibodies in SLE patients [42]. Moreover, an association between a DNase (DNaseI) and SLE had been previously reported [43]. TREX1 causes damage to the single-stranded DNA during caspase-independent apoptosis activated by granzyme A. Mutations of TREX1 cause Aicardi-Goutièrs (AGS1) syndrome, a rare progressive familiar encephalopathy with autosomal dominant inheritance, developing in pediatric age and characterized by high levels of IFN in the cerebrospinal fluid. Mutations associated with the AGS destroy the catalytic activity of TREX1. It is assumed that the loss of the enzyme activity causes the accumulation of altered DNA that can trigger a destructive autoimmune response [44]. TREX1 is also a potential candidate gene because there are recent reports of mutations in this gene in patients with familial chilblain lupus, a monogenic form of cutaneous lupus erythematosus [45,46].

BANK1 is a gene that encodes for a B lymphocyte-specific tyrosine kinase that is able to promote the phosphorylation of receptor for inositol 1,4,5-triphosphate. Some SNPs have recently been associated with susceptibility to SLE in patients of different geographic origin [47,48]. The B lymphocyte activation mediated by this receptor leads to phosphorylation of BANK1, which in turn is associated with the tyrosine kinases Lyn and to the calcium channel IP3R, leading to the phosphorylation of IP3R mediated by Lyn, and the consequent leakage of calcium from the endoplasmic reticulum. We know that the B lymphocyte activation is a key stage in the pathogenesis of SLE, leading to autoantibody production and the consequent development of autoreactive clones able to promote autoimmunity.

Two loci, C8orf13-BLK on chromosome 8 and ITGAM-ITGAX on chromosome 16, have been associated with SLE in genome-wide studies [16]. The most likely candidate genes within these loci are BLK and ITGAM. The family of tyrosine kinase Src-BLK is a new and interesting candidate gene locus for SLE. The expression of BLK is limited to the B cell line. The expression of BLK in mice is observed at the end of the cell cycle in pro-B cells and continues throughout the development of B cells, whereas it is consequently downregulated in plasma cells. It was hypothesized that BLK is a tyrosine kinase capable of transducing signals downstream of the B cell receptor and which has a redundant role in murine models (given the lack of a specific phenotype in mice-deficient BLK). The hypothesis is that impaired levels of BLK protein could affect the mechanisms of tolerance of B cells, predisposing to the development of systemic ADs. A similar mechanism has recently been shown for Ly108, a major genetic locus in the NZM2410 lupus mouse model. A haplotype of the C8orf13 gene, linked to BLK, has been associated with the disease, but the function of this gene is unknown. Variants of ITGAM/ITGAX were found associated with susceptibility to lupus in genome-wide association studies [49] and in replication studies [50–52]. ITGAM (also known as CD11b, Mac-1, and the complement receptor C3) is a molecule belonging to the family of alpha chain integrins, which is expressed by a variety of myeloid cells including dendritic cells, macrophages, monocytes, and neutrophils. ITGAM forms a heterodimer with the integrin beta-2 (ITGB2, or CD18) and mediates the adhesion between different immune system cells as well as the adhesion of myeloid cell to endothelium. ITGAM-deficient mice have a more rapid progression and worse disease outcome. ITGAM can suppress the differentiation of Th17 cells, thereby impairing the induction of autoimmune phenomena [53].

Among other non-HLA genes, several genes have been found associated with diseases susceptibility as well as with some specific disease features. For instance, polymorphisms of TRAF3 interacting protein 2 (TRAF3IP2), a gene localized on chromosome 6q21 that encodes for Act1, were found associated with the disease and the onset of pericarditis. Act1 is a negative regulator of humoral immunity as well as a positive signaling adaptor of IL-17–dependent NF-kB activation [54]. The activities mediated by Act1 are crucial to determine the events downstream of the signaling induced by IL-17 (e.g., the activation of NFκB, JNK, ERK) and the expression of proinflammatory genes (KC, GM-CSF, and IL-6) [55]. Studies on TRAF3IP2-deficient mice suggest that Act1 is a negative regulator of humoral immunity through its inhibitory effects on the signaling mediated by CD40 and the BAFFR [56]. It has been demonstrated that Act1-deficient Balb/c mice develop

Sjogren's syndrome in association with lupus nephritis and high titers of anti-SSA/Ro and anti-SSB/La antibodies as a result of hyper-functionality of B cells [57]. This is in agreement with another study that showed a reduced expression of TRAF3IP2 in peripheral B cell transcriptomas from quiescent lupus patients [58] (Fig. 12.1).

We can assume that a loss of function of the protein can lead to a hyperactivation of B cells (similar to what is observed in mouse models) or a dysregulation of the Th17 immune response.

STAT4 is another non-HLA gene associated with SLE. The STAT4 rs7574865 polymorphism, located within the third intron of the gene, shows the strongest association with several autoimmune conditions [59,60], such as SLE, RA, type 1 and 2 diabetes, systemic sclerosis (SSc), inflammatory bowel diseases, primary Sjogren's syndrome, juvenile idiopathic arthritis, primary antiphospholipid syndrome, autoimmune thyroid diseases, multiple sclerosis, psoriasis, granulomatosis with polyangiitis, and giant cell arteritis [60].

The STAT4 gene can be activated and phosphorylated on ligation of the type I IFN receptor by IFN-α, and subsequently induce downstream transcription of IFN-α–induced genes [61]. It has been recently showed that a great number of genes target for STAT4 are involved in functional pathways in the type I IFN system and have key roles in the inflammatory response. Thus, by participating in transcription complex with other cofactors, STAT4 harbors the potential of regulating a large number of target genes, which may contribute to their strong association with SLE [62].

STAT4 is a cytosolic factor, which, after activation by cytokines, is phosphorylated and accumulated in the nucleus. Activated STAT4 stimulates the transcription of specific genes including IFN-γ, which is in turn leads to differentiation of T cells into T helper 1 lymphocytes (Th1) [63]. STAT4 is also involved in the differentiation of CD4+ Th17 [64]. This activity depends partly by IL-23 [65]. The proinflammatory Th17 cells may play an important if not predominant role in chronic inflammation. STAT4-deficient mouse models are generally resistant to ADs. Moreover, targeting STAT4 with specific inhibitory oligodeoxynucleotides or antisense oligonucleotides can improve a disease model of arthritis [66], suggesting

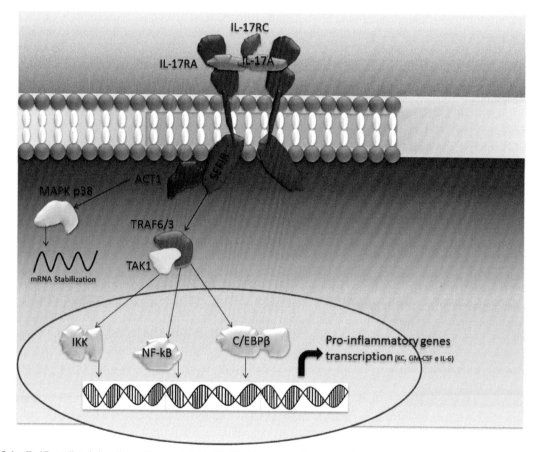

FIGURE 12.1   IL-17–mediated signaling pathways of Act 1. The IL-17R complex is composed of two subunits IL-17RA and IL-17RC. Both subunits encode for a SEFIR domain. On activation, the intracellular signaling pathways of IL-17 include an Act1-dependent path. The IL-17RA commits a domain SEFIR to recruit Act1. This protein contains a binding motif that can also bind TRAF3, TRAF6, and TAK1, resulting in the activation of the canonical NF-kB. Act1 is also required for the activation of p38 MAPK with the following stabilization of mRNA.

that STAT4 could be a therapeutic target. The rs7574865 polymorphism is associated with susceptibility to RA as well as to SLE [67]. The minor alleles are present in 27% of patients with RA, compared with 22% of controls [68]. The rs7574865 polymorphism is strongly associated with lupus, being the variant allele present in 31% of patients and in 22% of controls (OR for the risk allele = 1.55) [69].

It has been shown that the STAT4 SLE-risk allele rs7574865[T] is associated with increased IL-12–induced IFN-γ production in T cells from patients with SLE [70].

We also described an association with polymorphisms of HCP5 that are also associated with anti-SSA/Ro antibodies as well as with pericarditis [71]. The rs3099844 polymorphism has been previously described as involved in Steven Johnson Syndrome and Toxic Epidermal Necrolysis susceptibility [72,73], but also in another autoimmune condition, primary sclerosing cholangitis [74]. In this condition, anti-ENA including anti-SSA/Ro can be found in up to 11.5% of patients and anti-dsDNA at a lesser extent (1%–3% of patients). However, the most interesting study is a genome-wide association study showing an association between the rs3099844 and the cardiac manifestations of SLE [75]. As it is well known, this clinical condition is associated with the presence of anti-SSA/Ro antibodies [76–83]. Altogether, these data suggest a strong evidence of an association of such polymorphism with the anti-SSA/Ro antibodies, and further studies are awaited to clarify the specific underlying mechanisms. Moreover, in our study, we developed a risk model for pericarditis using the variant alleles of four SNPs: rs33980500 (TRAF3IP2 gene), rs1463335 (MIR1279 gene), rs7574865 (STAT4 gene), and rs2542151 (PTPN2 gene). Our model seems useful to define SLE patients more susceptible to develop such complication [84].

GENETICS OF SYSTEMIC SCLEROSIS

Systemic Sclerosis (SSc) is an AD characterized by vascular damage and fibrosis of the skin and internal organs. Various pathogenic factors contribute to its pathogenesis, such as viral infections, which act as trigger elements for the development of the clinical phenotype in genetically predisposed subjects. The most important risk factor for the development of the disease is having a first-degree relative affected. Over the past decade, more than 30 susceptibility genes have been associated with SSc; these include both HLA and non-HLA genes. Many of these genetic associations are shared with other ADs [85]. STAT4 in SSc may have important profibrotic properties acting on the activation and proliferation of T lymphocytes and on the release of proinflammatory cytokines. Knock-out mice for this gene, in fact, are protected by cutaneous fibrosis induced by bleomycin in experimental models [86]. Polymorphisms of the TNFSF4 gene (or OX40L, superfamily of the ligand of tumor necrosis factor 4) [87] have also been associated with the development of SSc. Several evidences have in fact shown higher levels of TNFSF4 in the peripheral blood of patients with SSc compared to healthy subjects [88]. IRAK1, a gene located on the X chromosome, is involved in both innate immunity and adaptive immunity and is the only gene present on a sex chromosome to be associated with the susceptibility to SSc, thus being able to explain the higher prevalence of the disease in females [89].

The BANK1 gene encodes a B cell membrane protein; two different studies have identified an allelic variant of SNP rs10516487 of this gene both as protective (less frequent in cases than controls) and as a risk factor (more frequent in cases than in controls) [90]. Given this contrasting result, the role of the allelic variant of BANK1 in susceptibility to SSc is unclear [90]. An allelic variant of the PTPN22 gene, coding for a tyrosine phosphatase, has been associated with numerous ADs, such as type 1 diabetes mellitus, SLE, RA, and subsequently also with the development of SSc in large cohorts of patients of different ethnic groups [91].

Genetic variants related to innate immunity and cytokines have been identified as associated with SSc, for example, genes of the IFN pathway family and of the toll-like receptors [92,93] and the MIF gene, which encodes by a factor of inhibition of macrophage migration and which induces the expression of adhesion molecules on the surface of endothelial cells, probably contributing to the vasculopathy of SSc [94].

GENETICS OF SJÖGREN'S SYNDROME

Sjögren's syndrome (SjS) is an autoimmune chronic and progressive exocrinopathy characterized by lymphocytic infiltration and destruction of salivary and lacrimal glands. The characteristic symptoms are represented by dry eyes and dry mouth, although any organ may be involved by the inflammatory process, making the clinical phenotype rather heterogeneous. Despite the high prevalence of the syndrome (0.5%–1%), its genetic and molecular bases have been little investigated compared to other ADs. The genetic factors primarily associated with SjS belong to the class II MHC [95]. For instance, the DR2-DQ1 haplotype is strongly correlated with the presence of anti-Ro/SSA antibodies, whereas the DR3-DQ2 haplotype seems to favor the production of both anti-Ro/SSA and anti-La/SSB antibodies. Also, SjS displays associations with SNPs shared with other ADs (PTPN22, STAT4, IL-1RN, IL-6, TNF, and IL-10) [96].

GENETICS OF PSORIATIC ARTHRITIS

Psoriatic arthritis (PsA) is a seronegative inflammatory arthritis, affecting approximately 30% of patients with cutaneous psoriasis [97]. It is a complex, multifactorial disease in which a quite strong genetic effect is evident. In fact, numerous studies have shown that 40% of subjects with PsA have a first-degree relative with the same pathology. The association between PsA and HLA alleles of class I, HLA-B16, HLA-B17, HLA-B27, HLA-B39, and Cw6, is well documented [98]. These alleles might also be used as prognostic markers of the progression of joint damage. HLA-B7 and HLA-B27 are also associated with other seronegative spondyloarthropathies, HLA-DR4 is found in the polyarticular forms of PsA, HLA-B39 and B27 are associated with the progression of the disease, and Cw6 is associated with psoriasis and early onset PsA [99]. Two loci seem to have a strong association with PsA but not with psoriasis: HLA-B27 and IL-13. Moreover, other important genes are HLA-C region, IL12B, TRAF3IP2, and FBXL19, and genes involved in the epidermal skin barrier [100].

REFERENCES

[1] Dallapiccola B, Novelli G. Genetica Medica Essenziale. CIC Edizioni Internazionali; 2012.

[2] Tsokos GC. Systemic lupus erythematosus. N Engl J Med December 1, 2011;365(22):2110–21.

[3] Perdriger A, Werner-Leyval S, Rollot-Elamrani K. The genetic basis for systemic lupus erythematosus. Joint Bone Spine March 2003;70(2):103–8.

[4] Tsao BP. Update on human systemic lupus erythematosus genetics. Curr Opin Rheumatol September 2004;16(5):513–21.

[5] Luo L, Peng G, Zhu Y, Dong H, Amos CI, Xiong M. Genome-wide gene and pathway analysis. Eur J Hum Genet 2010;18:1045–53.

[6] Teruel M, Alarcón-Riquelme ME. The genetic basis of systemic lupus erythematosus: what are the risk factors and what have we learned. J Autoimmun November 2016;74:161–75.

[7] Wiley GB, Kelly JA, Gaffney PM. Use of next-generation DNA sequencing to analyze genetic variants in rheumatic disease. Arthritis Res Ther 2014;16(6):490.

[8] Horton R, et al. Gene map of the extended human MHC. Nat Rev Genet 2004;5:889–99.

[9] Kaufman JF, Auffray C, Korman AJ, Shackelford DA, Strominger J. The class II molecules of the human and murine major histocompatibility complex. Cell 1984;36:1–13.

[10] Shiina T, Hosomichi K, Inoko H, Kulski JK. The HLA genomic loci map: expression, interaction, diversity and disease. J Hum Genet 2009;54:15–39.

[11] Klein J, Figueroa F. Evolution of the major histocompatibility complex. Crit Rev Immunol 1986;6:295–386.

[12] Trowsdale J, Knight JC. Major histocompatibility complex genomics and human disease. Annu Rev Genom Hum Genet 2013;14:301–23.

[13] Marsh SG, et al. Nomenclature for factors of the HLA system, 2010. Tissue Antigens 2010;75:291–455.

[14] Cruz-Tapias P, et al. Shared HLA class II in six autoimmune diseases in Latin America: a meta-analysis. Autoimmune Dis 2012:569728.

[15] Graham RR, Hom G, Ortmann W, Behrens TW. Review of recent genome-wide association scans in lupus. J Intern Med 2009;265:680–8.

[16] Hom G, Graham RR, Modrek B, Taylor KE, Ortmann W, Garnier S, Lee AT, Chung SA, Ferreira RC, Pant PV, Ballinger DG, Kosoy R, Demirci FY, Kamboh MI, Kao AH, Tian C, Gunnarsson I, Bengtsson AA, Rantapää-Dahlqvist S, Petri M, Manzi S, Seldin MF, Rönnblom L, Syvänen AC, Criswell LA, Gregersen PK, Behrens TW. Association of systemic lupus erythematosus with C8orf13-BLK and ITGAM-ITGAX. N Engl J Med 2008;358:900–9.

[17] Weening JJ, D'Agati VD, Schwartz MM, Seshan SV, Alpers CE, Appel GB, Balow JE, Bruijn JA, Cook T, Ferrario F, Fogo AB, Ginzler EM, Hebert L, Hill G, Hill P, Jennette JC, Kong NC, Lesavre P, Lockshin M, Looi LM, Makino H, Moura LA, Nagata M. International Society of Nephrology Working group on the Classification of lupus nephritis; renal Pathology Society Working group on the Classification of lupus nephritis. The classification of glomerulonephritis in systemic lupus erythematosus revisited. Kidney Int February 2004;65(2):521–30.

[18] Jeong DY, Lee SW, Park YH, Choi JH, Kwon YW, Moon G, Eisenhut M, Kronbichler A, Shin JI. Genetic variation and systemic lupus erythematosus: a field synopsis and systematic meta-analysis. Autoimmun Rev June 2018;17(6):553–66.

[19] David T, Ling SF, Barton A. Genetics of immune-mediated inflammatory diseases. Clin Exp Immunol July 2018;193(1):3–12.

[20] Graham RR, et al. Visualizing human leukocyte antigen class II risk haplotypes in human systemic lupus erythematosus. Am J Hum Genet 2002;71:543–53.

[21] Podrebarac TA, Boisert DM, Goldstein R. Clinical correlates, serum autoantibodies and the role of the major histocompatibility complex in French Canadian and non-French Canadian Caucasians with SLE. Lupus 1998;7:183–91.

[22] Bang SY, et al. Influence of susceptibility HLA-DRB1 alleles on the clinical subphenotypes of systemic lupus erythematosus in Koreans. Arthritis Rheumatol May 2016;68(5):1190–6.

[23] Niu Z, Zhang P, Tong Y. Value of HLA-DR genotype in systemic lupus erythematosus and lupus nephritis: a meta-analysis. Int J Rheum Dis 2015;18:17–28.

[24] Dieudé P, Wipff J, Guedj M, et al. BANK1 is a genetic risk factor for diffuse cutaneous systemic sclerosis and has additive effects with IRF5 and STAT4. Arthritis Rheum 2009;60:3447–54.

[25] Rueda B, Gourh P, Broen J, et al. BANK1 functional variants are associate with susceptibility to diffuse systemic sclerosis in Caucasians. Ann Rheum Dis 2010;69:700–5.

[26] Ceccarelli F, D'Alfonso S, Perricone C, Carlomagno Y, Alessandri C, Croia C, Barizzone N, Montecucco C, Galeazzi M, Sebastiani GD, Minisola G, Fiocco U, Valesini G. The role of eight polymorphisms in three candidate genes in determining the susceptibility, phenotype, and response to anti-TNF therapy in patients with rheumatoid arthritis. Clin Exp Rheumatol November–December 2012;30(6):939–44.

[27] Perricone C, Ceccarelli F, Valesini G. An overview on the genetic of rheumatoid arthritis: a never-ending story. Autoimmun Rev August 2011;10(10):599–608.

[28] Lundberg K, Bengtsson C, Kharlamova N, Reed E, Jiang X, Kallberg H, Pollak-Dorocic I, Israelsson L, Kessel C, Padyukov L, Holmdahl R, Alfredsson L, Klareskog L. Genetic and environmental determinants for disease risk in subsets of rheumatoid arthritis defined by the anticitrullinated protein/peptide antibody fine specificity profile. Ann Rheum Dis May 2013;72(5):652–8.

[29] Vang T, Miletic AV, Bottini N, Mustelin T. Protein tyrosine phosphatase PTPN22 in human autoimmunity. Autoimmunity September 2007;40(6):453–61.

[30] Dieudé P, Guedj M, Wipff J, et al. The PTPN22 620W allele conferssusceptibility to systemic sclerosis: findings of a large case-control studyof European Caucasians and a meta-analysis. Arthritis Rheum 2008;58:2183–8.

[31] Ciccacci C, Conigliaro P, Perricone C, Rufini S, Triggianese P, Politi C, Novelli G, Perricone R, Borgiani P. Polymorphisms in STAT-4, IL-10, PSORS1C1, PTPN2 and MIR146A genes are associated differently with prognostic factors in Italian patients affected by rheumatoid arthritis. Clin Exp Immunol November 2016;186(2):157–63.

[32] Conigliaro P, Ciccacci C, Politi C, Triggianese P, Rufini S, Kroegler B, Perricone C, Latini A, Novelli G, Borgiani P, Perricone R. Polymorphisms in STAT4, PTPN2, PSORS1C1 and TRAF3IP2 genes are associated with the response to TNF inhibitors in patients with rheumatoid arthritis. PLoS One January 20, 2017;12(1):e0169956.

[33] International Consortium for Systemic Lupus Erythematosus Genetics (SLEGEN), Harley JB, Alarcón-Riquelme ME, Criswell LA, Jacob CO, Kimberly RP, Moser KL, Tsao BP, Vyse TJ, Langefeld CD, Nath SK, Guthridge JM, Cobb BL, Mirel DB, Marion MC, Williams AH, Divers J, Wang W, Frank SG, Namjou B, Gabriel SB, Lee AT, Gregersen PK, Behrens TW, Taylor KE, Fernando M, Zidovetzki R, Gaffney PM, Edberg JC, Rioux JD, Ojwang JO, James JA, Merrill JT, Gilkeson GS, Seldin MF, Yin H, Baechler EC, Li QZ, Wakeland EK, Bruner GR, Kaufman KM, Kelly JA. Genome-wide association scan in women with systemic lupus erythematosus identifies susceptibility variants in ITGAM, PXK, KIAA1542 and other loci. Nat Genet February 2008;40(2):204–10.

[34] Taniguchi T, Ogasawara K, Takaoka A, Tanaka N. IRF family of transcription factors as regulators of host defense. Annu Rev Immunol 2001;19:623–55.

[35] Takaoka A, Yanai H, Kondo S, Duncan G, Negishi H, Mizutani T, Kano S, Honda K, Ohba Y, Mak TW, Taniguchi T. Integral role of IRF-5 in the gene induction programme activated by Toll-like receptors. Nature March 10, 2005;434(7030):243–9.

[36] Graham RR, Kozyrev SV, Baechler EC, Reddy MV, Plenge RM, Bauer JW, Ortmann WA, Koeuth T, González Escribano MF, Argentine and Spanish Collaborative Groups, Pons-Estel B, Petri M, Daly M, Gregersen PK, Martín J, Altshuler D, Behrens TW, Alarcón-Riquelme ME. A common haplotype of interferon regulatory factor 5 (IRF5) regulates splicing and expression and is associated with increased risk of systemic lupus erythematosus. Nat Genet May 2006;38(5):550–5.

[37] Feng D, Stone RC, Eloranta ML, Sangster-Guity N, Nordmark G, Sigurdsson S, Wang C, Alm G, Syvänen AC, Rönnblom L, Barnes BJ. Genetic variants and disease-associated factors contribute to enhanced interferon regulatory factor 5 expression in blood cells of patients with systemic lupus erythematosus. Arthritis Rheum February 2010;62(2):562–73.

[38] Gateva V, Sandling JK, Hom G, Taylor KE, Chung SA, Sun X, Ortmann W, Kosoy R, Ferreira RC, Nordmark G, Gunnarsson I, Svenungsson E, Padyukov L, Sturfelt G, Jönsen A, Bengtsson AA, Rantapää-Dahlqvist S, Baechler EC, Brown EE, Alarcón GS, Edberg JC, Ramsey-Goldman R, McGwin Jr G, Reveille JD, Vilá LM, Kimberly RP, Manzi S, Petri MA, Lee A, Gregersen PK, Seldin MF, Rönnblom L, Criswell LA, Syvänen AC, Behrens TW, Graham RR. A large-scale replication study identifies TNIP1, PRDM1, JAZF1, UHRF1BP1 and IL10 as risk loci for systemic lupus erythematosus. Nat Genet November 2009;41(11):1228–33.

[39] Subramanian S, Tus K, Li QZ, Wang A, Tian XH, Zhou J, Liang C, Bartov G, McDaniel LD, Zhou XJ, Schultz RA, Wakeland EK. A Tlr7 translocation accelerates systemic autoimmunity in murine lupus. Proc Natl Acad Sci USA June 27, 2006;103(26):9970–5.

[40] Edberg JC, Wu J, Langefeld CD, Brown EE, Marion MC, McGwin Jr G, Petri M, Ramsey-Goldman R, Reveille JD, Frank SG, Kaufman KM, Harley JB, Alarcón GS, Kimberly RP. Genetic variation in the CRP promoter: association with systemic lupus erythematosus. Hum Mol Genet April 15, 2008;17(8):1147–55.

[41] Russell AI, Cunninghame Graham DS, Shepherd C, Roberton CA, Whittaker J, Meeks J, Powell RJ, Isenberg DA, Walport MJ, Vyse TJ. Polymorphism at the C-reactive protein locus influences gene expression and predisposes to systemic lupus erythematosus. Hum Mol Genet January 1, 2004;13(1):137–47.

[42] Hur JW, Sung YK, Shin HD, Park BL, Cheong HS, Bae SC. TREX1 polymorphisms associated with autoantibodies in patients with systemic lupus erythematosus. Rheumatol Int June 2008;28(8):783–9.

[43] Bodaño A, González A, Ferreiros-Vidal I, Balada E, Ordi J, Carreira P, Gómez-Reino JJ, Conde C. Association of a non-synonymous single-nucleotide polymorphism of DNASEI with SLE susceptibility. Rheumatology July 2006;45(7):819–23.

[44] O'Driscoll M. TREX1 DNA exonuclease deficiency, accumulation of single stranded DNA and complex human genetic disorders. DNA Repair June 1, 2008;7(6):997–1003.

[45] Lee-Kirsch MA, Chowdhury D, Harvey S, Gong M, Senenko L, Engel K, Pfeiffer C, Hollis T, Gahr M, Perrino FW, Lieberman J, Hubner N. A mutation in TREX1 that impairs susceptibility to granzyme A-mediated cell death underlies familial chilblain lupus. J Mol Med (Berl) May 2007;85(5):531–7.

[46] Lee-Kirsch MA, Gong M, Chowdhury D, Senenko L, Engel K, Lee YA, de Silva U, Bailey SL, Witte T, Vyse TJ, Kere J, Pfeiffer C, Harvey S, Wong A, Koskenmies S, Hummel O, Rohde K, Schmidt RE, Dominiczak AF, Gahr M, Hollis T, Perrino FW, Lieberman J, Hübner N. Mutations in the gene encoding the 3′-5′ DNA exonuclease TREX1 are associated with systemic lupus erythematosus. Nat Genet September 2007;39(9):1065–7.

[47] Dam EM, Habib T, Chen J, Funk A, Glukhova V, Davis-Pickett M, Wei S, James R, Buckner JH, Cerosaletti K. The BANK1 SLE-risk variants are associated with alterations in peripheral B cell signaling and development in humans. Clin Immunol December 2016;173:171–80.

[48] Zhou XJ, Qi YY, Cheng FJ, Zhang H. Genetic interactions between BANK1 and BLK in Chinese patients with systemic lupus erythematosus. J Rheumatol October 2013;40(10):1772–3.

[49] Zhou XJ, Lu XL, Nath SK, Lv JC, Zhu SN, Yang HZ, Qin LX, Zhao MH, Su Y, Shen N, Li ZG, Zhang H. International Consortium on the genetics of systemic lupus erythematosus. Gene-gene interaction of BLK, TNFSF4, TRAF1, TNFAIP3, and REL in systemic lupus erythematosus. Arthritis Rheum January 2012;64(1):222–31.

[50] Roberts AL, Thomas ER, Bhosle S, Game L, Obraztsova O, Aitman TJ, Vyse TJ, Rhodes B. Resequencing the susceptibility gene, ITGAM, identifies two functionally deleterious rare variants in systemic lupus erythematosus cases. Arthritis Res Ther May 21, 2014;16(3):R114.

[51] Toller-Kawahisa JE, Vigato-Ferreira IC, Pancoto JA, Mendes-Junior CT, Martinez EZ, Palomino GM, Louzada-Júnior P, Donadi EA, Del Lama JE, Marzocchi-Machado CM. The variant of CD11b, rs1143679 within ITGAM, is associated with systemic lupus erythematosus and clinical manifestations in Brazilian patients. Hum Immunol February 2014;75(2):119–23.

[52] Anaya JM1, Kim-Howard X, Prahalad S, Cherñavsky A, Cañas C, Rojas-Villarraga A, Bohnsack J, Jonsson R, Bolstad AI, Brun JG, Cobb B, Moser KL, James JA, Harley JB, Nath SK. Evaluation of genetic association between an ITGAM non-synonymous SNP (rs1143679) and multiple autoimmune diseases. Autoimmun Rev February 2012;11(4):276–80. https://doi.org/10.1016/j.autrev.2011.07.007. Epub 2011 Aug 5.

[53] Deng Y, Tsao BP. Genetic susceptibility to systemic lupus erythematosus in the genomic era. Nat Rev Rheumatol December 2010;6(12):683–92.

[54] Liu C, Qian W, Qian Y, Giltiay NV, Lu Y, Swaidani S, Misra S, Deng L, Chen ZJ, Li X. Act1, a U-box E3 ubiquitin ligase for IL-17 signaling. Sci Signal October 13, 2009;2(92):ra63.

[55] May MJ. IL-17R signaling: new players get in on the Act1. Nat Immunol August 18, 2011;12(9):813–5.

[56] Giltiay NV, Lu Y, Allman D, Jørgensen TN, Li X. The adaptor molecule Act1 regulates BAFF responsiveness and self-reactive B cell selection during transitional B cell maturation. J Immunol July 1, 2010;185(1):99–109.

[57] Qian Y, Giltiay N, Xiao J, Wang Y, Tian J, Han S, Scott M, Carter R, Jorgensen TN, Li X. Deficiency of Act1, a critical modulator of B cell function, leads to development of Sjögren's syndrome. Eur J Immunol August 2008;38(8):2219–28.

[58] Pisitkun P, Claudio E, Ren N, Wang H, Siebenlist U. The adaptor protein CIKS/ACT1 is necessary for collagen-induced arthritis, and it contributes to the production of collagen-specific antibody. Arthritis Rheum November 2010;62(11):3334–44.

[59] Korman BD, Kastner DL, Gregersen PK, Remmers EF. STAT4: genetics, mechanisms, and implications for autoimmunity. Curr Allergy Asthma Rep 2008;8:398–403.

[60] Liang YL, Wu H, Shen X, Li PQ, Yang XQ, Liang L, et al. Association of STAT4 rs7574865 polymorphism with autoimmune diseases: a meta-analysis. Mol Biol Rep 2012;39:8873–82.

[61] Kariuki SN, Niewold TB. Genetic regulation of serum cytokines in systemic lupus erythematosus. Transl Res 2010;155:109–17.

[62] Wang C, Sandling JK, Hagberg N, Berggren O, Sigurdsson S, Karlberg O, et al. Genome-wide profiling of target genes for the systemic lupus erythematosus-associated transcription factors IRF5 and STAT4. Ann Rheum Dis 2013;72:96–103. https://doi.org/10.1136/annrheumdis-2012-201364.

[63] Murphy KM, Ouyang W, Farrar JD, Yang J, Ranganath S, Asnagli H, Afkarian M, Murphy TL. Signaling and transcription in T helper development. Annu Rev Immunol 2000;18:451–94.

[64] Guo L, Wei G, Zhu J, Liao W, Leonard WJ, Zhao K, Paul W. IL-1 family members and STAT activators induce cytokine production by Th2, Th17, and Th1 cells. Proc Natl Acad Sci USA August 11, 2009;106(32):13463–8.

[65] Watford WT, Hissong BD, Bream JH, Kanno Y, Muul L, O'Shea JJ. Signaling by IL-12 and IL-23 and the immunoregulatory roles of STAT4. Immunol Rev December 2004;202:139–56.

[66] Hildner KM, Schirmacher P, Atreya I, Dittmayer M, Bartsch B, Galle PR, Wirtz S, Neurath MF. Targeting of the transcription factor STAT4 by antisense phosphorothioate oligonucleotides suppresses collagen-induced arthritis. J Immunol March 15, 2007;178(6):3427–36.

[67] Remmers EF, Plenge RM, Lee AT, Graham RR, Hom G, Behrens TW, de Bakker PI, Le JM, Lee HS, Batliwalla F, Li W, Masters SL, Booty MG, Carulli JP, Padyukov L, Alfredsson L, Klareskog L, Chen WV, Amos CI, Criswell LA, Seldin MF, Kastner DL, Gregersen PK. STAT4 and the risk of rheumatoid arthritis and systemic lupus erythematosus. N Engl J Med September 6, 2007;357(10):977–86.

[68] Orozco G, Alizadeh BZ, Delgado-Vega AM, González-Gay MA, Balsa A, Pascual-Salcedo D, Fernández-Gutierrez B, González-Escribano MF, Petersson IF, van Riel PL, Barrera P, Coenen MJ, Radstake TR, van Leeuwen MA, Wijmenga C, Koeleman BP, Alarcón-Riquelme M, Martín J. Association of STAT4 with rheumatoid arthritis: a replication study in three European populations. Arthritis Rheum July 2008;58(7):1974–80.

[69] Hellquist A, Sandling JK, Zucchelli M, Koskenmies S, Julkunen H, D'Amato M, Garnier S, Syvänen AC, Kere J. Variation in STAT4 is associated with systemic lupus erythematosus in a Finnish family cohort. Ann Rheum Dis May 2010;69(5):883–6.

[70] Hagberg N, Joelsson M, Leonard D, Reid S, Eloranta ML, Mo J, Nilsson MK, Syvänen AC, Bryceson YT, Rönnblom L. The STAT4 SLE risk allele rs7574865[T] is associated with increased IL-12-induced IFN-γ production in T cells from patients with SLE. Ann Rheum Dis July 2018;77(7):1070–7.

[71] Ciccacci C, Perricone C, Ceccarelli F, Rufini S, Di Fusco D, Alessandri C, Spinelli FR, Cipriano E, Novelli G, Valesini G, Borgiani P, Conti F. A multilocus genetic study in a cohort of Italian SLE patients confirms the association with STAT4 gene and describes a new association with HCP5 gene. PLoS One November 4, 2014;9(11):e111991.

[72] Borgiani P, Di Fusco D, Erba F, Marazzi MC, Mancinelli S, Novelli G, et al. HCP5 genetic variant (rs3099844) contributes to Nevirapine-induced Stevens Johnsons Syndrome/Toxic Epidermal Necrolysis susceptibility in a population from Mozambique. Eur J Clin Pharmacol 2014;70:275–8. https://doi.org/10.1007/s00228-013-1622-5.

[73] Tohkin M, Kaniwa N, Saito Y, Sugiyama E, Kurose K, Nishikawa J, et al. Japan Pharmacogenomics Data Science Consortium. A whole-genome association study of major determinants for allopurinol-related Stevens-Johnson syndrome and toxic epidermal necrolysis in Japanese patients. Pharmacogenom J 2013;13:60–9.

[74] Génin E, Schumacher M, Roujeau JC, Naldi L, Liss Y, Kazma R, et al. Genome-wide association study of Stevens-Johnson syndrome and toxic epidermal necrolysis in Europe. Orphanet J Rare Dis 2011;6:52.

[75] Karlsen TH, Franke A, Melum E, Kaser A, Hov JR, Balschun T, et al. Genome-wide association analysis in primary sclerosing cholangitis. Gastroenterology 2010;138:1102–11.

[76] Clancy RM, Marion MC, Kaufman KM, Ramos PS, Adler A. International Consortium on Systemic Lupus Erythematosus Genetics. Identification of candidate loci at 6p21 and 21q22 in a genome-wide association study of cardiac manifestations of neonatal lupus. Arthritis Rheum 2010;62:3415–24.

[77] Julkunen H, Kurki P, Kaaja R, Heikkila R, Immonen I, Chan EK, et al. Isolated congenital heart block. Long-term outcome of mothers and characterization of the immune response to SS-A/Ro and to SS-B/La. Arthritis Rheum 1993;36:1588–98.

[78] Salomonsson S, Dorner T, Theander E, Bremme K, Larsson P, Wahren-Herlenius M. A serologic marker for fetal risk of congenital heart block. Arthritis Rheum 2002;46:1233–41.

[79] Fritsch C, Hoebeke J, Dali H, Ricchiuti V, Isenberg DA, Meyer O, et al. 52-kDa Ro/SSA epitopes preferentially recognized by antibodies from mothers of children with neonatal lupus and congenital heart block. Arthritis Res Ther 2006;8:R4.

[80] Eronen M, Miettinen A, Walle TK, Chan EK, Julkunen H. Relationship of maternal autoimmune response to clinical manifestations in children with congenital complete heart block. Acta Paediatr 2004;93:803–9.

[81] Salomonsson S, Dzikaite V, Zeffer E, Eliasson H, Ambrosi A, Bergman G, et al. A population-based investigation of the autoantibody profile in mothers of children with atrioventricular block. Scand J Immunol 2011;74:511–7.

[82] Perricone C, Ciccacci C, Ceccarelli F, Di Fusco D, Spinelli FR, Cipriano E, Novelli G, Valesini G, Conti F, Borgiani P. TRAF3IP2 gene and systemic lupus erythematosus: association with disease susceptibility and pericarditis development. Immunogenetics October 2013;65(10):703–9.

[83] Ceccarelli F, Perricone C, Borgiani P, Ciccacci C, Rufini S, Cipriano E, Alessandri C, Spinelli FR, Sili Scavalli A, Novelli G, Valesini G, Conti F. Genetic factors in systemic lupus erythematosus: contribution to disease phenotype. J Immunol Res 2015;2015:745647.

[84] Ciccacci C, Perricone C, Politi C, Rufini S, Ceccarelli F, Cipriano E, Alessandri C, Latini A, Valesini G, Novelli G, Conti F, Borgiani P. A polymorphism upstream MIR1279 gene is associated with pericarditis development in Systemic Lupus Erythematosus and contributes to definition of a genetic risk profile for this complication. Lupus July 2017;26(8):841–8.

[85] Mayes MD. The genetics of scleroderma: looking into the postgenomic era. Curr Opin Rheumatol November 2012;24(6):677–84.

[86] Tsou PS, Sawalha AH. Unfolding the pathogenesis of scleroderma through genomics and epigenomics. J Autoimmun September 2017;83:73–94.

[87] Zhao W, Yue X, Liu K, Zheng J, Huang R, Zou J, Riemekasten G, Petersen F, Yu X. The status of pulmonary fibrosis in systemic sclerosis is associated with IRF5, STAT4, IRAK1, and CTGF polymorphisms. Rheumatol Int August 2017;37(8):1303–10.

[88] Carmona FD, Cénit MC, Diaz-Gallo LM, Broen JC, Simeón CP, Carreira PE, Callejas-Rubio JL, Fonollosa V, López-Longo FJ, González-Gay MA, Hunzelmann N, Riemekasten G, Witte T, Kreuter A, Distler JH, Madhok R, Shiels P, van Laar JM, Schuerwegh AJ, Vonk MC, Voskuyl AE, Fonseca C, Denton CP, Herrick A, Worthington J, Arnett FC, Tan FK, Assassi S, Radstake TR, Mayes MD, Martín J, Spanish Scleroderma Group. New insight on the Xq28 association with systemic sclerosis. Ann Rheum Dis December 2013;72(12):2032–8.

[89] Coustet B, Dieudé P, Guedj M, Bouaziz M, Avouac J, Ruiz B, Hachulla E, Diot E, Cracowski JL, Tiev K, Sibilia J, Mouthon L, Frances C, Amoura Z, Carpentier P, Cosnes A, Meyer O, Kahan A, Boileau C, Chiocchia G, Allanore Y. C8orf13-BLK is a genetic risk locus for systemic sclerosis and has additive effects with BANK1: results from a large French cohort and meta-analysis. Arthritis Rheum July 2011;63(7):2091–6.

[90] Dawidowicz K, Dieudé P, Avouac J, Wipff J, Hachulla E, Diot E, Tiev K, Cracowski JL, Mouthon L, Amoura Z, Frances C, Carpentier P, Meyer O, Kahan A, Boileau C, Allanore Y. Association study of B-cell marker gene polymorphisms in European Caucasian patients with systemic sclerosis. Clin Exp Rheumatol September–October 2011;29(5):839–42.

[91] Diaz-Gallo LM, Gourh P, Broen J, Simeon C, Fonollosa V, Ortego-Centeno N, Agarwal S, Vonk MC, Coenen M, Riemekasten G, Hunzelmann N, Hesselstrand R, Tan FK, Reveille JD, Assassi S, García-Hernandez FJ, Carreira P, Camps MT, Fernandez-Nebro A, de la Peña PG, Nearney T, Hilda D, González-Gay MA, Airo P, Beretta L, Scorza R, Herrick A, Worthington J, Pros A, Gómez-Gracia I, Trapiella L, Espinosa G, Castellvi I, Witte T, de Keyser F, Vanthuyne M, Mayes MD, Radstake TR, Arnett FC, Martin J, Rueda B. Analysis of the influence of PTPN22 gene polymorphisms in systemic sclerosis. Ann Rheum Dis March 2011;70(3):454–62.

[92] Bossini-Castillo L, Broen JC, Simeon CP, Beretta L, Vonk MC, Ortego-Centeno N, Espinosa G, Carreira P, Camps MT, Navarrete N, González-Escribano MF, Vicente-Rabaneda E, Rodríguez L, Tolosa C, Román-Ivorra JA, Gómez-Gracia I, García-Hernández FJ, Castellví I, Gallego M, Fernández-Nebro A, García-Portales R, Egurbide MV, Fonollosa V, de la Peña PG, Pros A, González-Gay MA, Hesselstrand R, Riemekasten G, Witte T, Coenen MJ, Koeleman BP, Houssiau F, Smith V, de Keyser F, Westhovens R, De Langhe E, Voskuyl AE, Schuerwegh AJ, Chee MM, Madhok R, Shiels P, Fonseca C, Denton C, Claes K, Padykov L, Nordin A, Palm O, Lie BA, Airó P, Scorza R, van Laar JM, Hunzelmann N, Kreuter A, Herrick A, Worthington J, Radstake TR, Martin J, Rueda B. A replication study confirms the association of TNFSF4 (OX40L) polymorphisms with systemic sclerosis in a large European cohort. Ann Rheum Dis April 2011;70(4):638–41.

[93] Muskardin TLW, Niewold TB. Type I interferon in rheumatic diseases. Nat Rev Rheumatol March 21, 2018;14(4):214–28.

[94] Bossini-Castillo L, Campillo-Davó D, López-Isac E, Carmona FD, Simeon CP, Carreira P, Callejas-Rubio JL, Castellví I, Fernández-Nebro A, Rodríguez-Rodríguez L, Rubio-Rivas M, García-Hernández FJ, Madroñero AB, Beretta L, Santaniello A, Lunardi C, Airó P, Hoffmann-Vold AM, Kreuter A, Riemekasten G, Witte T, Hunzelmann N, Vonk MC, Voskuyl AE, de Vries-Bouwstra J, Shiels P, Herrick A, Worthington J, Radstake TRDJ, Martin J, Spanish Scleroderma Group. An MIF promoter polymorphism is associated with susceptibility to pulmonary arterial hypertension in diffuse cutaneous systemic sclerosis. J Rheumatol October 2017;44(10):1453–7.

[95] Teos LY, Alevizos I. Genetics of Sjögren's syndrome. Clin Immunol September 2017;182:41–7.

[96] Reksten TR, Lessard CJ, Sivils KL. Genetics in Sjögren syndrome. Rheum Dis Clin N Am August 2016;42(3):435–47.

[97] Chimenti MS, Perricone C, Novelli L, Caso F, Costa L, Bogdanos D, Conigliaro P, Triggianese P, Ciccacci C, Borgiani P, Perricone R. Interaction between microbiome and host genetics in psoriatic arthritis. Autoimmun Rev March 2018;17(3):276–83.

[98] Genetic Analysis of Psoriasis Consortium & the Wellcome Trust Case Control Consortium 2, Strange A, Capon F, Spencer CC, Knight J, Weale ME, Allen MH, Barton A, Band G, Bellenguez C, Bergboer JG, Blackwell JM, Bramon E, Bumpstead SJ, Casas JP, Cork MJ, Corvin A, Deloukas P, Dilthey A, Duncanson A, Edkins S, Estivill X, Fitzgerald O, Freeman C, Giardina E, Gray E, Hofer A, Hüffmeier U, Hunt SE, Irvine AD, Jankowski J, Kirby B, Langford C, Lascorz J, Leman J, Leslie S, Mallbris L, Markus HS, Mathew CG, McLean WH, McManus R, Mössner R, Moutsianas L, Naluai AT, Nestle FO, Novelli G, Onoufriadis A, Palmer CN, Perricone C, Pirinen M, Plomin R, Potter SC, Pujol RM, Rautanen A, Riveira-Munoz E, Ryan AW, Salmhofer W, Samuelsson L, Sawcer SJ, Schalkwijk J, Smith CH, Ståhle M, Su Z, Tazi-Ahnini R, Traupe H, Viswanathan AC, Warren RB, Weger W, Wolk K, Wood N, Worthington J, Young HS, Zeeuwen PL, Hayday A, Burden AD, Griffiths CE, Kere J, Reis A, McVean G, Evans DM, Brown MA, Barker JN, Peltonen L, Donnelly P, Trembath RC. A genome-wide association study identifies new psoriasis susceptibility loci and an interaction between HLA-C and ERAP1. Nat Genet November 2010;42(11):985–90.

[99] Tsoi LC, Spain SL, Knight J, Ellinghaus E, Stuart PE, Capon F, Ding J, Li Y, Tejasvi T, Gudjonsson JE, Kang HM, Allen MH, McManus R, Novelli G, Samuelsson L, Schalkwijk J, Ståhle M, Burden AD, Smith CH, Cork MJ, Estivill X, Bowcock AM, Krueger GG, Weger W, Worthington J, Tazi-Ahnini R, Nestle FO, Hayday A, Hoffmann P, Winkelmann J, Wijmenga C, Langford C, Edkins S, Andrews R, Blackburn H, Strange A, Band G, Pearson RD, Vukcevic D, Spencer CC, Deloukas P, Mrowietz U, Schreiber S, Weidinger S, Koks S, Kingo K, Esko T, Metspalu A, Lim HW, Voorhees JJ, Weichenthal M, Wichmann HE, Chandran V, Rosen CF, Rahman P, Gladman DD, Griffiths CE, Reis A, Kere J, Collaborative Association Study of Psoriasis (CASP), Genetic Analysis of Psoriasis Consortium, Psoriasis Association Genetics Extension, Wellcome Trust Case Control Consortium 2, Nair RP, Franke A, Barker JN, Abecasis GR, Elder JT, Trembath RC. Identification of 15 new psoriasis susceptibility loci highlights the role of innate immunity. Nat Genet December 2012;44(12):1341–8. https://doi.org/10.1038/ng.2467.

[100] Docampo E, Giardina E, Riveira-Muñoz E, de Cid R, Escaramís G, Perricone C, Fernández-Sueiro JL, Maymó J, González-Gay MA, Blanco FJ, Hüffmeier U, Lisbona MP, Martín J, Carracedo A, Reis A, Rabionet R, Novelli G, Estivill X. Deletion of LCE3C and LCE3B is a susceptibility factor for psoriatic arthritis: a study in Spanish and Italian populations and meta-analysis. Arthritis Rheum July 2011;63(7):1860–5.

Chapter 13

Epigenetics

Haijing Wu, Qianjin Lu

Department of Dermatology, Second Xiangya Hospital, Central South University, Hunan Key Laboratory of Medical Epigenomics, Changsha, China

The term "epigenetics" has been launched when it is realized that DNA sequence is completely the same in the somatic cells, whereas the gene expression patterns vary greatly among different cells types. The word "epigenetics" has become popular when genetic susceptibilities cannot explain all incidences, and the concordance rate of diseases, such as autoimmune diseases, is less than 50% in monozygotic twins [1]. The major disappointments from genome-wide association studies, which have identified thousands of gene polymorphisms, reveal that most susceptible loci are within the introns, which may not interfere the gene expression pattern. In contrary, epigenetic regulations, which heritably alter the gene expression but do not change the DNA sequence by chemical modifications of DNA and structural changes of chromatin, show critical importance in etiopathogenesis of diseases. In addition, epigenetics may partially explain the environmental factor–induced effects on the individuals, which cannot be explained by genetics.

Epigenetic modifications, including DNA methylation/demethylation, histone modification, and noncoding RNAs (ncRNAs), regulate gene expression and thereby play a key role in various biological processes and pathogenesis of disease [2]. This chapter aims to summarize the up-to-date knowledge of epigenetics, especially in the field of autoimmune diseases. The possible utilization of epigenetics modifications in the diagnosis and therapies will be also discussed, providing universal and novel insights of epigenetics for the better understanding of diseases and potential therapeutic targets.

DNA METHYLATION/DEMETHYLATION

As the most intensively studied field, DNA methylation is defined as a potentially heritable and relatively stable epigenetic alteration, which is the first recognized epigenetic modification of DNA. DNA methylation is a biochemical process in which a methyl group is added to a cytosine or adenine residue at the fifth position on the pyrimidine ring, locking the gene transcription in the "off" status [3]. Therefore, DNA methylation acts as a flag indicating the repression of gene transcription, which is a process involved in many important biological processes.

The CpG dinucleotides tend to cluster in regions called CpG islands, defined as regions of more than 200 bases with a G+C content of at least 50% and a ratio of observed to statistically expected CpG frequencies of at least 0.6. Approximate 60% of gene promoters are associated with CpG islands and are normally unmethylated, although some of them (about 6%) become methylated in a tissue-specific manner during early development or in differentiated tissues [4]. This may explain why all cells in an organism share the same genetic information but show different phenotypes. In general, CpG island methylation is associated with gene silencing. Methylation serves as a mark that indicates repression of gene expression, and DNA methylation is therefore involved in many biological processes, such as cell differentiations and immune responses.

DNA methylation inhibits gene expression via various mechanisms. For example, methyl-CpG-binding domain (MBD) proteins can be recruited by methylated DNA, and MBD family members recruit histone-modifying and chromatin-remodeling complexes to methylated sites in turn [5]. Moreover, DNA methylation can also directly inhibit transcription by precluding the recruitment of DNA-binding proteins from their target sites. However, DNA methylation does not occur exclusively at CpG islands, and CpG island shores, which refer to regions of lower density of CpG and lie close to CpG, are associated with transcriptional inactivation. Most tissue-specific DNA methylation occurs not at CpG islands but at CpG island shores [6]. In mammalian cells, DNA methylation is restricted to regions of CpG islands, which are typically present in promoter regions [7]. DNA methylation is mediated by methyltransferases, including DNMT1, DNMT3a, and DNMT3b. Notably, every methyltransferase shows distinguished capacities. During DNA replication, DNMT1 usually sustains the methylation status, whereas other two methyltransferases participate in de novo methylation [8].

DNA demethylation occurs during the programmed failure in transmission of a methylation pattern, which results in reactivation of transcription of silenced genes [9]. DNA demethylation occurs through the sequential iterative oxidation of 5-mC while the final modified group is removed by thymine-DNA glycosylase (TDG) to yield cytosine instead of 5-mC [9].

Mosaic of Autoimmunity. **https://doi.org/10.1016/B978-0-12-814307-0.00013-X**

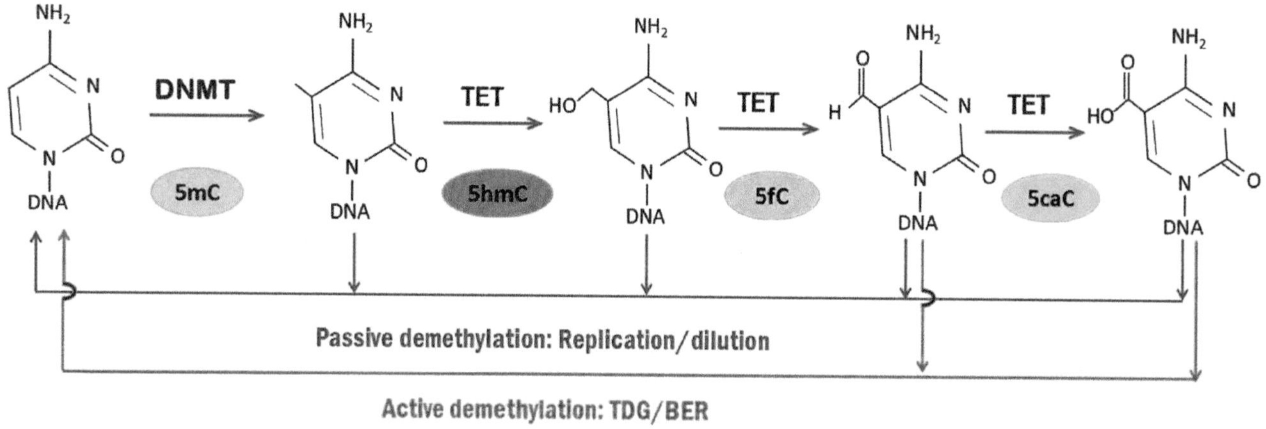

FIGURE 13.1 The process of DNA methylation and demethylation.

During this process, oxidation of 5-mC to 5-hydroxymethylcytosine (5-hmC) is mainly mediated by ten-eleven translocation (TET) family dioxygenase enzymes, including TET1, TET2, and TET3 [10], which can subsequently oxidize 5-hmC to 5-formylcytosine (5-fC) and 5-carboxylcytosine (5-CaC), thereby displaying the order of 5-mC, 5-hmC, 5-fC, and 5-CaC [11]. In addition, both 5-fC and 5-CaC could be removed by TDG, which can further trigger base excision repair [12,13] (Fig. 13.1).

Abnormal DNA Methylation in Autoimmunity

Systemic lupus erythematosus (SLE) is a typical autoimmune disease, and the DNA methylation status has been intensively studied in lupus. Not surprisingly, DNA demethylation has been observed in human lupus CD4+ T cells, indicating a more activated status of T cells with overexpressed Lymphocyte function-associated antigen 1 (LFA-1) and CD40L [14,15]. Genome-wide DNA methylation study revealed epigenetic accessibility and transcriptional poising of interferon-regulated genes in naïve CD4+ T cells from lupus patients [16], as well as from lupus patients with different clinical manifestations, such as malar rash versus discoid rash [17] and renal involvement versus nonrenal involvement [18]. Lupus-associated and inflammatory cytokine genes, such as IL4, IL6, IL10, and IL13, are demethylated in lupus T cells and may contribute to disease progression [19,20]. The upstream mechanism has been found to be related with certain proteins, such as RFX1 [21], DNA damage-inducible 45 alpha (Gadd45a) [22], and high mobility group box protein 1 (HMGB1) [23]. In addition, in a large-scale DNA methylation investigation, DNA hypomethylation was found in interferon-regulated genes in lupus naïve T cells, including IFI44L, IFIT1, IFIT3, MX1, STAT1, USP18, BST2, and TRIM22, suggesting abnormalities in T cell progenitors [16]. More important is that the DNA methylation level on IFI44L promoter is identified as a sensitive and specific biomarker for lupus diagnosis [24].

A genome-wide mapping of 5-hmC in CD4+ T cells has shown that 5-hmC marks transcriptional regulatory regions of T cell lineage-specific signature genes, and meanwhile, Tet2 protein is recruited to 5-hmC–enriched regions and promotes the expression of signature cytokines in Th1 and Th17 cells [25]. We recently have observed an increased 5-hmC level in genomic DNA in CD4þ T cells from patients with SLE compared with healthy controls, accompanied by the upregulated expression of TET2 and TET3. They have further confirmed that CTCF, a transcription activator, can bind to the promoter region of SOCS1 and contribute to overexpression of SOCS1 in SLE CD4+ T cells by mediating DNA hydroxymethylation and decreasing DNA methylation level at the locus [26]. Abnormal DNA methylation in other autoimmune diseases is summarized in Table 13.1.

HISTONE MODIFICATIONS

Histone modification is a covalent posttranslational modification that regulates gene expression via changing chromatin structure or recruiting other modifications, thereby involving numerous biological processes. It has been well established that nucleosome is formed by 146 base pairs (bp) corresponding to two turns of DNA wrapped around a histone core, which displays two repeated sets of H2A, H2B, H3, and H4. These histones possess small protein "tails" from the nucleosomes that are available for modifications, including acetylation, methylation, ubiquitination, phosphorylation, and sumoylation [55]. Acetylation and deacetylation can add or remove an acetyl group, which are mediated by histone acetyltransferases

TABLE 13.1 Alterations of DNA Methylation in Autoimmune Diseases: Systemic Lupus Erythematosus (SLE), Rheumatic Arthritis (RA), Systemic Sclerosis (SSc), Peripheral Blood Mononuclear Cells (PBMCs), and Primary Biliary Cirrhosis (PBC)

Disease	Cell Types	Alterations of DNA Methylation	References
SLE	Whole blood	IFI44L: decreases FOXP3 TSDR: increase	[24,26]
SLE	PBMCs	Global, ERa: decrease	[27,28]
SLE	T cells	X chromosome genes, *IL4, IL6*: decrease	[20,29,30]
SLE	CD4+ T cells	Global, IFN-regulated genes, IL-10, IL-13, CD11a, CD70, CD40L, perforin, PP2Aca, KIR2DL4: decrease	[31–38]
SLE	Naïve CD4+ T cells	IFN-regulated genes, MIR886, TRIM69, CHST12: decrease	[16–18]
SLE	B cells and monocytes	IFN-regulated genes: decrease	[32]
RA	PBMCs	IL6, ERa: decrease	[28,39,40]
RA	T cells	Global: decrease	[41,42]
RA	CD4+ T cells	CD40L: decrease	[40]
RA	Fibroblast-like synoviocytes	Global, L1 retrotransposon: decrease	[43,44]
RA	Synovial fibroblasts	Global, CXCL12: decrease	[45,46]
SSc	CD4+ T cells	Global, CD11a, CD70, CD40L: decrease	[47–50]
SSC	Dermal fibroblasts	Wnt pathway antagonist genes, the collagen suppressor gene FLI1, TGF-beta-related genes: increase	[51–53]
PBC	CD4+ T cells	CD40L, CXCR3: decrease	[51,54]

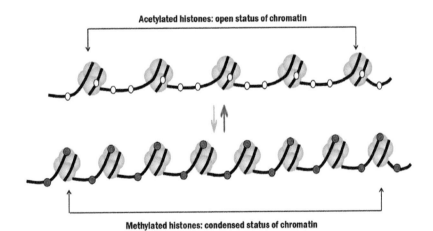

FIGURE 13.2 The regulation of open and condensed status of chromatin by histone acetylation.

and histone deacetylases (HDACs), respectively [56]. Histone methylation, defined as transferring 1, 2, or 3 methyl groups to arginine or lysine residues, is mainly mediated by histone methyltransferases and other enzymes, such as EZH2, G9a, SUV39-h1, ESET, and SETDB1, etc. The consequences of histone methylation depend on both modified residue and the number of methyl groups. Generally, acetylation promotes gene expression by opening the chromatin, while methylation switches the chromatin to the tight status, showing the opposite effects (Fig. 13.2). For example, H3K4me3 activates gene transcription, whereas H3K27me3 and H3K9me3 result in gene silencing [57,58]. Similar to methylation, ubiquitination on histones is implicated in both activation and repression of gene transcription [59]. Many enzymes have been identified to control the addition and removal of ubiquitin. The ubiquitination on H2A and H2B has been found to play an essential role in numerous biological processes, such as transcription initiation, elongation, repression, and DNA repair [60]. Phosphorylation can occur at all four histone tails that contain acceptor sites, which is mediated by protein kinases [61]. These four modifications can directly regulate histone–DNA interactions and also recruit nonhistone proteins to chromatin.

TABLE 13.2 Alterations of Histone Modifications in Autoimmune Diseases: Systemic Lupus Erythematosus (SLE), Rheumatic Arthritis (RA), Systemic Sclerosis (SSc), and Primary Biliary Cirrhosis (PBC)

Disease	Cell Types	Alterations of Histone Modifications	References
SLE	T cells	H3K18 deacetylation at *IL2* promoter, increased H3 acetylation of the *IL17* locus	[65,68,70,74]
SLE	CD4+ T cells	Site-specific H3 and H4 hypoacetylation, global H3K9 hypomethylation	[62]
SLE	Monocytes	Global H4 hyperacetylation, increased histone acetylation of TNF-α gene, broader peaks of H3K4me3 mainly enriched at immune response genes	[67,68,70,75]
RA	Synovial fibroblasts	Histone H3 hyperacetylation in the *IL6* promoter	[76]
SSc	Fibroblasts	Histone H3 and H4 hypoacetylation in the FLI1 gene promoter, a global increase of H3K27me3 enrichment	[52,77]
SSc	B cells	A global histone H4 hyperacetylation and H3K9 hypomethylation	[78]
PBC	T cells	Overexpression of barr1 associated with histone H4 hyperacetylation in promoters of CD40L, LIGHT, IL-17 and interferon-g, and histone H4 hypoacetylation in the promoters of TRAIL, Apo2, and HDAC7A	[79]

And the combinations of these modifications presenting on the same or the other histone tails have been reported as "histone codes," which is deciphered by proteins which present specific binding motifs for each modification [61].

Aberrant Histone Modifications in Autoimmunity

Unsurprisingly, histone modifications play a role in the pathogenesis of SLE. Global histone H3 and H4 hypoacetylation has been found in lupus CD4+ T cells [62], and aberrant histone modifications have been observed within the TNFSF7 promoter, leading to CD70 overexpression on T cells, which may contribute to the disease [63]. Treatment of healthy T cells with HDAC inhibitors resulted in decreased CD3ς chain expression, leading to abnormalities in T cells [64]. Tsokos et al. revealed that the transcription factor CREMα may participate in histone acetylation in active lupus T cells by silencing IL-2 expression through HDAC recruitment to Cre sites in the IL-2 promoter [65]. In addition to T cells, Dai et al. investigated an alteration of H3K4me3 in various key candidate genes in lupus PBMCs [66]. Global H4 acetylation was reportedly altered in lupus monocytes, and 63% of these H4 acetylated genes were potentially regulated by IFN regulatory factors [67].

On a more gene-specific level, histone modification also regulates lupus-related cytokine secretion, such as enhanced H3 acetylation at the IL-17 locus and elevated IL-10 production by chromatin remodeling regulated by Stat3 [68,69]. Furthermore, histone hyperacetylation has been found to be associated with an increased level of TNF-α and enhanced maturation of lupus monocytes [70]. However, it has not been elucidated whether histone modifications represent the cause or the consequence of lupus, despite the fact that the involvement of histone modifications in pathogenesis has been further suggested by mouse studies. Sirtuin-1 (Sirt-1), an HDAC, was found to be overexpressed in lupus-prone mice, MRL/lpr mice [71], and the downregulation of Sirt-1 resulted in short-term enhanced H3 and H4 acetylation, with reduced levels of anti-dsDNA, glomerular IgG deposition, and kidney damage [27]. Treatment of MRL/lpr mice with HDAC inhibitors also had therapeutic effects, with improvement of proteinuria, reduced renal damage, and downregulation of lupus-associated cytokine levels [72]. Recent progress has been made from a study that identifies candidate causal variants for 21 autoimmune diseases from genetic and epigenetic mapping in different subtypes of CD4+ T cells, including regulatory T cells, Th17, Th1, and Th2 cells [73]. In this outstanding study, distinct H3K27 peaks have been observed in the super-enhancer in IL-2RA locus preferentially in regulatory T cells and Th17 cells. The summary of aberrant histone modifications in other autoimmune diseases is shown in Table 13.2.

MicroRNAs

With a length of 21–25 bp, microRNAs (miRNAs) belong to ncRNAs that regulate posttranscriptional and posttranslational gene expression. miRNAs bind to the 3′-UTR of specific target mRNA, resulting in mRNA cleavage, degradation, or block translation [80–82] (Fig. 13.3). miRNAs, similar to other epigenetic regulations, involve numerous biological processes, including cell cycle, differentiation, apoptosis, and innate and adaptive immune responses. Increasing evidence has shown

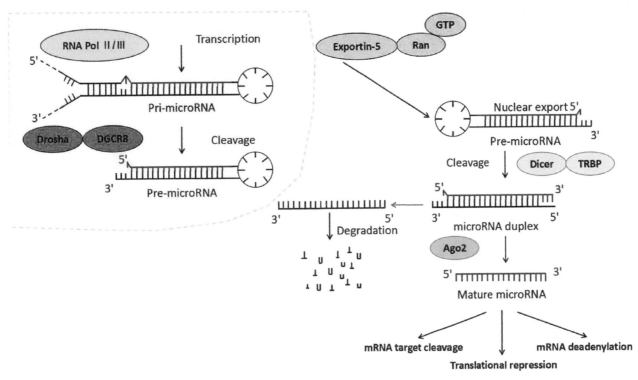

FIGURE 13.3 The pathway of miRNA regulation of gene expression.

that aberrant levels of miRNAs in different cell subtypes and tissues are associated with the pathogenesis of various diseases, facilitating them as potential noninvasive biomarkers for prediction and diagnosis, as well as potential treatment targets. To date, most work on ncRNAs in B cell differentiation and antibody response has mainly focused on miRNAs. Moreover, miRNAs cross-talk with histone modification and DNA methylation [83], synergically regulating biological processes.

The maturation of miRNAs includes the production of the primary miRNA transcript (pri-miRNA) by RNA polymerase II or III and cleavage of the pri-miRNA by the microprocessor complex Drosha–DGCR8 (Pasha) in the nucleus. Then the pre-miRNA hairpin is exported from the nucleus by Exportin-5–Ran-GTP. In the cytoplasm, the RNase Dicer in complex with the double-stranded RNA-binding protein TAR RNA binding protein (TRBP) cleaves the pre-miRNA hairpin to its mature length. The functional strand of the mature miRNA is loaded together with Argonaute (Ago2) proteins into the RNA-induced silencing complex (RISC), where it guides the RISC to silence target mRNAs through mRNA cleavage, translational repression, or deadenylation, whereas the passenger strand is degraded.

Dysregulated MicroRNAs and Their Targeting Genes in Autoimmunity

It has been demonstrated that each miRNA may bind to different targets but regulate the same gene. Although numerous miRNAs are found to be abnormally expressed in T cells, certain of them target lupus-related gene expression, including IL-10, IL-17, and DNMT1. For example, miR-21, miR-126, and miR148a were found to be decreased in SLE T cells and to target DNMT1, though they were bound to different regions [84,85]. Interestingly, the repression of miR-21, miR-148a, and miR-29b in SLE T cells was able to reverse pathogenic phenotypes to normal ones to some extent, suggesting their potential roles in SLE [85,86]. Moreover, miR-21 has been observed to suppress PDCD4 expression, thus enhancing cell proliferation and increasing CD40L and IL-10 expression in lupus T cells [87]. In addition, miR-142 [88] and miR-31 [89] have been reported to regulate T cell functions by inhibiting IL-4, IL-10, CD40L, and ICOS expression and enhancing IL-2 production, respectively. Based on our previous finding for miR-146a and -241-3p/5p, we recently reported that mycophenolic acid, which has been applied in clinical use for lupus, ameliorates the autoreactivity of lupus T cells by regulating these two miRNAs, indicating the involvement of miR-146a and -241-3p/5p in SLE pathogenesis [90].

Numerous circulating miRNAs have been identified to be correlated with lupus and have also been suggested to serve as biomarkers. Among them, miR-146a and miR-155 are the first-described miRNAs that are decreased in lupus serum and are regarded as biomarkers [91]. In subsequent studies, the serum levels of miR-200a, miR-200b, miR-200c, miR-429,

TABLE 13.3 Dysregulated microRNAs (miRNAs) in Autoimmune Diseases: Systemic Lupus Erythematosus (SLE), Rheumatic Arthritis (RA), Systemic Sclerosis (SSc), and Primary Biliary Cirrhosis (PBC)

Disease	Cell Types	Alterations of miRNAs	Targeting Genes	References
SLE	PBMCs	miR-155: decrease miR-146a: decrease	PP2Ac IFN-α and IFN-β	[95,96]
SLE	T cells	miR-21: increase miR-31: decrease	PDCD4 RhoA	[87,89]
SLE	CD4+ T cells	miR-142-3p/5p: decrease miR-21, 148a, 126 and 29b: increase	SAP, CD84, and IL-10 DNMT1	[84–86,88]
SLE	B cells	miR-30a: increase miR-1246: decrease	Lyn EBF1	[97,98]
RA	T cells	miR-223: decrease	IGF-1R	[99]
RA	CD4+ T cells	miR-146a: increase	FAF1	[100]
RA	Synovial fibroblasts	miR-155: increase	MMP-3	[101,102]
SSc	Fibroblasts	miR-21: increases miR-29a: decrease miR-196a: decrease	Smad7 Type I and III collagen Type I collagen	[103–106]
PBC	PBMCs	miR-155 and 146a: increase	–	[107]

miR-205, miR-192, miR-126, miR-16, miR-451, miR-223, miR-21, and miR-125a-3p [92,93] were found to be abnormally expressed in SLE and correlated with Systemic lupus erythematous disease activity index (SLEDAI). More inspiring is that miR-126 has been reported to regulate DNA methylation in lupus T cells by targeting DNMT1 [84], supporting the idea that lupus T cells are switched on by DNA hypomethylation via miRNAs [94]. Dysregulated miRNAs in other autoimmune disease are summarized in Table 13.3.

LONG NONCODING RNAs

In addition to miRNAs, a large number of long ncRNAs (lncRNAs), greater than 200 nt in length, have been identified, but only a minority of them has been assigned functions. Based on their genomic proximity to protein coding genes, lncRNAs are divided into five types: sense, antisense, intronic, intergenic, and bidirectional lncRNAs [108]. Unlike miRNAs, lncRNAs can both negatively and positively regulate gene expression and may function by forming lncRNA–RNA, lncRNA–protein, or lncRNA–chromatin interactions [109,110]. lncRNAs are currently the focus of intense research because multiple lines of evidence suggest that lncRNAs contribute to a range of human diseases, from neurodegeneration to cancer, by altering their primary structure, secondary structure, and expression levels [111,112].

Pathogenic Role of Long Noncoding RNAs in Autoimmunity

Studies of lncRNAs in patients with autoimmune diseases have not arisen until recent years, when a differential expression of lncRNAs in autoimmune diseases such as SLE, polymyositis/dermatomyositis, RA, type 1 diabetes mellitus, multiple sclerosis, and autoimmune thyroid disease has been revealed [113]. Growth arrest–specific transcript, also known as GAS5, is a lncRNA gene potentially implicated in the pathogenesis of SLE. This lncRNA plays essential roles in normal growth arrest, apoptosis, and cell cycle both in T cell lines and nontransformed lymphocytes [114]. The downregulated GAS5 may inhibit cell cycle and apoptosis and may thus contribute to the promotion of antigen exposure and production of autoantibodies [115]. Large intergenic ncRNAs (lincRNAs), a specific type of lncRNAs, can also regulate gene expression and is implicated in various physiological and disease conditions. Two lincRNAs, linc0949 and linc0597, have been identified to be significantly decreased in PBMCs from patients with SLE, compared to those from patients with RA and healthy controls [116]. Of note, the decreased expression level of linc0949 is correlated with complement component C3 level, SLE disease activity index, and the presence of lupus nephritis and cumulative organ damage and can increase significantly after effective treatment for lupus, suggesting its potential to serve as a biomarker for disease activity and therapeutic response in SLE [116,117].

CONCLUSION AND PERSPECTIVES

Accumulating evidence suggests the involvement of epigenetic mechanisms in immune regulation and the pathogenesis of autoimmune disorders. DNA hypomethylation, histone hypoacetylation and hyperacetylation, and decreased and/or enhanced expression of miRNAs have been identified to play a role in the pathogenesis of several autoimmune diseases. Moreover, recent studies have been focused on identifying the upstream and downstream factors that affect or impact epigenetic modifications. Efforts have been made, for example, to examine how environmental triggers promote epigenetic changes and contribute to lupus, explore the interaction of epigenetic modifications, and investigate the relationship between transcription factors and epigenetics. In a very recent report, 111 reference human epigenomes have been identified and analyzed, including 1821 histone modification data sets, 360 DNA accessibility data sets, 277 DNA methylation data sets, and 166 RNA-seq data sets [118], implying the real advent of the epigenomics era. Based on these findings and future expected results, researchers will continue to broaden and deepen our understanding of pathogenesis of autoimmune diseases and establish more individually optimized therapeutic strategies for patients.

REFERENCES

[1] Renaudineau Y, Garaud S, Le Dantec C, Alonso-Ramirez R, Daridon C, Youinou P. Autoreactive B cells and epigenetics. Clin Rev Allergy Immunol 2010;39(1):85–94.

[2] Wu H, Zhao M, Tan L, Lu Q. The key culprit in the pathogenesis of systemic lupus erythematosus: aberrant DNA methylation. Autoimmun Rev 2016;15(7):684–9.

[3] Bernstein BE, Meissner A, Lander ES. The mammalian epigenome. Cell 2007;128(4):669–81.

[4] Straussman R, Nejman D, Roberts D, Steinfeld I, Blum B, Benvenisty N, et al. Developmental programming of CpG island methylation profiles in the human genome. Nat Struct Mol Biol 2009;16(5):564–71.

[5] Esteller M. Epigenetic gene silencing in cancer: the DNA hypermethylome. Hum Mol Genet 2007;16:R50–9. Spec No 1.

[6] Doi A, Park IH, Wen B, Murakami P, Aryee MJ, Irizarry R, et al. Differential methylation of tissue- and cancer-specific CpG island shores distinguishes human induced pluripotent stem cells, embryonic stem cells and fibroblasts. Nat Genet 2009;41(12):1350–3.

[7] Bird A. DNA methylation patterns and epigenetic memory. Genes Dev 2002;16(1):6–21.

[8] Denis H, Ndlovu MN, Fuks F. Regulation of mammalian DNA methyltransferases: a route to new mechanisms. EMBO Rep 2011;12(7):647–56.

[9] Kohli RM, Zhang Y. TET enzymes, TDG and the dynamics of DNA demethylation. Nature 2013;502(7472):472–9.

[10] Tahiliani M, Koh KP, Shen Y, Pastor WA, Bandukwala H, Brudno Y, et al. Conversion of 5-methylcytosine to 5-hydroxymethylcytosine in mammalian DNA by MLL partner TET1. Science 2009;324(5929):930–5.

[11] Ito S, Shen L, Dai Q, Wu SC, Collins LB, Swenberg JA, et al. Tet proteins can convert 5-methylcytosine to 5-formylcytosine and 5-carboxylcytosine. Science 2011;333(6047):1300–3.

[12] He YF, Li BZ, Li Z, Liu P, Wang Y, Tang Q, et al. Tet-mediated formation of 5-carboxylcytosine and its excision by TDG in mammalian DNA. Science 2011;333(6047):1303–7.

[13] Maiti A, Drohat AC. Thymine DNA glycosylase can rapidly excise 5-formylcytosine and 5-carboxylcytosine: potential implications for active demethylation of CpG sites. J Biol Chem 2011;286(41):35334–8.

[14] Zhao M, Liu S, Luo S, Wu H, Tang M, Cheng W, et al. DNA methylation and mRNA and microRNA expression of SLE CD4+ T cells correlate with disease phenotype. J Autoimmun 2014;54:127–36.

[15] Lu Q, Wu A, Tesmer L, Ray D, Yousif N, Richardson B. Demethylation of CD40LG on the inactive X in T cells from women with lupus. J Immunol 2007;179(9):6352–8.

[16] Coit P, Jeffries M, Altorok N, Dozmorov MG, Koelsch KA, Wren JD, et al. Genome-wide DNA methylation study suggests epigenetic accessibility and transcriptional poising of interferon-regulated genes in naive CD4+ T cells from lupus patients. J Autoimmun 2013;43:78–84.

[17] Renauer P, Coit P, Jeffries MA, Merrill JT, McCune WJ, Maksimowicz-McKinnon K, et al. DNA methylation patterns in naive CD4+ T cells identify epigenetic susceptibility loci for malar rash and discoid rash in systemic lupus erythematosus. Lupus Sci Med 2015;2(1):e000101.

[18] Coit P, Renauer P, Jeffries MA, Merrill JT, McCune WJ, Maksimowicz-McKinnon K, et al. Renal involvement in lupus is characterized by unique DNA methylation changes in naive CD4+ T cells. J Autoimmun 2015;61:29–35.

[19] Liu Y, Chen Y, Richardson B. Decreased DNA methyltransferase levels contribute to abnormal gene expression in "senescent" CD4(+)CD28(-) T cells. Clin Immunol 2009;132(2):257–65.

[20] Zhao M, Tang J, Gao F, Wu X, Liang Y, Yin H, et al. Hypomethylation of IL10 and IL13 promoters in CD4+ T cells of patients with systemic lupus erythematosus. J Biomed Biotechnol 2010;2010:931018.

[21] Zhao M, Sun Y, Gao F, Wu X, Tang J, Yin H, et al. Epigenetics and SLE: RFX1 downregulation causes CD11a and CD70 overexpression by altering epigenetic modifications in lupus CD4+ T cells. J Autoimmun 2010;35(1):58–69.

[22] Li Y, Zhao M, Yin H, Gao F, Wu X, Luo Y, et al. Overexpression of the growth arrest and DNA damage-induced 45alpha gene contributes to autoimmunity by promoting DNA demethylation in lupus T cells. Arthritis Rheum 2010;62(5):1438–47.

[23] Li Y, Huang C, Zhao M, Liang G, Xiao R, Yung S, et al. A possible role of HMGB1 in DNA demethylation in CD4+ T cells from patients with systemic lupus erythematosus. Clin Dev Immunol 2013;2013:206298.

[24] Zhao M, Zhou Y, Zhu B, Wan M, Jiang T, Tan Q, et al. IFI44L promoter methylation as a blood biomarker for systemic lupus erythematosus. Ann Rheum Dis 2016;75:1998–2006.

[25] Ichiyama K, Chen T, Wang X, Yan X, Kim BS, Tanaka S, et al. The methylcytosine dioxygenase Tet2 promotes DNA demethylation and activation of cytokine gene expression in T cells. Immunity 2015;42(4):613–26.

[26] Zhao M, Wang J, Liao W, Li D, Li M, Wu H, et al. Increased 5-hydroxymethylcytosine in CD4(+) T cells in systemic lupus erythematosus. J Autoimmun 2016;69:64–73.

[27] Javierre BM, Fernandez AF, Richter J, Al-Shahrour F, Martin-Subero JI, Rodriguez-Ubreva J, et al. Changes in the pattern of DNA methylation associate with twin discordance in systemic lupus erythematosus. Genome Res 2010;20(2):170–9.

[28] Liu HW, Lin HL, Yen JH, Tsai WC, Chiou SS, Chang JG, et al. Demethylation within the proximal promoter region of human estrogen receptor alpha gene correlates with its enhanced expression: implications for female bias in lupus. Mol Immunol 2014;61(1):28–37.

[29] Hewagama A, Gorelik G, Patel D, Liyanarachchi P, McCune WJ, Somers E, et al. Overexpression of X-linked genes in T cells from women with lupus. J Autoimmun 2013;41:60–71.

[30] Mi XB, Zeng FQ. Hypomethylation of interleukin-4 and -6 promoters in T cells from systemic lupus erythematosus patients. Acta Pharmacol Sin 2008;29(1):105–12.

[31] Jeffries MA, Dozmorov M, Tang Y, Merrill JT, Wren JD, Sawalha AH. Genome-wide DNA methylation patterns in CD4+ T cells from patients with systemic lupus erythematosus. Epigenetics 2011;6(5):593–601.

[32] Absher DM, Li X, Waite LL, Gibson A, Roberts K, Edberg J, et al. Genome-wide DNA methylation analysis of systemic lupus erythematosus reveals persistent hypomethylation of interferon genes and compositional changes to CD4+ T-cell populations. PLoS Genet 2013;9(8):e1003678.

[33] Lu Q, Kaplan M, Ray D, Ray D, Zacharek S, Gutsch D, et al. Demethylation of ITGAL (CD11a) regulatory sequences in systemic lupus erythematosus. Arthritis Rheum 2002;46(5):1282–91.

[34] Oelke K, Lu Q, Richardson D, Wu A, Deng C, Hanash S, et al. Overexpression of CD70 and overstimulation of IgG synthesis by lupus T cells and T cells treated with DNA methylation inhibitors. Arthritis Rheum 2004;50(6):1850–60.

[35] Lu Q, Wu A, Richardson BC. Demethylation of the same promoter sequence increases CD70 expression in lupus T cells and T cells treated with lupus-inducing drugs. J Immunol 2005;174(10):6212–9.

[36] Kaplan MJ, Lu Q, Wu A, Attwood J, Richardson B. Demethylation of promoter regulatory elements contributes to perforin overexpression in CD4+ lupus T cells. J Immunol 2004;172(6):3652–61.

[37] Kozlowska A, Hrycaj P, Lacki JK, Jagodzinski PP. Perforin level in CD4+ T cells from patients with systemic lupus erythematosus. Rheumatol Int 2010;30(12):1627–33.

[38] Balada E, Castro-Marrero J, Felip L, Ordi-Ros J, Vilardell-Tarres M. Clinical and serological findings associated with the expression of ITGAL, PRF1, and CD70 in systemic lupus erythematosus. Clin Exp Rheumatol 2014;32(1):113–6.

[39] Nile CJ, Read RC, Akil M, Duff GW, Wilson AG. Methylation status of a single CpG site in the IL6 promoter is related to IL6 messenger RNA levels and rheumatoid arthritis. Arthritis Rheum 2008;58(9):2686–93.

[40] Liao J, Liang G, Xie S, Zhao H, Zuo X, Li F, et al. CD40L demethylation in CD4(+) T cells from women with rheumatoid arthritis. Clin Immunol 2012;145(1):13–8.

[41] Corvetta A, Della Bitta R, Luchetti MM, Pomponio G. 5-Methylcytosine content of DNA in blood, synovial mononuclear cells and synovial tissue from patients affected by autoimmune rheumatic diseases. J Chromatogr 1991;566(2):481–91.

[42] Richardson B, Scheinbart L, Strahler J, Gross L, Hanash S, Johnson M. Evidence for impaired T cell DNA methylation in systemic lupus erythematosus and rheumatoid arthritis. Arthritis Rheum 1990;33(11):1665–73.

[43] Nakano K, Whitaker JW, Boyle DL, Wang W, Firestein GS. DNA methylome signature in rheumatoid arthritis. Ann Rheum Dis 2013;72(1):110–7.

[44] Neidhart M, Rethage J, Kuchen S, Kunzler P, Crowl RM, Billingham ME, et al. Retrotransposable L1 elements expressed in rheumatoid arthritis synovial tissue: association with genomic DNA hypomethylation and influence on gene expression. Arthritis Rheum 2000;43(12):2634–47.

[45] Takami N, Osawa K, Miura Y, Komai K, Taniguchi M, Shiraishi M, et al. Hypermethylated promoter region of DR3, the death receptor 3 gene, in rheumatoid arthritis synovial cells. Arthritis Rheum 2006;54(3):779–87.

[46] Karouzakis E, Rengel Y, Jungel A, Kolling C, Gay RE, Michel BA, et al. DNA methylation regulates the expression of CXCL12 in rheumatoid arthritis synovial fibroblasts. Genes Immun 2011;12(8):643–52.

[47] Lei W, Luo Y, Lei W, Luo Y, Yan K, Zhao S, et al. Abnormal DNA methylation in CD4+ T cells from patients with systemic lupus erythematosus, systemic sclerosis, and dermatomyositis. Scand J Rheumatol 2009;38(5):369–74.

[48] Wang Y, Shu Y, Xiao Y, Wang Q, Kanekura T, Li Y, et al. Hypomethylation and overexpression of ITGAL (CD11a) in CD4(+) T cells in systemic sclerosis. Clin Epigenetics 2014;6(1):25.

[49] Jiang H, Xiao R, Lian X, Kanekura T, Luo Y, Yin Y, et al. Demethylation of TNFSF7 contributes to CD70 overexpression in CD4+ T cells from patients with systemic sclerosis. Clin Immunol 2012;143(1):39–44.

[50] Lian X, Xiao R, Hu X, Kanekura T, Jiang H, Li Y, et al. DNA demethylation of CD40l in CD4+ T cells from women with systemic sclerosis: a possible explanation for female susceptibility. Arthritis Rheum 2012;64(7):2338–45.

[51] Lleo A, Liao J, Invernizzi P, Zhao M, Bernuzzi F, Ma L, et al. Immunoglobulin M levels inversely correlate with CD40 ligand promoter methylation in patients with primary biliary cirrhosis. Hepatology 2012;55(1):153–60.

[52] Wang Y, Fan PS, Kahaleh B. Association between enhanced type I collagen expression and epigenetic repression of the FLI1 gene in scleroderma fibroblasts. Arthritis Rheum 2006;54(7):2271–9.

[53] Romero LI, Zhang DN, Cooke JP, Ho HK, Avalos E, Herrera R, et al. Differential expression of nitric oxide by dermal microvascular endothelial cells from patients with scleroderma. Vasc Med 2000;5(3):147–58.

[54] Lleo A, Zhang W, Zhao M, Tan Y, Bernuzzi F, Zhu B, et al. DNA methylation profiling of the X chromosome reveals an aberrant demethylation on CXCR3 promoter in primary biliary cirrhosis. Clin Epigenetics 2015;7:61.

[55] Rothbart SB, Strahl BD. Interpreting the language of histone and DNA modifications. Biochim Biophys Acta 2014;1839(8):627–43.

[56] Peserico A, Simone C. Physical and functional HAT/HDAC interplay regulates protein acetylation balance. J Biomed Biotechnol 2011;2011:371832.

[57] Renaudineau Y, Youinou P. Epigenetics and autoimmunity, with special emphasis on methylation. Keio J Med 2011;60(1):10–6.

[58] Black JC, Van Rechem C, Whetstine JR. Histone lysine methylation dynamics: establishment, regulation, and biological impact. Mol Cell 2012;48(4):491–507.

[59] Hochstrasser M. Origin and function of ubiquitin-like proteins. Nature 2009;458(7237):422–9.

[60] Weake VM, Workman JL. Histone ubiquitination: triggering gene activity. Mol Cell 2008;29(6):653–63.

[61] Rossetto D, Avvakumov N, Cote J. Histone phosphorylation: a chromatin modification involved in diverse nuclear events. Epigenetics 2012;7(10):1098–108.

[62] Hu N, Qiu X, Luo Y, Yuan J, Li Y, Lei W, et al. Abnormal histone modification patterns in lupus CD4+ T cells. J Rheumatol 2008;35(5):804–10.

[63] Zhou Y, Qiu X, Luo Y, Yuan J, Li Y, Zhong Q, et al. Histone modifications and methyl-CpG-binding domain protein levels at the TNFSF7 (CD70) promoter in SLE CD4+ T cells. Lupus 2011;20(13):1365–71.

[64] Nambiar MP, Warke VG, Fisher CU, Tsokos GC. Effect of trichostatin A on human T cells resembles signaling abnormalities in T cells of patients with systemic lupus erythematosus: a new mechanism for TCR zeta chain deficiency and abnormal signaling. J Cell Biochem 2002;85(3):459–69.

[65] Hedrich CM, Tsokos GC. Epigenetic mechanisms in systemic lupus erythematosus and other autoimmune diseases. Trends Mol Med 2011;17(12):714–24.

[66] Dai Y, Zhang L, Hu C, Zhang Y. Genome-wide analysis of histone H3 lysine 4 trimethylation by ChIP-chip in peripheral blood mononuclear cells of systemic lupus erythematosus patients. Clin Exp Rheumatol 2010;28(2):158–68.

[67] Zhang Z, Song L, Maurer K, Petri MA, Sullivan KE. Global H4 acetylation analysis by ChIP-chip in systemic lupus erythematosus monocytes. Genes Immun 2010;11(2):124–33.

[68] Apostolidis SA, Rauen T, Hedrich CM, Tsokos GC, Crispin JC. Protein phosphatase 2A enables expression of interleukin 17 (IL-17) through chromatin remodeling. J Biol Chem 2013;288(37):26775–84.

[69] Hedrich CM, Rauen T, Apostolidis SA, Grammatikos AP, Rodriguez Rodriguez N, Ioannidis C, et al. Stat3 promotes IL-10 expression in lupus T cells through trans-activation and chromatin remodeling. Proc Natl Acad Sci U S A 2014;111(37):13457–62.

[70] Sullivan KE, Suriano A, Dietzmann K, Lin J, Goldman D, Petri MA. The TNFalpha locus is altered in monocytes from patients with systemic lupus erythematosus. Clin Immunol 2007;123(1):74–81.

[71] Hu N, Long H, Zhao M, Yin H, Lu Q. Aberrant expression pattern of histone acetylation modifiers and mitigation of lupus by SIRT1-siRNA in MRL/lpr mice. Scand J Rheumatol 2009;38(6):464–71.

[72] Mishra N, Reilly CM, Brown DR, Ruiz P, Gilkeson GS. Histone deacetylase inhibitors modulate renal disease in the MRL-lpr/lpr mouse. J Clin Investig 2003;111(4):539–52.

[73] Farh KK, Marson A, Zhu J, Kleinewietfeld M, Housley WJ, Beik S, et al. Genetic and epigenetic fine mapping of causal autoimmune disease variants. Nature 2015;518(7539):337–43.

[74] Tenbrock K, Juang YT, Leukert N, Roth J, Tsokos GC. The transcriptional repressor cAMP response element modulator alpha interacts with histone deacetylase 1 to repress promoter activity. J Immunol 2006;177(9):6159–64.

[75] Zhang Z, Shi L, Dawany N, Kelsen J, Petri MA, Sullivan KE. H3K4 tri-methylation breadth at transcription start sites impacts the transcriptome of systemic lupus erythematosus. Clin Epigenetics 2016;8:14.

[76] Wada TT, Araki Y, Sato K, Aizaki Y, Yokota K, Kim YT, et al. Aberrant histone acetylation contributes to elevated interleukin-6 production in rheumatoid arthritis synovial fibroblasts. Biochem Biophys Res Commun 2014;444(4):682–6.

[77] Kramer M, Dees C, Huang J, Schlottmann I, Palumbo-Zerr K, Zerr P, et al. Inhibition of H3K27 histone trimethylation activates fibroblasts and induces fibrosis. Ann Rheum Dis 2013;72(4):614–20.

[78] Wang Y, Yang Y, Luo Y, Yin Y, Wang Q, Li Y, et al. Aberrant histone modification in peripheral blood B cells from patients with systemic sclerosis. Clin Immunol 2013;149(1):46–54.

[79] Hu Z, Huang Y, Liu Y, Sun Y, Zhou Y, Gu M, et al. beta-Arrestin 1 modulates functions of autoimmune T cells from primary biliary cirrhosis patients. J Clin Immunol 2011;31(3):346–55.

[80] Chen CZ, Li L, Lodish HF, Bartel DP. MicroRNAs modulate hematopoietic lineage differentiation. Science 2004;303(5654):83–6.

[81] Fabian MR, Sonenberg N, Filipowicz W. Regulation of mRNA translation and stability by microRNAs. Annu Rev Biochem 2010;79:351–79.

[82] Winter J, Jung S, Keller S, Gregory RI, Diederichs S. Many roads to maturity: microRNA biogenesis pathways and their regulation. Nat Cell Biol 2009;11(3):228–34.

[83] Sato F, Tsuchiya S, Meltzer SJ, Shimizu K. MicroRNAs and epigenetics. FEBS J 2011;278(10):1598–609.

[84] Zhao S, Wang Y, Liang Y, Zhao M, Long H, Ding S, et al. MicroRNA-126 regulates DNA methylation in CD4+ T cells and contributes to systemic lupus erythematosus by targeting DNA methyltransferase 1. Arthritis Rheum 2011;63(5):1376–86.

[85] Pan W, Zhu S, Yuan M, Cui H, Wang L, Luo X, et al. MicroRNA-21 and microRNA-148a contribute to DNA hypomethylation in lupus CD4+ T cells by directly and indirectly targeting DNA methyltransferase 1. J Immunol 2010;184(12):6773–81.

[86] Qin H, Zhu X, Liang J, Wu J, Yang Y, Wang S, et al. MicroRNA-29b contributes to DNA hypomethylation of CD4+ T cells in systemic lupus erythematosus by indirectly targeting DNA methyltransferase 1. J Dermatol Sci 2013;69(1):61–7.

[87] Stagakis E, Bertsias G, Verginis P, Nakou M, Hatziapostolou M, Kritikos H, et al. Identification of novel microRNA signatures linked to human lupus disease activity and pathogenesis: miR-21 regulates aberrant T cell responses through regulation of PDCD4 expression. Ann Rheum Dis 2011;70(8):1496–506.

[88] Ding S, Liang Y, Zhao M, Liang G, Long H, Zhao S, et al. Decreased microRNA-142-3p/5p expression causes CD4+ T cell activation and B cell hyperstimulation in systemic lupus erythematosus. Arthritis Rheum 2012;64(9):2953–63.

[89] Fan W, Liang D, Tang Y, Qu B, Cui H, Luo X, et al. Identification of microRNA-31 as a novel regulator contributing to impaired interleukin-2 production in T cells from patients with systemic lupus erythematosus. Arthritis Rheum 2012;64(11):3715–25.

[90] Tang Q, Yang Y, Zhao M, Liang G, Wu H, Liu Q, et al. Mycophenolic acid upregulates miR-142-3P/5P and miR-146a in lupus CD4+T cells. Lupus 2015.

[91] Wang G, Tam LS, Li EK, Kwan BC, Chow KM, Luk CC, et al. Serum and urinary cell-free MiR-146a and MiR-155 in patients with systemic lupus erythematosus. J Rheumatol 2010;37(12):2516–22.

[92] Wang G, Tam LS, Li EK, Kwan BC, Chow KM, Luk CC, et al. Serum and urinary free microRNA level in patients with systemic lupus erythematosus. Lupus 2011;20(5):493–500.

[93] Wang H, Peng W, Ouyang X, Li W, Dai Y. Circulating microRNAs as candidate biomarkers in patients with systemic lupus erythematosus. Transl Res 2012;160(3):198–206.

[94] Ceribelli A, Yao B, Dominguez-Gutierrez PR, Chan EK. Lupus T cells switched on by DNA hypomethylation via microRNA? Arthritis Rheum 2011;63(5):1177–81.

[95] Lashine YA, Salah S, Aboelenein HR, Abdelaziz AI. Correcting the expression of miRNA-155 represses PP2Ac and enhances the release of IL-2 in PBMCs of juvenile SLE patients. Lupus 2015;24(3):240–7.

[96] Tang Y, Luo X, Cui H, Ni X, Yuan M, Guo Y, et al. MicroRNA-146A contributes to abnormal activation of the type I interferon pathway in human lupus by targeting the key signaling proteins. Arthritis Rheum 2009;60(4):1065–75.

[97] Liu Y, Dong J, Mu R, Gao Y, Tan X, Li Y, et al. MicroRNA-30a promotes B cell hyperactivity in patients with systemic lupus erythematosus by direct interaction with Lyn. Arthritis Rheum 2013;65(6):1603–11.

[98] Luo S, Liu Y, Liang G, Zhao M, Wu H, Liang Y, et al. The role of microRNA-1246 in the regulation of B cell activation and the pathogenesis of systemic lupus erythematosus. Clin Epigenetics 2015;7:24.

[99] Lu MC, Yu CL, Chen HC, Yu HC, Huang HB, Lai NS. Increased miR-223 expression in T cells from patients with rheumatoid arthritis leads to decreased insulin-like growth factor-1-mediated interleukin-10 production. Clin Exp Immunol 2014;177(3):641–51.

[100] Li J, Wan Y, Guo Q, Zou L, Zhang J, Fang Y, et al. Altered microRNA expression profile with miR-146a upregulation in CD4+ T cells from patients with rheumatoid arthritis. Arthritis Res Ther 2010;12(3):R81.

[101] Stanczyk J, Ospelt C, Karouzakis E, Filer A, Raza K, Kolling C, et al. Altered expression of microRNA-203 in rheumatoid arthritis synovial fibroblasts and its role in fibroblast activation. Arthritis Rheum 2011;63(2):373–81.

[102] Stanczyk J, Pedrioli DM, Brentano F, Sanchez-Pernaute O, Kolling C, Gay RE, et al. Altered expression of MicroRNA in synovial fibroblasts and synovial tissue in rheumatoid arthritis. Arthritis Rheum 2008;58(4):1001–9.

[103] Zhu H, Luo H, Li Y, Zhou Y, Jiang Y, Chai J, et al. MicroRNA-21 in scleroderma fibrosis and its function in TGF-beta-regulated fibrosis-related genes expression. J Clin Immunol 2013;33(6):1100–9.

[104] Maurer B, Stanczyk J, Jungel A, Akhmetshina A, Trenkmann M, Brock M, et al. MicroRNA-29, a key regulator of collagen expression in systemic sclerosis. Arthritis Rheum 2010;62(6):1733–43.

[105] Xiao J, Meng XM, Huang XR, Chung AC, Feng YL, Hui DS, et al. miR-29 inhibits bleomycin-induced pulmonary fibrosis in mice. Mol Ther 2012;20(6):1251–60.

[106] Honda N, Jinnin M, Kajihara I, Makino T, Makino K, Masuguchi S, et al. TGF-beta-mediated downregulation of microRNA-196a contributes to the constitutive upregulated type I collagen expression in scleroderma dermal fibroblasts. J Immunol 2012;188(7):3323–31.

[107] Katsushima F, Takahashi A, Sakamoto N, Kanno Y, Abe K, Ohira H. Expression of micro-RNAs in peripheral blood mononuclear cells from primary biliary cirrhosis patients. Hepatol Res 2014;44(10):E189–97.

[108] Rinn JL, Chang HY. Genome regulation by long noncoding RNAs. Annu Rev Biochem 2012;81:145–66.

[109] Kretz M, Siprashvili Z, Chu C, Webster DE, Zehnder A, Qu K, et al. Control of somatic tissue differentiation by the long non-coding RNA TINCR. Nature 2013;493(7431):231–5.

[110] Johnsson P, Ackley A, Vidarsdottir L, Lui WO, Corcoran M, Grander D, et al. A pseudogene long-noncoding-RNA network regulates PTEN transcription and translation in human cells. Nat Struct Mol Biol 2013;20(4):440–6.

[111] Wapinski O, Chang HY. Long noncoding RNAs and human disease. Trends Cell Biol 2011;21(6):354–61.

[112] Li Z, Chao TC, Chang KY, Lin N, Patil VS, Shimizu C, et al. The long noncoding RNA THRIL regulates TNFalpha expression through its interaction with hnRNPL. Proc Natl Acad Sci U S A 2014;111(3):1002–7.

[113] Wu GC, Pan HF, Leng RX, Wang DG, Li XP, Li XM, et al. Emerging role of long noncoding RNAs in autoimmune diseases. Autoimmun Rev 2015;14(9):798–805.

[114] Mourtada-Maarabouni M, Hedge VL, Kirkham L, Farzaneh F, Williams GT. Growth arrest in human T-cells is controlled by the non-coding RNA growth-arrest-specific transcript 5 (GAS5). J Cell Sci 2008;121(Pt 7):939–46.

[115] Haywood ME, Rose SJ, Horswell S, Lees MJ, Fu G, Walport MJ, et al. Overlapping BXSB congenic intervals, in combination with microarray gene expression, reveal novel lupus candidate genes. Genes Immun 2006;7(3):250–63.

[116] Wu Y, Zhang F, Ma J, Zhang X, Wu L, Qu B, et al. Association of large intergenic noncoding RNA expression with disease activity and organ damage in systemic lupus erythematosus. Arthritis Res Ther 2015;17:131.

[117] Duarte JH. Connective tissue diseases: large intergenic noncoding RNA linked to disease activity and organ damage in SLE. Nat Rev Rheumatol 2015;11(7):384.

[118] Roadmap Epigenomics C, Kundaje A, Meuleman W, Ernst J, Bilenky M, Yen A, et al. Integrative analysis of 111 reference human epigenomes. Nature 2015;518(7539):317–30.

Chapter 14

Citrullination and Autoimmunity

Guido Valesini[1], Maria Chiara Gerardi[2], Cristina Iannuccelli[2], Viviana Antonella Pacucci[2], Monica Pendolino[2], Yehuda Shoenfeld[3,4]

[1]Rheumatology, Department of Internal Medicine, Sapienza University of Rome, Rome, Italy; [2]Department of Internal Medicine and Medical Specialties, Rheumatology, Sapienza University of Rome, Rome, Italy; [3]Zabludowicz Center for Autoimmune Diseases, Sheba Medical Center, affiliated to Sackler Faculty of Medicine, Tel Aviv University, Tel Aviv, Israel; [4]Laboratory of the Mosaics of Autoimmunity, Saint-Petersburg University, Saint-Petersburg, Russian Federation

INTRODUCTION

Autoimmune diseases are characterized by the body's own immune system attack to the self-tissues. Normally, the immune system does not react against self-antigens because of the processes of central and peripheral immune tolerance. In predisposed subjects, the abnormality in self-tolerance might be enabled by posttranslational modifications because these processes might promote generation of neo-(auto)antigens. During the last 10 years, great attention has been paid to citrullination because of its role in inducing anticitrullinated proteins/peptide antibodies (ACPA), a class of autoantibodies with diagnostic, predictive, and prognostic value for rheumatoid arthritis (RA).

Citrullination is the posttranslational modification of protein-bound arginine into the nonstandard amino acid citrulline, catalyzed by Ca^{2+}-dependent peptidylarginine deiminases (PAD) enzymes. Each converted molecule (arginine to citrulline) leads to a 0.984 Da mass increase and the loss of one positive charge [1]. This latter change determines a substantial effect on the acidity of the amino acid side chain, changing the isoelectric point (pI) from 11.41 for arginine to 5.91 for citrulline [2]. Moreover, it can influence the hydrogen bond–forming ability and the interaction with other amino acidic residues of the same protein or of another one. Thus, a conformational alteration may occur, and consequently a possible functional alteration and change in the protein half-life, so that a new protein is finally created. Noteworthy, the modifications of proteins can generate new epitopes, thus causing the formation of new autoantigens, different from that to which the self has apprehended to be tolerant. Indeed, it is well established that small modifications can enhance the immunogenicity of the proteins due to an enhanced protein unfolding and subsequent processing and exposure of the immunogenic epitopes [3]; to an increased uptake of the modified antigen by the antigen-presenting cells (APC) [4]; and to an improved presentation through enhanced recognition by the APC [5]. Interestingly, it seems that citrullinated peptides, but not Epstein–Barr virus derived citrullinated peptides, fit better in the HLA-DRB1 (DRB1*0401 or *0404) antigen-binding grooves—the so-called shared epitope (SE)—than the corresponding arginine-containing peptides [6]. This observation is confirmed by studies in rats immunized with citrullinated collagen type II which develop a more frequent and a more severe form of arthritis than do those immunized with unmodified collagen type II [7].

Peptidylarginine Deiminase Enzymes

The conversion of peptidylarginine into peptidylcitrulline is catalyzed by PAD [8]. To date, five isoforms of this enzyme have been identified with different tissue expressions and consequently different functions [9]. PAD1 is predominantly expressed in the epidermis and the uterus. PAD2 has been found in muscle tissues, central nervous system (CNS), and hematopoietic cells, including mast cells and macrophages. PAD3 is localized in the hair follicles, while PAD4, formerly known as PAD5, has been found in neutrophils and eosinophils, spleen, and secretory glands. Finally, PAD6 expression has been detected in eggs, ovaries, testis tissues, small intestine, spleen, lung, liver, skeletal muscle cells, and in early embryos [10,11].

PAD-induced citrullination has been studied in different physiological and pathological conditions. PAD1, physiologically implicated in the keratinization of the skin, has been demonstrated to be hypofunctional in psoriasis; on the other hand, PAD2, essential for myelin sheath stability and the plasticity of the brain, is hyperfunctional in multiple sclerosis. PAD4 reciprocally influences the expression of estrogen and p53 target genes, so it seems to play a role in tumorigenesis. Of note, citrullination catalyzed by PAD4, which physiologically alters the functions of chemokines and participates in antibacterial neutrophil extracellular traps (NETs) formation, is pathologically implicated in the generation of new auto-antigens in RA. Moreover, because PAD is not expressed in the thymus [12], the likelihood that citrullination occurs in the thymus is low and T cells reactive to citrullinated antigens could be not eliminated, generating a possible immune reaction against citrullinated antigens. Citrullination could be triggered by smoking or infections and lead to ACPA production in susceptible individuals with SE containing HLA molecules and/or general autoimmunity marker protein tyrosine phosphatase nonreceptor type 22 (PTPN22) [13].

Besides eukaryotes, PADs have been found only in one prokaryote, *Porphyromonas gingivalis* (PPAD), a major pathogen bacterium in periodontitis (PD). PPAD differs from human PADs in that it is not dependent on Ca^{2+}; furthermore, it is active at higher pH and preferentially citrullinates C-terminal arginines, both the peptide-bound and the free ones [14,15]. The citrullinated peptides generated by *P. Gingivalis* are produced by the combined action of arginine gingipains cleaving polypeptides in short peptides with C-terminal arginines followed by rapid citrullination by PPAD. It is plausible that this may trigger an immunological response to citrullinated proteins in a subset of RA patients with PD, who have the SE.

It has been recently demonstrated that PAD4 may undergo autocitrullination, a process that in one hand might inactivate the same enzyme, as a mechanism of control, but in the other modifies the structure of the enzyme, increasing its recognition by human autoantibodies [16]. In addition, anti-PAD4 antibodies have been reported to have predictive and prognostic value in RA patients [17]. Interestingly, also PPAD autocitrullinates and is a common antigenic target; so antibodies generated against autocitrullinated PPAD could perpetuate the immune response through epitope spreading and cross-reactivity with citrullinated human proteins [14]. Nonetheless, Konig and colleagues have recently reported data disproving this hypothesis because anti-PPAD antibodies do not correlate with ACPA levels and disease activity in RA and seem even to have a protective role for the development of PD in patients with RA [18].

Anticitrullinated Proteins/Peptide Antibodies

ACPA are a collection of partly cross-reactive antibodies recognizing citrulline-containing proteins and peptides. The ACPA response, often detected in assays capturing the vast majority of ACPA such as the cyclic citrullinated peptide (CCP) assay, can be divided into several partly cross-reactive fine specificities. Overall, ACPA binding to citrullinated proteins (i.e., citrullinated fibrinogen) cross-reacts with other citrullinated proteins (i.e., citrullinated vimentin) [19]. Presumably, these proteins contain multiple citrullinated residues [19]. Reactivity to a specific citrullinated peptide shows a more private recognition pattern, although these reactivities can also be partly cross-reactive. At present, it is not known whether the immune reactivity against CCP peptides or peptides with sequences derived from citrullinated proteins reflect the ability of these ACPA to recognize citrullinated proteins present in the inflamed joint, although often otherwise speculated.

During the last years, the autoantibodies directed against cyclic citrullinated proteins (anti-CCP) have been object of different studies aiming to find a serological marker able to early confirm clinical diagnosis of RA and to predict disease evolution. History of ACPA starts in 1964 when fluorescence of perinuclear keratohyalin granules of human buccal cells, defined as antiperinuclear factor antibodies (APF), was described. Subsequently, antikeratin antibodies were identified [20,21], showing, accordingly to APF, a high specificity for RA. Over the years, other candidate citrullinated autoantigens have been identified, such as fibrinogen, vimentin, fibronectin, and α-enolase [22–25]. More recently, van Beers and coworkers coined the term "citrullinome" referring to the whole citrullinated proteins, 53 in all, identified in sera and synovial fluid of RA patients [26].

ACPA are detectable in about 70% of RA patients [27]. First-generation CCP test (anti-CCP1) showed 68% sensitivity with 97%–98% specificity [28]; a higher sensitivity (80%) and superior specificity (98%) was next obtained with the second-generation CCP test (CCP2), developed through several citrulline-containing peptide libraries screening with RA sera pool [29]. Finally, even third-generation assays (CCP3) were developed, characterized by a significantly higher sensitivity in testing rheumatoid factor (RF)–negative RA and the total RA population [30]. Interestingly, a recent work carried out by Demoruelle and coworkers reported differences in the three test performances accordingly to the moment of the natural history of RA: in patients with established RA, CCP2 was more specific, whereas in subjects with undifferentiated inflammatory arthritis, CCP3 had a higher predictive value for development of RA [31]. Anyhow, given their specificity and sensitivity, an undisputed value in diagnosing RA has been attributed to this class of autoantibodies [32,33] so that ACPA positivity has been included in the new 2010 ACR/EULAR classification criteria for RA [34]. Furthermore, different studies have demonstrated that ACPA are present many years before the onset of RA [35] and can predict a worse evolution of the disease [36]: moreover, they are associated with poor remission rates and with the development of more erosive joint involvement and several extra-articular manifestations.

A number of studies on experimental models suggest the pathogenic role of ACPA. Immunizing DBA/1J mice with bovine type II collagen (CII), Kuhn and coworkers demonstrated the presence of antibodies directed against CII and CCP, before joint swelling was observed; moreover, the following tolerization to the same peptides determined a reduction in disease severity and incidence [37]. A couple of years later, Hill et al. reported that mice transgenic for human HLA-DRB1*0401 immunized with human citrullinated fibrinogen (cFb) developed arthritis but none of those animals immunized with the unmodified fibrinogen [38], neither wild-type C57BL/6 mice immunized with cFb. These data confirm the selective role in presenting citrullinated peptides and inducing the consequent autoimmune response. Finally, Willis et al. recently showed that the most potent PAD inhibitor Cl-amidine reduces both synovial citrullination and disease activity in collagen-induced arthritis but not in collagen antibody–induced arthritis, indicating that this effect is due to its ability to inhibit deimination (i.e., during gene regulation and immune functions) and to reduce epitope spreading [39].

Taken together, these findings support the diagnostic, predictive, and prognostic role, as well as the pathogenic value of ACPA in RA.

CITRULLINATION AND INFLAMMATION

The presence of citrullinated proteins, initially considered specific for the RA synovium, was later observed in non-RA inflammatory conditions. Citrullination has been reported to be a process present in a wide range of inflammatory tissues, suggesting that this is an inflammation-dependent rather than disease-dependent process. This is in agreement with the concept of inflammation as common soil of the multifactorial diseases, encompassing several chronic inflammatory rheumatic disorders [40].

In 2004, Vossenaar et al. first demonstrated that the presence of citrullinated proteins is not specific for rheumatoid synovial tissue because they can be observed in synovial tissue of patients with various inflammatory arthritides. Immunohistochemical staining of citrullinated proteins with the use of various antibodies was observed in the synovium of RA patients and in those from disease controls (inflammatory osteoarthritis, reactive arthritis, other inflammatory joint diseases, and trauma or joint disease of unknown origin). Of interest, in RA patients, the concentrations of ACPA corrected for the total amount of IgG were higher in synovial fluid than in serum suggesting a local production of these antibodies, as confirmed in a following Italian study [41,42]. According to these data, deiminated fibrin has been observed in the synovial tissue of RA patients and in patients with other inflammatory arthritides (spondyloarthropathies, psoriatic arthritis, reactive arthritis, undifferentiated spondyloarthropathy, systemic lupus erythematosus, osteoarthritis of the knee) [43]. Citrullinated proteins were detectable in all synovial biopsy specimens from RA patients, whereas only 3 of 10 healthy synovial biopsy specimens exhibited scarce amounts of citrullinated antigens [44]. Later, citrullinated proteins were also detected in inflammatory conditions other than arthritides; citrullination has been observed in muscle biopsy samples from patients with polymyositis, whereas healthy controls were totally negative. Colonic biopsy samples from patients with intestinal bowel disease presented various amounts of citrullination with no significant differences between macroscopically affected and nonaffected areas. Citrullinated proteins were detectable in tonsils from patients with chronic tonsillitis [44]. Citrullinated autoantigens have been identified also in multiple sclerosis and type 1 diabetes [45,46]. Taken together, these data demonstrated that increased citrullination is not a disease-related phenomenon but an inflammation-dependent process.

The role of *P. gingivalis* infections in RA is well known; in fact several studies demonstrated an increased incidence and severity of PD in RA [47–49]. RA-related autoantibody-positive patients resulted more likely to have moderate to severe PD than autoantibody-negative patients [50]. Conversely, in individuals with aggressive PD and without RA, autoantibodies to citrullinated filaggrin-derived peptides have been observed [51] and patients with PD presented higher serum ACPA titers than healthy donors [52]. Although RA and PD apparently have different etiology (the former autoimmune and the latter infective), the two diseases seem to have similar pathogenic mechanisms and immunologic pathways of bone and tissue destruction. In both diseases, adaptive and innate immune cells promote secretion of proinflammatory cytokines (i.e., IL-1, IL-6, and tumor necrosis factor) leading to the upregulation of matrix metalloproteinases and reactive oxygen species (ROS) that cause tissue destruction and erosion of periarticular and periodontal bone, respectively. Furthermore, RA and PD share genetic and environmental risk factors, such as MHC class II HLA-DRB1 epitope and smoking [53,54]. Interestingly, *P. gingivalis*, a major cause of PD, expresses a PAD enzyme capable of citrullinating human peptides/proteins, but with different properties from those of the human PADs; in fact, as given above, it is active at a higher pH, and it does not require calcium for its activity and also citrullinates C-terminal arginine residues and deiminates free arginine, whereas mammalian PADs do not. This microbe, citrullinating mucosal protein peptides such as vimentin, keratin, and α-enolase, seemingly generates neoepitopes that can then contribute to the loss of immune tolerance and eventually to the production of ACPA [55,56]. Particularly, human citrullinated enolase peptide-1 (CEP-1) shows 82% sequence similarity with *P. gingivalis* α-enolase and antibodies to CEP-1 cross-react with the equivalent epitope of *P. gingivalis*–derived enolase in RA patients [57]. Furthermore, in individuals at risk of RA, Mikuls et al. [58] observed an association between the concentrations of antibodies to *P. gingivalis* and serum RA-related autoantibodies; furthermore, inflamed gingival tissue has been demonstrated to express increased levels of PAD and citrullinated proteins [59,60]. A recent work has shown that infection with a strain of *P. gingivalis* exacerbated collagen-induced arthritis in a mouse model with an earlier onset, an accelerated progression, and enhanced severity of the disease [61].

As chronic exposure to citrullinated proteins at periodontal sites could contribute to the breakdown of immune tolerance to citrullinated epitopes, chronic inflammatory conditions in the lungs may also predispose susceptible individuals to the development of autoantibodies and the development of RA. Smoking and silica dust are well-known risk factors for RA and, in particular, cigarette smoking is a risk factor for ACPA-positive RA [62,63]. Recent studies suggested that the lung is involved in the citrullination of proteins and consequent generation of RA-related autoimmunity. Cigarette smoking has been shown to generate increased PAD expression and protein citrullination in bronchoalveolar lavage cells of smokers without arthritis in comparison to nonsmokers [64]. Recent findings have shown a higher prevalence of inflammatory airways disease detectable by computed tomographic imaging in individuals with ACPA and/or RF without arthritis compared with autoantibody-negative matched controls [65]. Moreover, Fischer et al. described imaging evidence of airways inflammation similar to that observed in RA-related lung disease in a cohort of patients with respiratory symptoms and ACPA positivity but without RA [66]. Recently, it has been reported that seronegative first-degree relative of RA patients had ACPA and/or RF in their sputum but not in their serum and patients with established RA and RA-autoantibody positive subjects without arthritis had higher levels of ACPA and/or RF in their sputum compared with their serum [66,67]. In line with the hypothesis of the lung as initial site of RA-autoantibody production, in a previous work, it has been reported that 14% of patients (6 of 43) with chronic obstructive pulmonary disease (COPD) but without RA were positive for serum anti–mutated citrullinated vimentin autoantibodies (anti-MCV) [68]. Furthermore, increased vimentin levels in the lungs of smokers and patients with COPD have been identified [69], and anti-MCV has been associated with severe extra-articular manifestations in RA patients [70], even if their additional diagnostic and prognostic role in comparison to anti-CCP in RA is controversial [71]. The potential role of the lung in the RA-autoimmunity development, as well as in other autoimmune diseases, is further validated by the study of Odoardi and colleagues. The authors, using a rat model of multiple sclerosis, demonstrated that myelin-specific autoimmune cells, before establishing disease in the CNS, home to the lung from where they move to the bronchus-associated lymphoid tissue and draining lymph nodes and then they reenter the blood circulation and reach the CNS. On the way from the lung to the CNS, the T cells deeply reprogram their gene expression profile, upregulate chemokine receptors and adhesion molecules that regulate their orientation toward inflamed tissues, and simultaneously get the capacity to breach endothelial barriers in the CNS [72]. While some sites of the human body have the *immune privilege* to tolerate the introduction of antigens without eliciting an inflammatory immune response, the lung seems to have a sort of *reverse immune privilege*. Thanks to its reverse immune privilege, the lung could have the capacity to license lung-resident autoreactive T cells to migrate to the target organ.

Even if evidence suggests that airborne particles exposure can elicit an autoimmune response and a previous Swedish work reported an elevated risk for RA in women living in the proximity of the road where traffic pollution is elevated, a recent study demonstrated that particulate matter, a measure of air pollution, is not associated with increased risk of developing RA in individuals at risk RA-autoantibody positive [73]. In the last years, nanomaterials have been introduced in everyday life and in a wide range of biomedical applications, but the potential risk to human health is still unknown. Mohamed and colleagues demonstrated that nanomaterials of distinct origin, morphology, and physicochemical properties (amorphous silicon dioxide, ultrafine carbon black, and single-walled carbon nanotubes [SWCNTs]) are able to induce protein citrullination via increased Ca^{2+}-mediated PAD activity in cultured human cells (lung epithelial and phagocytic cells) and in lung tissues of mice exposed to respirable SWCNTs [74]. In a following study, the same authors showed that SWCNTs are able to induce in vitro protein citrullination in lung epithelial cells prior to any detectable onset of inflammatory responses, suggesting that protein citrullination could be considered as a sign of early cellular damage [75]. In addition to citrullination, even carbamylation, a process which leads to the formation of carbamyl-lysine or homocitrulline and recently suggested to be implicated in the pathogenesis of RA, seems to be associated with inflammation rather than with a single disease [76].

CITRULLINATION AND CELL DEATH

During evolution, the eukaryotic cell develops different processes to adapt themselves to environmental changes and to die or to survive. These processes include apoptosis, autophagy, NETosis: citrullination is implicated in all of these physiological mechanisms as summarized in Table 14.1. The above-mentioned conditions, somehow extreme, are characterized by higher levels of calcium (as compared with physiologic conditions) and consequent PAD activation.

TABLE 14.1 The Role of Citrullination in Cell Death

	Apoptosis	Autophagy	NETosis
Morphology	Chromatin condensation; nuclear fragmentation; apoptotic bodies	Autophagic vacuoles	Extrusion of NET: DNA, histones, granular proteins (myeloperoxidase, elastase, lactoferrin, etc.), cytoplasmic proteins (calprotectin, catalase)
Triggers	Extrinsic pathway → death receptors (fasL)	Amino acid starvation; grown factor withdrawal; energy withdrawal; environmental stress (intracellular reactive oxygen species, etc.)	PMA, LPS, IL 8, TNF-α, LL-37, H_2O_2, LPS-activated, platelets, ANCAs, immune complexes, antineutrophil antibodies, activated endothelium, *Streptococcus* species, *Pseudomonas aeruginosa*, *Staphylococcus* species, *Candida albicans*, *Escherichia coli*, *Mycobacterium tuberculosis*, HIV
	Intrinsic pathway→viral infection, DNA damage, mitochondrial release of cytochrome *c*		
Mediators	Extrinsic pathway→caspase 8, 10	Autophagy proteins 1, 5, 6, 8, 12, 17, 13	MPO, elastase, NOX2, NADPH, PAD4, H_2O_2,
	Intrinsic pathway→caspase 9		
Inhibitors	Caspase inhibitors	Bcl-2 ?; anabolic metabolism (class I PI3K)	Catalase, Dnase, DPI
Citrullination	Citrullination is needed to prepare intracellular proteins for degradation during apoptosis with a complete loss of both polymerization competence of the intermediate filament protein and filament-forming ability	The presentation of the citrullinated peptides by the APC is associated with autophagy. Citrullination can be considered as a biochemical marker of autophagy	Citrullination of histones is responsible for chromatin decondensation that leads to the release of histones in the NET and prevents histone methylation and further transcription

ANCAs, antineutrophil cytoplasmic antibodies; *APC*, antigen-presenting cells; *Bcl-2*, B cell lymphoma 2; *DPI*, diphenyleneiodonium; *H_2O_2*, hydrogen peroxide; *HIV*, human immunodeficiency virus; *IL*, interleukin; *LL-37*, cathelicidin LL-37; *LPS*, lipopolysaccharides; *MPO*, myeloperoxidase; *NAPDH*, nicotinamide adenine dinucleotide phosphate; *NET*, neutrophil extracellular trap; *NOX2*, NADPH oxidase 2; *PAD4*, peptidylarginine deiminase 4; *PI3K*, phosphoinositide 3-kinase; *PMA*, phorbol 12-myristate 13-acetate; *TNF-α*, tumor necrosis factor alpha.

Apoptosis

Apoptosis is a physiologically programmed cell death finalized to control cell proliferation and to react to DNA injury. Two main pathways, converging toward the activation of effector caspases (caspase-9 and caspase-8, respectively), have been recognized.

The process of citrullination usually takes place in those cells that are going under the process of apoptosis. Unlimited influx of extracellular Ca^{2+} ions and consequent PAD enzymes activation start during cell death: these steps lead to the modification of peptidylarginine into peptidylcitrulline.

Citrullination is believed to prepare intracellular proteins for degradation during apoptosis with a complete loss both of polymerization competence of the intermediate filament protein and of filament-forming ability [77]. When generated, apoptotic bodies are rapidly engulfed by phagocytes, thus preventing inflammatory reactions. A dysregulation of apoptosis and/or an ineffective clearance of apoptotic material is suspected to be involved in the breach of self-tolerance with accumulation of dying cells and consequent exposition of nuclear antigens [78]. Thus, citrullinated proteins meet the immune system leading to autoantibodies generation [79].

Alteration of the mitochondrial pathway of apoptosis seems to occur in RA with a consequent resistance to receptor-mediated apoptosis [80]. Recently, it has been described that the impaired apoptosis of RA fibroblast-like synoviocytes is pivotal in the establishment of the inflammatory process [81].

Autophagy

Autophagy is a highly conserved pathway in eukaryotic organisms; this process can be defined as the physiological mechanism that promotes the turnover of cell macromolecules and organelles via the lysosomal degradative pathway. Autophagy, although detectable in surviving cells, can be dysregulated under adverse conditions, such as during cell senescence or in conditions of growth factors starvation and it can also lead to cell death by a sort of self-cannibalism.

Recent studies have also implicated autophagy in crucial immune mechanisms such as MHC class II presentation of intracellular antigens and, consequently, activation and regulation of CD4+ T cells by APC.

Thus, autophagy, as well as apoptosis, could be relevant in the induction, or loss, of self-tolerance to intracellular molecules and might act as a source of autoantigens in autoimmune diseases.

Autophagy has been shown to have a strict crosstalk with apoptosis [82]. The two processes are not mutually exclusive and for many aspects interfere with each other. Sometimes autophagy acts as a survival pathway, contrasting apoptosis, sometimes it acts as a death pathway, enhancing or replacing apoptosis.

A role for autophagy in the pathogenesis of autoimmune diseases is suspected, but it is not completely elucidated. Recently, Kato and colleagues [83] hypothesized a dual role of autophagy in stress-induced cell death in RA synovial fibroblasts: this pathway can promote cell death in the context of endoplasmic reticulum stress but can protect against cell death in the context of proteasome inhibition [83].

Yet little is known about the link between autophagy and citrullination even if a central role of autophagy in citrullination of peptides by APC has been hypothesized [84]. Ireland and Unanue demonstrated that APC presentation of the citrullinated peptides but not of the peptides unmodified is associated with autophagy. These findings suggest that the presentation of citrullinated peptide is a result and a biochemical marker of an autophagy response in APC. More studies are needed to elucidate the link between autophagy and autoreactivity through the generation of neoepitopes.

NETosis

A large body of evidence demonstrates how neutrophils contribute to host defense and inflammation by different mechanisms. These include phagocytosis, oxidative burst, and the release of lytic enzymes that destroy extracellular pathogens via nicotinamide adenine dinucleotide phosphate.

The process of NET generation, known as NETosis, is a specific type of cellular death that differs from apoptosis and necrosis [85,86]. NETs are produced on the influence of many inflammatory stimuli, such as the contact with various bacteria, lipopolysaccharide (LPS), phorbol 12-myristate 13-acetate, fungi, or activated platelets. This weapon can concentrate antibacterial substances and entrap invading microorganisms. Immunofluorescence studies demonstrated that NETosis consists in the extrusion of intracellular material composed by DNA and histones, granular proteins, and cytoplasmic proteins [85].

Two are the main biochemical events required for NET formation: production of ROS and chromatin unfolding [87]. ROS is considered being the conditio sine qua non for NET production. In fact, the formation of hydrogen peroxide (H_2O_2) turns the cellular balance toward the inactivation of the tyrosine phosphatase throughout the oxidation of a cysteine residue. This enzyme inactivation seems to participate to the dismantling of the nuclear envelope and in the mixing of the NET components.

The second step required for NET formation made up by elastase, myeloperoxidase, and cathelicidins (LL37) is the chromatin decondensation that leads to the release of histones [88,89]. On neutrophils activation by different stimuli, such as LPS, H_2O_2, or after calcium ionophore treatment in vitro, the PAD4 catalyzes; through this nuclear dominium in a calcium-dependent reaction, the conversion of arginine residues to citrulline in three of the four core histones [90,91]. The citrullination prevents histone methylation and further transcription and contributes to the chromatin decondensation [92].

NETs have been observed consistently in human autoimmune disorders and in related autoimmune inflammatory diseases such as small-vessel vasculitis, systemic lupus erythematosus, RA, and microscopic polyangiitis.

In particular, the citrullination that is indispensable for NETosis seems to join the formation of NETs in RA.

Polymorphonuclear leukocytes from RA patients were found to be significantly more prone to NETs formation [93]. Because the generation of ACPA is thought to play an important role in RA and citrullinated histones were found in RA synovial fluid, synovial tissues, and rheumatoid nodules, ACPA and citrullinated histones are supposed to be the source of autoantigens promoting aberrant immune responses and inflammation [93–95].

CONCLUSION

In the last years, great attention has been paid to citrullination because of its potential pathogenetic role in RA, an autoimmune condition characterized by an abnormal humoral response to citrullinated proteins. However, recent evidence suggests that citrullination is not a disease-related phenomenon but an inflammation-dependent process or, even, a sign of early cellular damage, as demonstrated by its involvement in apoptosis, autophagy, and NETosis. Hence, if inflammation or cellular deaths are able to induce citrullination, other factors contribute to the development of autoimmunity and further inflammation. The latter is the common soil of the multifactorial diseases, encompassing several chronic inflammatory rheumatic disorders.

Future studies to clarify the key events involved in the development of autoimmunity to citrullinated proteins are needed.

Take-Home Messages

- Citrullination is a posttranslational modification of protein-bound arginine into the nonstandard amino acid citrulline, catalyzed by Ca^{2+}-dependent PAD enzymes, which can generate new epitopes, thus causing the formation of new autoantigens, different from that to which the self has apprehended to be tolerant.
- Although ACPA are a class of autoantibodies with undisputed diagnostic, predictive, and prognostic value for RA, citrullination has been reported to be a process present in a wide range of inflammatory tissues.
- Environmental exposure to cigarette smoke and nanomaterials of air pollution may be able to induce citrullination in lung cells prior to any detectable onset of inflammatory responses, suggesting that protein citrullination could be considered as a sign of early cellular damage.
- Citrullination is implicated in all those paraphysiological processes, such as cellular death pathways, in which calcium concentration raises to higher levels than in physiologic conditions.
- Rather than being a disease-dependent process, citrullination is an inflammatory-dependent condition playing a central role in autoimmune diseases.

Soluble CXCL16 Chemokine Levels Are Upregulated in Active SLE Patients and Associated With Organ Involvement

Soluble C-X-C motif chemokine ligand 16 (sCXCL16) is a member of the chemokine superfamily which is overexpressed at tissue level and in the circulation in inflammation and autoimmunity. Growing evidence supports the notion that sCXCL16 is involved in the pathogenesis of systemic lupus erythematosus (SLE). The present cross-sectional study by Qin et al. *(Clin Rheumatol 2014;33:1595–1601)* investigated the clinical value of sCXCL16 as a serological marker of SLE. Serum levels of sCXCL16 were determined in 35 SLE patients, 16 patients with rheumatoid arthritis (RA), and 15 age/sex-matched healthy controls (HC), using commercially available ELISA, and the relationships between sCXCL16 and SLE disease activity index (SLEDAI), organ damage index (SDI), and presence/absence of specific organ involvement were studied. Serum levels of sCXCL16 were significantly elevated in patients with SLE than in patients with RA or in HC. Soluble CXCL16 was significantly higher in active SLE patients than in inactive ones, correlated with SLEDAI, SDI, SLE renal, and skin involvement and was responsive to conventional successful treatment. The authors proposed sCXCL16 as a serological marker of disease activity in SLE, particularly useful to evaluate treatment response in patients with renal or skin involvement.

Anna Ghirardello

REFERENCES

[1] Gyorgy B, Toth E, Tarcsa E, Falus A, Buzas EI. Citrullination: a posttranslational modification in health and disease. Int J Biochem Cell Biol 2006;38:1662–77.

[2] Orgovan G, Noszal B. The complete microspeciation of arginine and citrulline. J Pharm Biomed Anal 2011;54(5):965–71.

[3] Carrasco-Marin E, Paz-Miguel J, Lopez-Mato P, Alvarez-Dominguez C, Leyva-Cobian F. Oxidation of defined antigens allows protein unfolding and increases both proteolytic processing and exposes peptide epitopes which are recognized by specific T cells. Immunology 1998;95:314–21.

[4] Wallberg M, Bergquist J, Achour A, Breij E, Harris R. Malondialdehyde modification of myelin oligodendrocyte glycoprotein leads to increased immunogenicity and encephalitogenicity. Eur J Immunol 2007;37:1986–95.

[5] Allison M, Fearon D. Enhanced immunogenicity of aldehyde-bearing antigens: a possible link between innate and adaptive immunity. Eur J Immunol 2000;30:2881–7.

[6] Pratesi F, Petit Teixeira E, Sidney J, Michou L, Puxeddu I, Sette A, et al. HLA shared epitope and ACPA: just a marker or an active player? Autoimmun Rev 2013;12:1182–7.

[7] Lundberg K, Nijenhuis S, Vossenaar ER, Palmblad K, van Venrooij WJ, Klareskog L, et al. Citrullinated proteins have increased immunogenicity and arthritogenicity and their presence in arthritic joints correlates with disease severity. Arthritis Res Ther 2005;7:458–67.

[8] Vossenaar ER, Zendman AJ, van Venrooij WJ, Pruijn GJ. PAD, a growing family of citrullinating enzymes: genes, features and involvement in disease. Bioessays 2003;25:1106–18.

[9] Baka Z, György B, Géher P, Buzás EI, Falus A, Nagy G. Citrullination under physiological and pathological conditions. Joint Bone Spine 2012;79:431–6.

[10] Zhang J, Dai J, Zhao E, Lin Y, Zeng L, Chen J, et al. cDNA cloning, gene organization and expression analysis of human peptidylarginine deiminase type VI. Acta Biochim Pol 2004;51:1051–8.

[11] Chavanas S, Méchin M-C, Takahara H, Kawada A, Nachat R, Serre G, et al. Comparative analysis of the mouse and human peptidylarginine deiminase gene clusters reveals highly conserved non-coding segments and a new human gene, PADI6. Gene 2004;330:19–27.

[12] Suzuki A, Yamada R, Chang X, Tokuhiro S, Sawada T, Suzuki M, et al. Functional haplotypes of PADI4, encoding citrullinating enzyme peptidylarginine deiminase 4, are associated with rheumatoid arthritis. Nat Genet 2003;34:395–402.

[13] Klareskog L, Malmström V, Lundberg K, Padyukov L, Alfredsson L. Smoking, citrullination and genetic variability in the immunopathogenesis of rheumatoid arthritis. Semin Immunol 2011;23:92–8.

[14] Quirke AM, Lugli EB, Wegner N, Hamilton BC, Charles P, Chowdhury M, et al. Heightened immune response to autocitrullinated *Porphyromonas gingivalis* peptidylarginine deiminase: a potential mechanism for breaching immunologic tolerance in rheumatoid arthritis. Ann Rheum Dis 2014;73(1):263–9.

[15] Abdullah SN, Farmer EA, Spargo L, Logan R, Gully N. *Porphyromonas gingivalis* peptidylarginine deiminase substrate specificity. Anaerobe 2013;23:102–8.

[16] Andrade F, Darrah E, Gucek M, Cole RN, Rosen A, Zhu X. Autocitrullination of human peptidyl arginine deiminase type 4 regulates protein citrullination during cell activation. Arthritis Rheum 2010;62(6):1630–40.

[17] Zhao J, Zhao Y, He J, Jia R, Li Z. Prevalence and significance of anti-peptidylarginine deiminase 4 antibodies in rheumatoid arthritis. J Rheumatol 2008;35(6):969–74.

[18] Konig MF, Paracha AS, Moni M, Bingham CO, Andrade F. Defining the role of *Porphyromonas gingivalis* peptidylarginine deiminase (PPAD) in rheumatoid arthritis through the study of PPAD biology. Ann Rheum Dis 2015. [Epub ahead of print].

[19] Trouw LA, Huizinga TW, Toes RE. Autoimmunity in rheumatoid arthritis: different antigens — common principles. Ann Rheum Dis 2013;72(Suppl. 2):132–6.

[20] Nienhuis RL, Mandema E. A new serum factor in patients with rheumatoid arthritis; the antiperinuclear factor. Ann Rheum Dis 1964;23:302–5.

[21] Young BJ, Leslie RD, Clark CJ, Hamblin TJ. Anti-keratin antibodies in rheumatoid arthritis. Br Med J 1979;2:97–9.

[22] Sebbag M, Moinard N, Auger I, Clavel C, Arnaud J, Nogueira L, et al. Epitopes of human fibrin recognized by the rheumatoid arthritis-specific autoantibodies to citrullinated proteins. Eur J Immunol 2006;36:2250–63.

[23] Vossenaar ER, Despres N, Lapointe E, van der Heijden A, Lora M, Senshu T, et al. Rheumatoid arthritis specific anti-Sa antibodies target citrullinated vimentin. Arthritis Res Ther 2004;6:142–50.

[24] Masson-Bessiere C, Sebbag M, Girbal-Neuhauser E, Nogueira L, Vincent C, Senshu T, et al. The major synovial targets of the rheumatoid arthritis-specific antifilaggrin autoantibodies are deiminated forms of the alpha- and beta-chains of fibrin. J Immunol 2001;166:4177–84.

[25] Takizawa Y, Suzuki A, Sawada T, Ohsaka M, Inoue T, Yamada R, et al. Citrullinated fibrinogen detected as a soluble citrullinated autoantigen in rheumatoid arthritis synovial fluids. Ann Rheum Dis 2006;65:1013–20.

[26] van Beers JJ, Schwarte CM, Stammen-Vogelzangs J, Oosterink E, Božič B, Pruijn GJ. The rheumatoid arthritis synovial fluid citrullinome reveals novel citrullinated epitopes in apolipoprotein E, myeloid nuclear differentiation antigen, and β-actin. Arthritis Rheum 2013;65:69–80.

[27] Payet J, Goulvestre C, Bialé L, Avouac J, Wipff J, Job-Deslandre C, et al. Anticyclic citrullinated peptide antibodies in rheumatoid and nonrheumatoid rheumatic disorders: experience with 1162 patients. J Rheumatol 2014;41:2395–402.

[28] Schellekens GA, Visser H, de Jong BA, van den Hoogen FH, Hazes JM, Breedveld FC, et al. The diagnostic properties of rheumatoid arthritis recognizing a cyclic citrullinated peptide. Arthritis Rheum 2000;43:155–63.

[29] van Venrooij WJ, Hazes JM, Visser H. Anticitrullinated protein/peptide antibody and its role in the diagnosis and prognosis of early rheumatoid arthritis. Neth J Med 2002;60:383–8.

[30] Szekanecz Z, Szabó Z, Zeher M, Soós L, Dankó K, Horváth I, et al. Superior performance of the CCP3.1 test compared to CCP2 and MCV in the rheumatoid factor-negative RA population. Immunol Res 2013;56:439–43.

[31] Demoruelle MK, Parish MC, Derber LA, Kolfenbach JR, Hughes-Austin JM, Weisman MH, et al. Performance of anti-cyclic citrullinated peptide assays differs in subjects at increased risk of rheumatoid arthritis and subjects with established disease. Arthritis Rheum 2013;65:2243–52.

[32] Palazzi C, Buskila D, D'Angelo S, D'Amico E, Olivieri I. Autoantibodies in patients with chronic hepatitis C virus infection: pitfalls for the diagnosis of rheumatic diseases. Autoimmun Rev 2012;11:659–63.

[33] Olivieri I, Sarzi-Puttini P, Bugatti S, Atzeni F, d'Angelo S, Caporali R. Early treatment in early undifferentiated arthritis. Autoimmun Rev 2012;11:589–92.

[34] Aletaha D, Neogi T, Silman AJ, Funovits J, Felson DT, Bingham 3rd CO, et al. 2010 Rheumatoid arthritis classification criteria: an American College of Rheumatology/European League against rheumatism collaborative initiative. Arthritis Rheum 2010;62:2569–81.

[35] Nielen MM, van Schaardenburg D, Reesink HW, Twisk JW, van de Stadt RJ, van der Horst-Bruinsma IE, et al. Simultaneous development of acute phase response and autoantibodies in preclinical rheumatoid arthritis. Ann Rheum Dis 2006;65:535–7.

[36] López-Longo FJ, Sánchez-Ramón S, Carreño L. The value of anti-cyclic citrullinated peptide antibodies in rheumatoid arthritis: do they imply new risk factors? Drug News Perspect 2009;22:543–8.

[37] Kuhn KA, Kulik L, Tomooka B, Braschler KJ, Arend WP, Robinson WH, et al. Antibodies against citrullinated proteins enhance tissue injury in experimental autoimmune arthritis. J Clin Investig 2006;116:961–73.

[38] Hill JA, Bell DA, Brintnell W, Yue D, Wehrli B, Jevnikar AM, et al. Arthritis induced by posttranslationally modified (citrullinated) fibrinogen in DR4-IE transgenic mice. J Exp Med 2008;205:967–79.

[39] Willis VC, Gizinski AM, Banda NK, Causey CP, Knuckley B, Cordova KN, et al. N-α-benzoyl-N5-(2-chloro-1-iminoethyl)-L-ornithine amide, a protein arginine deiminase inhibitor, reduces the severity of murine collagen-induced arthritis. J Immunol 2011;186:4396–404.

[40] Scrivo R, Vasile M, Bartosiewicz I, Valesini G. Inflammation as "common soil" of the multifactorial diseases. Autoimmun Rev 2011;10:369–74.

[41] Vossenaar ER, Smeets TJ, Kraan MC, Raats JM, van Venrooij WJ, Tak PP. The presence of citrullinated proteins is not specific for rheumatoid synovial tissue. Arthritis Rheum 2004;50:3485–94.

[42] Spadaro A, Riccieri V, Alessandri C, Scrivo R, Valesini G. Usefulness of anti-cyclic citrullinate peptide antibody determination in synovial fluid analysis of patients with rheumatoid arthritis. Reumatismo 2006;58:116–20.

[43] Chapuy-Regaud S, Sebbag M, Baeten D, Clavel C, Foulquier C, De Keyser F, et al. Fibrin deimination in synovial tissue is not specific for rheumatoid arthritis but commonly occurs during synovitides. J Immunol 2005;174:5057–64.

[44] Makrygiannakis D, af Klint E, Lundberg IE, Löfberg R, Ulfgren AK, Klareskog L, et al. Citrullination is an inflammation-dependent process. Ann Rheum Dis 2006;65:1219–22.

[45] Bradford CM, Ramos I, Cross AK, Haddock G, McQuaid S, Nicholas AP, et al. Localisation of citrullinated proteins in normal appearing white matter and lesions in the central nervous system in multiple sclerosis. J Neuroimmunol 2014;273:85–95.

[46] Rondas D, Crèvecoeur I, D'Hertog W, Ferreira GB, Staes A, Garg AD, et al. Citrullinated glucose-regulated protein 78 is an autoantigen in type 1 diabetes. Diabetes 2015;64:573–86.

[47] De Pablo P, Dietrich T, McAlindon TE. Association of periodontal disease and tooth loss with rheumatoid arthritis in the US population. J Rheumatol 2008;35:70–6.

[48] Potikuri D, Dannana KC, Kanchinadam S, Agrawal S, Kancharla A, Rajasekhar L, et al. Periodontal disease is significantly higher in nonsmoking treatment-naive rheumatoid arthritis patients: results from a case–control study. Ann Rheum Dis 2012;71:1541–4.

[49] Pischon N, Pischon T, Kroger J, Gülmez E, Kleber BM, Bernimoulin JP, et al. Association among rheumatoid arthritis, oral hygiene, and periodontitis. J Periodontol 2008;79:979–86.

[50] Dissick A, Redman RS, Jones M, Rangan BV, Reimold A, Griffiths GR, et al. Association of periodontitis with rheumatoid arthritis: a pilot study. J Periodontol 2010;81:223–30.

[51] Hendler A, Mulli TK, Hughes FJ, Perrett D, Bombardieri M, Houri-Haddad Y, et al. Involvement of autoimmunity in the pathogenesis of aggressive periodontitis. J Dent Res 2010;89:1389–94.

[52] Lappin DF, Apatzidou D, Quirke AM, Oliver-Bell J, Butcher JP, Kinane DF, et al. Influence of periodontal disease, *Porphyromonas gingivalis* and cigarette smoking on systemic anti-citrullinated peptide antibody titres. J Clin Periodontol 2013;40:907–15.

[53] Liao F, Li Z, Wang Y, Shi B, Gong Z, Cheng X. *Porphyromonas gingivalis* may play an important role in the pathogenesis of periodontitis-associated rheumatoid arthritis. Med Hypotheses 2009;72:732–5.

[54] Berthelot J-M, Le Goff B. Rheumatoid arthritis and periodontal disease. Joint Bone Spine 2010;77:537–41.

[55] Wegner N, Wait R, Sroka A, Eick S, Nguyen KA, Lundberg K, et al. Peptidylarginine deiminase from *Porphyromonas gingivalis* citrullinates human fibrinogen and alpha-enolase: implications for autoimmunity in rheumatoid arthritis. Arthritis Rheum 2010;62:2662–72.

[56] McGraw WT, Potempa J, Farley D, Travis J. Purification, characterization, and sequence analysis of a potential virulence factor from *Porphyromonas gingivalis*, peptidylarginine deiminase. Infect Immun 1999;67:3248–56.

[57] Lundberg K, Kinloch A, Fisher BA, Wegner N, Wait R, Charles P, et al. Antibodies to citrullinated alpha-enolase peptide 1 are specific for rheumatoid arthritis and cross-react with bacterial enolase. Arthritis Rheum 2008;58:3009–19.

[58] Mikuls TR, Thiele GM, Deane KD, Payne JB, O'Dell JR, Yu F, et al. *Porphyromonas gingivalis* and disease-related autoantibodies in individuals at increased risk for future rheumatoid arthritis. Arthritis Rheum 2012;64:3522–30.

[59] Nesse W, Westra J, van der Wal JE, Abbas F, Nicholas AP, Vissink A, et al. The periodontium of periodontitis patients contains citrullinated proteins which may play a role in ACPA (anticitrullinated protein antibody) formation. J Clin Periodontol 2012;39:599–607.

[60] Harvey GP, Fitzsimmons TR, Dhamarpatni AA, Marchant C, Haynes DR, Bartold PM. Expression of peptidylarginine deiminase-2 and -4, citrullinated proteins and anticitrullinated protein antibodies in human gingiva. J Periodontal Res 2013;48:252–61.

[61] Maresz KJ, Hellvard A, Sroka A, Adamowicz K, Bielecka E, Koziel J, et al. *Porphyromonas gingivalis* facilitates the development and progression of destructive arthritis through its unique bacterial peptidylarginine deiminase (PAD). PLoS Pathog 2013;9:e1003627.

[62] Klareskog L, Stolt P, Lundberg K, Källberg H, Bengtsson C, Grunewald J, et al. A new model for an etiology of rheumatoid arthritis: smoking may trigger HLA–DR (shared epitope)–restricted immune reactions to autoantigens modified by citrullination. Arthritis Rheum 2006;54:38–46.

[63] Oliver JE, Silman AJ. Risk factors for the development of rheumatoid arthritis. Scand J Rheumatol 2006;35:169–74.

[64] Makrygiannakis D, Hermansson M, Ulfgren AK, Nicholas AP, Zendman AJ, Eklund A, et al. Smoking increases peptidylarginine deiminase 2 enzyme expression in human lungs and increases citrullination in BAL cells. Ann Rheum Dis 2008;67:1488–92.

[65] Demoruelle MK, Weisman MH, Simonian PL, Lynch DA, Sachs PB, Pedraza IF, et al. Brief report: airways abnormalities and rheumatoid arthritis-related autoantibodies in subjects without arthritis: early injury or initiating site of autoimmunity? Arthritis Rheum 2012;64:1756–61.

[66] Fischer A, Solomon JJ, du Bois RM, Deane KD, Olson AL, Fernandez-Perez ER, et al. Lung disease with anti-CCP antibodies but not rheumatoid arthritis or connective tissue disease. Respir Med 2012;106:1040–7.

[67] Willis VC, Demoruelle MK, Derber LA, Chartier-Logan CJ, Parish MC, Pedraza IF, et al. Sputa autoantibodies in patients with established rheumatoid arthritis and subjects at-risk for future clinically apparent disease. Arthritis Rheum 2013;65:2545–54.

[68] Gerardi MC, De Luca N, Alessandri C, Iannuccelli C, Valesini G, Di Franco M. Frequency of antibodies to mutated citrullinated vimentin in chronic obstructive pulmonary disease: comment on the article by Demoruelle et al. Arthritis Rheum 2013;65:1672–3.

[69] Milara J, Peiró T, Serrano A, Cortijo J. Epithelial to mesenchymal transition is increased in patients with COPD and induced by cigarette smoke. Thorax 2013;68:410–20.

[70] Turesson C, Mathsson L, Jacobsson LT, Sturfelt G, Rönnelid J. Antibodies to modified citrullinated vimentin are associated with severe extra-articular manifestations in rheumatoid arthritis. Ann Rheum Dis 2013;72:2047–8.

[71] Bartoloni E, Alunno A, Bistoni O, Bizzaro N, Migliorini P, Morozzi G, et al. Diagnostic value of anti-mutated citrullinated vimentin in comparison to anti-cyclic citrullinated peptide and anti-viral citrullinated peptide 2 antibodies in rheumatoid arthritis: an Italian multicentric study and review of the literature. Autoimmun Rev 2012;11:815–20.

[72] Odoardi F, Sie C, Streyl K, Ulaganathan VK, Schläger C, Lodygin D, et al. T cells become licensed in the lung to enter the central nervous system. Nature 2012;488:675–9.

[73] Gan RW, Deane KD, Zerbe GO, Demoruelle MK, Weisman MH, Buckner JH, et al. Relationship between air pollution and positivity of RA-related autoantibodies in individuals without established RA: a report on SERA. Ann Rheum Dis 2013;72:2002–5.

[74] Mohamed BM, Verma NK, Davies AM, McGowan A, Crosbie-Staunton K, Prina-Mello A, et al. Citrullination of proteins: a common post-translational modification pathway induced by different nanoparticles in vitro and in vivo. Nanomedicine (Lond) 2012;7:1181–95.

[75] Mohamed BM, Movia D, Knyazev A, Langevin D, Davies AM, Prina-Mello A, et al. Citrullination as early-stage indicator of cell response to single-walled carbon nanotubes. Sci Rep 2013;3:1124.

[76] Shi J, van Veelen PA, Mahler M, Janssen GM, Drijfhout JW, Huizinga TW, et al. Carbamylation and antibodies against carbamylated proteins in autoimmunity and other pathologies. Autoimmun Rev March 2014;13(3):225–30.

[77] Inagaki M, Takahara H, Nishi Y, Sugawara K, Sato C. Ca^{2+}-dependent deimination-induced disassembly of intermediate filaments involves specific modification of the amino-terminal head domain. J Biol Chem 1989;264:18119–27.

[78] Luban S, Li ZG. Citrullinated peptide and its relevance to rheumatoid arthritis: an update. Int J Rheumatol Dis 2010;13:284–7.

[79] Moeez S, John P, Bhatti A. Anti-citrullinated protein antibodies: role in pathogenesis of RA and potential as a diagnostic tool. Rheumatol Int 2013;33:1669–73.

[80] Baier A, Meineckel I, Gay S, Pap T. Apoptosis in rheumatoid arthritis. Curr Opin Rheumatol 2003;15:274–9.

[81] Li H, Wan A. Apoptosis of rheumatoid arthritis fibroblast-like synoviocytes: possible roles of nitric oxide and the thioredoxin 1. Mediat Inflamm 2013;2013:953462.

[82] Eisenberg-Lerner A, Bialik S, Simon HU, Kimchi A. Life and death partners: apoptosis, autophagy and the cross-talk between them. Cell Death Differ 2009;16:966–75.

[83] Kato M, Ospelt C, Gay RE, Gay S, Klein K. Dual role of autophagy in stress-induced cell death in rheumatoid arthritis synovial fibroblasts. Arthritis Rheumatol 2014;66:40–8.

[84] Ireland JM, Unanue ER. Processing of proteins in autophagy vesicles of antigen-presenting cells generates citrullinated peptides recognized by the immune system. Autophagy 2012;8:429–30.

[85] Galluzzi L, Vitale I, Abrams JM, Alnemri ES, Baehrecke EH, Blagosklonny MV, et al. Molecular definitions of cell death subroutines: recommendations of the Nomenclature Committee on Cell Death 2012. Cell Death Differ 2012;19:107–20.

[86] Brinkmann V, Reichard U, Goosmann C, Fauler B, Uhlemann Y, Weiss DS, et al. Neutrophil extracellular traps kill bacteria. Science 2004;303:1532–5.

[87] Amulic B, Hayes G. Neutrophil extracellular traps. Curr Biol 2011;21:R297–8.

[88] Mesa MA, Vasquez G. NETosis. Autoimmun Dis 2013;2013:651497.

[89] Fuchs TA, Abed U, Goosmann C, Hurwitz R, Schulze I, Wahn V, et al. Novel cell death program leads to neutrophil extracellular traps. J Cell Biol 2007;176:231–41.

[90] Mastronardi FG, Wood DD, Mei J, Raijmakers R, Tseveleki V, Dosch HM, et al. Increased citrullination of histone H3 in multiple sclerosis brain and animal models of demyelination: a role for tumor necrosis factor-induced peptidylarginine deiminase 4 translocation. J Neurosci 2006;26:11387–96.

[91] Leshner M, Wang S, Lewis C, Zheng H, Chen XA, Santy L, et al. PAD4 mediated histone hypercitrullination induces heterochromatin decondensation and chromatin unfolding to form neutrophil extracellular trap-like structures. Front Immunol 2012;3:307.

[92] Wang Y, Li M, Stadler S, Correll S, Li P, Wang D, et al. Histone hypercitrullination mediates chromatin decondensation and neutrophil extracellular trap formation. J Cell Biol 2009;184:205–13.

[93] Khandpur R, Carmona-Rivera C, Vivekanandan-Giri A, Gizinski A, Yalavarthi S, Knight JS, et al. NETs are a source of citrullinated autoantigens and stimulate inflammatory responses in rheumatoid arthritis. Sci Transl Med 2013;5:178ra40.

[94] Pratesi F, Dioni I, Tommasi C, Alcaro MC, Paolini I, Barbetti F, et al. Antibodies from patients with rheumatoid arthritis target citrullinated histone 4 contained in neutrophils extracellular traps. Ann Rheum Dis 2014;73:1414–22.

[95] Sakkas LI, Bogdanos DP, Katsiari C, Platsoucas CD. Anti-citrullinated peptides as autoantigens in rheumatoid arthritis-relevance to treatment. Autoimmun Rev 2014;13:1114–20.

Chapter 15

Cytokines and Chemokines

Yumi Tsuchida, Keishi Fujio

Department of Allergy and Rheumatology, Graduate School of Medicine, The University of Tokyo, Tokyo, Japan

To mount an effective response against pathogens, the immune system needs to coordinate the function and migration of immune cells in a time- and space-specific manner. Cytokines and chemokines are signaling molecules that play important roles in the communication among immune cells and are essential for the coordination of an effective immune response. Cytokines and chemokines are important in various processes and diseases, such as infections, autoimmune diseases, allergies, cancer, and atherosclerosis. In this chapter, we focus on the role of cytokines and chemokines in the normal immune system and in autoimmunity.

CYTOKINES: AN OVERVIEW

Cytokines are small proteins that are produced by various cells and modulate the function of cells that express their specific receptors. Many cytokines exert their effects by being secreted while others, for example, tumor necrosis factor (TNF) exist in membrane-anchored forms and exert their effect without becoming soluble. Cytokines generally bind to their specific receptors with high binding affinity and can exert their effects at very low concentrations. Cytokines generally modify function of cells nearby, in a paracrine manner, or act upon themselves, in an autocrine manner. Sometimes, cytokines exert their effects on distant cells in an endocrine manner.

The discovery of cytokines is generally attributed to the description of interferons as a substance that interferes with the replication of viruses by Issacs and Lindenmann in the 1950s [1]. Since then, numerous cytokines have been discovered, and now over 60 cytokines that are important in immune regulation have been described, including interferons, interleukins, TNF-α, and TGF-β [2]. As our understanding of cytokines evolves, the nomenclature of cytokines has changed, and many cytokines are called by several different names.

There are various methods for classifying cytokines. Cytokines may be classified based on their function on the inflammatory response, for example, either pro-inflammatory or anti-inflammatory. Cytokines may also be classified by the cells that produce them; for example, monokines are produced by monocytes, while lymphokines are produced by lymphocytes. Cytokines may also be classified by their function, structure, and receptors. In the following section, we will describe some of the major families of cytokines and their representative members.

The IL-1 Family

The IL-1 family of cytokines now consists of 11 members. Among them, IL-1α, IL-1β, IL-19, IL-33, IL-36α, IL-36β, and IL-36γ exhibit pro-inflammatory properties, and IL-1Ra, IL-36Ra, IL-37, and IL-38 show anti-inflammatory properties.

IL-1 was the first interleukin to be identified and consists of two proteins: IL-1α and IL-β. IL-1α and IL-1β, although encoded by different genes without much sequence homology, bind to the same receptor and have similar biological effects. IL-1α precursor is expressed by epithelial layers of various organs such as the gastrointestinal tract, and it is also expressed by endothelial cells and astrocytes. Upon necrosis of those cells, the precursor protein is released. IL-1β is mainly expressed by hematopoietic cells, such as monocytes, macrophages, and dendritic cells. The IL-1β precursor protein does not exhibit biological activity and needs to be cleaved by caspase-1 in the inflammasome to become active [3]. IL-1 was originally reported as a pyrogen, a substance that induces fever [2], but it has much more effects. For example, it induces the production of acute phase proteins in the liver, such as the C-reactive protein and complement components. It also induces endothelial cells to express chemokines and adhesion molecules, aiding leukocyte recruitment. IL-1 also promotes survival and effector function of neutrophils and monocytes. In addition to activating the innate immune system, IL-1 helps to coordinate the adaptive immune response, for example, by inducing Th17 cells [3]. Excessive inflammation can cause tissue damage, and to avoid excessive inflammatory response, negative regulators of IL-1 are present. IL-1Rα and IL-1R2 are receptors that competitively bind to IL-1 and inhibit the inflammatory response by IL-1 [4].

The Common γ Chain Cytokines

The common γ chain cytokines are cytokines whose receptors include the common cytokine receptor γ chain (γ_c or CD132; encoded by the *IL2RG* gene), and this family consists of IL-2, IL-4, IL-7, IL-9, IL-15, and IL-21. Common γ chain cytokines have a similar structure with four α-helices [5]. Mutations in the *IL2RG* gene cause X-SCID, which is characterized by severe immunodeficiency, demonstrating the importance of those cytokines [6,7].

IL-2 is mainly produced by activated T cells, but CD8+ T cells, natural killer cells (NK cells), and NK T cells also produce IL-2 [5]. Its receptor consists of three components: IL-2Rα (CD25), IL-2Rβ (CD122), and γc. IL-2 induces the proliferation of effector T cells, as well as NK cells, and it is necessary for the development, survival, and function of Foxp3+ regulatory T cells (Tregs) [8]. IL-2 induces proliferation and antibody production in B cells [9].

IL-4 is a Th2 signature cytokine, along with other cytokines such as IL-5 and IL-13, and produced by Th2 cells. It is also produced by type 2 ILCs, basophils, mast cells, and eosinophils. It induces B cell class switching to IgE, and T cell differentiation into Th2 cells. IL-4 is involved in the control of parasite infection and has been implicated in various allergic diseases, along with other Th2 cytokines, such as IL-5 and IL-13 [5].

IL-9 is produced mainly by Th9 cells, a subset of helper T cells that has recently been recognized. Unlike other Th subsets that are characterized by lineage specific transcription factors, for example, T-bet in Th1 cells, no lineage specific transcription factor has been identified in Th9 cells, and some people question whether Th9 cells really represents a unique Th subset. Th9 cells are induced by IL-4 and TGF-β. IL-9 plays an important role in allergic reactions by promoting the survival and proliferation of mast cells [10].

IL-21 is produced mainly by follicular helper T cells (Tfh) and is also produced by Th17 cells and NK T cells [11]. IL-21 is essential for B cell differentiation, inducing them to differentiate into plasmablasts and plasma cells [11,12]. IL-21 also promotes class switching. In addition, IL-21 induces the differentiation of human Th17 cells [13]. IL-21 has also been implicated in the differentiation of Tfh cells, thus having an autocrine function [11].

The IL-10 Family

The IL-10 family consists of IL-10, IL-19, IL-20, IL-22, IL-24, IL-26, IL-28, and IL-29.

IL-10 is an anti-inflammatory cytokine that plays an important role in immunoregulation. Among T cells, IL-10 is produced by a subset of regulatory T cells called type 1 Tregs (Tr1) [14]. They are characterized by the expression of transcription factor EGR2 and cell surface expression of LAG3 [15]. IL-10 is also produced by a subset of B cells with a regulatory function called regulatory B cells (Bregs) [16]. IL-10 is generally known as an anti-inflammatory cytokine and inhibits the activation of T cells by macrophages and dendritic cells (DCs) by reducing the expression of co-stimulatory molecules and pro-inflammatory cytokines by those cells [17]. Although generally known as an inhibitory cytokine, IL-10 promotes IgG class switching and IgG production by B cells [18].

Among the IL-10 family, IL-19, IL-20, IL-22, IL-24, and IL-26 are sometimes grouped as the IL-20 subfamily because of the common usage of receptor subunits and similarities in their function. They are involved in the homeostasis of the skin and stimulate proliferation of epithelial cells and the production of antimicrobial proteins by epithelial cells. They play important roles in would healing and in shaping the microbiota [2,19]. IL-19 is expressed by activated monocytes, as well as B cells. IL-20 is produced by monocytes and DCs, as well as epithelial and endothelial cells. IL-22 is produced by a subset of T cells including Th17 cells and Th22 cells, as well as γδ T cells. IL-22 is also produced by type 3 ILCs [2,20]. IL-24 is a cytokine produced by melanocytes, T cells, and monocytes. IL-26 is produced by Th17 cells, as well as NK cells.

The IL-12 Family

The IL-12 family consists of four cytokines that partially share common receptor and ligand chains: IL-12, IL-23, IL-27, and IL-35. IL-12 consists of two subunits: p35 and p40. It is produced mainly by DCs and macrophages and is involved in the differentiation of Th1 cells and IFN-γ production by Th1 cells. IL-12 also induces IFN-γ production by NK cells and type 1 ILCs. IL-23 consists of the IL-12p40 subunit and IL-23p19 subunit, and it is also produced by macrophages and DCs. IL-23 activates NK cells and is involved in the differentiation and maintenance of Th17 cells [21]. IL-27 consists of EBI3 and the p28 subunits. It promotes inflammation by inducing the production of IFN-γ by NK cells and differentiation of Th1 cells, but it may also exert anti-inflammatory effects by inducing Tr1 cells [17]. IL-35 consists of EBI3 and the p35 subunit of IL-12 and is generally known as an anti-inflammatory cytokine [2].

The IL-17 Family

IL-17A, also called IL-17, was the first member to be reported in this family. It is mainly produced by Th17 cells, which is characterized by the master transcription factor RORγt/RORC2 [22]. It is also produced by NK cells, NK T cells, γδ T cells, and type 3 ILCs [23]. IL-17A promotes inflammation by inducing the production of pro-inflammatory cytokines and chemokines, such as IL-8, IL-6, G-CSF, GM-CSF, and MCP-1, and by inducing the recruitment of neutrophils [24]. Other members of the IL-17 family include IL-17B, IL-17C, IL-17D, and IL-17F. IL-17F has the greatest homology with IL-17A and is also produced by Th17 cells.

IL-6 Type Family

The IL-6 type family of cytokines, also called the IL-6 superfamily, includes IL-6, leukemia inhibitory factor (LIF), ciliary neurotrophic factor (CNTF), and oncostatin M (OSM) [2].

IL-6 is produced by various cells, including monocytes, macrophages, B cells, endothelial cells, and fibroblasts. The IL-6 receptor consists of IL-6Rα and gp130 and exists in membrane-bound and soluble forms. IL-6 induces the production of acute phase proteins, such as the C reactive protein, serum amyloid protein A, and complement C3. IL-6 is also involved in hematopoiesis and induces neutrophilia and thrombocytosis associated with inflammation. IL-6 also promotes the differentiation of B cells into plasma cells. In T cells, IL-6, along with other cytokines such as TGF-β, induces the differentiation of Th17 cells [25].

The TNF Superfamily

The TNF superfamily consists of 19 proteins that have both pro-inflammatory and anti-inflammatory effects. Member of the TNF superfamily are unique in that many of them exist as transmembrane proteins, thus limiting their range of action. Members of the TNF superfamily generally exert their effect by inducing the clustering of their receptor subunits.

TNF-α, the prototype of this superfamily, was originally reported to induce necrosis of tumors and cachexia. It is mainly produced by macrophages and is also produced by fibroblasts, activated T cells, and B cells. TNF-α, along with IL-1 and IL-6 in many cases, induces the production of pro-inflammatory cytokines and fever. It also induces the recruitment of neutrophils [26].

Receptor activator of nuclear factor kappa-B ligand (RANKL), also known as s tumor necrosis factor ligand superfamily member 11 (TNFSF11), is a member of the TNF superfamily mainly expressed by osteoblasts and T cells. Its receptor, RANK, is expressed on osteoclast precursors and osteoclasts, and RANKL acts through RANK to induces osteoclast maturation and bone resorption [27].

B-cell activating factor (BAFF, also known as BLyS) and anti-proliferation inducing ligand (APRIL) are members of the TNF superfamily that are important in the homeostasis of B cells. BAFF and APRIL exert their effect by binding to transmembrane activator and CAML interactor (TACI) and B cell maturation antigen (BCMA). BAFF can also bind to BAFF-R. Both BAFF and APRIL promote survival of B cells and production of antibodies [28].

Many members of the TNF superfamily are therapeutic targets in autoimmune diseases, which will be discussed later in this chapter.

The TGF Superfamily

The TGF superfamily consists of TGF, bone morphogenic proteins (BMPs), and activins and is involved in various processes including cell development and differentiation [29]. Among the TGF superfamily, TGF-β1 has mainly gained attention in immunology although there is increasing evidence that other members such as TGF-β3 and BMPs are also important in immunology [30]. TGF-β1 is generally known as an inhibitory cytokine although its action is highly context dependent, and TGF-β1 exhibits immunostimulatory effects in certain situations. Among CD4+ T cells, TGF-β1 induces the expression of Foxp3 and differentiation of Foxp3+ regulatory T cells [31,32]. However, when present with other inflammatory cytokines such as IL-6, TGF-β1 induces the differentiation of Th17 cells [13,33,34]. TGF-β1 is expressed on the cell surface of Foxp3+ regulatory T cells and is involved in the suppressive function of Foxp3+ Tregs [35]. TGF-β1 induces apoptosis of B cells and inhibits B cell proliferation, as well as antibody production; however, in certain situations, TGF-β1 induces proliferation of B cells and class switching to IgA [36]. It inhibits the secretion of pro-inflammatory cytokines by dendritic cells and the expression of co-stimulatory molecules by dendritic cells, and TGF-β1 also inhibits the action of NK cells [37].

Interferons

Interferons were originally reported as a substance that inhibits the replication of viruses. They are divided into three types: type I, type II, and type III.

Type I interferon family is the largest family with IFN-α being the prototype. Virtually all nucleated cell of the body can produce IFN-α in response to infection, but the main source of IFN-α is plasmacytoid DCs. Activation of Toll-like receptor (TLR)7 and TLR9 induce the production of type I interferons in DCs [38]. IFN-α signals through IFNAR1/IFNAR2 and affects the function of various immune cells. For example, in B cells, IFN-α induces differentiation, class switching, and antibody production. In addition, IFN-α induces the expression of MHC class II molecules and co-stimulatory molecules on DCs. Furthermore, IFN-α promotes the survival of activated CD4+ T cells as well as memory CD8+ T cells [39].

IFN-γ is the only member of type II interferon family. It is produced mainly by Th1 cells, CD8+ T cells, and NK cells [38]. IFN-γ signals through its receptors, IFNGR1 and IFNGR2, to activates macrophages and promotes Th1 responses [40]. IFN-γ signaling is necessary for granuloma formation and for controlling infections with intracellular pathogens, such as mycobacterial species. Polymorphisms and mutations in this pathway have been associated with mycobacterial infections [41,42].

Type III interferon family is the most recently described family and consists of IFNλ-1 (also called IL-29), IFNλ-2 (IL-28A), IFNλ-3 (IL-28B), and IFNλ-4. It is produced by antigen-presenting cells and epithelial cells [38]. Although there are subtle differences, type III interferons exhibit similar functions as type I interferons [43].

THE JAK-STAT PATHWAY

When cytokines bind to their respective receptors, they rapidly activate signal molecules associated with the receptors, initiating a cascade of events leading to their function. Many important cytokines, including the common γ chain cytokines, interferons, and IL-6, utilize the JAK-STAT pathway.

The JAK (Janus kinase) family, in mammals, consists of JAK1, JAK2, JAK3, and TYK2. They are tyrosine kinases associated with the cytoplasmic tail of type I and type II cytokine receptors. Binding of the cognate ligand to the receptors brings the JAKs in close proximity, allowing them to phosphorylate and activate each other. The JAKs, in turn, phosphorylate the receptors, which creates binding sites for the STAT proteins. STAT proteins bind to the receptor and are phosphorylated by JAKs. STAT proteins are transcription factors, and upon phosphorylation by JAKs, they dimerize, translocated to the nucleus, and induce changes in the transcription of their target genes [44] (Fig. 15.1). There are seven STAT proteins in mammals: STAT1, STAT2, STAT3, STAT4, STAT5A, STAT5B, and STAT6. JAKs and STAT proteins activated by cytokines important in autoimmunity is summarized in Table 15.1.

The JAK-STAT pathway is regulated by various mechanisms. For example, there are many phosphatases that hydrolyze phosphorylated tyrosines in JAKs, such as SHP1, SHP2, and DUSP2. Another mechanism involves the protein inhibitor of activated STAT (PIAS). PIAS modifies STAT-mediated regulation of transcription, generally through physical

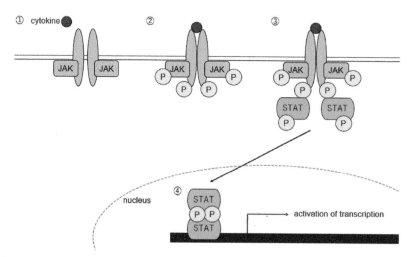

FIGURE 15.1 The JAK-STAT Pathway. ① The cytokine receptors consist of at least two chains associated with JAKs. ② Binding of the cytokine to the receptor causes the receptor chains to dimerize, allowing the JAKs to phosphorylate each other and the receptor. ③ STAT proteins bind to the receptors and are phosphorylated. ④ The phosphorylated STAT proteins move to the nucleus and induce transcription of the target genes.

TABLE 15.1 JAKs and STAT Proteins Activated by Cytokines

Cytokine	JAK	STAT
IL-2	JAK1, JAK3	STAT5
IL-4	JAK1, JAK3	STAT6
IL-6	JAK1, JAK2, TYK2	STAT1, STAT3
IL-10	JAK1, TYK2	STAT3
IL-12	JAK2, TYK2	STAT4
IL-21	JAK1, JAK3	STAT3
IFN-α	JAK1, TYK2	STAT1, STAT2
IFN-γ	JAK1, JAK2	STAT1

Based on Narazaki M, Tanaka T, Kishimoto T. The role and therapeutic targeting of IL-6 in rheumatoid arthritis. Expert Rev Clin Immunol 2017;13(6):535–51; Luo S, Wang Y, Zhao M, Lu Q. The important roles of type I interferon and interferon-inducible genes in systemic lupus erythematosus. Int Immunopharmacol 2016;40:542–9; Schwartz DM, Kanno Y, Villarino A, Ward M, Gadina M, O'Shea JJ. JAK inhibition as a therapeutic strategy for immune and inflammatory diseases. Nat Rev Drug Discov 2017;16(12):843–62; Carey AJ, Tan CK, Ulett GC. Infection-induced IL-10 and JAK-STAT: a review of the molecular circuitry controlling immune hyperactivity in response to pathogenic microbes. Jakstat 2012;1(3):159–67; Mahmud SA, Manlove LS, Farrar MA. Interleukin-2 and STAT5 in regulatory T cell development and function. Jakstat 2013;2(1):e23154.

interactions with the STAT proteins in the nucleus. The JAK-STAT pathway is also regulated by the SOCS (suppressor of cytokine signaling) family. In mammals there are four members of the SOCS family: SOCS1, SOCS2, SOCS3, and CISH. The transcription of SOCS is induced by the STAT proteins they inhibit, allowing them to work as a negative feedback loop [45]. Using those mechanisms, the action of cytokines and JAK-STAT signaling is controlled in a time- and space-specific manner.

CYTOKINES IN AUTOIMMUNE DISEASES

Cytokines play important roles in the pathophysiology of autoimmune diseases. The dysregulation of cytokines in autoimmune diseases is presumed, at least in part, to be due to genetic predisposition as many GWAS SNPs of autoimmune diseases are in or near genes encoding cytokines, their receptors, signal transduction molecules, or regulators of the signal transduction pathway. In this section, we will discuss the role of cytokines in the pathogenesis of several autoimmune diseases.

Rheumatoid Arthritis

Many GWAS SNPs associated with rheumatoid arthritis (RA) are in or near genes encoding cytokines or signal transduction molecules, for example, IL-2, IL-21, STAT4, and TYK2, suggesting the importance of cytokine signaling in the pathogenesis of RA [46,47]. The success of cytokine-targeted therapies in RA also illustrates the importance of cytokines in the pathophysiology of RA. RA is characterized by increased levels of various pro-inflammatory cytokines, including TNF-α, IL-1, IL-6, and IL-17.

TNF-α is abundant in the synovial fluid of RA patients and is produced by activated macrophages, as well as synovial fibroblasts and activated lymphocytes. TNF-α activates synovial fibroblasts and induces the production of connective tissue growth factor (CTGF), which promotes activation of osteoclasts and joint destruction. Furthermore, TNF-α induces the production of other pro-inflammatory cytokines, chemokines, and proteases including matrix metalloproteinases.

IL-1 is produced by activated macrophages and monocytes, as well as synovial fibroblasts in RA. It contributes to arthritis and joint destruction by inducing the production of pro-inflammatory cytokines and chemokines and by promoting RANKL induced osteoclastogenesis.

IL-6 is produced by various cells including activated macrophages, synovial fibroblasts, and activated lymphocytes. IL-6 promotes the production of pro-inflammatory cytokines, antibody production by B cells, and angiogenesis. Furthermore, IL-6 contributes to the pathogenesis of RA by inducing the differentiation of Th17 cells, and IL-17A, produced by Th17 cells, induces RANKL mediated osteoclastogenesis, as well as the production of pro-inflammatory cytokines, chemokines, and matrix metalloproteinases [48,49].

Blocking the action of those cytokines has been shown to improve arthritis in RA patients, demonstrating the importance of those cytokines in the pathophysiology of RA.

Systemic Lupus Erythematosus

SLE GWAS SNPs also include genes involved in cytokine and its signaling, such as *TYK2*, *IL10*, and *STAT4* [50]. Levels of various cytokines, such as type I interferons, TNF-α, IL-4, IL-6, IL-10, and BAFF, are increased in systemic lupus erythematosus (SLE). Type I interferons, especially IFN-α, is one of the key mediators of autoimmunity in SLE. Impaired clearance of apoptotic material, such as nuclear antigens, leads to the stimulation of Toll-like receptors (TLR) and the production of IFN-α by plasmacytoid DCs in SLE. Neutrophil extracellular traps (NETs) produced during NETosis, a form of neutrophil death, also contributes to the abnormal production of IFN-α in SLE. Increased levels of IFN-α contributes to the pathogenesis of SLE in several ways. For example, IFN-α induces the differentiation of myeloid DCs and increases the expression of MHC molecules on the cell surface of DCs, promoting antigen presentation. In addition, IFN-α induces the production of BAFF, which induces B cell proliferation and the production of autoantibodies. IFN-α impairs the function of regulatory T cells, thus inducing autoimmunity [38,51].

CYTOKINE-MODIFYING THERAPIES FOR AUTOIMMUNE DISEASES

As cytokines play an important role in the pathophysiology of many autoimmune diseases, modification of their production or action can be therapeutic. For example, steroids, used for the treatment of many autoimmune diseases, decrease the production of pro-inflammatory cytokines. The introduction of biologics in the late 1990s has allowed us to control cytokines in a more specific manner. Biologics, also called biologic agents or biologic therapy, are genetically engineered proteins that block the function of a specific component of the immune system. Many of them block either cytokines or cytokine receptors. Recently, small compounds that block the activity of JAKs have been introduced, allowing us to modify the signal transduction of cytokines. In this section, we will discuss some of the key drugs that modify the action of cytokines.

TNF Inhibitors

TNF inhibitors were among the first biologics to be used for autoimmune diseases. Now, five TNF inhibitors are available: infliximab, etanercept, adalimumab, certolizumab, and golimumab. In addition, biosimilars, products with the same primary amino acid sequence as the original drugs but not under patent, are also available for infliximab, etanercept, and adalimumab. Etanercept is a fusion protein with two p75 TNF receptors bound to the Fc portion of IgG. The other four TNF inhibitors are monoclonal antibodies directed against TNF-α. Etanercept can only block TNF-α in the serum while the other TNF inhibitors can also inhibit TNF-α expressed on the cell surface. Although there are some differences among the different reagents, TNF-α inhibitors are effective for various autoimmune diseases including RA [52], JIA, ankylosing spondylitis (AS) [53], psoriatic arthritis (PsA) [54], ulcerative colitis [55], Crohn's disease [56], Bechet disease [57], and Takayasu arteritis [58]. Paradoxically, anti-TNF inhibitors can induce autoimmune phenomenon, including SLE [59] and multiple sclerosis [60], presumably due to enhancement of type I IFN activity.

Tocilizumab

Tocilizumab is an anti-human IL-6 receptor antibody and blocks the action of IL-6. It is effective for the treatment of RA [61], systemic JIA [62], adult onset Still's disease [63], giant cell arthritis (GCA) [64], Takayasu arteritis [65], and systemic sclerosis [66]. IL-6 is tightly linked to the production of serum amyloid A protein (SAA) and secondary amyloidosis due to autoimmune diseases, and treatment with tocilizumab has been reported to improve amyloidosis in autoimmune diseases [67].

IL-1 Inhibitors

Three IL-1 inhibitors are now available. Anakinra is a recombinant human IL-1Ra and inhibits the action of IL-1 by competitively binding to the IL-1 receptor. Anakinra is effective for systemic JIA [62] and adult onset Still's disease [68]. It is also effective for autoinflammatory disorders such as cryopyrin-associated periodic syndromes (CAPS) [69] and tumor necrosis factor receptor-1 associated periodic syndromes (TRAPS) [70]. Anakinra is modestly effective in RA [71], but because other biologics such as TNF inhibitors are more effective, anakinra is seldom used for RA. Other IL-1 inhibitors include canakinumab and rilonacept, which are used for the treatment of autoinflammatory disorders including CAPS.

IL-17 Inhibitors

There are several IL-17 inhibitors now available. Secukinumab and ixekizumab are monoclonal antibodies against IL-17A, and brodalumab is an anti-IL-17 receptor antibody [54,72,73]. IL-17 inhibitors are effective for psoriasis and PsA. Secukinumab is also effective for ankylosing spondylitis [53].

IL-12/IL-23 Inhibitor

Ustekinumab is a monoclonal antibody against the p40 subunit that is shared by IL-12 and IL-23. Ustekinumab is used for the treatment of PsA [74]. It is also effective for Crohn's disease [75] and may be effective for giant cell arteritis and Takayasu arteritis [58].

BAFF Inhibitor

Belimumab is a monoclonal antibody against BAFF and is effective for SLE [76]. It is the first biologic to be introduced for SLE, and its efficacy has especially been shown for musculoskeletal and mucocutaneous symptoms of SLE. There is increasing evidence that it may improve other symptoms of SLE, such as lupus nephritis [77].

Fresolimumab

TGF-β mediated fibrosis has been implicated to play an important role in the pathogenesis of systemic sclerosis, and a clinical trial with fresolimumab, a neutralizing antibody for all TGF-β isoforms, has been performed, showing reduced skin thickening compared to placebo [78].

Denosumab

Denosumab, a monoclonal antibody against RANKL, reduces osteoclastogenesis. It has been used for the treatment for osteoporosis. In addition, it prevents bone destruction in RA [27,79].

JAK Inhibitors

JAK inhibitors are small compounds that inhibit the activity of JAKs. Unlike biologics, they are administered orally. Tofacitinib was the first JAK inhibitor to be introduced for the treatment of rheumatoid arthritis and inhibits mainly JAK1 and JAK3, although it also inhibits other JAKs to a certain extent. It is used for the treatment of RA [52] and has also been reported to improve arthritis in PsA [80,81]. Baricitinib, which inhibits JAK1 and JAK2, has been recently introduced to the treatment of RA [82].

CYTOKINES AS THERAPEUTIC AGENTS FOR AUTOIMMUNE DISEASES

Cytokines themselves may be used for the treatment of autoimmune diseases. One example that is already in clinical application is the use of IFN-1β-1b [83] and IFN-1β-1a [84] for the treatment of relapsing remitting multiple sclerosis. IFN-1β works through several mechanisms. First it decreases the production of pro-inflammatory cytokines. Also, it reduces immune cell trafficking across the blood-brain barrier, and it increases the production of nerve growth factors [85].

Attempts to use cytokines as therapy for other autoimmune diseases has been reported. For example, IL-2 is important for the expansion of regulatory T cells, and the administration of low-dose IL-2 may theoretically ameliorate autoimmunity by inducing the expansion of regulatory T cells. Attempts to treat SLE patients with low-dose IL-2 therapy has been reported with some small clinical trials reporting its efficacy; however, this therapy remains controversial and more studies are needed to assess its efficacy and safety [86].

CHEMOKINES: AN OVERVIEW

Chemokines are small peptides, usually about 8-10 kDa in size, that regulate the migration of immune cells. Some chemokines are expressed constitutively and called homeostatic chemokines. Others are expressed only under inflammatory conditions and called inflammatory chemokines. They are essential, not only for immune cell trafficking, but also for various cellular processes including angiogenesis and wound healing. Here, we focus on the role of chemokines in the normal immune system and in autoimmunity.

Chemokines have a conserved motif consisting of cysteine residues, and they are grouped into four families based on the relative location of the cysteine residues: CXC, CC, CX$_3$C, and (X)C. Chemokines exhibit their action by binding to G protein-coupled surface receptors, and the receptors are grouped into CXCR, CCR, CX$_3$CR, and CR, according to their respective ligands. Some receptors are activated by several chemokines while others are activated by only one (Table 15.2).

In general, most CXC chemokines are involved in the recruitment of neutrophils, although some of them act as chemoattractants for monocytes and lymphocytes. CC chemokines generally act as chemoattractants for monocytes, and some CC chemokines recruit lymphocytes as well. In the following section, we will examine the role of some important chemokines.

CXCL4

CXCL4, also known as platelet factor-4 (PF-4), is a chemokine released by activated platelets, and its receptor is CXCR3. CXCL4 induces the binding of monocytes to endothelial cells. CXCL4 also induces the differentiation of monocytes to a specific phenotype called "M4" that is associated with atherosclerosis. CXCL4 influences the proliferation and differentiation of T cell subsets [87], and CXCL4 has been reported as a marker of systemic sclerosis [88].

CXCL8

Recruitment of neutrophils to the site of infection is often the first and the most important step in controlling infection, and the interaction between CXCL8 and CXCR1 plays an important role in this process. Macrophages resident in the tissues release CXCL8 upon encountering pathogens. Neutrophils express CXCR1, the receptor for CXCL8, and are recruited to the site of infection [89]. CXCL8 is also called IL-8 because it was originally reported as an interleukin.

CXCL10

CXCL10 is produced by lymphocytes including CD4+ T cells and CD8+ T cells, and it may also be produced by neutrophils, monocytes, and keratinocytes. Its production is induced by IFN-γ, and CXCL10, through its receptor CXCR3, promotes Th1 responses, thus, creating a positive feedback loop. CXCL10, in addition to promoting Th1 responses among CD4+ T cells, acts as a chemoattractant for neutrophils [90,91].

CXCL12

CXCL12 is a chemokine that plays an important role in the germinal center reaction along with CXCL13. When B cells are activated, they move to the follicles of secondary lymphoid organs, where they proliferate and form germinal centers. The germinal center is divided into the light zone and the dark zone, and the cycling between those regions is important for affinity maturation. In the dark zone, B cells undergo rapid proliferation and somatic hypermutation, and eventually some B cells decrease their rate of proliferation, move to the light zone, and undergo antigen-driven selection. B cells that can bind to antigens return to the dark zone where they undergo another round of proliferation and somatic hypermutation. CXCL12 is expressed by the stromal cells of the dark zone. B cells in the dark zone express CXCR4, the receptor for CXCL12, and the interaction between CXCL12 and CXCR4 helps to retain B cells in the dark zone while they are proliferating and undergoing somatic hypermutation [92] (Fig. 15.2).

CXCL13

CXCL13, along with CXCL12, plays an important role in the germinal center reaction. CXCL13 is expressed by follicular dendritic cells of the light zone. When the B cells move from the dark zone to the light zone, they decrease the expression of CXCR4, and CXCR5, the receptor for CXCL13 expressed constitutively by B cells, helps to direct B cells to the light zone [92]. CXCR5 is also expressed by follicular helper T cells, which may help them enter the follicle and interact with B cells [93].

CCL2 (MCP1)

When an infection occurs, neutrophils are generally the first to be recruited, followed by monocytes several hours later. This recruitment of monocytes is mediated by CCL2, also known as MCP1, which is produced by various cells including monocytes, macrophages, endothelial cells, and epithelial cells. Monocytes express CCR2, the receptor for CCL2, and is thereby recruited to the site of infection [94].

TABLE 15.2 Chemokines and Their Receptors

	Chemokines	Receptors
CXC-chemokines	CXCL1 (GROα)	CXCR2
	CXCL2 (GROβ)	CXCR2
	CXCL3 (GROγ)	CXCR2
	CXCL4 (PF4)	CXCR3
	CXCL5 (ENA78)	CXCR2
	CXCR6 (GCP2)	CXCR1, CXCR2
	CXCL7 (NAP2)	CXCR2
	CXCL8 (IL-8)	CXCR1, CXCR2
	CXCL9 (MIG)	CXCR3
	CXCL10 (IP10)	CXCR3
	CXCL11 (ITAC)	CXCR3
	CXCL12 (SDF-1α/β)	CXCR4
	CXCL13 (BCA1)	CXCR5
	CXCL14 (BRAK)	unknown
	CXCL16 (SR-PSOX)	CXCR6
	CXCL17	GPR35/CXCR8
CC Chemokines	CCL1 (I-309)	CCR8
	CCL2 (MCP1)	CCR2, CCR4
	CCL3 (MIP-1α)	CCR1, CCR4, CCR5
	CCL3L1 (LD78)	CCR5
	CCL4 (MIP-1β)	CCR1, CCR5, CCR8
	CCL5 (RANTES)	CCR1, CCR3, CCR5, CCR5
	CCL7 (MCP3)	CCR1, CCR2, CCR3
	CCL8 (MCP2)	CCR1, CCR2, CCR5, CCR11
	CCL9 (MRP1γ, CCL10)	CCR1
	CCL11 (Eotaxin1)	CCR3
	CCL12 (MCP5)	CCR2
	CCL13 (MCP4)	CCR1, CCR2, CCR3
	CCL14 (HCC1)	CCR1, CCR5, CCR11
	CCL15 (HCC2)	CCR1, CCR3
	CCL16 (HCC4)	CCR1, CCR2
	CCL17 (TARC)	CCR4, CCR8
	CCL18 (PARC, DC-CK1)	CCR8
	CCL19 (MIP-3β, ELC)	CCR7
	CCL20 (MIP-3α)	CCR6
	CCL21 (SLC)	CCR7
	CCL22 (MDC)	CCR4
	CCL23 (MPIF1)	CCR1, CCR12

Continued

TABLE 15.2 Chemokines and Their Receptors—cont'd

	Chemokines	Receptors
	CCL24 (Eotaxin2)	CCR3
	CCL25 (TECK)	CCR9
	CCL26 (Eotaxin3)	CCR3
	CCL27 (CTACK)	CCR10
	CCL28 (MEC)	CCR3, CCR10
C-chemokines	XCL1 (Lymphotactin-α)	XCR1
	XCL2 (Lymphotactin-β)	XCR1
CX3C-chemokine	CX3CL1 (Fractalkine)	CX3CR1

Adapted from Bernardini G, Benigni G, Scrivo R, Valesini G, Santoni A. The Multifunctional Role of the Chemokine System in Arthritogenic Processes. Curr Rheumatol Rep 2017;19(3):11; Nanki T, Imai T, Kawai S. Fractalkine/CX3CL1 in rheumatoid arthritis. Mod Rheumatol 2017;27(3):392–7.

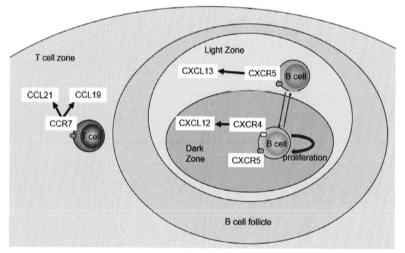

FIGURE 15.2 Chemokines in the Secondary Lymphoid Organs. CCL19 and CCL21 are expressed in the T cell zone, and CCR7, their receptor, is expressed by naïve T cells. B cells in the dark zone express CXCR4, and CXCL12, the ligand for CXCR4, is expressed in the dark zone, which helps to retain B cells in the dark zone while they are proliferating. B cells eventually downregulated the expression of CXCR4, and the interaction between CXCR5, which is expressed constitutively by B cells, and CXCL13, the ligand for CXCR5, helps the B cells move to the light zone.

CCL5 (RANTES)

CCL5 was originally reported as a substance released from TCR-activated T cells several days after stimulation and therefore also referred to as RANTES (regulated on activation, normal T cell expressed and secreted). Activated platelets are also an important source of CCL5. CCL5 mainly activates CCR5 and can also signal through CCR1 and CCR3. CCL5 induces the binding of monocytes to the inflamed endothelium. CCL5 also acts as a chemoattractant for CD4+ T cells, NK cells, basophils, and eosinophils [95].

CCL11 (Eotaxin1)

CCL11, also referred to as eotaxin1, acts as a chemoattractant for eosinophils. Two other members of the eotaxin family, have also been identified: CCL24 (eotaxin2) and CCL26 (eotaxin3). They are important in Th2 cell responses and allergies [96].

CCL17 (TARC)

CCL17 is also referred to as TARC (thymus and activation-regulated chemokine) and is expressed by DCs, endothelial cells, keratinocytes, and fibroblasts. It is also expressed in the thymus. It activates CCR4 and is known as a Th2 chemokine, playing an important role in various diseases such as atopic dermatitis [97].

CCL21

Activation of naïve T cells by antigen presenting cells in secondary lymphoid organs, such as the lymph nodes and the spleen is an important process in the adaptive immune response, and the interaction between CCL21 and CCR7 are essential for this process. CCL21 is expressed by high endothelial venules, specialized vessels through which the T cells enter secondary lymphoid organs, and by stromal cells in the T cell zones of the secondary lymphoid organs. Naïve T cells express CCR7, the receptor for CCL21, allowing them to enter secondary lymphoid organs. CCL19 also plays a role in this process, although CCL21 is generally considered to play a more prominent role [98,99]. DCs also express CCR7 when they encounter pathogens, which allows them to move to secondary lymphoid organs and to interact with T cells [100].

CX3CL1 (Factalkine)

CX_3CL1 (Fractalkine) is the only CX_3CL chemokine and exists in both membrane-bound and soluble forms. CX_3CL1 is expressed by vascular endothelial cells and its expression is upregulated by pro-inflammatory cytokines such as TNF-α. CX_3CR1 is the receptor for CX_3CL1 and is expressed monocytes and a subset of T cells [101].

CHEMOKINE RECEPTORS AND CELL CLASSIFICATION

Chemokine receptors are often tightly linked to cell function, and chemokine receptors on the cell surface are useful in classifying immune cells. For example, among the memory CD4+ T cell subsets, CXCR3 is a marker of Th1 cells, and CCR6 is a marker of Th17 cells [102]. CCR4 is expressed by Th2 cells [103] and Th17 cells [104], as well as Foxp3+ Tregs [105]. Follicular helper T cells are characterized by cell surface expression of CXCR5 [93], and Th22 cells are characterized by the expression of CCR10 [106].

The analysis of chemokine receptors on immune cells in different autoimmune diseases have provided clues regarding the immune cell subsets important for the pathogenesis of autoimmune diseases. In addition, many autoimmune diseases are very heterogenous, making it difficult to predict disease course and treatment response, and the analysis of chemokine receptors on immune cells using flow cytometry may aid in subgrouping patients and predicting disease course, as well as treatment response [107,108].

CHEMOKINES IN RHEUMATOID ARTHRITIS

Next, we will examine the role of chemokines in the pathophysiology in rheumatoid arthritis. Chemokines contribute to the pathogenesis of rheumatoid arthritis in several ways. They recruit immune cells to joints, activate synovial fibroblasts, and induce angiogenesis. The RA joint is characterized by infiltration of mononuclear cells, such as macrophages, monocytes, and T cells. The expression of various chemokines such as CCL5 [109] are reported to be elevated in the RA joint, promoting the recruitment of monocytes to the joints. In addition, RA patients may have increased expression of chemokine receptors on monocytes of the peripheral blood, which may further promote the migration of monocytes to the joints [109,110]. Fibroblasts are major constituents of the pannus, and their proliferation is stimulated in an autocrine manner in RA by CX_3CL1. Osteoclast activation, which plays an important role in bone destruction, is mediated by various cytokines such as CCL20, CXCL12, and CX_3CL1. CXCL12 and CX_3CL1 also promote the formation of pannus and joint destruction by recruiting endothelial precursors and promoting angiogenesis [111]. Several inhibitors of chemokine receptors have been undergone clinical trials in RA; however, due to limited efficacy, they are not used in clinical practice [112]. Other inhibitors of chemokines are under trial [101].

CONCLUSION

In this chapter, we focused on cytokines and chemokines, signal molecules that are essential for the immune cells to work at the right time at the right place. Proper function of cytokines and chemokines are essential for the normal immune system, and dysregulation of cytokine and chemokine activity can lead to autoimmunity. Manipulation of cytokine activity can be therapeutic for autoimmune diseases.

REFERENCES

[1] Isaacs A, Lindenmann J. Virus interference. I. The interferon. Proc R Soc Lond B Biol Sci 1957;147(927):258–67.

[2] Akdis M, Aab A, Altunbulakli C, Azkur K, Costa RA, Crameri R, et al. Interleukins (from IL-1 to IL-38), interferons, transforming growth factor beta, and TNF-alpha: Receptors, functions, and roles in diseases. J Allergy Clin Immunol 2016;138(4):984–1010.

[3] Garlanda C, Dinarello CA, Mantovani A. The interleukin-1 family: back to the future. Immunity 2013;39(6):1003–18.

[4] Palomo J, Dietrich D, Martin P, Palmer G, Gabay C. The interleukin (IL)-1 cytokine family–balance between agonists and antagonists in inflammatory diseases. Cytokine 2015;76(1):25–37.

[5] Lin JX, Leonard WJ. The common cytokine receptor gamma chain family of cytokines. Cold Spring Harb Perspect Biol 2017.

[6] Puck JM, Deschenes SM, Porter JC, Dutra AS, Brown CJ, Willard HF, et al. The interleukin-2 receptor gamma chain maps to Xq13.1 and is mutated in X-linked severe combined immunodeficiency, SCIDX1. Hum Mol Genet 1993;2(8):1099–104.

[7] Noguchi M, Yi H, Rosenblatt HM, Filipovich AH, Adelstein S, Modi WS, et al. Interleukin-2 receptor gamma chain mutation results in X-linked severe combined immunodeficiency in humans. Cell 1993;73(1):147–57.

[8] Zheng SG, Wang J, Wang P, Gray JD, Horwitz DA. IL-2 is essential for TGF-beta to convert naive CD4+CD25- cells to CD25+ Foxp3+ regulatory T cells and for expansion of these cells. J Immunol 2007;178(4):2018–27.

[9] Armitage RJ, Macduff BM, Spriggs MK, Fanslow WC. Human B cell proliferation and Ig secretion induced by recombinant CD40 ligand are modulated by soluble cytokines. J Immunol 1993;150(9):3671–80.

[10] Li J, Chen S, Xiao X, Zhao Y, Ding W, Li XC. IL-9 and Th9 cells in health and diseases-From tolerance to immunopathology. Cytokine Growth Factor Rev 2017;37:47–55.

[11] Gensous N, Schmitt N, Richez C, Ueno H, Blanco P. T follicular helper cells, interleukin-21 and systemic lupus erythematosus. Rheumatology (Oxford) 2017;56(4):516–23.

[12] Ding BB, Bi E, Chen H, Yu JJ, Ye BH. IL-21 and CD40L synergistically promote plasma cell differentiation through upregulation of Blimp-1 in human B cells. J Immunol 2013;190(4):1827–36.

[13] Yang L, Anderson DE, Baecher-Allan C, Hastings WD, Bettelli E, Oukka M, et al. IL-21 and TGF-beta are required for differentiation of human Th17 cells. Nature 2008;454(7202):350–2.

[14] Kleinewietfeld M, Hafler DA. Regulatory T cells in autoimmune neuroinflammation. Immunol Rev 2014;259(1):231–44.

[15] Okamura T, Fujio K, Sumitomo S, Yamamoto K. Roles of LAG3 and EGR2 in regulatory T cells. Ann Rheum Dis 2012;71(Suppl. 2):i96–100.

[16] Mauri C, Menon M. Human regulatory B cells in health and disease: therapeutic potential. J Clin Investig 2017;127(3):772–9.

[17] Fujio K, Okamura T, Yamamoto K. The Family of IL-10-secreting CD4+ T cells. Adv Immunol 2010;105:99–130.

[18] Malisan F, Briere F, Bridon JM, Harindranath N, Mills FC, Max EE, et al. Interleukin-10 induces immunoglobulin G isotype switch recombination in human CD40-activated naive B lymphocytes. J Exp Med 1996;183(3):937–47.

[19] Rutz S, Wang X, Ouyang W. The IL-20 subfamily of cytokines–from host defence to tissue homeostasis. Nat Rev Immunol 2014;14(12):783–95.

[20] Nikoopour E, Bellemore SM, Singh B. IL-22, cell regeneration and autoimmunity. Cytokine 2015;74(1):35–42.

[21] Zwirner NW, Ziblat A. Regulation of NK Cell Activation and Effector Functions by the IL-12 Family of Cytokines: The Case of IL-27. Front Immunol 2017;8:25.

[22] Unutmaz D. RORC2: the master of human Th17 cell programming. Eur J Immunol 2009;39(6):1452–5.

[23] Chizzolini C, Dufour AM, Brembilla NC. Is there a role for IL-17 in the pathogenesis of systemic sclerosis? Immunol Lett 2017.

[24] Li D, Guo B, Wu H, Tan L, Chang C, Lu Q. Interleukin-17 in systemic lupus erythematosus: A comprehensive review. Autoimmunity 2015;48(6):353–61.

[25] Narazaki M, Tanaka T, Kishimoto T. The role and therapeutic targeting of IL-6 in rheumatoid arthritis. Expert Rev Clin Immunol 2017;13(6):535–51.

[26] Kalliolias GD, Ivashkiv LB. TNF biology, pathogenic mechanisms and emerging therapeutic strategies. Nat Rev Rheumatol 2016;12(1):49–62.

[27] Tanaka S, Tanaka Y, Ishiguro N, Yamanaka H, Takeuchi T. RANKL: A therapeutic target for bone destruction in rheumatoid arthritis. Mod Rheumatol 2017:1–8.

[28] Samy E, Wax S, Huard B, Hess H, Schneider P. Targeting BAFF and APRIL in systemic lupus erythematosus and other antibody-associated diseases. Int Rev Immunol 2017;36(1):3–19.

[29] Kamato D, Burch ML, Piva TJ, Rezaei HB, Rostam MA, Xu S, et al. Transforming growth factor-beta signalling: role and consequences of Smad linker region phosphorylation. Cell Signal 2013;25(10):2017–24.

[30] Fujio K, Komai T, Inoue M, Morita K, Okamura T, Yamamoto K. Revisiting the regulatory roles of the TGF-beta family of cytokines. Autoimmun Rev 2016;15(9):917–22.

[31] Chen W, Jin W, Hardegen N, Lei KJ, Li L, Marinos N, et al. Conversion of peripheral CD4+CD25- naive T cells to CD4+CD25+ regulatory T cells by TGF-beta induction of transcription factor Foxp3. J Exp Med 2003;198(12):1875–86.

[32] Peng Y, Laouar Y, Li MO, Green EA, Flavell RA. TGF-beta regulates in vivo expansion of Foxp3-expressing CD4+CD25+ regulatory T cells responsible for protection against diabetes. Proc Natl Acad Sci U S A 2004;101(13):4572–7.

[33] Banchereau J, Pascual V, O'Garra A. From IL-2 to IL-37: the expanding spectrum of anti-inflammatory cytokines. Nat Immunol 2012;13(10):925–31.

[34] Wilson NJ, Boniface K, Chan JR, McKenzie BS, Blumenschein WM, Mattson JD, et al. Development, cytokine profile and function of human interleukin 17-producing helper T cells. Nat Immunol 2007;8(9):950–7.

[35] Nakamura K, Kitani A, Strober W. Cell contact-dependent immunosuppression by CD4(+)CD25(+) regulatory T cells is mediated by cell surface-bound transforming growth factor beta. J Exp Med 2001;194(5):629–44.

[36] Dullaers M, Li D, Xue Y, Ni L, Gayet I, Morita R, et al. A T cell-dependent mechanism for the induction of human mucosal homing immunoglobulin A-secreting plasmablasts. Immunity 2009;30(1):120–9.

[37] Marcais A, Viel S, Grau M, Henry T, Marvel J, Walzer T. Regulation of mouse NK cell development and function by cytokines. Front Immunol 2013;4:450.

[38] Chasset F, Arnaud L. Targeting interferons and their pathways in systemic lupus erythematosus. Autoimmun Rev 2017.

[39] Luo S, Wang Y, Zhao M, Lu Q. The important roles of type I interferon and interferon-inducible genes in systemic lupus erythematosus. Int Immunopharmacol 2016;40:542–9.

[40] Green DS, Young HA, Valencia JC. Current prospects of type II interferon gamma signaling and autoimmunity. J Biol Chem 2017;292(34):13925–33.

[41] Pacheco AG, Cardoso CC, Moraes MO. IFNG +874T/A, IL10 -1082G/A and TNF -308G/A polymorphisms in association with tuberculosis susceptibility: a meta-analysis study. Hum Genet 2008;123(5):477–84.

[42] van de Vosse E, van Dissel JT. IFN-gammaR1 defects: Mutation update and description of the IFNGR1 variation database. Hum Mutat 2017;38(10):1286–96.

[43] Zanoni I, Granucci F, Broggi A. Interferon (IFN)-lambda Takes the Helm: Immunomodulatory Roles of Type III IFNs. Front Immunol 2017;8:1661.

[44] Schwartz DM, Kanno Y, Villarino A, Ward M, Gadina M, O'Shea JJ. JAK inhibition as a therapeutic strategy for immune and inflammatory diseases. Nat Rev Drug Discov 2017;16(12):843–62.

[45] Villarino AV, Kanno Y, O'Shea JJ. Mechanisms and consequences of Jak-STAT signaling in the immune system. Nat Immunol 2017;18(4):374–84.

[46] Yamamoto K, Okada Y, Suzuki A, Kochi Y. Genetics of rheumatoid arthritis in Asia–present and future. Nat Rev Rheumatol 2015;11(6):375–9.

[47] Okada Y, Wu D, Trynka G, Raj T, Terao C, Ikari K, et al. Genetics of rheumatoid arthritis contributes to biology and drug discovery. Nature 2014;506(7488):376–81.

[48] Brzustewicz E, Bryl E. The role of cytokines in the pathogenesis of rheumatoid arthritis–practical and potential application of cytokines as biomarkers and targets of personalized therapy. Cytokine 2015;76(2):527–36.

[49] Sharma J, Bhar S, Devi CS. A review on interleukins: the key manipulators in rheumatoid arthritis. Mod Rheumatol 2017;27(5):723–46.

[50] Teruel M, Alarcon-Riquelme ME. The genetic basis of systemic lupus erythematosus: What are the risk factors and what have we learned. J Autoimmun 2016;74:161–75.

[51] Tsokos GC, Lo MS, Costa Reis P, Sullivan KE. New insights into the immunopathogenesis of systemic lupus erythematosus. Nat Rev Rheumatol 2016;12(12):716–30.

[52] Nam JL, Takase-Minegishi K, Ramiro S, Chatzidionysiou K, Smolen JS, van der Heijde D, et al. Efficacy of biological disease-modifying antirheumatic drugs: a systematic literature review informing the 2016 update of the EULAR recommendations for the management of rheumatoid arthritis. Ann Rheum Dis 2017;76(6):1113–36.

[53] van der Heijde D, Ramiro S, Landewe R, Baraliakos X, Van den Bosch F, Sepriano A, et al. 2016 update of the ASAS-EULAR management recommendations for axial spondyloarthritis. Ann Rheum Dis 2017;76(6):978–91.

[54] Ramiro S, Smolen JS, Landewe R, van der Heijde D, Dougados M, Emery P, et al. Pharmacological treatment of psoriatic arthritis: a systematic literature review for the 2015 update of the EULAR recommendations for the management of psoriatic arthritis. Ann Rheum Dis 2016;75(3):490–8.

[55] Bressler B, Marshall JK, Bernstein CN, Bitton A, Jones J, Leontiadis GI, et al. Clinical practice guidelines for the medical management of nonhospitalized ulcerative colitis: the Toronto consensus. Gastroenterology 2015;148(5):1035–58.e3.

[56] Peyrin-Biroulet L, Deltenre P, de Suray N, Branche J, Sandborn WJ, Colombel JF. Efficacy and safety of tumor necrosis factor antagonists in Crohn's disease: meta-analysis of placebo-controlled trials. Clin Gastroenterol Hepatol 2008;6(6):644–53.

[57] Arida A, Fragiadaki K, Giavri E, Sfikakis PP. Anti-TNF agents for Behcet's disease: analysis of published data on 369 patients. Semin Arthritis Rheum 2011;41(1):61–70.

[58] Koster MJ, Matteson EL, Warrington KJ. Recent advances in the clinical management of giant cell arteritis and Takayasu arteritis. Curr Opin Rheumatol 2016;28(3):211–7.

[59] Shovman O, Tamar S, Amital H, Watad A, Shoenfeld Y. Diverse patterns of anti-TNF-alpha-induced lupus: case series and review of the literature. Clin Rheumatol 2017.

[60] Kaltsonoudis E, Voulgari PV, Konitsiotis S, Drosos AA. Demyelination and other neurological adverse events after anti-TNF therapy. Autoimmun Rev 2014;13(1):54–8.

[61] Singh JA, Beg S, Lopez-Olivo MA. Tocilizumab for rheumatoid arthritis: a cochrane systematic review. J Rheumatol 2011;38(1):10–20.

[62] Horneff G, Schulz AC, Klotsche J, Hospach A, Minden K, Foeldvari I, et al. Experience with etanercept, tocilizumab and interleukin-1 inhibitors in systemic onset juvenile idiopathic arthritis patients from the BIKER registry. Arthritis Res Ther 2017;19(1):256.

[63] Ma Y, Wu M, Zhang X, Xia Q, Yang J, Xu S, et al. Efficacy and safety of tocilizumab with inhibition of interleukin-6 in adult-onset Still's disease: a meta-analysis. Mod Rheumatol 2017:1–25.

[64] Stone JH, Tuckwell K, Dimonaco S, Klearman M, Aringer M, Blockmans D, et al. Trial of Tocilizumab in giant-cell arteritis. N Engl J Med 2017;377(4):317–28.

[65] Nakaoka Y, Isobe M, Takei S, Tanaka Y, Ishii T, Yokota S, et al. Efficacy and safety of tocilizumab in patients with refractory Takayasu arteritis: results from a randomised, double-blind, placebo-controlled, phase 3 trial in Japan (the TAKT study). Ann Rheum Dis 2017.

[66] Khanna D, Denton CP, Lin CJ, van Laar JM, Frech TM, Anderson ME, et al. Safety and efficacy of subcutaneous tocilizumab in systemic sclerosis: results from the open-label period of a phase II randomised controlled trial (faSScinate). Ann Rheum Dis 2017.

[67] Lane T, Gillmore JD, Wechalekar AD, Hawkins PN, Lachmann HJ. Therapeutic blockade of interleukin-6 by tocilizumab in the management of AA amyloidosis and chronic inflammatory disorders: a case series and review of the literature. Clin Exp Rheumatol 2015;33(6 Suppl. 94):S46–53.

[68] Giampietro C, Ridene M, Lequerre T, Costedoat Chalumeau N, Amoura Z, Sellam J, et al. Anakinra in adult-onset Still's disease: long-term treatment in patients resistant to conventional therapy. Arthritis Care Res (Hoboken) 2013;65(5):822–6.

[69] Hoffman HM, Rosengren S, Boyle DL, Cho JY, Nayar J, Mueller JL, et al. Prevention of cold-associated acute inflammation in familial cold auto-inflammatory syndrome by interleukin-1 receptor antagonist. Lancet 2004;364(9447):1779–85.

[70] Gattorno M, Pelagatti MA, Meini A, Obici L, Barcellona R, Federici S, et al. Persistent efficacy of anakinra in patients with tumor necrosis factor receptor-associated periodic syndrome. Arthritis Rheum 2008;58(5):1516–20.

[71] Fleischmann RM, Schechtman J, Bennett R, Handel ML, Burmester GR, Tesser J, et al. Anakinra, a recombinant human interleukin-1 receptor antagonist (r-metHuIL-1ra), in patients with rheumatoid arthritis: a large, international, multicenter, placebo-controlled trial. Arthritis Rheum 2003;48(4):927–34.

[72] Mease PJ, van der Heijde D, Ritchlin CT, Okada M, Cuchacovich RS, Shuler CL, et al. Ixekizumab, an interleukin-17A specific monoclonal antibody, for the treatment of biologic-naive patients with active psoriatic arthritis: results from the 24-week randomised, double-blind, placebo-controlled and active (adalimumab)-controlled period of the phase III trial SPIRIT-P1. Ann Rheum Dis 2017;76(1):79–87.

[73] Mease PJ, Genovese MC, Greenwald MW, Ritchlin CT, Beaulieu AD, Deodhar A, et al. Brodalumab, an anti-IL17RA monoclonal antibody, in psoriatic arthritis. N Engl J Med 2014;370(24):2295–306.

[74] Kavanaugh A, Ritchlin C, Rahman P, Puig L, Gottlieb AB, Li S, et al. Ustekinumab, an anti-IL-12/23 p40 monoclonal antibody, inhibits radiographic progression in patients with active psoriatic arthritis: results of an integrated analysis of radiographic data from the phase 3, multicentre, randomised, double-blind, placebo-controlled PSUMMIT-1 and PSUMMIT-2 trials. Ann Rheum Dis 2014;73(6):1000–6.

[75] Hibi T, Imai Y, Murata Y, Matsushima N, Zheng R, Gasink C. Efficacy and safety of ustekinumab in Japanese patients with moderately to severely active Crohn's disease: a subpopulation analysis of phase 3 induction and maintenance studies. Intest Res 2017;15(4):475–86.

[76] Navarra SV, Guzman RM, Gallacher AE, Hall S, Levy RA, Jimenez RE, et al. Efficacy and safety of belimumab in patients with active systemic lupus erythematosus: a randomised, placebo-controlled, phase 3 trial. Lancet 2011;377(9767):721–31.

[77] Tesar V, Hruskova Z. Belimumab in the management of systemic lupus erythematosus - an update. Expert Opin Biol Ther 2017;17(7):901–8.

[78] Rice LM, Padilla CM, McLaughlin SR, Mathes A, Ziemek J, Goummih S, et al. Fresolimumab treatment decreases biomarkers and improves clinical symptoms in systemic sclerosis patients. J Clin Investig 2015;125(7):2795–807.

[79] Cohen SB, Dore RK, Lane NE, Ory PA, Peterfy CG, Sharp JT, et al. Denosumab treatment effects on structural damage, bone mineral density, and bone turnover in rheumatoid arthritis: a twelve-month, multicenter, randomized, double-blind, placebo-controlled, phase II clinical trial. Arthritis Rheum 2008;58(5):1299–309.

[80] Gladman D, Rigby W, Azevedo VF, Behrens F, Blanco R, Kaszuba A, et al. Tofacitinib for Psoriatic Arthritis in Patients with an Inadequate Response to TNF Inhibitors. N Engl J Med 2017;377(16):1525–36.

[81] Mease P, Hall S, FitzGerald O, van der Heijde D, Merola JF, Avila-Zapata F, et al. Tofacitinib or Adalimumab versus Placebo for Psoriatic Arthritis. N Engl J Med 2017;377(16):1537–50.

[82] Taylor PC, Keystone EC, van der Heijde D, Weinblatt ME, Del Carmen Morales L, Reyes Gonzaga J, et al. Baricitinib versus placebo or adalimumab in rheumatoid arthritis. N Engl J Med 2017;376(7):652–62.

[83] Interferon beta-1b is effective in relapsing-remitting multiple sclerosis. I. Clinical results of a multicenter, randomized, double-blind, placebo-controlled trial. The IFNB Multiple Sclerosis Study Group. Neurology 1993;43(4):655–61.

[84] Jacobs LD, Cookfair DL, Rudick RA, Herndon RM, Richert JR, Salazar AM, et al. Intramuscular interferon beta-1a for disease progression in relapsing multiple sclerosis. The Multiple Sclerosis Collaborative Research Group (MSCRG). Ann Neurol 1996;39(3):285–94.

[85] Kieseier BC. The mechanism of action of interferon-beta in relapsing multiple sclerosis. CNS Drugs 2011;25(6):491–502.

[86] Mizui M, Tsokos GC. Low-Dose IL-2 in the treatment of Lupus. Curr Rheumatol Rep 2016;18(11):68.

[87] Domschke G, Gleissner CA. CXCL4-induced macrophages in human atherosclerosis. Cytokine 2017.

[88] Volkmann ER, Tashkin DP, Roth MD, Clements PJ, Khanna D, Furst DE, et al. Changes in plasma CXCL4 levels are associated with improvements in lung function in patients receiving immunosuppressive therapy for systemic sclerosis-related interstitial lung disease. Arthritis Res Ther 2016;18(1):305.

[89] Godaly G, Bergsten G, Hang L, Fischer H, Frendeus B, Lundstedt AC, et al. Neutrophil recruitment, chemokine receptors, and resistance to mucosal infection. J Leukoc Biol 2001;69(6):899–906.

[90] Antonelli A, Ferrari SM, Giuggioli D, Ferrannini E, Ferri C, Fallahi P. Chemokine (C-X-C motif) ligand (CXCL)10 in autoimmune diseases. Autoimmun Rev 2014;13(3):272–80.

[91] Ferrari SM, Ruffilli I, Colaci M, Antonelli A, Ferri C, Fallahi P. CXCL10 in psoriasis. Adv Med Sci 2015;60(2):349–54.

[92] Allen CD, Ansel KM, Low C, Lesley R, Tamamura H, Fujii N, et al. Germinal center dark and light zone organization is mediated by CXCR4 and CXCR5. Nat Immunol 2004;5(9):943–52.

[93] Morita R, Schmitt N, Bentebibel SE, Ranganathan R, Bourdery L, Zurawski G, et al. Human blood CXCR5(+)CD4(+) T cells are counterparts of T follicular cells and contain specific subsets that differentially support antibody secretion. Immunity 2011;34(1):108–21.

[94] Yadav A, Saini V, Arora S. MCP-1: chemoattractant with a role beyond immunity: a review. Clin Chim Acta 2010;411(21–22):1570–9.

[95] Krensky AM, Ahn YT. Mechanisms of disease: regulation of RANTES (CCL5) in renal disease. Nat Clin Pract Nephrol 2007;3(3):164–70.

[96] Foster PS, Maltby S, Rosenberg HF, Tay HL, Hogan SP, Collison AM, et al. Modeling TH 2 responses and airway inflammation to understand fundamental mechanisms regulating the pathogenesis of asthma. Immunol Rev 2017;278(1):20–40.

[97] Saeki H, Tamaki K. Thymus and activation regulated chemokine (TARC)/CCL17 and skin diseases. J Dermatol Sci 2006;43(2):75–84.

[98] Gregor CE, Foeng J, Comerford I, McColl SR. Chemokine-Driven CD4(+) T Cell Homing: new concepts and recent advances. Adv Immunol 2017;135:119–81.

[99] Cyster JG. Chemokines, sphingosine-1-phosphate, and cell migration in secondary lymphoid organs. Annu Rev Immunol 2005;23:127–59.

[100] Platt AM, Randolph GJ. Dendritic cell migration through the lymphatic vasculature to lymph nodes. Adv Immunol 2013;120:51–68.

[101] Nanki T, Imai T, Kawai S. Fractalkine/CX3CL1 in rheumatoid arthritis. Mod Rheumatol 2017;27(3):392–7.

[102] Maecker HT, McCoy JP, Nussenblatt R. Standardizing immunophenotyping for the Human Immunology Project. Nat Rev Immunol 2012;12(3):191–200.

[103] Annunziato F, Galli G, Cosmi L, Romagnani P, Manetti R, Maggi E, et al. Molecules associated with human Th1 or Th2 cells. Eur Cytokine Netw 1998;9(3 Suppl.):12–6.

[104] Zhao F, Hoechst B, Gamrekelashvili J, Ormandy LA, Voigtlander T, Wedemeyer H, et al. Human CCR4+ CCR6+ Th17 cells suppress autologous CD8+ T cell responses. J Immunol 2012;188(12):6055–62.

[105] Iellem A, Mariani M, Lang R, Recalde H, Panina-Bordignon P, Sinigaglia F, et al. Unique chemotactic response profile and specific expression of chemokine receptors CCR4 and CCR8 by CD4(+)CD25(+) regulatory T cells. J Exp Med 2001;194(6):847–53.

[106] Eyerich S, Eyerich K, Pennino D, Carbone T, Nasorri F, Pallotta S, et al. Th22 cells represent a distinct human T cell subset involved in epidermal immunity and remodeling. J Clin Investig 2009;119(12):3573–85.

[107] Kubo S, Nakayamada S, Yoshikawa M, Miyazaki Y, Sakata K, Nakano K, et al. Peripheral Immunophenotyping Identifies Three Subgroups Based on T Cell Heterogeneity in Lupus Patients. Arthritis Rheumatol 2017;69(10):2029–37.

[108] Tanaka Y. Psoriatic arthritis in Japan: difference in clinical features and approach to precision medicine. Clin Exp Rheumatol 2016;34(4 Suppl. 98): 49–52.

[109] Haringman JJ, Smeets TJ, Reinders-Blankert P, Tak PP. Chemokine and chemokine receptor expression in paired peripheral blood mononuclear cells and synovial tissue of patients with rheumatoid arthritis, osteoarthritis, and reactive arthritis. Ann Rheum Dis 2006;65(3):294–300.

[110] Katschke Jr KJ, Rottman JB, Ruth JH, Qin S, Wu L, LaRosa G, et al. Differential expression of chemokine receptors on peripheral blood, synovial fluid, and synovial tissue monocytes/macrophages in rheumatoid arthritis. Arthritis Rheum 2001;44(5):1022–32.

[111] Bernardini G, Benigni G, Scrivo R, Valesini G, Santoni A. The Multifunctional Role of the Chemokine System in Arthritogenic Processes. Curr Rheumatol Rep 2017;19(3):11.

[112] Asquith DL, Bryce SA, Nibbs RJ. Targeting cell migration in rheumatoid arthritis. Curr Opin Rheumatol 2015;27(2):204–11.

[113] Carey AJ, Tan CK, Ulett GC. Infection-induced IL-10 and JAK-STAT: a review of the molecular circuitry controlling immune hyperactivity in response to pathogenic microbes. Jakstat 2012;1(3):159–67.

[114] Mahmud SA, Manlove LS, Farrar MA. Interleukin-2 and STAT5 in regulatory T cell development and function. Jakstat 2013;2(1):e23154.

[115] Nanki T. Treatment for rheumatoid arthritis by chemokine blockade. Nihon Rinsho Meneki Gakkai Kaishi 2016;39(3):172–80.

Chapter 16

Autophagy and Autoimmunity

Tania Colasanti*, Marta Vomero*, Cristiana Barbati, Annacarla Finucci, Fabrizio Conti,
Cristiano Alessandri, Guido Valesini
Rheumatology, Department of Internal Medicine, Sapienza University of Rome, Rome, Italy

INTRODUCTION

Autophagy is a lysosomal degradation mechanism in eukaryotic organisms and has a crucial role in cell homeostasis by controlling organelles and proteins turnover and sustaining survival in cellular stress conditions such as nutrients deprivation [1]. Cytoplasmic material, sequestered within characteristic double-membrane vesicles, known as autophagosomes, is degraded into autophagolysosome to recycle components for energy supply [2]. Recently, the Nobel Prize assigned to the Japanese biologist Yoshinori Ohsumi for his studies on molecular mechanism of autophagy in yeast, brought to light the importance of the process as a therapeutic target in human diseases. In this regard, autophagy was found to be dysregulated in several disorders, such as cancer and neurodegeneration, as well as in other diseases [3]. Moreover, immune system development and function appeared to be strictly linked to autophagy activation. Autophagy orchestrates innate and adaptive immune responses to intracellular pathogens and contributes to MHC class II-mediated presentation of intracellular antigens to CD4$^+$ T lymphocytes [4]. Indeed, B and T lymphocytes, key players in autoimmune diseases pathogenesis, seem to be particularly dependent on autophagy for their development, survival, and proliferation. Starting from these considerations, interesting data on the role of autophagy in the pathogenesis of autoimmune diseases were obtained, suggesting a treatment intervention based on autophagy modulation. In this chapter, we analyze only the role of macroautophagy (autophagy) in autoimmune diseases.

AUTOPHAGY MECHANISMS

Autophagy is a lysosome-mediated catabolic process, highly conserved in eukaryotes, that allows cellular degradation of cytoplasmic constituents and nutrients recycle, in a regulated manner [5]. It differs from other cell degradation systems, and particularly from the ubiquitin–proteasome system, due to its unlimited degradative ability. Lipids, nucleic acids, proteins, macromolecules, proteic aggregates, and whole organelles can be eliminated through autophagy [6]. Indeed, the autophagic process can be selective when it degrades specific damaged cellular organelles, or may occur in a casual way in the cytoplasm. Depending on the way the substrate is delivered to the lysosomes, different types of autophagy can be distinguished:

- *macroautophagy or autophagy* is the most studied and it is characterized by the formation of double-membrane vesicles, named autophagosomes, that sequester cytoplasmic constituents and deliver them to lysosomes, forming autophagolysosomes, to degrade and recycle engulfed material;
- *microautophagy* involves the direct engulfment of cytoplasmic material into the lysosome through protrusions or invaginations of its membrane [7];
- *chaperone-mediated autophagy* is a very complex and specific pathway, which involves the recognition of misfolded proteins, through a characteristic sequence (KFERQ), by a system of chaperones, such as HSP70; it mediates the misfolded protein bond with the lysosomal membrane and its passage in the lumen by LAMP2A [8];
- *mitophagy* is the selective degradation of mitochondria by autophagy; it prevents the accumulation of dysfunctional mitochondria, which can lead to cellular degeneration [9].

Autophagy provides degradation of the transported material in the autophagolysosomes and consists of several phases: (1) initiation, which involves the formation of the initial membrane portion, called phagophorus; (2) elongation of this membrane; (3) formation and maturation of the autophagosome, which thus encompasses cytoplasmic material; (4) fusion of

---

* These authors equally contributed to this work.

Mosaic of Autoimmunity. https://doi.org/10.1016/B978-0-12-814307-0.00016-5

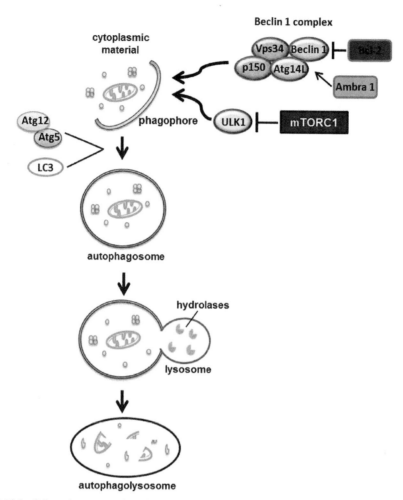

FIGURE 16.1 Schematic representation of signaling pathways involved in autophagy regulation and progression.

autophagosome with lysosome; and finally (5) degradation of the embedded material by lysosomal hydrolases (Fig. 16.1). This complex process is controlled by the autophagy-related genes (Atg) described in detail in several reviews [10].

The initial signal to autophagosomes formation is directed by the Beclin-1-interacting complex, consisting of Beclin-1/Atg6, class III phosphatidylinositol 3-Kinase PI3K (hVps34), the regulatory protein kinase p150 (hVps15), and Atg14L. Activation of this complex generates phosphatidylinositol 3-phosphate (PI3P), which promotes autophagosomal membrane nucleation. The B-cell lymphoma 2 (Bcl-2) family members, such as Bcl-2 and Bcl-X_L, are able to bind Beclin-1, negatively regulating this process, preventing Beclin-1 from binding to the PI3K complex, and thereby inhibiting autophagy. In response to starvation, the constitutive Bcl-2/Beclin-1 interaction is disrupted, with consequent release of Beclin-1 and autophagy induction. Vesicle elongation and completion are mediated by two ubiquitin-like systems: the microtubule-associated protein 1 light chain 3 (LC3) and Atg12–Atg5. LC3 is cleaved by Atg4 to produce the cytosolic form LC3-I, which becomes LC3-II, after conjugation to phosphatidylethanolamine (PE). The initial cleavage of LC3 by Atg4 determines the exposure of a glycine residue at the C-terminal domain, which allows the formation of the covalent bond with the PE. Therefore LC3-II, the only protein stably associated with the autophagosome during its maturation, is the most commonly used marker to assay autophagic activity [11].

Autophagy pathway is negatively regulated by the mammalian target of rapamycin (mTOR), a nutrient-sensing kinase pathway that acts as a key regulator of cell growth, survival, metabolism, and proliferation [12]. It inhibits autophagy by integrating different signals that are generated by growth factors, energy depletion, and various stressors, including hypoxia and DNA damage. mTOR is the catalytic subunit of two distinct complexes called mTOR complex 1 (mTORC1) and mTORC2. mTORC1 contains mTOR and regulatory-associated protein of mTOR (Raptor), whereas the mTORC2 complex contains mTOR and rapamycin-insensitive companion of mTOR (Rictor). A major signaling cascade controlling mTORC1 is the class I PI3K/Akt pathway. In response to insulin and other growth factors signaling, the activation of class I PI3K leads to phosphorylation and activation of Akt. In turn, Akt phosphorylates and inhibits the mTOR repressor tuberous sclerosis complex 2 (TSC2; tuberin), which forms the TSC with TSC1 (hamartin), thus leading to activation of mTORC1. mTORC1 negatively regulates the induction of autophagy by phosphorylating and inactivating unc-51-like kinase 1 (ULK1), a proximal component of the autophagy signal transduction cascade.

Another important regulator of autophagy process is the activating molecule in Beclin-1-regulated autophagy 1 (Ambra1) [13], recently renamed by the HUGO Nomenclature Committee as autophagy/Beclin-1 regulator 1.

Under basal conditions Ambra1, together with Beclin-1 and PI3KIII, is bound to the dynein light chains (DLC1 and DLC2) of the dynein motor complex [14]. During autophagy induction, ULK1 mediates the release of Ambra1 from the dynein complex that translocates, together with Beclin-1 and PI3KIII, to the endoplasmic reticulum (ER), where autophagosomes form. Recently, it has been shown that Ambra1 regulates the activity and the stability of ULK1, by promoting the ubiquitylation of ULK1 through Lys63-linked ubiquitin chains; this modification is essential for the self-association of ULK1 and is mediated by the E3 ligase TNF receptor-associated factor 6 (TRAF6), which interacts with the Ambra1–ULK1 complex. In addition, Ambra1 acts as an essential cofactor for new other E3 ligases, such as cullin 5. Indeed, cullin 5 has recently been observed to be associated with Ambra1 [15]. Here, in the early stages of autophagy induction, Ambra1 interacts with elongin B (also known as TCEB2), to suppress cullin 5 activity, which then allows the stabilization of DEP-domain-containing mTOR-interacting protein (DEPTOR), a starvation-inducible inhibitor of mTORC1 activity. Increased expression of DEPTOR is required to establish a negative-feedback loop of mTORC1 to maintain autophagy activation [16].

AUTOPHAGY IN INNATE AND ADAPTIVE IMMUNITY

Autophagy contributes to many aspects of innate and adaptive immunity, controlling the activation of immune and inflammatory response. In innate immunity, autophagy is involved in the protection of the environment from the colonization by intracellular pathogens, by mediating their degradation through a selective mechanism known as xenophagy [17]. Viruses, bacteria, and parasites, either free in the cytosol or contained within vesicles, are sequestered into autophagosomes, where subsequently they are degraded. These steps involve different molecules, such as p62 and NBR1, which belong to sequestosome (p62/SQSTM1)-like receptors (SLRs) [18]. SLRs recognize proteins with ubiquitination tags and, thanks to a specific LC3-interacting region (LIR), lead them to autophagosome for degradation. It has been demonstrated that this mode of action is used to destroy different microorganisms, including *Mycobacterium tuberculosis* (MT), causal agent of tubercular infection, whose reactivation is common in patients affected by autoimmune diseases treated with TNF inhibitors [19]. According to these data, several in vitro and in vivo studies demonstrated that autophagy activator molecules are required for MT degradation [20]. Moreover, specific polymorphisms in genes encoding autophagy-related proteins, such as IRGM, IFN-γ receptor, and Toll-like receptor (TLR) 8, were found in MT patients, suggesting that an autophagy defect could be associated with the development of this infection [21].

Autophagy-dependent antigen presentation holds a crucial role in the maintenance of immunological tolerance. Characterization of the MHC class II-bound peptides reveals that 20%–30% of them comes from cytosolic antigens, and several lines of evidence suggest that this phenomenon depends on autophagy activation [22]. Several years ago, Brazil and colleagues found that the autophagy inhibitor 3-methyladenine (3-MA) blocked the MHC class II presentation of endogenous C5 mouse complement protein [23]. More recently, it has been demonstrated that autophagy is constitutively activated in antigen-presenting cells (APC), such as dendritic cells (DCs), macrophages, and B cells [24]. In detail, LC3 colocalizes with MHC class II loading compartments markers in professional APCs, suggesting a prominent role of autophagy in delivery of antigens for MHC class II presentation and for CD4+ T-cell stimulation. Indeed, in absence of autophagy, a reduction in Epstein–Barr virus nuclear antigen 1 (EBNA-1)-specific CD4+ T cells was detected. Moreover, Jagannath and colleagues found that autophagy activation by rapamycin enhanced presentation of MT-derived peptides by DCs [25].

AUTOPHAGY IN B AND T LYMPHOCYTES

B and T lymphocytes are key players in autoimmune disease pathogenesis, and they seem to be particularly depending on autophagy for their development, survival, and proliferation. It has been demonstrated that CD4+ T cells defective for Beclin-1 were more susceptible to apoptosis and showed increased levels in proapoptotic proteins, such as Bim, suggesting a new mechanism by which autophagy contributes to cell survival [26]. Studies on Atg5-deficient mice revealed that these animals died within 24 h of birth, due to their inability to survive in a period of nutrient deprivation, and was also noticed a reduction in peripheral blood T-cells population [27]. This phenomenon could be directly related to an increase in apoptotic rates observed in Atg5$^{-/-}$ CD8+ T cells, suggesting that peripheral immune cells depend on autophagy for their survival.

T cell-specific deletion of Vps34 (protein involved in the early stage of autophagy) caused a reduction of the percentage of both CD4+ and CD8+ T cells in the spleen, lymph nodes, and peripheral blood [28].

It has been shown that autophagy promotes the survival of B cells and controls the development and maturation from the lymphoid progenitors. Considering these aspects, Miller and colleagues [29] demonstrated that B lymphocytes from Atg5−/− mice showed an arrest in the transition from pro-B to pre-B cells in the bone marrow. This defect of maturation is associated with a high rate of cell death by apoptosis, suggesting that autophagy is essential for the survival of B cells during development. Moreover, the deletion of Atg5 led to a significant reduction of B-1a cells in the peritoneum, but this had no effect on of peripheral B and B-1 cells population. It was also shown that Beclin-1 is required for the maintenance of B lymphocytes progenitors [30]. In mature B lymphocytes, a massive formation of autophagosomes is induced, not only following the activation of B-cell receptor but also when the activated B cells undergo apoptosis [31]. Therefore, these experimental results suggest that autophagy is involved in the maintenance of immune repertoire and in the elimination of autoreactive B cells.

As far as antibodies production is concerned, autophagy seems to be the "lead character" of plasma cells differentiation program, since Atg transcripts increased during this mechanism [32]. To analyze this aspect, a group of investigators used Atg5-deficient B cells demonstrating that they were well differentiated, but presented a much more abundant ER structure, compared with wild-type counterpart that is able to secret a larger amount of antibodies (Abs) [33]. These results suggest that autophagy can act as "physiological brake" of Abs secretion by the elimination ER structure.

AUTOPHAGY IN SYSTEMIC LUPUS ERYTHEMATOSUS

Systemic lupus erythematosus (SLE) is a multifactorial and highly polymorphic systemic autoimmune disorder that affects multiple organs, including skin, joints, kidneys, muscles, and heart. The etiology of SLE remains still unknown; it is likely that the complex interaction between genetic, environmental (e.g., infectious agents, UV light, drugs), and hormonal factors promotes the immune dysfunction underlying the pathogenesis of the disease [34]. SLE is characterized by auto-antibody production, dysregulated B cells, and aberrant immune cell activation due to abnormal APC function. It is also characterized by target organ infiltration by inflammatory T cells, the major contributors to the disease that participate in the initiation, progression, and perpetration of SLE. This is due to increased cell activation and abnormal cell death by apoptosis and to the production of pathogenic autoantibodies in a T cell-dependent process [35]. More recently, autophagy has been reported to play a key role. Indeed, genetic studies have linked some mutations of autophagy regulators with SLE pathogenesis and a dysregulation of autophagy has been described either in T cells from lupus-prone mice or from patients with SLE. In addition, the activation of mTOR has been documented in SLE T cells. Furthermore, it was discovered that serum IgG from patients with SLE was able to induce autophagy in T lymphocytes from healthy donors, suggesting a role for anti-lymphocyte antibodies as autophagy inducers [36]. On the other hand, whereas treatment of T lymphocytes from healthy donors with serum IgG from patients with SLE resulted in a twofold increase in LC3-II levels, T lymphocytes from SLE patients were resistant to autophagic induction and also displayed an upregulation of genes negatively regulating autophagy, e.g., α-synuclein [36]. Alpha-synuclein is primarily found in neuronal tissue, and its involvement in some neurodegenerative diseases includes the ability of hindering autophagy in neuronal cells. Since α-synuclein can be also found in other cell types, including peripheral blood lymphocytes, the implication of α-synuclein in the autophagic process in primary human T lymphocytes was investigated [37]. In particular, in this study some evidences were provided: knocking down of the α-synuclein gene resulted in increased autophagy; autophagy induction by energy deprivation was associated with a significant decrease of α-synuclein levels; autophagy inhibition by 3-MA or by ATG5 knocking down led to a significant increase of α-synuclein levels; defective autophagy, constitutive in T lymphocytes from patients with SLE, was associated with abnormal accumulation of α-synuclein aggregates. Considering all these results, α-synuclein could be considered as an autophagy-related marker of peripheral blood lymphocytes, potentially suitable for use in the clinical practice [37].

Even though it is well known that the majority of patients with SLE develop autoantibodies to lymphocyte surface antigens able to inhibit T-cell activation and proliferation, few data are available, so far as concerns the antigenic target of these antibodies. In this regard, in another study, it has been identified the small GTPase family inhibitor D4GDI as a possible key antigenic determinant implicated in the pathogenesis of the disease [38]. In this study, D4GDI was characterized as a peripheral blood lymphocyte antigen recognized by serum autoantibodies from a large percentage of patients with SLE. The authors found a significant association between the presence of anti-D4GDI Abs and hematologic manifestations (i.e., leukopenia and thrombocytopenia) occurring in SLE patients [38]. The mechanisms underlying the activity of these autoantibodies appeared to be associated with increased levels of the GTP-bound form of Rac and Rho small GTPases and increased activity of Rho GTPases on their subcellular target. To assess the possible implication of these autoantibodies in the pathogenetic mechanisms of SLE, T lymphocytes were analyzed for their susceptibility to autophagy. The results showed that only T cells from healthy subjects and from patients that were negative for autoantibodies specific to D4GDI appeared to be susceptible to autophagy induction by anti-D4GDI Abs, whereas those obtained from patients that were positive to these antibodies were refractory. So far, the authors hypothesized that D4GDI-specific autoantibodies could be capable of triggering important responses in T cells, such as cytoskeleton remodeling and autophagy pathway and that, in SLE patients, the chronic exposure to these specific autoantibodies could lead to the selection of autophagy-resistant T cell clones, contributing to the pathogenesis of the disease [38]. Several drugs that have been demonstrated to act as autophagy modulators are already used or are under preclinical development in SLE (Table 16.1) [39,40]. Among these drugs hydroxychloroquine (HCQ), the first-line treatment for patients with mild SLE, has been shown to interfere with the acidification of lysosomes and to inhibit the phagosome function, by inhibiting in this way, autophagy pathway. In addition, rapamycin is a US Food and Drug Administration (FDA)-approved immunosuppressive agent in solid organ transplantation and it has been demonstrated as an effective therapeutic treatment, both in animal models of lupus and in patients with SLE (Table 16.1) [41]. Rapamycin binds the small protein 12-kDa FK506-binding protein (FKBP12) and, in turn, rapamycin-FKBP12 binds and inhibits mTORC1, which is required for transducing T-cell activation, increasing autophagy. Recently, the spliceosomal P140 peptide (IPP-201101), a 21-mer fragment of the spliceosomal U1-70K small nuclear ribonucleo-protein, has been demonstrated to display protective properties in patients with SLE, by decreasing the stability of MHC class II molecules in antigen-presenting B cells, in association with a downregulation of autophagic flux (Table 16.1) [42]. These data reveal a very unique property of P140 peptide that alters the autophagy pathway. So, this molecule could be an interesting candidate as therapeutic target in SLE.

TABLE 16.1 Autophagy Regulation in Autoimmune Diseases

Disease	Drug/Molecule for Therapy	Effects	Mechanism of Action
Systemic Lupus Erythematosus	Chloroquine and hydroxychloroquine	Inhibition	Acidification of lysosomes and inhibition of the phagosome function
	Rapamycin	Induction	Inhibition of mTORC1, required for transducing T-cell activation
	P140 peptide	Inhibition	Downregulation of autophagy flux
Rheumatoid Arthritis	Chloroquine and hydroxychloroquine	Inhibition	Autophagosomes accumulation by increasing lysosomal pH
Multiple Sclerosis	CB2R (cannabinoid receptor type 2) activators	Induction	Events leading to the inhibition of the NLRP3 inflammasome
	1,25(OH)2D3	Impairment	Elevated expression of Beclin-1, increased Bcl-2/Bax ratio, and decreased LC3-II accumulation
Sjögren's Syndrome	Chloroquine and hydroxychloroquine	Inhibition	Acidification of lysosomes and inhibition of the phagosome function
Inflammatory Bowel Disease	3-methyladenine, chloroquine, bafilomycin A1, Beclin-1 siRNA	Inhibition	Abolishment of the inhibitory effects of andrographolide (a diterpenoids extracted from a kind of herb called andrographolide) on the NLRP3 inflammasome
	Celastrol	Induction	Inhibition of the PI3K/Akt/mTOR signaling pathway
	CB2R (cannabinoid receptor type 2) activators	Induction	Enhancement of autophagy through the AMPK-mTOR-P70S6K signaling pathway and inhibition of the NLRP3 inflammasome activation
	1,25(OH)2D3 (Vitamin D)	Impairment	Deficiency in vitamin D can lead to the reduction of ATG16L1 and, thus, the level of autophagy
	Glutamine	Induction	Enhancement of autophagy level through the regulation of the mTOR and p38 MAPK signaling pathway

In the Table, several agents in use or proposed for the therapy, their effect (if known) on autophagy process, and their presumed mechanism of action are reported

AUTOPHAGY IN RHEUMATOID ARTHRITIS

Rheumatoid arthritis (RA) is a chronic autoimmune disorder that particularly affects the joints, but extraarticular manifestations, including cardiovascular, pulmonary, and bone alterations, reflect the systemic origin of the disease. RA is a consequence of autoimmune response versus autologous proteins, leading to the production of autoantibodies, such as rheumatoid factor and anti-cyclic citrullinated peptide antibodies (anti-CCP), which are considered the most important diagnostic markers of the disease [43]. Many genetic and environmental factors are involved in the pathogenesis and progression of the disease; recently, it has been demonstrated that cooking salt affected Th17/regulatory T cells (Treg) balance ex vivo in patients with RA and SLE, suggesting that a reduction of sodium intake may have beneficial effect in autoimmune diseases [44]. Inflammation is the result of the combined activation of innate and adaptive immune cells (T and B cells, macrophages, synovial fibroblasts, chondrocytes, and osteoclasts), and the release of cytokines (TNF-α, IL-6, IL-1) that sustain the progression of the disease [45].

Recent studies have demonstrated how autophagy takes part in different aspects of RA pathogenesis. RA fibroblast-like synoviocytes (FLS) turn into aggressive and invasive phenotype and appear to be resistant to apoptosis induction, in particular Fas-mediated apoptosis pathway [46,47]. Moreover, a reduction of several apoptosis-related molecules has been found at synovial level, suggesting how the low capacity of undergoing apoptosis holds a central role in the extension of RA-FLS life span [48]. In this context, it was well documented how autophagy is actively involved in RA-FLS apoptosis resistance. Shin and colleagues found that RA-FLS subjected to ER stress were protected from apoptosis thanks to autophagy activation [49]. Similarly, Kato and colleagues showed that, following inhibition of proteasome compartment, osteoarthritis (OA) synovial fibroblasts were more susceptible to apoptosis compared with RA synovial fibroblasts [50]. Moreover, synovial tissue from RA patients displayed higher levels of autophagic markers LC3-II and Beclin-1 compared to those obtained from OA patients. Furthermore, an inverse correlation between autophagy and the percentage of apoptosis cells was found in RA synovial tissue [51]. As recently demonstrated, increased autophagy in RA synoviocytes seemed to be strictly associated with RA progression, whereas autophagy inhibition improved inflammatory status. Indeed, the treatment of RA-FLS with autophagy inhibitors 3-MA and chloroquine (CQ) caused the reduction of IL-6 expression after hypoxia-induced autophagy, leading to the suppression of inflammatory potential [52]. In synovial tissue from active RA patients, a positive correlation between LC3-II levels and several disease activity parameters was detected, emphasizing the importance of autophagy in all RA clinical aspects [53].

Activation of osteoclastogenesis is a crucial mechanism for RA progression, and recent studies suggested an involvement of autophagy in this process. In leukemic monocyte-macrophage hypoxia, stimulus for osteoclast differentiation, induced an increase in autophagic flux and autophagy inhibition blocked this phase of maturation [54]. Moreover, in the same cell line, it has been recently demonstrated that the autophagy protein p62 was directly involved in RANKL-induced osteoclastogenesis [55]. By genetic and pharmacologic approaches for induction/inhibition of autophagy, Lin and colleagues demonstrated that autophagy was able to influence osteoclasts differentiation and thus bone erosion in transgenic arthritic mouse model overexpressing human TNF-α [56]. Furthermore, osteoclasts from RA patients synovial tissue displayed increased levels of Atg7 and Beclin-1 compared with OA patients, showing how autophagy was hyperactivated in these cells.

Despite most of RA pathogenic events occur at synovial level, also peripheral immune cells participate in the progression of disease sustaining chronic inflammation. Data on lymphocytes autophagy in RA context are limited and contrasting. Yang and colleagues found that naive CD4$^+$ T cells from RA patients showed a defect in aerobic glycolysis due to a reduction of the glycolytic enzyme 6-phosphofructo-2-kinase/fructose-2,6-bisphosphatase 3 (PFKFB3) levels, and this metabolic impairment was also associated with autophagy downregulation [57]. Opposite results come from a recent work showing an increased LC3-II levels in CD4$^+$ T cells from RA patients, compared with healthy donors [58]. To test whether inhibition of autophagy could be beneficial in RA, the researchers treated collagen-induced arthritis mice with HCQ, demonstrating that suppression of autophagy lead to a reduction of disease score. More studies are needed to better investigate the involvement of autophagy in lymphocytes homeostasis in RA pathogenesis and progression.

Because immune response against citrullinated proteins has a central role in autoimmunity and anti-CCP Abs are important diagnostic marker of RA [59], the study of the relationship between autophagy and generation of citrullinated peptides is fundamental to provide a direct involvement of autophagy in RA development. Moreover, as already discussed, autophagy is involved in presentation of self and nonself antigens to lymphocytes, contributing to the creation of immune repertoire. Recent works demonstrated that the presentation of citrullinated peptides was dependent on autophagy activation, and that the peptidyl arginine deiminases (PAD), the enzyme class that catalyzes citrullination, were detected in autophagosomes purified from APC [60]. Furthermore, the inhibition of autophagy by Atg5 knockdown or 3-MA treatment repressed autophagy-mediated presentation of citrullinated peptides in both B cell lymphoma and DCs. In this regard, a recent study demonstrated that the induction of autophagy by different stimuli, including the mTOR activator rapamycin, caused the activation of PAD4 and the generation of citrullinated peptides in FLSs from RA patients [61]. Interestingly, monocytes from anti-CCP positive RA patients displayed higher levels of autophagic marker LC3-II compared to anti-CCP negative patients, and significant direct association between autophagy and anti-CCP Abs serum levels was found [62].

Taking together, these data indicate that autophagy seems to be dysregulated in many cell types involved in RA pathogenesis. Although the studies are still limited and more experimental evidences are needed, a clinical approach based on autophagy modulation may be a therapeutic choice in RA. In this regard, CQ and HCQ, drugs that cause autophagosomes accumulation by increasing lysosomal pH, are used in clinical practice because of their effectiveness in RA. mTOR inhibition could be another approach to modulate autophagy in RA, although currently studies are limited. In a multicenter study, it has been demonstrated that response to therapy in RA patients was significantly higher in the group treated with the mTOR inhibitor everolimus plus methotrexate than with methotrexate alone (Table 16.1) [63].

AUTOPHAGY IN MULTIPLE SCLEROSIS

Multiple sclerosis (MS) is an autoimmune disease involving the central nervous system (CNS), with a neurological impairment typical of chronic inflammatory demyelinating disorder. It is known that autophagy participates in the progress of MS or experimental autoimmune encephalomyelitis (EAE, a mouse model of MS).

Deficiency of basal autophagy in neurons leads to protein aggregation, resulting in a neurodegenerative phenotype. Neuroinflammation is negatively regulated by autophagy to avoid its harm to the CNS. Because the progression of MS and EAE involves many cell types, autophagy seems to function differently depending on the cell type, so different cell types in the lesion site might show different patterns of autophagy [64].

Microglia, the resident immune cells in the CNS, play important roles in the initiation and sustenance of neuroinflammation to clear pathogens. They produce proinflammatory and neurotoxic factors including reactive oxygen species (ROS) and nitric oxide (NO). Subsequently activated astrocytes amplify the inflammation to produce more proinflammatory factors, chemokines, and NO, which have toxic effects on primary neurons. Autophagy may be a stress response to the negative-feedback regulation of neuroinflammation.

Autophagy is also closely linked to demyelination and remyelination. During demyelination, cell debris is mainly phagocytized by microglia, and this process requires autophagy-related genes. Impairment of autophagy in microglia may hinder debris clearance, leading to damaged remyelination and augmentation of persistent neuroinflammation. The rapid activation of microglia produces proinflammatory cytokines and free radicals and acts as the major APC. Proinflammatory factors, such as IL-1β, can trigger microglial autophagy, suggesting links between autophagy and inflammation activation. mTOR plays a pivotal role in autophagy suppression and promotes inflammation in microglia, and rapamycin may have a beneficial effect in the treatment of MS. mTOR inhibitors reduce neuroinflammation by inhibiting microglial activation or viability, decreasing proinflammatory cytokines [64].

Many studies describe MS as an autoimmune disease wherein autoreactive T cells target the myelin sheath in the CNS, leading to impairments in neuronal function. It has been shown that survival of autoreactive T cells in EAE depends on autophagy-related protein BECN-1, suggesting a role for autophagy in the progression of MS [65]. In agreement, ATG-5 expression is increased in circulating immune cells of mice with EAE, as well as T cells from blood and brain tissue of MS patients. Moreover, several autophagy-related genes including *atg-16L2*, *atg-9A*, and *ULK-1* are upregulated in blood samples of patients diagnosed with MS, which suggests that an overactivation of autophagy may underlie MS pathology, through the modulation of T lymphocyte survival [65]. On the other hand, ATG-7 modulates antigen presentation by DCs, which influences T cell activation in EAE. Thus, DC-specific deletion of ATG-7 reduces antigen presentation by DCs to T cells and alleviates EAE pathology. Additionally, treatment with the lysosomal inhibitor CQ, before or after EAE onset, delays progression or reduces the severity of disease, respectively, suggesting that the autophagy machinery may facilitate antigen presentation by DCs, eliciting T cell priming and autoimmunity in EAE, and possibly in MS. Overall, autophagy-related genes seem to affect DC-mediated activation of T cells, as well as the survival of autoreactive T lymphocytes, playing a deleterious role in MS pathology through the promotion of T cell-mediated demyelination and neurodegeneration [65].

Moreover, in MS lesions, LAMP2 expression is reduced, implying an impairment of autophagy. The mTOR signaling pathway that inhibits autophagy restores the regrowth of axons in the CNS, which is important for remyelination in MS. In acute and chronic EAE, protein aggresomes in the spinal cord and a reduced LC3-II/LC3-I ratio suggest that the protein turnover mechanism through autophagy is impaired. In fact, the mechanism of autophagy in the pathogenesis of MS in the CNS is still superficially understood.

Finally, dysfunction of mitochondria is one of the important factors in the pathogenesis of MS.

Patergnani and colleagues [66] found an increase for both ATG5 and Parkin, a mitophagic marker, in cerebral spinal fluid (CSF) of patients with MS, indicating a pathological role of autophagy/mitophagy in CNS of patients with MS. Therefore, the correlations between both ATG5 and Parkin levels and TNF-α concentrations in CSF seem to confirm the in vivo association among autophagic/mitophagic activity and inflammatory stimuli. Again, the positive correlation between ATG5 and Parkin concentrations suggests that autophagic and mitophagic mechanisms are reciprocally associated in CSF and serum of patients with MS.

Even if one of the major focuses of the research on MS is the identification of biomarkers in biological fluids, such as CSF or blood, we have to consider the difficulties in obtaining spinal fluid samples and the necessity for lumbar puncture to make a diagnosis. Since currently there are no clearly established MS blood-based biomarkers, other processes may provide increasingly important tools for clinical practice [67]. Activating the cannabinoid receptor type 2 (CB2R) has been reported to contribute to the alleviation of EAE through the increase of autophagy, which in turn led to the inhibition of the NLRP3 inflammasome [68]. Interestingly, the protective effect of 1,25(OH)2D3 (vitamin D) was associated with significantly elevated expression of Beclin-1, increased Bcl-2/Bax ratio, and decreased LC3-II accumulation. Thus, 1,25(OH)2D3 may represent a promising new MS treatment (Table 16.1) [69].

So far, little is known about the exact mechanism of autophagy in MS. It is still controversial whether autophagy leads to cell death in MS or is a rescue mechanism activated as part of an endogenous neuroprotective response, since autophagy plays opposite functions in inflammation and cell survival, depending on the inflammatory context.

AUTOPHAGY IN SJÖGREN'S SYNDROME

Primary Sjögren's syndrome (pSS) is a systemic autoimmune disease characterized by infiltration of exocrine glands by T and B lymphocytes that regulate the chronic inflammatory process, by producing chemokines and cytokines [70,71].

Follicular T-helper cells seem to be relevant biomarkers of pSS and cytokines, such as IL-21 and IL-23, play a major role in their modulation [72].

In animal models, it has been shown that activation of the autophagosomal pathway is involved in preventing or alleviating salivary and lacrimal gland dysfunctions [73 75]. Katsiougiannis et al. [76] demonstrated that, in human salivary glands cells, ER stress induced autophagy and apoptosis in both patients with SS and controls.

In a recent study, an autophagy dysregulation in both salivary and peripheral T lymphocytes from pSS patients was demonstrated [77]. A positive correlation was found between autophagy level and CD4+ T-lymphocyte infiltration in salivary glands of pSS patients. Additionally, the level of autophagy in peripheral blood T lymphocytes positively correlated with pSS disease activity indexes.

However, there are few studies involving autophagy in Sjögren's syndrome. It seems that in salivary human submandibular gland cells, the alteration of autophagy process increases the apoptotic effect of ER stress–inducing agents, dropping Ca^{2+} levels, to promote cell survival.

AUTOPHAGY IN INFLAMMATORY BOWEL DISEASE

Intestinal mucosal barrier, mainly composed of the intestinal mucus layer and the epithelium, plays a critical role in nutrient absorption and protection from pathogenic microorganisms. The damage of intestinal mucosal barrier or the disturbance of microorganism balance in the intestinal tract contributes to the pathogenesis and progression of inflammatory bowel disease (IBD), which mainly includes Crohn's disease and ulcerative colitis [68,78].

Regarding the role of autophagy in the pathogenesis and progression of IBD, it has been reported that Atgs like *Atg16l1* and *IRGM* contributes to the susceptibility of IBD, suggesting that autophagy possibly mediated the pathophysiology of IBD [79].

Evidence has shown that impaired autophagy disturbs the function of intestinal epithelial cells and influences the innate and adaptive immune responses, ROS production, and ER stress, leading to abnormal inflammatory reaction, and ultimately promoting the occurrence and development of IBD [79]. It should be also considered the crosstalk between autophagy and the damage-associated molecular pattern molecules (DAMPs) release and degradation in IBD. DAMPs are endogenous molecules including the S100A calgranulins, chromatin-associated high-mobility group box 1 (HMGB1), HSPs, IL-1 family members, histones, ATP, DNA, RNA, uric acid, hyaluronan, and heparin sulfate, which are released by dead, dying, injured, or stressed cells [79]. Previous studies demonstrated that the regulation of IBD progression by DAMPs occurs through several approaches, including the decrease of the levels of DAMPs by autophagy, through the promotion of DAMPs degradation [78,79]. It was also underlined that conditions such as starvation or the stimulation of cytotoxic drugs not only induce autophagy, but could also lead to the release of DAMPs.

Furthermore, the specific mechanism of IBD still remains partially unknown. Only few literatures have reported the effects of autophagy inducers in the clinical treatment of IBD (Table 16.1). Finally, although inducing autophagy contributes to the alleviation of IBD, it seems that the induction of autophagy may also lead to inverse effects. To this, autophagy inducers may lead side effects, inducing the enhancement of colorectal cancer cells tolerance to antitumor drugs [78,79].

CONCLUSION

Autophagy has an important role in many biological processes, including cell development, metabolism, immunity, and aging. Of note, dysfunction in the autophagy pathway has been implicated in an increasing number of human diseases, including autoimmune diseases such as SLE, RA, MS, pSS, and IBD. Further understanding of the molecular mechanisms underlying this process and their involvement in the etiopathogenesis of these diseases could lead to the development of new appealing diagnostic and therapeutic strategies.

REFERENCES

[1] Levine B, Klionsky DJ. Development by self-digestion: molecular mechanisms and biological functions of autophagy. Dev Cell 2004;6:463–77.

[2] Yin Z, Pascual C, Klionsky DJ. Autophagy: machinery and regulation. Microb Cell 2016;3:588–96.

[3] Meijer AJ, Codogno P. Signalling and autophagy regulation in health, aging and disease. Mol Asp Med 2006;27:411–25.

[4] Pierdominici M, Vomero M, Barbati C, Colasanti T, Maselli A, Vacirca D, et al. Role of autophagy in immunity and autoimmunity, with a special focus on systemic lupus erythematosus. FASEB J 2012;26(4):1400–12.

[5] de Duve C. The separation and characterization of subcellular particles. Harvey Lect 1965;59:49–87.

[6] Klionsky DJ, Abdelmohsen K, Abe A, Abedin MJ, Abeliovich H, Acevedo Arozena A, et al. Guidelines for the use and interpretation of assays for monitoring autophagy (3rd ed.). Autophagy 2016;12:1–222.

[7] Mijaljica D, Prescott M, Devenish RJ. Microautophagy in mammalian cells: revisiting a 40-year-old conundrum. Autophagy 2011;7:673–82.

[8] Cuervo AM. Chaperone-mediated autophagy: selectivity pays off. Trends Endocrinol Metab 2010;21:142–50.

[9] Galluzzi L, Bravo-San Pedro J, Kroemer G. Mitophagy: permitted by prohibitin. Curr Biol 2017;27:R73–6.

[10] Mizushima N, Yoshimori T, Oshumi Y. The role of Atg proteins in autophagosome formation. Annu Rev Cell Dev Biol 2011;27:107–32.

[11] Tanida I, Ueno T, Kominami E. LC3 and autophagy. Methods Mol Biol 2008;445:77–88.

[12] Fernandez D, Perl A. mTOR signaling: a central pathway to pathogenesis in systemic lupus erythematosus? Discov Med 2010;9:173–8.

[13] Nazio F, Cecconi F. mTOR, AMBRA1, and autophagy: an intricate relationship. Cell Cycle 2013;12:2524–5.

[14] Fimia GM, Stoykova A, Romagnoli A, Giunta L, Di Bartolomeo S, Nardacci R, et al. Ambra1 regulates autophagy and development of the nervous system. Nature 2007;447:1121–5.

[15] Nazio F, Strappazzon F, Antonioli M, Bielli P, Cianfanelli V, Bordi M, et al. mTOR inhibits autophagy by controlling ULK1 ubiquitylation, self-association and function through AMBRA1 and TRAF6. Nat Cell Biol 2013;15:406–16.

[16] Catena V, Fanciulli M. Deptor: not only a mTOR inhibitor. J Exp Clin Cancer Res 2017;36:12.

[17] Levine B, Deretic V. Unveiling the roles of autophagy in innate and adaptive immunity. Nat Rev Immunol 2007;7:767–76.

[18] Deretic V. Autophagy in immunity and cell-autonomous defense against intracellular microbes. Immunol Rev 2011;240:92–104.

[19] Deretic V, Delgado M, Vergne I, Master S, De Haro S, Ponpuak M, et al. Autophagy in immunity against *Mycobacterium tuberculosis*: a model system to dissect immunological roles of autophagy. Curr Top Microbiol Immunol 2009;335:169–88.

[20] Castillo EF, Dekonenko A, Arko-Mensah J, Mandell MA, Dupont N, Jiang S, et al. Autophagy protects against active tuberculosis by suppressing bacterial burden and inflammation. Proc Natl Acad Sci USA 2012;109:E3168–76.

[21] Songane M, Kleinnijenhuis J, Netea MG, van Crevel R. The role of autophagy in host defence against *Mycobacterium tuberculosis* infection. Tuberculosis 2012;92:388–96.

[22] Dengjel J, Schoor O, Fischer R, Reich M, Kraus M, Müller M, et al. Autophagy promotes MHC class II presentation of peptides from intracellular source proteins. Proc Natl Acad Sci USA 2005;102:7922–7.

[23] Brazil MI, Weiss S, Stockinger B. Excessive degradation of intracellular protein in macrophages prevents presentation in the context of major histocompatibility complex class II molecules. Eur J Immunol 1997;27:1506–14.

[24] Schmid D, Pypaert M, Munz C. Antigen-loading compartments for major histocompatibility complex class II molecules continuously receive input from autophagosomes. Immunity 2007;26:79–92.

[25] Jagannath C, Lindsey DR, Dhandayuthapani S, Xu Y, Hunter Jr RL, Eissa NT. Autophagy enhances the efficacy of BCG vaccine by increasing peptide presentation in mouse dendritic cells. Nat Med 2009;15:267–76.

[26] Kovacs JR, Li C, Yang Q, Li G, Garcia IG, Ju S, et al. Autophagy promotes T-cell survival through degradation of proteins of the cell death machinery. Cell Death Differ 2012;19:144–52.

[27] Pua HH, Dzhagalov I, Chuck M, Mizushima N, He YW. A critical role for the autophagy gene Atg5 in T cell survival and proliferation. J Exp Med 2007;204:25–31.

[28] Parekh VV, Wu L, Boyd KL, Williams JA, Gaddy JA, Olivares-Villagómez D, et al. Impaired autophagy, defective T cell homeostasis and a wasting syndrome in mice with a T cell-specific deletion of Vps34. J Immunol 2013;190:5086–101.

[29] Miller BC, Zhao Z, Stephenson LM, Cadwell K, Pua HH, Lee HK, et al. The autophagy gene Atg5 plays an essential role in B lymphocyte development. Autophagy 2008;4:309–14.

[30] Arsov I, Adebayo A, Kucerova-Levisohn M, Haye J, MacNeil M, Papavasiliou FN, et al. A role for autophagic protein beclin1 early in lymphocyte development. J Immunol 2011;186:2201–9.

[31] Watanabe K, Ichinose S, Hayashizaki K, Tsubata T. Induction of autophagy by B cell antigen receptor stimulation and its inhibition by costimulation. Biochem Biophys Res Commun 2008;374:274–81.

[32] Cenci S. Autophagy, a new determinant of plasma cell differentiation and antibody responses. Mol Immunol 2014;62:289–95.

[33] Pengo N, Scolari M, Oliva L, Milan E, Mainoldi F, Raimondi A, et al. Plasma cells require autophagy for sustainable immunoglobulin production. Nat Immunol 2013;14:298–305.

[34] Rahman A, Isenberg DA. Systemic lupus erythematosus. N Engl J Med 2008;3:929–39.

[35] Gualtierotti R, Biggioggero M, Penatti AE, Meroni PL. Updating on the pathogenesis of systemic lupus erythematosus. Autoimmun Rev 2010;10:3–7.

[36] Alessandri C, Barbati C, Vacirca D, Piscopo P, Confaloni A, Sanchez M, et al. T lymphocytes from patients with systemic lupus erythematosus are resistant to induction of autophagy. FASEB J 2012;26:4722–32.

[37] Colasanti T, Vomero M, Alessandri C, Barbati C, Maselli A, Camperio C, et al. Role of alpha-synuclein in autophagy modulation of primary human T lymphocytes. Cell Death Dis 2014;5:e1265.

[38] Barbati C, Alessandri C, Vomero M, Vona R, Colasanti T, Vacirca D, et al. Autoantibodies specific to D4GDI modulate Rho GTPase mediated cytoskeleton remodeling and induce autophagy in T lymphocytes. J Autoimmun 2015;58:78–89.

[39] Ramos-Barrón A, Piñera-Haces C, Gómez-Alamillo C, Santiuste-Torcida I, Ruiz JC, Buelta-Carrillo L, et al. Prevention of murine lupus disease in (NZBxNZW) F1 mice by sirolimus treatment. Lupus 2007;16:775–81.

[40] Wang F, Muller S. Manipulating autophagic processes in autoimmune diseases: a special focus on modulating chaperone-mediated autophagy, an emerging therapeutic target. Front Immunol 2015;6:252.

[41] Fernandez D, Bonilla E, Mirza N, Niland B, Perl A. Rapamycin reduces disease activity and normalizes T cell activation-induced calcium fluxing in patients with systemic lupus erythematosus. Arthritis Rheum 2006;54:2983–8.

[42] Muller S, Monneaux F, Schall N, Rashkov RK, Oparanov BA, Wiesel P, et al. Spliceosomal peptide P140 for immunotherapy of systemic lupus erythematosus: results of an early phase II clinical trial. Arthritis Rheum 2008;58(12):3873–83.

[43] McInnes IB, Schett G. The pathogenesis of rheumatoid arthritis. N Engl J Med 2011;201(365):2205–19.

[44] Scrivo R, Massaro L, Barbati C, Vomero M, Ceccarelli F, Spinelli FR, et al. The role of dietary sodium intake on the modulation of T helper 17 cells and regulatory T cells in patients with rheumatoid arthritis and systemic lupus erythematosus. PLoS One 2017;12:e0184449.

[45] Firestein GS, McInnes IB. Immunopathogenesis of rheumatoid arthritis. Immunity 2017;46:183–96.

[46] Pap T, Müller-Ladner U, Gay RE, Gay S. Fibroblast biology. Role of synovial fibroblasts in the pathogenesis of rheumatoid arthritis. Arthritis Res 2000;2:361–7.

[47] Nakajima T, Aono H, Hasunuma T, Yamamoto K, Shirai T, Hirohata K, et al. Apoptosis and functional Fas antigen in rheumatoid arthritis synoviocytes. Arthritis Rheum 1995;38:485–91.

[48] Pope RM. Apoptosis as a therapeutic tool in rheumatoid arthritis. Nat Rev Immunol 2002;2:527–35.

[49] Shin YJ, Han SH, Kim DS, Lee GH, Yoo WH, Kang YM, et al. Autophagy induction and CHOP under-expression promotes survival of fibroblasts from rheumatoid arthritis patients under endoplasmic reticulum stress. Arthritis Res Ther 2010;12:R19.

[50] Kato M, Ospelt C, Gay RE, Gay S, Klein K. Dual role of autophagy in stress-induced cell death in rheumatoid arthritis synovial fibroblasts. Arthritis Rheumatol 2014;66:40–8.

[51] Xu K, Xu P, Yao JF, Zhang YG, Hou WK, Lu SM. Reduced apoptosis correlates with enhanced autophagy in synovial tissues of rheumatoid arthritis. Inflamm Res 2013;62:229–37.

[52] Yang R, Zhang Y, Wang L, Hu J, Wen J, Xue L, et al. Increased autophagy in fibroblast-like synoviocytes leads to immune enhancement potential in rheumatoid arthritis. Oncotarget 2017;8(9):15420–30.

[53] Zhu L, Wang H, Wu Y, He Z, Qin Y, Shen Q. The autophagy level is increased in the synovial tissues of patients with active rheumatoid arthritis and is correlated with disease severity. Mediat Inflamm 2017;2017:7623145.

[54] Zhao Y, Chen G, Zhang W, Xu N, Zhu JY, Jia J, et al. Autophagy regulates hypoxia-induced osteoclastogenesis through the HIF-1a/BNIP3 signaling pathway. J Cell Physiol 2012;227:639–48.

[55] Li RF, Chen G, Ren JG, Zhang W, Wu ZX, Liu B, et al. The adaptor protein p62 is involved in RANKL-induced autophagy and osteoclastogenesis. J Histochem Cytochem 2014;62:879–88.

[56] Lin NY, Beyer C, Giessl A, Kireva T, Scholtysek C, Uderhardt S, et al. Autophagy regulates TNFα-mediated joint destruction in experimental arthritis. Ann Rheum Dis 2013;72:761–8.

[57] Yang Z, Fujii H, Mohan SV, Goronzy JJ, Weyand CM. Phosphofructokinase deficiency impairs ATP generation, autophagy, and redox balance in rheumatoid arthritis T cells. J Exp Med 2013;210:2119–34.

[58] van Loosdregt J, Rossetti M, Spreafico R, Moshref M, Olmer M, Williams GW, et al. Increased autophagy in CD4+ T cells of rheumatoid arthritis patients results in T-cell hyperactivation and apoptosis resistance. Eur J Immunol 2016;46:2862–70.

[59] Valesini G, Gerardi MC, Iannuccelli C, Pacucci VA, Pendolino M, Shoenfeld Y. Citrullination and autoimmunity. Autoimmun Rev 2015;14:490–7.

[60] Ireland JM, Unanue ER. Autophagy in antigen presenting cells results in presentation of citrullinated peptides to CD4 T cells. J Exp Med 2011;208:2625–32.

[61] Ireland JM, Unanue ER. Processing of proteins in autophagy vesicles of antigen-presenting cells generates citrullinated peptides recognized by the immune system. Autophagy 2012;8:429–30.

[62] Sorice M, Iannuccelli C, Manganelli V, Capozzi A, Alessandri C, Lococo E, et al. Autophagy generates citrullinated peptides in human synoviocytes: a possible trigger for anti-citrullinated peptide antibodies. Rheumatology 2016;55:1374–85.

[63] Bruyn GA, Tate G, Caeiro F, Maldonado-Cocco J, Westhovens R, Tannenbaum H, et al. Everolimus in patients with rheumatoid arthritis receiving concomitant methotrexate: a 3-month, double-blind, randomised, placebo-controlled, parallel-group, proof-of-concept study. Ann Rheum Dis 2008;67:1090–5.

[64] Liang P, Le W. Role of autophagy in the pathogenesis of multiple sclerosis. Neurosci Bull 2015;31:435–44.

[65] Plaza-Zabala A, Sierra-Torre V, Sierra A. Autophagy and microglia: novel partners in neurodegeneration and aging. Int J Mol Sci 2017;18:598.

[66] Patergnani S, Castellazzi M, Bonora M, Marchi S, Casetta I, Pugliatti M, et al. Autophagy and mitophagy elements are increased in body fluids of multiple sclerosis-affected individuals. J Neurol Neurosurg Psychiatry 2017. pii:jnnp-2017-316234. Letter.

[67] D'Ambrosio A, Pontecorvo S, Colasanti T, Zamboni S, Francia A, Margutti P. Peripheral blood biomarkers in multiple sclerosis. Autoimmun Rev 2015;14:1097–110.

[68] Ke P, Shao BZ, Xu ZQ, Chen XW, Liu C. Intestinal autophagy and its pharmacological control in inflammatory bowel disease. Front Immunol 2017;7:695.

[69] Zhen C, Feng X, Li Z, Wang Y, Li B, Li L, et al. Suppression of murine experimental autoimmune encephalomyelitis development by 1,25-dihydroxyvitamin D3 with autophagy modulation. Neuroimmunology 2015;280:1–7.

[70] Astorri E, Scrivo R, Bombardieri M, Picarelli G, Pecorella I, Porzia A, et al. CX3CL1 and CX3CR1 expression in tertiary lymphoid structures in salivary gland infiltrates: fractalkine contribution to lymphoid neogenesis in Sjogren's syndrome. Rheumatology (Oxf) 2014;53:611–20.

[71] Barone F, Bombardieri M, Rosado MM, Morgan PR, Challacombe SJ, De Vita S, et al. CXCL13, CCL21, and CXCL12 expression in salivary glands of patients with Sjögren's syndrome and MALT lymphoma: association with reactive and malignant areas of lymphoid organization. J Immunol 2008;1:5130–40.

[72] Gong YZ, Nititham J, Taylor K, Miceli-Richard C, Sordet C, Wachsmann D, et al. Differentiation of follicular helper T cells by salivary gland epithelial cells in primary Sjögren's syndrome. J Autoimmun 2014;51:57–66.

[73] Morgan-Bathke M, Lin HH, Chibly AM, Zhang W, Sun X, Chen CH, et al. Deletion of ATG5 shows a role of autophagy in salivary homeostatic control. J Dent Res. 2013;92:911–7.

[74] Morgan-Bathke M, Hill GA, Harris ZI, Lin HH, Chibly AM, Klein RR, et al. Autophagy correlates with maintenance of salivary gland function following radiation. Sci Rep 2014;4:5206.

[75] Seo Y, Ji YW, Lee SM, Shim J, Noh H, Yeo A, et al. Activation of HIF-1alpha (hypoxia inducible factor-1alpha) prevents dry eye-induced acinar cell death in the lacrimal gland. Cell Death Dis 2014;5:e1309.

[76] Katsiougiannis S, Tenta R, Skopouli FN. Endoplasmic reticulum stress causes autophagy and apoptosis leading to cellular redistribution of the autoantigens Ro/Sjögren's syndrome-related antigen A (SSA) and La/SSB in salivary gland epithelial cells. Clin Exp Immunol 2015;181:244–52.

[77] Alessandri C, Ciccia F, Priori R, Astorri E, Guggino G, Alessandro R, et al. CD4 T lymphocyte autophagy is upregulated in the salivary glands of primary Sjögren's syndrome patients and correlates with focus score and disease activity. Arthritis Res Ther 2017;19(1):178.

[78] Lassen KG, Xavier RJ. Genetic control of autophagy underlies pathogenesis of inflammatory bowel disease. Mucosal Immunol 2017;10:589–97.

[79] Zhang Q, Kang R, Zeh 3rd HJ, Lotze MT, Tang D. DAMPs and autophagy: cellular adaptation to injury and unscheduled cell death. Autophagy 2013;9:451–8.

Chapter 17

Laboratory Diagnostics

Nicola Bizzaro[1,2], Renato Tozzoli[1,2]

[1]Laboratory of Clinical Pathology, Azienda Sanitaria Universitaria Integrata di Udine, San Antonio Hospital, Tolmezzo, Italy; [2]Laboratory of Clinical Pathology, Department of Laboratory Medicine, S. Maria degli Angeli Hospital, Pordenone, Italy

Laboratory diagnostics provide two pieces in the mosaic of autoimmunity: the *autoantibody tests* and the *immunological methods* used to measure antibodies. Using the most appropriate autoantibody test for each clinical setting and the methods that provide the best diagnostic accuracy for clinical use is a duty of the autoimmunology laboratory.

This task has become even more complex today because the scenario has deeply changed since 10–15 years ago: in this time interval, new autoantibody–autoantigen systems (both systemic and organ-specific) have been discovered; new diagnostic technologies have become available and changes in organizational processes have occurred, mainly because of introduction of advanced information technology and test automation [1–3]. Given the wide number of tests and methods currently available and the different roles recognized to many antibodies, the choice of the most appropriate test and method involves organizational and strategic issues that depend on the type of clinical context and the purpose of antibody research [4].

Currently available autoantibody tests contribute significantly to the diagnosis of autoimmune diseases, both for screening purposes when the tests have high sensitivity and for disease classification when the tests are highly specific. However, the search for new antibodies is still needed (1) to find immuno-serological markers in diseases whose autoimmune pathogenesis has only recently been highlighted; (2) to close as far as possible the gap in those diseases in which the already available antibodies display an insufficient diagnostic sensitivity; and (3) to finding antibodies that can be used to monitor therapy.

Just to mention only a few of them, new antibody tests have been proposed for deamidated gliadin in celiac disease, carbamylated proteins and 3-14-3η protein in rheumatoid arthritis (RA), anti-PLA$_2$R in primary membranous nephropathy, anti-NMDA receptor in limbic encephalitis, antiamphiphysin and anti-Tr antibodies in paraneoplastic neurological syndromes, anti-beta 2 GPI domain I in antiphospholipid syndrome (APS), antimuscle specific kinase (MuSK) in miastenia gravis, and antiaquaporin 4 antibodies in neuromyelitis optica. Some of these antibodies have been already introduced in clinical practice; for others there is still a need to undertake clinical validation studies before considering routine diagnostic use.

In parallel with the new antibodies introduced in the diagnostics, over the years there has been an awareness that antibodies that are already measured daily in many laboratories have characteristics that can be used for different clinical purposes [5]. Here, then, the notion has emerged that antibodies can have not only diagnostic but also prognostic meaning (when they are pathogenetic or involved in the mechanism that causes the disease), can be predictive of disease onset, and ultimately can also be protective, ie., capable to counteract the development of some autoimmune diseases.

THE DIAGNOSTIC AND PROGNOSTIC VALUE OF AUTOANTIBODIES

The detection of serum autoantibodies against a wide number of structural and functional molecules present in ubiquitous or tissue-specific cells is used for the diagnosis and classification of autoimmune diseases (Table 17.1). Autoantibodies that are well-recognized criteria of some autoimmune diseases are antinuclear antibodies (ANA), anti-dsDNA, anti-Sm and antiphospholipid antibodies (aPL) for systemic lupus erythematous (SLE), rheumatoid factor for RA, anti-Ro for Sjögren's syndrome, anti-U$_1$RNP for mixed connective tissue disease, antitopoisomerase and anticentromere B protein for systemic sclerosis (SSc), and antimitochondrial antibodies (AMA) for primary biliary cholangitis (PBC). More recently, other antibodies have been included among classification/diagnosis criteria for specific autoimmune disorders, namely anticitrullinated protein antibodies (ACPA) for RA [6], anti-RNA polymerase III antibodies for SSc [7], anti–tissue transglutaminase antibodies (tTG) for celiac disease [8], anti–soluble liver antigen (SLA) for type 1 autoimmune hepatitis [9], and anti-TSH receptor (TRAb) for Graves' disease [10].

Mosaic of Autoimmunity. https://doi.org/10.1016/B978-0-12-814307-0.00017-7

TABLE 17.1 Diagnostic/Classificative Role of Autoantibodies

Antibody	Disease
ANA, anti-dsDNA, anti-Sm, aPL	Systemic lupus erythematosus
Rheumatoid factor	Rheumatoid arthritis
Anti-Ro	Sjögren's syndrome
Anti-U1RNP	Mixed connective tissue disease
Antitopoisomerase, anticentromere B protein	Systemic sclerosis
Antimitochondrial	Primary biliary cholangitis
Anticitrullinated protein	Rheumatoid arthritis
Anti-RNA polymerase III	Systemic sclerosis
Antitissue transglutaminase	Celiac disease
Antisoluble liver antigen	Type 1 autoimmune hepatitis
Anti-TSH receptor	Graves' disease

TABLE 17.2 Prognostic Role of Autoantibodies

Antibody	Disease	Clinical Aspect
Anticitrullinated protein	Rheumatoid arthritis	Clinical progression
Different antibodies	Systemic lupus erythematosus	Nephritis, neonatal lupus, congenital heart block
Antiribosomal P protein	Systemic lupus erythematosus	Cerebritis, psychosis, depression
aPL	Systemic lupus erythematosus	Stroke
aCL, antiprothrombin	Systemic lupus erythematosus	Thrombotic event
Antitopoisomerase I, anticentromere	Systemic sclerosis	Activity and severity
Anti-RNA polymerase III	Systemic sclerosis	Cutaneous thickening, renal crisis
Anti-C1q, anti-dsDNA	Systemic lupus erythematosus	Renal flares
Anti-TSH receptor	Graves' disease	Remission/recurrence
Anti–alpha actinin	Type 1 autoimmune hepatitis	Response to therapy
Anti-Ro52, soluble liver antigen	Type 1 autoimmune hepatitis	Poor prognosis

In addition, as autoantibodies may reflect the presence, nature, and intensity of the immune response, it is possible to use them as prognostic markers of disease activity and severity in patients who already have been diagnosed with an auto-immune disease (Table 17.2).

In RA, the presence of ACPA antibodies is an important independent predictor of the clinical progression [11–16]. In SLE, certain antibodies have been found to be correlated with nephritis, whereas others (i.e., anti-Ro antibodies) were found to represent a significant risk factor for neonatal lupus and congenital heart block in the patient's sibling. Antiribosomal p protein antibodies have been associated with cerebritis, psychosis, and depression. In addition, aPL have been found to predict stroke in SLE patients [17], and around 50% of SLE patients with anticardiolipin antibodies (aCL) [18] or with antiprothrombin antibodies [19] have a clinical thrombotic event (venous or arterial or recurrent spontaneous abortions) prior to diagnosis.

Reports have highlighted the close relationship between anti–DNA-topoisomerase I and anticentromere antibody concentration and SSc activity and severity [20]. SSc patients with anti-RNA polymerase III antibodies have the most severe cutaneous thickening and the highest frequency of renal crisis [21]. It has been shown that active nephritis in SLE is associated with higher concentrations of anti-C1q antibodies and that this type of autoantibody is a predictor of renal flares with a specificity superior or similar to that of anti-dsDNA antibodies [22,23]. Antineutrophil cytoplasmic antibodies (ANCA) are considered sensitive markers of disease activity in patients with small-vessel vasculitides, with a moderate ability to predict relapse and guide therapeutic decisions [24,25].

Antibody prediction in prognosis is not restricted to rheumatic diseases but extends to organ-specific autoimmune diseases. In patients with Graves' disease, TRAb can predict remission or recurrence in patients undergoing antithyroid drug treatment [26]; antismooth muscle antibodies predict development of autoimmune hepatitis in patients with normal liver function [27], and anti–alpha actinin antibodies may predict response to therapy in patients with type 1 autoimmune hepatitis [28]. In addition, anti-Ro52 antibodies associated to SLA antibodies indicate a poor prognosis in type 1 autoimmune hepatitis [29].

THE PREDICTIVE VALUE OF AUTOANTIBODIES

Besides their diagnostic and prognostic role, many specific autoantibodies are early screening indicators, as they can be detected in the sera of asymptomatic subjects who later eventually develop overt systemic [30–32] or organ-specific [33,34] autoimmune diseases (Table 17.3). Studies highlighting the predictive value of autoantibodies are important because they redefined the natural history of autoimmune diseases as a group of human diseases characterized by a long latency period and by the appearance of autoantibodies when clinical manifestations are still absent.

Among autoimmune rheumatic diseases, antibodies to U_1RNP, Sm, dsDNA, cardiolipin, Ro, and La have a positive predictive value (PPV) for SLE ranging from 94% to 100%. According to the type of antibody, the appearance can precede clinical diagnosis by 7–10 years with a frequency that varies from 32% to 78% at the moment of diagnosis [35]. Moderate or high levels of aCL are present in 18% of asymptomatic individuals up to 7 years before SLE diagnosis [18]. In subjects with scleroderma, anticentromere and antitopoisomerase I antibodies are detectable up to 11 years before clinical manifestations, with a PPV of 100%. In RA, rheumatoid factor has a predictivity between 52% and 88%, whereas for ACPA the predictivity is much higher, reaching 97%. These two antibodies have been detected in serum up to 14 years before patients manifest the first symptoms of the disease [36,37].

Anti-Ro and anti-La antibodies have been detected on average 5 years before diagnosis in 73% of asymptomatic mothers who had given birth to a child with autoantibody-associated congenital heart block and who later developed Sjögren's syndrome [38,39]. Antisynthetase antibodies may be found in patients with idiopathic inflammatory myositis years before disease onset [40], and antinucleosome antibodies were found to be present in 67% of patients with APS up to 11 years before the development of SLE [41].

TABLE 17.3 Predictive Value of Autoantibodies

Antibody	Disease
Anti-U_1RNP, anti-dsDNA, anti-Sm, aCL, anti-Ro, anti-La	Systemic lupus erythematosus
Rheumatoid factor, citrullinated protein	Rheumatoid arthritis
Anti-Ro, anti-La	Sjögren's syndrome
Anti-TPO	Postpartum thyroiditis
Parietal cells	Autoimmune gastritis
Antimitochondrial	Primary biliary cholangitis
Anti-insulin, anti-GAD, anti-IA-2, anti-zinc transporter 8	Type 1 diabetes mellitus
Adrenal cortex	Addison's disease
Anti-*Saccharomyces cerevisiae*	Crohn's disease
Antitissue transglutaminase, antiendomysial	Celiac disease

In organ-specific autoimmune diseases, the predictive value of each antibody characteristic for a specific disease is similar to that found for the autoantibodies in autoimmune rheumatic diseases. Antithyroid peroxidase antibodies (anti-TPO) have been shown to be a good predictor of postpartum thyroid dysfunction. A high anti-TPO antibody level immediately postpartum can predict thyroiditis with 97% sensitivity, 91% specificity, and a PPV of 92% [42]. The presence of antiparietal cell antibodies predicts the development of autoimmune gastritis [43]. In AMA-positive subjects without clinical or biochemical signs of hepatic damage, AMA can be detected up to 25 years before the clinical manifestation of PBC [44]. Their PPV is higher of 95% [45]. Pancreatic islet cells antibodies and antibodies to insulin, to 65-kD glutamic acid decarboxylase (GAD), and to tyrosine phosphatase-like (IA-2) protein are predictive markers of type 1 diabetes mellitus (T1DM) [46]. Their PPV is 43%, 55%, 42%, and 29%, respectively [47]. The risk of developing the disease in first-degree relatives of patients with diabetes grows progressively with the duration of the follow-up and with the number of positive autoantibodies, being 2%, 25%, and 70%, with one, two, and three or four positive antibodies [47]. Recently, antibodies to the zinc transporter 8 (ZnT8) were shown to predict diabetes independently of antiislet cell antibodies [48] and antibodies to GAD could predict development of thyroid autoimmune diseases in adult patients with T1DM [49]. Adrenal cortex autoantibodies may precede Addison's disease onset by up to 10 years and their PPV is about 70% [50]. Anti-*Saccharomyces cerevisiae* antibodies as markers for Crohn's disease have been detected in the sera of apparently healthy subjects, on average 3 years before the disease became manifest. Their diagnostic sensitivity was 31%, but specificity and predictive value were both 100% [51]. The predictive value for celiac disease onset of anti-tTG and antiendomysial antibodies is 50%–60%. If the patient carries the HLA-DQ2 or DQ8 antigens, known to be genetic markers for celiac disease susceptibility, the PPV of autoantibodies approaches 100% [52].

THE PROTECTIVE ROLE OF AUTOANTIBODIES

Natural polyreactive autoantibodies, mostly of the IgM isotype, are found in the sera of healthy individuals and react with both self and nonself antigens. Nonspecific and low-affinity binding of these natural autoantibodies to self-antigens may prevent autoreactive clones from reacting with self-antigens by masking their antigenic determinants [53]. Protective autoantibodies are thought to play a role in preventing many autoimmune diseases, such as SLE. Indeed, IgM anti-dsDNA antibodies were found to be significantly associated with milder disease activity and have a negative correlation with the severity of glomerulonephritis in SLE [54,55]; in addition, their administration into SLE-prone mice prevented the development of nephritis. Interestingly, the presence of antinuclear and anti-dsDNA antibodies is associated with a better prognosis of cancer suggesting that these autoantibodies may function as potential antineoplastic agents [56]. IgM antibodies to oxidized low density lipoproteins (LDL) have been suggested to prevent the clinical manifestations of atherosclerosis [57] and the presence of rheumatoid factor in SLE to be protective against the development of lupus nephritis.

THE METHODS TO DETECT AUTOANTIBODIES

Compared with the methods used 10 years ago, the mosaic has further expanded. Although, for the time being, the method of indirect immunofluorescence (IIF) maintains its basic role in autoimmune diagnostics, to cope with increased antibody request and at the same time continue to exploit the high sensitivity of IIF, automated systems have been developed for reading and interpretation of IIF tests for ANA. Although their performance needs to be further improved, these systems already allow for automated classification of samples, with a high efficiency in discriminating between positive and negative ANA and an acceptable correlation with manual microscope reading [58]. Automated quantification of autoantibodies [59,60] and implementation of a quantitative internal QC system [61] are possible further advantageous applications of this IIF method innovation.

In addition, the availability of these systems suggests that automation of cell-based IIF testing may improve standardization of antibody testing and help to reduce variability among autoimmunology laboratories. Automated systems have been developed also for the detection of anti-dsDNA antibodies on *Crithidia luciliae* substrate [62] and for ANCA [63,64]. Efforts are in progress to extend this technology to tissues for the detection of antibodies to gastric parietal cells, smooth muscle, mitochondrial, and endomysial antigens.

Besides these recent improvements in IIF, a wide number of different immunoassays (monoplex and multiplex) have been introduced and are currently used for single or multiple measurements of autoantibodies [65]. A classification of these methods is shown in Table 17.4.

While immunoenzymatic methods (ELISA) are progressively abandoned in clinical laboratories, fully automated random access chemiluminescence (CLIA) instruments are emerging as a promising technology and are destined for further development [66]. Current chemiluminescent immunoassays consist of tests that measure one autoantibody at a time.

TABLE 17.4 Classification of Immunoassay Methods for the Detection of Autoantibodies

First-Generation Monoplex	Abbreviation
Double immunodiffusion	ID
Complement fixation	CF
Indirect immunofluorescence	IIF
Passive agglutination	PHA
Radioimmunoprecipitation	RIPA
Western blot/immunodot	WB/IB
Second–Third Generation Monoplex	**Abbreviation**
Radioimmunoassay–immunoradiometric assay	RIA-IRMA
Radioreceptor assay	RRA
Immunoenzymatic assay–immunoenzymometric assay	ELISA-IEMA
Immunoblot	IB
Immunodot	DB
Chemiluminescence immunoassay	CLIA-ILMA
Fluorescence immunoassay	FIA-IFMA
Multiplex	**Abbreviation**
Nonplanar (addressable microbeads) immunoassay	NPMIA
Planar (membranes, glass slides) immunoassay	PMIA

However, the need is emerging for multiparametric tests that can identify all the components of the immunological picture in a single analytical step, efficiently and at reasonable cost. Use of the *two-dimensional resolution for CL multiplex immunoassay* [67,68] and of the ultrasensitive *chemiluminescence magnetic nanoparticles immunoassay* technology will further increase the analytic sensitivity of the CLIA method [69,70] and might open doors for the setting up of multiparametric CLIA tests enabling significantly reduction in the analysis time [71].

Also, planar and nonplanar autoantigenic arrays have found application for research on autoantibody profiling of autoimmune diseases [72–74]. Planar array systems are made up of microspots on glass slides or on polystyrene microplates and linear immunoblot systems on nitrocellulose membranes. Among the nonplanar arrays there have been developed systems in suspension that use microparticles recognized by laser nephelometry or laser fluorimetry in flow cytometry [75]. Many of these systems are already used in diagnostics; others are still in the early stages of development and need clinical validation, but their ease of use and speed of analysis suggest them as valid alternatives to current immunometric methods.

ORGANIZATION OF THE AUTOIMMUNE LABORATORY

The progressive increase in requests of autoantibody tests that occurred in recent years has brought to the introduction of subtotal and total automation in the clinical immunology laboratory [76,77]. Currently, all stages of the analytical procedure for detection and quantification of autoantibodies are automated. The third generation of laboratory systems now encompasses most of the analytical steps of the laboratory workflow, enabling the clinical pathologists to focus on "value-added" work, such as result validation and production of narrative reports for clinical interpretation [3].

Automation technology has many advantages: it can reduce labor requirements; improve turnaround time; achieve higher quality of testing (precision, limits of detections, dynamic range, etc.); reduce pre-, post-, and analytical errors; and increase throughput and productivity.

The choice of the best strategy depends on many factors: the tests requested (screening, diagnostic confirmation, monitoring); the pathology to be investigated (rheumatic disease, liver disease, celiac disease, etc.); technologies available to the laboratory; diagnostic accuracy; and cost of test and methods.

A final note concerns the possibility that new technologies offer today to respond in a very short time to the request of autoantibody tests. Although in most cases this is not clinically justified, real-time measurement of autoantibodies may clearly benefit the rheumatology or the nephrology practice in emergency and urgent care settings.

Furthermore, the availability of automated analyzers with reduced assay times as well of manual point-of-care systems enables real-time antibody measurement in the same day of the request or even in *stat mode*, avoiding delay and improving compliance [78]. This also responds to the increasing need for faster diagnosis owing to shorter period of hospitalization.

In conclusion, in recent years major changes have occurred in the laboratory diagnostics of autoimmune diseases. Physicians need to fully understand these changes for appropriate test requests; the laboratory autoimmunologist needs to acquire a higher clinical expertise and a complete knowledge of the pros and cons of new analytical methods, far superior to the one required only a few years ago, for optimal clinical governance.

REFERENCES

[1] Tozzoli R. Recent advances in diagnostic technologies and their impact in autoimmune diseases. Autoimmun Rev 2007;6:334–40.

[2] Tozzoli R, Bonaguri C, Melegari A, Antico A, Bassetti D, Bizzaro N. Current state of diagnostic technologies in the autoimmunology laboratory. Clin Chem Lab Med 2013;51:129–38.

[3] Bizzaro N, Tozzoli R, Villalta D. Autoimmune diagnostics: the technology, the strategy and the clinical governance. Immunol Res 2015;61:126–34.

[4] Tozzoli R, Bizzaro N. The clinical autoimmunologist and laboratory autoimmunologist: the two sides of the coin. Autoimmun Rev 2012;11:766–70.

[5] Damoiseaux J, Andrade LE, Fritzler MJ, Shoenfeld Y. Autoantibodies 2015: from diagnostic biomarkers toward prediction, prognosis and prevention. Autoimmun Rev 2015;14:555–63.

[6] Aletaha D, Neogi T, Silman AJ, Funovits J, Felson DT, Bingham 3rd CO, et al. 2010 rheumatoid arthritis classification criteria: an American College of Rheumatology/European League against Rheumatism collaborative initiative. Arthritis Rheum 2010;62:2569–81.

[7] van den Hoogen F, Khanna D, Fransen J, Johnson SR, Baron M, Tyndall A, et al. 2013 classification criteria for systemic sclerosis: an American College of Rheumatology/European League against Rheumatism collaborative initiative. Ann Rheum Dis 2013;72:1747–55.

[8] Husby S, Koletzko S, Korponay-Szabó IR, Mearin ML, Phillips A, Shamir R. European society for pediatric gastroenterology, hepatology, and nutrition guidelines for the diagnosis of coeliac disease. Pediatr Gastroenterol Nutr 2012;54:136–60.

[9] Hennes EM, Zeniya M, Czaja AJ, Parés A, Dalekos GN, Krawitt EL, et al. Simplified criteria for the diagnosis of autoimmune hepatitis. Hepatology 2008;48:169–74.

[10] Ross DS, Burch HB, Cooper DS, Greenlee MC, Laurberg P, Maia AL, et al. 2016 American thyroid association guidelines for diagnosis and management of hyperthyroidism and other causes of thyrotoxicosis. Thyroid 2016;26:1343–421.

[11] Forslind K, Ahlmèn M, Eberhardt HI, Svensson B. Prediction of radiological outcome in early rheumatoid arthritis in clinical practice: role of antibodies to citrullinated peptides (anti-CCP). Ann Rheum Dis 2004;63:1090–5.

[12] Ronnelid J, Wick MC, Lampa J, Lindblad S, Nordmark B, Klareskog L, et al. Longitudinal analysis of cytrullinated protein/peptide antibodies (anti-CP) during 5 years follow up in early rheumatoid arthritis: anti-CP status predicts worse disease activity and greater radiological progression. Ann Rheum Dis 2005;64:1744–9.

[13] Meyer O, Nicaise-Roland P, Santos MD, Labarre C, Dougados M, Goupille P, et al. Serial determination of cyclic citrullinated peptide autoantibodies predicted five-year radiological outcomes in a prospective cohort of patients with early rheumatoid arthritis. Arthritis Res Ther 2006;26:8.

[14] Schoels M, Bombardier C, Aletaha D. Diagnostic and prognostic value of antibodies and soluble biomarkers in undifferentiated peripheral inflammatory arthritis: a systematic review. J Rheumatol Suppl 2011;87:20–5.

[15] Bizzaro N, Bartoloni E, Morozzi G, Manganelli S, Riccieri V, Sabatini P, et al. Anti-cyclic citrullinated peptide antibody titer predicts time to rheumatoid arthritis onset in patients with undifferentiated arthritis: results from a 2-year prospective study. Arthritis Res Ther 2013;15. R16.

[16] Koga T, Okada A, Fukuda T, Hidaka T, Ishii T, Ueki Y, et al. Anti-citrullinated peptide antibodies are the strongest predictor of clinically relevant radiographic progression in rheumatoid arthritis patients achieving remission or low disease activity: a post hoc analysis of a nationwide cohort in Japan. PLoS One 2017;12. e0175281.

[17] Ruiz-Irastorza G, Egurbide MV, Martinez-Berriotxoa A, Ugalde J, Aguirre C. Antiphospholipid antibodies predict early damage in patients with systemic lupus erythematosus. Lupus 2004;13:900–5.

[18] McClain MT, Arbuckle MR, Heinlen LD, Dennis GJ, Roebuck J, Rubertone MV, et al. The prevalence, onset, and clinical significance of antiphospholipid antibodies prior to diagnosis of systemic lupus erythematosus. Arthritis Rheum 2004;50:1226–32.

[19] Bizzaro N, Ghirardello A, Zampieri S, Iaccarino L, Tozzoli R, Ruffatti A, et al. Anti-prothrombin antibodies predict thrombosis in patients with systemic lupus erythematosus: a 15-year longitudinal study. J Thromb Haemost 2007;5:1158–64.

[20] Hu PQ, Fertig N, Medsger TA, Wright TM. Correlation of serum DNA topoisomerase I antibody levels with disease severity and activity in systemic sclerosis. Arthritis Rheum 2003;48:1363–73.

[21] Steen VD. Autoantibodies in systemic sclerosis. Semin Arthritis Rheum 2005;35:35–42.

[22] Oelzner P, Deliyska B, Funfstuck R, Hein G, Herrmann D, Stein G. Anti-C1q antibodies and antiendothelial cell antibodies in systemic lupus erythematosus – relationship with disease activity and renal involvement. Clin Rheumatol 2003;22:271–8.

[23] Marto N, Bertolaccini ML, Calabuig E, Hughes GRV, Khamashta MA. Anti-C1q antibodies in nephritis and renal disease activity and positive predictive value in systemic lupus erythematosus. Ann Rheum Dis 2005;64:444–8.

[24] Birck R, Schmitt WH, Kaelsh IA, van der Woude FJ. Serial ANCA determinations for monitoring disease activity in patients with ANCA-associated vasculitis: systematic review. Am J Kidney Dis 2006;47:15–23.

[25] Tomasson G, Grayson PC, Mahr AD, Lavalley M, Merkel PA. Value of ANCA measurements during remission to predict a relapse of ANCA-associated vasculitis–a meta-analysis. Rheumatology (Oxford) 2012;51:100–9.

[26] Giuliani C, Cerrone D, Harii N, Thornton M, Kohn LD, Dagia NM, et al. A TSHR-LH/CGR chimera that measures functional thyroid-stimulating autoantibodies (TSAb) can predict remission or recurrence in Graves' patients undergoing antithyroid drug (ATD) treatment. J Clin Endocrinol Metab 2012;97:E1080–7.

[27] Healey R, Corless L, Gordins P, Holding S. Do anti-smooth muscle antibodies predict development of autoimmune hepatitis in patients with normal liver function? - A retrospective cohort review. Autoimmun Rev 2016;15:668–72.

[28] Zachou K, Oikonomou K, Renaudineau Y, Chauveau A, Gatselis N, Youinou P, et al. Anti-α actinin antibodies as new predictors of response to treatment in autoimmune hepatitis type 1. Aliment Pharmacol Ther 2012;35:116–25.

[29] Montano-Loza AJ, Shums Z, Norman GL, Czaja AJ. Prognostic implications of antibodies to Ro/SSA and soluble liver antigen in type 1 autoimmune hepatitis. Liver Int 2012;32:85–92.

[30] Scofield RH. Autoantibodies as predictors of disease. Lancet 2004;363:1544–6.

[31] Bizzaro N, Tozzoli R, Shoenfeld Y. Are we at a stage to predict autoimmune rheumatic diseases? Arthritis Rheum 2007;56:1736–44.

[32] Bizzaro N. Autoantibodies as predictors of disease: the clinical and experimental evidence. Autoimmun Rev 2007;6:325–33.

[33] Bizzaro N. The predictive significance of autoantibodies in organ-specific autoimmune diseases. Clin Rev Allergy Immunol 2007;34:326–31.

[34] Tozzoli R. The diagnostic role of autoantibodies in the prediction of organ-specific autoimmune diseases. Clin Chem Lab Med 2008;46:577–87.

[35] Arbuckle MR, McClain MT, Rubertone MV, Scofield RH, Dennis GJ, James JA, et al. Development of autoantibodies before the clinical onset of systemic lupus erythematosus. N Engl J Med 2003;349:1526–33.

[36] Rantapää-Dahlqvist S, de Jong BAW, Berglin E, Hallmans G, Wadell G, Stenlund H, et al. Antibodies against cyclic citrullinated peptide and IgA rheumatoid factor predict the development of rheumatoid arthritis. Arthritis Rheum 2003;48:2741–9.

[37] Nielen MM, van Schaardenburg D, Reesink HW, van de Stadt RJ, van der Horst-Bruinsma IE, de Koning MHM, et al. Specific autoantibodies precede the symptoms of rheumatoid arthritis: a study of serial measurements in blood donors. Arthritis Rheum 2004;50:380–6.

[38] McCune AB, Weston WL, Lee LA. Maternal and fetal outcome in neonatal lupus erythematosus. Ann Intern Med 1987;106:518–23.

[39] Waltuck J, Buyon JP. Autoantibody-associated congenital heart block: outcome in mothers and children. Ann Intern Med 1994;120:544–52.

[40] Sarkar K, Miller FW. Autoantibodies as predictive and diagnostic markers of idiopathic inflammatory myopaties. Autoimmunity 2004;37:291–4.

[41] Abraham-Simon J, Rojas-Serrano J, Cabiedes J, Alcocer-Varela J. Antinucleosome antibodies may help predict development of systemic lupus erythematosus in patients with primary antiphospholipid syndrome. Lupus 2004;13:177–81.

[42] Kita M, Goulis DG, Avramides A. Post-partum thyroiditis in a Mediterranean population: a prospective study of a large cohort of thyroid antibody positive women at the time of delivery. J Endocrinol Investig 2002;25:513–9.

[43] Tozzoli R, Kodermaz G, Perosa AR, Tampoia M, Zucano A, Antico A, Bizzaro N. Autoantibodies to parietal cells as predictors of atrophic body gastritis: a five-year prospective study in patients with autoimmune thyroid diseases. Autoimmun Rev 2010;10:80–3.

[44] Metcalf JV, Mitchison HC, Palmer JM, Jones DE, Bassendine MF, James OFW. Natural history of early primary biliary cirrhosis. Lancet 1996;348:1399–402.

[45] Prince MI, Chetwynd A, Craig WL, Metcalf JV, James OFW. Asymptomatic primary biliary cirrhosis: clinical features, prognosis, and symptom progression in a large population based cohort. Gut 2004;53:865–70.

[46] Bonifacio E, Ziegler AG. Advances in the prediction and natural history of type 1 diabetes. Endocrinol Metab Clin North Am 2010;39:513–25.

[47] Kulmala P, Savola K, Petersen JS, Vähäsalo P, Karjalainen J, Löppönen T, et al. Prediction of insulin-dependent diabetes mellitus in siblings of children with diabetes. A population-based study. J Clin Investig 1998;101:327–36.

[48] Yu L, Boulware DC, Beam CA, Hutton JC, Wenzlau JM, Greenbaum CJ, et al. Type 1 diabetes TrialNet study group. Zinc transporter-8 autoantibodies improve prediction of type 1 diabetes in relatives positive for the standard biochemical autoantibodies. Diabetes Care 2012;35:1213–8.

[49] Jin P, Huang G, Lin J, Yang L, Xiang B, Zhou W, et al. High titre of antiglutamic acid decarboxylase autoantibody is a strong predictor of the development of thyroid autoimmunity in patients with type 1 diabetes and latent autoimmune diabetes in adults. Clin Endocrinol (Oxf) 2011;74:587–92.

[50] Betterle C, Zanette F, Zanchetta R, Pedini B, Trevisan A, Mantero T, et al. Complement-fixing adrenal autoantibodies as a marker for predicting onset of idiopathic Addison's disease. Lancet 1983;1:1238–41.

[51] Israeli E, Grotto I, Gilburd B, Balicer RD, Goldin E, Wiik A, et al. Anti-Saccharomyces cerevisiae and antineutrophil cytoplasmic antibodies as predictors of inflammatory bowel disease. Gut 2005;54:1232–6.

[52] Berglin E, Padyukov L, Sundin U, Hallmans G, Stenlund H, van Venrooij WJ, et al. A combination of autoantibodies to cyclic citrullinated peptide (CCP) and HLA-DRBl locus antigens is strongly associated with future onset of rheumatoid arthritis. Arthritis Res Ther 2004;6:R303–8.

[53] Shoenfeld Y, Toubi E. Protective autoantibodies. Role in homeostasis, clinical importance, and therapeutic potential. Arthritis Rheum 2005;52:2599–606.

[54] Bootsma H, Spronk PE, Ter Borg EJ, Hummel EJ, de Boer G, Limburg PC, Kallenberg CG. The predictive value of fluctuations in IgM and IgG class anti-dsDNA antibodies for relapses in systemic lupus erythematosus. A prospective long-term observation. Ann Rheum Dis 1997;56:661–6.

[55] Grönwall C, Akhter E, Oh C, Burlingame RW, Petri M, Silverman GJ. IgM autoantibodies to distinct apoptosis-associated antigens correlate with protection from cardiovascular events and renal disease in patients with SLE. Clin Immunol 2012;142:390–8.

[56] Toubi E, Shoenfeld Y. Protective autoimmunity in cancer. Oncol Rep 2007;17:245–51.

[57] van Leeuwen M, Damoiseaux J, Duijvestijn A, Tervaert JW. The therapeutic potential of targeting B cells and anti-oxLDL antibodies in atherosclerosis. Autoimmun Rev 2009;9:53–7.

[58] Bizzaro N, Antico A, Platzgummer S, Tonutti E, Bassetti D, Pesente F, et al. Automated antinuclear immunofluorescence antibody screening: a comparative study of six computer-aided diagnostic systems. Autoimmun Rev 2013;13:292–8.

[59] Bertin D, Jourde-Chiche N, Bongrand P, Bardin N. Original approach for automated quantification of antinuclear autoantibodies by indirect immunofluorescence. Clin Dev Immunol 2013:182172.

[60] Peng X, Tang J, Wu Y, Yang B, Hu J. Novel method for ANA quantitation using IIF imaging system. J Immunol Methods 2014;404:52–8.

[61] Maenhout TM, Bonroy C, Verfaillie SV, Devreese K. Automated indirect immunofluorescence microscopy enables the implementation of a quantitative internal quality control system for anti-nuclear antibody (ANA) analysis. Clin Chem Lab Med 2014;52:989–98.

[62] Buzzulini F, Rigon A, Soda P, Onofri L, Infantino M, Arcarese L, et al. The classification of Crithidia luciliae immunofluorescence test (CLIFT) using a novel automated system. Arthritis Res Ther 2014;16:R71.

[63] Knütter I, Hiemann R, Brumma T, Büttner T, Großmann K, Cusini M. Automated interpretation of ANCA patterns a new approach in the serology of ANCAassociated vasculitis. Arthritis Res Ther 2012;14:R271.

[64] Sowa M, Grossmann K, Knutter I, Hiemann R, Rober N, Anderer U, et al. Simultaneous automated screening and confirmatory testing for vasculitis-specific ANCA. PLoS One 2014;9. e107743.

[65] Tozzoli R, Sorrentino MC, Bizzaro N. Detecting multiple autoantibodies to diagnose autoimmune comorbidity (multiple autoimmune syndromes and overlap syndromes): a challenge for the autoimmunologist. Immunol Res 2013;56:425–31.

[66] Cinquanta L, Fontana DE, Bizzaro N. Chemiluminescent immunoassay technology: what does it change in autoantibody detection? Autoimmun Highlights 2017;8:9.

[67] Fu ZF, Liu H, Ju HX. Flow-through multianalyte chemiluminescent immunosensing system with designed substrate zone-resolved technique for sequential detection of tumor markers. Anal Chem 2006;78:6999–7005.

[68] Liu H, Fu ZF, Yang ZJ, Yan F, Ju HX. Sampling-resolution strategy for one-way multiplexed immunoassay with sequential chemiluminescent detection. Anal Chem 2008;80:5654–9.

[69] Du L, Ji W, Zhang Y, Zhang C, Liu G, Wang S. An ultrasensitive detection of 17β-estradiol using a gold nanoparticle-based fluorescence immunoassay. Analyst 2015;140:2001–7.

[70] Tao X, Jiang H, Yu X, Zhu J, Wang X, Wang Z, et al. An ultrasensitive chemiluminescence immunoassay of chloramphenicol based on gold nanoparticles and magnetic beads. Drug Test Anal 2013;53:46–52.

[71] Wang C, Wu J, Zong C, Xu J, Ju HX. Chemiluminescent immunoassay and its applications. Chin J Anal Chem 2012;40:3–10.

[72] Tozzoli R, Bizzaro N. Novel diagnostic methods for autoantibody detection. In: Shoenfeld Y, Gershwin ME, Meroni PL, editors. Autoantibodies. Amsterdam: Elsevier; 2006. p. 77–82.

[73] Villalta D, Girolami E, Alessio MG, Sorrentino MC, Tampoia M, Brusca I, et al. Autoantibody profiling in a cohort of pediatric and adult patients with autoimmune hepatitis. J Clin Lab Anal 2016;30:41–6.

[74] Villalta D, Sorrentino MC, Girolami E, Tampoia M, Alessio MG, Brusca I, et al. Autoantibody profiling of patients with primary biliary cirrhosis using a multiplexed line-blot assay. Chim Clin Acta 2015;438:135–8.

[75] Fulton RJ, McDade RL, Smith PL, Kienker LJ, Kettman JRJ. Advanced multiplexed analysis with the FluoMetrix system. Clin Chem 1997;43:1749–56.

[76] Armbruster DA, Overcash DR, Reyes J. Clinical chemistry laboratory automation in the 21st century – Amat Victoria curam (victory loves careful preparation). Clin Biochem Rev 2014;35:143–53.

[77] Tozzoli R, D'Aurizio F, Villalta D, Bizzaro N. Automation, consolidation, and integration in autoimmune diagnostics. Autoimmun Highlights July 3, 2015. https://doi.org/10.1007/s13317-015-0067-5.

[78] Kostantinov KN, Tzamaloukas A, Rubin RL. Detection of autoantibodies in a point-of-care rheumatology setting. Autoimmun Highlights 2013;4:55–61.

Chapter 18

Diagnostic: Imaging

Fulvia Ceccarelli, Ramona Lucchetti, Enrica Cipriano, Guido Valesini, Carlo Perricone
Rheumatology, Department of Internal Medicine, Sapienza University of Rome, Rome, Italy

INTRODUCTION

The diagnosis of autoimmune diseases derives from a complex path in which imaging plays a central role. It is important to know the resources and the limits of the different imaging tools available to the specialist: the most frequently used in clinical practice are conventional radiography (CR), ultrasonography (US), magnetic resonance (MR), and computed tomography (CT). Thanks to the improvement of hardware and software of these techniques, new applications have been developed, such as single-photon emission CT and positron emission tomography (PET) [1–5].

CR represents the landmark in the diagnosis of rheumatic conditions and still maintains an incontrovertible value, thanks to the wide availability and reliability due to the traditional application in the assessment of structural damage in inflammatory and degenerative diseases, such as rheumatoid arthritis (RA) and osteoarthritis (OA). However, the higher sensitivity and specificity of other imaging techniques, such as US and MR, in comparison with CR have been widely demonstrated. This is true especially in the assessment of early disease stages and inflammatory modifications: in these conditions the exclusive use of CR could determine false-negative results [1–5]. Table 18.1 summarizes the main advantages and disadvantages of CR, US, MR, and CT.

According to their technical characteristics, imaging tools could have a diverse performance in the assessment of different articular and periarticular structures, as summarized in Table 18.2.

The knowledge of the performance in the study of different structures is mandatory to be able to choose the best imaging tool according to the clinical suspicion and disease duration.

Traditionally, the use of imaging tools in rheumatic diseases was confined to the assessment of patients affected by inflammatory or degenerative arthropathies in terms of diagnosis and follow-up. More recently, the spectrum of application of imaging has become more extensive, with application of different tools to study other organs and tissues involved in autoimmune conditions [5,6].

THE PAST: IMAGING IN THE ASSESSMENT OF INFLAMMATORY AND DEGENERATIVE ARTHROPATHIES

Conventional Radiography

CR is an inexpensive and easily available imaging tool, allowing wide coverage of affected regions and reasonable level of reproducibility. However, as demonstrated by several evidences, CR plays a restricted role in the early diagnosis of inflammatory arthritis, such as RA [7,8]. Periarticular soft tissue swelling and juxtaarticular osteopenia represent the earliest findings identified by CR in these conditions, while early erosions typically occur at the junction between the cartilage and periosteal synovial membrane insertion. The joint space could initially appear widened because of the presence of a joint effusion or synovitis; at a later stage, a cartilage destruction occurs, with a joint space narrowing (JSN). A joint subluxation or bony fusion could appear in more aggressive phenotype. In clinical practice, hands X-ray are typically obtained at disease onset to assess the disease severity. The identification of erosive damage at this stage represents a negative prognostic factor and could address the physician in the treatment choice. Moreover, CR can be used as an outcome measure to assess the progression of arthritis and to evaluate the treatment efficacy [7,8].

Fig. 18.1 represents a case of a long-standing RA with severe erosive X-ray detected damage at level of proximal interphalangeal joints.

The wide application of CR in RA patients leads to the development of scoring systems able to estimate the disease progression. Fig. 18.2 represents the timeline of development of most frequently used X-ray score systems, underlining the modifications occurring during the years [9–16].

TABLE 18.1 Main Advantages and Disadvantages of CR, US, MR, CT

Imaging Technique	Advantages	Disadvantages
CR	Low cost	Two-dimensional representation of a three-dimensional lesion
	Wide availability and easy access	Ionizing radiation
	Standardization available	Low sensitivity to early bone damage
	Easy reproducibility	Low sensitivity to assess soft tissues
US	Valid assessment methods	
	Noninvasive method	Operator dependence
	Relatively low cost	Low reproducibility
	Absence of ionizing radiation	No standardization
	Detection of inflammatory and destructive features	Difficult visualization of some joints (i.e., wrists)
	Guide for diagnostic and therapeutic procedures	
MR	Absence of ionizing radiation	High costs
	High sensitivity	Limited availability of the equipment
	Assessment of all structures affected	Requirement of extended periods of time
	Differential diagnosis of undifferentiated polyarthritis	Limited to one joint per exam
	Detection of bone edema as independent predictor of bone erosion	Questionable correlation with clinical prognosis
CT	Widely available	High costs
	Fast scan acquisition times	Ionizing radiation
	High sensitivity in the bone assessment	

CR, conventional radiography; *CT*, computed tomography; *MR*, magnetic resonance; *US*, ultrasonography.

TABLE 18.2 Performance of Imaging Tools in the Assessment of Articular and Periarticular Structures

	CR	US	MR	CT
Cartilage	+	++	++++	+++
Joint space narrowing	++	+	+++	+++
Bone marrow lesion	−	−	++++	++
Erosions, osteophytes	++	++	++++	++++
Subchondral cysts, sclerosis	++	−	+++	++++
Joint inflammation	−	+++	++++	++++
Periarticular structure	−	+++	++++	++

CR, conventional radiography; *CT*, computed tomography; *MR*, magnetic resonance; *US*, ultrasonography.

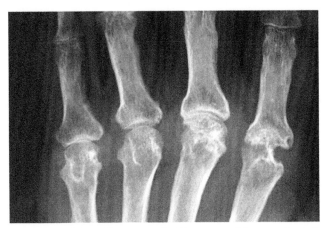

FIGURE 18.1 Long-standing rheumatoid arthritis with severe erosive X-ray detected damage at level of proximal interphalangeal joints.

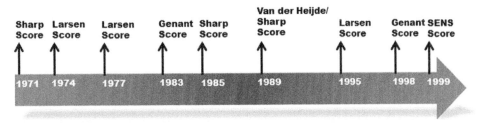

FIGURE 18.2 Timeline of X-ray scoring systems proposed for rheumatoid arthritis.

The first scoring system was proposed by Larsen in 1971 and suggested six stages reflecting gradual, progressive deterioration, as follows: grade 0 = normal; grade 1 = slight abnormalities (periarticular soft tissue swelling and osteoporosis, slight JSN); grade 2 = definite early abnormalities; grade 3 = medium destructive abnormalities; grade 4 = severe definite abnormalities; and grade 5 = mutilating abnormalities [9]. Starting from this first system, numerous scores have been suggested in the following years [9–16].

Fig. 18.3 summarizes the joints evaluated in the different scoring: the main difference is related to the evaluation of the wrist, considered as a single joint, or divided into four quadrants, or by evaluating the different bone structures. Moreover, some systems separately evaluated erosions and JSN, whereas other scores provided a total score including the two parameters [9–16]. To date, the most frequently used scoring system in RA patients is the Sharp score modified by van der Heijde in 1989; however, in 1999, the same research group proposed the simple erosion narrowing score (SENS) method, a simplified X-ray scoring, in which the number of joints with erosions and/or JSN was recorded instead of grading. Erosion is considered in 32 joints in the hands and 12 in the feet, as well as JSN in 30 and 12 joints, respectively. Thus, the total SENS score ranges from 0 to 86 [13,16].

Scoring systems allow the evaluation of disease progression: therefore, they have been used in several randomized controlled trials (RCTs) to evaluate drug's efficacy in the prevention of erosive damage [17–19]. This outcome represents one of the most important targets in the EULAR recommendations for the RA patients' treatment [20].

The imaging represents a fundamental diagnostic tool also for patients affected by spondyloarthritis (SpA), with particular regard to the evaluation of sacroiliac joints (SIJs). Therefore, SIJs X-ray assessment is recommended as the first imaging tool to diagnose sacroiliitis, according to the Assessment of Spondyloarthritis International Society (ASAS) and EULAR recommendations [21]. The modified New York criteria identified five stages of radiographic changes in the SIJs (Table 18.3): in the first step, changes with poor definition of the joint outlines could be identified because of the presence of erosions and to the formation of new bone bridges. Erosions appear as scalloped–dentate contours in the caudal portion of the joint. If the process of erosion is marked, an impression of pseudo-widening of the joint space could be observed. The development of sclerosis could occur, typically involving the caudal portion of the joint, extending into the middle portion. This is normally broad and is predominant in the iliac side. A partial or total ankylosis is the result of the progression of these lesions, particularly the bone bridging [22].

CR is both sensitive and specific in the established and long-standing ankylosing spondylitis (AS): more than 95% of patients show radiographic changes in the SIJs, whereas approximately 50%–70% of patients show spinal involvement

X-ray score		HANDS						WRIST	FOOT		RANGE SCORE
		DIP	PIP	MCP	CMC	IP	MCB		MTP	IP	
Sharp, 1971	E	X	X	X		X	X	All except radiocarpal			0-216
	JSN	X	X	X	X	X		All except pisiform/trapezoid			0-216
Sharp, 1985	E		X	X			X(1)	All except capitate/hamate/radiocarpal			0-170
	JSN		X	X	X(3-5)			All except pisiform/hamate			0-144
Larsen, 1977	E+JSN	X	X	X		X		As 1 unit, score multiplied by five)	X	X	0-250
Larsen, 1995	E+JSN		X (2-5)	X (2-5)		X		Divided into 4 quadrant	X (2-5)		0-250
Genant, 1998	E		X	X	X (1)	X		Scafoid/radio-ulnar			0-98
	JSN		X	X	X(3-5)	X		Scafoid/lunate/capitate/radio-carpal			0-100
Van der Heijde/Sharp, 1989	E		X	X		X	X(1)	All except triquetral, pisiform	X	X	0-160
	JSN		X	X	X(3-5)			All except triquetral, pisiform, hamate, radioulnar	X	X	0-168
SENS, 1999	E		X	X		X	X(1)	All except triquetral, pisiform, capitate, hamate, radiocarpal	X	X	0-86
	JSN		X	X	X(3-5)			All except triquetral, pisiform, hamate, radioulnar	X	X	

FIGURE 18.3 Joints counted in the different X ray scoring systems. *CMC*, carpometacarpal; *DIP*, distal interphalangeal; *E*, erosion; *FOOT IP*, interphalangeal; *HANDS IP*, interphalangeal joint of thumb; *JSN*, joint space narrowing; *MCB*, metacarpal base; *MCP*, metacarpophalangeal; *MTP*, metatarsophanageal; *PIP*, proximal interphalangeal.

TABLE 18.3 Grading of X-Ray Sacroliitis According to Modified New York Criteria

Grade	X-Ray Feature
0	Normal
1	Suspicious changes
2	Minimal abnormality (small localized areas with erosion or sclerosis, without changes in joint width)
3	Unequivocal abnormality (moderate or advanced sacroiliitis with one or more: erosions, evidence of sclerosis, widening, narrowing, or partial ankylosis)
4	Severe abnormality (total ankylosis)

with syndesmophytes and/or ankylosis of small vertebral joints. Moreover, CR should be used in long-term monitoring of established structural changes (in particular new bone formation) at level of SIJs and/or spine in axial SpA patients. In particular, it is superior to MR in the detection of spinal syndesmophytes at cervical and lumbar spine, well recognized as negative predictor in terms of severity [23].

As known, AS represents the prototype of axial SpA: the SIJs involvement is usually bilateral and symmetric and gradually progressive. The disease typically starts in the SIJs with tiny serrated erosions, resembling the appearance of the edge of a postage stamp and starting on the iliac side of the joint. During the disease progression, the definition of the joint is lost and proliferative changes became predominant, with areas of subchondral sclerosis and new bone formation with narrowing and complete fusion of the joint in the final stages. However, SpA is a group of different conditions, characterized by not only several similarities but also specific features. In patients affected by psoriatic arthritis (PsA), the incidence of sacroiliitis is high but typically unilateral. In reactive arthritis, the SIJs involvement is generally asymmetric and bilateral, even though can be unilateral in the early disease stages. Finally, in enteropathic arthritis, the pattern is symmetric, similar to AS [24].

Spine could be involved in approximately 50% of AS patients: the earliest changes generally occur in the thoracolumbar and lumbosacral regions; as the disease progresses, the mid-lumbar, mid-thoracic, and cervical regions are affected. This well-ordered progression in spine involvement represents an AS peculiar feature not identified in the other SpA. The earliest changes in the spine appear as a result of enthesitis at the edges of the discovertebral joints. Three types of changes were described by Cawley and colleagues [25]:

- **Type I lesions**, localized central lesions in the vertebral endplate (Andersson type A lesions), mild and focal and stable for months or years, usually occurring in the thoracolumbar spine. Typically found in the first decade of the disease and radiographically identified as endplate erosions, in most cases asymptomatic.

- **Type II lesions**, localized peripheral erosive lesions (*Romanus* lesions) with reactive sclerosis (*shiny corner*) at the anterior corner of vertebral endplates, mainly localized in the lumbar region. The resolution of *Romanus* lesions leads to the formation of syndesmophytes, representing the ossification of the outer fibers of the annulus fibrosus, where Sharpey's fibers attach to the vertebral bodies. Periosteal proliferation and new bone formation at the anterosuperior and inferior vertebral margins, resulting in squaring of vertebral borders. Progressive growth of syndesmophytes, extending anteriorly along the deep layer of the anterior intervertebral ligament (prediscal type) and involving the paravertebral soft tissue, bridging the intervertebral space causing ankylosis, producing a smooth, undulating spinal contour called the *bamboo spine*.

- **Type II lesions** (Andersson type B), extensive central and peripheral lesions, representing a failure to regenerate intervertebral disk fracture in the context of multisegmental ankylosis; rare and typically developing in late disease stages. Changes in the apophyseal joints as mixed result of arthritis and enthesitis. Ligament ossifications typical of late stages, and involving the interspinal ligaments (dagger sign) and the iliolumbar ligaments [25].

Fig. 18.4 represents the case of a patients affected by AS with X-ray detected syndesmophytes localized at cervical region of spine (A) and bilateral grade III sacroiliitis (B).

The joint extra-axial manifestations of AS mainly include the lower extremities in an asymmetric way, with frequent involvement of hips and knees. From a radiographic point of view, a combination of erosive and proliferative processes could be identified, with early erosion development and subsequent new bone formation. PsA patients typically show the involvement of distal interphalangeal (DIP) joints of the hands and feet, with presence of asymmetric lesions and an oligoarticular distribution, progressing to polyarticular. Early changes, often difficult to detect, consist of speculated or woolly *foci* of epiphyseal ossification on the distal phalanges, acroosteolysis, and layered periosteal ossifications on the shafts of the tubular bones. These changes are followed by the typical bone destruction–proliferation sequence of the seronegative arthritis, with irregularity of the joint lines, erosions, destruction of bone, specular ossifications at joint margins (especially at the bases of the distal phalanges), and eventually ankylosis [26].

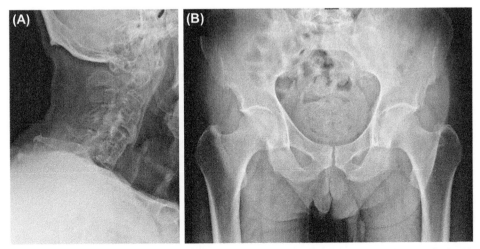

FIGURE 18.4 X-ray of a patients affected by ankylosing spondylitis with syndesmophytes localized at cervical region of spine (A) and bilateral grade III sacroiliitis (B).

Moreover, in AS patients, enthesitis typically involved ischial tuberosities, trochanter, plantar calcaneal surface, triceps insertion, and patella. Other possible locations for inflammatory changes are the symphysis pubis and manubriosternal synchondrosis, with erosions, sclerosis, and soft tissue swelling [24].

CR finds wide application also in the assessment of patients affected by microcrystal arthritis, especially gout. In the early disease stages, during an acute gout attack, no bone changes are present, but signs of joint swelling and effusion can be identified on plain X-ray. In the advanced disease phases, tophaceous deposits may cause an increase in the radiodensity of periarticular tissues. The most characteristic findings in the advanced stages of gouty arthritis are well-defined deep bony erosions with sharp overhanging edges and a sclerotic rim [27].

Finally, X-ray is the gold standard for the assessment of OA, allowing the identification of JSN, subchondral sclerosis, marginal osteophytes, and geode or subchondral cyst. All these X-ray detected abnormalities have a specific anatomical correspondence (i.e., loss cartilage tissue, bone thickening and proliferation, subchondral microfractures) [28]. The Kellgren score, firstly proposed in 1957, represents an attempt to standardize the X-ray assessment in OA patients and includes the above-mentioned abnormalities, which could be scored in a five-point scale (0=none, 1=doubtful, 2=minimal, 3=moderate, 4=severe) [29]. According to the EULAR recommendations published in 2017, CR should be used before other modalities when imaging is needed. However, the EULAR experts underline that imaging is not required to make the diagnosis in OA patients with typical presentation (i.e., usage-related pain, short duration morning stiffness, age>40 years, symptoms affecting one or a few joints) [30].

Magnetic Resonance

MR has proved to be the most sensitive of all the available modalities in making an early diagnosis in patients affected by RA. Its excellent soft tissue contrast, multiplanar imaging evaluation, and the use of gadolinium-based contrast allow the differentiation of synovitis from joint effusion or tenosynovitis as well as the identification of bone marrow edema and erosions. MR imaging is more sensitive than clinical examination and X-ray in the detection of inflammatory and destructive joint changes in early RA patients. It is, however, an expensive and time-consuming modality, sometimes not well tolerated by patients [31].

To standardize the MR procedure, OMERACT developed standardized techniques, joint pathology definitions, and scoring systems for the application of this imaging tool in RA patients [32]. According to these definitions, synovitis is an area localized in the synovial compartment, showing above normal postgadolinium enhancement, with increased thickness compared with normal synovium. A joint effusion may be seen in association with synovial thickening, but without enhancement after intravenous gadolinium. The application of contrast medium increases the sensitivity in detection of synovitis, tenosynovitis, and bone marrow edema [32].

In clinical practice, the administration of gadolinium is often omitted, with a reliance on fat-suppressed T2-weighted sequences or short tau inversion recovery imaging for the assessment of synovitis. It has been shown that not using intravenous contrast results in a decrease in sensitivity, specificity, and intra- and interreader reliability with regard to synovitis. This is a very important issue in the light of prognostic value exerted by the identification of this specific feature [32].

Next to the synovitis, tenosynovitis is commonly identified in patients with early RA, often with a bilateral distribution. The tendons most typically involved are flexor and extensor digitorum at the wrist level, and index and middle flexor in the fingers. On MR imaging, tenosynovitis is demonstrated as thickening of the synovial sheath or fluid within the sheath, with high signal on T2-weighted images [33].

Moving on to bone modifications, the MR signal alterations in the subchondral bone marrow of RA patients seem to match with histologically detected inflammatory infiltrates, including lymphocytes and osteoclasts [34]. On MR imaging, bone marrow edema is identified as a poorly defined area of low signal within bone on T1-weighted images, with high signal on T2-weighted fat-suppressed or short tau inversion recovery images. The presence of bone marrow edema in RA is associated with a high risk of progression to bone erosions and thus irreversible joint damage over time. Bone edema scored on MR imaging scans of the dominant carpus at presentation has been shown to predict radiographic joint damage of the hands and feet in patients with RA after 5–6 years follow-up. Moreover, bone marrow edema resulted associated with a 6.5-fold risk of erosions development within 1 year [35]. According to this literature data, bone marrow edema can be used as a marker to predict medium-term functional disability and can therefore help to identify RA patients requiring early and aggressive treatment to prevent joint damage and disability.

Moreover, the MR identification of bone edema plays an important role in SpA diagnosis, allowing the early identification of affected patients. In particular, in 2009, the classification criteria developed by the ASAS introduced a specific new entity, the so-called nonradiographic axial SpA (nr-axSpA). This condition includes patients without CR signs of sacroiliitis but satisfying clinical criteria for diagnosis for axSpA (i.e., presence of HLA-B27 and two other SpA features), as well as

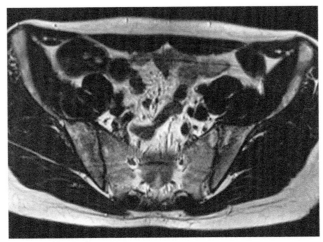

FIGURE 18.5 The case of a patient with nonradiographic axial SpA: magnetic resonance assessment demonstrates the presence of bone edema and erosions at level of sacroiliac joints.

patients with active inflammation in the SIJs detected by MR [36,37]. Fig. 18.5 represents the case of a patient with nr-axSpA: MR assessment demonstrates the presence of bone edema and erosions at level of SIJs.

Nr-axSpA can be considered an early stage of axial SpA: progression to radiographic form is reported in approximately 10% of cases over 2 years [38]. Three main features seem to differentiate radiographic from nonradiographic form: in particular, an opposite male-to female ratio, the presence of objective evidences of inflammation (i.e., C-reactive protein [CRP] levels and/or positive MR imaging findings, with presence of bone edema), and the degree of limitation in spinal mobility. Moreover, a progression toward the radiographic phenotype occurs more frequently in the presence of objective inflammatory evidence (i.e., high CRP levels and/or positive MR findings) [38].

Concerning erosions in MR, they are defined as a sharply marginated lesion, with a juxtaarticular location and typical signal characteristics, visible in at least 2 planes with a cortical break seen in at least 1 plane. On T1-weighted images, the low signal intensity of cortical bone is lost and the normal fatty marrow signal is replaced. Rapid gadolinium enhancement suggests the presence of active, hypervascularized synovial tissue within the erosion. Several studies identified for MR higher sensitivity in the erosions detection compared with X-ray and can visualize lesions 6–12 months before they show up on radiographs [39,40].

MRI measures might be useful for evaluating RA joint damage in RCTs, even though a major validation is needed. For this purpose, the RAMRIS score was proposed [41].

This measures RA joint inflammation and erosions regardless of patient age, disease duration, disease activity, and treatment status/response. Evidence of content validity is provided by seven studies describing that RAMRIS can measure synovitis, osteitis, and erosions in early and established RA. Furthermore, these data describe RAMRIS responsiveness and sensitivity to change together with evidence that this system could discriminate efficacy among therapies. Currently, MRI plays a role in improving diagnostic confidence, in predicting the progression of the disease to definitive RA rather than to undifferentiated inflammatory arthritis, in detecting evidence of persistent inflammation in the setting of clinical remission and in predicting treatment response.

As MRI is the gold standard for the detection of bone marrow edema, it is recommended to be used for independent prediction of subsequent bone damage.

Ultrasonography

In the last decades, US assessment has acquired an ever-increasing role in the assessment of patients affected by inflammatory arthritis, focusing on early diagnosis, monitoring, and prognosis. The growing application in RA patients was demonstrated by ACR/EULAR classification criteria suggesting the use of this imaging technique in detecting synovitis in clinically asymptomatic articular sites to increase the number of involved joints needed to fulfill the criteria [42]. In addition, several studies demonstrated that RA patients assessed by US are likely to fulfill these criteria at an earlier disease stage than those assessed using conventional imaging tools [42–45]. In patients at risk to develop RA (i.e., patients with arthralgia but without clinically detected synovitis or patients positive for rheumatoid factor or anticitrullinated peptide antibodies without clinical signs of inflammation), ultrasound-detected abnormalities have shown to be a prognostic marker of RA development [46].

In order to improve the reliability of US in RA, the OMERACT proposed punctual definitions [47]. In agreement with these, joint effusion appears as an anechoic and compressible feature, without Doppler signal, while synovitis is defined as a hypoechogenic, thickened intraarticular tissue, nondisplaceable and poorly compressible, which may exhibit Doppler signals. This aspect is very important because of the well-established correlation between increased Doppler signal and disease activity [48]. Moreover, a high concordance between Doppler US imaging and contrast-enhanced MR imaging has been demonstrated for the detection of synovitis in RA wrist and finger joints, indicating that the imaging findings reflect a similar pathologic phenomenon [49]. Both US and MR are more sensitive than clinical assessment to detect inflammatory status at joint level, and both can demonstrate the presence of subclinical synovitis. The absence of signs of synovitis in the peripheral joints in both modalities has a strong negative predictive value for RA diagnosis. On US imaging, tenosynovitis is demonstrated as hypoechoic thickening of the synovial sheath that could exhibit Doppler signal. Conversely, tendinosis is demonstrated as tendon thickening with hypoechoic change and loss of the normal fibrillar pattern. From a prognostic point of view, both gray scale (GS) synovitis and Doppler signal seem to be predictive, but at different levels: both modalities have the same sensitivity that clinical examination and laboratory markers in detecting overtime changes in RA patients [50–53]. Interestingly, the US-detected response seems to be fast, showing a significant decrease in a combined GS and Doppler score after 7 days of treatment. Moreover, synovial hypertrophy measured by GS alone showed a statistically significant change, as compared with baseline, after 2 weeks [54].

To evaluate treatment response by using US, some systems have been proposed: they differ for qualitative, quantitative, or semiquantitative scoring applied and articular site evaluated. Moreover, the studies published so far are heterogeneous in terms of treatments and follow-up durations [50–53].

Because sustained remission is the ultimate goal of the modern RA treatments, a punctual definition of this state is very important and flares predict overtime erosive progression and functional disability development. However, patients classified as in remission according to different clinical criteria showed a subclinical synovitis in both GS and Doppler modalities in more than 30% of the cases, regardless the treatment administered (synthetic of biological DMARDs). Saleem and colleagues observed that the presence of subclinical synovitis with Doppler signal was associated with disease flare. Moreover, an US-detected synovitis in patients treated by synthetic DMARDs is associated with radiographic progression [55,56].

Moreover, recently published studies argue the added value of ultrasound for achieving a remission state in the context of a tight control in early RA. The studies showed that in an early population, both the clinical and the US tight controls permit to achieve remission without any superiority of an ultrasound approach. Nonetheless, the ultrasound arm seemed to produce a better structural outcome with a lower percentage of radiographic progression as compared with the clinical arm [57].

Moreover, US could play a role in the assessment of SpA patients: in particular, this imaging tool could be very helpful in the evaluation of enthesitis, as demonstrated by its higher sensitivity in comparison with clinical examination [58]. However, it should be considered that enthesis involvement, especially at level of lower limbs, may be related to inflammatory lesions or degenerative microtraumatic changes. Therefore, it is important to avoid overdiagnosis of SpA based only on US findings.

US-detected abnormalities on enthesis include tendon and ligament thickening and loss of the normal tendon/ligament echostructure with hypoechogenicity. The increase of Doppler signal seems to play an important role in the light of the association with disease activity. The concomitant presence of new bone formation such as enthesophytes with erosive changes suggests the diagnosis of an inflammatory enthesis [59]. Also for this specific disease features, some scoring systems have been proposed, characterized by different entheseal sites evaluated [58,60].

Moreover, typical US findings could be identified in peripheral SpA, including digital tenosynovitis and dactylitis. Inflammation of fatty tissue (i.e., the Kager fat pad) can also be encountered in peripheral SpA. Synovitis is frequently present, especially at DIP level, with asymmetric distribution [61]. Some attempts have been made to evaluate the application of US in the study of SIJs: the study published by Spadaro and colleagues suggested that US could be useful in the assessment of SIJs involvement in SpA, resulting in images that are fast and inexpensive and may complete the physical examination [62].

Furthermore, US may contribute to assessment of patients affected by gouty arthritis, thanks to the presence of specific features related to the presence of monosodium urate (MSU) crystals. In particular, in the joint effusion, it is possible to identify the presence of material with homogeneous low echogenicity or dense highly echogenicity, with multiple hyperechoic spots with different shapes and sizes, with or without posterior acoustic shadowing. Moreover, the presence of microaggregates, showed as echogenic foci within the erosions, may help distinguish gout from other erosive conditions. Gouty erosions are typically seen in a juxtaarticular distribution, with a predilection for the first metatarsophalangeal joint. In chronic gout, the presence of tophi, tendon pathology, and bone erosions can be detected by US. Finally, MSU crystals can precipitate on the articular surface of hyaline cartilage, forming a hyperechoic, bright band parallel to hyperechoic bony cortex. This specific feature is called "double contour" [63,64].

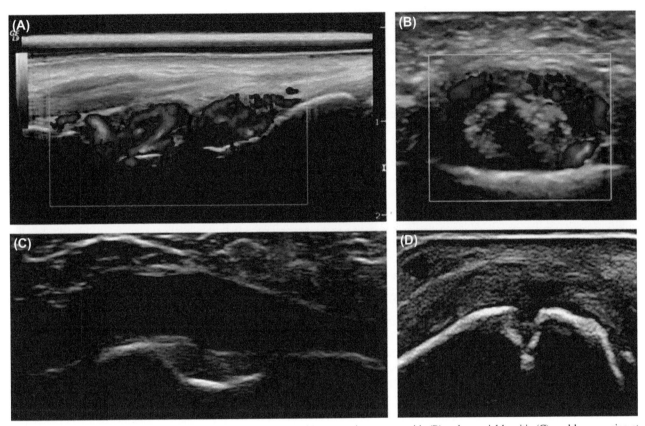

FIGURE 18.6 Ultrasonography-detected features: active joint synovitis (A), active tenosynovitis (B), subacromial bursitis (C), and bone erosion at metacarpophalangeal level (D).

The first attempt to include US assessment in classification criteria was made for polymyalgia rheumatica (PMR), an inflammatory condition characterized by pain and stiffness at shoulder and hip girdle and neck [65]. The musculoskeletal US evaluation of patients affected by PMR shows some characteristic pattern, such as subdeltoid bursitis, biceps tenosynovitis, small glenohumeral effusions, hip synovitis, and trochanteric bursitis. This finding leads to the incorporation of US in the EULAR/ACR classification criteria for the PMR [66].

Fig. 18.6 reports images representing different US features: in particular, active joint synovitis (A) and tenosynovitis (B), subacromial bursitis (C), and bone erosion at metacarpophalangeal level (D).

THE PRESENT: OTHER THAN ARTHRITIS

Musculoskeletal involvement is a frequent manifestation in almost every connective tissue disease. In particular, a prevalence ranging from 69% to 95% was observed in patients affected by systemic lupus erythematosus (SLE) [67,68] and up to 50% in Sjögren syndrome (SS) [69,70]. Different degree of severity, ranging from arthralgia to severe deforming or erosive arthritis, could be experienced by these patients, with possible development of disability significantly impacting the quality of life [71,72]. In light of these considerations, the application of imaging techniques is very important to early diagnose this manifestation and to follow disease progression and response to treatment.

Similarly to inflammatory arthritis, US has been frequently used in clinical practice to define the presence and severity of articular and periarticular inflammation [73].

In the past decade, several studies have demonstrated the usefulness of US in the assessment of SLE and SS patients with musculoskeletal manifestation [74–80]. Taken together, these studies demonstrate a higher prevalence of arthritis in both SLE and SS when US was applied in comparison with the clinical examination.

Moving on to SLE, US-detected synovitis was described in almost 60% of the patients evaluated and tenosynovitis in 4%–57%; an erosive bone damage was reported in 2%–47% of patients [74–77]. Only one study tried to discriminate the different subtypes of SLE joint manifestation, identifying US-detect erosions in 87% of Ruphus patients, in which SLE overlapped with RA [75]. Concerning SS, the majority of the studies published so far investigated joint involvement through the physical examination, without finding any correlation with immunological or other clinical features. Few studies investigated US inflammatory abnormalities, showing a prevalence of mild-moderate synovitis lower than 30% [78–80].

As suggested by the last EULAR recommendations, US could be applied to evaluate other tissues and organs involved in autoimmune diseases [81]. In particular, SS is characterized by inflammation and lymphocytic infiltration of exocrine glands, causing dryness of the mucous membranes [82]. The standard tests traditionally used to evaluate the salivary glands involvement were represented by scintigraphy and contrast sialography. Scintigraphy has a sensitivity of almost 80% but a very low specificity because the alteration in the uptake and excretion of 99mTc pertechnetate is not pathognomonic for SS [83]. Similarly, parotid sialography shows a sensitivity reaching 95%, but the SS, parotitis, and lymphoepithelial lesion could share a similar phenotype [84]. Thus, US assessment was proposed as an alternative imaging technique to evaluate salivary glands in SS patients: the results of the studies published so far demonstrated a reproducibility comparable with the sialography [85,86]. If healthy gland tissue is represented as a homogeneous granular structure, with echogenicity similar to thyroid gland, SS salivary glands are characterized by hypoechoic areas, surrounded by hyperechoic region. During disease flare, an intense blood flow could be observed in microvascular system. However, only evident inhomogeneity with multiple scattered hypoechoic areas or multiple cyst-like lesions can have a real diagnostic value. In chronic disease, the tissue can be replaced by adipose tissue and in the late stages fibrosis with sparse blood flow could develop [86–88]. Some studies have investigated possible role of US as surrogate of minor salivary gland biopsy, in the light of its non-invasivity. In comparison with biopsy, US demonstrated a sensitivity of 43%–93% and a specificity of 64%–100% [89,90].

Moreover, US assessment was applied to evaluate skin involvement in systemic sclerosis (SSc), a disease characterized by fibrosis involving primarily not only skin but also internal organs. In the different SSC subsets, cutaneous changes are the spy for disease classification and activity and represent a prognostic marker [91,92]. Therefore, the identification and the quantification of cutaneous involvement are fundamental to follow the disease progression. The degree of skin involvement is generally evaluated with modified Rodnan skin score (mRss), a physical examination estimating skin thickness and its diffusion. Despite the standardization of mRss, this tool could be dependent by the examiner skills and experience. To bypass these disadvantages, the possible use of US to assess epidermis, dermis, and subcutaneous fat has been suggested [93,94]. Thus, US seems to be able to identify different skin layers and to measure dermal thickness with a good intra- and interobserver reliability [6]. Some of these studies also find a correlation between US findings and global mRss [94,95].

The lung involvement represents the third most frequent manifestation in SSc patients. Lungs could be affected by interstitial lung disease (ILD), fibrosis, or vascular involvement, leading to pulmonary arterial hypertension, associated with severe morbidity and mortality [96]. This involvement does not correlate with the extent or severity of skin manifestation and it may also occur in SSc patients without cutaneous changes [97,98].

The high-resolution computerized tomography (HRCT) has been proposed as gold standard to early diagnose ILD and to define the distribution and pattern of lung fibrosis [99]. However, in the light of disadvantages of CT, researchers are looking for an easy, rapid, cheap, and radiation free technique for the routine follow-up of SSc patients. Thus, the use of transthoracic US to assess lung involvement in SSc patients has been proposed. The main US feature in ILD is the B-lines, or comet-tail images [100,101]. These lines, visible when the air content is decreased or the interstitial space is expanded, are characterized by laser-like vertical hyperechoic reverberation artifacts that move with the breath acts [102,103]. The data from different studies demonstrate a correlation between B-lines number and the presence of HRCT-detected fibrosis [104]. Despite these efforts, to date an US-validated score is still lacking and HRCT remains the best technique to diagnose ILD in a very early phase. In 1991, Warrick and colleagues proposed an HRCT score. This is a semiquantitative score, allowing to differentiate lung's lesions according to extent and severity of pulmonary damage. It considers five types of elementary lesions, receiving a score from 1 to 5 according to severity. The elementary lesions are as follows: 1—ground glass opacities, 2—irregularities in the pleural margins, 3—septal lines due to thickening of the interlobular septa and subpleural lines, 4—honeycombing, 5—thin-walled subpleural cystic areas. Moreover, the Warrick score takes in account the number of segment (1 to more than 9) involved by each type of lesions, assigning a score from 1 to 3: score 1 is assigned if the lesion is present in less than 3 segments, score 2 if it is present in 4–9 segments, and score 3 if it is present in more than 9 segments [105]. In the study conducted by Gargani and colleagues, the number of US-detected B-lines was correlated with the HRCT Warrick score [106].

In the last years, US assessment found a place in the evaluation of patients affected by vasculitis, n heterogeneous group of diseases characterized by the presence of inflammatory infiltrate in the vessel wall, leading to structural damage, bleeding, stenosis, and aneurysms. Depending on the type of vasculitis, the inflammation can involve different sizes of vessels in different areas of the body. In fact, vasculitis is primarily classified according to the predominant diameter of the affected vessels. Because vasculitis could represent life-threatening diseases, their prompt recognition is mandatory. Many different imaging techniques, such as US, CT, MRI, and PET, have been proposed in the standard approach to screen patients suspected to have large vessel vasculitis (LVV) [107].

In the evaluation of patients affected by giant cell arteritis (GCA), US allows to detect the inflammation of the wall, appearing as a concentric thickening. In healthy condition, the intima–media complex has a homogenous hypoechoic structure, delineated by two hyperechoic margins with a thickness of about 0.2 mm [107]. During an inflammatory condition, the edema causes thickening and reduction of echogenicity of the artery wall, increasing wall thickness up to 0.5–0.8 mm. These features are called the "halo sign" [108]. Moreover, the wall swelling is incompressible with the probe, in contrast to the preserved compressibility of the normal artery wall [109]. The normalization of US-detected abnormalities could be evident after about 3 weeks from the beginning of glucocorticoid treatment [110,111]. Furthermore, US allows check vessels damage such as stenosis and aneurysms and provides a guide to perform a targeted biopsy. Notably, US has been proven to be more sensitive than biopsy alone in the GCA diagnosis, allowing to explore a larger anatomical area [112].

Because almost 40% of patients affected by GCA do not show any involvement of temporal arteries, it has been suggested that all patients with a suspected GCA should perform US assessment at level of superficial temporal arteries, frontal and parietal branches, and axillary arteries [113]. This is particularly relevant in younger female patients and to prevent a delayed diagnosis [114,115].

Regarding the axillary arteries, the thickness of healthy intima-media complex is about 0.6 mm, but in case of vasculitis it could reach 1.5 mm or more [113].

Furthermore, CT and CT angiography (CTA) technology is particularly useful in LVV assessment in the light of their ability to measure vessels diameter, to detect mural calcifications, and to evaluate the wall and the lumen of large arteries [116]. In early disease phases, CTA can show the wall thickening with mural enhancement and low attenuation ring on delayed images [107]. Thanks to the application of these imaging tools, a high prevalence (up to 67.5%) of aorta and tributaries involvement in newly diagnosed patients has been observed [117,118]. The earliest alteration is the mural contrast enhancement, which disappear after the beginning of the therapy; conversely, the arterial wall thickening is still present after more than 12 months in 68% of patients [118,119].

The application of MR allows to investigate the wall abnormalities of the deep and large vessels without the disadvantages of ionizing radiation exposure; moreover, MR angiography provides information about luminal stenosis, occlusion, or dilatation [116]. Specifically, T1 sequences allow the visualization of mural contrast enhancement as early sign of inflammation, while T2 and fat-suppressed sequences to distinguish vessel wall thickness, with a diffuse circumferential pattern, and edema [107]. In GCA patients, MR assessment is able to detect sign of inflammation in multiple cranial arteries, identifying the involvement of occipital arteries in the 29.9% of cases [120]. Moreover, MR is sensitive to change and is able to identify modification after 6 days of glucocorticoid treatment [120].

Recently some studies proposed the use of PET to evaluate the extent of the disease in LVV [121–123]. During a phase of activity, PET is able to show an increased uptake of ^{18}F-fluorodeoxyglucose in the artery wall, with a smooth linear pattern, even in smaller vessel, larger than 4 mm [121,124]. Different authors show a PET sensitivity between 80% and 90.5% and specificity between 89% and 98% in the GCA diagnosis [121–126], especially in patients with less typical manifestations at the onset. PET performance declined rapidly after the onset of therapy [127]. To date, a validated interpretation of PET scan is not yet available.

MR could be useful in the assessment of neuropsychiatric involvement in patients affected by autoimmune diseases: in particular, SLE patients experience this heterogeneous feature in up to 75% of cases [128,129].

To date, MR is the best technique in the investigation of central nervous system (CNS), thanks to its ability to acquire multiplanar images and the excellent resolution for the soft tissue contrast. In general, MR abnormalities can be observed in 19%–70% of SLE patients, with or without CNS involvement, losing in terms of specificity [130,131]. Moreover, about 50% of neuropsychiatric events occur in SLE patients without the appearance of neuroimaging abnormalities [132,133]. In the light of these issues, the EULAR suggested a specific protocol to assess SLE patients with neuropsychiatric involvement, including T1 and T2 scans, postgadolinium sequences, fluid attenuated inversion recovery imaging, gradient recalled echo, and diffusion weighted imaging (DWI) [134].

MR imaging in SLE patients could identify several and heterogeneous abnormalities such as white or gray matter hyperintensities, focal or diffuse brain atrophy, infarcts, lacunes, hemorrhages, inflammatory type lesions, and also posterior reversible encephalopathy syndrome [135]. However, the most frequent MR-detected abnormalities are the cortical atrophy (15%–20%) and multiple small white matter lesions (30%–75%) [132]. The severity of cortical atrophy seems to be associated with several different factors, such as disease duration, age; presence of antiphospholipid antibodies, cumulative organ damage, and use of glucocorticoid [136–138]. Instead white matter lesions can be associated with some risk factors not necessarily related to the disease, such as age, dyslipidemia, diabetes, and hypertension [136–138].

The MR technique allows the application of advanced methods offering, beside the anatomical visualization, physiologic data, and information about chemical brain composition. Among these, DWI sequence allows the differentiation between acute, subacute, or chronic infarction, whereas diffusion tensor imaging (DTI) could be used to study neurocognitive dysfunction showing a loss of streamline density and pairwise connectivity in childhood SLE onset [139,140]. MR with spectroscopy is able to evaluate the concentration of different molecules in brain tissue: in particular, N-acetylaspartate, marker for neuronal and axonal integrity, was reduced in SLE patients with chronic brain lesions [130,132]. Instead choline (Cho) is a marker for the membrane cell turnover; its level increases in presence of an inflammatory condition and was associated with development of gliosis, vasculopathy, and edema [141].

Some attempts to classify MR findings in neuropsychiatric SLE have been performed: Sibbitt and colleagues proposed to distinguish acute and chronic CNS lesions, whereas Sarbu et al. suggested three different groups of abnormalities: large vessel disease, small vessel disease, and inflammatory-like lesions [132,142].

CONCLUSIONS

Imaging tools play a key role in diagnosis and follow-up of autoimmune diseases. Next to the traditional assessment of musculoskeletal manifestations, imaging techniques could be used to evaluate the involvement of other organs and tissues, helping the physician in the more appropriate treatment choice. The knowledge of main faces of different tools is needed to avoid false-positive or false-negative results.

REFERENCES

[1] Vasanth LC, Pavlov H, Bykerk V. Imaging of rheumatoid arthritis. Rheum Dis Clin North Am 2013;39:547–66.
[2] Iagnocco A, Ceccarelli F, Perricone C, Valesini G. The role of ultrasound in rheumatology. Semin Ultrasound CT MR 2011;32:66–73.
[3] De Leonardis F, Orzincolo C, Prandini N, Trotta F. The role of conventional radiography and scintigraphy in the third millennium. Best Pract Res Clin Rheumatol 2008;22:961–79.
[4] Barile A, Arrigoni F, Bruno F, Guglielmi G, Zappia M, Reginelli A, et al. Computed tomography and MR imaging in rheumatoid arthritis. Radiol Clin North Am 2017;55:997–1007.
[5] D'Agostino MA, Haavardsholm EA, van der Laken CJ. Diagnosis and management of rheumatoid arthritis; what is the current role of established and new imaging techniques in clinical practice? Best Pract Res Clin Rheumatol 2016;30:586–607.
[6] Cutolo M, Damjanov N, Ruaro B, Zekovic A, Smith V. Imaging of connective tissue diseases: beyond visceral organ imaging? Best Pract Res Clin Rheumatol 2016;30:670–87.
[7] Kainberger F, Peloschek P, Langs G, Boegl K, Bischof H. Differential diagnosis of rheumatic diseases using conventional radiography. Best Pract Res Clin Rheumatol December 2004;18(6):783–811.
[8] Boonen A, van der Heijde D. Conventional x-ray in early arthritis. Rheum Dis Clin North Am 2005;31:681–98.
[9] Sharp JT, Lidsky MD, Collins LC, Moreland J. Method of scoring the progression of radiologic changes in rheumatoid arthritis. Arthritis Rheum 1971;14:706–20.
[10] Larsen A, Dale K, Eek M. Radiographic evaluation of rheumatoid arthritis and related conditions by reference films. Acta Radiol Diagn 1977;18:481–91.
[11] Genant HK. Methods of assessing radiographic change in rheumatoid arthritis. Am J Med 1983;75:35–47.
[12] Sharp JT, Young DY, Bluhm GB, Brook A, Brower AC, Corbett M, et al. How many joints in the hands and wrists should be included in a score of radiologic abnormalities used to assess rheumatoid arthritis? Arthritis Rheum 1985;28:1326–35.
[13] Van der Heijde D, Van Riel PL, Nuver-Zwart IH, Gribnau FW, Van de Putte L. Effects of hydroxychloroquine and sulfasalazine on progression of joint damage in rheumatoid arthritis. Lancet 1989;i:1036–8.
[14] Larsen A. How to apply Larsen score in evaluating radiographs of rheumatoid arthritis in long-term studies. J Rheumatol 1995;22:1974–5.
[15] Genant HK, Jiang Y, Peterfy C, Lu Y, Redei J, Countryman PJ. Assessment of rheumatoid arthritis using a modified scoring method on digitized and original radiographs. Arthritis Rheum 1998;41:1583–90.
[16] Van der Heijde D, Dankert T, Nieman F, Rau R, Boers M. Reliability and sensitivity to change of a simplification of the Sharp/van der Heijde radiological assessment in rheumatoid arthritis. Rheumatology 1999;38:941–7.
[17] Mary J, De Bandt M, Lukas C, Morel J, Combe B. Triple oral therapy versus antitumor necrosis factor plus methotrexate (MTX) in patients with rheumatoid arthritis and inadequate response to MTX: a systematic literature review. J Rheumatol 2017;44:773–9.
[18] Huizinga TW, Conaghan PG, Martin-Mola E, Schett G, Amital H, Xavier RM, et al. Clinical and radiographic outcomes at 2 years and the effect of tocilizumab discontinuation following sustained remission in the second and third year of the ACT-RAY study. Ann Rheum Dis 2015;74:35–43.
[19] Ciubotariu E, Gabay C, Finckh A. Physicians of the Swiss clinical quality management program for rheumatoid arthritis. Joint damage progression in patients with rheumatoid arthritis in clinical remission: do biologics perform better than synthetic antirheumatic drugs? J Rheumatol 2014;41:1576–82.
[20] Smolen JS, Landewé R, Bijlsma J, Burmester G, Chatzidionysiou K, Dougados M, et al. EULAR recommendations for the management of rheumatoid arthritis with synthetic and biological disease-modifying antirheumatic drugs: 2016 update. Ann Rheum Dis 2017;76(6):960–77.
[21] Mandl P, Navarro-Compán V, Terslev L, Aegerter P, van der Heijde D, D'Agostino MA, et al. EULAR recommendations for the use of imaging in the diagnosis and management of spondyloarthritis in clinical practice. Ann Rheum Dis 2015;74(7):1–13.
[22] van der Linden S, Valkenburg HA, Cats A. Evaluation of diagnostic criteria for ankylosing spondylitis. A proposal for modification of the New York criteria. Arthritis Rheum 1984;27:361–8.

[23] Poddubnyy D, Sieper J. Radiographic progression in ankylosing spondylitis/axial spondyloarthritis: how fast and how clinically meaningful? Curr Opin Rheumatol 2012;24:363–9.

[24] Kataria RK, Brent LH. Spondyloarthropathies. Am Fam Phys 2004;69:2853–60.

[25] Cawley MI, Chalmers TM, Ball J. Destructive lesions of vertebral bodies in ankylosing spondylitis. Ann Rheum Dis 1971;30:539–40.

[26] Rahman P, Gladman DD, Cook RJ, Zhou Y, Young G, Salonen D. Radiological assessment in psoriatic arthritis. Br J Rheumatol 1998;37:760–5.

[27] Jacques T, Michelin P, Badr S, Nasuto M, Lefebvre G, Larkman N, et al. Conventional radiology in crystal arthritis: gout, calcium pyrophosphate deposition, and basic calcium phosphate crystals. Radiol Clin North Am 2017;55:967–84.

[28] Hayashi D, Roemer FW, Jarraya M, Guermazi A. Imaging in osteoarthritis. Radiol Clin North Am 2017;55:1085–102.

[29] Kellgren JH, Lawrence JS. Radiological assessment of osteoarthritis. Ann Rheum Dis 1957;16:494.

[30] Sakellariou G, Conaghan PG, Zhang W, Bijlsma JWJ, Boyesen P, D'Agostino MA, et al. EULAR recommendations for the use of imaging in the clinical management of peripheral joint osteoarthritis. Ann Rheum Dis 2017;76:1484–94.

[31] McQueen FM. A vital clue to deciphering bone pathology: MRI bone oedema in rheumatoid arthritis and osteoarthritis. Ann Rheum Dis 2007;66:1549–52.

[32] Boers M, Kirwan JR, Wells G, Beaton D, Gossec L, d'Agostino MA, et al. Developing core outcome measurement sets for clinical trials: OMERACT filter 2.0. J Clin Epidemiol 2014;67:745–53.

[33] Ostendorf B, Peters R, Dann P, Becker A, Scherer A, Wedekind F, et al. Magnetic resonance imaging and miniarthroscopy of metacarpophalangeal joints: sensitive detection of morphologic changes in rheumatoid arthritis. Arthritis Rheum 2001;44:2492–502.

[34] McQueen FM, GaoA OM, King A, Shalley G, Robinson E, et al. High-grade MRI bone oedema is common within the surgical field in rheumatoid arthritis patients undergoing joint replacement and is associated with osteitis in subchondral bone. Ann Rheum Dis 2007;66:1581–7.

[35] McQueen FM, Stewart N, Crabbe J, Robinson E, Yeoman S, Tan PL, et al. Magnetic resonance imaging of the wrist in early rheumatoid arthritis reveals a high prevalence of erosions at four months after symptom onset. Ann Rheum Dis 1998;57:350–6.

[36] Rudwaleit M, Landewe R, van der Heijde D, Listing J, Brandt J, Braun J, et al. The development of Assessment of SpondyloArthritis international Society classification criteria for axial spondyloarthritis (part I): classification of paper patients by expert opinion including uncertainty appraisal. Ann Rheum Dis 2009;68:770–6.

[37] Rudwaleit M, van der Heijde D, Landewe R, Listing J, Akkoc N, Brandt J, et al. The development of Assessment of SpondyloArthritis international Society classification criteria for axial spondyloarthritis (part II): validation and final selection. Ann Rheum Dis 2009;68:777–83.

[38] Baraliakos X, Braun J. Non-radiographic axial spondyloarthritis and ankylosing spondylitis: what are the similarities and differences? RMD Open 2015;1(Suppl. 1):e000053.

[39] Boyesen P, Haavardsholm EA, Ostergaard M, van der Heijde D, Sesseng S, Kvien TK. MRI in early rheumatoid arthritis: synovitis and bone marrow oedema are independent predictors of subsequent radiographic progression. Ann Rheum Dis 2011;70:428–33.

[40] Dohn UM, Ejbjerg BJ, Hasselquist M. Detection of bone erosions in rheumatoid arthritis wrist joints with magnetic resonance imaging, computed tomography and radiography. Arthritis Res 2008;10:R25.

[41] Woodworth TG, Morgacheva O, Pimienta OL, Troum OM, Ranganath VK, Furst DE. Examining the validity of the rheumatoid arthritis magnetic resonance imaging score according to the OMERACT filter—a systematic literature review. Rheumatology 2017;56(7):1177–88.

[42] Nakagomi D, Ikeda K, Okubo A, Iwamoto T, Sanayama Y, Takahashi K, et al. Ultrasound can improve the accuracy of the 2010 American College of Rheumatology/European League against rheumatism classification criteria for rheumatoid arthritis to predict the requirement for methotrexate treatment. Arthritis Rheum 2013;65:890–8.

[43] Nam JL, Hensor EM, Hunt L, Conaghan PG, Wakefield RJ, Emery P. Ultrasound findings predict progression to inflammatory arthritis in anti-CCP antibody-positive patients without clinical synovitis. Ann Rheum Dis 2016;75:2060–7.

[44] Filer A, de Pablo P, Allen G, Nightingale P, Jordan A, Jobanputra P, et al. Utility of ultrasound joint counts in the prediction of rheumatoid arthritis in patients with very early synovitis. Ann Rheum Dis 2011;70:500–7.

[45] Rakieh C, Nam JL, Hunt L, Hensor EM2, Das S1, Bissell LA, et al. Predicting the development of clinical arthritis in anti-CCP positive individuals with non-specific musculoskeletal symptoms: a prospective observational cohort study. Ann Rheum Dis 2015;74:1659–66.

[46] Stadt LA, Bos WH, Meursinge Reynders M, Wieringa H, Turkstra F, van der Laken CJ, et al. The value of ultrasonography in predicting arthritis in auto-antibody positive arthralgia patients: a prospective cohort study. Arthritis Res Ther 2010;12:R98.

[47] Wakefield RJ, Balint PV, Szkudlarek M, Filippucci E, Backhaus M, D'Agostino MA, et al. Musculoskeletal ultrasound including definitions for ultrasonographic pathology. J Rheumatol 2005;32:2485–7.

[48] Aletaha D, Ward MM, Machold KP, Nell VP, Stamm T, Smolen JS. Remission and active disease in rheumatoid arthritis: defining criteria for disease activity states. Arthritis Rheum 2005;52:2625–36.

[49] Szkudlarek M, Klarlund M, Narvestad E, Court-Payen M, Strandberg C, Jensen KE, et al. Ultrasonography of the metacarpophalangeal and proximal interphalangeal joints in rheumatoid arthritis: a comparison with magnetic resonance imaging, conventional radiography and clinical examination. Arthritis Res Ther 2006;8:R52.

[50] Iagnocco A, Finucci A, Ceccarelli F, Perricone C, Iorgoveanu V, Valesini G. Power Doppler ultrasound monitoring of response to anti-tumour necrosis factor alpha treatment in patients with rheumatoid arthritis. Rheumatology (Oxford) 2015;54:1890–6.

[51] Perricone C, Ceccarelli F, Modesti M, Vavala C, Di Franco M, Valesini G, et al. The 6-joint ultrasonographic assessment: a valid, sensitive-to-change and feasible method for evaluating joint inflammation in RA. Rheumatology (Oxford) 2012;51:866–73.

[52] Iagnocco A, Filippucci E, Perella C, Ceccarelli F, Cassarà E, Alessandri C, et al. Clinical and ultrasonographic monitoring of response to adalimumab treatment in rheumatoid arthritis. J Rheumatol 2008;35:35–40.

[53] Iagnocco A, Perella C, Naredo E, Meenagh G, Ceccarelli F, Tripodo E, et al. Etanercept in the treatment of rheumatoid arthritis: clinical follow-up over one year by ultrasonography. Clin Rheumatol 2008;27:491–6.

[54] Naredo E, Rodríguez M, Campos C, Rodríguez-Heredia JM, Medina JA, Giner E, et al. Validity, reproducibility, and responsiveness of a twelve-joint simplified power Doppler ultrasonographic assessment of joint inflammation in rheumatoid arthritis. Arthritis Rheum 2008;59:515–22.

[55] Saleem B, Brown AK, Keen H, Nizam S, Freeston J, Karim Z, et al. Disease remission state in patients treated with the combination of tumor necrosis factor blockade and methotrexate or with disease-modifying antirheumatic drugs: a clinical and imaging comparative study. Arthritis Rheum 2009;60:1915–22.

[56] Naredo E, Möller I, Cruz A, Carmona L, Garrido J. Power Doppler ultrasonographic monitoring of response to anti-tumor necrosis factor therapy in patients with rheumatoid arthritis. Arthritis Rheum 2008;58:2248–56.

[57] Wakefield RJ, D'Agostino MA, Naredo E, Buch MH, Iagnocco A, Terslev L, et al. After treat-to-target: can a targeted ultrasound initiative improve RA outcomes? Ann Rheum Dis June 2012;71(6):799–803.

[58] Zabotti A, Bandinelli F, Batticciotto A, Scirè CA, Iagnocco A, Sakellariou G. Musculoskeletal Ultrasound Study Group of the Italian Society of Rheumatology. Musculoskeletal ultrasonography for psoriatic arthritis and psoriasis patients: a systematic literature review. Rheumatology (Oxford) 2017;56:1518–32.

[59] Micu MC, Fodor D. Concepts in monitoring enthesitis in patients with spondylarthritis–the role of musculoskeletal ultrasound. Med Ultrason 2016;18:82–9.

[60] Kaeley GS. Review of the use of ultrasound for the diagnosis and monitoring of enthesitis in psoriatic arthritis. Curr Rheumatol Rep 2011;13:338–45.

[61] Baraliakos X, Maksymowych WP. Imaging in the diagnosis and management of axial spondyloarthritis. Best Pract Res Clin Rheumatol 2016;30:608–23.

[62] Spadaro A, Iagnocco A, Baccano G, Ceccarelli F, Sabatini E, Valesini G. Sonographic-detected joint effusion compared with physical examination in the assessment of sacroiliac joints in spondyloarthritis. Ann Rheum Dis 2009;68:1559–63.

[63] Naredo E, Iagnocco A. One year in review 2017: ultrasound in crystal arthritis. Clin Exp Rheumatol May–June 2017;35(3):362–7.

[64] Dalbeth N, Doyle A, McQueen FM. Imaging in gout: insights into the pathological features of disease. Curr Opin Rheumatol 2012;24:132–8.

[65] Muratore F, Pazzola G, Pipitone N, Salvarani C. Recent advances in the diagnosis and treatment of polymyalgia rheumatica. Expert Rev Clin Immunol 2016;12:1037–45.

[66] Dasgupta B, Cimmino MA, Maradit-Kremers H, Schmidt WA, Schirmer M, Salvarani C, et al. 2012 provisional classification criteria for polymyalgia rheumatica: a European league against Rheumatism/American College of Rheumatology collaborative initiative. Ann Rheum Dis 2012;71:484–92.

[67] Cervera R, Khamashta MA, Font J, Sebastiani GD, Gil A, Lavilla P, et al. Systemic lupus erythematosus: clinical and immunologic patterns of disease expression in a cohort of 1,000 patients. The European Working Party on Systemic Lupus Erythematosus. Medicine (Baltim) 1993;72:113–24.

[68] Petri M. Musculoskeletal complications of systemic lupus erythematosus in the Hopkins Lupus Cohort: an update. Arthritis Care Res 1995;8:137–45.

[69] Pease CT, Shattles W, Barrett NK, Maini RN. The arthropathy of Sjögren's syndrome. Br J Rheumatol 1993;32:609–13.

[70] Baldini C, Pepe P, Quartuccio L, Priori R, Bartoloni E, Alunno A, et al. Primary Sjogren's syndrome as a multi-organ disease: impact of the serological profile on the clinical presentation of the disease in a large cohort of Italian patients. Rheumatology (Oxford) 2014;53:839–44.

[71] Castro-Poltronieri A, Alarcón-Segovia D. Articular manifestations of primary Sjögren's syndrome. J Rheumatol 1983;10:485–8.

[72] Ceccarelli F, Perricone C, Cipriano E, Massaro L, Natalucci F, Capalbo G, et al. Joint involvement in systemic lupus erythematosus: from pathogenesis to clinical assessment. Semin Arthritis Rheum 2017;47:53–64.

[73] Plagou A, Teh J, Grainger AJ, Schueller-Weidekamm C, Sudoł-Szopińska I, Rennie W, et al. Recommendations of the ESSR arthritis subcommittee on ultrasonography in inflammatory joint disease. Semin Musculoskelet Radiol 2016;20:496–506.

[74] Ball EM, Gibson DS, Bell AL, Rooney MR. Plasma IL-6 levels correlate with clinical and ultrasound measures of arthritis in patients with systemic lupus erythematosus. Lupus 2014;23:46–56.

[75] Gabba A, Piga M, Vacca A, Porru G, Garau P, Cauli A, Mathieu A. Joint and tendon involvement in systemic lupus erythematosus: an ultrasound study of hands and wrists in 108 patients. Rheumatology (Oxford) 2012;51:2278–85.

[76] Iagnocco A, Ceccarelli F, Rizzo C, Truglia S, Massaro L, Spinelli FR, et al. Ultrasound evaluation of hand, wrist and foot joint synovitis in systemic lupus erythematosus. Rheumatology (Oxford) 2014;53:465–72.

[77] Mosca M, Tani C, Carli L, Vagnani S, Possemato N, Delle Sedie A, et al. The role of imaging in the evaluation of joint involvement in 102 consecutive patients with systemic lupus erythematosus. Autoimmun Rev 2015;14:10–5.

[78] Yoon HS, Kim KJ, Baek IW, Park YJ, Kim WU, Yoon CH, et al. Ultrasonography is useful to detect subclinical synovitis in SLE patients without musculoskeletal involvement before symptoms appear. Clin Rheumatol 2014;33:341–8.

[79] Iagnocco A, Modesti M, Priori R, Alessandri C, Perella C, Takanen S, et al. Subclinical synovitis in primary Sjögren's syndrome: an ultrasonographic study. Rheumatology (Oxford) 2010;49:1153–7.

[80] Amezcua-Guerra LM, Hofmann F, Vargas A, Rodriguez-Henriquez P, Solano C, Hernández-Díaz C, et al. Joint involvement in primary Sjögren's syndrome: an ultrasound "target area approach to arthritis". BioMed Res Int 2013;2013:640265.

[81] Möller I, Janta I, Backhaus M, Ohrndorf S, Bong DA, Martinoli C, et al. The 2017 EULAR standardised procedures for ultrasound imaging in rheumatology. Ann Rheum Dis 2017;76:1974–9.

[82] Moutsopoulos HM. Sjögren's syndrome: autoimmune epithelitis. Clin Immunol Immunopathol 1994;72:162–5.

[83] Håkansson U, Jacobsson L, Lilja B, Manthorpe R, Henriksson V. Salivary gland scintigraphy in subjects with and without symptoms of dry mouth and/or eyes, and in patients with primary Sjögren's syndrome. Scand J Rheumatol 1994;23:326–33.

[84] Kalk WW, Vissink A, Spijkervet FK, Bootsma H, Kallenberg CG, Roodenburg JL. Parotid sialography for diagnosing Sjögren syndrome. Oral Surg Oral Med Oral Pathol Oral Radiol Endod 2002;94:131–7.

[85] Takagi Y, Kimura Y, Nakamura H, Sasaki M, Eguchi K, Nakamura T. Salivary gland ultrasonography: can it be an alternative to sialography as an imaging modality for Sjogren's syndrome? Ann Rheum Dis 2010;69:1321–4.

[86] Milic V, Petrovic R, Boricic I, Radunovic G, Marinkovic-Eric J, Jeremic P, et al. Ultrasonography of major salivary glands could be an alternative tool to sialoscintigraphy in the American-European classification criteria for primary Sjogren's syndrome. Rheumatology (Oxford) 2012;51:1081–5.

[87] Zhang X, Zhang S, He J, Hu F, Liu H, Li J, Zhu J, Li Z. Ultrasonographic evaluation of major salivary glands in primary Sjögren's syndrome: comparison of two scoring systems. Rheumatology (Oxford) 2015;54:1680–7.

[88] Takagi Y, Kimura Y, Nakamura H, Sasaki M, Eguchi K, Nakamura T. Salivary gland ultrasonography: can it be an alternative to sialography as an imaging modality for Sjogren's syndrome? Ann Rheum Dis 2010;69:1321–4.

[89] De Vita S, Lorenzon G, Rossi G, Sabella M, Fossaluzza V. Salivary gland echography in primary and secondary Sjögren's syndrome. Clin Exp Rheumatol 1992;10:351–6.

[90] Milic VD, Petrovic RR, Boricic IV, Marinkovic-Eric J, Radunovic GL, Jeremic PD, et al. Diagnostic value of salivary gland ultrasonographic scoring system in primary Sjogren's syndrome: a comparison with scintigraphy and biopsy. J Rheumatol 2009;36:1495–500.

[91] Clements PJ, Lachenbruch PA, Ng SC, Simmons M, Sterz M, Furst DE. Skin score. A semiquantitative measure of cutaneous involvement that improves prediction of prognosis in systemic sclerosis. Arthritis Rheum 1990;33:1256–63.

[92] Czirják L, Foeldvari I, Müller-Ladner U. Skin involvement in systemic sclerosis. Rheumatology (Oxford) 2008;47(Suppl. 5):44–5.

[93] Moore TL, Lunt M, McManus B, Anderson ME, Herrick AL. Seventeen-point dermal ultrasound scoring system–a reliable measure of skin thickness in patients with systemic sclerosis. Rheumatology (Oxford) 2003;42:1559–63.

[94] Kaloudi O, Bandinelli F, Filippucci E, Conforti ML, Miniati I, Guiducci S, et al. High frequency ultrasound measurement of digital dermal thickness in systemic sclerosis. Ann Rheum Dis 2010;69:1140–3.

[95] Delle Sedie A, Riente L. Ultrasound in connective tissue diseases. Clin Exp Rheumatol 2014;32(1 Suppl. 80):S53–60.

[96] Scleroderma SRM. Clinical problems. The lungs. Rheum Dis Clin North Am 1996;22:825–40.

[97] Diot E, Boissinot E, Asquier E, Guilmot JL, Lemarié E, Valat C, et al. Relationship between abnormalities on high-resolution CT and pulmonary function in systemic sclerosis. Chest 1998;114:1623–9.

[98] Ostojic P, Damjanov N. Improvement of lung function in patients with systemic sclerosis after 6 months cyclophosphamide pulse therapy. Clin Rheumatol 2006;25:819–21.

[99] Lynch DA, Godwin JD, Safrin S, Starko KM, Hormel P, Brown KK, et al. High-resolution computed tomography in idiopathic pulmonary fibrosis: diagnosis and prognosis. Am J Respir Crit Care Med 2005;172:488–93.

[100] Lichtenstein D, Mézière G, Biderman P, Gepner A, Barré O. The comet-tail artifact. An ultrasound sign of alveolar-interstitial syndrome. Am J Respir Crit Care Med 1997;156:1640–6.

[101] Delle Sedie A, Carli L, Cioffi E, Bombardieri S, Riente L. The promising role of lung ultrasound in systemic sclerosis. Clin Rheumatol 2012;31:1537–41.

[102] Volpicelli G, Melniker LA, Cardinale L, Lamorte A, Frascisco MF. Lung ultrasound in diagnosing and monitoring pulmonary interstitial fluid. Radiol Med 2013;118:196–205.

[103] Soldati G, Inchingolo R, Smargiassi A, Sher S, Nenna R, Inchingolo CD, et al. Ex vivo lung sonography: morphologic-ultrasound relationship. Ultrasound Med Biol 2012;38:1169–79.

[104] Song G, Bae SC, Lee YH. Diagnostic accuracy of lung ultrasound for interstitial lung disease in patients with connective tissue diseases: a meta-analysis. Clin Exp Rheumatol 2016;34:11–6.

[105] Warrick JH, Bhalla M, Schabel SI, Silver RM. High resolution computed tomography in early scleroderma lung disease. J Rheumatol 1991;18:1520–8.

[106] Gargani L, Doveri M, D'Errico L, Frassi F, Bazzichi ML, Delle Sedie A, et al. Ultrasound lung comets in systemic sclerosis: a chest sonography hallmark of pulmonary interstitial fibrosis. Rheumatology (Oxford) 2009;48:1382–7.

[107] Muratore F, Pipitone N, Salvarani C, Schmidt WA. Imaging of vasculitis: state of the art. Best Pract Res Clin Rheumatol 2016;30:688–706.

[108] Schmidt WA, Kraft HE, Vorpahl K, Völker L, Gromnica-Ihle EJ. Color duplex ultrasonography in the diagnosis of temporal arteritis. N Engl J Med 1997;337:1336–42.

[109] Aschwanden M, Imfeld S, Staub D, Baldi T, Walker UA, Berger CT, et al. The ultrasound compression sign to diagnose temporal giant cell arteritis shows an excellent interobserver agreement. Clin Exp Rheumatol 2015;33(2 Suppl. 89). S-113-5.

[110] Hauenstein C, Reinhard M, Geiger J, Markl M, Hetzel A, Treszl A, et al. Effects of early corticosteroid treatment on magnetic resonance imaging and ultrasonography findings in giant cell arteritis. Rheumatology (Oxford) 2012;5:1999–2003.

[111] Diamantopoulos AP, Myklebust G. Long-term inflammation in the temporal artery of a giant cell arteritis patient as detected by ultrasound. Ther Adv Musculoskelet Dis 2014;6:102–3.

[112] Luqmani RA. Disease assessment in systemic vasculitis. Nephrol Dial Transplant 2015;30(Suppl. 1). i76–82.

[113] Schmidt WA, Seifert A, Gromnica-Ihle E, Krause A, Natusch A. Ultrasound of proximal upper extremity arteries to increase the diagnostic yield in large-vessel giant cell arteritis. Rheumatology (Oxford) 2008;47:96–101.

[114] Germanò G, Muratore F, Cimino L, Lo Gullo A, Possemato N, Macchioni P, et al. Is colour duplex sonography-guided temporal artery biopsy useful in the diagnosis of giant cell arteritis? A randomized study. Rheumatology (Oxford) 2015;54:400–4.

[115] Czihal M, Piller A, Schroettle A, Kuhlencordt P, Bernau C, Schulze-Koops H, et al. Impact of cranial and axillary/subclavian artery involvement by color duplex sonography on response to treatment in giant cell arteritis. J Vasc Surg 2015;61:1285–91.

[116] Pipitone N, Salvarani C. Role of imaging in vasculitis and connective tissue diseases. Best Pract Res Clin Rheumatol 2008;22:1075–91.

[117] Muratore F, Pazzola G, Pipitone N, Boiardi L, Salvarani C. Large-vessel involvement in giant cell arteritis and polymyalgia rheumatica. Clin Exp Rheumatol 2014;32(3 Suppl. 82):S106–11.

[118] Prieto-González S, Arguis P, García-Martínez A, Espígol-Frigolé G, Tavera-Bahillo I, Butjosa M, et al. Large vessel involvement in biopsy-proven giant cell arteritis: prospective study in 40 newly diagnosed patients using CT angiography. Ann Rheum Dis 2012;7:1170–6.

[119] Prieto-González S, Arguis P, Alba MA, García-Martínez A, Espígol-Frigolé G, Grau JM, et al. Evaluation of aortic inflammation using computed tomographic angiography: vasculitis, atherosclerosis, or both. J Am Geriatr Soc 2015;63:415–6.

[120] Klink T, Geiger J, Both M, Ness T, Heinzelmann S, Reinhard M, et al. Giant cell arteritis: diagnostic accuracy of MR imaging of superficial cranial arteries in initial diagnosis-results from a multicenter trial. Radiology 2014;273:844–52.

[121] Besson FL, Parienti JJ, Bienvenu B, Prior JO, Costo S, Bouvard G, et al. Diagnostic performance of ^{18}F-fluorodeoxyglucose positron emission tomography in giant cell arteritis: a systematic review and meta-analysis. Eur J Nucl Med Mol Imaging 2011;38:1764–72.

[122] Brodmann M, Lipp RW, Passath A, Seinost G, Pabst E, Pilger E. The role of 2-18F-fluoro-2-deoxy-D-glucose positron emission tomography in the diagnosis of giant cell arteritis of the temporal arteries. Rheumatology (Oxford) 2004;43:241–2.

[123] Meller J, Strutz F, Siefker U, Scheel A, Sahlmann CO, Lehmann K, et al. Early diagnosis and follow-up of aortitis with [(18)F]FDG PET and MRI. Eur J Nucl Med Mol Imag 2003;30:730–6.

[124] Brodmann M, Lipp RW, Passath A, Seinost G, Pabst E, Pilger E. The role of 2-18F-fluoro-2-deoxy-D-glucose positron emission tomography in the diagnosis of giant cell arteritis of the temporal arteries. Rheumatology (Oxford) 2004;43:241–2.

[125] Treglia G, Mattoli MV, Leccisotti L, Ferraccioli G, Giordano A. Usefulness of whole-body fluorine-18-fluorodeoxyglucose positron emission tomography in patients with large-vessel vasculitis: a systematic review. Clin Rheumatol 2011;30:1265–75.

[126] Soussan M, Nicolas P, Schramm C, Katsahian S, Pop G, Fain O, et al. Management of large-vessel vasculitis with FDG-PET: a systematic literature review and meta-analysis. Medicine (Baltim) 2015;94:e622.

[127] Fuchs M, Briel M, Daikeler T, Walker UA, Rasch H, Berg S, et al. The impact of 18F-FDG PET on the management of patients with suspected large vessel vasculitis. Eur J Nucl Med Mol Imag 2012;39:344–53.

[128] Steup-Beekman GM, Zirkzee EJ, Cohen D, Gahrmann BM, Emmer BJ, Steens SC, et al. Neuropsychiatric manifestations in patients with systemic lupus erythematosus: epidemiology and radiology pointing to an immune-mediated cause. Ann Rheum Dis 2013;72(Suppl. 2). ii76-9.

[129] Govoni M, Bortoluzzi A, Padovan M, Silvagni E, Borrelli M, Donelli F, et al. The diagnosis and clinical management of the neuropsychiatric manifestations of lupus. J Autoimmun 2016;74:41–72.

[130] Appenzeller S, Vasconcelos Faria A, Li LM, Costallat LT, Cendes F. Quantitative magnetic resonance imaging analyses and clinical significance of hyperintense white matter lesions in systemic lupus erythematosus patients. Ann Neurol 2008;64:635–43.

[131] Postal M, Costallat LT, Appenzeller S. Neuropsychiatric manifestations in systemic lupus erythematosus: epidemiology, pathophysiology and management. CNS Drugs 2011;25(9):721–36.

[132] Sarbu N, Alobeidi F, Toledano P, Espinosa G, Giles I, Rahman A, et al. Brain abnormalities in newly diagnosed neuropsychiatric lupus: systematic MRI approach and correlation with clinical and laboratory data in a large multicenter cohort. Autoimmun Rev 2015;14:153–9.

[133] Jones JT, DiFrancesco M, Zaal AI, Klein-Gitelman MS, Gitelman D, Ying J, et al. Childhood-onset lupus with clinical neurocognitive dysfunction shows lower streamline density and pairwise connectivity on diffusion tensor imaging. Lupus 2015;24:1081–6.

[134] Bertsias GK, Ioannidis JP, Aringer M, Bollen E, Bombardieri S, Bruce IN, et al. EULAR recommendations for the management of systemic lupus erythematosus with neuropsychiatric manifestations: report of a task force of the EULAR standing committee for clinical affairs. Ann Rheum Dis 2010;69:2074–82.

[135] Luyendijk J, Steens SC, Ouwendijk WJ, Steup-Beekman GM, Bollen EL, van der Grond J, et al. Neuropsychiatric systemic lupus erythematosus: lessons learned from magnetic resonance imaging. Arthritis Rheum 2011;63:722–32.

[136] Muscal E, Brey RL. Antiphospholipid syndrome and the brain in pediatric and adult patients. Lupus 2010;19:406–11.

[137] Sanna G, Piga M, Terryberry JW, Peltz MT, Giagheddu S, Satta L, et al. Central nervous system involvement in systemic lupus erythematosus: cerebral imaging and serological profile in patients with and without overt neuropsychiatric manifestations. Lupus 2000;9:573–83.

[138] Ainiala H, Dastidar P, Loukkola J, Lehtimäki T, Korpela M, Peltola J, et al. Cerebral MRI abnormalities and their association with neuropsychiatric manifestations in SLE: a population-based study. Scand J Rheumatol 2005;34:376–82.

[139] Hughes M, Sundgren PC, Fan X, Foerster B, Nan B, Welsh RC, et al. Diffusion tensor imaging in patients with acute onset of neuropsychiatric systemic lupus erythematosus: a prospective study of apparent diffusion coefficient, fractional anisotropy values, and eigenvalues in different regions of the brain. Acta Radiol 2007;48:213–22.

[140] Corrêa DG, Zimmermann N, Pereira DB, Doring TM, Netto TM, Ventura N, et al. Evaluation of white matter integrity in systemic lupus erythematosus by diffusion tensor magnetic resonance imaging: a study using tract-based spatial statistics. Neuroradiology 2016;58:819–25.

[141] Appenzeller S, Li LM, Costallat LT, Cendes F. Neurometabolic changes in normal white matter may predict appearance of hyperintense lesions in systemic lupus erythematosus. Lupus 2007;16:963–71.

[142] Sibbitt Jr WL, Brooks WM, Kornfeld M, Hart BL, Bankhurst AD, Roldan CA. Magnetic resonance imaging and brain histopathology in neuropsychiatric systemic lupus erythematosus. Semin Arthritis Rheum 2010;40:32–52.

The Classical Factors Associated With Autoimmunity

Chapter 19

Hormones and Autoimmunity

Roberta Gualtierotti[1,2], Carolina Artusi[1], Guia Maria Vannucchi[3], Irene Campi[3,4], Luca Persani[2,3], Pier Luigi Meroni[5]

[1]Lupus Clinic, Department of Clinical Rheumatology and Medical Sciences, ASST Pini-CTO, Milan, Italy; [2]Department of Clinical Sciences and Community Health, University of Milan, Milan, Italy; [3]Division of Endocrine and Metabolic Diseases, Laboratory of Endocrine and Metabolic Research, IRCCS Istituto Auxologico Italiano, Milan, Italy; [4]Department of Pathophysiology and Transplantation, University of Milan, Milan, Italy; [5]Immunorheumatology Research Laboratory, IRCCS Istituto Auxologico Italiano, Milan, Italy

INTRODUCTION

The etiology of autoimmune diseases (ADs) has not been completely clarified, although it is evident that it is the result of a complex interaction of the immune system with environmental and genetic factors. The clear disparity between the immune responses of females and males accounts for the well-established concept of sexual dimorphism observed in both human and animal models [1]. A number of ADs, such as rheumatoid arthritis (RA) and systemic lupus erythematosus (SLE), show a striking female predominance, with female to male prevalence ratios of 2–3:1 and 7–9:1, respectively [2].

Cells of the immune system express estrogen and androgen receptors. Estrogens enhance the response to antigen of peripheral blood mononuclear cells (PBMCs) obtained from women [3] and target the immune system toward Th2 dominance with consequent activation of B cells and antibody production [4] and a stronger interferon (IFN) response [5]. The changes of serum sex hormone levels, which are involved in pregnancy, postpartum breastfeeding, and menopause, as well as in the case of exogenous sex steroids such as oral contraceptives or hormone replacement therapy (HRT), highly influence the life of women. Several lines of evidence also indicate the fluctuation during the menstrual cycle of disease severity of ADs. Notably, SLE and multiple sclerosis (MS) appear to worsen in the premenstrual phase of the menstrual cycle, whereas RA worsens during menstruation [6]. Further evidence for the influence of sex hormones on the development of ADs comes from the changes in disease severity during pregnancy. Also in this case, pregnancy has opposite effects on RA and SLE [7]. A protective role of pregnancy on RA has long been recognized [8] and later other diseases, such as MS, were added to the group in which symptoms are reduced during gestation [9]. On the other hand, many studies have indicated that pregnancy and estrogens make the symptoms of SLE and related diseases more severe [10]. The different effect of pregnancy on ADs suggests that the role of sex hormones in these diseases may not be always the same or that pregnancy and sex hormones might differ in their abilities to exacerbate disease in some instances.

Apart from estrogens and androgens, other hormones, neuropeptides, and cytokines released by cells in the immune-neuroendocrine system are involved in the regulation of the immune response [11–14]. The rupture of this homeostatic-molecular balance may lead to the development of autoimmunity and the pathogenesis of ADs [13–15]. Furthermore, sexual dimorphism in ADs is not fully explained by a dichotomous behavior driven by sex hormones, but other mechanisms such as epigenetics and microbiome may be involved [16]. In this chapter we will focus on the effects of sex hormones and prolactin (PRL) on AD pathogenesis and evolution. For further reading, we suggest the review by Coronel-Restrepo et al. and by Rubtsova et al. [15,16].

SEX HORMONES

Estrogens

Estrogens bind to two functionally distinct estrogen receptors (ERs), ERa and ERb, forming homo- and heterodimers. When bound, ERs translocate to the nucleus where they bind to estrogen-responsive elements in gene promoters, controlling gene transcription [17]. ERs are expressed not only in the female reproductive tract but also on B and T cells, dendritic cells, neutrophils, macrophages, natural killer (NK) cells, thymic stromal cells, bone marrow, and endothelial cells [18–20]. Estrogens affect the immune system by influencing the maturation of T and B cells [19,21], by decreasing B cell lymphopoiesis throughout the downregulation of interleukin (IL)-7 production by bone marrow stromal cells [21], by reducing the B cell receptor signal strength and regulation of CD22 expression [22–24], and by promoting extramedullary hematopoiesis [25]. In addition, estrogens induce the transcriptional activation of activation-induced deaminase in nonimmune tissues, promoting DNA instability [26] or altering signaling and/or apoptotic pathways [27], thus allowing production of autoantibodies. Exposure to estrogens decreases the number of developing thymic CD4+/CD8+ T cells and promotes lymphopoiesis in the liver, allowing cells to escape negative selection, potentially leading to accumulation of autoreactive cells [25,28]. Estrogens may also support survival of autoreactive T cell clones by increasing Bcl2 expression [25] and promoting Th2 responses resulting in increased levels of IL-4, IL-5, and IL-10 [18,19,29].

The regulation of Th1 and Th2 responses by estrogens is typically biphasic during the menstrual cycle: low doses of estrogens, accompanying menstruation, and the luteal phase invoke Th1-mediated immunity, whereas higher doses in the follicular phase invoke Th2-mediated immunity [30]. Estrogens act in a dose-dependent manner: low doses seem to stimulate proinflammatory cytokines such as tumor necrosis factor (TNF) or IL-1 beta and NK cells [31], whereas high doses, such as in pregnancy, lead to antiinflammatory effects by suppressing the signaling of proinflammatory cytokines and by inducing the expression of antiinflammatory cytokines (Th2) [4].

Progesterone

Progesterone binds both cell surface and intracellular receptors. Intracellular progesterone receptors (iPRs) are ligand-sensitive transcription factors of the nuclear receptor superfamily [32]. Structurally unrelated to iPRs, membrane progesterone receptors (mPRs: mPR-α, mPR-β, mPR-γ) are linked to inhibitory G-coupled proteins, explaining some of progesterone's rapid nontranscriptional actions [33]. The expression of a number of PRs in some cell subsets supports the idea that progesterone can directly regulate the immune system.

In vivo and in vitro evidence indicates that progesterone has some capacity to suppress CD4+ T cell proliferation and Th1/Th17 differentiation and effector functions. Progesterone stimulates a switch from a predominantly proinflammatory to an antiinflammatory immune response favoring Treg differentiation [34]. This is accompanied by decreased numbers of IFN-γ–producing CD4+ T cells [35]. Postpartum immune response returns to Th1, which together with the elevated levels of PRL observed during lactation may explain exacerbations in RA patients [35].

Androgens

Androgen receptors are found on B [36] and T cells [37]. Androgens enhance a Th1 response, specifically leading to increased IL-2 production and augment activation of CD8+ T cells [18–20,29]. The androgen receptor has been shown to play a role in B cell homeostasis and tolerance [36]. Several studies indicate that testosterone has suppressive effects on the immune system by inhibiting proinflammatory cytokine production, Th1 differentiation, immunoglobulin production, and NK cell cytotoxic activity and by potentiating the expression of antiinflammatory cytokines [38].

PROLACTIN AND AUTOIMMUNITY

The role of PRL goes well beyond the regulation of biological processes linked to reproduction and lactation. PRL acts by binding PRL receptors (PRLR), belonging to the hematopoietic cytokine receptor superfamily, which is widely expressed in different tissues. Derangements of the physiological production of PRL and its receptors have been associated with human diseases such as ADs and cardiovascular diseases [1,2]. Extrapituitary secretion has been found in several tissues of the immune system such as thymus, spleen, tonsil, and lymph nodes [39,40]. PRLRs are expressed on monocytes, macrophages, T and mainly B cells and NK cells, granulocytes, and thymus epithelial cells [41]. PRL decreases the apoptosis of transitional B cells mediated by anti-IgM and may be important in the breakdown of B cell tolerance to self and the development of autoimmunity [42]. This in vitro antiapoptotic effect of PRL has been demonstrated in animal models and in human myeloma cell lines [43]. PRL stimulates antigen-presenting cells expressing major histocompatibility complex (MHC) class II and promotes co-stimulatory molecules expression [44] and antibody secretion [45]. Indeed, PRL supports proliferation and survival of T cells [46]. However, it is also associated with tissue repair: an antiapoptotic effect of a local or systemic treatment with PRL has been demonstrated in the cartilage in a mouse model of RA [47]. Besides this protective role on chondrocytes, PRL also inhibits osteoclastogenesis and bone loss in inflammatory arthritis reducing cytokine-induced expression of receptor activator of nuclear factor kappa-B ligand in joints and synovial fibroblasts [47]. Finally, PRL may be involved in the sexual

TABLE 19.1 Clinical Trials With Dopamine Agonists in Several Autoimmune Diseases

Authors	Disease	N pts (Controls)	Treatment	Study Design	Findings
Bissay V. et al. [50]	MS	15	BCR 2.5 mg/day	Open	No benefit
Qian Q. et al. [51]	SLE	38 (38)	BCR 2.5 mg oral, twice a day for 14 days versus no treatment	RCT	Benefit in preventing disease relapse
Jara L.J. et al. [52]	SLE	10 (10)	PDN 10 mg/day with or without BCR 2.5 mg/day	RCT	Benefit in preventing maternal-fetal complications and active disease
McMurray R.W. et al. [53]	SLE	7	BCR 2.5 mg/day	Open	Improvement of SLE activity. Increased disease activity after BCR discontinuation
Hrycek A. et al. [54]	SLE	25	QNG 12.5 µg/day for a month, and 25–50 µg/day for 2 months	Open	IL-6 and SLEDAI score improved during therapy
Salesi M. et al. [55]	RA	40 (38)	MTX + BCR (5 mg/day) or placebo	RCT	Not significant improvement
Alvarez-Nemegyei J. et al. [56]	SLE	36 (30)	BCR 2.5 mg/day versus placebo	RCT	SLEDAI score decreased in the BCR group

BCR, bromocriptine; *IL-6*, interleukin-6; *MS*, multiple sclerosis; *MTX*, methotrexate; *PDN*, prednisone; *pts*, patients; *QNG*, quinagolide; *RA*, rheumatoid arthritis; *RCT*, randomized clinical trial; *SLE*, systemic lupus erythematosus; *SLEDAI*, SLE disease activity index.

dimorphism typical of several ADs because of its influence on gonadotropins [48]. Clinical evidence is controversial. Some patients may present with hyperprolactinemia (HPRL) before the development of ADs such as Graves' disease, dermatomyositis, and SLE. A group of SLE patients with prolactinoma has been described and a subset of these patients presented HPRL 5 years before SLE diagnosis [12,49]. However, a study conducted in patients with a recent diagnosis of RA untreated with both steroids and disease-modifying anti-rheumatic drugs showed no difference in PRL serum concentrations after hypothalamic stimulation with the releasing hormone [71]. One possible explanation for this discrepancy is that PRL plays its role with a paracrine/autocrine mechanism of action at a tissue level, which is not easily measurable, in blood. Moreover, PRLR may also bind growth hormone (GH) and human placental lactogen; thus it could be difficult to determine the specific effects of PRL in vivo. Finally, the results of clinical trials in several ADs with dopamine agonists (bromocriptine or the selective D2 receptor agonist quinagolide) are not conclusive, as some authors failed to find any improvement in the patients treated compared with the control group (Table 19.1) [50–56].

HORMONAL CONTRACEPTION AND AUTOIMMUNITY

Oral contraceptives are used by over 100 million women worldwide [57].

Although a definite pathogenic mechanism linking hormonal contraceptives (HCs) or HRT to the pathogenesis of ADs has not been identified yet, the exposure to sex hormones has been reckoned as one of the environmental factors involved in the susceptibility of ADs [15,16]. Sex hormone activity is very complex and still not completely clarified with different effects on susceptibility/disease activity among the various ADs. Consequently, as ADs often affect women in fertile age, contraception is an important issue. For example, patients with SLE may experience negative offspring or maternal outcomes when pregnancy occurs in the course of high disease activity, and the intake of potentially teratogenic drugs such as methotrexate, mycophenolate mofetil, or alkylating agents requires mandatory effective contraceptive methods [58]. Finally, HCs and HRT may be associated with a higher risk of thrombotic events suggesting a careful use in patients with antiphospholipid antibodies (aPL). Therefore, a tailored counseling should be performed in each patient of childbearing age depending on the AD is suffering from.

Combined and Progestin-Only Contraceptives

The first available combined HCs had 3–5 times the estrogen content of current oral contraceptives, containing low-dose synthetic estrogen (ethinylestradiol or mestranol, 20–50 mg) and a progestin (17-α-ethinyl analogues of 19-nortestosterone). Second-generation progestins include norethindrone and levonorgestrel; third-generation progestins have less androgenic side effects and include norgestimate and desogestrel; drospirenone is an analogue of spironolactone and is considered a fourth-generation progestin [59]. Serious complications associated with HC use include venous thromboembolism (VTE), stroke, and myocardial infarction (MI) because of an overall net prothrombotic effect on the hemostatic system.

For patients who have contraindications for estrogens, progestin-only contraceptives containing norethindrone or norgestrel present an alternative option. They have beneficial effects such as decreased menstrual bleeding and amelioration of endometriosis symptoms but may be burdened by more frequent side effects, such as irregular vaginal bleeding and weight gain; furthermore, they must be taken at the same time each day to ensure stable serum levels [59]. Depot medroxyprogesterone acetate (DMPA) allows reaching more stable serum levels through intramuscular or subcutaneous injection every 3 months. Unlike other progestin methods, DMPA suppresses ovulation and may cause reversible bone loss. Therefore, in patients with a history of fragility fracture, overt osteoporosis, or strong risk factors for osteoporosis (such as long-term corticosteroid use), use of DMPA is generally contraindicated [60]. The risk for thromboembolism with progestin-only contraceptives is lower than that for combined HCs, but is still present [61].

Levonorgestrel is contained in some intrauterine devices (IUD). Levonorgestrel-containing IUD generally reduce dysmenorrhea and menstrual bleeding. The progestin effect of the levonorgestrel-IUD is mainly local, with only a small proportion of patients reporting systemic side effects [62].

Emergency contraception is widely available to prevent unwanted pregnancy after unprotected intercourses. Rheumatic diseases, cardiovascular diseases, and thrombophilia are not contraindications to the use of emergency contraception [63].

Susceptibility to Autoimmunity

The use of combined HCs as a risk for the development of RA is controversial, with studies showing no or a protective effect [64–68], whereas in a case-control study in patients positive for antibodies to citrullinated proteins, an increased risk was observed [69].

Regarding SLE, a significantly increased risk for development was shown for "ever use" of combined HCs in two studies [70,71], for current use in one study [72] and for past use in one study [70]. None of the studies showed a decreased risk.

As far as other ADs are concerned, in inflammatory bowel diseases (IBDs), current use of HCs is associated with an increased risk of developing Crohn's disease (CD), but not ulcerative colitis (UC) [73]. None of the primary studies showed a significantly decreased risk; one meta-analysis gave a significantly increased risk for "ever use" of combined HCs for CD [74]. The risk of developing IBDs with HRT use in menopausal patients is still debated [75]. For MS, data are controversial with significantly increased risk for the development of MS observed with current or past use of HCs in several studies [76,77] and a delayed onset of MS in HC users observed in others [78,79]. In autoimmune thyroid diseases, the use of HCs seems to play a protective role on the development of Graves' disease but not on Hashimoto's disease [80], and the use of HRT is not linked to subclinical hypothyroidism or the presence of anti-thyroperoxidase (TPO) antibodies [81].

Risk of Disease Flare

Another aspect to be considered in patients with ADs taking HCs is the risk of disease flare.

Despite the risk of disease flare or of thrombotic events, the effective contraception provided by HCs is often required in patients with systemic ADs treated with disease-modifying drugs with teratogenic potential.

Studies have been performed evaluating whether the use of HCs impacts on the clinical course of RA but failed to show the marked positive effects typically observed during pregnancy [82,83]. Reports on the risk of disease flare-ups in SLE women treated with HCs and HRT are conflicting [84–88]. Several reports have suggested that combined HCs may induce flares of SLE [89–91] and a multicenter survey has reported mild musculoskeletal disease flares [84]. Actually, two well-designed randomized clinical trials (RCTs) found no differences in disease activity or incidence of severe flares [92,93]. However, subjects included in the RCTs had clinically inactive or stable active SLE and were negative for aPL, and therefore, results should be interpreted with caution and not extrapolated for all SLE patients. Progestin-only contraceptives and HRT in postmenopausal women do not seem to be associated with disease flares in SLE [94]. Based on this background, the management of contraception in SLE and aPL syndrome (APS) is particularly complex and should be tailored to a given patient with a detailed counseling. The European League Against Rheumatism (EULAR) developed evidence-based recommendations on the management of family planning and women's health issues in SLE and/or APS [95].

As far as other ADs are concerned, evidence suggests that HCs do not negatively affect MS disease course [96–98] and two retrospective cohort studies suggest even a positive effect on disease progression [96,98].

Thrombotic Effects of Hormonal Contraception

Both estrogen and progestin components contribute to increased thrombotic risk. The overall risk of VTE in women on current combined HCs is increased by a factor of 3–5 from the baseline annual risk in healthy women of 1 in 10,000 [99]. Nonoral preparations may confer higher risk than some of the oral preparations [100]. Thrombotic risk is higher during the first year of use and is influenced by other thrombophilic factors such as smoking, age greater than 35 years, obesity, and genetic and acquired thrombophilia including aPL positivity [101]. Therefore, it is of paramount importance that all SLE patients are screened for aPL before starting combined HCs [102]. The earlier combined HCs were burdened by the highest relative risk. Currently, the lower estrogen content of HCs has reduced the risk of oral preparations, whereas the type of progestin now accounts for most of the variability in VTE risk among different combined HCs. Third-generation progestins confer greater risk than second-generation progestins do because of a greater activated protein C resistance [103]. Arterial thrombosis risk is also increased with combined HC use. The risk of MI and ischemic strokes is increased twofold and depends on the presence of additional risk factors such as older age, smoking, hypertension, diabetes mellitus, hyperlipidemia, and obesity [104,105]. The likelihood of stroke associated with use of third-generation progestins is no higher than that associated with second-generation progestins and may be slightly lower [106]. In patients with positivity for aPL, progestin-only pill may be considered, as it carries a lower thromboembolic risk compared to combined HCs [58].

A similar thrombotic risk profile has been reported by several studies conducted in postmenopausal SLE patients taking HRT [107,108]. Therefore, risks and benefits from HRT should be discussed with each patient on an individual basis.

Each patient with SLE or APS should be evaluated for individual risk factors—such as hypertension, overweight, smoke, family history of hormone-dependent cancers—and disease-related risk factors, particularly disease activity and thrombotic risk, including the aPL profile (single vs. double/triple positivity, presence of lupus anticoagulant) or previous vascular APS manifestations [95].

EPIGENETIC INFLUENCE ON SEX DISPARITIES IN AUTOIMMUNE DISEASES: THE EXAMPLE OF SLE AND RA

Against a simplified hypothesis of a prevalent influence of hormones or of genetics on the greater prevalence of ADs in females, many studies have highlighted the importance of epigenetic-related mechanisms in the pathogenesis of ADs [109–113]. Epigenetics is the discipline that studies heritable changes in gene expression that are not due to alteration of the DNA sequence. Epigenetic mechanisms regulate multiple aspects of chromatin structure and function, including the regulation of transcriptionally repressive and permissive configurations for gene expression. In particular, epigenetic modifications may represent the link between genetic and environmental factors influencing the development and the course of ADs [109,114].

Striking examples of this complex interaction of factors are SLE and RA. SLE is a chronic relapsing-remitting AD affecting several organs. SLE is a typical female disease, with peak disease prevalence between menarche and menopause. Its genetic background is not yet fully understood, but epigenetic modulation is emerging as an important mechanism to understand how the susceptibility genes for SLE may interact with environmental factors to cause a full-blown disease. The rate of concordance in monozygotic twins is up to 40% supporting this thesis, and suggesting that environmental and epigenetic factors, as well as genetic–epigenetic interaction, play a critical role in the susceptibility for SLE. For all these reasons SLE can be considered a well-supported example for gender studies.

There is evidence that the balance between estrogen and progesterone may account for the female prevalence and for the disease flares during pregnancy and chronic estrogen exposure in SLE. However, oral contraceptives containing low-dose estrogen, progesterone, or both and HRT in older patients with milder disease did not show a significant increase in disease flares. These results suggest that sex hormones alone cannot explain the female predominance of SLE, indicating that other gender-associated factors contribute to the higher female prevalence [7,115].

DNA methylation, histone modification, and altered micro-RNA (miRNA) profiling are widely accepted as the key epigenetic mechanisms with a critical role in SLE. Table 19.2 shows the main epigenetic mechanisms and their evidence in the development of SLE. Although differences in DNA methylation, histone modifications, and miRNA profiling were found between SLE patients and normal subjects, the specificity of these findings, in comparison with nonlupus systemic ADs, has not been addressed in a systematic way [116].

Lupus patients display impaired DNA methylation on the inactive X-chromosome; as a consequence, reactivation of genes typically suppressed on the inactive X-chromosomes of female lupus patients was suggested to contribute to the

TABLE 19.2 Main Epigenetic Mechanisms in Systemic Lupus Erythematosus (SLE) [95]

SLE Mechanism	Evidence
DNA methylation	• DNA hypomethylation in SLE CD4+ T cells • UV- and drug-induced DNA hypomethylation • DNA hypomethylation correlates with disease activity
Histone modifications including methylation and acetylation/deacetylation	• Global H3/H4 hypoacetylation in SLE CD4+ T cells • Abnormal histone acetylation close to IL-17 locus
miRNA regulation	• Abnormal miRNA profile in PBMC in CD4+ T cells in plasma and kidney from SLE patients

miRNA, micro-RNA; *PBMC*, peripheral blood mononuclear cells; *SLE*, systemic lupus erythematosus; *UV*, ultraviolet radiations.

female predominance of SLE [117]. Further evidence for the role of the naturally inactivated sex chromosome in SLE susceptibility comes from the observation that SLE is much more frequent in Klinefelter's syndrome, a genetic disorder that occurs in men who have an extra X chromosome [118].

The different epigenetic mechanisms may interact with each other [119]. For example, the transcription factor cyclic adenosine monophosphate (cAMP) responsive element modulator (CREM) α downregulates IL-2 expression in T cells from SLE patients through both histone deacetylation and CpG-DNA methylation [120]. Comparable interaction was also reported for some miRNAs, which target DNA methyltransferase (DNMT)1 directly or indirectly through the modulation of extracellular signal–regulated kinases signaling [121,122].

There are limited data on genetic influences on sex disparities in RA. In contrast to SLE, RA has been described very rarely in patients with Klinefelter's syndrome, suggesting that the extra X chromosome does not confer an added risk for RA. One study showed an association between RA and single-nucleotide polymorphisms of the X-encoded genes of tissue inhibitors of metalloproteinase 1, which inhibits matrix metalloproteinases and prevents cartilage degradation, and IL-9 receptor (IL9R), which is involved in IL-9 signaling and in early T cell development. Moreover, the IL9R polymorphism was significantly more common among males compared with females with RA. In a cohort of patients with SLE or RA and their parents, there was no association between maternal or paternal history of disease and patient sex, suggesting that transmission of the X chromosome from mother versus father is unlikely to account for sex differences in disease prevalence [123,124].

Alterations in DNA methylation, histone modifications, and miRNA expression have been also found both in immune and in stromal cells of RA patients. These changes in the epigenome in RA patients influence key inflammatory and matrix-degrading pathways and are suspected to play a major role in the pathogenesis of RA. Methylation signatures of fibroblast-like synoviocytes distinguish not only RA from osteoarthritis but also early RA from late RA or juvenile idiopathic arthritis. Methylation patterns are also specific to individual joint locations, which might explain the distribution of joint involvement in some rheumatic diseases [125].

The examples of SLE and RA show that sex differences in ADs result from a complex interaction of hormonal, genetic, and epigenetic factors. Further insight into how epigenetic modifications are involved in the pathogenesis and activity of ADs will hopefully allow us to understand how various risk factors interact differently in men and in women in the development of ADs.

LIST OF ABBREVIATIONS

ADs Autoimmune diseases
BCR Bromocriptine
CD Crohn's disease
DMPA Depot medroxyprogesterone acetate
ER Estrogen receptor
GH Growth hormone
HCs Hormonal contraceptives
HRT Hormonal replacement therapy
IBD Inflammatory bowel disease
IFN Interferon
IL Interleukin

IUD Intrauterine device
MHC Major histocompatibility complex
MI Myocardial infarction
MS Multiple sclerosis
PR Progesterone receptor
PRL Prolactin
QNG Quinagolide
RA Rheumatoid arthritis
RCT Randomized clinical trial
SLE Systemic lupus erythematosus
TNF Tumor necrosis factor
UC Ulcerative colitis
VTE Venous thromboembolism

REFERENCES

[1] Nalbandian G, Kovats S. Understanding sex biases in immunity: effects of estrogen on the differentiation and function of antigen-presenting cells. Immunol Res 2005;31(2):91–106.

[2] Fish EN. The X-files in immunity: sex-based differences predispose immune responses. Nat Rev Immunol 2008;8(9):737–44.

[3] Young NA, Wu LC, Burd CJ, Friedman AK, Kaffenberger BH, Rajaram MV, et al. Estrogen modulation of endosome-associated toll-like receptor 8: an IFNalpha-independent mechanism of sex-bias in systemic lupus erythematosus. Clin Immunol 2014;151(1):66–77.

[4] McCarthy M. The "gender gap" in autoimmune disease. Lancet 2000;356(9235):1088.

[5] Shen H, Panchanathan R, Rajavelu P, Duan X, Gould KA, Choubey D. Gender-dependent expression of murine Irf5 gene: implications for sex bias in autoimmunity. J Mol Cell Biol 2010;2(5):284–90.

[6] Oertelt-Prigione S. Immunology and the menstrual cycle. Autoimmun Rev 2012;11(6–7):A486–92.

[7] Hughes GC, Choubey D. Modulation of autoimmune rheumatic diseases by oestrogen and progesterone. Nat Rev Rheumatol 2014;10(12):740–51.

[8] Hench PS. Effect of Jaundice on rheumatoid arthritis. Br Med J 1938;2(4050):394–8.

[9] Confavreux C, Hutchinson M, Hours MM, Cortinovis-Tourniaire P, Moreau T. Rate of pregnancy-related relapse in multiple sclerosis. Pregnancy in Multiple Sclerosis Group. N Engl J Med 1998;339(5):285–91.

[10] Jara LJ, Medina G, Cruz-Dominguez P, Navarro C, Vera-Lastra O, Saavedra MA. Risk factors of systemic lupus erythematosus flares during pregnancy. Immunol Res 2014;60(2–3):184–92.

[11] Besedovsky HO, del Rey A. Immune-neuro-endocrine interactions: facts and hypotheses. Endocr Rev 1996;17(1):64–102.

[12] Jara LJ, Navarro C, Medina G, Vera-Lastra O, Blanco F. Immune-neuroendocrine interactions and autoimmune diseases. Clin Dev Immunol 2006;13(2–4):109–23.

[13] Tait AS, Butts CL, Sternberg EM. The role of glucocorticoids and progestins in inflammatory, autoimmune, and infectious disease. J Leukoc Biol 2008;84(4):924–31.

[14] Di Comite G, Grazia Sabbadini M, Corti A, Rovere-Querini P, Manfredi AA. Conversation galante: how the immune and the neuroendocrine systems talk to each other. Autoimmun Rev 2007;7(1):23–9.

[15] Coronel-Restrepo N, Posso-Osorio I, Naranjo-Escobar J, Tobon GJ. Autoimmune diseases and their relation with immunological, neurological and endocrinological axes. Autoimmun Rev 2017;16(7):684–92.

[16] Rubtsova K, Marrack P, Rubtsov AV. Sexual dimorphism in autoimmunity. J Clin Invest 2015;125(6):2187–93.

[17] Cunningham M, Gilkeson G. Estrogen receptors in immunity and autoimmunity. Clin Rev Allergy Immunol 2011;40(1):66–73.

[18] Bouman A, Heineman MJ, Faas MM. Sex hormones and the immune response in humans. Hum Reprod Update 2005;11(4):411–23.

[19] Ackerman LS. Sex hormones and the genesis of autoimmunity. Arch Dermatol 2006;142(3):371–6.

[20] Heldring N, Pike A, Andersson S, Matthews J, Cheng G, Hartman J, et al. Estrogen receptors: how do they signal and what are their targets. Physiol Rev 2007;87(3):905–31.

[21] Hill L, Jeganathan V, Chinnasamy P, Grimaldi C, Diamond B. Differential roles of estrogen receptors alpha and beta in control of B-cell maturation and selection. Mol Med 2011;17(3–4):211–20.

[22] Grimaldi CM, Michael DJ, Diamond B. Cutting edge: expansion and activation of a population of autoreactive marginal zone B cells in a model of estrogen-induced lupus. J Immunol 2001;167(4):1886–90.

[23] Grimaldi CM, Cleary J, Dagtas AS, Moussai D, Diamond B. Estrogen alters thresholds for B cell apoptosis and activation. J Clin Invest 2002;109(12):1625–33.

[24] Venkatesh J, Peeva E, Xu X, Diamond B. Cutting Edge: hormonal milieu, not antigenic specificity, determines the mature phenotype of autoreactive B cells. J Immunol 2006;176(6):3311–4.

[25] Verthelyi D. Sex hormones as immunomodulators in health and disease. Int Immunopharmacol 2001;1(6):983–93.

[26] Pauklin S, Sernandez IV, Bachmann G, Ramiro AR, Petersen-Mahrt SK. Estrogen directly activates AID transcription and function. J Exp Med 2009;206(1):99–111.

[27] Goodnow CC. Multistep pathogenesis of autoimmune disease. Cell 2007;130(1):25–35.

[28] Grimaldi CM, Hill L, Xu X, Peeva E, Diamond B. Hormonal modulation of B cell development and repertoire selection. Mol Immunol 2005;42(7):811–20.

[29] Zandman-Goddard G, Peeva E, Shoenfeld Y. Gender and autoimmunity. Autoimmun Rev 2007;6(6):366–72.

[30] Pernis AB. Estrogen and CD4+ T cells. Curr Opin Rheumatol 2007;19(5):414–20.

[31] Straub RH. The complex role of estrogens in inflammation. Endocr Rev 2007;28(5):521–74.

[32] Baker ME. Origin and diversification of steroids: co-evolution of enzymes and nuclear receptors. Mol Cell Endocrinol 2011;334(1–2):14–20.

[33] Thomas P. Characteristics of membrane progestin receptor alpha (mPRalpha) and progesterone membrane receptor component 1 (PGMRC1) and their roles in mediating rapid progestin actions. Front Neuroendocrinol 2008;29(2):292–312.

[34] Tan IJ, Peeva E, Zandman-Goddard G. Hormonal modulation of the immune system – a spotlight on the role of progestogens. Autoimmun Rev 2015;14(6):536–42.

[35] Hughes GC. Progesterone and autoimmune disease. Autoimmun Rev 2012;11(6–7):A502–14.

[36] Altuwaijri S, Chuang KH, Lai KP, Lai JJ, Lin HY, Young FM, et al. Susceptibility to autoimmunity and B cell resistance to apoptosis in mice lacking androgen receptor in B cells. Mol Endocrinol 2009;23(4):444–53.

[37] Benten WP, Lieberherr M, Giese G, Wrehlke C, Stamm O, Sekeris CE, et al. Functional testosterone receptors in plasma membranes of T cells. FASEB J 1999;13(1):123–33.

[38] Trigunaite A, Dimo J, Jorgensen TN. Suppressive effects of androgens on the immune system. Cell Immunol 2015;294(2):87–94.

[39] Leite De Moraes MC, Touraine P, Gagnerault MC, Savino W, Kelly PA, Dardenne M. Prolactin receptors and the immune system. Ann Endocrinol (Paris) 1995;56(6):567–70.

[40] Dardenne M, de Moraes Mdo C, Kelly PA, Gagnerault MC. Prolactin receptor expression in human hematopoietic tissues analyzed by flow cytofluorometry. Endocrinology 1994;134(5):2108–14.

[41] Bole-Feysot C, Goffin V, Edery M, Binart N, Kelly PA. Prolactin (PRL) and its receptor: actions, signal transduction pathways and phenotypes observed in PRL receptor knockout mice. Endocr Rev 1998;19(3):225–68.

[42] Krumenacker JS, Buckley DJ, Leff MA, McCormack JT, de Jong G, Gout PW, et al. Prolactin-regulated apoptosis of Nb2 lymphoma cells: pim-1, bcl-2, and bax expression. Endocrine 1998;9(2):163–70.

[43] Buckley AR. Prolactin, a lymphocyte growth and survival factor. Lupus 2001;10(10):684–90.

[44] Matera L, Mori M, Galetto A. Effect of prolactin on the antigen presenting function of monocyte-derived dendritic cells. Lupus 2001;10(10):728–34.

[45] Lahat N, Miller A, Shtiller R, Touby E. Differential effects of prolactin upon activation and differentiation of human B lymphocytes. J Neuroimmunol 1993;47(1):35–40.

[46] Carreno PC, Sacedon R, Jimenez E, Vicente A, Zapata AG. Prolactin affects both survival and differentiation of T-cell progenitors. J Neuroimmunol 2005;160(1–2):135–45.

[47] Adan N, Guzman-Morales J, Ledesma-Colunga MG, Perales-Canales SI, Quintanar-Stephano A, Lopez-Barrera F, et al. Prolactin promotes cartilage survival and attenuates inflammation in inflammatory arthritis. J Clin Invest 2013;123(9):3902–13.

[48] Szawka RE, Ribeiro AB, Leite CM, Helena CV, Franci CR, Anderson GM, et al. Kisspeptin regulates prolactin release through hypothalamic dopaminergic neurons. Endocrinology 2010;151(7):3247–57.

[49] Walker SE, Jacobson JD. Roles of prolactin and gonadotropin-releasing hormone in rheumatic diseases. Rheum Dis Clin N Am 2000;26(4):713–36.

[50] Bissay V, De Klippel N, Herroelen L, Schmedding E, Buisseret T, Ebinger G, et al. Bromocriptine therapy in multiple sclerosis: an open label pilot study. Clin Neuropharmacol 1994;17(5):473–6.

[51] Qian Q, Liuqin L, Hao L, Shiwen Y, Zhongping Z, Dongying C, et al. The effects of bromocriptine on preventing postpartum flare in systemic lupus erythematosus patients from South China. J Immunol Res 2015;2015:316965.

[52] Jara LJ, Cruz-Cruz P, Saavedra MA, Medina G, Garcia-Flores A, Angeles U, et al. Bromocriptine during pregnancy in systemic lupus erythematosus: a pilot clinical trial. Ann N Y Acad Sci 2007;1110:297–304.

[53] McMurray RW, Weidensaul D, Allen SH, Walker SE. Efficacy of bromocriptine in an open label therapeutic trial for systemic lupus erythematosus. J Rheumatol 1995;22(11):2084–91.

[54] Hrycek A, Pochopien-Kenig G, Scieszka J. Selected acute phase proteins and interleukin-6 in systemic lupus erythematosus patients treated with low doses of quinagolide. Autoimmunity 2007;40(3):217–22.

[55] Salesi M, Sadeghihaddadzavareh S, Nasri P, Namdarigharaghani N, Farajzadegan Z, Hajalikhani M. The role of bromocriptine in the treatment of patients with active rheumatoid arthritis. Int J Rheum Dis 2013;16(6):662–6.

[56] Alvarez-Nemegyei J, Cobarrubias-Cobos A, Escalante-Triay F, Sosa-Munoz J, Miranda JM, Jara LJ. Bromocriptine in systemic lupus erythematosus: a double-blind, randomized, placebo-controlled study. Lupus 1998;7(6):414–9.

[57] Petitti DB. Clinical practice. Combination estrogen-progestin oral contraceptives. N Engl J Med 2003;349(15):1443–50.

[58] Lateef A, Petri M. Hormone replacement and contraceptive therapy in autoimmune diseases. J Autoimmun 2012;38(2–3):J170–6.

[59] Lobo RA, Gershenson DM, Lentz GM, Valea FA. Comprehensive gynecology e-book. Elsevier Health Sciences; 2016.

[60] Sammaritano LR. Contraception in patients with rheumatic disease. Rheum Dis Clin N Am 2017;43(2):173–88.

[61] Hennessy S, Berlin JA, Kinman JL, Margolis DJ, Marcus SM, Strom BL. Risk of venous thromboembolism from oral contraceptives containing gestodene and desogestrel versus levonorgestrel: a meta-analysis and formal sensitivity analysis. Contraception 2001;64(2):125–33.

[62] Hidalgo M, Bahamondes L, Perrotti M, Diaz J, Dantas-Monteiro C, Petta C. Bleeding patterns and clinical performance of the levonorgestrel-releasing intrauterine system (Mirena) up to two years. Contraception 2002;65(2):129–32.

[63] Armstrong C. ACOG Recommendations on emergency contraception. Am Fam Physician 2010;82(10):1278.

[64] Reduction in incidence of rheumatoid arthritis associated with oral contraceptives. Royal College of General Practitioners' Oral Contraception Study. Lancet 1978;1(8064):569–71.

[65] Vandenbroucke JP, Valkenburg HA, Boersma JW, Cats A, Festen JJ, Huber-Bruning O, et al. Oral contraceptives and rheumatoid arthritis: further evidence for a preventive effect. Lancet 1982;2(8303):839–42.

[66] Hazes JM, Dijkmans BA, Vandenbroucke JP, De Vries RR, Cats A. Oral contraceptives and rheumatoid arthritis; further evidence for a protective effect independent of duration of pill use. Br J Rheumatol 1989;28(Suppl. 1:34):42–5. discussion.

[67] Doran MF, Crowson CS, O'Fallon WM, Gabriel SE. The effect of oral contraceptives and estrogen replacement therapy on the risk of rheumatoid arthritis: a population based study. J Rheumatol 2004;31(2):207–13.

[68] Adab P, Jiang CQ, Rankin E, Tsang YW, Lam TH, Barlow J, et al. Breastfeeding practice, oral contraceptive use and risk of rheumatoid arthritis among Chinese women: the Guangzhou Biobank Cohort Study. Rheumatology (Oxford) 2014;53(5):860–6.

[69] Pedersen M, Jacobsen S, Klarlund M, Pedersen BV, Wiik A, Wohlfahrt J, et al. Environmental risk factors differ between rheumatoid arthritis with and without auto-antibodies against cyclic citrullinated peptides. Arthritis Res Ther 2006;8(4):R133.

[70] Costenbader KH, Feskanich D, Stampfer MJ, Karlson EW. Reproductive and menopausal factors and risk of systemic lupus erythematosus in women. Arthritis Rheum 2007;56(4):1251–62.

[71] Sanchez-Guerrero J, Karlson EW, Liang MH, Hunter DJ, Speizer FE, Colditz GA. Past use of oral contraceptives and the risk of developing systemic lupus erythematosus. Arthritis Rheum 1997;40(5):804–8.

[72] Bernier MO, Mikaeloff Y, Hudson M, Suissa S. Combined oral contraceptive use and the risk of systemic lupus erythematosus. Arthritis Rheum 2009;61(4):476–81.

[73] Khalili H, Higuchi LM, Ananthakrishnan AN, Richter JM, Feskanich D, Fuchs CS, et al. Oral contraceptives, reproductive factors and risk of inflammatory bowel disease. Gut 2013;62(8):1153–9.

[74] Godet PG, May GR, Sutherland LR. Meta-analysis of the role of oral contraceptive agents in inflammatory bowel disease. Gut 1995;37(5):668–73.

[75] Garcia Rodriguez LA, Gonzalez-Perez A, Johansson S, Wallander MA. Risk factors for inflammatory bowel disease in the general population. Aliment Pharmacol Ther 2005;22(4):309–15.

[76] Hellwig K, Chen LH, Stancyzk FZ, Langer-Gould AM. Oral contraceptives and multiple sclerosis/clinically isolated syndrome susceptibility. PLoS One 2016;11(3):e0149094.

[77] Kotzamani D, Panou T, Mastorodemos V, Tzagournissakis M, Nikolakaki H, Spanaki C, et al. Rising incidence of multiple sclerosis in females associated with urbanization. Neurology 2012;78(22):1728–35.

[78] Nielsen NM, Jorgensen KT, Stenager E, Jensen A, Pedersen BV, Hjalgrim H, et al. Reproductive history and risk of multiple sclerosis. Epidemiology 2011;22(4):546–52.

[79] Magyari M. Role of socio-economic and reproductive factors in the risk of multiple sclerosis. Acta Neurol Scand 2015;132(199):20–3.

[80] Vestergaard P, Rejnmark L, Weeke J, Hoeck HC, Nielsen HK, Rungby J, et al. Smoking as a risk factor for Graves' disease, toxic nodular goiter, and autoimmune hypothyroidism. Thyroid 2002;12(1):69–75.

[81] Massoudi MS, Meilahn EN, Orchard TJ, Foley Jr TP, Kuller LH, Costantino JP, et al. Prevalence of thyroid antibodies among healthy middle-aged women. Findings from the thyroid study in healthy women. Ann Epidemiol 1995;5(3):229–33.

[82] Bijlsma JW, Huber-Bruning O, Thijssen JH. Effect of oestrogen treatment on clinical and laboratory manifestations of rheumatoid arthritis. Ann Rheum Dis 1987;46(10):777–9.

[83] Camacho EM, Lunt M, Farragher TM, Verstappen SM, Bunn DK, Symmons DP. The relationship between oral contraceptive use and functional outcome in women with recent-onset inflammatory polyarthritis: results from the Norfolk Arthritis Register. Arthritis Rheum 2011;63(8):2183–91.

[84] Buyon JP, Kalunian KC, Skovron ML, Petri M, Lahita R, Merrill J, et al. Can women with systemic lupus erythematosus safely use exogenous estrogens? J Clin Rheumatol 1995;1(4):205–12.

[85] Julkunen H. Hormone replacement therapy in women with rheumatic diseases. Scand J Rheumatol 2000;29(3):146–53.

[86] Lakasing L, Khamashta M. Contraceptive practices in women with systemic lupus erythematosus and/or antiphospholipid syndrome: what advice should we be giving? J Fam Plan Reprod Health Care 2001;27(1):7–12.

[87] Schwarz EB, Lohr PA. Oral contraceptives in women with systemic lupus erythematosus. N Engl J Med 2006;354(11):1203–4. author reply-4.

[88] Gompel A, Piette JC. Systemic lupus erythematosus and hormone replacement therapy. Menopause Int 2007;13(2):65–70.

[89] Jungers P, Dougados M, Pelissier C, Kuttenn F, Tron F, Lesavre P, et al. Influence of oral contraceptive therapy on the activity of systemic lupus erythematosus. Arthritis Rheum 1982;25(6):618–23.

[90] Julkunen HA, Kaaja R, Friman C. Contraceptive practice in women with systemic lupus erythematosus. Br J Rheumatol 1993;32(3):227–30.

[91] Petri M, Robinson C. Oral contraceptives and systemic lupus erythematosus. Arthritis Rheum 1997;40(5):797–803.

[92] Sanchez-Guerrero J, Uribe AG, Jimenez-Santana L, Mestanza-Peralta M, Lara-Reyes P, Seuc AH, et al. A trial of contraceptive methods in women with systemic lupus erythematosus. N Engl J Med 2005;353(24):2539–49.

[93] Petri M, Kim MY, Kalunian KC, Grossman J, Hahn BH, Sammaritano LR, et al. Combined oral contraceptives in women with systemic lupus erythematosus. N Engl J Med 2005;353(24):2550–8.

[94] Chabbert-Buffet N, Amoura Z, Scarabin PY, Frances C, Levy DP, Galicier L, et al. Pregnane progestin contraception in systemic lupus erythematosus: a longitudinal study of 187 patients. Contraception 2011;83(3):229–37.

[95] Andreoli L, Bertsias GK, Agmon-Levin N, Brown S, Cervera R, Costedoat-Chalumeau N, et al. EULAR recommendations for women's health and the management of family planning, assisted reproduction, pregnancy and menopause in patients with systemic lupus erythematosus and/or antiphospholipid syndrome. Ann Rheum Dis 2017;76(3):476–85.

[96] Gava G, Bartolomei I, Costantino A, Berra M, Venturoli S, Salvi F, et al. Long-term influence of combined oral contraceptive use on the clinical course of relapsing-remitting multiple sclerosis. Fertil Steril 2014;102(1):116–22.

[97] Pozzilli C, De Giglio L, Barletta VT, Marinelli F, Angelis FD, Gallo V, et al. Oral contraceptives combined with interferon beta in multiple sclerosis. Neurol Neuroimmunol Neuroinflamm 2015;2(4):e120.

[98] Sena A, Couderc R, Vasconcelos JC, Ferret-Sena V, Pedrosa R. Oral contraceptive use and clinical outcomes in patients with multiple sclerosis. J Neurol Sci 2012;317(1–2):47–51.

[99] Martinelli I. Risk factors in venous thromboembolism. Thromb Haemost 2001;86(1):395–403.

[100] Stam-Slob MC, Lambalk CB, van de Ree MA. Contraceptive and hormonal treatment options for women with history of venous thromboembolism. BMJ 2015;351:h4847.

[101] Tanis BC, Rosendaal FR. Venous and arterial thrombosis during oral contraceptive use: risks and risk factors. Semin Vasc Med 2003;3(1):69–84.

[102] Urbanus RT, Siegerink B, Roest M, Rosendaal FR, de Groot PG, Algra A. Antiphospholipid antibodies and risk of myocardial infarction and ischaemic stroke in young women in the RATIO study: a case-control study. Lancet Neurol 2009;8(11):998–1005.

[103] van Hylckama Vlieg A, Helmerhorst FM, Vandenbroucke JP, Doggen CJ, Rosendaal FR. The venous thrombotic risk of oral contraceptives, effects of oestrogen dose and progestogen type: results of the MEGA case-control study. BMJ 2009;339:b2921.

[104] Lewis MA, Heinemann LA, Spitzer WO, MacRae KD, Bruppacher R. The use of oral contraceptives and the occurrence of acute myocardial infarction in young women. Results from the Transnational Study on Oral Contraceptives and the Health of Young Women. Contraception 1997;56(3):129–40.

[105] Kemmeren JM, Tanis BC, van den Bosch MA, Bollen EL, Helmerhorst FM, van der Graaf Y, et al. Risk of Arterial Thrombosis in Relation to Oral Contraceptives (RATIO) study: oral contraceptives and the risk of ischemic stroke. Stroke 2002;33(5):1202–8.

[106] Lidegaard O, Lokkegaard E, Jensen A, Skovlund CW, Keiding N. Thrombotic stroke and myocardial infarction with hormonal contraception. N Engl J Med 2012;366(24):2257–66.

[107] Buyon JP, Petri MA, Kim MY, Kalunian KC, Grossman J, Hahn BH, et al. The effect of combined estrogen and progesterone hormone replacement therapy on disease activity in systemic lupus erythematosus: a randomized trial. Ann Intern Med 2005;142(12 Pt 1):953–62.

[108] Sanchez-Guerrero J, Gonzalez-Perez M, Durand-Carbajal M, Lara-Reyes P, Jimenez-Santana L, Romero-Diaz J, et al. Menopause hormonal therapy in women with systemic lupus erythematosus. Arthritis Rheum 2007;56(9):3070–9.

[109] Meda F, Folci M, Baccarelli A, Selmi C. The epigenetics of autoimmunity. Cell Mol Immunol 2011;8(3):226–36.

[110] Pedre X, Mastronardi F, Bruck W, Lopez-Rodas G, Kuhlmann T, Casaccia P. Changed histone acetylation patterns in normal-appearing white matter and early multiple sclerosis lesions. J Neurosci 2011;31(9):3435–45.

[111] Kellermayer R. Epigenetics and the developmental origins of inflammatory bowel diseases. Can J Gastroenterol 2012;26(12):909–15.

[112] Zhang Z, Zhang R. Epigenetics in autoimmune diseases: pathogenesis and prospects for therapy. Autoimmun Rev 2015;14(10):854–63.

[113] Wang B, Shao X, Song R, Xu D, Zhang JA. The emerging role of epigenetics in autoimmune thyroid diseases. Front Immunol 2017;8:396.

[114] Vojdani A, Pollard KM, Campbell AW. Environmental triggers and autoimmunity. Autoimmune Dis 2014;2014:798029.

[115] Schwartzman-Morris J, Putterman C. Gender differences in the pathogenesis and outcome of lupus and of lupus nephritis. Clin Dev Immunol 2012;2012:604892.

[116] Meroni PL, Penatti AE. Epigenetics and systemic lupus erythematosus: unmet needs. Clin Rev Allergy Immunol 2016;50(3):367–76.

[117] Lu Q, Wu A, Tesmer L, Ray D, Yousif N, Richardson B. Demethylation of CD40LG on the inactive X in T cells from women with lupus. J Immunol 2007;179(9):6352–8.

[118] Scofield RH, Bruner GR, Namjou B, Kimberly RP, Ramsey-Goldman R, Petri M, et al. Klinefelter's syndrome (47,XXY) in male systemic lupus erythematosus patients: support for the notion of a gene-dose effect from the X chromosome. Arthritis Rheum 2008;58(8):2511–7.

[119] Richardson BC, Patel DR. Epigenetics in 2013. DNA methylation and miRNA: key roles in systemic autoimmunity. Nat Rev Rheumatol 2014;10(2):72–4.

[120] Rauen T, Hedrich CM, Tenbrock K, Tsokos GC. cAMP responsive element modulator: a critical regulator of cytokine production. Trends Mol Med 2013;19(4):262–9.

[121] Pan W, Zhu S, Yuan M, Cui H, Wang L, Luo X, et al. MicroRNA-21 and microRNA-148a contribute to DNA hypomethylation in lupus CD4+ T cells by directly and indirectly targeting DNA methyltransferase 1. J Immunol 2010;184(12):6773–81.

[122] Zhao TY, Tu J, Wang Y, Cheng DW, Gao XK, Luo H, et al. The efficacy of aspirin in preventing the recurrence of colorectal adenoma: a renewed meta-analysis of randomized trials. Asian Pac J Cancer Prev 2016;17(5):2711–7.

[123] Tedeschi SK, Bermas B, Costenbader KH. Sexual disparities in the incidence and course of SLE and RA. Clin Immunol 2013;149(2):211–8.

[124] Somers EC, Antonsen S, Pedersen L, Sorensen HT. Parental history of lupus and rheumatoid arthritis and risk in offspring in a nationwide cohort study: does sex matter? Ann Rheum Dis 2013;72(4):525–9.

[125] Hammaker D, Firestein GS. Epigenetics of inflammatory arthritis. Curr Opin Rheumatol 2018 Mar;30(2):188–96.

Chapter 20

Human Microbiota and Autoimmune Diseases

Gustavo Resende[1], Jozélio Freire de Carvalho[2,3]

[1]Rheumatology Division, Clinical Hospital, Federal University of Minas Gerais, Belo Horizonte, Brazil; [2]Institute for Health Sciences, Federal University of Bahia, Salvador, Brazil; [3]Rheumatology Division, Aliança Medical Center, Salvador, Brazil

INTRODUCTION

Microbiota is the name given to the set of microorganisms that cohabit a multicellular organism. The concept of human microbiota encompasses unicellular eukaryotic microbes such as fungi and protozoa; prokaryotes such as bacteria and archaea; and even acellular organisms such as viruses. The relations between hosts and microbes are called mutualism, commensalism, or parasitism when they result, respectively, in benefits, indifference, or damage to the host. When this damage is sufficient to alter host homeostasis, the disease state [1] appears. Helminths, although they also establish similar relations with us, are not included in the concept of microbiota because they are much larger multicellular organisms. Microbioma, which is often used as a synonym for microbiota, refers, in a broader sense, to the biological unit made up of the microbiota and the host environment in which it is housed, its habitat [2]. To the genome of this community, it is called metagenome. In the human microbiota, the number of bacteria exceeds that of eukaryotes and archaea by 2–3 orders of magnitude and, therefore, often refers to the bacterial flora as the microbiota [3]. In one of the attempts already made to catalog the human intestinal microbiota, 99% of the sequenced genes were bacteria belonging to approximately 1150 different species, each individual in this cohort harboring at least 160 different species [4]. Historically, it has been estimated that in an adult human body there would be 10 times more cells of microorganisms than human cells. More recently, the review of these calculations establishes this much closer to 1:1 ratio [5]. However, the number of genes in the human metagenome, which exceeds 3 million [4], exceeds the human genome by more than 150 times, with around 20,000 [6].

MICROBIOTA EVALUATION METHODS

Until the emergence of genetic sequencing identification methods, the microbiome composition studies were limited to cell culture–dependent techniques for microbiological identification, thus excluding an expressive proportion (greater than 50% in the case of fecal samples) of noncultivars of the human microbiota [7,8]. With the advent of high-throughput techniques, the decrease in sequencing costs seen in the last decade was inversely proportional to the increase in the number of studies published on the subject [2].

For didatical reasons, the microbiota is classified using method of structural classification, It is possible, for the purpose of didactic, to divide the main processes used for the study of microbiota in methods of structural classification, which aim to determine the taxonomic composition of the flora, and functional classification methods, that seek to define which biological activities this same flora has potential to play (and which actually plays) both locally and systemically [2,9].

Among the structural classification procedures, a strategy called target-directed can be utilized, in which a genetic marker is applied, which preferably must be present on the whole population and be able to distinguish (only and always) species with different genomes. The most commonly used marker is the 16S rRNA gene (the ribosomal RNA gene of the small 16S bacterial ribosome unit) that contains highly conserved phylogenetically and other hypervariable regions. The latter is used to discriminate the genus or species present and their abundance in a given sample. In another approach, called metagenomics, the whole genome of the microbiota (metagenome) is sequenced. Obviously, there are advantages and disadvantages between these tools and the detailed description of their methods goes beyond the scope of this chapter.

Simply put, the target-directed strategy involves the processes of DNA extraction, amplification of the gene of interest (16S rRNA) with specific primers and sequencing of one or more of their hypervariable regions, for later bioinformatic analysis, which ultimately aggregates readings, and representatives of each genus or species found in the sample, depending on the level

Mosaic of Autoimmunity. https://doi.org/10.1016/B978-0-12-814307-0.00020-7

of specificity chosen (97% or 99%, for example). It has already proved robust enough for gender discrimination, but some factors, such as the choice of primers or depth of sequencing, can introduce bias into the results. Already a basic metagenomic protocol includes DNA extraction from the sample, genomic fragmentation, and shotgun sequencing of small fragments, which are then "assembled" and compared with databases of known genes. Although more expensive and less accessible, the metagenome allows to know all the genetic inventories present and, therefore, to infer about its functional potential [7–9].

As for the methods, which allow a functional evaluation, one can also sequence only the expressed part of the metagenome (already transcribed in mRNA), called the transcriptome. For this, the total RNA is extracted from the sample, the rRNA (ribosome) is deleted and not provided functional information, the "purified" mRNA converted to cDNA is converted by reverse transcriptase, and the results are analyzed in a similar manner to metagenomics. The great advantage of this more complex method is the possibility of measuring changes in gene expression occurring in the course of alterations (experimental or otherwise) in the conditions of the microenvironment. More specifically, and with the advantage of excluding posttranscriptional interferences, one can also evaluate the effects of the transcriptome on microbiome metabolism by directly measuring the proteins and metabolites (peptides, oligosaccharides, and lipids) in a sample, composing the proteome and or metabolome, respectively [2,7,8].

An important aspect to be analyzed in the methods of the microbiota studies is the definition of the type of sample used. For example, to study the intestinal microbiome, both fecal specimens and biopsy specimens of the intestinal mucosa could be used, which determines in probably incomparable results because even different microbiomes can be treated. While fecal samples represent the entire microbiota inhabiting the intestinal lumen, samples from mucosal biopsies make only the resident microbiota in close contact with the mucus, epithelium, and local immune system. The same is true for cutaneous microbiome studies, which depend on the collection sites chosen and vary greatly from their findings.

All these details need to be considered when comparing results from different studies and especially when considering to find some pathogenic sense in associations found between disease states and microbiome alterations.

CONSTITUTION OF THE MICROBIOTA

At birth, a human baby begins the process, which will persist throughout his life, colonization by microbes, each of the niches of his body. Although a small prenatal microbial exposure has been revealed, based on the presence of low bacterial load on amniotic fluid, cord blood, and meconium, massive and rapid population of the skin, digestive, respiratory, and genitourinary tracts will occur only after birth, giving rise to very different microbiomes [10]. Several factors influence how this happens in each of these sites. Conditions such as gestational age at birth; the delivery route and whether or not the hospital was delivered; if there was breastfeeding and how long it was kept; the age at which other diets were introduced and what these diets were; and the use of antibiotics and immunizations play a relevant role in this dynamic process [9]. By the end of the second year of life, this microbiota becomes less variable, already assuming a pattern similar to that of the adult individual [11–13]. During these first 2 years of life, as a general rule, there is an increase in alpha diversity or variety of species in the same individual. At the same time, there is a reduction of the beta diversity or the distinction between microbiotas of different individuals [14].

In 2011, the discovery of three "enterotypes," which are groupings of genus found in the intestinal flora of healthy individuals, was published. Each enterotype had a dominant genus (*Bacteroides*, *Prevotella*, or *Ruminococcus*), indicating that the variability should be distributed in categories and not in a continuum [3]. However, this concept has been challenged, supported by results that suggest a continuous gradient of diversity in the gut and also in other niches and demonstrate how the method of analysis used may affect the identification of "types" [15,16]. Even in adult individuals, small seasonal variations in the microbiota [17,18] can be detected even in a single day [19] and also in response to changes in diet, even after a few days [20]. The use of antibiotics in any age group causes changes in this composition, often transient, returning to patterns of distribution similar to the preantibiotic stage, demonstrating what is called microbiotic resilience. Similarly, the use of immunosuppressants and other immunodepression states also contributes to shaping the microbiota. Especially in the smaller age groups, before the final maturation of the microbiota, these effects are more likely to be permanent, reinforcing the concept of an early, critical "window" of host microbial programming in the postnatal period [9,10]. Some "proofs of concept" of this theory have already been produced: in migration studies among countries with different incidences of asthma [21] and multiple sclerosis (MS) [22,23], the descendants of immigrants have higher frequencies than their progeny, but only when displaced before a certain age (5 years for asthma, 15 years for MS). When displacement occurred above these ages, a protective effect of the original environment was observed. Another data in this same direction are the apparent protective role of breastfeeding in the family prevalence of ankylosing spondylitis, observed in a recent case-control study [24].

Although some attempts have already been made to define what will become a "normal" microbiota, including analysis of several niches of a few hundred healthy people [4,18], this problem still persists without a definitive answer. Therefore, the difficulty of defining rigorously what is its imbalance, called dysbiosis [18,25], persists.

MICROBIOTA AND IMMUNE SYSTEM

Selective pressure throughout evolution favored efficient microbiota compositions both in surviving host defense mechanisms and in offering advantages to this host. In other words, there is an evolutionary tendency to the transformation of parasites into symbionts to minimize conflicts among members of the ecosystem [26]. As an example of benefit to the host, it is possible to emphasize the collaboration of bacteria to digest some macronutrients, with release of energy and/or micronutrients previously inaccessible.

Another advantage is the greater protection or resistance against pathogens, conferred both by direct competition among species and by the modulation of host epithelial and immune responses by the commensal microbiota [26,27]. Contact with intestinal germs plays a critical role in the full development of lymphoid structures, as demonstrated by the absence of isolated lymphoid follicles in the small intestine of germ-free mice. The microbiota also contributes to the balance among T cell subtypes in the intestinal lamina propria. Segmented filamentous bacteria induce Th17 accumulation and to a lesser extent Th1, while certain *Clostridium* species do so with T cells regulators (Treg) [27]. The state of colonization influences the appearance or intensity of some autoimmune conditions. In experimental animal models of arthritis, encephalomyelitis, and enterocolitis, the rule is a marked attenuation of the pathological phenotype in germ-free animals, in which the subsequent microbial exposure can "rescue" the severity of the autoimmune disease [27–30]. Thus, it is reasonable to assume an indirect causal relationship between the contact with the germs and the appearance of autoimmunity in these models because there is only complete development of the immune system through the interaction with the flora. This idea seems as appropriate as interpreting that the symptoms of immune reconstitution inflammatory syndrome in a patient with AIDS and occult opportunistic infection are indirectly caused by antiretroviral therapy through the immune reconstitution it provides.

On the other hand, in an animal model of type 1 diabetes (T1D), animals colonized by microbiota have a lower incidence of T1D when compared with germ-free animals, revealing a protective role of the microbiota [31]. In addition, according to the hypothesis of hygiene, sanitary changes and expansion of the use of antibiotics, with consequent reduction in the frequency of infections, observed mainly in developed countries during the 19th and 20th centuries, have led to an increase in the incidence of allergic and autoimmune diseases, theoretically, by abbreviating exposure to certain microbes, with protective role of autoimmunity, so-called "old friends" [32,33].

DYSBIOSIS AND AUTOIMMUNE DISEASES

Dysbiosis is any loss of the microbial state of equilibrium in a given ecosystem. In the case of the human microbiome, it can be translated by qualitative and/or quantitative perturbations of the commensal species of each site. The rarefaction of once dominant species or the overgrowth of others, usually minority or absent, exemplifies dysbiotic conditions. Several autoimmune and autoinflammatory diseases have been associated with dysbiosis. A summary, with examples of some of these associations, is shown in Table 20.1 (Animal Models) and Table 20.2 (Human Studies).

There is great disagreement between outcomes as to what occurs with alpha diversity in dysbiosis associated with immune-mediated diseases. In the intestinal microbiota studies in MS, the results seem to converge to avoid differences in the diversity of patients in relation to the controls (see Table 20.2); in diseases such as Crohn's and ulcerative colitis, there is a general tendency to loss of diversity (less abundance of species) [4,34]; and in others, such as spondyloarthritis (SpA), systemic lupus erythematosus, and rheumatoid arthritis (RA), the comments are controversial (see Table 20.2). Moreover, the results of studies that assume some pathogenetic role for specific species are even more variable (if not contradictory), which may be partly justified by the small size of the samples used, most of them not exceeding some dozens of participants, and by the fact that the vast majority of studies cited are cross-sectional evaluations, with great limitations on the interpretation of the temporal relations existing between changes in the microbiota and the pathogenesis of said diseases.

Hypothetically, when there is a predominance of species whose modulation on the immune system of the host tends to inflammation and autoimmunity, to the detriment of species that promote immunoregulation and tolerance, there is an environmental pressure that genetically susceptible individuals can influence the appearance or aggravation of autoimmune and autoinflammatory conditions. Other mechanisms have already been proposed to explain possible roles of the microbiome in the etiology of these diseases, such as changes in intestinal permeability, leading to greater translocation of bacteria and toxins, access to the central immune system [35], and molecular mimicry, which could justify the break of self-tolerance in some cases [36].

In some conditions, the causal relationship between the onset of symptoms and an infection (sometimes subclinical) is much better defined, as is the case of reactive arthritis, a subtype of SpA, in which some species of enterobacteria of the genus *Shigella*, *Salmonella*, *Campylobacter*, and *Yersinia* have already been implicated in their epidemiological model of intestinal infection [37] and *Chlamydia trachomatis* in the urogenital [38]. Another example is the well-defined association between periodontal infection and RA, from which accumulating evidence supporting some causality such as patients with RA have periodontal disease more frequently and severely than healthy controls [39–42]. *Porphyromonas gingivalis*

TABLE 20.1 Associations Between Autoimmunity and Dysbiosis in Animal Models

Disease	Used Models	Most Relevant Findings
MS	MOG$_{35-55}$ induced EAE in C57BL6 mice	Improved clinical score (protection) and exchange of a proinflammatory profile for an antiinflammatory reduction of Th1/Th17/IL17 and increase of Treg/IL-10 when raised in a germ-free environment [30,48] and after oral administration of broad-spectrum antibiotics [49–51].
	Spontaneous EAE in SJL mice	
RA	K/BxN mice	Reduction of Th17 in the lamina propria and less severe arthritis when raised under germ-free conditions. Phenotype is restored after introduction of bacteria [29].
	Zymosan-induced arthritis in mice	Fecal samples from RA patients, but not from controls, aggravate arthritis in rats raised in germ-free conditions [52].
	Collagen-induced arthritis (CIA) in mice	Dysbiosis after ATB increase IL17A + cells in mesenteric lymph nodes and worsen signs of arthritis [53]. Infection (prior or concomitant to the induction of arthritis) by *Porphyromonas gingivalis* (orally, subcutaneously, or intraperitoneally) aggravates the signs of arthritis and is associated with higher titers of ACPA and more bone erosion [54–58].
SpA	HLA-B27 and human β2-microglobulin transgenic rats	Absence of intestinal and articular phenotype when raised in a germ-free environment [28]. Development of colitis and arthritis with exposure to conventional flora [59]. HLA-B27tg rats have different cecal microbiota and metabolome of the wild type [60,61]. Increased expression of inflammatory cytokines, antimicrobial peptides, and IgA precedes intestinal inflammation and dysbiosis [62].
	B10.BR (H-2^k) male mice	They do not develop ankylosing disease (ANKENT) in a germ-free environment, but after conventional colonization and with specific species [63,64].
	BALB/c ZAP-70W163C–mutant (SKG) mice injected with *curdlan*	Germ-free conditions attenuate the joint (peripheral and axial) phenotype and suppress ileitis (including ileal expression of IL23 and IL17) [65].

ACPA, anticitrullinated protein antibodies; *EAE*, experimental autoimmune encephalomyelitis; *MS*, multiple sclerosis; *RA*, rheumatoid arthritis; *SpA*, spondyloarthritis.

infection and periodontal inflammation support the development of anticitrullinated protein antibodies [43–45]; levels of anti-Porphyromonas antibodies are detected years before the appearance of RA symptoms [46]; and the nonsurgical treatment (scaling, root planning, and oral hygiene instructions) of periodontal disease improved RA symptoms [47].

However, in other conditions, considering the relationship between microbiota and the bidirectional immune system, the problem that dysbiosis may not be a cause but a consequence of these diseases (its microbial phenotype) still persists without definitive solution.

MICROBIOTA THERAPEUTIC MANIPULATION

Given the large amount of evidence of microbioma participation in various clinical conditions, the manipulation of this ecosystem in favor of the rescue of beneficial functions or the suppression of harmful activities presents itself as an attractive therapeutic alternative. Fig. 20.1 illustrates the main strategies for restoring the structural and functional balance of the intestinal microbiota with potential use in immune-mediated diseases.

Since the use of antibiotics, with the disadvantage of less specificity and possibility of resistance selection, even the use of bacteriophages (viruses with a more restricted tropism) represents, at least theoretically, options to modify the intestinal flora and to bring benefits under conditions of overgrowth or bacterial imbalance. On the other hand, the stimulus to rebalance the microbiome could be tried through nutritional therapy, the use of probiotics (live microorganisms administered in sufficient amounts to bring health benefits), prebiotics (food compounds not digestible by the host, but with a capacity to stimulate the growth of specific members of the microbiota), or symbiotic (probiotics and prebiotics administered simultaneously). Finally, another way to permanently change the diseased microbiota is fecal microbiota transplantation from healthy donors, although it is still an expensive technique (by donor screening costs), poorly available, with a low yield of prolonged grafting and with some risk of infection.

Table 20.3 brings together results from clinical studies in some of the conditions discussed in this chapter. Most of the studies found to date are of poor methodological quality or have not achieved satisfactory results. There are few randomized control trials with sufficient samples that show promising results, evidencing an abyss between the better understanding of the human microbiome's relations with immune-mediated diseases and the therapeutic use of this knowledge.

TABLE 20.2 Changes in Microbiota in Patients Versus Healthy Controls

Disease	Most Relevant Findings
MS	No difference in the abundance (richness) of intestinal microbiota species of patients and controls [66–68]. Qualitative changes in the intestinal microbiota of patients in relation to controls and even between treated and untreated patients, which include increase in the proportion of *Methanobrevibacter* species [68,69] and *Akkermansia* [69,70] and the reduction of *Clostridium* [67,68,71] and *Faecalibacterium* [67,68,70] (both genus belonging to the *Clostridiaceae* family), as well as *Botelloides* species [66,68], *Prevotella* [66,67,69] and *Butyricimonas* [68,69] (the latter belonging to the order *Bacteroidal*)
RA	Relative reduction of *Haemophilus* (negatively correlated with serum autoantibodies) and increase of *Lactobacillus salivarius* in fecal, salivary, and dental samples (plaques) of rheumatoid arthritis patients compared with controls. Changes were partially reversed after treatment [72].
	In patients with early RA (<6 months of symptoms) and without DMARD treatment, statistically fewer *Bacteroides*, *Porphyromonas*, and *Prevotella* (of the order *Bacteroidales*) were observed; *Eubacterium* and *Clostridium* (from the order *Clostridiales*); and *Bifidobacteria* in fecal samples when compared with controls with fibromyalgia [73]. Another study with similar population has already found a relative increase in *Prevotella copri* and reduction in *Bacteroides* [74], with reduced alpha diversity. When only the *Lactobacillus* community was studied, the observed alpha diversity was higher in patients than in controls [75]. Already in alveolar bronchial lavage samples, a lower diversity (similar to patients with sarcoidosis) was also seen when compared with healthy controls. It observed a smaller representation of several genus and greater abundance of *Pseudonocardia* in these samples [76].
SpA	When fecal samples were used, there was a reduction of alpha diversity (richness) in patients with spondyloarthritis compared with controls, in addition to some specific alterations such as reduction of *Bacteroides*, *Prevotella*, and *Clostridium* and increase of *Bifidobacterium* [77,78] and *Ruminococcus* [79]. The latter correlated with disease activity in patients with a history of associated inflammatory bowel disease. Conversely, when mucosal samples (ileal or colonic biopsies) were used, there was an increase in alpha diversity in patients with ankylosing spondylitis [80,81], with qualitative changes including an increase of five families: *Lachnospiraceae*, *Ruminococcaceae*, *Rikenellaceae*, *Porphyromonadaceae*, and *Bacteroidaceae*; and reduction of two families: *Veillonellaceae* and *Prevotellaceae* [81]. There was also a higher frequency of *Dialister* in patients with spondyloarthritis and inflammation of the intestinal mucosa than in controls and patients without inflammation. Their presence was also correlated with the activity of axial joint disease [80].
	In psoriatic disease, considering the skin microbiota, there is no consensus between alpha diversity data [82], while compositional results converge to a reduction of *Propionibacterium* [83–85] and increase of *Streptococcus* [83,85,86]. Regarding the intestinal microbiota, a reduction of *Coprococcus* was found in psoriatic patients with and without arthritis (PsA), whereas a reduction in the *Akkermansia*, *Ruminococcus*, and *Pseudobutyrivibrio* genus was associated only in patients with PsA [87]. In juvenile spondyloarthritis (enthesitis-related arthritis), a study observed in fecal samples lower abundance of *Faecalibacterium* and relative increase of *Akkermansia* and *Bifidobacterium* in relation to healthy controls [88]; another found *Prevotella* reduction and *Bacteroides* increase [89].

DMARD, disease-modifying antirheumatic drugs; *MS*, multiple sclerosis; *RA*, rheumatoid arthritis; *SpA*, spondyloarthritis.

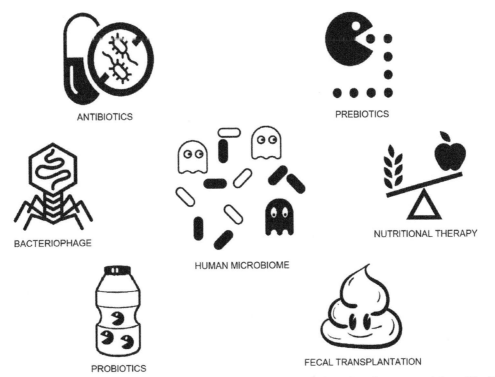

FIGURE 20.1 Potential strategies for therapeutic manipulation of the microbiome. *EAE*, experimental autoimmune encephalomyelitis; *MS*, multiple sclerosis; *RA*, rheumatoid arthritis; *SpA*, spondyloarthritis. (*Illustration modified by the author from icons of authorship of IQON, Martin Jasinski, Omar Vargas, Viktor Vorobyev, Shmidt Sergey, Ralf Schmitzer, Thomas Helbig, Andreas Flores and Parkjisun, published by Noun project (https://thenounproject.com/).*)

TABLE 20.3 Clinical Trials With Manipulation of the Microbiota in Immune-Mediated Diseases

Disease	Trial, Number of Participants	Type of Probiotics, Dosage	Outcomes
JIA	Noncontrolled, N=10 [90]	Probiotics—*Lactobacillus rhamnosus* GG, daily for 14 days	No clinically beneficial effect.
RA	RCT, N=109, placebo=110 [91,92]	Antibiotics—oral minocycline 200 mg daily for 48 weeks	Significant differences in tender/swelling joint counts, ESR and RF levels at week 48. But no differences in radiographic progression at week 104.
	RCT, N=44, Placebo=22 [93]	Antibiotics—oral doxycycline 20 mg, 100 mg or placebo twice daily with MTX, for 2 years	Significant difference in ACR50 response, without differences between doses.
	RCT, N=8, placebo=13 [94]	Probiotics—*L. rhamnosus* GG, twice daily for 12 months	No significant differences.
	RCT, N=22, placebo=22 [95]	Probiotics—*Bacillus coagulans*, daily for 60 days	No significant differences.
	RCT, N=15, placebo=11 [96]	Probiotics—*L. rhamnosus*, *Lactobacillus reuteri*, twice daily for 12 weeks	No significant differences.
	RCT, N=22, placebo=24 [97]	Probiotics—*Lactobacillus casei*, maltodextrin, daily for 8 weeks	Significant decreases in serum CRP, IL-12, TNF-α, tender/swollen joints counts, DAS28 score and significant increase in serum IL-10.
	RCT, N=30, placebo=30 [98]	Probiotics—*L. casei*, *Lactobacillus acidophilus*, *Bifidobacterium bifidum* daily for 8 weeks	Significant decreases in serum CRP, insulin levels, and DAS28 score.
	Noncontrolled, N=24 [99]	Vegan, low-fat diet, ad libitum for 4 weeks	Significant decrease in patient pain VAS and tender/swollen joints counts. No significant differences in ESR, CRP, and RF levels.
	Nonrandomized, N=75, controls=55 [100]	Mediterranean diet for 6 months	No significant changes in ESR, CRP, or IL-6 levels; significant improvement in global patient and pain assessments.
	Single-blinded, N=29, controls=27 [101]	Mediterranean diet or standard hospital meals for 3 weeks and then Mediterranean diet for 9 weeks	Significant decrease in serum CRP, swollen joint counts, DAS28 score, HAQ, patient pain VAS.
	Nonrandomized, fasting, N=22 Mediterranean, N=28 [102]	2 Weeks Mediterranean diet or fasting (calorie restriction)	No change in CRP, decrease in DAS28 score in both groups.
SpA	RCT, N=32, placebo=31 [103]	Probiotics—*Streptococcus salivarius*, *Bifidobacterium lactis*, *L. acidophilus* twice daily for 12 weeks	No significant differences.
	RCT, N=65, placebo=69 [104]	Probiotics—*Lactobacillus* spp., *Bifidobacterium* spp. daily for 12 weeks	No significant differences.

TABLE 20.3 Clinical Trials With Manipulation of the Microbiota in Immune-Mediated Diseases—cont'd

Disease	Trial, Number of Participants	Type of Probiotics, Dosage	Outcomes
IBD	Nonrandomized, open-label, N=30, controls=30 (UC) [105]	Probiotic—*L. salivarius*, *L. acidophilus*, *Bifidobacterium bifidus*, and mesalazine 1200 mg daily for 2 years	Significant decrease in modified Mayo index from 6 months to 2 years.
	RCT, N=28, placebo=28 (UC) [106]	Probiotic—*Bifidobacterium longum* (BB536) for 8 weeks	Significant differences between groups in decrease of UCDAI and endoscopic index, but no significant differences in remission rates at week 8.
	RCT, N=20, placebo=20 (pediatric UC) [107]	Probiotics—rectal enema of *L. reuteri* ATCC 55730 for 8 weeks	Significant differences between groups in decrease of Mayo score, histological score, IL-1β, TNF-α, and IL-8 mucosal levels and increase in IL-10 at week 8.
	RCT, N=59, placebo=60 (CD after ileocolonic resection and re-anastomosis) [108]	Probiotics—*Lactobacillus*, *Bifidobacterium*, *S. salivarius* (VSL#3) for 90 days	No clinical differences.
	RCT, N=80, placebo=79 (CD under remission) [109]	Probiotics—*Saccharomyces boulardii* (1 g/day) for 52 weeks	No significant differences in remission rates, time to relapse and CDAI.
	RCT, N=54, placebo=49 (CD) [110]	Prebiotics—fructooligosaccharides for 4 weeks	No clinical benefit.
	Noncontrolled, N=30 (UC) [111]	FMT by colonoscopic administration (500 mL into terminal ileum)	13 of the 30 (43.3%) patients achieved clinical and endoscopic remission at the week 12.
	Noncontrolled, N=41 (UC) [112]	FMT by colonoscopic administration	Significant decrease in full Mayo score, Mayo clinical score, but not in Mayo endoscopic score at week 8. No patient achieved clinical remission.
	Noncontrolled, N=7 (UC) [113]	FMT by colonoscopic administration	One of five patients achieved 50% donor similarity at week 4. One patient (40% donor similarity) achieved clinical and histologic remission at day 30, lost at day 60–90. No patients remained in remission at 3 months.
	RCT, N=38, placebo=37 (UC) [114]	FMT by colonoscopic administration (50 mL once weekly for 6 weeks)	Significant difference in remission at week 7. No difference in adverse events. Significant greater microbial diversity in FMT group than placebo.
	RCT, N=23, controls (autologous FMT)=25 [115]	FMT by nasoduodenal tube at weeks 0 and 3	No significant difference in clinical and endoscopic remission at week 12.
	Open-label, N=9 (pediatric CD) [116]	FMT by nasogastric tube	Engraftment in seven of nine patients. Five of nine patients who did not receive additional medical therapy were in remission at week 12.
	Open-label, N=4 (pediatric UC) [117]	FMT by nasogastric tube	No clinical or laboratory benefit at week 12.

CD, Crohn's disease; *CRP*, C-reactive protein; *ESR*, erythrocyte sedimentation rate; *FMT*, fecal microbiota transplantation; *IBD*, inflammatory bowel disease; *IPAA*, ileal pouch–anal anastomosis; *JIA*, juvenile idiopathic arthritis; *RA*, rheumatoid arthritis; *RCT*, randomized control trials; *SpA*, spondyloarthritis; *UC*, ulcerative colitis; *VAS*, visual analogue scale.

REFERENCES

[1] Casadevall A, Pirofski LA. What is a host? Incorporating the microbiota into the damage-response framework. Infect Immun 2015;83(1):2–7.

[2] Young VB. The role of the microbiome in human health and disease: an introduction for clinicians. BMJ 2017;356. j831.

[3] Arumugam M, Raes J, Pelletier E, Le Paslier D, Yamada T, Mende DR, et al. Enterotypes of the human gut microbiome. Nature 2011;473(7346):174–80.

[4] Qin J, Li R, Raes J, Arumugam M, Burgdorf KS, Manichanh C, et al. A human gut microbial gene catalogue established by metagenomic sequencing. Nature 2010;464(7285):59–65.

[5] Sender R, Fuchs S, Milo R. Are we really vastly outnumbered? Revisiting the ratio of bacterial to host cells in humans. Cell 2016;164(3):337–40.

[6] Ezkurdia I, Juan D, Rodriguez JM, Frankish A, Diekhans M, Harrow J, et al. Multiple evidence strands suggest that there may be as few as 19,000 human protein-coding genes. Hum Mol Genet 2014;23(22):5866–78.

[7] Morgan XC, Huttenhower C. Chapter 12: human microbiome analysis. PLoS Comput Biol 2012;8(12):e1002808.

[8] Lawley B, Tannock GW. Nucleic acid-based methods to assess the composition and function of the bowel microbiota. Gastroenterol Clin N Am 2012;41(4):855–68.

[9] Arrieta M-C, Stiemsma LT, Amenyogbe N, Brown EM, Finlay B. The intestinal microbiome in early life: health and disease. Front Immunol 2014;5(427).

[10] Nogacka AM, Salazar N, Arboleya S, Suarez M, Fernandez N, Solis G, et al. Early microbiota, antibiotics and health. Cell Mol Life Sci 2018;75(1):83–91.

[11] Palmer C, Bik EM, DiGiulio DB, Relman DA, Brown PO. Development of the human infant intestinal microbiota. PLoS Biol 2007;5(7):e177.

[12] Dominguez-Bello MG, Costello EK, Contreras M, Magris M, Hidalgo G, Fierer N, et al. Delivery mode shapes the acquisition and structure of the initial microbiota across multiple body habitats in newborns. Proc Natl Acad Sci USA 2010;107(26):11971–5.

[13] Kostic AD, Gevers D, Siljander H, Vatanen T, Hyotylainen T, Hamalainen AM, et al. The dynamics of the human infant gut microbiome in development and in progression toward type 1 diabetes. Cell Host Microbe 2015;17(2):260–73.

[14] Backhed F, Roswall J, Peng Y, Feng Q, Jia H, Kovatcheva-Datchary P, et al. Dynamics and stabilization of the human gut microbiome during the first year of life. Cell Host Microbe 2015;17(5):690–703.

[15] Koren O, Knights D, Gonzalez A, Waldron L, Segata N, Knight R, et al. A guide to enterotypes across the human body: meta-analysis of microbial community structures in human microbiome datasets. PLoS Comput Biol 2013;9(1):e1002863.

[16] Knights D, Ward TL, McKinlay CE, Miller H, Gonzalez A, McDonald D, et al. Rethinking "enterotypes". Cell Host Microbe 2014;16(4):433–7.

[17] Costello EK, Lauber CL, Hamady M, Fierer N, Gordon JI, Knight R. Bacterial community variation in human body habitats across space and time. Science 2009;326(5960):1694–7.

[18] Human Microbiome Project C. Structure, function and diversity of the healthy human microbiome. Nature 2012;486(7402):207–14.

[19] Thaiss CA, Levy M, Korem T, Dohnalova L, Shapiro H, Jaitin DA, et al. Microbiota diurnal rhythmicity programs host transcriptome oscillations. Cell 2016;167(6):1495–510. e12.

[20] Wu GD, Chen J, Hoffmann C, Bittinger K, Chen YY, Keilbaugh SA, et al. Linking long-term dietary patterns with gut microbial enterotypes. Science 2011;334(6052):105–8.

[21] Kuehni CE, Strippoli MP, Low N, Silverman M. Asthma in young south Asian women living in the United Kingdom: the importance of early life. Clin Exp Allergy J Br Soc Allergy Clin Immunol 2007;37(1):47–53.

[22] Dean G, Elian M. Age at immigration to England of Asian and Caribbean immigrants and the risk of developing multiple sclerosis. J Neurol Neurosurgery Psychiatry 1997;63(5):565–8.

[23] Gale CR, Martyn CN. Migrant studies in multiple sclerosis. Prog Neurobiol 1995;47(4–5):425–48.

[24] Montoya J, Matta NB, Suchon P, Guzian MC, Lambert NC, Mattei JP, et al. Patients with ankylosing spondylitis have been breast fed less often than healthy controls: a case-control retrospective study. Ann Rheum Dis 2016;75(5):879–82.

[25] Hanage WP. Microbiology: microbiome science needs a healthy dose of scepticism. Nature 2014;512(7514):247–8.

[26] Costello EK, Stagaman K, Dethlefsen L, Bohannan BJ, Relman DA. The application of ecological theory toward an understanding of the human microbiome. Science 2012;336(6086):1255–62.

[27] Hooper LV, Littman DR, Macpherson AJ. Interactions between the microbiota and the immune system. Science 2012;336:1268–73.

[28] Taurog JD, Richardson JA, Croft JT, Simmons WA, Zhou M, Fernández-Sueiro JL, et al. The germfree state prevents development of gut and joint inflammatory disease in HLA-B27 transgenic rats. J Exp Med 1994;180:2359–64.

[29] Wu HJ, Ivanov II, Darce J, Hattori K, Shima T, Umesaki Y, et al. Gut-residing segmented filamentous bacteria drive autoimmune arthritis via T helper 17 cells. Immunity 2010;32(6):815–27.

[30] Lee YK, Menezes JS, Umesaki Y, Mazmanian SK. Proinflammatory T-cell responses to gut microbiota promote experimental autoimmune encephalomyelitis. Proc Natl Acad Sci USA 2011;108(Suppl. 1):4615–22.

[31] King C, Sarvetnick N. The incidence of type-1 diabetes in NOD mice is modulated by restricted flora not germ-free conditions. PLoS One 2011;6(2):e17049.

[32] Dunne DW, Cooke A. A worm's eye view of the immune system: consequences for evolution of human autoimmune disease. Nat Rev Immunol 2005;5(5):420–6.

[33] Bach JF. The hygiene hypothesis in autoimmunity: the role of pathogens and commensals. Nat Rev Immunol 2018;18(2):105–20.

[34] Huttenhower C, Kostic Aleksandar D, Xavier Ramnik J. Inflammatory bowel disease as a model for translating the microbiome. Immunity 2014;40(6):843–854. https://doi.org/10.1016/j.immuni.2014.05.013. Review. PubMed PMID: 24950204; PubMed Central PMCID: PMC4135443.

[35] Mu Q, Kirby J, Reilly CM, Luo XM. Leaky gut as a danger signal for autoimmune diseases. Front Immunol 2017;8:598.

[36] Pianta A, Arvikar SL, Strle K, Drouin EE, Wang Q, Costello CE, et al. Two rheumatoid arthritis-specific autoantigens correlate microbial immunity with autoimmune responses in joints. J Clin Investig 2017;127(8):2946–56.

[37] Hill Gaston JS, Lillicrap MS. Arthritis associated with enteric infection. Best Pract Res Clin Rheumatol 2003;17(2):219–39.

[38] Zeidler H, Kuipers J, Kohler L. Chlamydia-induced arthritis. Curr Opin Rheumatol 2004;16(4):380–92.

[39] Mikuls TR, Payne JB, Yu F, Thiele GM, Reynolds RJ, Cannon GW, et al. Periodontitis and Porphyromonas gingivalis in patients with rheumatoid arthritis. Arthritis Rheumatol 2014;66(5):1090–100.

[40] Kharlamova N, Jiang X, Sherina N, Potempa B, Israelsson L, Quirke AM, et al. Antibodies to Porphyromonas gingivalis indicate interaction between oral infection, smoking, and risk genes in rheumatoid arthritis etiology. Arthritis Rheumatol 2016;68(3):604–13.

[41] Schmickler J, Rupprecht A, Patschan S, Patschan D, Muller GA, Haak R, et al. Cross-sectional evaluation of periodontal status and microbiologic and rheumatoid parameters in a large cohort of patients with rheumatoid arthritis. J Periodontol 2017;88(4):368–79.

[42] Ayravainen L, Leirisalo-Repo M, Kuuliala A, Ahola K, Koivuniemi R, Meurman JH, et al. Periodontitis in early and chronic rheumatoid arthritis: a prospective follow-up study in Finnish population. BMJ Open 2017;7(1):e011916.

[43] Shimada A, Kobayashi T, Ito S, Okada M, Murasawa A, Nakazono K, et al. Expression of anti-Porphyromonas gingivalis peptidylarginine deiminase immunoglobulin G and peptidylarginine deiminase-4 in patients with rheumatoid arthritis and periodontitis. J Periodontal Res 2016;51(1):103–11.

[44] Bello-Gualtero JM, Lafaurie GI, Hoyos LX, Castillo DM, De-Avila J, Munevar JC, et al. Periodontal disease in individuals with a genetic risk of developing arthritis and early rheumatoid arthritis: a cross-sectional study. J Periodontol 2016;87(4):346–56.

[45] Terao C, Asai K, Hashimoto M, Yamazaki T, Ohmura K, Yamaguchi A, et al. Significant association of periodontal disease with anti-citrullinated peptide antibody in a Japanese healthy population - the Nagahama study. J Autoimmun 2015;59:85–90.

[46] Johansson L, Sherina N, Kharlamova N, Potempa B, Larsson B, Israelsson L, et al. Concentration of antibodies against Porphyromonas gingivalis is increased before the onset of symptoms of rheumatoid arthritis. Arthritis Res Ther 2016;18.201.

[47] Khare N, Vanza B, Sagar D, Saurav K, Chauhan R, Mishra S. Nonsurgical periodontal therapy decreases the severity of rheumatoid arthritis: a case-control study. J Contemp Dent Pract 2016;17(6):484–8.

[48] Berer K, Mues M, Koutrolos M, Rasbi ZA, Boziki M, Johner C, et al. Commensal microbiota and myelin autoantigen cooperate to trigger autoimmune demyelination. Nature 2011;479(7374):538–41.

[49] Yokote H, Miyake S, Croxford JL, Oki S, Mizusawa H, Yamamura T. NKT cell-dependent amelioration of a mouse model of multiple sclerosis by altering gut flora. Am J Pathol 2008;173(6):1714–23.

[50] Ochoa-Reparaz J, Mielcarz DW, Ditrio LE, Burroughs AR, Foureau DM, Haque-Begum S, et al. Role of gut commensal microflora in the development of experimental autoimmune encephalomyelitis. J Immunol 2009;183(10):6041–50.

[51] Ochoa-Reparaz J, Mielcarz DW, Haque-Begum S, Kasper LH. Induction of a regulatory B cell population in experimental allergic encephalomyelitis by alteration of the gut commensal microflora. Gut Microbes 2010;1(2):103–8.

[52] Maeda Y, Kurakawa T, Umemoto E, Motooka D, Ito Y, Gotoh K, et al. Dysbiosis contributes to arthritis development via activation of autoreactive T cells in the intestine. Arthritis Rheumatol 2016;68(11):2646–61.

[53] Dorozynska I, Majewska-Szczepanik M, Marcinska K, Szczepanik M. Partial depletion of natural gut flora by antibiotic aggravates collagen induced arthritis (CIA) in mice. Pharmacol Rep 2014;66(2):250–5.

[54] Maresz KJ, Hellvard A, Sroka A, Adamowicz K, Bielecka E, Koziel J, et al. Porphyromonas gingivalis facilitates the development and progression of destructive arthritis through its unique bacterial peptidylarginine deiminase (PAD). PLoS Pathog 2013;9(9).e1003627.

[55] Marchesan JT, Gerow EA, Schaff R, Taut AD, Shin S-Y, Sugai J, et al. Porphyromonas gingivalis oral infection exacerbates the development and severity of collagen-induced arthritis. Arthritis Res Ther 2013;15(6):R186.

[56] Chukkapalli S, Rivera-Kweh M, Gehlot P, Velsko I, Bhattacharyya I, Calise SJ, et al. Periodontal bacterial colonization in synovial tissues exacerbates collagen-induced arthritis in B10.RIII mice. Arthritis Res Ther 2016;18(1):161.

[57] Sandal I, Karydis A, Luo J, Prislovsky A, Whittington KB, Rosloniec EF, et al. Bone loss and aggravated autoimmune arthritis in HLA-DRβ1-bearing humanized mice following oral challenge with Porphyromonas gingivalis. Arthritis Res Ther 2016;18(1):249.

[58] Gully N, Bright R, Marino V, Marchant C, Cantley M, Haynes D, et al. Porphyromonas gingivalis peptidylarginine deiminase, a key contributor in the pathogenesis of experimental periodontal disease and experimental arthritis. PLoS One 2014;9(6):e100838.

[59] Rath HC, Herfarth HH, Ikeda JS, Grenther WB, Hamm Jr TE, Balish E, et al. Normal luminal bacteria, especially Bacteroides species, mediate chronic colitis, gastritis, and arthritis in HLA-B27/human beta2 microglobulin transgenic rats. J Clin Investig 1996;98(4):945–53.

[60] Lin P, Bach M, Asquith M, Lee AY, Akileswaran L, Stauffer P, et al. HLA-B27 and human beta2-microglobulin affect the gut microbiota of transgenic rats. PLoS One 2014;9(8):e105684.

[61] Asquith M, Davin S, Stauffer P, Michell C, Janowitz C, Lin P, et al. Intestinal metabolites are profoundly altered in the context of HLA-B27 expression and functionally modulate disease in a rat model of spondyloarthritis. Arthritis Rheumatol 2017;69(10):1984–95.

[62] Asquith MJ, Stauffer P, Davin S, Mitchell C, Lin P, Rosenbaum JT. Perturbed mucosal immunity and dysbiosis accompany clinical disease in a rat model of spondyloarthritis. Arthritis Rheumatol 2016;68(9):2151–62.

[63] Rehakova Z, Capkova J, Stepankova R, Sinkora J, Louzecka A, Ivanyi P, et al. Germ-free mice do not develop ankylosing enthesopathy, a spontaneous joint disease. Hum Immunol 2000;61(6):555–8.

[64] Sinkorova Z, Capkova J, Niederlova J, Stepankova R, Sinkora J. Commensal intestinal bacterial strains trigger ankylosing enthesopathy of the ankle in inbred B10.BR (H-2(k)) male mice. Hum Immunol 2008;69(12):845–50.

[65] Rehaume LM, Mondot S, Aguirre de Carcer D, Velasco J, Benham H, Hasnain SZ, et al. ZAP-70 genotype disrupts the relationship between microbiota and host, leading to spondyloarthritis and ileitis in SKG mice. Arthritis Rheumatol 2014;66(10):2780–92.

[66] Chen J, Chia N, Kalari KR, Yao JZ, Novotna M, Soldan MM, et al. Multiple sclerosis patients have a distinct gut microbiota compared to healthy controls. Sci Rep 2016;6:28484.

[67] Miyake S, Kim S, Suda W, Oshima K, Nakamura M, Matsuoka T, et al. Dysbiosis in the gut microbiota of patients with multiple sclerosis, with a striking depletion of species belonging to Clostridia XIVa and IV clusters. PLoS One 2015;10(9):e0137429.

[68] Tremlett H, Fadrosh DW, Faruqi AA, Zhu F, Hart J, Roalstad S, et al. Gut microbiota in early pediatric multiple sclerosis: a case-control study. Eur J Neurol 2016;23(8):1308–21.

[69] Jangi S, Gandhi R, Cox LM, Li N, von Glehn F, Yan R, et al. Alterations of the human gut microbiome in multiple sclerosis. Nat Commun 2016;7:12015.

[70] Cantarel BL, Waubant E, Chehoud C, Kuczynski J, DeSantis TZ, Warrington J, et al. Gut microbiota in multiple sclerosis: possible influence of immunomodulators. J Investig Med 2015;63(5):729–34.

[71] Rumah KR, Linden J, Fischetti VA, Vartanian T. Isolation of *Clostridium perfringens* type B in an individual at first clinical presentation of multiple sclerosis provides clues for environmental triggers of the disease. PLoS One 2013;8(10):e76359.

[72] Zhang X, Zhang D, Jia H, Feng Q, Wang D, Liang D, et al. The oral and gut microbiomes are perturbed in rheumatoid arthritis and partly normalized after treatment. Nat Med 2015;21(8):895–905.

[73] Vaahtovuo J, Munukka E, Korkeamaki M, Luukkainen R, Toivanen P. Fecal microbiota in early rheumatoid arthritis. J Rheumatol 2008;35(8):1500–5.

[74] Scher JU, Sczesnak A, Longman RS, Segata N, Ubeda C, Bielski C, et al. Expansion of intestinal *Prevotella copri* correlates with enhanced susceptibility to arthritis. eLife 2013;2:e01202.

[75] Liu X, Zou Q, Zeng B, Fang Y, Wei H. Analysis of fecal Lactobacillus community structure in patients with early rheumatoid arthritis. Curr Microbiol 2013;67(2):170–6.

[76] Scher JU, Joshua V, Artacho A, Abdollahi-Roodsaz S, Ockinger J, Kullberg S, et al. The lung microbiota in early rheumatoid arthritis and autoimmunity. Microbiome 2016;4(1):60.

[77] Stebbings S, Munro K, Simon MA, Tannock G, Highton J, Harmsen H, et al. Comparison of the faecal microflora of patients with ankylosing spondylitis and controls using molecular methods of analysis. Rheumatology 2002;41(12):1395–401.

[78] Wen C, Zheng Z, Shao T, Liu L, Xie Z, Le Chatelier E, et al. Quantitative metagenomics reveals unique gut microbiome biomarkers in ankylosing spondylitis. Genome Biol 2017;18(1):142.

[79] Breban M, Tap J, Leboime A, Said-Nahal R, Langella P, Chiocchia G, et al. Faecal microbiota study reveals specific dysbiosis in spondyloarthritis. Ann Rheum Dis 2017;76(9):1614–22.

[80] Tito RY, Cypers H, Joossens M, Varkas G, Van Praet L, Glorieus E, et al. Brief report: dialister as a microbial marker of disease activity in spondyloarthritis. Arthritis Rheumatol 2017;69(1):114–21.

[81] Costello ME, Ciccia F, Willner D, Warrington N, Robinson PC, Gardiner B, et al. Brief report: intestinal dysbiosis in ankylosing spondylitis. Arthritis Rheumatol 2015;67(3):686–91.

[82] Yan D, Issa N, Afifi L, Jeon C, Chang HW, Liao W. The role of the skin and gut microbiome in psoriatic disease. Curr Dermatol Rep 2017;6(2):94–103.

[83] Fahlen A, Engstrand L, Baker BS, Powles A, Fry L. Comparison of bacterial microbiota in skin biopsies from normal and psoriatic skin. Arch Dermatol Res 2012;304(1):15–22.

[84] Drago L, De Grandi R, Altomare G, Pigatto P, Rossi O, Toscano M. Skin microbiota of first cousins affected by psoriasis and atopic dermatitis. Clin Mol Allergy 2016,14(1).2.

[85] Gao Z, Tseng CH, Strober BE, Pei Z, Blaser MJ. Substantial alterations of the cutaneous bacterial biota in psoriatic lesions. PLoS One 2008;3(7):e2719.

[86] Alekseyenko AV, Perez-Perez GI, De Souza A, Strober B, Gao Z, Bihan M, et al. Community differentiation of the cutaneous microbiota in psoriasis. Microbiome 2013;1(1):31.

[87] Scher JU, Ubeda C, Artacho A, Attur M, Isaac S, Reddy SM, et al. Decreased bacterial diversity characterizes the altered gut microbiota in patients with psoriatic arthritis, resembling dysbiosis in inflammatory bowel disease. Arthritis Rheumatol 2015;67(1):128–39.

[88] Stoll ML, Kumar R, Morrow CD, Lefkowitz EJ, Cui X, Genin A, et al. Altered microbiota associated with abnormal humoral immune responses to commensal organisms in enthesitis-related arthritis. Arthritis Res Ther 2014;16(6):486.

[89] Aggarwal A, Sarangi AN, Gaur P, Shukla A, Aggarwal R. Gut microbiome in children with enthesitis-related arthritis in a developing country and the effect of probiotic administration. Clin Exp Immunol 2017;187(3):480–9.

[90] Malin M, Verronen P, Korhonen H, Syvaoja EL, Salminen S, Mykkanen H, et al. Dietary therapy with Lactobacillus GG, bovine colostrum or bovine immune colostrum in patients with juvenile chronic arthritis: evaluation of effect on gut defence mechanisms. Inflammopharmacology 1997;5(3):219–36.

[91] Tilley BC, Alarcon GS, Heyse SP, Trentham DE, Neuner R, Kaplan DA, et al. Minocycline in rheumatoid arthritis. A 48-week, double-blind, placebo-controlled trial. MIRA Trial Group. Ann Intern Med 1995;122(2):81–9.

[92] Bluhm GB, Sharp JT, Tilley BC, Alarcon GS, Cooper SM, Pillemer SR, et al. Radiographic results from the minocycline in rheumatoid arthritis (MIRA) trial. J Rheumatol 1997;24(7):1295–302.

[93] O'Dell JR, Elliott JR, Mallek JA, Mikuls TR, Weaver CA, Glickstein S, et al. Treatment of early seropositive rheumatoid arthritis: doxycycline plus methotrexate versus methotrexate alone. Arthritis Rheum 2006;54(2):621–7.

[94] Hatakka K, Martio J, Korpela M, Herranen M, Poussa T, Laasanen T, et al. Effects of probiotic therapy on the activity and activation of mild rheumatoid arthritis–a pilot study. Scand J Rheumatol 2003;32(4):211–5.

[95] Mandel DR, Eichas K, Holmes J. Bacillus coagulans: a viable adjunct therapy for relieving symptoms of rheumatoid arthritis according to a randomized, controlled trial. BMC Compl Alternative Med 2010;10:1.

[96] Pineda Mde L, Thompson SF, Summers K, de Leon F, Pope J, Reid G. A randomized, double-blinded, placebo-controlled pilot study of probiotics in active rheumatoid arthritis. Med Sci Mon Int Med J Exp Clin Res 2011;17(6). CR347-54.

[97] Alipour B, Homayouni-Rad A, Vaghef-Mehrabany E, Sharif SK, Vaghef-Mehrabany L, Asghari-Jafarabadi M, et al. Effects of Lactobacillus casei supplementation on disease activity and inflammatory cytokines in rheumatoid arthritis patients: a randomized double-blind clinical trial. Int J Rheum Dis 2014;17(5):519–27.

[98] Zamani B, Golkar HR, Farshbaf S, Emadi-Baygi M, Tajabadi-Ebrahimi M, Jafari P, et al. Clinical and metabolic response to probiotic supplementation in patients with rheumatoid arthritis: a randomized, double-blind, placebo-controlled trial. Int J Rheum Dis 2016;19(9):869–79.

[99] McDougall J, Bruce B, Spiller G, Westerdahl J, McDougall M. Effects of a very low-fat, vegan diet in subjects with rheumatoid arthritis. J Alternative Compl Med 2002;8(1):71–5.

[100] McKellar G, Morrison E, McEntegart A, Hampson R, Tierney A, Mackle G, et al. A pilot study of a Mediterranean-type diet intervention in female patients with rheumatoid arthritis living in areas of social deprivation in Glasgow. Ann Rheum Dis 2007;66(9):1239–43.

[101] Skoldstam L, Hagfors L, Johansson G. An experimental study of a Mediterranean diet intervention for patients with rheumatoid arthritis. Ann Rheum Dis 2003;62(3):208–14.

[102] Abendroth A, Michalsen A, Ludtke R, Ruffer A, Musial F, Dobos GJ, et al. Changes of intestinal microflora in patients with rheumatoid arthritis during fasting or a mediterranean diet. Forschende Komplementärmed 2010;17(6):307–13.

[103] Jenks K, Stebbings S, Burton J, Schultz M, Herbison P, Highton J. Probiotic therapy for the treatment of spondyloarthritis: a randomized controlled trial. J Rheumatol 2010;37(10):2118–25.

[104] Brophy S, Burrows CL, Brooks C, Gravenor MB, Siebert S, Allen SJ. Internet-based randomised controlled trials for the evaluation of complementary and alternative medicines: probiotics in spondyloarthropathy. BMC Muscoskel Disord 2008;9:4.

[105] Palumbo VD, Romeo M, Marino Gammazza A, Carini F, Damiani P, Damiano G, et al. The long-term effects of probiotics in the therapy of ulcerative colitis: a clinical study. Biomedical papers of the Medical Faculty of the University Palacky, Olomouc. Czechoslovakia 2016;160(3):372–7.

[106] Tamaki H, Nakase H, Inoue S, Kawanami C, Itani T, Ohana M, et al. Efficacy of probiotic treatment with Bifidobacterium longum 536 for induction of remission in active ulcerative colitis: a randomized, double-blinded, placebo-controlled multicenter trial. Dig Endosc 2016;28(1):67–74.

[107] Oliva S, Di Nardo G, Ferrari F, Mallardo S, Rossi P, Patrizi G, et al. Randomised clinical trial: the effectiveness of Lactobacillus reuteri ATCC 55730 rectal enema in children with active distal ulcerative colitis. Alimentary Pharmacol Ther 2012;35(3):327–34.

[108] Fedorak RN, Feagan BG, Hotte N, Leddin D, Dieleman LA, Petrunia DM, et al. The probiotic VSL#3 has anti-inflammatory effects and could reduce endoscopic recurrence after surgery for Crohn's disease. Clin Gastroenterol Hepatol 2015;13(5):928–35. e2.

[109] Bourreille A, Cadiot G, Le Dreau G, Laharie D, Beaugerie L, Dupas JL, et al. *Saccharomyces boulardii* does not prevent relapse of Crohn's disease. Clin Gastroenterol Hepatol 2013;11(8):982–7.

[110] Benjamin JL, Hedin CR, Koutsoumpas A, Ng SC, McCarthy NE, Hart AL, et al. Randomised, double-blind, placebo-controlled trial of fructo-oligosaccharides in active Crohn's disease. Gut 2011;60(7):923–9.

[111] Uygun A, Ozturk K, Demirci H, Oger C, Avci IY, Turker T, et al. Fecal microbiota transplantation is a rescue treatment modality for refractory ulcerative colitis. Medicine 2017;96(16):e6479.

[112] Nishida A, Imaeda H, Ohno M, Inatomi O, Bamba S, Sugimoto M, et al. Efficacy and safety of single fecal microbiota transplantation for Japanese patients with mild to moderately active ulcerative colitis. J Gastroenterol 2017;52(4):476–82.

[113] Damman CJ, Brittnacher MJ, Westerhoff M, Hayden HS, Radey M, Hager KR, et al. Low level engraftment and improvement following a single colonoscopic administration of fecal microbiota to patients with ulcerative colitis. PLoS One 2015;10(8):e0133925.

[114] Moayyedi P, Surette MG, Kim PT, Libertucci J, Wolfe M, Onischi C, et al. Fecal microbiota transplantation induces remission in patients with active ulcerative colitis in a randomized controlled trial. Gastroenterology 2015;149(1):102–9. e6.

[115] Rossen NG, Fuentes S, van der Spek MJ, Tijssen JG, Hartman JH, Duflou A, et al. Findings from a randomized controlled trial of fecal transplantation for patients with ulcerative colitis. Gastroenterology 2015;149(1):110–8. e4.

[116] Suskind DL, Brittnacher MJ, Wahbeh G, Shaffer ML, Hayden HS, Qin X, et al. Fecal microbial transplant effect on clinical outcomes and fecal microbiome in active Crohn's disease. Inflamm Bowel Dis 2015;21(3):556–63.

[117] Suskind DL, Singh N, Nielson H, Wahbeh G. Fecal microbial transplant via nasogastric tube for active pediatric ulcerative colitis. J Pediatr Gastroenterol Nutr 2015;60(1):27–9.

Chapter 21

Infections: Viruses and Bacteria

Dimitrios P. Bogdanos, Lazaros I. Sakkas

Department of Rheumatology and Clinical Immunology, Faculty of Medicine, School of Health Sciences, University of Thessaly, Larissa, Greece

Autoimmune diseases are a heterogeneous group of immune-mediated disorders caused by inflammatory processes targeting host tissues, ultimately leading to full-blown disease. A remarkable increase of the incidence of most autoimmune diseases in Northern Europe and North America over the last three decades has challenged the understanding of the pathogenesis of autoimmunity. Genetic studies and data stemming from cohorts of twins clearly indicate that the genetic makeup of the affected patients is not per se the most important cause of the disease. Environmental factors, including the widespread use of antibiotics, immunization, westernized diet habits and way of life, exposure to infections and pollution, and other factors, are shaping up an orchestrated attack of our immune system, which in genetically susceptible individuals with compromised defense mechanisms cannot tolerate the autoimmune attack and immunological breakdown, which leads to initiation of innate and adaptive immune responses against self-antigens, persistent inflammation, cell destruction, tissue damage, and establishment of autoimmune disorders.

Autoimmune diseases comprise a heterogeneous group of more than 80 disorders. They currently affect approximately 20% of North America's population and their incidence has increased dramatically over the last three decades. The mechanisms responsible for the induction of autoimmune diseases are perplexed and involve genetic, epigenetic, and environmental factors which act in isolation or in concert to break immunological tolerance and to induce cell destruction, tissue injury, and clinically overt autoimmune disease [1,2]. The studies conducted over the years in experimental models of autoimmune diseases provided a lot of information regarding the influence of the factors contributing to the induction of autoimmunity and helped us to appreciate the influence of genetic and environmental factors in the pathogenesis of autoimmunity. Twin studies showed low concordance rates among monozygotic twins, further underlying that genes per se are not the most influential factor [3].

Among the environmental factors initiating autoimmune inflammatory processes, infectious agents have been considered the most likely triggers in such an extent that Noel and Shoenfeld raised the question as to whether "autoimmune diseases are infectious unless proven otherwise."

If infections are triggers of autoimmunity, the question is which are the ones to blame and how they can achieve it.

MICROBE–HOST INTERACTIONS: A CHESS GAME PLAYED BY TWO

To better understand the close interplay between microbes and the host, we need to get an insight of the complex host–microbe interactions.

Although no one can deny the adaptation of core defense mechanisms the host acquired over the years to preserve its survival, there is also no doubt that microbes—and more remarkably viruses—have evolved effective means to challenge the host's safeguard mechanisms to continue to exist.

A typical example is that of Epstein–Barr virus (EBV), a human herpes virus 4 (HHV4), which encodes a mimic of human IL-10, with a remarkable amino acid similarity with the human cytokine (Fig. 21.1) [4]. Such mimicry instigated from the virus has been regarded for many years as a testimony of EBV (and related herpesviruses) to manipulate our immune system to avoid elimination.

The processes taking place during immune system's exposure to infections have been considered as a "war" between the host and the microbe. Over the years, many battles are taking places, some won from the host, while others are gained by the pathogens. The ultimate goal of our immune system is the ending of the war in favor of the host. Others stochastically considered this host–microbe interaction as a "chess game." There are a lot of parallelisms between chess game and the game played between the virus/microbe and the host. In a simplistic way, this may hold true as chess is after all a war game against two opponents (i.e., an army of two), only one of whom is going to win. As this is a strategy board game played by only two players under strict rules that none of the opponents can circumvent, it becomes apparent that the cleverness of the opponent

Score	Expect	Method	Identities	Positives	Gaps
237 bits(605)	2e-86	Compositional matrix adjust.	131/142(92%)	136/142(95%)	0/142(0%)

```
Query   36   NLPNMLRDLRDAFSRVKTFFQMKDQLDNLLLKESLLEDFKGYLGCQALSEMIQFYLEEVM    95
             N P MLRDLRDAFSRVKTFFQ KD++DNLLLKESLLEDFKGYLGCQALSEMIQFYLEEVM
Sbjct    4   NFPQMLRDLRDAFSRVKTFFQTKDEVDNLLLKESLLEDFKGYLGCQALSEMIQFYLEEVM    63

Query   96   PQAENQDPDIKAHVNSLGENLKTLRLRLRRCHRFLPCENKSKAVEQVKNAFNKLQEKGIY   155
             PQAENQDP+ K HVNSLGENLKTLRLRLRRCHRFLPCENKSKAVEQ+KNAFNKLQEKGIY
Sbjct   64   PQAENQDPEAKDHVNSLGENLKTLRLRLRRCHRFLPCENKSKAVEQIKNAFNKLQEKGIY   123

Query  156   KAMSEFDIFINYIEAYMTMKIR   177
             KAMSEFDIFINYIEAYMT+K R
Sbjct  124   KAMSEFDIFINYIEAYMTIKAR   145
```

FIGURE 21.1   Epstein–Barr virus encodes a viral product highly homologous to human IL-10, which shares 95% local amino acid homology with human IL-10.

regarding the strategic movements that will follow is going to govern the fate of the game, the same way we as hosts—and the strategy our immune system decides to follow—will determine whether we are going to win or lose the fight we are giving against the microbes. In chess, each of the players begins with the same 16 pieces of army, a king and a queen, two knights, two bishops, two rooks, and eight pawns. Thus, none of the opponents can claim that is superior to the other. Chess is played on a square board of eight rows and eight columns. By convention, the game pieces are divided into white and black sets and are set out at specific squares. Each piece has its own way of moving which is highly restricted. They are moved to either an unoccupied square or one occupied by an opponent's piece, which is captured and removed from play. A player may not make any move that would put or leave the player's own king under attack. A player cannot "pass"; at each turn one must make a legal move. If the player to move has no legal move, the game is over. A white piece always starts the game, followed by the move of a black piece and so forth. The king can move in every direction he desires but only for a square. For reasons that we may never learn the most powerful piece, in terms of the plasticity and extent of movements allowed, is the queen, and the least powerful (as expected) is the pawn. Those who play chess understand from the very start that no single pawn or piece can stand-alone; the whole chess army needs to exercise teamwork as a unit to meet the glory, i.e., to win the game. At times the players of a chess game may sacrifice one piece (even if this is the queen). Such sacrifices could be part of the tactic they use to misguide the opponent and to win the game. This may parallel the orchestrated maneuvers of our immune system to fight viral infections without sacrificing tissue's integrity. The battle is won if the king is placed under an unavoidable treat or capture by the movement of an opponent's piece, also known as "checkmate." The opponent can also voluntary resigns if, because of the excessive lost material, the checkmate appears unavoidable. In the battle that we give against infections, neither we start with the same number of pieces nor we continue the game in equal terms, as at times we as hosts have weak ability to overcome specific fatal infections. Patients suffered from immunodeficiencies are a typical example of that. On the other hand, most of the time our immune system is so well equipped with an endless number of effective constituents that we are more than sure that we will eliminate or at least control the microbial infection, irrespectively of its arsenal. At the end of the day, our immune system's very existence is to defend us from the invaders (the microbes, parasites, etc.), and it will be rather unexpected to be unable to do that, if we consider that we have prevailed for thousands of years, or not?

The tactics our immune system uses to control infection and those applied by infectious agents to overcome our immune system are the ones that will be decisive for the fate of the game. In chess, you wish to post your pieces at squares where they can accomplish something assisting either your defense or attack tactics. You ultimately want to keep your king safe from sudden moves and attacks (strikes) of the opponent and to avoid many losses especially at the start, as this will weaken both your defense and attack strategy. Using an aggressive-attacking strategy to make threats when developing the pieces usually limits the opponent's freedom of choice and dictates the game's course in your favor but only if your threads are meaningful. Develop and threaten is a good chess strategy but whether this is also the proper tactic to be used against microbes is a matter of debate. Conservative movements with wise defense tactics and passive game may also achieve the goal of the player, who nevertheless needs to be patient and persistent. We now know that the tactics used by microbes to survive are endless. In general they modulate innate responses, the first line of defense, and the more sophisticated adaptive immune responses to accomplish survival, colonization, and persistent infection at the expense of the host.

Chess movements are dynamic and the opponent learns from the other's tactic. Evolution has made microbe's arsenal able to escape elimination using an arsenal able to put forward tactics working at various levels. While some make use of stealth strategies at early stages, others prefer to operate in this way later on. They try to avoid pattern recognition, to evade death by polymorphonuclear cells, to avoid death within macrophages, to diminish inflammatory signals, to sabotage antigen-presenting functions mainly of dendritic cells, to inactivate effective immune cells, and finally to target and if possible destroy adaptive immune effector cell mechanisms [5]. If they succeed, microbes achieve confrontation by humoral defense mechanisms, interference with antigen presentation, inhibition of antimicrobial cytokine and chemokine recruitment, inhibition of T (CD8 and CD4), B, and NK cell functions, and induction of apoptosis or anergy of immune cells [5].

Chess players gain their experience mainly during the game against skilled opponents. Several studies are now documenting that our immune system requires intestinal microbiota for its maturation and the prompt response during the encounter with aggressive pathogens.

GERM-FREE ANIMALS REVEAL THE NEED FOR MICROBIOTA TO ACHIEVE GUT IMMUNE HOMEOSTASIS

We learned more about the role of microbiota in shaping our immune system from studies using germ-free animals. These animals have never been exposed to any pathogens as they have been raised in a sterile environment. It appears that these animals have developmental defects including (1) a defective gut-associated lymphoid tissue, which is a first-class line of defense for intestinal pathogens; (2) fewer and smaller Peyer's patches; (3) smaller mesenteric lymph nodes with less cellular composition; and (4) less cellular lamina propria of the small intestine. Several immune cells are decreased or functionally impaired in germ-free animals [6]. The intestinal epithelial cells are fewer and show a significant reduction of Toll-like receptors (TLRs) and class II major histocompatibility complex molecules compared with those animals that are not germ-free. Moreover, in germ-free mice $CD4^+$ T cells in the lamina propria are reduced and intestinal intraepithelial lymphocytes are numerically fewer and their cytotoxic potential is impaired. The maturity of isolated lymphoid follicles, which are dedicated intestinal structures mainly composed by dendritic cells and B cell aggregates, is also highly dependent by the encounter with the gut microbiome [6]. All these are highly suggestive of a decisive role of microbiota in developing the intestinal barrier and its defense mechanisms in terms of pathogen sensing and antigen presentation [7]. Thus, microbiota educates our immune system and the timing of microbial entry governs the extent of genes, which are exchanged between microbes and humans. This exchange plays an important role in the counterattack of the host against pathogens. We may understand that better from an evolutionary perspective [8,9]. Microbes populated this planet billion of years before any eukaryotic life. This simply means that most of them had the ability to survive without us. In a sense, we are the ones that we invaded their world; to consider them as invaders of our world could be unfair. To them, humans and other animals represent nutrient-rich ecosystems. For us, microbes are tools to help us digest complex carbohydrates providing us with necessary nutrients.

HOST–MICROBE INTERACTIONS: A WAR OF WORLDS OR A WORLD WAR?

If the game we play with microbes looks like chess, it becomes apparent that we as hosts every minute of our lives play countless chess games, given the exhaustive number of microbes we are exposed to at a given time point. Our immune system is programmed in such a way that can deal with hundreds of foreign invaders at the same time. Thus, it is not inaccurate to say that a "war of worlds" is taking place rather than just a single battle; a war of our world against their worlds and their worlds are rather too many. Of interest, microbes do not only fight for their survival against our immune system but also compete for their existence with other neighboring microbes. That may explain some of the evolutionary tactics microbes acquired over time. Microbes compete with other pathogens for nutrients and space, and this could be serious causes for their professional maneuvers during their encounter with our immune system.

Over time human's coevolution of trillions of microbes that inhabited our bodies (known as microbiome) has led to a harmonic cohabitation, a state of symbiosis. This state is dynamic and is influenced by a variety of internal and external parameters. When the balance is lost and the pathogens prevail against the symbionts, dysbiosis is established, inflammation persists, and tissue injury is established. Ongoing studies are focused on distinguishing "healthy" from "unhealthy/disease-related" microbiomes, the former being those, which are noted, in various heterogeneous diseases, including autoimmune disorders. These attempts may have a profound therapeutic effect or help us preventing disease induction. Herpesviruses are part of the microbiome because they can establish lifelong infection of the human host. Unlike bacteria and fungi, though, this tenacious state is retained through latent genomic persistence within the host cell nucleus.

DISCRIMINATING BETWEEN THE "GOOD" AND "BAD" MICROBIOME

The task to discriminate the bad from the good microbiome has become extremely difficult, as it was soon documented an inter- and intrapersonal diversity of the microbiomes not only within affected individuals but also among healthy people. Changes of the microbiome composition, which have been considered pathogenic in one disease, appear to be beneficial (prophylactic) in another autoimmune disease, suggesting the complexity of the pathophysiological processes. Environmental factors such as diet habits with high salt, fat and carbohydrates, misuse of antibiotics, smoking, vaccination, and other factors profoundly affect the microbiome and establish dysbiosis states which could be the "original sin" for breaking of immunological tolerance in a stepwise fashion [10–13].

The concept of infectome and autoinfectome was introduced in 2003 to describe the cumulative infections we are exposed to throughout life, which contribute directly or indirectly to the induction of autoimmune diseases [14–16]. The affected individual is exposed to hundreds of pathogens but only few of those trigger autoimmune phenomena. If we consider the induction of autoimmunity as an "offense scene," autoinfectomics is a tool to dissect those who are responsible for the offense of our immune system and the breakdown of immunological tolerance [17].

The genetic makeup of the susceptible individual is an important component of its potency to be affected by the pathogen stimuli [15]. These infections initiate immune responses which through various mechanisms, such as that of molecular mimicry, bystander activation, cryptic epitope recognition, and neoantigen formulation, can lead to induction of organ- and non–organ-specific autoantibodies and autoreactive CD4 and CD8 T cell responses against autoantigens critical for the induction of tissue destruction [18,19]. To study these mechanisms, such as that of molecular mimicry, in humans has been difficult. To be convincing, studies need to be conducted long before the induction of any autoimmune phenomena. Biological material needs to be obtained before and after the exposure to the pathogen and arguably before and after the induction of autoantibodies or autoantigen-specific T cells [16]. Indirect attempts to tackle this hurdle have been made. Studies can be performed in biomaterial obtained before and after vaccination, and if immunological cross-reactivity is only witnessed after vaccination, an indirect proof that microbial/self-mimicry is operated in man can be considered likely [20,21]. Evidence that adjuvants rather than molecular mimicry are the likely causes of vaccine-related autoimmune phenomena, also known as ASIA, has been obtained [22–24]. Outside murine models of autoimmune diseases, molecular mimicry and other mechanisms of autoimmunity can be studied in animals suffering from microbial-triggered diseases that resemble autoimmune diseases, such as the model of mycobacterium avium paratuberculosis in ruminants, also known as Jone's disease, which shares striking features of Crohn's disease [25–27].

We largely divide the infectious triggers of autoimmunity to two categories, those with convincing data and those with circumstantial associations. Experimental models of organ-specific autoimmune diseases such as multiple sclerosis, insulin-dependent mellitus, and primary biliary cholangitis have helped us understand the role of infectious triggers of autoimmunity. A wealth of data also stems from the study of non–organ-specific autoimmune diseases, the best examples being those of autoimmune rheumatic diseases (AIRDs).

AUTOIMMUNE RHEUMATIC DISEASES AS MODELS TO STUDY INTERACTIONS BETWEEN VIRAL PATHOGENS AND MICROBIOME

AIRDs such as rheumatoid arthritis (RA), Sjogren's syndrome (SS), systemic lupus erythematosus (SLE), and systemic sclerosis (SSc) are systemic autoimmune diseases with well-defined clinical phenotypes but poorly understood immunopathogeneses. The best-studied triggers of autoimmunity are those of DNA viruses and in particular EBV and human cytomegalovirus (CMV), as those two have been considered the most likely triggers for a plethora of autoimmune diseases, including AIRDs [28,29]. Viruses may also explain the frequent coexistence of several autoimmune disorders [30,31]. Other viruses or microbial pathogens have been considered relevant for the pathogenesis of ARDs (Fig. 21.2) [32].

Herpes simplex virus 1 (HSV1) genetic material has been detected in salivary glands of SS patients [33]. Molecular mimicry between HSV1 proteins and human autoantigens related to AIRDs has been reported. The immediate-early protein of HSV1 contains epitopes with a significant degree of amino acid similarity with centromere protein B (CENP-B) and Sm autoantigens [32], targeting antigens in SSc and SLE, respectively.

EBV has been linked with various AIRDs. EBV DNA viral load has been isolated from peripheral blood samples of patients with RA [34] and EBV DNA is isolated from bone marrow of RA patients. In fact, those patients appear to have better response under rituximab treatment compared with those with undetectable EBV [35]. Also, CD8 T cells specific for EBV antigens were detected in synovial fluid of patients with RA [36]. In addition, the EBV gp110, expressed on the budding virion during EBV replication, contains the QKRAA amino acid sequence, which is also present on HLA-DRB1*SE [37]. HLA-DRB1*0404, an HLA-DRB1*SE allele, is associated with low T cell responses to EBV gp110. In contrast, HLA-DRB1*07, an allele which protects from RA, is associated with high T cell reactivity to EBV gp110. More importantly, clinical phenotypes of RA are associated with low T cell responses to gp110 [38].

Anticitrullinated peptide antibodies (ACPAs) are the serological markers of RA, and infectious agents that can act as antigenic sources of citrullinated peptides can be considered likely triggers of RA [39,40]. Citrullination is a posttranslational modification of proteins in which arginine residues are converted to citrulline via the action of en enzyme called peptidylarginine deiminase. EBV has been proved to be an inducer of citrullinated peptides and has reasonably been

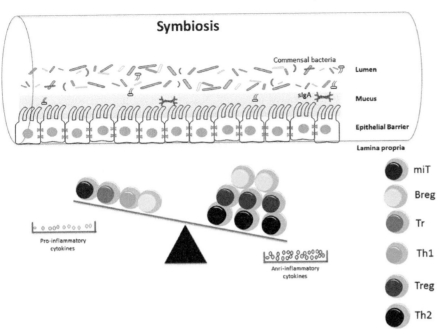

FIGURE 21.2 The same virus can be involved as triggering factor in more than one disease. *A. act, Aggregatibacter actinomycetemcomitans; ADV,* adenovirus; *CMV,* cytomegalovirus; *EBV,* Epstein–Barr virus; *HSV1,* herpes simplex virus; *P. cop, Prevotella copri; P. int, Prevotella intermedia; PB19,* parvo B19 virus; *RA,* rheumatoid arthritis; *SSc,* systemic sclerosis; *VZV,* varicella zoster virus.

considered a trigger of ACPAs. Citrullinated peptides originated from EBV are targeted by ACPAs and can be detected in serum samples of patients with RA suggesting that EBV infection can be a source of RA-specific citrullinated peptides. This makes EBV a potential trigger of ACPAs and potentially of the disease. The best-studied microbial trigger of ACPAs is that of *Porphyromonas gingivalis* (*P. gingivalis*), which is a major component of oral microbiome and a usual cause of periodontal disease (PD). *P. gingivalis* can citrullinate various antigens and is a likely inducer of neoantigens, a precondition for the breakdown of immunological tolerance and the induction of disease-specific autoreactive responses. This may explain the apparent link between PD, *P. gingivalis*, ACPA, and RA. Herpesvirus DNA is detected in saliva at variable levels (from 10^6 to 10^9 per mL) and has been associated with symptomatic PD including aggressive periodontitis [41]. *Aggregatibacter actinomycetemcomitans* (*A. actinomycetemcomitans*), another causative agent of PD, induces ACPA and may be a trigger of RA [49].

EBV-citrullinated peptides arise from EBNA-1 [42] and EBNA-2 [43]. Antibodies against the viral specific citrullinated peptides appear to be cross-reactive with ACPAs targeting the immunodominant citrullinated fibrin peptide [44]. Moreover, ACPA-producing plasma cells in the synovial membrane of RA patients co-express BFRF1, a protein of early EBV lytic phase [45], suggesting that posttranslationally modified EBV antigens in germinal center (GC)–like structures in RA synovial membranes may trigger ACPA production via cross-reactivity or other less understood immunological mechanisms. More recently, antibody reactivity against novel citrullinated peptides, not associated with antibodies to *P. gingivalis*, is associated with antibodies to a *Prevotella* species, constituents of the oral of gut microbiome, such as that of *Prevotella intermedia* and *Prevotella copri* suggesting that infection with these pathogens may drive the generation of ACPA in a way distinct of that of *P gingivalis* [46–49].

Additional data from independent studies underline the role played by *Prevotella* as a trigger of ACPAs and ultimately RA. A hypothesis has been formulated linking gut and joint inflammation, *Prevotella* playing a key role. A state of dysbiosis weakens the mucosal barrier and leads to a leaky gut. Such a leakage of commensal microorganisms leads to activation of T and B lymphocytes that specifically target microbial antigens. A characteristic example is that of *Prevotella*, as not only antibodies but also *Prevotella*-specific T cell responses have been documented in patients with RA. Evidence of T cell cross-reactivity involving these microbial peptides and self-epitopes belonging to proteins expressed in joints has been provided, especially in those patients with SE alleles. Tissue-resident lymphocytes T may then home to inflamed joints and cross-react with homologous self-antigens. When commensal organisms or their remnants overexpress antigen-presenting cells reaching the joints, perpetuation of inflammation is secured and tissue destruction is inevitable.

The EBV's tropism for salivary and lacrimal glands [50] may explain why this virus has long been considered a trigger of SS, a disease characterized by lymphocytic infiltration of salivary and lacrimal glands. Antibodies specific for EBV early antigen and EBNA correlate with SS-A Ro-52 antibodies in patients with SS [51]. B cells and plasma cells from GC-like structure contained in salivary glands from patients with SS express latent and lytic proteins of EBV [52]. When GC-like structures contained in SS salivary glands are removed and transplanted into SCID mice, plasma cells of those can produce not only anti-Ro52 antibodies but also EBV-specific antibodies [52]. Besides autoimmunity, EBV also affects salivary gland function.

In patients with SLE, up to 100-fold higher EBV DNA is detected in sera of SLE patients compared with controls. At the site of tissue inflammation, i.e., in renal biopsies from lupus nephritis SLE patients, EBV latent membrane protein-1 (LMP-1), a CD40 mimic, was detected [53,54]. EBV-encoded RNA-1 (EBER-1), a small RNA that is the most abundant RNA in EBV latent phase, was also detected in such biopsy material [53].

In addition, several studies have shown that IgM, IgG, and IgA antibodies against various EBV antigens are higher in SLE compared with controls [28,29,55]. Higher titers of antibodies against EBV lytic early antigen diffuse were detected in SLE patients [56,57]. Furthermore, EBV LMP-1 positivity in lupus nephritis patients was associated with anti-Sm antibodies [53]. As expected, molecular mimicry and immunological cross-reactivity has been considered a likely mechanism for SLE-specific autoantibody induction and a large number of peptides have been reported to share amino acid similarities between EBV and disease-related autoantigens [32,58]. The notorious PPPGMRPP Sm B/B′ sequence is homologous to a peptide from EBNA-1 sequence PPPGRRP, which is also recognized by sera from SLE patients but not from EBV-positive healthy individuals, which rather suggests its disease specificity and potential pathophysiological significance. Cross-reactivity was also found between Sm D1 and EBNA-1 [28,59]. It is not unexpected that rodents immunized with EBNA-1 PPPGRRP peptide develop lupus-related autoantibodies, as well as lupus-like disease [28]. It also appears that high anti-EBV antibodies inversely correlate with SLE disease activity [60].

EBV has also been linked to SSc. EBV antigens such as the early EBV lytic transactivator BZLF1 that drives EBV replication, latent genes, and early lytic protein is isolated not only from peripheral blood mononuclear cells but also from skin fibroblasts and endothelial cells of patients with SSc [61]. When EBV infects, fibroblasts induce overexpression of TLR8 and IFN-regulated genes and establish a profibrotic phenotype which is one of the first noted features of SSc [61]. TGFβ1 expression was upregulated in fibroblasts expressing high levels of EBV BZFL1 [61]. Recent data show that peripheral blood monocytes from SSc patients and skin macrophages also express BZLF1, as well as BFRF1, an EBV early lytic protein [62]. Molecular mimicry between EBV immunodominant antigens and SSc autoantigens has been demonstrated and cross-reactivity has been witnessed in serum samples from patients with SSc.

A recent study by Gianella et al. [63] has studied the effect of CMV and EBV on intestinal mucosal gene expression and microbiome composition of HIV-infected patients and compared that with HIV uninfected. HIV-infected individuals demonstrated less detectable CMV but when detected CMV was more frequently detected in terminal ileum than in colon. EBV was more frequently detectable in HIV-infected patients compared with uninfected individuals. Of interest higher CMV was associated with a lower relative abundance of *Actinobacteria* in the ileum in HIV-infected participants while EBV had no effect on microbiome composition. The results of this study further indicate how complex is the interplay between three viruses (HIV, CMV, and EBV) and the gut microbiome and suggest a role particularly for CMV on the microbiome homeostasis in HIV-infected patients.

Early exposure to the one but not the other virus may play a role in pathogen-induced autoimmunity in susceptible individuals. Latent CMV infection, as detected by CMV seropositivity, was associated with more severe joint damage in RA [64]. Cytotoxic CD4+ CD28− T cells are closely associated with CMV seropositivity and appear expanded in patients with RA [65,66]. A study by Davis et al. found that ex vivo T cell responses to CMV lysates were associated with more severe joint damage [67] and drug-induced clinical response in patients with RA [68]. In the same study, a higher baseline anti-CMV response predicted inadequate clinical response. On the contrary, another study demonstrated association between low anti-EBV/anti-B19 antibody levels and ACPA-positive RA, in particular when HLA-DRB1 SE was present but not with low or high anti-CMV. These data are provocative as could theoretically indicate that high antiviral antibody levels or the factors leading to such levels would play be protective role against the induction of ACPA in RA.

CMV DNA was detected in the synovial membrane from 11 out of 83 patients with RA compared to 2 out of 64 patients with other joint disorders [69]. The prevalence of IgG anti-CMV antibodies was found to be lower in SS than in controls [51]. CMV may be implicated in the pathogenesis of SLE. IgA and IgG antibodies to CMV pp52 early lytic antigen were significantly higher in SLE compared with healthy controls and were positively associated with lymphocyte counts [57]. There are similarities between CMV vasculopathy and the vascular damage seen in SSc [70], and this has been considered an indirect proof that CMV may cause SSc. In a murine model of vasculopathy, which has with SSc vasculopathy, it was noted that though CMV infection alone cannot cause neointima formation, this is possible if CMV infection is operating at a state of immune dysregulation. Irradiated murine CMV-infected mice lacking the IFNγ receptor (IFNγR−/−) develop extensive adventitial and medial inflammatory infiltrates, and neointima formation in arteries, with proliferation of myofibroblasts and upregulation of TGFβ and platelet-derived growth factor A and B [71]. Serological evidence of antibodies against specific CMV antigens including antibodies against UL94, pp65, and UL57 being more prevalent in SSc than in controls has been obtained but per se cannot be considered a marker of viral involvement in disease's pathogenesis [72,73]. On the other hand, there are multiple peptide homologies between CMV and CENP-B, which could support a molecular mimicry between CMV and humans [32]. In addition, topoisomerase I shares a pentapeptide homology with the CMV UL70 protein [74]. The immune response to CMV can cause vascular injury and fibrosis. For instance, antibodies to CMV-encoded UL94 protein cross-react with the cell membrane tetraspanin transmembrane 4 superfamily member 7 (TM4SF7 or NAG-2) molecule and induce apoptosis of endothelial cells and activation of fibroblasts [75,76]. Such mimicries may be able to induce autoantigen-specific antibodies but no evidence has been provided so far that this can be possible in animal models. Others have been unable to demonstrate immunological cross-reactivity between CMV antigens and SSc-specific autoantigens, further indicating that molecular mimicry is not a likely trigger of SSc-specific autoreactive responses [73]. Gastrointestinal (GI) manifestations are frequently found in patients with SSc. This makes studies investigating the microbiome of the gut in patients with SSc difficult to be carried out properly. Nevertheless, interesting data have been reported. The fecal microbiota of patients with SSc and GI involvement subjects was characterized by higher levels of *Lactobacillus*, *Eubacterium*, and *Acinetobacter* compared with healthy controls, as well as lower proportions of *Roseburia*, *Clostridium*, and *Ruminococcus*. On the other hand, the intestinal microbiota of SSc patients without GI involvement was more analogous to that of patients with microbiota of healthy individuals [77].

For autoreactive responses to be developed and maintained, a state of immune dysregulation, i.e., a functional impairment of not only regulatory T but also B lymphocytes and Th17 lymphocyte predominance must be present [78–80]. We believe that the hierarchy of events which lead to virus-triggered autoimmunity largely depends on early changes of the microbiome which are imperative for the induction of autoimmunity. The "multiple hits" mechanism that we believe is taking place consists of the following hits: (1) an environmental trigger alters microbiome composition and induces dysbiosis. This hit can be due to antibiotic treatment, smoking or diet, vaccination, or vitamin D deficiency; (2) the second hit is subsequent to the first, as alterations of the microbiome promote the growth of proinflammatory and the inhibition of antiinflammatory or beneficial tolerogenic microbiota; (3) the third hit is due to a direct or indirect effect on the functional capacity of regulatory lymphocyte subsets (autoregulome) which are important for the control/suppression of proinflammatory/autoreactive responses. This could be from microbiota or environmental factors that change the microbiota or both; and finally (4) the fourth hit consists of a series of events which under the state of dysregulation take place and are not other than viral or microbial infections acting over time and induce autoantibody or autoreactive T cells, thus promoting disease development by various mechanisms (such as molecular mimicry). Thus, from a state of symbiosis (Fig. 21.3) to a state of dysbiosis (Fig. 21.4), multiple interconnected hits may be responsible for the establishment of autoimmunity.

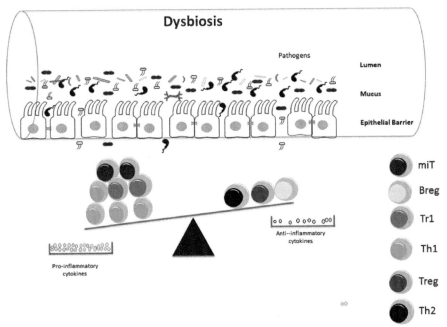

FIGURE 21.3 Symbiosis is characterized by a predominance of commensal bacteria and symbionts and an abundance of pathogens. The intestinal barrier is intact and the mucosal homeostasis is preserved due to tolerance to commensal bacteria, largely because of the protective action of soluble IgA and the dominance of antiinflammatory cells (Tregs, Bregs, and presumably invariant T cells associated to mucosa) over proinflammatory Th1 and Th17 cells.

FIGURE 21.4   A model of a multiple (four) hit mechanism which is causing dysbiosis and attenuates autoimmune disease. Hit 1: environmental changes alter microbiome homeostasis; Hit 2: proinflammatory immune cells and cytokines prevail; Hit 3: microbiome changes and immune cell alterations induce directly or indirectly immune dysregulation and impairment of Tregs/Bregs with a shift toward Th17 dominance; Hit 4: breakdown of immunological tolerance possibly because of molecular mimicry and immunological cross-reactivity mechanisms lead to overt autoimmune disease.

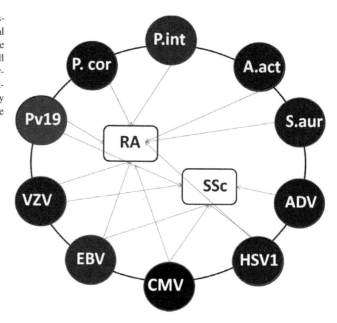

LIST OF ABBREVIATIONS

AIRD Autoimmune rheumatic diseases
CMV Cytomegalovirus
EBNA Epstein–Barr nuclear antigen
HHV Human herpes virus
HSV Herpes simplex virus
SS Sjogren's syndrome
SSc Systemic sclerosis

REFERENCES

[1] Smyk D, Rigopoulou EI, Baum H, Burroughs AK, Vergani D, Bogdanos DP. Autoimmunity and environment: am I at risk? Clin Rev Allergy Immunol 2012;42(2):199–212.

[2] Sakkas LI, Bogdanos DP. Infections as a cause of autoimmune rheumatic diseases. Auto Immun Highlights 2016;7(1):13.

[3] Bogdanos DP, Smyk DS, Rigopoulou EI, Mytilinaiou MG, Heneghan MA, Selmi C, et al. Twin studies in autoimmune disease: genetics, gender and environment. J Autoimmun 2012;38(2–3):J156–69.

[4] Hsu DH, de Waal Malefyt R, Fiorentino DF, Dang MN, Vieira P, de Vries J, et al. Expression of interleukin-10 activity by Epstein-Barr virus protein BCRF1. Science 1990;250(4982):830–2.

[5] Sansonetti PJ, Di Santo JP. Debugging how bacteria manipulate the immune response. Immunity 2007;26(2):149–61.

[6] Smith K, McCoy KD, Macpherson AJ. Use of axenic animals in studying the adaptation of mammals to their commensal intestinal microbiota. Semin Immunol 2007;19(2):59–69.

[7] Hill DA, Artis D. Intestinal bacteria and the regulation of immune cell homeostasis. Annu Rev Immunol 2010;28:623–67.

[8] Backhed F, Ley RE, Sonnenburg JL, Peterson DA, Gordon JI. Host-bacterial mutualism in the human intestine. Science 2005;307(5717):1915–20.

[9] Koropatnick TA, Engle JT, Apicella MA, Stabb EV, Goldman WE, McFall-Ngai MJ. Microbial factor-mediated development in a host-bacterial mutualism. Science 2004;306(5699):1186–8.

[10] Shamriz O, Mizrahi H, Werbner M, Shoenfeld Y, Avni O, Koren O. Microbiota at the crossroads of autoimmunity. Autoimmun Rev 2016;15(9):859–69.

[11] Perricone C, Versini M, Ben-Ami D, Gertel S, Watad A, Segel MJ, et al. Smoke and autoimmunity: the fire behind the disease. Autoimmun Rev 2016;15(4):354–74.

[12] Smyk DS, Rigopoulou EI, Muratori L, Burroughs AK, Bogdanos DP. Smoking as a risk factor for autoimmune liver disease: what we can learn from primary biliary cirrhosis. Ann Hepatol 2012;11(1):7–14.

[13] Wilck N, Matus MG, Kearney SM, Olesen SW, Forslund K, Bartolomaeus H, et al. Salt-responsive gut commensal modulates TH17 axis and disease. Nature 2017;551(7682):585–9.

[14] Bogdanos DP, Sakkas LI. From microbiome to infectome in autoimmunity. Curr Opin Rheumatol 2017;29(4):369–73.

[15] Bogdanos DP, Smyk DS, Invernizzi P, Rigopoulou EI, Blank M, Pouria S, et al. Infectome: a platform to trace infectious triggers of autoimmunity. Autoimmun Rev 2013;12(7):726–40.

[16] Bogdanos DP, Smyk DS, Invernizzi P, Rigopoulou EI, Blank M, Sakkas L, et al. Tracing environmental markers of autoimmunity: introducing the infectome. Immunol Res 2013;56(2–3):220–40.

[17] Bogdanos DP, Smyk DS, Rigopoulou EI, Sakkas LI, Shoenfeld Y. Infectomics and autoinfectomics: a tool to study infectious-induced autoimmunity. Lupus 2015;24(4–5):364–73.

[18] Ehser J, Holdener M, Christen S, Bayer M, Pfeilschifter JM, Hintermann E, et al. Molecular mimicry rather than identity breaks T-cell tolerance in the CYP2D6 mouse model for human autoimmune hepatitis. J Autoimmun 2013;42:39–49.

[19] Bogdanos DP, Choudhuri K, Vergani D. Molecular mimicry and autoimmune liver disease: virtuous intentions, malign consequences. Liver 2001;21(4):225–32.

[20] Bogdanos D, Pusl T, Rust C, Vergani D, Beuers U. Primary biliary cirrhosis following Lactobacillus vaccination for recurrent vaginitis. J Hepatol 2008;49(3):466–73.

[21] Bogdanos DP, Smith H, Ma Y, Baum H, Mieli-Vergani G, Vergani D. A study of molecular mimicry and immunological cross-reactivity between hepatitis B surface antigen and myelin mimics. Clin Dev Immunol 2005;12(3):217–24.

[22] Polymeros D, Tsiamoulos ZP, Koutsoumpas AL, Smyk DS, Mytilinaiou MG, Triantafyllou K, et al. Bioinformatic and immunological analysis reveals lack of support for measles virus related mimicry in Crohn's disease. BMC Med 2014;12:139.

[23] Shoenfeld Y, Agmon-Levin N. 'ASIA' - autoimmune/inflammatory syndrome induced by adjuvants. J Autoimmun 2011;36(1):4–8.

[24] Perricone C, Colafrancesco S, Mazor RD, Soriano A, Agmon-Levin N, Shoenfeld Y. Autoimmune/inflammatory syndrome induced by adjuvants (ASIA) 2013: unveiling the pathogenic, clinical and diagnostic aspects. J Autoimmun 2013;47:1–16.

[25] Liaskos C, Spyrou V, Athanasiou LV, Orfanidou T, Mavropoulos A, Rigopoulou EI, et al. Crohn's disease-specific anti-CUZD1 pancreatic antibodies are absent in ruminants with paratuberculosis. Clin Res Hepatol Gastroenterol 2015;39(3):384–90.

[26] Liaskos C, Spyrou V, Roggenbuck D, Athanasiou LV, Orfanidou T, Mavropoulos A, et al. Crohn's disease-specific pancreatic autoantibodies are specifically present in ruminants with paratuberculosis: implications for the pathogenesis of the human disease. Autoimmunity 2013;46(6):388–94.

[27] Polymeros D, Bogdanos DP, Day R, Arioli D, Vergani D, Forbes A. Does cross-reactivity between mycobacterium avium paratuberculosis and human intestinal antigens characterize Crohn's disease? Gastroenterology 2006;131(1):85–96.

[28] Toussirot E, Roudier J. Epstein-Barr virus in autoimmune diseases. Best Pract Res Clin Rheumatol 2008;22(5):883–96.

[29] Barzilai O, Sherer Y, Ram M, Izhaky D, Anaya JM, Shoenfeld Y. Epstein-Barr virus and cytomegalovirus in autoimmune diseases: are they truly notorious? A preliminary report. Ann NY Acad Sci 2007;1108:567–77.

[30] Rigopoulou EI, Smyk DS, Matthews CE, Billinis C, Burroughs AK, Lenzi M, et al. Epstein-Barr virus as a trigger of autoimmune liver diseases. Adv Virol 2012;2012:987471.

[31] Muratori L, Bogdanos DP, Muratori P, Lenzi M, Granito A, Ma Y, et al. Susceptibility to thyroid disorders in hepatitis C. Clin Gastroenterol Hepatol 2005;3(6):595–603.

[32] Douvas A, Sobelman S. Multiple overlapping homologies between two rheumatoid antigens and immunosuppressive viruses. Proc Natl Acad Sci USA 1991;88(14):6328–32.

[33] Perrot S, Calvez V, Escande JP, Dupin N, Marcelin AG. Prevalences of herpesviruses DNA sequences in salivary gland biopsies from primary and secondary Sjogren's syndrome using degenerated consensus PCR primers. J Clin Virol 2003;28(2):165–8.

[34] Balandraud N, Meynard JB, Auger I, Sovran H, Mugnier B, Reviron D, et al. Epstein-Barr virus load in the peripheral blood of patients with rheumatoid arthritis: accurate quantification using real-time polymerase chain reaction. Arthritis Rheum 2003;48(5):1223–8.

[35] Magnusson M, Brisslert M, Zendjanchi K, Lindh M, Bokarewa MI. Epstein-Barr virus in bone marrow of rheumatoid arthritis patients predicts response to rituximab treatment. Rheumatology (Oxf) 2010;49(10):1911–9.

[36] Scotet E, David-Ameline J, Peyrat MA, Moreau-Aubry A, Pinczon D, Lim A, et al. T cell response to Epstein-Barr virus transactivators in chronic rheumatoid arthritis. J Exp Med 1996;184(5):1791–800.

[37] Roudier J, Petersen J, Rhodes GH, Luka J, Carson DA. Susceptibility to rheumatoid arthritis maps to a T-cell epitope shared by the HLA-Dw4 DR beta-1 chain and the Epstein-Barr virus glycoprotein gp110. Proc Natl Acad Sci USA 1989;86(13):5104–8.

[38] Balandraud N, Roudier J, Roudier C. Epstein-Barr virus and rheumatoid arthritis. Autoimmun Rev 2004;3(5):362–7.

[39] Sakkas LI, Daoussis D, Liossis SN, Bogdanos DP. The infectious basis of ACPA-positive rheumatoid arthritis. Front Microbiol 2017;8:1853.

[40] Sakkas LI, Bogdanos DP, Katsiari C, Platsoucas CD. Anti-citrullinated peptides as autoantigens in rheumatoid arthritis-relevance to treatment. Autoimmun Rev 2014;13(11):1114–20.

[41] Saygun I, Nizam N, Keskiner I, Bal V, Kubar A, Acikel C, et al. Salivary infectious agents and periodontal disease status. J Periodontal Res 2011;46(2):235–9.

[42] Pratesi F, Tommasi C, Anzilotti C, Chimenti D, Migliorini P. Deiminated Epstein-Barr virus nuclear antigen 1 is a target of anti-citrullinated protein antibodies in rheumatoid arthritis. Arthritis Rheum 2006;54(3):733–41.

[43] Pratesi F, Tommasi C, Anzilotti C, Puxeddu I, Sardano E, Di Colo G, et al. Antibodies to a new viral citrullinated peptide, VCP2: fine specificity and correlation with anti-cyclic citrullinated peptide (CCP) and anti-VCP1 antibodies. Clin Exp Immunol 2011;164(3):337–45.

[44] Cornillet M, Verrouil E, Cantagrel A, Serre G, Nogueira L. ACPA-positive RA patients, antibodies to EBNA35-58Cit, a citrullinated peptide from the Epstein-Barr nuclear antigen-1, strongly cross-react with the peptide beta60-74Cit which bears the immunodominant epitope of citrullinated fibrin. Immunol Res 2015;61(1–2):117–25.

[45] Croia C, Serafini B, Bombardieri M, Kelly S, Humby F, Severa M, et al. Epstein-Barr virus persistence and infection of autoreactive plasma cells in synovial lymphoid structures in rheumatoid arthritis. Ann Rheum Dis 2013;72(9):1559–68.

[46] Pianta A, Arvikar S, Strle K, Drouin EE, Wang Q, Costello CE, et al. Evidence of the immune relevance of *Prevotella copri*, a gut microbe, in patients with rheumatoid arthritis. Arthritis Rheumatol 2017;69(5):964–75.

[47] Pianta A, Arvikar SL, Strle K, Drouin EE, Wang Q, Costello CE, et al. Two rheumatoid arthritis-specific autoantigens correlate microbial immunity with autoimmune responses in joints. J Clin Investig 2017;127(8):2946–56.

[48] Sato K, Takahashi N, Kato T, Matsuda Y, Yokoji M, Yamada M, et al. Aggravation of collagen-induced arthritis by orally administered Porphyromonas gingivalis through modulation of the gut microbiota and gut immune system. Sci Rep 2017;7(1):6955.

[49] Kaur G, Mohindra K, Singla S. Autoimmunity-Basics and link with periodontal disease. Autoimmun Rev 2017;16(1):64–71.

[50] Fox RI, Pearson G, Vaughan JH. Detection of Epstein-Barr virus-associated antigens and DNA in salivary gland biopsies from patients with Sjogren's syndrome. J Immunol 1986;137(10):3162–8.

[51] Kivity S, Arango MT, Ehrenfeld M, Tehori O, Shoenfeld Y, Anaya JM, et al. Infection and autoimmunity in Sjogren's syndrome: a clinical study and comprehensive review. J Autoimmun 2014;51:17–22.

[52] Croia C, Astorri E, Murray-Brown W, Willis A, Brokstad KA, Sutcliffe N, et al. Implication of Epstein-Barr virus infection in disease-specific auto-reactive B cell activation in ectopic lymphoid structures of Sjogren's syndrome. Arthritis Rheumatol 2014;66(9):2545–57.

[53] Yu XX, Yao CW, Tao JL, Yang C, Luo MN, Li SM, et al. The expression of renal Epstein-Barr virus markers in patients with lupus nephritis. Exp Ther Med 2014;7(5):1135–40.

[54] Ding Y, He X, Liao W, Yi Z, Yang H, Xiang W. The expression of EBV-encoded LMP1 in young patients with lupus nephritis. Int J Clin Exp Med 2015;8(4):6073–8.

[55] Draborg A, Izarzugaza JM, Houen G. How compelling are the data for Epstein-Barr virus being a trigger for systemic lupus and other autoimmune diseases? Curr Opin Rheumatol 2016;28(4):398–404.

[56] Fattal I, Shental N, Molad Y, Gabrielli A, Pokroy-Shapira E, Oren S, et al. Epstein-Barr virus antibodies mark systemic lupus erythematosus and scleroderma patients negative for anti-DNA. Immunology 2014;141(2):276–85.

[57] Rasmussen NS, Draborg AH, Nielsen CT, Jacobsen S, Houen G. Antibodies to early EBV, CMV, and HHV6 antigens in systemic lupus erythematosus patients. Scand J Rheumatol 2015;44(2):143–9.

[58] Capone G, Calabro M, Lucchese G, Fasano C, Girardi B, Polimeno L, et al. Peptide matching between Epstein-Barr virus and human proteins. Pathog Dis 2013;69(3):205–12.

[59] Riemekasten G, Marell J, Trebeljahr G, Klein R, Hausdorf G, Haupl T, et al. A novel epitope on the C-terminus of SmD1 is recognized by the major-ity of sera from patients with systemic lupus erythematosus. J Clin Investig 1998;102(4):754–63.

[60] Draborg AH, Sandhu N, Larsen N, Lisander Larsen J, Jacobsen S, Houen G. Impaired cytokine responses to Epstein-Barr virus antigens in systemic lupus erythematosus patients. J Immunol Res 2016;2016:6473204.

[61] Farina A, Cirone M, York M, Lenna S, Padilla C, McLaughlin S, et al. Epstein-Barr virus infection induces aberrant TLR activation pathway and fibroblast-myofibroblast conversion in scleroderma. J Investig Dermatol 2014;134(4):954–64.

[62] Farina A, Peruzzi G, Lacconi V, Lenna S, Quarta S, Rosato E, et al. Epstein-Barr virus lytic infection promotes activation of Toll-like receptor 8 innate immune response in systemic sclerosis monocytes. Arthritis Res Ther 2017;19(1):39.

[63] Gianella S, Chaillon A, Mutlu EA, Engen PA, Voigt RM, Keshavarzian A, et al. Effect of cytomegalovirus and Epstein-Barr virus replication on intestinal mucosal gene expression and microbiome composition of HIV-infected and uninfected individuals. AIDS 2017;31(15):2059–67.

[64] Pierer M, Rothe K, Quandt D, Schulz A, Rossol M, Scholz R, et al. Association of anticytomegalovirus seropositivity with more severe joint destruc-tion and more frequent joint surgery in rheumatoid arthritis. Arthritis Rheum 2012;64(6):1740–9.

[65] Hooper M, Kallas EG, Coffin D, Campbell D, Evans TG, Looney RJ. Cytomegalovirus seropositivity is associated with the expansion of CD4+CD28- and CD8+CD28- T cells in rheumatoid arthritis. J Rheumatol 1999;26(7):1452–7.

[66] Broadley I, Pera A, Morrow G, Davies KA, Kern F. Expansions of cytotoxic CD4+CD28- T cells drive excess cardiovascular mortality in rheumatoid arthritis and other chronic inflammatory conditions and are triggered by CMV infection. Front Immunol 2017;8:195.

[67] Davis 3rd JM, Knutson KL, Skinner JA, Strausbauch MA, Crowson CS, Therneau TM, et al. A profile of immune response to herpesvirus is associ-ated with radiographic joint damage in rheumatoid arthritis. Arthritis Res Ther 2012;14(1):R24.

[68] Davis JM, Knutson KL, Strausbauch MA, Green AB, Crowson CS, Therneau TM, et al. Immune response profiling in early rheumatoid arthritis: discovery of a novel interaction of treatment response with viral immunity. Arthritis Res Ther 2013;15(6):R199.

[69] Einsele H, Steidle M, Muller CA, Fritz P, Zacher J, Schmidt H, et al. Demonstration of cytomegalovirus (CMV) DNA and anti-CMV response in the synovial membrane and serum of patients with rheumatoid arthritis. J Rheumatol 1992;19(5):677–81.

[70] Kahaleh MB, LeRoy EC. Autoimmunity and vascular involvement in systemic sclerosis (SSc). Autoimmunity 1999;31(3):195–214.

[71] Hamamdzic D, Harley RA, Hazen-Martin D, LeRoy EC. MCMV induces neointima in IFN-gammaR-/- mice: intimal cell apoptosis and persistent proliferation of myofibroblasts. BMC Musculoskelet Disord 2001;2:3.

[72] Marou E, Liaskos C, Efthymiou G, Dardiotis E, Daponte A, Scheper T, et al. Increased immunoreactivity against human cytomegalovirus UL83 in systemic sclerosis. Clin Exp Rheumatol 2017;106(4):31–4. Sep-Oct;35 Suppl.

[73] Marou E, Liaskos C, Simopoulou T, Efthymiou G, Dardiotis E, Katsiari C, et al. Human cytomegalovirus (HCMV) UL44 and UL57 specific anti-body responses in anti-HCMV-positive patients with systemic sclerosis. Clin Rheumatol 2017;36(4):863–9.

[74] Muryoi T, Kasturi KN, Kafina MJ, Cram DS, Harrison LC, Sasaki T, et al. Antitopoisomerase I monoclonal autoantibodies from scleroderma patients and tight skin mouse interact with similar epitopes. J Exp Med 1992;175(4):1103–9.

[75] Lunardi C, Bason C, Navone R, Millo E, Damonte G, Corrocher R, et al. Systemic sclerosis immunoglobulin G autoantibodies bind the human cytomegalovirus late protein UL94 and induce apoptosis in human endothelial cells. Nat Med 2000;6(10):1183–6.

[76] Traggiai E, Lunardi C, Bason C, Dolcino M, Tinazzi E, Corrocher R, et al. Generation of anti-NAG-2 mAb from patients' memory B cells: implications for a novel therapeutic strategy in systemic sclerosis. Int Immunol 2010;22(5):367–74.

[77] Patrone V, Puglisi E, Cardinali M, Schnitzler TS, Svegliati S, Festa A, et al. Gut microbiota profile in systemic sclerosis patients with and without clinical evidence of gastrointestinal involvement. Sci Rep 2017;7(1):14874.

[78] Mavropoulos A, Liaskos C, Simopoulou T, Bogdanos DP, Sakkas LI. IL-10-producing regulatory B cells (B10 cells), IL-17+ T cells and autoantibodies in systemic sclerosis. Clin Immunol Nov 2017;184:26–32.

[79] Mavropoulos A, Simopoulou T, Varna A, Liaskos C, Katsiari CG, Bogdanos DP, et al. Breg cells are numerically decreased and functionally impaired in patients with systemic sclerosis. Arthritis Rheumatol 2016;68(2):494–504.

[80] Mavropoulos A, Varna A, Zafiriou E, Liaskos C, Alexiou I, Roussaki-Schulze A, et al. IL-10 producing Bregs are impaired in psoriatic arthritis and psoriasis and inversely correlate with IL-17- and IFNgamma-producing T cells. Clin Immunol 2017;184:33–41.

Section IV

The Novel Environmental Factors Associated With Autoimmunity

Chapter 22

Geoepidemiology of Autoimmune Diseases

Elena Generali[1], Carlo Selmi[1,2]

[1]Division of Rheumatology and Clinical Immunology, Humanitas Research Hospital, Rozzano, Italy; [2]BIOMETRA Department, University of Milan, Milan, Italy

INTRODUCTION

The idea of autoimmunity, or an immune response directed toward the self, can be dated back to 1890, which coincides with the beginning of the modern era of immunology. Before 1890, it was already known that the body can protect from the dangers of the outer world, the environment, and that it can learn from the experience, adaptive immunity; however, only at the beginning of the 20th century, serum sickness, blood group reactions, and anaphylaxis were described, supporting the idea of autoimmunity [1]. Furthermore, in 1901 the idea of autoantibodies was firstly described by Paul Ehrlich, although it took several years and the development of more modern technology (i.e., electrophoresis, radioactivity, chromatography) to identify other autoantibodies [2]. Across 1930s and 1940s, Eric Waaler and Harry Rose simultaneously described what we now call rheumatoid factor (RF) in rheumatoid arthritis (RA) patients [3]. In 1948 "lupus erythematosus (LE) cell" were described in systemic lupus erythematosus (SLE) patients and later antibodies directed toward cells nuclei. Between the 1960s and 1970s, rheumatologic diseases were drawn together and autoantibodies were recognized as the first manifestation.

There are now well over 100 human diseases considered to be autoimmune in their etiopathogenesis and all share a hereditary component. Nonetheless, genetic factors are insufficient to explain the susceptibility to immune tolerance breakdown and the clinical variability observed in autoimmunity, as well supported by the largely incomplete concordance rates of autoimmune diseases between monozygotic twins, which share identical genome. Genome-wide association studies have identified numerous genetic polymorphisms associated with autoimmune diseases, in some cases within genes shared among diseases, thus suggesting a common mechanistic pathway, which may indicate a genetic susceptibility resulting from the additive effects of several common risk variants [4,5].

The association between autoimmunity and environmental factors has been suspected for many years, particularly with epidemiological evidences, i.e., the "hygiene hypothesis" has been gathered by clinical epidemiology data linking infections or the Westernized lifestyle and the risk of autoimmunity and showing the increasing incidence of autoimmune and chronic inflammatory diseases in modern times [6]. In the recent past, the impact of environmental factors, not only infectious agents, in autoimmunity has been the focus of the National Institute of Environmental Health Sciences (NIEHS) expert panel workshop, which has critically evaluated the epidemiology and laboratory studies associated with autoimmunity in the 1980–2010 scientific literature and resulted in a comprehensive overview of the criteria and mechanisms of environmentally induced autoimmunity [7]. In this view, the concept of "exposome" has been introduced to collate and possibly measure the effects of environmental factors as the term encompasses all putative nonhereditary factors, both exogenous and endogenous [8]. Subsequently, the microbiota, the ecological community of commensal, symbiotic, and pathogenic microorganisms living in exquisite relationship with us, has been identified as an influencer of autoimmunity. From both experimental and theoretical models, the infections by viruses, bacteria, parasites, and fungi are ideal triggers for autoimmunity, also due to the individual susceptibility to develop acute and chronic infections [9] and to the parallel geoepidemiology of autoimmunity and infections worldwide [10]. Within the exposome, infections have been cumulatively defined as "infectome" as the part referring to the collection of an individual infectious exposures that are associated with autoimmune diseases [8].

Despite the significant progress in our tools and understanding of genetics, epigenetics, immunology, and epidemiology, it remains unclear why autoimmunity affects up to 5% of the general population [11] with a striking female predominance [12]. Geoepidemiology of autoimmune and chronic inflammatory diseases means the study of the distribution of these conditions and the determinants of disease gradients across multiple regions and populations [13,14]. For certain diseases in fact, geoepidemiology might uncover genetic risk factors by observing a gradient of disease rates corresponding to the distribution of certain HLA alleles, i.e., HLA-B27 and spondyloarthritis (SpA) [15,16], or conversely allow to identify geographical clusters of autoimmune diseases in areas that contain an environmental trigger, such as pollutants or infections [17,18]. Moreover, geoepidemiology might show the complex interplay between genes and environmental factors, for example, by comparing ethnic migrant populations with the native population and with the same ethnic group in their region of origin [19,20].

However, there is a paucity of reliable and up-to-date studies of the incidence and prevalence of autoimmune diseases, mostly derived from Europe and the United States through small studies with methodological differences. In the present chapter, we will review the available evidence regarding geoepidemiology of autoimmune and chronic inflammatory diseases.

RHEUMATOID ARTHRITIS

RA is a chronic inflammatory joint disease, characterized by joint destruction and systemic manifestations [21]. RA affects most frequently women in postmenopausal age and it is associated with the presence of disease-specific autoantibodies, i.e., RF and anticitrullinated peptides antibodies (ACPA) [22]. The incidence of RA varies across populations. In North America and Northern Europe, the estimated incidence of RA is around 20–50 cases per 100,000 population/year, with a point prevalence of 0.5%–1.1% [23,24]. In Mediterranean countries, lower incidences of 9–24 cases per 100,000 population have been reported [25,26], while estimates are not available for developing countries [27]. The onset of RA is most frequently reported around 40–50 years of age; however, a recent study showed that in tropical countries, RA onset occurs 8 years earlier compared to northern latitudes [28].

It is well recognized that RA develops in genetically predisposed individuals, among other and across all ethnic groups HLA-DR4 [29,30], and is triggered by environmental factors, smoking, and infections (Table 22.1). Periodontitis, an oral infection caused by *Porphyromonas gingivalis*, is the only human pathogen known to express peptidylarginine deiminase (PAD), the enzyme that generates citrullinated epitopes recognized by RA autoantibodies [31,32]. In fact, *P. gingivalis* expresses a PAD enzyme capable of citrullinating self-proteins (fibrinogen and enolase), which act as neoantigens and can bind with high affinity to major histocompatibility complex class II HLA-DR4 shared epitopes, leading in turn to ACPA production and RA development [33–35]. Autoantibodies directed toward post-translational modifications (PTM) proteins are able to bind both the native and the modified form. In RA, collagen type II is an autoantigen involved in the pathogenesis, and studies from our group have also shown different B and T cell epitopes on the molecule [36]. The B and T cell epitopes may undergo citrullination and glycosylation in vivo and thus induce the activation of immune cells in genetic predisposed subjects [36]. Interestingly, the risk of periodontitis is lower in population dwelling in suburban and rural area, compared to those who lived in urban area, while the higher income group has the higher risk of periodontitis compared with lower income group [37], which reflect the epidemiology of RA. In fact, urbanization has been associated with an increased prevalence of RA [38].

Other infections have been linked to RA development. Parvovirus B19 infection may also cause erosive arthritis and trigger RF appearance in the serum [39,40], thus mimicking seropositive RA [41–43]. Moreover, B19 infection is associated with the HLA-DR4 antigen and HLA-DRB1*01 and *04 alleles [44–46]. Parvovirus B19 infection has been reported to activate monocytes, T cells, and natural killer cells leading to the upregulation of proinflammatory cytokines (i.e., IL-1, IL-6, and IFN-γ) [47], which in predisposed individuals may also trigger RA. Lastly, anti-B19 IgM are detected only in a minority of patients, and IgG show no difference between patients with RA and controls [41,48] while viral DNA is detected in the synovial tissue of up to 75% of RA cases, even in the absence of serum antibodies, compared with 17% of other chronic arthritides [49].

SYSTEMIC LUPUS ERYTHEMATOSUS

SLE is an autoimmune disease involving several organs with various clinical manifestations and immunological alterations [50]. The global distribution of SLE is relatively homogeneous, and in the US population, SLE incidence is around 5–20 per 100,000 population/year, with higher SLE incidence in African Americans and Native Americans in particular, in which disease course and outcome are different [51]. There are, however, some exceptions in certain African regions where the incidence rate is low, as well as in Brazil where the incidence rate is high [52]. SLE is characterized by a striking female predominance (9:1 female to male ratio). Nevertheless, the geoepidemiology of SLE demonstrates the ethnic variance, which is explained by genetic susceptibility and environmental factors, including infections (Table 22.1), ultraviolet (UV) radiation, and pollutants [53,54].

TABLE 22.1 Infectious Agents (Viruses, Bacteria, Fungi) Proposed for the Initiation of Autoimmune and Chronic Inflammatory Diseases

	Pathogen	Disease	References
Viruses			
	Parvovirus B19	Rheumatoid arthritis, systemic lupus erythematosus	[65,124,125]
	Epstein–Barr virus	Rheumatoid arthritis, systemic lupus erythematosus, Sjögren's syndrome, primary biliary cholangitis, autoimmune hepatitis	[55–58,126–128]
	Cytomegalovirus	Systemic lupus erythematosus	[129,130]
	Betaretrovirus	Primary biliary cholangitis	[131]
	Hepatitis A virus	Autoimmune hepatitis	[132]
Bacteria			
	Porphyromonas gingivalis	Rheumatoid arthritis	[31]
	Segmented filamentous bacteria	Rheumatoid arthritis	[133]
	Yersinia enterocolitica	Rheumatoid arthritis, spondyloarthritis, reactive arthritis	[134,135]
	Salmonella typhi	Spondyloarthritis, reactive arthritis, systemic lupus erythematosus	[136,137]
	Shigella flexneri	Reactive arthritis	[138]
	Proteus mirabilis	Rheumatoid arthritis	[139]
	Campylobacter jejuni	Reactive arthritis	[140,141]
	Klebsiella pneumoniae	Ankylosing spondylitis, reactive arthritis	[142,143]
	Clostridium difficile	Reactive arthritis	[144]
	Staphylococcus aureus	Rheumatoid arthritis	[145]
	Streptococcus pyogenes	Rheumatic fever, psoriasis, psoriatic arthritis	[146–149]
	Chlamydia spp.	Reactive arthritis, primary biliary cholangitis	[150–152]
	Mycoplasma spp.	Reactive arthritis, rheumatoid arthritis, juvenile idiopathic arthritis, primary biliary cholangitis	[153–157]
	Mycobacterium tuberculosis	Spondyloarthritis	[158]
	Mycobacterium gordonae	Primary biliary cholangitis	[159,160]
	Novosphingobium aromaticivorans	Primary biliary cholangitis	[161]
	Borrelia burgdorferi	Lyme arthritis, spondyloarthritis, reactive arthritis, primary biliary cholangitis	[162–164]
	Escherichia coli	Reactive arthritis, primary biliary cholangitis	[165–168]
Fungi			
	Candida albicans	Arthritis	[169]

Epstein–Barr virus (EBV) has been reported in association with not only SLE [55] but also other autoimmune diseases, i.e., RA [56], Sjögren's syndrome [57], primary biliary cholangitis, and autoimmune hepatitis [58], among others. In SLE, it has been shown that EBV infection stimulates the production of EBV nuclear antigen 1 (EBNA-1) antibodies, which predispose to the development of cross-reactive autoantibodies, with further progression to clinical SLE [8,59,60]. This is supported by the evidence that a recent EBV infection or reactivation is more frequent in subjects with serum antinuclear antibodies (ANA); in particular, anti–EBV-VCA and EA IgG concentrations are significantly higher in the presence of

TABLE 22.2 Xenobiotics Associated With Autoimmune Diseases

Xenobiotic	Disease	References
Mercury	Glomerulonephritis, immune complex formation	[170,171]
Iodine	Autoimmune thyroiditis	[172]
Vinyl chloride	Scleroderma-like disease	[173]
Aromatic amines	Drug-related lupus	[174]
Hydrazines	Systemic lupus erythematosus	[175]
Silica	Rheumatoid arthritis, systemic lupus erythematosus, systemic sclerosis	[176,177]
Organic solvents	Systemic sclerosis, primary biliary cholangitis	[177,178]
Halothane	Hepatitis	[179]
Canavanine	Systemic lupus erythematosus–like symptoms	[180]
Toxic oil	Scleroderma-like disease	[181]

ANA positivity [61]. Moreover, anti–EBNA-1 antibodies can bind specific SLE antigens, i.e., Sm and Ro [60]. EBV infection has also been associated with disease flares in SLE, especially in the winter season [62].

Acute parvovirus B19 infection may clinically mimic SLE, as symptoms significantly overlap (fever, rash, arthralgia, myalgia, lymphadenopathy, anemia, cytopenias, hepatitis, production of ANA), or may trigger its onset or exacerbate preexisting SLE [63–66]. Furthermore, parvovirus B19 infection may trigger autoantibodies development, in particular ANA, anticardiolipin, and anti-beta2-glycoprotein I antibodies with the same specificity observed in SLE [67–69].

Cytomegalovirus (CMV) is a herpesvirus with a worldwide distribution, and several studies have supported its association with SLE. The presence of both anti-CMV IgM and CMV-DNA has been detected at disease onset in a subgroup of SLE cases [70,71] and the infection has been associated with SLE vascular manifestations with no renal involvement [72]. CMV may also trigger autoantibodies production, as reported for high-titer anti-Sm/RNP in SLE and Sjogren's syndrome (SjS) [57,73] while being protective or neutral with regard to RA [57,74].

Interestingly, although UV radiation is a well-known cause of SLE flare [75], it could also be the link between the increased susceptibility to SLE in African Americans or Hispanics living in the United States or Europe because of reduced exposure to sunlight and people living in countries near the Equator. In this view, low vitamin D levels could be key players in the development of SLE [76,77]. Moreover, experimental studies suggest that UV radiation results in the induction of reactive oxygen species, leading to DNA damage, resulting in the production of novel forms of autoantigens and autoreactive T cells [78–80], while conversely it may have immunomodulatory effects on T cells and cytokines [81].

Silica and other chemical agents cumulatively coined xenobiotics, i.e., industrial solvents have been implicated in triggering SLE and autoimmunity (Table 22.2) [82–84], as can induce protein alterations and neoantigen formation [85] and lead to autoantibody response also in healthy subjects [86]. The association between silica exposure and increased SLE risk has been observed in occupational, residential, rural, and urban settings [87,88], and it has a dose response as it increases with exposure [75]. The mechanisms behind the break of tolerance induced by silica are not well elucidated. Experimental studies suggest that crystalline silica acts as an immune adjuvant that induces apoptosis and release of intracellular antigens, increasing proinflammatory cytokines, oxidative stress, and T cell responses and decreasing the number of regulatory T cells [89].

SPONDYLOARTHRITIS

SpA are a heterogeneous group of inflammatory joint diseases, including psoriatic arthritis (PsA), ankylosing spondylitis (AS), reactive arthritis, arthritis associated with inflammatory bowel disease, i.e., IBD-associated or enteropathic, and undifferentiated SpA. SpA affects with equal frequency both sexes, albeit with differences in the clinical manifestations, i.e., axial involvement being more frequent in men [90]. The incidence rates of SpA vary between 0.48 and 63 per 100,000 individuals, whereas the prevalence rate ranges from 0.01% to 2.5%, with geographical variations, which have been linked to HLA-B27. In fact, HLA-B27 positivity varies throughout the world with a wide ethnic and geographical variation. The estimated prevalence of AS in Caucasians ranges from 0.1% to 1.4%. A definite exception to this range is the prevalence of AS in Haida and Bella Indians, where the estimated prevalence is much higher, reaching 6.1% [91]. In the United States, the incidence of AS was found to be approximately 1 per 10 000 males per year and one-third of that in females [92], with similar results also in Norwegian and Finnish populations [16,93]. Conversely, in Mediterranean and Asian countries, the incidence and prevalence are much lower, suggesting a North–South gradient in the epidemiology of AS [94]. With regard to PsA, there are few studies assessing disease prevalence, while there are also methodological differences because of the different criteria used for PsA diagnosis [95]. Northern European studies estimated PsA prevalence around 0.05%–0.1% [96], whereas in the United States, most recent studies have estimated an increased prevalence of PsA, ranging from 0.158% to 0.25% [97,98]; lower prevalence have been reported in Mediterranean countries [99,100]. Interestingly, in Japan, PsA prevalence has been reported to be 0.00001% [94], whereas in China it is similar to the rest of the world [101]. The prevalence of PsA in psoriasis patients conversely is much higher, being reported between 6% and 42% [102,103].

Genetics play a predominant role in SpA pathogenesis and HLA-B27 is thought to have a direct pathogenic role in SpA development, and different theories have been proposed, mostly related to intracellular protein misfolding [104]. Accumulation of unconventional forms of HLA-B27, such as free heavy chains (FHCs), was recently reported in the gut and synovial tissue of SpA patients, as well as in HLA-B27 transgenic rats. Animal studies have shown that FHCs may accumulate in the endoplasmic reticulum (ER) and in turn trigger the unfolded protein response [105,106], which leads to the production of IL-23 [107]. In human dendritic cells, ER stress was also shown to increase IL-23 production after Toll-like receptor stimulation [108]. Nonetheless, HLA accounts only for 40% of the genetic risk for SpA, and also other polymorphisms in non-HLA genes, involved in innate immune recognition and cytokine signaling pathways, are linked with SpA. Such genes include tumor necrosis factor and IL-23 [109], which are also shared with IBD and psoriasis [110].

As the development of SpA cannot be fully explained by genetic factors, it has been proposed that many environmental components, including smoking, trauma, infections, and microbiota, are critically involved in the induction of the disease in genetically predisposed individuals. Infections have been recognized as triggers for SpA since a long time, as ReA (previously including Reiter syndrome, an eponym now abandoned for the connections of the late Dr. Reiter to Nazifascism) was described in 1916, with the classic triad of symptoms in a soldier following a digestive infection, and attributed to *Treponema pallidum* infection [111]. ReA follows an infection of the digestive or genitourinary tract caused by different microorganisms, including *Chlamydia trachomatis*, *Shigella flexneri*, *Salmonella enteritidis*, *Salmonella typhimurium*, *Salmonella muenchen*, *Yersinia enterocolitica*, *Yersinia pseudotuberculosis*, *Campylobacter jejuni*, *Campylobacter fetus*, *Ureaplasma urealyticum*, and *Clostridium difficile*. Other less common microorganisms involved in ReA include *Neisseria gonorrhoeae*, *Borrelia burgdorferi*, *Chlamydia pneumoniae*, and *Escherichia coli* [112]. The exact mechanism on how these bacteria trigger ReA is not known yet. Cross-reactivity has been hypothesized because of the association with HLA-B27. Contrary to the historical definition of ReA, *Chlamydia* DNA and RNA have been found in the joints of patients affected by ReA, *Chlamydia trachomatis* and *Chlamydia pneumoniae* represent the most frequent causes of ReA, and can be found in the synovial fluid and tissue of the affected joints [113–116].

Trauma, injury, and heavy lifting have been associated with SpA development, in particular for PsA [117,118], given the long observed Koebner phenomenon in psoriasis [119], where psoriatic plaques develop in areas of physical trauma [120]. These observations have been recently confirmed by a large real-life observational study, in which physical trauma at bone and joint level has been found to be associated with PsA development in psoriasis [121]. In this view, enthesitis, the inflammation of fibrocartilaginous enthesis, represents the common denominator between SpA, and subclinical enthesitis may be the primary pathology that triggers secondary joint synovitis through the release of proinflammatory mediators [122].

CONCLUSIONS AND FUTURE PERSPECTIVES

The geoepidemiology of autoimmune and chronic inflammatory diseases can allow us to identify genetic and environmental influences that finally lead to the disease development. Albeit numerous studies have been published, big methodological issues may fault the results and give a wrong picture of the pathogenesis of diseases. First, older studies are difficult to compare with the newest because of the change in diagnostic criteria, as well as diagnostic advances, changing methodological standards. Second, the access to medical care and other socioeconomic factors can vary between developed and developing world regions and can represent a source of bias when comparing epidemiological data. Finally, comparing community- and hospital-based studies constitutes a major source of bias. In this view, technology gives us a helping hand, and the most recent studies assess geoepidemiology using big data, as Google-driven search, which can give access to numbers of patients that with difficulty could be retrieved also in international registries [123]. With this approach, future studies will be able to capture data also from parts of the world usually excluded from traditional clinical research and the identification of potential new environmental factors.

Lupoid hepatitis was introduced by our unit in 195CiL to describe cases of active chronic hepatitis associate with a positive LE cell test and occasionally minor manifestations of systemic lupus erythema.

REFERENCES

[1] Plotz PH. Autoimmunity: the history of an idea. Arthritis Rheumatol 2014;66(11):2915–20.

[2] Silverstein AM. Paul Ehrlich's passion: the origins of his receptor immunology. Cell Immunol 1999;194(2):213–21.

[3] Fraser KJ. The Waaler-Rose test: anatomy of the eponym. Semin Arthritis Rheum 1988;18(1):61–71.

[4] Theofilopoulos AN, Kono DH, Baccala R. The multiple pathways to autoimmunity. Nat Immunol 2017;18(7):716–24.

[5] Gutierrez-Arcelus M, Rich SS, Raychaudhuri S. Autoimmune diseases - connecting risk alleles with molecular traits of the immune system. Nat Rev Genet 2016;17(3):160–74.

[6] Stiemsma LT, Reynolds LA, Turvey SE, Finlay BB. The hygiene hypothesis: current perspectives and future therapies. Immunotargets Ther 2015;4:143–57.

[7] Selmi C, Leung PS, Sherr DH, Diaz M, Nyland JF, Monestier M, et al. Mechanisms of environmental influence on human autoimmunity: a National Institute of Environmental Health Sciences expert panel workshop. J Autoimmun 2012;39(4):272–84.

[8] Bogdanos DP, Smyk DS, Invernizzi P, Rigopoulou EI, Blank M, Pouria S, et al. Infectome: a platform to trace infectious triggers of autoimmunity. Autoimmun Rev 2013;12(7):726–40.

[9] Sakkas LI, Bogdanos DP. Infections as a cause of autoimmune rheumatic diseases. Auto Immun Highlights 2016;7(1):13.

[10] Shoenfeld Y, Selmi C, Zimlichman E, Gershwin ME. The autoimmunologist: geoepidemiology, a new center of gravity, and prime time for autoimmunity. J Autoimmun 2008;31(4):325–30.

[11] Cooper GS, Bynum ML, Somers EC. Recent insights in the epidemiology of autoimmune diseases: improved prevalence estimates and understanding of clustering of diseases. J Autoimmun 2009;33(3–4):197–207.

[12] Selmi C. Autoimmunity in 2016. Clin Rev Allergy Immunol 2017;53(1):126–39.

[13] Shapira Y, Agmon-Levin N, Shoenfeld Y. Defining and analyzing geoepidemiology and human autoimmunity. J Autoimmun 2010;34(3):J168–77.

[14] Shapira Y, Agmon-Levin N, Shoenfeld Y. Geoepidemiology of autoimmune rheumatic diseases. Nat Rev Rheumatol 2010;6(8):468–76.

[15] Mathieu A, Paladini F, Vacca A, Cauli A, Fiorillo MT, Sorrentino R. The interplay between the geographic distribution of HLA-B27 alleles and their role in infectious and autoimmune diseases: a unifying hypothesis. Autoimmun Rev 2009;8(5):420–5.

[16] Ehrenfeld M. Geoepidemiology: the environment and spondyloarthropathies. Autoimmun Rev 2010;9(5):A325–9.

[17] Silman AJ, Howard Y, Hicklin AJ, Black C. Geographical clustering of scleroderma in south and west London. Br J Rheumatol 1990;29(2):93–6.

[18] Piga M, Mathieu A. The origin of Behcet's disease geoepidemiology: possible role of a dual microbial-driven genetic selection. Clin Exp Rheumatol 2014;32(4 Suppl. 84):S123–9.

[19] Ehehalt S, Popovic P, Muntoni S, Muntoni S, Willasch A, Hub R, et al. Incidence of diabetes mellitus among children of Italian migrants substantiates the role of genetic factors in the pathogenesis of type 1 diabetes. Eur J Pediatr 2009;168(5):613–7.

[20] McLeod JG, Hammond SR, Kurtzke JF. Migration and multiple sclerosis in United Kingdom and Ireland immigrants to Australia: a reassessment. II. Characteristics of early (pre-1947) compared to later migrants. J Neurol 2012;259(4):684–93.

[21] Deane KD, Demoruelle MK, Kelmenson LB, Kuhn KA, Norris JM, Holers VM. Genetic and environmental risk factors for rheumatoid arthritis. Best Pract Res Clin Rheumatol 2017;31(1):3–18.

[22] Falkenburg WJJ, van Schaardenburg D. Evolution of autoantibody responses in individuals at risk of rheumatoid arthritis. Best Pract Res Clin Rheumatol 2017;31(1):42–52.

[23] Symmons DP, Barrett EM, Bankhead CR, Scott DG, Silman AJ. The incidence of rheumatoid arthritis in the United Kingdom: results from the Norfolk Arthritis Register. Br J Rheumatol 1994;33(8):735–9.

[24] Pedersen JK, Kjaer NK, Svendsen AJ, Horslev-Petersen K. Incidence of rheumatoid arthritis from 1995 to 2001: impact of ascertainment from multiple sources. Rheumatol Int 2009;29(4):411–5.

[25] Alamanos Y, Voulgari PV, Drosos AA. Incidence and prevalence of rheumatoid arthritis, based on the 1987 American College of Rheumatology criteria: a systematic review. Semin Arthritis Rheum 2006;36(3):182–8.

[26] Guillemin F, Briancon S, Klein JM, Sauleau E, Pourel J. Low incidence of rheumatoid arthritis in France. Scand J Rheumatol 1994;23(5):264–8.

[27] Tobon GJ, Youinou P, Saraux A. The environment, geo-epidemiology, and autoimmune disease: rheumatoid arthritis. J Autoimmun 2010;35(1):10–4.

[28] Group G-R. Latitude gradient influences the age of onset of rheumatoid arthritis: a worldwide survey. Clin Rheumatol 2017;36(3):485–97.

[29] Lee HS, Korman BD, Le JM, Kastner DL, Remmers EF, Gregersen PK, et al. Genetic risk factors for rheumatoid arthritis differ in Caucasian and Korean populations. Arthritis Rheum 2009;60(2):364–71.

[30] Zhu H, Xia W, Mo XB, Lin X, Qiu YH, Yi NJ, et al. Gene-based genome-wide association analysis in European and Asian populations identified novel genes for rheumatoid arthritis. PLoS One 2016;11(11):e0167212.

[31] Potempa J, Mydel P, Koziel J. The case for periodontitis in the pathogenesis of rheumatoid arthritis. Nat Rev Rheumatol 2017 Oct;13(10):606–20.

[32] Sakkas LI, Daoussis D, Liossis SN, Bogdanos DP. The infectious basis of ACPA-positive rheumatoid arthritis. Front Microbiol 2017;8:1853.

[33] McGraw WT, Potempa J, Farley D, Travis J. Purification, characterization, and sequence analysis of a potential virulence factor from Porphyromonas gingivalis, peptidylarginine deiminase. Infect Immun 1999;67(7):3248–56.

[34] Wegner N, Wait R, Sroka A, Eick S, Nguyen KA, Lundberg K, et al. *Peptidylarginine deiminase* from *Porphyromonas gingivalis* citrullinates human fibrinogen and alpha-enolase: implications for autoimmunity in rheumatoid arthritis. Arthritis Rheum 2010;62(9):2662–72.

[35] Hill JA, Southwood S, Sette A, Jevnikar AM, Bell DA, Cairns E. Cutting edge: the conversion of arginine to citrulline allows for a high-affinity peptide interaction with the rheumatoid arthritis-associated HLA-DRB1*0401 MHC class II molecule. J Immunol 2003;171(2):538–41.

[36] De Santis M, Ceribelli A, Cavaciocchi F, Generali E, Massarotti M, Isailovic N, et al. Effects of type II collagen epitope carbamylation and citrullination in human leucocyte antigen (HLA)-DR4(+) monozygotic twins discordant for rheumatoid arthritis. Clin Exp Immunol 2016;185(3):309–19.

[37] Yu HC, Su NY, Huang JY, Lee SS, Chang YC. Trends in the prevalence of periodontitis in Taiwan from 1997 to 2013: a nationwide population-based retrospective study. Medicine (Baltim) 2017;96(45):e8585.

[38] Chou CT, Pei L, Chang DM, Lee CF, Schumacher HR, Liang MH. Prevalence of rheumatic diseases in Taiwan: a population study of urban, suburban, rural differences. J Rheumatol 1994;21(2):302–6.

[39] Murai C, Munakata Y, Takahashi Y, Ishii T, Shibata S, Muryoi T, et al. Rheumatoid arthritis after human parvovirus B19 infection. Ann Rheum Dis 1999;58(2):130–2.

[40] Jobanputra P, Davidson F, Graham S, O'Neill H, Simmonds P, Yap PL. High frequency of parvovirus B19 in patients tested for rheumatoid factor. BMJ 1995;311(7019):1542.

[41] Cohen BJ, Buckley MM, Clewley JP, Jones VE, Puttick AH, Jacoby RK. Human parvovirus infection in early rheumatoid and inflammatory arthritis. Ann Rheum Dis 1986;45(10):832–8.

[42] Taylor HG, Borg AA, Dawes PT. Human parvovirus B19 and rheumatoid arthritis. Clin Rheumatol 1992;11(4):548–50.

[43] Tyndall A, Jelk W, Hirsch HH. Parvovirus B19 and erosive polyarthritis. Lancet 1994;343(8895):480–1.

[44] Kerr JR, Mattey DL, Thomson W, Poulton KV, Ollier WE. Association of symptomatic acute human parvovirus B19 infection with human leukocyte antigen class I and II alleles. J Infect Dis 2002;186(4):447–52.

[45] Gendi NS, Gibson K, Wordsworth BP. Effect of HLA type and hypocomplementaemia on the expression of parvovirus arthritis: one year follow up of an outbreak. Ann Rheum Dis 1996;55(1):63–5.

[46] Klouda PT, Corbin SA, Bradley BA, Cohen BJ, Woolf AD. HLA and acute arthritis following human parvovirus infection. Tissue Antigens 1986;28(5):318–9.

[47] Wagner AD, Goronzy JJ, Matteson EL, Weyand CM. Systemic monocyte and T-cell activation in a patient with human parvovirus B19 infection. Mayo Clin Proc 1995;70(3):261–5.

[48] Harrison B, Silman A, Barrett E, Symmons D. Low frequency of recent parvovirus infection in a population-based cohort of patients with early inflammatory polyarthritis. Ann Rheum Dis 1998;57(6):375–7.

[49] Naides SJ, Scharosch LL, Foto F, Howard EJ. Rheumatologic manifestations of human parvovirus B19 infection in adults. Initial two-year clinical experience. Arthritis Rheum 1990;33(9):1297–309.

[50] La Paglia GMC, Leone MC, Lepri G, Vagelli R, Valentini E, Alunno A, et al. One year in review 2017: systemic lupus erythematosus. Clin Exp Rheumatol 2017;35(4):551–61.

[51] Peschken CA, Esdaile JM. Systemic lupus erythematosus in North American Indians: a population based study. J Rheumatol 2000;27(8):1884–91.

[52] Stojan G, Petri M. Epidemiology of systemic lupus erythematosus: an update. Curr Opin Rheumatol 2017 Sep;3(3):164–72.

[53] Borchers AT, Naguwa SM, Shoenfeld Y, Gershwin ME. The geoepidemiology of systemic lupus erythematosus. Autoimmun Rev 2010;9(5):A277–87.

[54] Gulati G, Brunner HI. Environmental triggers in systemic lupus erythematosus. Semin Arthritis Rheum 2018 Apr;47(5):710–17.

[55] Chougule D, Nadkar M, Rajadhyaksha A, Pandit-Shende P, Surve P, Dawkar N, Khadilkar P, Patwardhan M, Kaveri S, Ghosh K, Pradhan V. J Med Virol 2018 Mar;90(3):559–63.

[56] Pratesi F, Tommasi C, Anzilotti C, Chimenti D, Migliorini P. Deiminated Epstein-Barr virus nuclear antigen 1 is a target of anti-citrullinated protein antibodies in rheumatoid arthritis. Arthritis Rheum 2006;54(3):733–41.

[57] Kivity S, Arango MT, Ehrenfeld M, Tehori O, Shoenfeld Y, Anaya JM, et al. Infection and autoimmunity in Sjogren's syndrome: a clinical study and comprehensive review. J Autoimmun 2014;51:17–22.

[58] Rigopoulou EI, Smyk DS, Matthews CE, Billinis C, Burroughs AK, Lenzi M, et al. Epstein-barr virus as a trigger of autoimmune liver diseases. Adv Virol 2012;2012:987471.

[59] Harley JB, Harley IT, Guthridge JM, James JA. The curiously suspicious: a role for Epstein-Barr virus in lupus. Lupus 2006;15(11):768–77.

[60] Harley JB, James JA. Epstein-Barr virus infection induces lupus autoimmunity. Bull NYU Hosp Jt Dis 2006;64(1–2):45–50.

[61] Cuomo L, Cirone M, Di Gregorio AO, Vitillo M, Cattivelli M, Magliocca V, et al. Elevated antinuclear antibodies and altered anti-Epstein-Barr virus immune responses. Virus Res 2015;195:95–9.

[62] Watad A, Azrielant S, Bragazzi NL, Sharif K, David P, Katz I, et al. Seasonality and autoimmune diseases: the contribution of the four seasons to the mosaic of autoimmunity. J Autoimmun 2017;82:13–30.

[63] Cope AP, Jones A, Brozovic M, Shafi MS, Maini RN. Possible induction of systemic lupus erythematosus by human parvovirus. Ann Rheum Dis 1992;51(6):803–4.

[64] Chassagne P, Mejjad O, Gourmelen O, Moore N, Le Loet X, Deshayes P. Exacerbation of systemic lupus erythematosus during human parvovirus B19 infection. Br J Rheumatol 1993;32(2):158–9.

[65] Hemauer A, Beckenlehner K, Wolf H, Lang B, Modrow S. Acute parvovirus B19 infection in connection with a flare of systemic lupus erythematodes in a female patient. J Clin Virol 1999;14(1):73–7.

[66] Trapani S, Ermini M, Falcini F. Human parvovirus B19 infection: its relationship with systemic lupus erythematosus. Semin Arthritis Rheum 1999;28(5):319–25.

[67] Loizou S, Cazabon JK, Walport MJ, Tait D, So AK. Similarities of specificity and cofactor dependence in serum antiphospholipid antibodies from patients with human parvovirus B19 infection and from those with systemic lupus erythematosus. Arthritis Rheum 1997;40(1):103–8.

[68] Kalt M, Gertner E. Antibodies to beta 2-glycoprotein I and cardiolipin with symptoms suggestive of systemic lupus erythematosus in parvovirus B19 infection. J Rheumatol 2001;28(10):2335–6.

[69] Kerr JR, Boyd N. Autoantibodies following parvovirus B19 infection. J Infect 1996;32(1):41–7.

[70] Hayashi T, Lee S, Ogasawara H, Sekigawa I, Iida N, Tomino Y, et al. Exacerbation of systemic lupus erythematosus related to cytomegalovirus infection. Lupus 1998;7(8):561–4.

[71] Nawata M, Seta N, Yamada M, Sekigawa I, Lida N, Hashimoto H. Possible triggering effect of cytomegalovirus infection on systemic lupus erythematosus. Scand J Rheumatol 2001;30(6):360–2.

[72] Stratta P, Canavese C, Ciccone G, Santi S, Quaglia M, Ghisetti V, et al. Correlation between cytomegalovirus infection and Raynaud's phenomenon in lupus nephritis. Nephron 1999;82(2):145–54.

[73] Newkirk MM, van Venrooij WJ, Marshall GS. Autoimmune response to U1 small nuclear ribonucleoprotein (U1 snRNP) associated with cytomegalovirus infection. Arthritis Res 2001;3(4):253–8.

[74] Sherina N, Hreggvidsdottir HS, Bengtsson C, Hansson M, Israelsson L, Alfredsson L, et al. Low levels of antibodies against common viruses associate with anti-citrullinated protein antibody-positive rheumatoid arthritis; implications for disease aetiology. Arthritis Res Ther 2017;19(1):219.

[75] Parks CG, de Souza Espindola Santos A, Barbhaiya M, Costenbader KH. Understanding the role of environmental factors in the development of systemic lupus erythematosus. Best Pract Res Clin Rheumatol 2017;31(3):306–20.

[76] Ponsonby AL, McMichael A, van der Mei I. Ultraviolet radiation and autoimmune disease: insights from epidemiological research. Toxicology 2002;181–182:71–8.

[77] Shoenfeld N, Amital H, Shoenfeld Y. The effect of melanism and vitamin D synthesis on the incidence of autoimmune disease. Nat Clin Pract Rheumatol 2009;5(2):99–105.

[78] Runger TM, Epe B, Moller K. Processing of directly and indirectly ultraviolet-induced DNA damage in human cells. Recent Results Cancer Res 1995;139:31–42.

[79] Andrade F, Casciola-Rosen LA, Rosen A. Generation of novel covalent RNA-protein complexes in cells by ultraviolet B irradiation: implications for autoimmunity. Arthritis Rheum 2005;52(4):1160–70.

[80] Yung R, Powers D, Johnson K, Amento E, Carr D, Laing T, et al. Mechanisms of drug-induced lupus. II. T cells overexpressing lymphocyte function-associated antigen 1 become autoreactive and cause a lupuslike disease in syngeneic mice. J Clin Investig 1996;97(12):2866–71.

[81] Aubin F. Mechanisms involved in ultraviolet light-induced immunosuppression. Eur J Dermatol 2003;13(6):515–23.

[82] Somers EC, Richardson BC. Environmental exposures, epigenetic changes and the risk of lupus. Lupus 2014;23(6):568–76.

[83] Gilbert KM, Reisfeld B, Zurlinden TJ, Kreps MN, Erickson SW, Blossom SJ. Modeling toxicodynamic effects of trichloroethylene on liver in mouse model of autoimmune hepatitis. Toxicol Appl Pharmacol 2014;279(3):284–93.

[84] Lerner A, Matthias T. Changes in intestinal tight junction permeability associated with industrial food additives explain the rising incidence of autoimmune disease. Autoimmun Rev 2015;14(6):479–89.

[85] Mao TK, Davis PA, Odin JA, Coppel RL, Gershwin ME. Sidechain biology and the immunogenicity of PDC-E2, the major autoantigen of primary biliary cirrhosis. Hepatology (Baltimore, Md) 2004;40(6):1241–8.

[86] Vojdani A, Kharrazian D, Mukherjee PS. Elevated levels of antibodies against xenobiotics in a subgroup of healthy subjects. J Appl Toxicol 2015;35(4):383–97.

[87] Parks CG, Cooper GS, Nylander-French LA, Storm JF, Archer JD. Assessing exposure to crystalline silica from farm work: a population-based study in the Southeastern United States. Ann Epidemiol 2003;13(5):385–92.

[88] Finckh A, Cooper GS, Chibnik LB, Costenbader KH, Watts J, Pankey H, et al. Occupational silica and solvent exposures and risk of systemic lupus erythematosus in urban women. Arthritis Rheum 2006;54(11):3648–54.

[89] Pollard KM. Silica, silicosis, and autoimmunity. Front Immunol 2016;7:97.

[90] Eder L, Thavaneswaran A, Chandran V, Gladman DD. Gender difference in disease expression, radiographic damage and disability among patients with psoriatic arthritis. Ann Rheum Dis 2013;72(4):578–82.

[91] Benevolenskaya LI, Boyer GS, Erdesz S, Templin DW, Alexeeva LI, Lawrence RC, et al. Spondylarthropathic diseases in indigenous circumpolar populations of Russia and Alaska. Rev Rhum Engl Ed 1996;63(11):815–22.

[92] Carbone LD, Cooper C, Michet CJ, Atkinson EJ, O'Fallon WM, Melton 3rd LJ. Ankylosing spondylitis in Rochester, Minnesota, 1935-1989. Is the epidemiology changing? Arthritis Rheum 1992;35(12):1476–82.

[93] Bakland G, Nossent HC, Gran JT. Incidence and prevalence of ankylosing spondylitis in Northern Norway. Arthritis Rheum 2005;53(6):850–5.

[94] Hukuda S, Minami M, Saito T, Mitsui H, Matsui N, Komatsubara Y, et al. Spondyloarthropathies in Japan: nationwide questionnaire survey performed by the Japan Ankylosing Spondylitis Society. J Rheumatol 2001;28(3):554–9.

[95] Chandran V, Raychaudhuri SP. Geoepidemiology and environmental factors of psoriasis and psoriatic arthritis. J Autoimmun 2010;34(3):J314–21.

[96] O'Neill T, Silman AJ. Psoriatic arthritis. Historical background and epidemiology. Bailliere's Clin Rheumatol 1994;8(2):245–61.

[97] Wilson FC, Icen M, Crowson CS, McEvoy MT, Gabriel SE, Kremers HM. Time trends in epidemiology and characteristics of psoriatic arthritis over 3 decades: a population-based study. J Rheumatol 2009;36(2):361–7.

[98] Gelfand JM, Gladman DD, Mease PJ, Smith N, Margolis DJ, Nijsten T, et al. Epidemiology of psoriatic arthritis in the population of the United States. J Am Acad Dermatol 2005;53(4):573.

[99] Alamanos Y, Papadopoulos NG, Voulgari PV, Siozos C, Psychos DN, Tympanidou M, et al. Epidemiology of psoriatic arthritis in northwest Greece, 1982-2001. J Rheumatol 2003;30(12):2641–4.

[100] Trontzas P, Andrianakos A, Miyakis S, Pantelidou K, Vafiadou E, Garantziotou V, et al. Seronegative spondyloarthropathies in Greece: a population-based study of prevalence, clinical pattern, and management. The ESORDIG study. Clin Rheumatol 2005;24(6):583–9.

[101] Zeng QY, Chen R, Darmawan J, Xiao ZY, Chen SB, Wigley R, et al. Rheumatic diseases in China. Arthritis Res Ther 2008;10(1):R17.

[102] Ibrahim G, Waxman R, Helliwell PS. The prevalence of psoriatic arthritis in people with psoriasis. Arthritis Rheum 2009;61(10):1373–8.

[103] Gladman DD, Antoni C, Mease P, Clegg DO, Nash P. Psoriatic arthritis: epidemiology, clinical features, course, and outcome. Ann Rheum Dis 2005;64. Suppl 2:ii14-7.

[104] Colbert RA, DeLay ML, Layh-Schmitt G, Sowders DP. HLA-B27 misfolding and spondyloarthropathies. Prion 2009;3(1):15–26.

[105] Colbert RA, DeLay ML, Klenk EI, Layh-Schmitt G. From HLA-B27 to spondyloarthritis: a journey through the ER. Immunol Rev 2010;233(1):181–202.

[106] Turner MJ, Sowders DP, DeLay ML, Mohapatra R, Bai S, Smith JA, et al. HLA-B27 misfolding in transgenic rats is associated with activation of the unfolded protein response. J Immunol 2005;175(4):2438–48.

[107] DeLay ML, Turner MJ, Klenk EI, Smith JA, Sowders DP, Colbert RA. HLA-B27 misfolding and the unfolded protein response augment interleukin-23 production and are associated with Th17 activation in transgenic rats. Arthritis Rheum 2009;60(9):2633–43.

[108] Goodall JC, Wu C, Zhang Y, McNeill L, Ellis L, Saudek V, et al. Endoplasmic reticulum stress-induced transcription factor, CHOP, is crucial for dendritic cell IL-23 expression. Proc Natl Acad Sci U S A 2010;107(41):17698–703.

[109] Ambarus C, Yeremenko N, Tak PP, Baeten D. Pathogenesis of spondyloarthritis: autoimmune or autoinflammatory? Curr Opin Rheumatol 2012;24(4):351–8.

[110] Nestle FO, Kaplan DH, Barker J. Psoriasis N Engl J Med 2009;361(5):496–509.

[111] Wu IB, Schwartz RA. Reiter's syndrome: the classic triad and more. J Am Acad Dermatol 2008;59(1):113–21.

[112] Generali E, Ceribelli A, Massarotti M, Cantarini L, Selmi C. Seronegative reactive spondyloarthritis and the skin. Clin Dermatol 2015;33(5):531–7.

[113] Gerard HC, Schumacher HR, El-Gabalawy H, Goldbach-Mansky R, Hudson AP. Chlamydia pneumoniae present in the human synovium are viable and metabolically active. Microb Pathog 2000;29(1):17–24.

[114] Gerard HC, Branigan PJ, Schumacher Jr HR, Hudson AP. Synovial *Chlamydia trachomatis* in patients with reactive arthritis/Reiter's syndrome are viable but show aberrant gene expression. J Rheumatol 1998;25(4):734–42.

[115] Pavlica L, Draskovic N, Kuljic-Kapulica N, Nikolic D. Isolation of *Chlamydia trachomatis* or *Ureaplasma urealyticum* from the synovial fluid of patients with Reiter's syndrome. Vojnosanit Pregl 2003;60(1):5–10.

[116] Kumar P, Khanna G, Batra S, Sharma VK, Rastogi S. *Chlamydia trachomatis* elementary bodies in synovial fluid of patients with reactive arthritis and undifferentiated spondyloarthropathy in India. Int J Rheum Dis 2016;19(5):506–11.

[117] Love TJ, Zhu Y, Zhang Y, Wall-Burns L, Ogdie A, Gelfand JM, et al. Obesity and the risk of psoriatic arthritis: a population-based study. Ann Rheum Dis 2012;71(8):1273–7.

[118] Van Mechelen M, Lories RJ. Microtrauma: no longer to be ignored in spondyloarthritis? Curr Opin Rheumatol 2016;28(2):176–80.

[119] Liang Y, Sarkar MK, Tsoi LC, Gudjonsson JE. Psoriasis: a mixed autoimmune and autoinflammatory disease. Curr Opin Immunol 2017;49:1–8.

[120] Veale DJ, FitzGerald O. Psoriatic arthritis–pathogenesis and epidemiology. Clin Exp Rheumatol 2002;20(6 Suppl. 28):S27–33.

[121] Thorarensen SM, Lu N, Ogdie A, Gelfand JM, Choi HK, Love TJ. Physical trauma recorded in primary care is associated with the onset of psoriatic arthritis among patients with psoriasis. Ann Rheum Dis 2017;76(3):521–5.

[122] McGonagle D. Enthesitis: an autoinflammatory lesion linking nail and joint involvement in psoriatic disease. J Eur Acad Dermatol Venereol 2009;23(Suppl. 1):9–13.

[123] Ramos-Casals M, Brito-Zeron P, Kostov B, Siso-Almirall A, Bosch X, Buss D, et al. Google-driven search for big data in autoimmune geoepidemiology: analysis of 394,827 patients with systemic autoimmune diseases. Autoimmun Rev 2015;14(8):670–9.

[124] Kerr JR, Cartron JP, Curran MD, Moore JE, Elliott JR, Mollan RA. A study of the role of parvovirus B19 in rheumatoid arthritis. Br J Rheumatol 1995;34(9):809–13.

[125] Chang M, Pan MR, Chen DY, Lan JL. Human cytomegalovirus pp65 lower matrix protein: a humoral immunogen for systemic lupus erythematosus patients and autoantibody accelerator for NZB/W F1 mice. Clin Exp Immunol 2006;143(1):167–79.

[126] Cornillet M, Verrouil E, Cantagrel A, Serre G, Nogueira L. ACPA-positive RA patients, antibodies to EBNA35-58Cit, a citrullinated peptide from the Epstein-Barr nuclear antigen-1, strongly cross-react with the peptide beta60-74Cit which bears the immunodominant epitope of citrullinated fibrin. Immunol Res 2015;61(1–2):117–25.

[127] Croia C, Astorri E, Murray-Brown W, Willis A, Brokstad KA, Sutcliffe N, et al. Implication of Epstein-Barr virus infection in disease-specific autoreactive B cell activation in ectopic lymphoid structures of Sjogren's syndrome. Arthritis Rheumatol 2014;66(9):2545–57.

[128] James JA, Neas BR, Moser KL, Hall T, Bruner GR, Sestak AL, et al. Systemic lupus erythematosus in adults is associated with previous Epstein-Barr virus exposure. Arthritis Rheum 2001;44(5):1122–6.

[129] Barzilai O, Sherer Y, Ram M, Izhaky D, Anaya JM, Shoenfeld Y. Epstein-Barr virus and cytomegalovirus in autoimmune diseases: are they truly notorious? A preliminary report. Ann N Y Acad Sci 2007;1108:567–77.

[130] Hrycek A, Kusmierz D, Mazurek U, Wilczok T. Human cytomegalovirus in patients with systemic lupus erythematosus. Autoimmunity 2005;38(7):487–91.

[131] Mason AL. The evidence supports a viral aetiology for primary biliary cirrhosis. J Hepatol 2011;54(6):1312–4.

[132] Vento S, Cainelli F. Is there a role for viruses in triggering autoimmune hepatitis? Autoimmun Rev 2004;3(1):61–9.

[133] Wu HJ, Ivanov II , Darce J, Hattori K, Shima T, Umesaki Y, et al. Gut-residing segmented filamentous bacteria drive autoimmune arthritis via T helper 17 cells. Immunity 2010;32(6):815–27.

[134] Bech K, Clemmensen O, Larsen JH, Thyme S, Bendixen G. Cell-mediated immunity of Yersinia enterocolitica serotype 3 in patients with thyroid diseases. Allergy 1978;33(2):82–8.

[135] Kaarela K, Jantti JK, Kotaniemi KM. Similarity between chronic reactive arthritis and ankylosing spondylitis. A 32-35-year follow-up study. Clin Exp Rheumatol 2009;27(2):325–8.

[136] McColl GJ, Diviney MB, Holdsworth RF, McNair PD, Carnie J, Hart W, et al. HLA-B27 expression and reactive arthritis susceptibility in two patient cohorts infected with Salmonella Typhimurium. Aust N Z J Med 2000;30(1):28–32.

[137] Gerona JG, Navarra SV. Salmonella infections in patients with systemic lupus erythematosus: a case series. Int J Rheum Dis 2009;12(4):319–23.

[138] Hannu T, Mattila L, Siitonen A, Leirisalo-Repo M. Reactive arthritis attributable to Shigella infection: a clinical and epidemiological nationwide study. Ann Rheum Dis 2005;64(4):594–8.

[139] Rashid T, Ebringer A, Wilson C. The link between *Proteus mirabilis*, environmental factors and autoantibodies in rheumatoid arthritis. Clin Exp Rheumatol 2017 Sep–Oct;35(5):865–71.

[140] Pope JE, Krizova A, Garg AX, Thiessen-Philbrook H, Ouimet JM. Campylobacter reactive arthritis: a systematic review. Semin Arthritis Rheum 2007;37(1):48–55.

[141] Soderlin MK, Kautiainen H, Puolakkainen M, Hedman K, Soderlund-Venermo M, Skogh T, et al. Infections preceding early arthritis in southern Sweden: a prospective population-based study. J Rheumatol 2003;30(3):459–64.

[142] Puccetti A, Dolcino M, Tinazzi E, Moretta F, D'Angelo S, Olivieri I, et al. Antibodies directed against a peptide epitope of a Klebsiella pneumoniae-Derived protein are present in ankylosing spondylitis. PLoS One 2017;12(1):e0171073.

[143] Rashid T, Ebringer A, Wilson C. The link between Klebsiella and ankylosing spondylitis in worldwide geographical locations. Curr Rheumatol Rev 2016;12(3):223–31.

[144] Legendre P, Lalande V, Eckert C, Barbut F, Fardet L, Meynard JL, et al. *Clostridium difficile* associated reactive arthritis: case report and literature review. Anaerobe 2016;38:76–80.

[145] Liu ZQ, Deng GM, Foster S, Tarkowski A. Staphylococcal peptidoglycans induce arthritis. Arthritis Res 2001;3(6):375–80.

[146] Perez-Lorenzo R, Zambrano-Zaragoza JF, Moo-Castillo K, Luna-Vazquez DL, Ruiz-Guillermo L, Garcia-Latorre E. IgG class antibodies to heat shock-induced streptococcal antigens in psoriatic patients. Int J Dermatol 2003;42(2):110–5.

[147] Williamson DA, Smeesters PR, Steer AC, Steemson JD, Ng AC, Proft T, et al. M-protein analysis of *Streptococcus pyogenes* isolates associated with acute rheumatic fever in New Zealand. J Clin Microbiol 2015;53(11):3618–20.

[148] Rantakokko K, Rimpilainen M, Uksila J, Jansen C, Luukkainen R, Toivanen P. Antibodies to streptococcal cell wall in psoriatic arthritis and cutaneous psoriasis. Clin Exp Rheumatol 1997;15(4):399–404.

[149] Gudjonsson JE, Thorarinsson AM, Sigurgeirsson B, Kristinsson KG, Valdimarsson H. Streptococcal throat infections and exacerbation of chronic plaque psoriasis: a prospective study. Br J Dermatol 2003;149(3):530–4.

[150] Schmitt SK. Reactive arthritis. Infect Dis Clin N Am 2017;31(2):265–77.

[151] Abdulkarim AS, Petrovic LM, Kim WR, Angulo P, Lloyd RV, Lindor KD. Primary biliary cirrhosis: an infectious disease caused by Chlamydia pneumoniae? J Hepatol 2004;40(3):380–4.

[152] Liu HY, Deng AM, Zhang J, Zhou Y, Yao DK, Tu XQ, et al. Correlation of *Chlamydia pneumoniae* infection with primary biliary cirrhosis. World J Gastroenterol 2005;11(26):4108–10.

[153] Ataee RA, Golmohammadi R, Alishiri GH, Mirnejad R, Najafi A, Esmaeili D, et al. Simultaneous detection of *Mycoplasma pneumoniae*, *Mycoplasma hominis* and *Mycoplasma arthritidis* in synovial fluid of patients with rheumatoid arthritis by multiplex PCR. Arch Iran Med 2015;18(6):345–50.

[154] Rigante D, Bosco A, Esposito S. The etiology of juvenile idiopathic arthritis. Clin Rev Allergy Immunol 2015;49(2):253–61.

[155] Selmi C, Gershwin ME. Diagnosis and classification of reactive arthritis. Autoimmun Rev 2014;13(4–5):546–9.

[156] da Rocha Sobrinho HM, Jarach R, da Silva NA, Shio MT, Jancar S, Timenetsky J, et al. Mycoplasmal lipid-associated membrane proteins and *Mycoplasma arthritidis* mitogen recognition by serum antibodies from patients with rheumatoid arthritis. Rheumatol Int 2011;31(7):951–7.

[157] Berg CP, Kannan TR, Klein R, Gregor M, Baseman JB, Wesselborg S, et al. Mycoplasma antigens as a possible trigger for the induction of antimitochondrial antibodies in primary biliary cirrhosis. Liver Int 2009;29(6):797–809.

[158] van Tok MN, Satumtira N, Dorris M, Pots D, Slobodin G, van de Sande MG, et al. Innate immune activation can trigger experimental spondyloarthritis in HLA-B27/Hubeta2m transgenic rats. Front Immunol 2017;8:920.

[159] Bogdanos DP, Pares A, Baum H, Caballeria L, Rigopoulou EI, Ma Y, et al. Disease-specific cross-reactivity between mimicking peptides of heat shock protein of *Mycobacterium gordonae* and dominant epitope of E2 subunit of pyruvate dehydrogenase is common in Spanish but not British patients with primary biliary cirrhosis. J Autoimmun 2004;22(4):353–62.

[160] Vilagut L, Vila J, Vinas O, Pares A, Gines A, Jimenez de Anta MT, et al. Cross-reactivity of anti-*Mycobacterium gordonae* antibodies with the major mitochondrial autoantigens in primary biliary cirrhosis. J Hepatol 1994;21(4):673–7.

[161] Bogdanos DP, Vergani D. Bacteria and primary biliary cirrhosis. Clin Rev Allergy Immunol 2009;36(1):30–9.

[162] Arvikar SL, Steere AC. Diagnosis and treatment of Lyme arthritis. Infect Dis Clin N Am 2015;29(2):269–80.

[163] Arvikar SL, Crowley JT, Sulka KB, Steere AC. Autoimmune arthritides, rheumatoid arthritis, psoriatic arthritis, or peripheral spondyloarthritis following lyme disease. Arthritis Rheumatol 2017;69(1):194–202.

[164] Bogdanos DP, Koutsoumpas A, Baum H, Vergani D. *Borrelia Burgdorferi*: a new self-mimicking trigger in primary biliary cirrhosis. Dig Liver Dis 2006;38(10). 781-2; author reply 2–3.

[165] Singh Sangha M, Wright ML, Ciurtin C. Strongly positive anti-CCP antibodies in patients with sacroiliitis or reactive arthritis post-*E. coli* infection: a mini case-series based review. Int J Rheum Dis 2018 Jan;21(1):315–21.

[166] Nishizaki Y, Yamagami S, Inoue H, Uehara Y, Kobayashi S, Daida H. Reactive arthritis caused by urinary tract infection. Intern Med 2016;55(9):1195–8.

[167] Smyk DS, Bogdanos DP, Kriese S, Billinis C, Burroughs AK, Rigopoulou EI. Urinary tract infection as a risk factor for autoimmune liver disease: from bench to bedside. Clin Res Hepatol Gastroenterol 2012;36(2):110–21.

[168] Parikh-Patel A, Gold EB, Worman H, Krivy KE, Gershwin ME. Risk factors for primary biliary cirrhosis in a cohort of patients from the united states. Hepatology 2001;33(1):16–21.

[169] Hermann E, Mayet WJ, Klein O, Lohse AW, Trautwein C, Michiels I, et al. Candida arthritis: cellular immune responses of synovial fluid and peripheral blood lymphocytes to *Candida albicans*. Ann Rheum Dis 1991;50(10):697–701.

[170] Havarinasab S, Hultman P. Organic mercury compounds and autoimmunity. Autoimmun Rev 2005;4(5):270–5.

[171] Rowley B, Monestier M. Mechanisms of heavy metal-induced autoimmunity. Mol Immunol 2005;42(7):833–8.

[172] Rose NR, Bonita R, Burek CL. Iodine: an environmental trigger of thyroiditis. Autoimmun Rev 2002;1(1–2):97–103.

[173] Rieger R, Gershwin ME. The X and why of xenobiotics in primary biliary cirrhosis. J Autoimmun 2007;28(2–3):76–84.

[174] Reidenberg MM. Aromatic amines and the pathogenesis of lupus erythematosus. Am J Med 1983;75(6):1037–42.

[175] Yung RL, Richardson BC. Drug-induced lupus. Rheum Dis Clin N Am 1994;20(1):61–86.

[176] Steenland K, Goldsmith DF. Silica exposure and autoimmune diseases. Am J Ind Med 1995;28(5):603–8.

[177] Rubio-Rivas M, Moreno R, Corbella X. Occupational and environmental scleroderma. Systematic review and meta-analysis. Clin Rheumatol 2017;36(3):569–82.

[178] Gershwin ME, Selmi C, Worman HJ, Gold EB, Watnik M, Utts J, et al. Risk factors and comorbidities in primary biliary cirrhosis: a controlled interview-based study of 1032 patients. Hepatology 2005;42(5):1194–202.

[179] Liu ZX, Kaplowitz N. Immune-mediated drug-induced liver disease. Clin Liver Dis 2002;6(3):755–74.

[180] Montanaro A, Bardana Jr EJ. Dietary amino acid-induced systemic lupus erythematosus. Rheum Dis Clin N Am 1991;17(2):323–32.

[181] Posada de la Paz M, Philen RM, Borda AI. Toxic oil syndrome: the perspective after 20 years. Epidemiol Rev 2001;23(2):231–47.

Chapter 23

Seasonality and Autoimmune Diseases

Abdulla Watad[1,2,3], Kassem Sharif[1,2,3], Nicola Luigi Bragazzi[4], Benjamin Lichtbroun[2], Howard Amital[1,2,3], Yehuda Shoenfeld[5,6]

[1]Department of Medicine 'B', Sheba Medical Center, Tel-Hashomer, Israel; [2]Zabludowicz Center for Autoimmune Diseases, Sheba Medical Center, Tel-Hashomer, Israel; [3]Sackler Faculty of Medicine, Tel Aviv University, Tel Aviv, Israel; [4]Postgraduate School of Public Health, Department of Health Sciences (DISSAL), University of Genoa, Genoa, Italy; [5]Zabludowicz Center for Autoimmune Diseases, Sheba Medical Center, affiliated to Sackler Faculty of Medicine, Tel Aviv University, Tel Aviv, Israel; [6]Laboratory of the Mosaics of Autoimmunity, Saint-Petersburg University, Saint-Petersburg, Russian Federation

INTRODUCTION

Autoimmune diseases (ADs) are chronic conditions that result from the loss of immunological tolerance toward self-antigens, causing an immune response against self-tissues [1]. The pathogenesis of ADs comprises a series of complex interactions between genetic, environmental, and hormonal factors [2,3]. Various environmental variables, either conferring protective or deteriorating effects, can be associated with ADs. Levels of vitamin D, exposure to ultraviolet (UV) radiation, levels of melatonin, and infections exhibit a seasonal variation pattern [4,5].

Body levels of vitamin D are documented to fluctuate with changing seasons because of the influence of UV radiation exposure during different times of the year. Moreover, melatonin is a hormone responsible for the circadian rhythms of different physiological functions. Its secretion from the pineal gland changes according to daylight time and night length and with seasons [6]. Melatonin has anti-inflammatory properties mediated by its inhibition of inflammatory cytokines and its influences on different arms of the immune system [7,8].

In this review, we report the current knowledge on the association between seasonal factors and relevant ADs (Table 23.1).

MULTIPLE SCLEROSIS AND SEASONALITY

The relationship between multiple sclerosis (MS) and seasonality has been described. A higher susceptibility to developing MS was observed in individuals who were born in the spring, as contrasted to births during the winter months [9]. These findings were also replicated and supported by later studies that demonstrated a higher observed-to-expected ratio of MS in individuals born in April (odds ratio, OR, 1.21 [95% confidence interval (CI), 1.08–1.36]) [10]. In addition, higher levels of circulating vitamin D were associated with lower risk for developing MS as compared with low levels of vitamin D [11]. Ascherio et al. [12] documented a decrease in the active lesions and a decrease in the number of relapses per year in patients with higher levels of vitamin D.

Looking from another angle, the role of melatonin in influencing MS disease onset and progression remains disputable [13]. Melatonin levels were inversely associated with the length of disease since diagnosis ($P < .05$) [14]. Farez et al. [15] showed that increased melatonin levels correlated with decreased relapses in MS. These results seem to suggest a possible immunosuppressive role of melatonin on the disease process. Infectious role has also been proposed. In a prospective longitudinal study, MS relapses were found to be correlated with upper respiratory tract infections, which are more prevalent during winter [16]. In an additional study, Sibley et al. [17] reported the role of viral infections in MS precipitation/relapse, which occurs more frequently during winter [17].

SYSTEMIC LUPUS ERYTHEMATOSUS AND SEASONALITY

Recent studies showed the presence of seasonal variation patterns in systemic lupus erythematosus (SLE) presentation, a pattern that is best explained by changes in vitamin D and the amount of UV radiation exposure.

In a large prospective cohort, it has been demonstrated that photosensitive rash showed a significant increase in occurrence during the period between April–September ($P < .0001$). Secondly, arthritis exhibited seasonal variation with more episodes occurring during May to October ($P = .0057$). Thirdly, a decrease of renal flares could be noticed during

TABLE 23.1 Interaction Between Seasonal Factors and Autoimmune Diseases

Season	Influence of Disease
Spring	Month of birth ↑ risk for MS, UC, and GD for females
	⇊ Melatonin levels → ↑ IBD risk ↑ MS relapses
Summer	↑Vit.D ⇊ MS, ⇊ T1DM risk
	↑Vit.D ↓ IBD and MS relapses
	↑ *Escherichia coli* → ↑ PBC risk of onset
	↑ *Coxsackievirus* → ↑ T1DM onset
Autumn	Autumn births: ↑ GD in females
Winter	Winter births: ↑ GD in males
	↑ Melatonin levels → ↑ SLE relapses
	⇊ Vit.D → ↑ MS, IBD relapses
	↑ URTI → ↑ MS relapses ↑ EBV → ↑ SLE risk ↑ Rotavirus → ↑ T1DM

ALD, autoimmune liver diseases; *CD*, Crohn's disease; *EBV*, Epstein–Barr virus; *GD*, Grave's disease; *HD*, Hashimoto's disease; *IBD*, inflammatory bowel disease; *MS*, multiple sclerosis; *PBC*, primary biliary cholangitis; *SLE*, systemic lupus erythematosus; *T1DM*, type 1 diabetes mellitus; *UC*, ulcerative colitis; *Vit.D*, vitamin D.

summer ($P = .0397$). Fourthly, anti-DNA levels were significantly elevated during the months of October and November ($P < .0001$) [18].

Low levels of vitamin D in SLE patients were reported by Ben-Zvi et al. [19], who documented an inverse relationship between plasma vitamin D levels and disease activity ($P = .002$). Amital et al. [20] supported the previous relationship by reporting a higher disease activity in 378 SLE patients with lower vitamin D levels ($P = .018$).

Melatonin involvement in SLE was also described. Campillo et al. [21] evaluated the effect of melatonin on cells extracted from SLE patients, showing the critical anti-inflammatory actions of melatonin on these cells. Melatonin appeared to function in two major pathways, namely the Th1 cell inhibition and the Treg cell induction, both of which favor an anti-inflammatory environment [21].

Finally, UV light has been shown to play a contributory role in the disease process. Sanders et al. [22] demonstrated that 93% of SLE patients showed clinical and histological signs of photosensitivity after exposure to light radiation [22]. A Swedish study also reported that people who had serious sunburns were more likely to develop SLE when compared with healthy controls (OR 2.2 [95% CI 1.2–4.1]) [23]. These results support the notion that UV radiation leads to aggravation of cutaneous lupus. UV radiation is known to be higher during summer, a result that goes in concordance with the previously mentioned seasonal variation of cutaneous symptoms of the SLE spectrum.

TYPE 1 DIABETES AND SEASONALITY

Type 1 diabetes mellitus (T1DM) is another AD that shows seasonal variation. The process of seroconversion or the first appearance of autoantibodies in T1DM was found to be higher during autumn and winter versus spring and summer (79% vs. 21%, $P < .001$) [24]. These finding can be ascribed to seasonal variation of daylight hours and viral infections.

Vitamin D was shown to confer a protective role against T1DM (OR 0.67 [95% CI 0.53–0.86]) [25]. A Finnish birth cohort study also showed that children who received recommended supplemental vitamin D doses had a decreased risk for T1DM development as compared with control children who did not consume vitamin D (rate ratio, RR, 0.12 [95% CI 0.03–0.51]) [26]. Viral infections especially with *Enteroviruses* were postulated to be one of the environmental factors for the etiopathogenesis of T1DM [27,28]. This hypothesis was supported by data showing temporal concordance of *Enterovirus* infection and formation of autoantibodies [29]. The well-known Finnish DIPP study supported the temporal association with results confirming a prior *Enterovirus* infection in 57% of patients with T1DM as compared with healthy controls (OR 3.7 [95% CI 1.2–11.4]) [30]. Interestingly, two prospective studies, namely the BABYDIAB study conducted in Germany and the DAISY study conducted in Denver, failed to support such association [31,32].

Not all strains of *Enteroviruses* can cause T1DM; a crucial factor is given by the tropism of viruses to B islet cells of pancreas, which leads to cell damage and destruction [33]. For example, *Coxsackievirus* A and B, *Echovirus,* and *Rotavirus* tend to target and destroy islet beta cells [33,34]. In particular, *Coxsackievirus* is usually recognized to affect children in late summer and early autumn, whereas *Rotavirus* is known to have a peak during winter months [35], corresponding with the peaks in T1DM seroconversions.

INFLAMMATORY BOWEL DISEASE AND SEASONALITY

In inflammatory bowel disease (IBD), month of birth has been implicated in risk of disease development. In a case-control study in the United Kingdom with patients diagnosed with Crohn's disease (CD) and ulcerative colitis (UC), a peak in April (OR 1.06) and a trough in October (OR 0.93) were shown in UC patients, when compared with the general population. Individuals born in April had a 6.5% higher risk of developing UC than the ones born in October, whereas CD patients showed no seasonality [36]. A Canadian case-control study that compared seasons of birth among 11,145 individuals with IBD and 108,633 controls showed similar results: it demonstrated that 27% of CD patients were born from April to June, compared with only 25.6% of the controls (OR 1.07).

From another angle, vitamin D deficiency can lead to exacerbation and progression of IBD, and vitamin D normalization is associated with reduced risk of relapses, reduced risk of IBD-related surgeries, and improvement in quality of life [37,38].

In a prospective study carried out in Romania, which included 47 IBD patients, it was shown that UC patients tended to have lower levels of vitamin D during winter. The researchers also noticed that patients with moderate to severe disease tended to have lower levels of vitamin D than patients with a mild disease and those on remission [39].

As the risk of infections can vary according to climate, environmental events, and changes in the biorhythm, it is possible that there is a seasonal variation in the natural history of IBD, especially with relation to seasonal infections [40]. For example, low humidity is a seasonal factor that causes dry nasal passages and consequently a higher risk for cold viruses; the tendency to stay indoors during winter and the physical proximity to others during this time can contribute to the spreading of respiratory viral infections that are more common during winter and fall.

On the contrary, infections caused by *Enterovirus, Salmonella,* and *Campylobacter* have a peak of incidence/prevalence during fall and summer [41].

RHEUMATOID ARTHRITIS AND SEASONALITY

In 1973, Jacoby et al. [42] studied the early stages and prognosis of patients diagnosed with classical rheumatoid arthritis (RA); their results highlighted an increased disease onset in the winter semester as compared with other seasons with 43% of the patients presenting between December to February [42]. In another study, 1663 patients were examined for signs of flares and changes in disease activity. Among the subjects, a peak of disease activity was noted during spring, accompanied by a decrease in disease activity during fall, a result that was statistically significant for all of the criteria tested [43].

In a large metaanalysis on the levels of vitamin D and RA disease activity, RA patients were noted for having a significantly lower levels of vitamin D as compared with health controls. Moreover, disease activity score in 28 joints showed an inverse relationship between vitamin D plasma levels and disease activity (r=−0.12 [95% CI −0.23 to 0.00]) [44].

Infectious agents especially *Proteus mirabilis, E. coli,* and Epstein–Barr virus have been associated with the onset of RA [45]. Multiple studies showed significantly increased levels of *P. mirabilis* in the blood and urine of patients with RA compared with healthy controls [46]. No studies have been carried out so far to study the temporal relationship between these infectious agents and RA [47].

AUTOIMMUNE LIVER DISEASES AND SEASONALITY

Primary biliary cholangitis (PBC) showed an interesting pattern in terms of temporality of disease presentation. In PBC, patients attributed symptoms onset to spring and early summer ($P<.01$) [48]. Similarly, in 2011, McNally et al. [49] studied 1030 patients with PBC and demonstrated the presence of diagnostic peak during the month of June ($P=.001$). *E. coli* has been suggested to play an essential role in PBC etiopathogenesis. A cohort study that was done to assess the influence of environmental risk factors in PBC pathogenesis highlighted the increased associated risk in PBC development in patients with recurrent urinary tract infection as compared with healthy controls (OR 2.12 [95% CI 1.10–4.07]) [50]. In a population-based study, Hasan et al. [51] reported a 35% increased incidence ratio of *E. coli* infections during the warmest month of the year (June to September) compared with the rest of the year [51].

Higher incidence of *E. coli* infections in summer correlates with the temporal peak of PBC incidence during the same period. The mechanism by which *E. coli* is postulated to initiate PBC is through cross-reactivity and molecular mimicry of certain mitochondrial antigens, resulting in increased immune response against those peptides and a subsequent autoimmune destruction of self-tissues [52].

Concerning vitamin D levels in autoimmune liver diseases (ALDs), Efe et al. [53] demonstrated that patients with autoimmune hepatitis (AIH) had lower levels of vitamin D ($P < .0001$). Furthermore, they documented an increased disease activity which is manifested by higher rates of fibrosis noted on biopsies in patients with lower vitamin D levels [53]. Additionally, lower plasma vitamin D levels were also reported in patients with primary sclerosing cholangitis (PSC) and a higher degree of fibrosis in patients vitamin D deficiency as compared with patients with normal vitamin D levels and insufficient vitamin D levels ($P = .04$) [53]. A similar trend was also documented in patient with PBC and vitamin D deficiency ($P = .029$).

AUTOIMMUNE THYROID DISEASES AND SEASONALITY

A population-based study compared the month of birth of patients with autoimmune thyroid diseases (AITD) and the general population. With respect to Graves' disease development, male patients were more likely to be born in winter when compared with the general population ($P < .01$). On the contrary, female patient's month of birth distribution demonstrated a two-peaked dispersal with higher births during spring and autumn ($P < .01$). Male patients with Hashimoto thyroiditis had a bimodal distribution with a summer and winter peak ($P < .01$). Conversely, female patients had a significantly higher month of birth during winter ($P < .01$). The study attributed such finding to variations in vitamin D levels and precedent or concurrent viral infections during pregnancy in susceptible fetuses. These infections possess, indeed, a peak during winter [54].

Based on a large-scale quantitative metaanalysis, Wang et al. [55] demonstrated significantly lower levels of vitamin D in AITD patients when compared with healthy controls. Additionally, other studies demonstrated a statistically significant inverse relationship between levels of vitamin D and thyroid antibody levels (antithyroglobulin and antithyroid peroxidase) [56,57]. Other studies, including a recently published study by Zhou et al. [58], refuted such correlation between AITD and vitamin D.

SYSTEMIC SCLEROSIS AND SEASONALITY

Various studies have described that systemic sclerosis (SSc) patients are likely to have low vitamin D levels [59,60]. The authors also found that the lower the vitamin D levels, the higher the activity of disease score, the acute-phase reactants measurement, and the systolic pulmonary artery pressure [61].

It has been suggested that vitamin D levels play a role in disease etiology, in fibroblasts taken from SSc patients, and in SSc murine models; vitamin D receptor (VDR) expression was decreased and, moreover, the knockdown of VDR raised the response of the fibroblasts to TGF-β, causing more fibrosis.

The vitamin level is likely to increase during summer and decrease during winter. It could lead to the hypothesis that SSc may present a seasonal variation, with more activity rates during the cold seasons. Further studies on the topic are needed to support the idea of clinical fluctuations of SSc related to vitamin D serum levels.

SSc symptoms may vary according to the period of the year both in terms of recurrence and severity. A prospective study with 18 SSc patients showed that in winter the attacks of Reynaud's phenomenon (RP) were more severe, more frequent, and each attack lasted longer, when compared with episodes occurring in the summer [62]. Another study with SSc patients from the United States and France also reported that the cold may act as a trigger of SSc, contributing to the hypothesis that it is more common/severe during winter. RP is not the only SSc symptom that was related to seasonality [63]. A study with 19 progressive SSc patients looked for seasonal fluctuations on the diffusing capacity of the lung and its components. The study found significantly higher monoxide diffusion capacity, diffusing capacity of the membrane, and capillary blood volume from mid-March to mid-October. The authors suggested that it may reflect fluctuation in the amount of pulmonary interstitial fluid and/or pulmonary vasomotor tone during the different seasons [64]. For this reason, pulmonary symptoms may worsen during the cold seasons. Further studies are necessary to support this hypothesis.

CONCLUSION

On a final note, our understanding of ADs etiopathogenesis and natural history remains substantially limited by the multitudinous clinical manifestations and progression trends of these diseases. Environmental and genetic factors remain the governing factors that provide possible explanations for these disease etiopathology. While possibly ADs can be divided to both organ-specific, such as T1DM, AITD, celiac disease, ALD, and nonorgan-specific, exampled by RA and SLE among others, evidence gathered supports the role of the seasonal factors variation on the disease activity of both organ-specific and nonorgan-specific subgroups.

REFERENCES

[1] Valesini G, Gerardi MC, Iannuccelli C, Pacucci VA, Pendolino M, Shoenfeld Y. Citrullination and autoimmunity. Autoimmun Rev 2015;14(6):490–7.

[2] Arango M-T, Perricone C, Kivity S, Cipriano E, Ceccarelli F, Valesini G, et al. HLA-DRB1 the notorious gene in the mosaic of autoimmunity. Immunol Res 2016;65(1):82–98.

[3] Perricone C, Agmon-Levin N, Shoenfeld Y. Novel pebbles in the mosaic of autoimmunity. BMC Med 2013;11(1).

[4] Pludowski P, Holick MF, Pilz S, Wagner CL, Hollis BW, Grant WB, et al. Vitamin D effects on musculoskeletal health, immunity, autoimmunity, cardiovascular disease, cancer, fertility, pregnancy, dementia and mortality—a review of recent evidence. Autoimmun Rev 2013;12(10):976–89.

[5] Watad A, Azrielant S, Soriano A, Bracco D, Abu Much A, Amital H. Association between seasonal factors and multiple sclerosis. Eur J Epidemiol 2016;31(11):1081–9.

[6] Bartness TJ, Goldman BD. Mammalian pineal melatonin: a clock for all seasons. Experientia 1989;45(10):939–45.

[7] Galbo H, Kall L. Circadian variations in clinical symptoms and concentrations of inflammatory cytokines, melatonin, and cortisol in polymyalgia rheumatica before and during prednisolone treatment: a controlled, observational, clinical experimental study. Arthritis Res Ther 2016;18(1).

[8] Torres-Ruiz J, Sulli A, Cutolo M, Shoenfeld Y. Air travel, circadian rhythms/hormones, and autoimmunity. Clin Rev Allergy Immunol 2017.

[9] Shimura MKT, Miura T. Season of birth in some neurological disorders: multiple sclerosis, ALS senile dementia. Prog Biometerorol 1987;6:163–8.

[10] Balbuena LD, Middleton RM, Tuite-Dalton K, Pouliou T, Williams KE, Noble GJ. Sunshine, sea, and season of birth: MS incidence in wales. PLoS One 2016;11(5):e0155181.

[11] Munger KL, Levin LI, Hollis BW, Howard NS, Ascherio A. Serum 25-hydroxyvitamin D levels and risk of multiple sclerosis. JAMA 2006;296(23):2832.

[12] Ascherio A, Munger KL, White R, Köchert K, Simon KC, Polman CH, et al. Vitamin D as an early predictor of multiple sclerosis activity and progression. JAMA Neurol 2014;71(3):306.

[13] Carrillo-Vico A, Guerrero JM, Lardone PJ, Reiter RJ. A review of the multiple actions of melatonin on the immune system. Endocrine 2005;27(2):189–200.

[14] Sandyk R, Awerbuch GI. Nocturnal plasma melatonin and alpha-melanocyte stimulating hormone levels during exacerbation of multiple sclerosis. Int J Neurosci 1992;67(1–4):173–86.

[15] Farez Mauricio F, Mascanfroni Ivan D, Méndez-Huergo Santiago P, Yeste A, Murugaiyan G, Garo Lucien P, et al. Melatonin contributes to the seasonality of multiple sclerosis relapses. Cell 2015;162(6):1338–52.

[16] Tremlett H, van der Mei IAF, Pittas F, Blizzard L, Paley G, Mesaros D, et al. Monthly ambient sunlight, infections and relapse rates in multiple sclerosis. Neuroepidemiology 2008;31(4):271–9.

[17] Sibley W. Clinical viral infections and multiple sclerosis. Lancet 1985;325(8441):1313–5.

[18] Duarte-GarcÍa A, Fang H, To CH, Magder LS, Petri M. Seasonal variation in the activity of systemic lupus erythematosus. J Rheumatol 2012;39(7):1392–8.

[19] Ben-Zvi I, Aranow C, Mackay M, Stanevsky A, Kamen DL, Marinescu LM, et al. The impact of vitamin D on dendritic cell function in patients with systemic lupus erythematosus. PLoS One 2010;5(2):e9193.

[20] Amital H, Szekanecz Z, Szucs G, Danko K, Nagy E, Csepany T, et al. Serum concentrations of 25-OH vitamin D in patients with systemic lupus erythematosus (SLE) are inversely related to disease activity: is it time to routinely supplement patients with SLE with vitamin D? Ann Rheum Dis 2010;69(6):1155–7.

[21] Medrano-Campillo P, Sarmiento-Soto H, Alvarez-Sanchez N, Alvarez-Rios AI, Guerrero JM, Rodriguez-Prieto I, et al. Evaluation of the immunomodulatory effect of melatonin on the T-cell response in peripheral blood from systemic lupus erythematosus patients. J Pineal Res 2015;58(2):219–26.

[22] Sanders CJ, Van Weelden H, Kazzaz GA, Sigurdsson V, Toonstra J, Bruijnzeel-Koomen CA. Photosensitivity in patients with lupus erythematosus: a clinical and photobiological study of 100 patients using a prolonged phototest protocol. Br J Dermatol 2003;149(1):131–7.

[23] Bengtsson AA, Rylander L, Hagmar L, Nived O, Sturfelt G. Risk factors for developing systemic lupus erythematosus: a case-control study in southern Sweden. Rheumatology (Oxf Engl) 2002;41(5):563–71.

[24] Kimpimaki T, Kupila A, Hamalainen AM, Kukko M, Kulmala P, Savola K, et al. The first signs of beta-cell autoimmunity appear in infancy in genetically susceptible children from the general population: the Finnish type 1 diabetes prediction and prevention study. J Clin Endocrinol Metab 2001;86(10):4782–8.

[25] Vitamin D supplement in early childhood and risk for Type I (insulin-dependent) diabetes mellitus. The EURODIAB Substudy 2 Study Group. Diabetologia 1999;42(1):51–4.

[26] Hypponen E, Laara E, Reunanen A, Jarvelin MR, Virtanen SM. Intake of vitamin D and risk of type 1 diabetes: a birth-cohort study. Lancet (Lond Engl) 2001;358(9292):1500–3.

[27] Hyoty H, Hiltunen M, Knip M, Laakkonen M, Vahasalo P, Karjalainen J, et al. A prospective study of the role of coxsackie B and other enterovirus infections in the pathogenesis of IDDM. Childhood Diabetes in Finland (DiMe) Study Group. Diabetes 1995;44(6):652–7.

[28] Rodriguez-Calvo T, Sabouri S, Anquetil F, von Herrath MG. The viral paradigm in type 1 diabetes: who are the main suspects? Autoimmun Rev 2016;15(10):964–9.

[29] Hiltunen M, Hyoty H, Knip M, Ilonen J, Reijonen H, Vahasalo P, et al. Islet cell antibody seroconversion in children is temporally associated with enterovirus infections. Childhood Diabetes in Finland (DiMe) Study Group. J Infect Dis 1997;175(3):554–60.

[30] Lonnrot M, Korpela K, Knip M, Ilonen J, Simell O, Korhonen S, et al. Enterovirus infection as a risk factor for beta-cell autoimmunity in a prospectively observed birth cohort: the Finnish diabetes prediction and prevention study. Diabetes 2000;49(8):1314–8.

[31] Graves PM, Rotbart HA, Nix WA, Pallansch MA, Erlich HA, Norris JM, et al. Prospective study of enteroviral infections and development of beta-cell autoimmunity. Diabetes autoimmunity study in the young (DAISY). Diabetes Res Clin Pract 2003;59(1):51–61.

[32] Fuchtenbusch M, Irnstetter A, Jager G, Ziegler AG. No evidence for an association of coxsackie virus infections during pregnancy and early childhood with development of islet autoantibodies in offspring of mothers or fathers with type 1 diabetes. J Autoimmun 2001;17(4):333–40.

[33] Fohlman J, Friman G. Is juvenile diabetes a viral disease? Ann Med 1993;25(6):569–74.

[34] Honeyman MC, Coulson BS, Stone NL, Gellert SA, Goldwater PN, Steele CE, et al. Association between rotavirus infection and pancreatic islet autoimmunity in children at risk of developing type 1 diabetes. Diabetes 2000;49(8):1319–24.

[35] Fisman D. Seasonality of viral infections: mechanisms and unknowns. Clin Microbiol Infect 2012;18(10):946–54.

[36] Disanto G, Chaplin G, Morahan JM, Giovannoni G, Hyppönen E, Ebers GC, et al. Month of birth, vitamin D and risk of immune-mediated disease: a case control study. BMC Med 2012;10(1).

[37] Cosnes J, Gower–Rousseau C, Seksik P, Cortot A. Epidemiology and natural history of inflammatory bowel diseases. Gastroenterology 2011;140(6):1785–94.e4.

[38] Reich KM. Vitamin D improves inflammatory bowel disease outcomes: basic science and clinical review. World J Gastroenterol 2014;20(17):4934.

[39] Serum DG. 25-hydroxyvitamin D concentration and inflammatory bowel disease characteristics in Romania. World J Gastroenterol 2014;20(9):2392.

[40] Amre DK, Lambrette P, Law L, Krupoves A, Chotard V, Costea F, et al. Investigating the hygiene hypothesis as a risk factor in pediatric onset crohn's disease: a case-control study. Am J Gastroenterol 2006;101(5):1005–11.

[41] Dowell SF. Seasonal variation in host susceptibility and cycles of certain infectious diseases. Emerg Infect Dis 2001;7(3):369–74.

[42] Jacoby RK, Jayson MIV, Cosh JA. Onset, early stages, and prognosis of rheumatoid arthritis: a clinical study of 100 patients with 11-year follow-up. Br Med J 1973;2(5858):96–100.

[43] Iikuni N, Nakajima A, Inoue E, Tanaka E, Okamoto H, Hara M, et al. What's in season for rheumatoid arthritis patients? Seasonal fluctuations in disease activity. Rheumatology 2007;46(5):846–8.

[44] Lin J, Liu J, Davies ML, Chen W. Serum vitamin D level and rheumatoid arthritis disease activity: review and meta-analysis. PLoS One 2016;11(1).

[45] McInnes IB, Schett G. The pathogenesis of rheumatoid arthritis. N Engl J Med 2011;365(23):2205–19.

[46] Senior BW, Anderson GA, Morley KD, Kerr MA. Evidence that patients with rheumatoid arthritis have asymptomatic 'non-significant' *Proteus mirabilis* bacteriuria more frequently than healthy controls. J Infect 1999;38(2):99–106.

[47] Matveikov AG, Artishevskaia NI, Bezkrovnaia VG. [The chronobiological aspects of lysosomal enzyme activity in the synovial fluid and of remission in rheumatoid inflammation]. Ter Arkh 1994;66(5):13–7.

[48] Hamlyn AN, Macklon AF, James O. Primary biliary cirrhosis: geographical clustering and symptomatic onset seasonality. Gut 1983;24(10):940–5.

[49] McNally RJ, James PW, Ducker S, James OF. Seasonal variation in the patient diagnosis of primary biliary cirrhosis: further evidence for an environmental component to etiology. Hepatology (Baltim Md) 2011;54(6):2099–103.

[50] Parikh-Patel A, Gold EB, Worman H, Krivy KE, Gershwin ME. Risk factors for primary biliary cirrhosis in a cohort of patients from the United States. Hepatology (Baltim Md) 2001;33(1):16–21.

[51] Al-Hasan MN. Seasonal variation in *Escherichia coli* bloodstream infection: a population-based study. Clin Microbiol Infect 2009;15(10):947–50.

[52] Bogdanos DP, Baum H, Vergani D, Burroughs AK. The role of *E. coli* infection in the pathogenesis of primary biliary cirrhosis. Dis Markers 2010;29(6):301–11.

[53] Efe C, Kav T, Aydin C, Cengiz M, Imga NN, Purnak T, et al. Low serum vitamin D levels are associated with severe histological features and poor response to therapy in patients with autoimmune hepatitis. Dig Dis Sci 2014;59(12):3035–42.

[54] Krassas GE, Tziomalos K, Pontikides N, Lewy H, Laron Z. Seasonality of month of birth of patients with Graves' and Hashimoto's diseases differ from that in the general population. Eur J Endocrinol 2007;156(6):631–6.

[55] Wang J, Lv S, Chen G, Gao C, He J, Zhong H, et al. Meta-analysis of the association between vitamin D and autoimmune thyroid disease. Nutrients 2015;7(4):2485–98.

[56] Schwalfenberg GK. Solar radiation and vitamin D: mitigating environmental factors in autoimmune disease. J Environ Public Health 2012;2012:1–9.

[57] Unal AD, Tarcin O, Parildar H, Cigerli O, Eroglu H, Demirag NG. Vitamin D deficiency is related to thyroid antibodies in autoimmune thyroiditis. Cent Eur J Immunol 2014;39(4):493–7.

[58] Zhou P, Cai J, Markowitz M. Absence of a relationship between thyroid hormones and vitamin D levels. J Pediatr Endocrinol Metab 2016;29(6).

[59] Braun-Moscovici Y, Furst DE, Markovits D, Rozin A, Clements PJ, Nahir AM, et al. Vitamin D, parathyroid hormone, and acroosteolysis in systemic sclerosis. J Rheumatol 2008;35(11):2201.

[60] Orbach H, Zandman-Goddard G, Amital H, Barak V, Szekanecz Z, Szucs G, et al. Novel biomarkers in autoimmune diseases: prolactin, ferritin, vitamin D, and TPA levels in autoimmune diseases. Ann NY Acad Sci 2007;1109(1):385–400.

[61] Vacca A, Cormier C, Piras M, Mathieu A, Kahan A, Allanore Y. Vitamin D deficiency and insufficiency in 2 independent cohorts of patients with systemic sclerosis. J Rheumatol 2009;36(9):1924–9.

[62] Watson HR, Robb R, Belcher G, Belch JJ. Seasonal variation of Raynaud's phenomenon secondary to systemic sclerosis. J Rheumatol 1999;26(8):1734–7.

[63] Maricq HR, Carpentier PH, Weinrich MC, Keil JE, Palesch Y, Biro C, et al. Geographic variation in the prevalence of Raynaud's phenomenon: a 5 region comparison. J Rheumatol 1997;24(5):879–89.

[64] Emmanuel G, Saroja D, Gopinathan K, Gharpure A, Stuckey J. Environmental factors and the diffusing capacity of the lung in progressive systemic sclerosis. Chest 1976;69(2):304–7.

Chapter 24

Ultraviolet Radiation: Both Friend and Foe in Systemic Autoimmune Diseases?

Marina Venturini[1], Laura Andreoli[2], Mariachiara Arisi[1], Mariateresa Rossi[1], Franco Franceschini[2], Piergiacomo Calzavara-Pinton[1], Angela Tincani[2]

[1]Dermatology Unit, Spedali Civili, and Department of Clinical and Experimental Sciences, University of Brescia, Brescia, Italy; [2]Rheumatology and Clinical Immunology Unit, Spedali Civili, and Department of Clinical and Experimental Sciences, University of Brescia, Brescia, Italy

INTRODUCTION

Systemic autoimmune diseases (SADs) such as systemic lupus erythematosus (SLE), dermatomyositis (DM), and systemic sclerosis (SSc) are complex and multifactorial disorders. Despite the heterogeneity in the clinical phenotype, three common themes can be identified in the induction and perpetuation of autoimmunity: genetic predisposition, environmental factors, and immune regulation [1]. Among environmental factors, the ultraviolet radiation (UVR) has been claimed to play a role in the exacerbation of both cutaneous and systemic manifestations of SADs, although a clinically evident photosensitivity is not always present, being rather the hallmark of selected variants of lupus, such as lupus tumidus (LT) and subacute cutaneous lupus erythematosus (SCLE) [2]. Conversely, the increasing knowledge of the different immunologic effects of different wavebands of UVR, both locally in the skin and systemically, has been exploited to treat patients with UVA1 phototherapy and extracorporeal photopheresis [3]. This chapter will discuss the principles of photobiology and give insights into how and when UVR can be harmful or helpful in the management of patients with SADs.

EFFECT OF ULTRAVIOLET RADIATION ON HUMAN SKIN

The sun emits the full spectrum of nonionizing electromagnetic radiation. The UVR includes photons with wavelengths ranging from 100 to 400 nm. According to the photophysical and photobiological properties, UV radiation has been subdivided into UVC (100–280 nm), UVB (280–320 nm), and UVA (320–400 nm). The UVA portion is commonly further divided, resulting in the UVA2 (320–340 nm) and UVA1 (340–400 nm) wavebands. Solar UVC is absorbed by the ozone layer in the troposphere and therefore does not reach ground level, thus not being harmful for human beings. The environmental UVA/UVB ratio at sea level is usually referenced as being around 20:1 in the central hours of the day. However, the ratio increases in seasonal and environmental conditions leading to the increase of the distance that the solar rays travel through the atmosphere, e.g., lower latitudes, higher altitudes, winter and hours with a solar angle <60 degrees. In addition, atmospheric conditions modify UVR exposure. Heavily overcast skies may offer some protection from solar UVR, particularly UVB, whereas light or thin clouds have little or no effect. Wind and rain increase the irradiance because they remove aerosolized particles that scatter and reflect the solar rays and polluting gases that absorb them. Finally, reflective surfaces, i.e., snow, sand, rocks, and water, may enhance the intensity of incident UVR by up to 70% [4].

When the photons hit the human skin, they can be reflected, scattered, or absorbed. The penetration depth increases with increasing wavelength: almost all UVB are blocked by the absorbing molecules (also called chromophore) that are present on skin surface, e.g., urocanic acid, or in the epidermal cell populations (keratinocytes, melanocytes, immune cells), whereas a significant amount of UVA, particularly UVA1, penetrates into the papillary dermis and targets cell populations that are resident or trafficking in the upper dermis, e.g., stem cells of the bulge area and matrix of the hair follicle, fibroblasts, immune cells, endothelial cells, and blood cells. Intracellular chromophores, such as nucleic acids, lipids, and proteins, have a specific absorption spectrum that is the plot of their capacity to absorb photons with specific wavelengths [4]. The absorption of the quantum energy of the incident photon causes a cascade of photochemical reactions leading to a wide variety of different biochemical, immunological, pathological, and clinical acute and chronic effects on the skin. The most known acute clinical responses of human skin to UVR are phototoxic erythema, exacerbation of viral diseases, tanning, and triggering of flares of photosensitive disorders, whereas long-term clinical effects include photoaging and photocarcinogenesis.

Mosaic of Autoimmunity. https://doi.org/10.1016/B978-0-12-814307-0.00024-4

The main targets of DNA photodamage are the pyrimidine bases, particularly the quantitatively minor 5-methylcytosine, cytosine, and thymine. Their peak of absorption is in the UVB waveband, although they can also absorb UVA, albeit with an approximately 1000 times lower efficiency [5].

UVB photons have enough quantum energy to trigger a direct anaerobic photochemical reaction on DNA absorption. The most frequent DNA photoproducts are cyclobutane pyrimidine dimers (CPDs), mainly thymine dimers, and pyrimidine-pyrimidone (6–4) photoproducts (6–4PPs), which make up 65% and 35%, respectively, of the UVB-induced DNA lesions [6]. Other common photoproducts are Dewar isomers, cytosine hydrates, and DNA strand breaks.

If the nucleotide excision repair system fails to restore genomic integrity after the formation of a CPD, C (cytosine) to T (thymine) mutations and CC to TT tandem mutations occur. Once these were considered UVB fingerprint mutations, but the dogma that C to T mutations are only caused by UVB has been recently challenged by experimental evidence that they can also be generated, albeit with a much lower efficiency, by UVA through various molecular mechanisms. CPDs may form directly [7] or after the formation of oxidative DNA damage that is mediated by both UVB- and UVA-induced highly reactive oxygen species, such as singlet oxygen, superoxide anion, hydroxyl anion, and peroxide [7–11], or via energy transfer from oxidized endogenous chromophores [5], including porphyrins, flavins, and NADH/NADPH [12].

In addition, both UVA and UVB induce oxidative DNA damage with a mutagenic potential, such as 8-hydroxydeoxyguanosine that causes G-T transversions [7,13], protein-DNA cross-links, and thymine glycol formation [8,9,13], as well as single- and double-DNA strand breaks [14].

The effectiveness of UV to induce erythema declines rapidly in the 310–320 spectral area and UVA wavelengths are approximately 1000 times less effective than UVB wavelengths [15]. The action spectrum of erythema is practically superimposable to the absorption spectrum of DNA, demonstrating that it is mainly related to the cascade of molecular events following the DNA photodamage and therefore that UVB is much more (about 1000 times) erythemogenic than UVA [5]. At histological level, the development of apoptotic keratinocytes (sunburn cells) and a variable degree of inflammatory infiltrate are seen [16,17]. UVB-induced erythema occurs approximately 4 h after exposure, peaks around 8–24 h, and fades over a day or so. UVA-induced erythema is biphasic: erythema is often evidenced immediately at the end of the irradiation period; it fades in several hours, followed by a delayed erythema starting at 6 h and reaching its peak at 24 h.

Besides its deleterious proinflammatory effects, UVR has local and systemic immunosuppressive properties as well, leading to the reduction of the immunological surveillance against tumor and viral antigens. However, UV-induced immunosuppression may be helpful to prevent autoimmune responses to cutaneous neoantigens resulting from UV-mediated damage (e.g., UV-damaged DNA). For a long time, UVB has been thought to be the major immunosuppressive waveband. However, more recently, the substantial contribution of UVA to immune suppression in humans has been demonstrated, now being estimated to contribute about 75% of the whole effect [18,19].

More direct evidence of the ability of UVR to impair immune responses is derived from some experiments in animal models. Mice chronically exposed to UV radiation develop UV-induced tumors; when these tumors are removed and transplanted to the skin of genetically identical recipient mice, the tumors regress because a host immune response develops against the tumors. On the other hand, when the same tumors are transplanted to genetically identical recipients that have received subcarcinogenic doses of UVB radiation, the tumors grow progressively and ultimately kill their host [20]. These findings were confirmed in the model of contact hypersensitivity (CHS) [21] reporting that application of a contact allergen to the skin that had been exposed to low UVB doses failed to induce CHS in an antigen-specific manner (phenomenon termed "immunotolerance").

The molecular and pathological bases of photoimmunosuppression in human skin are complex [22] because UVR interferes with all skin cell populations with acquired and/or innate immunological activity; UV wavebands have different relative efficiency for different immunological effects and different UV doses may cause even opposite effects. UVB and UVA exposures, even at suberythemogenic doses, decrease the number of effector T cells and impair their activation by directly damaging antigen-presenting Langerhans cells, which leads to suppressed immune response [23,24]. The effects of UV-induced immunosuppression on the skin are summarized in Table 24.1.

Constitutive skin pigmentation is the main defense mechanisms against the damaging effects of UV, and facultative pigmentation (tanning) is the most adaptive response of our skin to UV damages. Tanning proceeds in several distinct steps. The first step is the immediate pigment darkening (IPD), a transient phenomenon which occurs within minutes of UV exposure, appearing as a grayish coloration of the skin that gradually fades to a brown color over a period of minutes to days, depending on the UV dose and the individual skin color. IPD is independent by the synthesis of new melanin, and it is caused by the photooxidation of preexisting melanin and the intracellular redistribution of melanosomes. The action spectrum of IPD shows a broad peak in the UVA region and is only marginally photoprotective. IPD is followed within hours after UV exposure by a more prolonged skin darkening phenomenon that persists up to 3–5 days called persistent pigment darkening (PPD). Also PPD, which is light brown to brown, is thought to result from the oxidation of melanin

TABLE 24.1 The Effects of UV-Induced Immunosuppression on the Skin

UV Target	UV-Induced Effect
Effector T cells (Teffs)	• Reduction of CD4+ and CD8+ T cells • Th2 predominance in Th1/Th2 ratio
Regulatory T cells (Tregs)	• Increase of Tregs (↓ Teffs/Tregs ratio)
Langerhans cells (LCs)	• Depletion and dysfunctional APC activity
Monocytes/macrophages	• Increase of infiltration into the epidermis by UV-induced overexpression of ELAM-1 on vascular endothelium
Cytokines	• Increase secretion of immunosuppressive cytokines (IL-10) and Th2 cytokines (IL-4, IL-5, IL-6) by Tregs, macrophages, keratinocytes, and NKT cells (↓ Th1/Th2 cytokines ratio) • Overexpression of IL-1ra by UV-stimulated keratinocytes
Trans-UCA	• Photoisomerization of *trans*-UCA to *cis*-UCA inducing depletion of LC and NKT cells, increase of IL-10 and histamine release
Neuropeptides	• Increased release of substance P, CGRP, α-MSH, beta-endorphins, and POMC with antiinflammatory properties (increase of IL-10, LC migration, and ↓ Th1/Th2 ratio)

APC, antigen-presenting cells; *CGRP*, calcitonin gene–related peptide; *ELAM-1*, endothelial leukocyte adhesion molecule-1; *IL-1ra*, IL-1 receptor antagonist; *NKT*, natural killer T; *POMC*, proopiomelanocortin; *UCA*, urocanic acid; *α-MSH*, alpha–melanocyte-stimulating hormone.

and it is elicited more strongly by UVA than by UVB. The last phase of skin tanning is the delayed tanning (DT) response. It can be induced by both UVB and UVA and becomes visually evident not before 2–3 days after the UV exposure. DT results from the stimulation of melanin synthesis and involves increases in the number and activity of functional melanocytes, increased number and length of dendrites, increased tyrosinase activity (the rate-limiting enzyme in the melanogenic pathway), increased synthesis of melanin in the melanosomes, and increased transfer of melanosomes to keratinocytes. UVB-induced DT is photoprotective (it is estimated to have an SPF of 3 in darker skin types), whereas UVA-induced DT is not considered to be as much photoprotective because it is not accompanied by a concomitant increase of the stratum corneum, which has another important adaptive response of the skin to UV. DT is maximal from 10 days to 3–4 weeks, depending on the UV dose and the individual's skin color. It may take several weeks or months for the skin to return to its base constitutive color [25].

Despite many negative effects of UVR on human skin, there are also some positive effects such as the cutaneous synthesis of vitamin D induced by UVB, which covers approximately 90% of the vitamin D requirements of the human body. During exposure to sunlight, 7-dehydrocholesterol (provitamin D3) in the skin absorbs UVB and is photolyzed to previtamin D3 and then thermoisomerized to vitamin D3 (cholecalciferol) in the bilayer of the plasma membrane. In the liver, vitamin D3 is hydroxylated to form 25-hydroxyvitamin D3, which in turn is transported to the kidney where it is converted into the biologically active form 1α,25-dihydroxyvitamin D3 (calcitriol) [26]. A growing number of experimental and clinical evidences have recently emphasized the immunological activities of vitamin D, besides its long-term well-known activities on bone metabolism.

THE ROLE OF ULTRAVIOLET RADIATION IN TRIGGERING AND EXACERBATING SYSTEMIC AUTOIMMUNE DISEASES

Systemic Lupus Erythematosus

SLE is the prototypic SAD characterized by a plethora of clinical manifestations and autoantibodies, many of which affect the skin [27]. Photosensitivity defined as "a skin rash as a result of unusual reaction to sunlight" is one of the classification criteria of SLE [28]. However, this criterion is often overrated because it does not specify if the reaction should be quantitatively (a low phototoxic threshold) or qualitatively (the development of a rash) unusual and, in the second case, if the reaction must be clinically and histologically pathognomonic of lupus. Epidemiologic studies have focused on linking UVR to both prevalent and incident SLE ("established" and "new" cases of SLE). In addition, photosensitivity varies in different lupus subgroups: it is present in almost all patients with LT and SCLE, whereas a few patients with SLE do not present photosensitivity, and phototesting does not always trigger a positive response. Although most chronic cutaneous lupus erythematosus (CCLE) develops on sun-exposed skin, very few patients complain of photosensitivity, and phototesting is usually negative. Although it is well established that UVR exposure may exacerbate preexisting SLE, it remains unclear whether UVR is a risk factor for developing SLE [29]. In fact, there are several challenges in interpreting the current literature due to methodological issues: (1) the assessment and quantification of individual UVR exposure; (2) seasonality according to geographical location; (3) use of sunscreen lotions with high solar protection factor indices; and (4) the role of vitamin D (induced by UVB exposure) as a possible protective factor because of its immunomodulatory properties [30]. Epidemiologic studies should be designed to investigate the unanswered questions related to a potential role of UVR in the development of SLE: (1) when is the relevant susceptibility window (childhood vs. adulthood)? and (2) UVR triggers SLE onset very soon after exposure or is cumulative lifetime exposure relevant for SLE risk? [29].

Systemic Sclerosis

The hallmark of SSc is the progressive, and sometimes rapid, thickening of the skin, along with the involvement of other organs such as the heart, lungs, and kidneys. The pathogenic features of this disease can be identified as (1) structural and functional vascular lesions yielding an obliterative vasculopathy; (2) perivascular and tissue infiltration of mononuclear inflammatory cells; and (3) excessive deposition of extracellular matrix, resulting in fibrotic destruction of internal organs [31]. There is a growing evidence that environmental factors have an impact in SSc onset and progression. For instance, occupational exposure to crystalline silica and several organic solvents has been linked to SSc. Conversely, there is insufficient evidence that exposure to UVR is a causative factor of SSc [32].

Dermatomyositis

DM is a heterogeneous and multifactorial disease characterized by inflammatory myopathy and a variety of skin manifestations (Gottron papules, heliotrope rash on the upper eyelids, rash at the face, trunk, and limbs) [33,34]. DM lesions usually located on sun-exposed skin support the role of UVR in the pathogenesis of the disease. However, only a fraction of DM patients were shown to have a lower UV minimal erythemal dose (MED) threshold as compared with normal control subjects [35]. The intensity of UVR (proximity to the equator) was significantly associated with the relative proportion of DM and particularly with a subset characterized by anti-Mi-2 antibodies (autoantibodies associated with the typical photosensitive rash of DM) [36]. This effect of UVR in modulating the clinical and immunologic expression of DM holds true for women but not for men in a nationwide study conducted in the United States [37].

PHOTOTHERAPY FOR THE TREATMENT OF SYSTEMIC AUTOIMMUNE DISEASES

Photodiagnostic Methods

Standardized photodiagnostic methods are used to investigate photosensitivity (1) to determine threshold dose and wavelength dependence and (2) to reproduce skin lesions by photoprovocative phototest procedures.

First, phototesting for the assessment of the individual MED is performed exposing squared $1 \, cm \times 1 \, cm$ areas of unexposed skin of the buttocks or inner side of the forearm to an incremental series of UVB or UVA radiations. Increases are made geometrically by multiplying with $\sqrt{2}$. The induced erythema is graded $24 \pm 2 \, h$ after irradiation using an established 5-point scale:

0: absence of erythema
(+): just perceptible erythema (diffuse mild erythema without defined borders)
+: uniform erythema with sharply defined borders
++: bright red color with induration on palpation (sign of edema)
+++: bright red color and pronounced induration raised above the surrounding skin

Dose (+), corresponding to a just perceptible erythema without defined borders, must be considered as MED because it can be determined with the greatest precision [38].

Different ultraviolet sources are used for phototesting. Polychromatic UVA or UVB sources are emitted with high irradiance from metal halide lamp (e.g., UVA-SUN 3000, Mutzhas, Munich, Germany) appropriately filtered in the UVA range with strict cutoffs. Fluorescent lamps can be used for UVB phototest (Philips UV 21, Eindhoven, Netherlands). Sometimes, a solar simulator (e.g., Multiport 601, Solar Light, Glenside, PA) is also needed.

Secondly, a provocative phototest is used to induce the development of skin lesions in patients with suspected autoimmune photosensitivity. The test should be performed better in early spring when the skin is not tanned. Test sites are larger than in MED testing, typically around 5 cm × 5 cm, and they should be performed on healthy but previously affected skin (usually on the upper back).

Polychromatic UVA and UVB light sources are used to expose the same site subdivided into three squared areas. An area is exposed to UVA, the second to UVB, and the third to both UVA and UVB. Light doses are 70–100 J/cm^2 of UVA (or 1,5-2 MEDs UVA in light skin types) and 1.5–2 MED UVB and irradiations are repeated from 2 to 5 consecutive days until the appearance of skin lesions [39]. A skin biopsy on photoprovocative area can be taken for histological analysis if the photoprovocative results are unclear. Once individual erythema thresholds and the threshold for a photoprovocative test are assessed, the initial UVB or UVA dose can be chosen [40].

Phototherapy: Sources and Protocols

Phototherapy describes the use of specific wavelengths of UVR in a therapeutic setting. It utilizes either UVA (320–400 nm) or UVB (290–320 nm), which is delivered directly to the skin by lamps. The administered wavelengths and dosages of UVR vary based on indications.

There are two types of UVB phototherapy: broad band (290–320 nm) and narrow band (311 ± 2 nm). Conventional "broadband" UVB (BB-UVB) lamps emit light in a broad range over the UVB spectrum, including both the therapeutic wavelengths specific to the treatment of skin diseases, plus the shorter wavelengths responsible for sunburning (erythema). Sunburning has a negative therapeutic benefit, increases the risk of skin cancer, causes patient discomfort, and limits the amount of therapeutic UVB that can be taken.

"Narrowband" UVB (NB-UVB) lamps, on the other hand, are fluorescent tubes that emit light over a short range of wavelengths around 311±2 nm. These wavelengths have a lower erythemogenic activity than radiations <310 nm and therefore NB-UVB phototherapy has replaced BB-UVB as a first-line treatment for psoriasis, atopic dermatitis, and vitiligo [41,42]. UVB phototherapy is usually administered two to three times weekly at increasing dosage according to skin phototype. The main mechanisms of action of UVB phototherapy are DNA damage, alteration of inflammatory cytokines, induction of cellular apoptosis, and promotion of immunosuppression.

UVA1 phototherapy uses the 340–400 nm waveband, thus reducing the risk of sunburn reactions associated with the shorter wavelength belonging to the UVA2 and UVB wavebands. Targets of UVA1 phototherapy are dermal dendritic cells, fibroblasts, endothelial cells, DNA components, and mast cells. UVA1 can also induce the apoptosis and depletion of skin-infiltrating T cells and stimulating the expression of collagenase-1 in dermal fibroblasts [43]. UVA1 phototherapy is delivered by fluorescent tubes, excimer lamps, or high-output metal halide bulbs. Conventionally, UVA1 phototherapy is divided into three different pattern of dosage: high-dose protocol applying doses >60 J/cm^2 for each session; medium-dose protocol admitting single doses between 30 and 59 J/cm^2; low-dose protocol administering single UVA1 doses of ≤29 J/cm^2 [44]. Treatment times can range from 10 min to 1 h per treatment session, depending on the irradiance of the UVA1 phototherapy unit. Sessions are typically repeated 3–5 times per week.

Psoralen photochemotherapy (PUVA) combines the use of oral 5- or 8-methoxypsoralen (P) and long-wave UV radiation (UVA). This combination results in a potent phototoxic effect, which cannot be produced by the two components alone. Psoralens are natural furocoumarins that can be found in a wide number of plants and can be synthetically derived. After entering the cells, psoralens intercalate between DNA base pairs and, after UVA exposure, they absorb photons, become chemically activated, and covalently bind to DNA forming cross-links. These have antiproliferative, antiangiogenetic, apoptotic, and immunosuppressive effects [43]. PUVA acts on pathologically altered keratinocyte differentiation and strongly suppresses infiltrating lymphocytes and presenting cells [45]. Psoralen can be administered orally or applied topically in the form of solutions or baths (bath PUVA) before UVA exposure. Bath PUVA is characterized by absent/reduced systemic side effects that are mainly gastrointestinal (nausea and vomiting) and ocular.

UVA photoactivation of psoralens can also be used in the irradiation of leukocyte-enriched blood in extracorporeal photopheresis (ECP). Initially, when this methodology was first developed, psoralen was administered orally to reach an effective plasma concentration. By the time, to reduce side effects risk and the individual variability in psoralen plasma concentration, the procedure was modified to use a liquid form of 8-methoxypsoralen, which is added directly to the plasma concentrate, which is then irradiated outside the body in the process of plasmapheresis and then returned to circulation. This technique is very potent in induction of T cell apoptosis and modification of their cytokine production [46]. For the reliability of phototherapy and photodiagnostic procedures, a careful dosimetry is recommended through regularly calibrated UV spectrophotometer (e.g., MACAM SR9910, MACAM, Livingston, UK) that allows to define, at 0.5 nm intervals, the light source irradiation spectrum and the absolute or relative power for each spectral range.

Phototherapy for Systemic Lupus Erythematosus

Phototherapy has been used for treatment of skin involvement of SLE patients, although, at a first glance, this could seem counterproductive because of the potential photosensitivity of the disease [28].

Before phototherapy, the eventual photosensitivity status of lupus patients should not be excluded solely on the basis of patient history but careful phototesting is highly recommended. Photoprovocative test must be performed, after MED determination, on previously affected skin areas (trunk or upper forearms). Doses of 60–100 J/cm^2 UVA and a UVB dose corresponding to 1.5 times the individual MED are administered for 3–5 consecutive days [47]. Usually threshold doses for erythema and pigmentation are within normal range. Positivity is found in the majority of LT and SCLE patients, in 42% of CCLE patients, and in 25% of SLE patients [48]. The action spectrum of the induced lesions is usually within both UVB and UVA wavebands (55%), less commonly in the UVB (33%) or UVA range alone (14%). Test sites should be followed up to 4 weeks because LE lesions may develop after a prolonged delay. Patients must be informed that photoprovoked skin lesions persist for weeks or even months [49].

Among different wavelengths, UVB, both broad band and narrow band, and UVA2 are not used for the treatment of lupus because they damage DNA causing release of TNF-α and trigger translocation of nuclear antigens to cell surface, thus inducing the exacerbation of SLE skin involvement.

The phototherapy of choice is UVA1 phototherapy because it can improve SLE through several concurrent mechanisms: (1) the promotion of the repair of UVB and UVA2-induced DNA damage (photoreactivation) and (2) immediate and delayed apoptosis of T and B lymphocytes. It has been hypothesized that UVA1 irradiation may not stimulate the adaptive immunity and therefore may be an appropriate therapy for SLE patients through cell-mediated immunosuppression, release of TNF-α and apoptosis [50]. UVA1 also can reduce levels of IL-4, IL-10, and interferon-γ [51]. The first study on UVA1 phototherapy in subacute cutaneous lupus was published in 1993 [52]. In this study a cumulative dose of 186 J/cm^2 was administered in 9-week series of UVA1 leading to an impressive improvement of skin lesions. To date, six other studies analyzed the in vivo effect of UVA1 on SLE with a global improvement in skin scores and normalization of serological tests [53–59]. In all these studies patients were exposed to low doses of UVA1 (between 6 and 15 J/cm^2) for 2–5 days per week without doses increments. Decreased levels of circulating Th1 and TC1 cells in UVA1-treated SLE patients suggest a potential mechanism of action, as these cells produce interferon-γ, which has been implicated in SLE pathogenesis [60]. Increased apoptosis of skin-infiltrating white blood cells had also been reported following UVA1 radiation [61]. Furthermore, reduction in B cell immunoglobulin production and lower anti-dsDNA titers in SLE were found with UVA1 exposure in vitro [62]. UVA1 interferes with the translocation of extractable nuclear antigens (e.g., Ro/SSA) on human keratinocytes, decreasing also anti-Ro/SSA antibody levels [63].

Based on these findings, UVA1 phototherapy appears to be a useful and relatively safe modality for the treatment of skin lesions in SLE (Fig. 24.1). However, UVA1 is not a common therapeutic choice because of its limited diffusion in dermatology offices.

ECP is postulated to downregulate T cell activity and to induce T cell apoptosis. These two actions added to the DNA damage induced by UVA could explain the beneficial effects in T cell–mediated diseases including SLE [64]. Five clinical uncontrolled studies of small samples series have been reported so far [64–68]. The largest clinical trial included eight patients with SLE, of which six experienced resolution of cutaneous lesions and showed reduction in clinical activity scores [65].

Although these reports indicate a positive response, at this time there is no sufficient evidence to recommend the use of ECP in patients with SLE.

Phototherapy for Systemic Sclerosis and Localized Scleroderma

In 1995, topical PUVA was used for the first time to treat a patient affected by SSc with clinical and histological improvement [69].

After that, bath PUVA and oral PUVA were widely used in patients with SSc until UVA1 phototherapy became available and demonstrated several therapeutic advantages.

Unlike UVB, UVA and particularly UVA1 wavelengths can penetrate into the dermis targeting fibroblasts, dermal immune cells, and microvessels. UVA induces the synthesis of specific m-RNA levels of various matrix metalloproteinases in cultured fibroblasts and decreases the synthesis of procollagen. Furthermore, it increases interstitial collagenase m-RNA levels, several cytokines, and soluble factors (e.g., IL-1, IL-6) stimulating the synthesis of collagenase [70,71].

Transforming growth factor beta (TGF-β) plays a role in initiating and propagating fibrosis in scleroderma: UVR can reduce TGF-β levels and its receptor in human skin decreasing fibrosis.

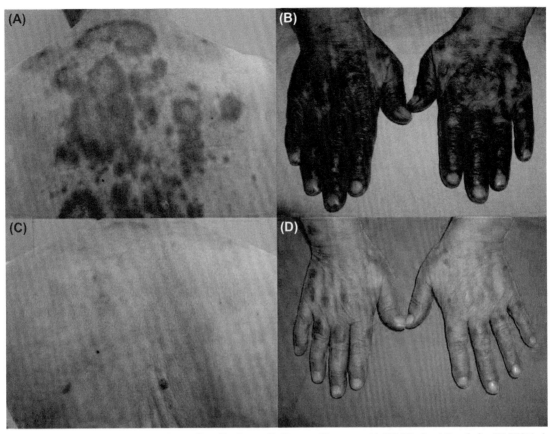

FIGURE 24.1   Clinical response to UVA1 in patients affected by lupus. (1) 52-year-old woman with SCLE before (A) and after (B) UVA1 phototherapy (3 sessions per week for a total of 24 sessions and a cumulative dose of 480 J/cm²); (2) 69-year-old woman with SLE: skin lesions before (C) and after (D) UVA1 phototherapy (3 sessions per week for a total of 21 sessions and a cumulative dose of 420 J/cm²). *SCLE*, subacute cutaneous lupus erythematosus; *SLE*, systemic lupus erythematosus.

Additionally, UVA irradiation is able to induce apoptotic cell death in dermal T cells [72] and it might exert a modulatory effect on impaired endothelial cells [73].

Many studies reported positive effects of UVA1 phototherapy in SSc without significant adverse events [74–76]. Medium-dose (30–59 J/cm²) and low-dose (≤29 J/cm²) UVA1 treatments resulted in statistically significant changes in skin scores comparing to placebo. Treatments with medium doses resulted in a longer duration of improvement as assessed by ultrasound measurement. In studies comparing high-dose and low-dose UVA1, high-dose regimen (>60 J/cm²) showed statistically significant changes in skin scores, ultrasound, and histological features [75]. The largest randomized trial included 62 patients with localized scleroderma randomized to low-dose UVA1, medium-dose UVA1, and NB-UVB. Modified skin scores were significantly reduced in all treatment group, but changes in skin thickness and percentage of body involvement showed that medium-dose UVA1 was more effective than NB-UVB [75]. Recurrence rate of sclerosing skin lesions is equal for both medium- and high-dose UVA1 [76]. Fig. 24.2 reports a case of localized scleroderma treated with UVA1.

Different studies investigated the effect of PUVA in SSc reporting positive clinical outcomes in term of skin sclerosis and joint mobility and improvement in histological and serological features with both oral- and bath PUVA [69,77].

Some studies reported the use of UVA1 phototherapy or PUVA together with other immunosuppressive drugs (e.g., corticosteroids, methotrexate, cyclosporine, or azathioprine) or antifibrotic treatment (e.g., pentoxifylline) showing good results [78,79]. Immunosuppressive side effects and skin cancer remain a concern and therefore none or short maintenance therapy is suggested.

Despite a number of pilot studies, the role of ECP in scleroderma remains controversial. Different randomized sham ECP or immunosuppressive therapy controlled trials showed that ECP was not superior in the treatment of SSc [80,81]. European Dermatology Forum guidelines [46] propose that ECP should be considered a second-line or adjuvant therapy to treat only skin lesions in scleroderma as this therapy failed in treating visceral involvement.

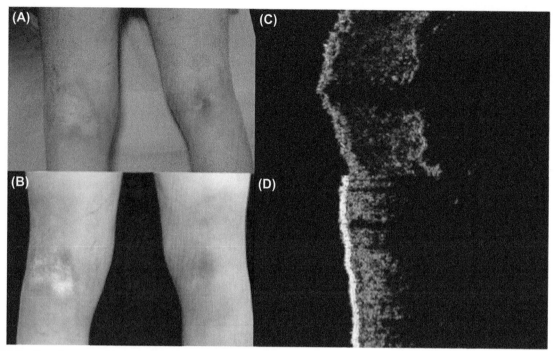

FIGURE 24.2 Sixty-three-year-old woman with localized scleroderma lesions (morphea) before (A) and after (B) UVA1 phototherapy (3 sessions per week for a total of 18 sessions and a cumulative dose of 1100 J/cm²). High-frequency ultrasound (50 MHz) analysis showed increment of echogenicity and thickness reduction after UVA1 phototherapy (D) compared with baseline (C) (DUB Skin Scanner, Taberna Pro Medicum, Im Dorf, Lüneburg).

Phototherapy for Dermatomyositis

Phototherapy is not commonly used in patients affected by DM because of the risk of photosensitivity. Only one study described the use of ECP in a patient with juvenile DM in addition to methotrexate. After 20 months of treatment, the patient's skin lesions remained unchanged [82].

There is one isolated report of a patient with a systemic sclerosis–DM overlap syndrome who was treated with bath PUVA photochemotherapy three times weekly at an initial dose of 0.1 J/cm² and a maximum dose of 8 J/cm². After 29 weeks of treatment, an appreciable skin improvement was described with no recurrence at 5-month follow-up [83,84].

Considering the well-documented photosensitivity related to this disease, it is reasonable to perform a photodiagnostic procedure to establish the MED to UVA before starting irradiation.

Side Effects and Limitations of Phototherapy

Sunburn is the most common side effect due to UVB phototherapy and typically occurs 24 h after irradiation and can be easily prevented by the determination of the individual MED before the treatment.

Acute phototoxic reactions to UVA1 are usually fewer and never clinically severe [85]. The most common side effects are dryness and itching that are usually responsive to the application of emollient creams.

Short-term side effects due to oral assumption of psoralens are nausea and vomiting. Hyperpigmentation can occur with repeated treatments. Toxic effects on the central nervous system including headache, dizziness, or depression are exceedingly rare [43].

All phototherapies can induce the relapse of an idiopathic photodermatosis (e.g., polymorphous light eruption and solar urticaria) and drug-induced photosensitivity.

Chronic side effects of PUVA therapy include freckling, photoaging, and induction of precancerous skin lesions (actinic keratosis) or tumors of the keratinocytic lineage such as basal cell carcinoma and squamous cell carcinoma and melanoma, and they have been extensively reviewed [86]. Although theoretically possible, the occurrence of these adverse effects with NB-UVB phototherapy and UVA1 phototherapy has never been found by registries and epidemiological studies [87]. However, the avoidance of prolonged treatment cycles and maintenance treatment and a close follow-up of patients are recommended.

REFERENCES

[1] Floreani A, Leung PS, Gershwin ME. Environmental basis of autoimmunity. Clin Rev Allergy Immunol 2016;50(3):287–300.

[2] Artukovic M, Ikic M, Kustelega J, Artukovic IN, Kaliterna DM. Influence of UV radiation on immunological system and occurrence of autoimmune diseases. Coll Antropol 2010;34(Suppl. 2):175–8.

[3] Elmets CA, Cala CM, Xu H. Photoimmunology. Dermatol Clin 2014;32(3):277–90. vii.

[4] Schuch AP, Garcia CC, Makita K, Menck CF. DNA damage as a biological sensor for environmental sunlight. Photochem Photobiol Sci 2013;12(8):1259–72.

[5] Young AR, Chadwick CA, Harrison GI, Nikaido O, Ramsden J, Potten CS. The similarity of action spectra for thymine dimers in human epidermis and erythema suggests that DNA is the chromophore for erythema. J Investig Dermatol 1998;111(6):982–8.

[6] Cadet J, Sage E, Douki T. Ultraviolet radiation-mediated damage to cellular DNA. Mutat Res 2005;571(1–2):3–17.

[7] Jiang Y, Rabbi M, Kim M, Ke C, Lee W, Clark RL, et al. UVA generates pyrimidine dimers in DNA directly. Biophys J 2009;96(3):1151–8.

[8] Runger TM, Kappes UP. Mechanisms of mutation formation with long-wave ultraviolet light (UVA). Photodermatol Photoimmunol Photomed 2008;24(1):2–10.

[9] Reid TM, Loeb LA. Tandem double CC-->TT mutations are produced by reactive oxygen species. Proc Natl Acad Sci USA 1993;90(9):3904–7.

[10] Drobetsky EA, Turcotte J, Chateauneuf A. A role for ultraviolet A in solar mutagenesis. Proc Natl Acad Sci USA 1995;92(6):2350–4.

[11] Kappes UP, Luo D, Potter M, Schulmeister K, Runger TM. Short- and long-wave UV light (UVB and UVA) induce similar mutations in human skin cells. J Investig Dermatol 2006;126(3):667–75.

[12] Kielbassa C, Roza L, Epe B. Wavelength dependence of oxidative DNA damage induced by UV and visible light. Carcinogenesis 1997;18(4):811–6.

[13] Ravanat JL, Di Mascio P, Martinez GR, Medeiros MH, Cadet J. Singlet oxygen induces oxidation of cellular DNA. J Biol Chem 2000;275(51):40601–4.

[14] Helleday T, Lo J, van Gent DC, Engelward BP. DNA double-strand break repair: from mechanistic understanding to cancer treatment. DNA Repair 2007;6(7):923–35.

[15] Parrish JA, Jaenicke KF, Anderson RR. Erythema and melanogenesis action spectra of normal human skin. Photochem Photobiol 1982;36(2):187–91.

[16] Murphy G, Young AR, Wulf HC, Kulms D, Schwarz T. The molecular determinants of sunburn cell formation. Exp Dermatol 2001;10(3):155–60.

[17] Sheehan JM, Cragg N, Chadwick CA, Potten CS, Young AR. Repeated ultraviolet exposure affords the same protection against DNA photodamage and erythema in human skin types II and IV but is associated with faster DNA repair in skin type IV. J Investig Dermatol 2002;118(5):825–9.

[18] Damian DL, Matthews YJ, Phan TA, Halliday GM. An action spectrum for ultraviolet radiation-induced immunosuppression in humans. Br J Dermatol 2011;164(3):657–9.

[19] Halliday GM, Byrne SN, Damian DL. Ultraviolet A radiation: its role in immunosuppression and carcinogenesis. Semin Cutan Med Surg 2011;30(4):214–21.

[20] Kripke ML. Antigenicity of murine skin tumors induced by ultraviolet light. J Natl Cancer Inst 1974;53(5):1333–6.

[21] Toews GB, Bergstresser PR, Streilein JW. Epidermal Langerhans cell density determines whether contact hypersensitivity or unresponsiveness follows skin painting with DNFB. J Immunol (Baltim Md 1950) 1980;124(1):445–53.

[22] Ullrich SE. Mechanisms underlying UV-induced immune suppression. Mutat Res 2005;571(1–2):185–205.

[23] Matos TR, Sheth V. The symbiosis of phototherapy and photoimmunology. Clin Dermatol 2016;34(5):538–47.

[24] Schwarz T. The dark and the sunny sides of UVR-induced immunosuppression: photoimmunology revised. J Investig Dermatol 2010;130(1):49–54.

[25] Brenner M, Hearing VJ. The protective role of melanin against UV damage in human skin. Photochem Photobiol 2008;84(3):539–49

[26] Holick MF, MacLaughlin JA, Clark MB, Holick SA, Potts Jr JT, Anderson RR, et al. Photosynthesis of previtamin D3 in human skin and the physiologic consequences. Science (New York NY) 1980;210(4466):203–5.

[27] Zhang YP, Wu J, Han YF, Shi ZR, Wang L. Pathogenesis of cutaneous lupus erythema associated with and without systemic lupus erythema. Autoimmun Rev 2017;16(7):735–42.

[28] Petri M, Orbai AM, Alarcon GS, Gordon C, Merrill JT, Fortin PR, et al. Derivation and validation of the Systemic Lupus International Collaborating Clinics classification criteria for systemic lupus erythematosus. Arthritis Rheum 2012;64(8):2677–86.

[29] Barbhaiya M, Costenbader KH. Ultraviolet radiation and systemic lupus erythematosus. Lupus 2014;23(6):588–95.

[30] Cutolo M, Plebani M, Shoenfeld Y, Adorini L, Tincani A. Vitamin D endocrine system and the immune response in rheumatic diseases. Vitam Horm 2011;86:327–51.

[31] Desbois AC, Cacoub P. Systemic sclerosis: an update in 2016. Autoimmun Rev 2016;15(5):417–26.

[32] Marie I, Gehanno JF. Environmental risk factors of systemic sclerosis. Semin Immunopathol 2015;37(5):463–73.

[33] Thompson C, Piguet V, Choy E. The pathogenesis of dermatomyositis. Br J Dermatol 2017.

[34] Gao S, Luo H, Zhang H, Zuo X, Wang L, Zhu H. Using multi-omics methods to understand dermatomyositis/polymyositis. Autoimmun Rev 2017;16(10):1044–8.

[35] Dourmishev L, Meffert H, Piazena H. Dermatomyositis: comparative studies of cutaneous photosensitivity in lupus erythematosus and normal subjects. Photodermatol Photoimmunol Photomed 2004;20(5):230–4.

[36] Okada S, Weatherhead E, Targoff IN, Wesley R, Miller FW. Global surface ultraviolet radiation intensity may modulate the clinical and immunologic expression of autoimmune muscle disease. Arthritis Rheum 2003;48(8):2285–93.

[37] Love LA, Weinberg CR, McConnaughey DR, Oddis CV, Medsger Jr TA, Reveille JD, et al. Ultraviolet radiation intensity predicts the relative distribution of dermatomyositis and anti-Mi-2 autoantibodies in women. Arthritis Rheum 2009;60(8):2499–504.

[38] Lock-Andersen J, Wulf HC. Threshold level for measurement of UV sensitivity: reproducibility of phototest. Photodermatol Photoimmunol Photomed 1996;12(4):154–61.

[39] European Dermatology Forum Guidelines on Phototesting. http://www.euroderm.org/edf/index.php/edf-guidelines/category/3-guidelines-on-photo-dermatoses; 2017.

[40] Photo(Chemo)Therapy for Psoriasis. In: Krutmann J, Hönigsmann H, Elmets CA, editors. Dermatological Phototherapy and photodiagnostic methods. 2nd ed. Berlin, Heidelberg: Springer-Verlag; 2009.

[41] Bulat V, Situm M, Dediol I, Ljubicic I, Bradic L. The mechanisms of action of phototherapy in the treatment of the most common dermatoses. Coll Antropol 2011;35(Suppl. 2):147–51.

[42] Ozawa M, Ferenczi K, Kikuchi T, Cardinale I, Austin LM, Coven TR, et al. 312-nanometer ultraviolet B light (narrow-band UVB) induces apoptosis of T cells within psoriatic lesions. J Exp Med 1999;189(4):711–8.

[43] Vangipuram R, Feldman SR. Ultraviolet phototherapy for cutaneous diseases: a concise review. Oral Diseases 2016;22(4):253–9.

[44] Kerr AC, Ferguson J, Attili SK, Beattie PE, Coleman AJ, Dawe RS, et al. Ultraviolet A1 phototherapy: a British Photodermatology Group workshop report. Clin Exp Dermatol 2012;37(3):219–26.

[45] Gozali MV, Zhou BR, Luo D. Update on treatment of photodermatosis. Dermatol Online J 2016;22(2).

[46] European Dermatology Forum. Guideline in Extracorporeal Photopheresis. 2017. http://www.euroderm.org/edf/index.php/edf-guidelines/category/5-guidelines-miscellaneous.

[47] Ruland V, Haust M, Stilling RM, Metze D, Amler S, Ruzicka T, et al. Updated analysis of standardized photoprovocation in patients with cutaneous lupus erythematosus. Arthritis Care Res 2013;65(5):767–76.

[48] Kind P, Lehmann P, Plewig G. Phototesting in lupus erythematosus. J Investig Dermatol 1993;100(1):53s–7s.

[49] Sanders CJ, Van Weelden H, Kazzaz GA, Sigurdsson V, Toonstra J, Bruijnzeel-Koomen CA. Photosensitivity in patients with lupus erythematosus: a clinical and photobiological study of 100 patients using a prolonged phototest protocol. Br J Dermatol 2003;149(1):131–7.

[50] Cohen MR, Isenberg DA. Ultraviolet irradiation in systemic lupus erythematosus: friend or foe? Br J Rheumatol 1996;35(10):1002–7.

[51] Smit N, Musson R, Romijn F, van Rossum H, van Pelt J. Effects of ultraviolet A-1 radiation on calcineurin activity and cytokine production in (skin) cell cultures. Photochem Photobiol 2010;86(2):360–6.

[52] Sonnichsen N, Meffert H, Kunzelmann V, Audring H. [UV-A-1 therapy of subacute cutaneous lupus erythematosus]. Der Hautarzt; Zeitschrift fur Dermatologie, Venerologie, und verwandte Gebiete 1993;44(11):723–5.

[53] McGrath Jr H. Ultraviolet-A1 irradiation decreases clinical disease activity and autoantibodies in patients with systemic lupus erythematosus. Clin Exp Rheumatol 1994;12(2):129–35.

[54] McGrath H, Martinez-Osuna P, Lee FA. Ultraviolet-A1 (340-400 nm) irradiation therapy in systemic lupus erythematosus. Lupus 1996;5(4):269–74.

[55] Polderman MC, le Cessie S, Huizinga TW, Pavel S. Efficacy of UVA-1 cold light as an adjuvant therapy for systemic lupus erythematosus. Rheumatology (Oxf Engl) 2004;43(11):1402–4.

[56] Polderman MC, Huizinga TW, Le Cessie S, Pavel S. UVA-1 cold light treatment of SLE: a double blind, placebo controlled crossover trial. Ann Rheum Dis 2001;60(2):112–5.

[57] Molina JF, McGrath Jr H. Longterm ultraviolet-A1 irradiation therapy in systemic lupus erythematosus. J Rheumatol 1997;24(6):1072–4.

[58] McGrath Jr H. Elimination of anticardiolipin antibodies and cessation of cognitive decline in a UV-A1-irradiated systemic lupus erythematosus patient. Lupus 2005;14(10):859–61.

[59] Jabara B, Dahlgren M, McGrath Jr H. Interstitial lung disease and pulmonary hypertension responsive to low-dose ultraviolet A1 irradiation in lupus. Journal of clinical rheumatology. Pract Rep Rheum Musculoskelet Dis 2010;16(4):188–9.

[60] Wolska H, Blaszczyk M, Jablonska S. Phototests in patients with various forms of lupus erythematosus. Int J Dermatol 1989;28(2):98–103.

[61] Pavel S. Light therapy (with UVA-1) for SLE patients: is it a good or bad idea? Rheumatology (Oxf Engl) 2006;45(6):653–5.

[62] Polderman MC, van Kooten C, Smit NP, Kamerling SW, Pavel S. Ultraviolet-A (UVA-1) radiation suppresses immunoglobulin production of activated B lymphocytes in vitro. Clin Exp Immunol 2006;145(3):528–34.

[63] Jones SK. The effects of hormonal and other stimuli on cell-surface Ro/SSA antigen expression by human keratinocytes in vitro: their possible role in the induction of cutaneous lupus lesions. Br J Dermatol 1992;126(6):554–60.

[64] Boeckler P, Liu V, Lipsker D. Extracorporeal photopheresis in recalcitrant lupus erythematosus. Clin Exp Dermatol 2009;34(7):e295–6.

[65] Knobler RM, Graninger W, Graninger W, Lindmaier A, Trautinger F, Smolen JS. Extracorporeal photochemotherapy for the treatment of systemic lupus erythematosus. A pilot study. Arthritis Rheum 1992;35(3):319–24.

[66] Wollina U, Looks A. Extracorporeal photochemotherapy in cutaneous lupus erythematosus. J Eur Acad Dermatol Venereol 1999;13(2):127–30.

[67] Morruzzi C, Liu V, Bohbot A, Cribier B, Lipsker D. [Four cases of photopheresis treatment for cutaneous lupus erythematosus refractory to standard therapy]. Ann Dermatol Venereol 2009;136(12):861–7.

[68] Richard MA, Saadallah S, Lefevre P, Poullin P, Buscaylet S, Grob JJ. [Extracorporeal photochemotherapy in therapy-refractory subacute lupus]. Ann Dermatol Venereol 2002;129(8–9):1023–6.

[69] Morita A, Sakakibara S, Sakakibara N, Yamauchi R, Tsuji T. Successful treatment of systemic sclerosis with topical PUVA. J Rheumatol 1995;22(12):2361–5.

[70] Petersen M, Hamilton T, Li HL. Regulation and inhibition of collagenase expression by long-wavelength ultraviolet radiation in cultured human skin fibroblasts. Photochem Photobiol 1995;62(3):444–8.

[71] Wlaschek M, Heinen G, Poswig A, Schwarz A, Krieg T, Scharffetter-Kochanek K. UVA-induced autocrine stimulation of fibroblast-derived collagenase/MMP-1 by interrelated loops of interleukin-1 and interleukin-6. Photochem Photobiol 1994;59(5):550–6.

[72] von Kobyletzki G, Heine O, Stephan H, Pieck C, Stucker M, Hoffmann K, et al. UVA1 irradiation induces deoxyribonuclease dependent apoptosis in cutaneous T-cell lymphoma in vivo. Photodermatol Photoimmunol Photomed 2000;16(6):271–7.

[73] Konttinen YT, Mackiewicz Z, Ruuttila P, Ceponis A, Sukura A, Povilenaite D, et al. Vascular damage and lack of angiogenesis in systemic sclerosis skin. Clin Rheumatol 2003;22(3):196–202.

[74] Fett N, Werth VP. Update on morphea: part II. Outcome measures and treatment. J Am Acad Dermatol 2011;64(2):231–42. Quiz 43–44.

[75] Kreuter A, Hyun J, Stucker M, Sommer A, Altmeyer P, Gambichler T. A randomized controlled study of low-dose UVA1, medium-dose UVA1, and narrowband UVB phototherapy in the treatment of localized scleroderma. J Am Acad Dermatol 2006;54(3):440–7.

[76] Vasquez R, Jabbar A, Khan F, Buethe D, Ahn C, Jacobe H. Recurrence of morphea after successful ultraviolet A1 phototherapy: a cohort study. J Am Acad Dermatol 2014;70(3):481–8.

[77] Kanekura T, Fukumaru S, Matsushita S, Terasaki K, Mizoguchi S, Kanzaki T. Successful treatment of scleroderma with PUVA therapy. J Dermatol 1996;23(7):455–9.

[78] Rose RF, Turner D, Goodfield MJ, Goulden V. Low-dose UVA1 phototherapy for proximal and acral scleroderma in systemic sclerosis. Photodermatol Photoimmunol Photomed 2009;25(3):153–5.

[79] Luftl M, Degitz K, Plewig G, Rocken M. Psoralen bath plus UV-A therapy. Possibilities and limitations. Arch Dermatol 1997;133(12):1597–603.

[80] Rook AH, Freundlich B, Jegasothy BV, Perez MI, Barr WG, Jimenez SA, et al. Treatment of systemic sclerosis with extracorporeal photochemotherapy. Results of a multicenter trial. Arch Dermatol 1992;128(3):337–46.

[81] Knobler RM, French LE, Kim Y, Bisaccia E, Graninger W, Nahavandi H, et al. A randomized, double-blind, placebo-controlled trial of photopheresis in systemic sclerosis. J Am Acad Dermatol 2006;54(5):793–9.

[82] De Wilde A, DiSpaltro FX, Geller A, Szer IS, Klainer AS, Bisaccia E. Extracorporeal photochemotherapy as adjunctive treatment in juvenile dermatomyositis: a case report. Arch Dermatol 1992;128(12):1656–7.

[83] Mohanna M, Distler O, Sprott H, Kundig T, French LE, Hofbauer G. Skin lesions in anti-Pm-Scl-70 positive systemic sclerosis-dermatomyositis overlap syndrome improve during local PUVA phototherapy. Eur J Dermatol 2013;23(5):730–1.

[84] Adamski J, Kinard T, Ipe T, Cooling L. Extracorporeal photopheresis for the treatment of autoimmune diseases. Transfus Apher Sci 2015;52(2):171–82.

[85] Zandi S, Kalia S, Lui H. UVA1 phototherapy: a concise and practical review. Skin Ther Lett 2012;17(1):1–4.

[86] Patel RV, Clark LN, Lebwohl M, Weinberg JM. Treatments for psoriasis and the risk of malignancy. J Am Acad Dermatol 2009;60(6):1001–17.

[87] Calzavara-Pinton P, Monari P, Manganoni AM, Ungari M, Rossi MT, Gualdi G, et al. Merkel cell carcinoma arising in immunosuppressed patients treated with high-dose ultraviolet A1 (320–400 nm) phototherapy: a report of two cases. Photodermatol Photoimmunol Photomed 2010;26(5):263–5.

Chapter 25

Vitamin D

Daniela Boleixa[1,2], Andreia Bettencourt[3,4], António Marinho[2,4], Ana Martins Silva[1,4], Cláudia Carvalho[3,4], Berta Martins Silva[3,4], Carlos Vasconcelos[2,4]

[1]Department of Neurology, Centro Hospitalar do Porto-Hospital de Santo António (CHP-HSA), Porto, Portugal; [2]Unidade de Imunologia Clínica (UIC), Centro Hospitalar do Porto-Hospital de Santo António (CHP-HSA); [3]Immunogenetics Laboratory, Abel Salazar Institute of Biomedical Sciences (ICBAS), University of Porto (UP), Porto, Portugal; [4]Unit for Multidisciplinary Research in Biomedicine (UMIB), Abel Salazar Institute of Biomedical Sciences (ICBAS), University of Porto (UP), Porto, Portugal

THE PHYSIOLOGY OF VITAMIN D

Vitamin D is a fat-soluble vitamin and a steroid hormone that plays a central role in maintaining calcium and phosphorus levels and bone homeostasis in close interaction with parathyroid hormone (PTH), acting on its classical target tissues, namely, bone, kidney, intestine, and parathyroid glands. Vitamin D endocrine system regulates several genes (about 3% of the human genome) involved in cell differentiation, cell cycle control, and cell function and exerts noncalcemic/pleiotropic effects on extraskeletal target tissues, such as immune and cardiovascular system, pancreatic endocrine cells, and muscle and adipose tissue. Several studies have suggested the role of vitamin D supplementation in the prevention/treatment of various autoimmune diseases (AIDs) and improvement of glucose metabolism, muscle, and adipose tissue function [1].

Synthesis, Sources, and Metabolism

Vitamin D is found in two forms: vitamin D2 and vitamin D3. Vitamin D3 is synthetized in the skin by ultraviolet radiation (UVR) or consumed in the diet through products such as eggs and milk (10%–20%). On the contrary, vitamin D2 cannot be formed by UVR; it is only acquired through food. Nevertheless exposure to sunlight is the major source of vitamin D. Sunlight mediates the conversion of 7-dehydrocholesterol (previtamin D3) to cholecalciferol (vitamin D3) in the skin, which is then hydroxylated in the liver to form metabolic inactive 25-hydroxyvitamin D [25(OH)D] or calcidiol, known to be the major circulating metabolite of vitamin D [2]. In the kidney, 25(OH)D is further hydroxylated, mainly by 1α-hydroxylase, to 1,25-dihydroxyvitamin D [$1,25(OH)_2D_3$], or calcitriol, the biologically active metabolite of vitamin D. This second hydroxylation is carefully regulated by PTH, phosphate, and vitamin D itself [3]. The PTH stimulates hydroxylation, whereas phosphate and vitamin D inhibit it. The fat solubility of vitamin D and its metabolites makes it necessary to be transported in blood bound to vitamin D–binding proteins (DBPs), furthermore making it also possible to leave DBP and freely diffuse across cell membranes and bind to cytosolic vitamin D receptors (VDRs) [3], to regulate not only calcium metabolism but also differentiation and division of several cell types [4]. The 25(OH)D serum concentration is widely accepted as the best indicator of the vitamin D status of an individual in vivo [2,4]. It covers not only the endocrine but also the paracrine biological pathways of vitamin D, whereas the active hormone $1,25(OH)_2D_3$ does not provide information on the vitamin D status and is often normal or increased as a result of secondary hyperparathyroidism associated with vitamin D deficiency [4]. Also, calcidiol has an almost 1000-fold greater concentration than $1,25(OH)_2D$; and because it has a longer half-life (20 days), it is more stable in the circulation [2]. Vitamin D metabolism is outlined in Fig. 25.1.

Vitamin D Receptor

Vitamin D acts in target tissues and cells via binding to an intranuclear receptor, vitamin D receptor (VDR), which belongs to the superfamily of transacting transcriptional regulatory factors [6].

Calcitriol enters the cell bound to the DBP. The rapid nongenomic actions of calcitriol include opening of Ca^{2+} channels and activation of second messenger pathways that engage in cross talk with the nucleus. Ligand activation results in VDR phosphorylation and translocation to the cell nucleus, where the VDR homodimerises or heterodimerises with Retinoid X receptor (RXR) to interact with vitamin D response elements (VDREs)—a short stretch of DNA that is a signature of genes

Mosaic of Autoimmunity. https://doi.org/10.1016/B978-0-12-814307-0.00025-6

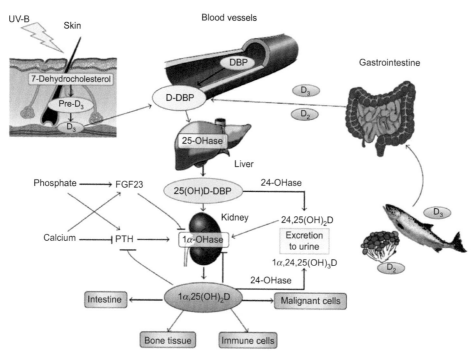

FIGURE 25.1 Vitamin D metabolism. *(Adapted from Obi Y, Hamano T, Isaka Y. Prevalence and prognostic implications of vitamin D deficiency in chronic kidney disease. Dis Markers 2015;2015:868961.)*

regulated by vitamin D—in vitamin D responsive genes (promoter regions). Depending on the target gene either coactivators or corepressors are attracted to the VDR/RXR complexes to induce or repress gene transcription [7,8], thus influencing the rate of transcription [9,10]. The net result is regulation of expression of proteins involved in calcium homeostasis and cell growth regulatory pathways [7]. Ligand-induced VDR/RXR heterodimerization is thought to enhance interaction with DNA [11].

Vitamin D Receptor Gene Polymorphisms

In humans, VDR gene is located on chromosome 12q13.1, extends over 100 kb, and includes eight protein-coding exons, six untranslated exons, eight introns, and two promoter regions [12]. Various single nucleotide polymorphisms (SNPs) have been described in the VDR gene [13], where four of which were extensively investigated: FokI C>T (rs2228570), BsmI A>G (rs1544410), ApaI G>T (rs7975232), and TaqI C>T (rs731236).

The FokI polymorphism, found in the coding region of the VDR gene, is caused by a T to C substitution in the translation initiation site in exon 2. It leads to the production of a VDR protein three amino acids shorter, suggesting a potential functional consequence [14]. Individuals with the C allele (F) initiate translation at the second ATG site, thereby lacking the three NH_2-terminal amino acid of the full length VDR protein (424 amino acid). In contrast, individuals with the T (f) allele initiate translation at the first ATG site and synthesize the full length VDR protein (427 amino acid) [15]. Although the short "F" isoform has been associated with a higher transcriptional activity [16,17], not all studies could replicate these results [18]. Therefore, this polymorphism seems to have consequences for both VDR protein structure and transcriptional activity [17].

The BsmI and ApaI polymorphisms are located in intron 8 and are in linkage disequilibrium (LD) with each other and with the TaqI polymorphism found in exon 9. Given that these polymorphisms do not seem to result in structural changes of the VDR protein, it is very unlikely that they have functional consequences. However, LD with other polymorphism(s) within VDR gene might underlie a potential effect. An example is the known LD with the 3′untranslated region of the VDR gene, a region that is involved in the regulation of mRNA stability and, in consequence, gene expression [19].

Vitamin D Receptor Gene Polymorphisms in Multiple Sclerosis

Patient-control and transmission studies have been used to study the association of VDR gene polymorphisms and multiple sclerosis (MS). The first studies were from Japan and reported an association with BsmI and ApaI [20,21]. The association with ApaI was reproduced in an Australian population and an association with TaqI was also found [22]. Although a British study showed a trend toward an underexpression of the ff FokI genotype [23], and a Canadian study showed marginally distorted transmission in HLA-DR15–negative patients [24], no other study reported associations of these polymorphisms and MS [25–30]. A possible hypothesis to explain the lack of association in studies performed in areas more remote from the equator is that an association of a VDR gene polymorphism with MS might be only penetrant in a population with sufficient vitamin D status [27].

In Portuguese patients an association between FokI ff genotype and MS susceptibility was found, but not with disease form or progression. Additional clinical and experimental studies should take the FokI VDR polymorphism into account and further clarify the role of vitamin D, its metabolites, and its receptor in MS [31].

Vitamin D Receptor Gene Polymorphisms in Systemic Lupus Erythematosus

The association between VDR polymorphisms and systemic lupus erythematosus (SLE) has been extensively studied, but no consistent conclusion has been reached so far. Previous studies in Asian populations reported a positive association between BsmI and FokI VDR polymorphisms and susceptibility to SLE [32–36]. The results from a metaanalysis show that BB genotype may be associated with elevated SLE risk among Asian population, as well as B allele. Nevertheless, no significance was found in both Caucasian subgroup and overall analysis [37].

It has also been observed that VDR SNPs may influence clinical manifestation such as nephropathy, serositis, antinuclear antibodies, anti-dsDNA, anti-Sm and antihistone antibodies [32,35,37–39]. In a Portuguese study from 2015, a positive association was found between VDR polymorphisms and SLE severity (chronic damage). The presence of Ff genotype of FokI and TT genotype of TaqI seems to confer a worse prognosis and may constitute a risk factor for higher long-term cumulative damage in SLE patients [40].

VITAMIN D DEFICIENCY

The environmental, hormonal, genetic, and nutritional conditions will influence the serum levels of vitamin D. Much debate has taken place over the definition of vitamin D deficiency. Most agree that a 25(OH)D concentration <50 nmol/L, or 20 ng/mL, is an indication of vitamin D deficiency, whereas a 25(OH)D concentration of 51–74 nmol/L, or 21–29 ng/mL, is considered to indicate insufficiency; concentrations >75 nmol/L, or 30 ng/mL, are considered to be adequate and recommended for bone and muscle function [4,41–43]. On this assumption several studies have described inadequacy of vitamin D levels all over the Europe, although the vitamin D status within different European countries shows a high variation [44–46]. Different studies showed mean serum 25(OH)D levels of 12–55 nmol/L in Southern European countries [47–51] and 45–63 nmol/L in Northern Europe [52–56], and that this concentration is dependent on season [48,49,57–59].

Nevertheless, in a recent study from Australia, where researchers sought to identify the 25(OH)D level below which abnormal bone physiology becomes evident, the authors believe their data justify a cutoff of 30 nmol/L (12 ng/mL) for deficiency [60]. Based on this lower cutoff levels some authors argue that much of the reported high prevalence of vitamin D deficiency/insufficiency in healthy populations of the world is artificial, created by unjustified high cutoff values of serum 25(OH)D [61].

THE EMERGING ROLE OF VITAMIN D IN IMMUNOMODULATION

The identification of VDRs in all cells of the immune system and the discovery that dendritic cells (DCs) can produce the metabolically active form of vitamin D, have led to the suggestion that vitamin D could act as an immunomodulator [40,62,63].

Vitamin D is actively involved in the regulation of innate and adaptive immune responses [64–67]. Direct genomic signaling by $1,25(OH)_2D_3$ occurs through its receptor, which is present in multiple cells of the immune system including activated $CD4^+$ and $CD8^+$ T lymphocytes, B cells, circulating monocytes, neutrophils, and antigen presenting cells, such as macrophages and DCs. Active vitamin D, i.e., $1,25(OH)_2D_3$, is recognized by target tissues that possess VDR. This receptor is also expressed widely in the intestine, skin, bone, kidneys, pituitary, parathyroid, pancreatic beta cells, gonads, skeletal muscles, and in neurons and glial cells in the human brain [68].

Vitamin D and Innate Immunity

Differentiation of monocytes, either into macrophages or DCs, is accompanied by a decrease in VDR-expression, making these cells less sensitive to $1,25(OH)_2D_3$ when they mature. Nevertheless, they can be influenced by $1,25(OH)_2D_3$.

It can modulate the activation of DCs by inhibiting the differentiation, maturation, survival, and immunostimulatory capacity of these cells. Furthermore, $1,25(OH)_2D_3$ can also alter DCs' ability to present antigens [42,69] by decreasing the expression of MHC II molecules as well as of CD40, CD80, and CD86 [70–72]. In addition, $1,25(OH)_2D_3$ decreases the synthesis of IL-12 [71,73] and simultaneously increases the production of IL-5 and IL-10 by DCs [71]. Although $1,25(OH)_2D_3$ primarily has inhibitory effects on the adaptive immune response, some of its effects on innate immune cells are stimulatory. For example, $1,25(OH)_2D_3$ can stimulate human monocyte proliferation in vitro [74] and has been shown to increase the production of both IL-1 and the bactericidal peptide cathelicidin by monocytes and macrophages (important for mycobacteria infection control, for example) [42].

Vitamin D and Adaptive Immunity

Although naive T cells only display very low VDR levels, this receptor is present in large quantities on T cell activation [66,75]. In T cells, $1,25(OH)_2D_3$ signaling is known to block the production of Th1 cytokines, particularly IFN-γ, while promoting Th2 cell differentiation [76,77] and directly by enhancing IL-4 production [72]. The activity of $1,25(OH)_2D_3$ on T cell differentiation is further enhanced by its capacity to block IL-12 production in DCs [71,73]. Furthermore, $1,25(OH)_2D_3$ also inhibits Th17 cell responses, probably owing in part to its capacity to inhibit IL-6 and IL-23 production, while inducing the differentiation and/or expansion of regulatory T cells (Tregs) [78,79]. FOXP3 (forkhead box P3) is a protein involved in immune system responses [80]. A member of the FOX protein family, FOXP3, appears to function as a master regulator of the regulatory pathway in the development and function of Tregs [81–83]. Regulatory T cells generally suppress the immune system, turning the immune response down. In cancer, an excess of regulatory T cell activity can prevent the immune system from destroying cancer cells. In AIDs, a deficiency of regulatory T cells activity can allow autoreactive cells to attack the body's own tissues [84,85]. The FOXP3 gene has a VDRE in its promoter region, being important for its cellular expression [86]. The assessment of the immunomodulatory effect by the imbalance of FoxP3+/IL-17A CD4+ T lymphocytes is widely recognized.

In addition to its activity on T cells, $1,25(OH)_2D_3$ also influences B cells activity by inducing its apoptosis, inhibiting its proliferation and generation of memory and plasma cells [62,69,77,87,88]. However, it has been suggested that the effect of $1,25(OH)_2D_3$ on B cells might be indirectly mediated through its effect on T helper cell differentiation [89]. Indeed, there are conflicting reports concerning the expression of VDR by B cells [88,90,91], leaving it unclear whether $1,25(OH)_2D_3$ can act directly on B cells. The effects of vitamin D on cells of the immune system are summarized in Fig. 25.2.

GENETIC AND EPIGENETIC EFFECTS OF VITAMIN D

SLE and other AIDs can be a conceptual form of resistance to vitamin D effect. This resistant state has multiple steps including the epigenetic mechanisms (also regulation of metabolic pathways), gene regulation in different cell types, and VDR polymorphisms (the transcriptome).

Vitamin D and Epigenetic Mechanisms

Epigenetic mechanisms play a crucial role in regulating gene expression as shown earlier with the VDRE in noncoding sequences of MHC II [93,94]. The main mechanisms involve methylation of DNA and covalent modifications of histones by methylation, acetylation, phosphorylation, or ubiquitination. Vitamin D interacts with the epigenome on multiple levels:

1. Critical genes in the vitamin D signaling system, such as those coding for VDR and the enzymes 25-hydroxylase (CYP2R1), 1α-hydroxylase (CYP27B1), and 24-hydroxylase (CYP24A1) have large 5′-C-phosphate-G-3' (CpG) islands in their promoter regions and therefore can be silenced by DNA methylation.
2. VDR protein physically interacts with coactivator and corepressor proteins, which in turn are in contact with chromatin modifiers and with chromatin remodelers.
3. A number of genes encoding for chromatin modifiers and remodelers are primary targets of VDR and its ligands.
4. There is evidence that certain VDR ligands (1,25-dihydroxyvitamin D3) have DNA demethylating effects [95].

SLE and other AIDs, such as cancer, are a state of DNA hypermethylation. The disease itself can mute key enzymes of its metabolism and create a state of 25(OH)D deficiency. Conversely, the "DNA demethylating" effect can be important to the maintenance of key enzymes and their target genes, maintaining immune system homeostasis. Once again, the replacement of cholecalciferol is not established and is likely to need very high levels or greater affinity analogues to overpass this resistance. This particular field lacks evidence.

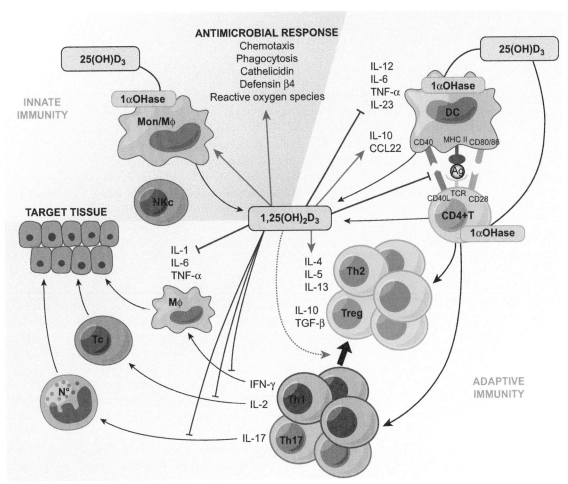

FIGURE 25.2 Effects of vitamin D on cells of the immune system. *(Adapted from Verstuyf A, Carmeliet G, Bouillon R, Mathieu C. Vitamin D: a pleiotropic hormone. Kidney Int 2010;78(2):140–5.)*

MicroRNAs

Given the strong genomic actions of $1,25(OH)_2D_3$ it is likely that it also regulates the expression of some of the remaining genome that includes microRNAs (miRNAs). Recently, a number of miRNAs have been identified as $1,25(OH)_2D_3$ targets [96]. Calcitriol regulates the expression of miRNAs through both direct mechanism that involves VDRE and indirect mechanism that affects the genesis of mature miRNA. Through the regulation of miRNA expression, $1,25(OH)_2D_3$ modulates cell proliferation, differentiation, apoptosis, and migration in many cancer cell types [97–99]. Considering these properties, an inflammatory profile in patients with vitamin D deficiency must be considered.

VITAMIN D AND AUTOIMMUNE DISEASES

As outlined in this book, autoimmune diseases are triggered by a multitude of factors. In this regard, vitamin D is a hormone that might be involved in AIDs development.

The importance of vitamin D in several autoimmune disorders has been reported and vitamin D deficiency has been associated with the pathogenesis and severity of MS, type I diabetes mellitus, rheumatoid arthritis (RA), systemic sclerosis, and SLE, among others [100].

The Danish National Patient Register (median follow-up time 10.8 years) identified 525 cases of incident AID, and it found statistically significant inverse associations between vitamin D status and development of any AID and thyrotoxicosis in particular [101].

Patients with AID showed low levels of vitamin D, although if cause or consequence is still matter of debate. The quality of the published studies, regarding number of patients, methods, and other factors preclude a definitive conclusion [102].

Other studies did not find correlation between vitamin D levels and some AIDs, such as Sjögren's Syndrome and Behçet disease (BD) [103,104].

Systemic Lupus Erythematosus

Considering SLE and vitamin D, many questions have been postulated in the last 10 years and some experimental works were performed.

Vitamin D insufficiency may be an important factor in SLE susceptibility during early life, based on vitamin D effect in autoreactive T-lymphocytes central deletion [93,94]. We can look for autoimmune susceptibility as an "early life" condition in which vitamin D insufficiency is also a determining factor for an autoreactive profile. As stated before, VDREs have been found in the promoter region of the MS-associated allele HLA-DRB1*15:01 [93,94], suggesting that with low vitamin D availability, VDREs are incapable of inducing DRB1*15:01 expression allowing early life autoreactive T cells to escape central thymic deletion. These findings have been found in MS; in SLE no data are available concerning these findings.

Taking all this information into account, retrospective genetic susceptibility studies, which do not have controlled vitamin D population levels in childhood, may have no valid results. The susceptibility studies related with polymorphisms of VDR are such an example, with different susceptibility profiles in different populations, but without controlled vitamin D levels in the studied population [105,106].

Usually, patients with established SLE lack vitamin D and its levels seem to correlate inversely with SLE disease activity index (SLEDAI) scores [107]. The reduced sun exposure, the use of sunscreens, the gut malabsorption (example: secondary to drugs such as corticosteroids), among others, are all significant factors for this steroid hormone insufficiency [108]. However, sun exposure, the most important factor for vitamin D precursor synthesis at the skin level, is also one of the strong activators of SLE flares, possibly because the UV wavelengths of sunlight potentiates the stimulator of interferon genes–dependent activation of the IRF3 in response to cytosolic DNA and cyclic dinucleotides in keratinocytes and other human cells [109]. This phenomenon, being well recognized, is also ignored in the supplementation strategies, which are based on the general population guidelines. SLE patients need treatment strategies based on serum levels of 25(OH)D and not standard supplementation strategies, even though serum levels of 30 ng/mL are validated to metabolic bone disease but not for immunological effects [87].

In Portugal, 25(OH)D levels on patients with SLE were shown to be lower than those in the general population, especially in the summer period ($P = .0003$) (not published, in preparation). Furthermore, it was possible to observe a higher number of flares in those patients with low baseline 25(OH)D levels ($P = .045$) as well as that patients with three or more flares were those with significantly lower baseline 25(OH)D levels ($P = .004$) (not published, in preparation). In a retrospective evaluation, the mean 25(OH)D levels of 68 patients in the previous 10 years of disease were lower in those with more severe flares, although not statistically significant ($P = .178$); however, if we consider two subgroups (patients with three or more and less than three severe flares), the difference reaches significance ($P = .044$) (not published, in preparation). Some genetic studies focused in VDR polymorphisms in a group of SLE Portuguese patients demonstrated that SLE damage, according to SLICC values, was higher in patients with FokI Ff and TaqI TT genotypes ($P = .031$ and $P = .046$ respectively) [40]. Despite this higher long-term cumulative damage, these effects seem to be unrelated to vitamin D levels. Lower baseline 25(OH)D levels at SLE diagnosis (before supplementation) and mean 25(OH)D levels in a 10-year follow-up, correlate negatively with disease severity (resulting in more aggressive SLE phenotypes) (not published, in preparation).

Multiple Sclerosis

The evidence for a neurobiological effect of vitamin D came in 1991 when the regulatory effect of 1,25-dihydroxyvitamin D3 on nerve growth factor was first reported [110]. Studies have since shown that bioactive vitamin D may modulate the production of neurotrophins, growth factors, and neurotransmitters in the mammalian brain [111].

Different studies have analyzed the serum concentrations of vitamin D metabolites in patients with MS. These studies showed that patients with MS had significantly lower 25-hydroxyvitamin D levels than controls [112–115]. There are also two longitudinal studies based on 25(OH)D concentrations before the onset of MS. One of the studies used a nested case-control design and comprised over 7 million individuals who served in the US military and had at least two serum samples stored in the US department of defense serum repository. The study concluded that serum concentration of 25(OH)D, in healthy young white adults, is an important risk predictor for MS, independently from their place of birth and latitude of residence during childhood [116]. The other study was a prospective study performed in nurses, where dietary vitamin D intake was assessed at baseline and updated every 4 years thereafter. During the follow-up, 173 cases of MS with onset of symptoms after baseline were confirmed. They concluded that women who took vitamin D (≥400 international units/day) had a 40% lower risk of MS than women who did not use vitamin D supplements [116]. Also there are some studies that found a negative correlation between serum 25(OH)D and MS clinical disease activity [10,117,118].

In accordance with the majority of the literature, low serum 25(OH)D levels were also associated with susceptibility and disability in MS patients from Portugal. Lower serum 25(OH)D levels were also found in patients with a recent disease onset, supporting vitamin D levels as a risk factor for MS [119].

Other Autoimmune Diseases

In RA patients, a metaanalysis involving 24 reports and a total of 3489 patients allowed the conclusion that these patients presented lower vitamin D values than healthy controls and also that there was a negative association between disease activity and vitamin D levels [120]. In fact, a cross-sectional study promoted by the European League Against Rheumatism showed that vitamin D insufficiency/deficiency is frequent in RA patients. This study involved the measurement of serum 25(OH)D level in samples collected during winter time of 625 RA patients and 276 age- and sex-matched healthy subjects from 13 European countries and found significant differences in vitamin D levels between countries not clearly explained by latitude. It was also observed that vitamin D serum concentrations correlate negatively and significantly with the D-PRO Global Risk Score, clinimetric indexes for quality of life, disease activity, and disability [121].

A project comparing the risk of cardiovascular events in 775 patients with RA, 738 with ankylosing spondylitis and 721 psoriatic arthritis (PsA) patients, and 667 patients with other nonchronic inflammatory rheumatic diseases (CARMA project) only found a statistically significant positive association between RA and 25(OH)D deficiency [122].

Remission was higher in patients with early-onset rheumatoid arthritis without 25(OH)D deficiency. Those with deficiency at baseline had higher Health Assessment Questionnaire and Physician Global Disease Activity Assessment scores, fatigue levels, erythrocyte sedimentation rate, and morning stiffness, but no radiographic progression was associated to hypovitaminosis D after 36-month follow-up. It was also found that patients with BB–Bb genotype polymorphism of VDR gene had lower 25(OH)D levels and a propensity to a more severe disease, which led the authors to propose a role of vitamin D as a clinical biomarker for RA [123]. Even in inactive RA patients the prevalence of vitamin D was lower in RA patients than in controls [124].

A metaanalysis from 2017 suggests that low serum 25(OH)D levels may be associated with comorbidities in psoriasis (PS) patients, including metabolic syndrome and cardiovascular risk [125]. However, the literature does not show significant differences between the PS and PsA groups in terms of serum 25(OH)D levels and a prevalence of vitamin D deficiency [126].

In SSc, an Italian group found hypovitaminosis D statistically associated with autoimmune thyroiditis, whereas calcinosis was more frequently observed in patients without 25(OH)D supplementation in comparison with those with supplementation. The authors also described a significantly higher percentage of serum anticentromere antibodies in patients of the last group with 25(OH)D level ≥30 ng/mL (P = .017) [127].

In patients with Sjögren's syndrome, low vitamin D is associated with extraglandular manifestations, such as lymphoma or neuropathy [128].

In a small study of 19 patients with BD in comparison with 95 controls, it was found that BD patients were significantly less likely to have 25(OH)D deficiency or insufficiency, which for the authors suggest a possible role for 25(OH)D in modifying the inflammatory response in BD [104].

In a case-control study, with 100 patients with and without noninfectious uveitis, lower vitamin D levels were associated with an increased risk of noninfectious anterior uveitis [129].

Moreover, in autoinflammatory syndrome induced by adjuvant (ASIA), a study with 131 patients in relation to silicone implant incompatibility found autoantibodies in 18% of them, from which the majority (78%) had vitamin D deficiency or insufficiency, which suggest it as a risk factor to the production of autoantibodies [130].

Vitamin D Supplementation

Most of the studies with vitamin D supplementation in AIDs have been inconclusive. One of the reasons could be related to measuring the metabolite 25(OH)D instead of the active form calcitriol [131].

Many studies address vitamin D therapy in real practice. There are some considerations that should be taken into account for real practice:

- Can vitamin D supplementation prevent SLE flares?
- Can vitamin D levels predict flares?
- What is the optimal dosage in SLE?
- Is there a window of opportunity for supplementation?

There are a large number of studies addressing this issue; however, the evidence is sparse. Birmingham et al. studied 46 SLE patients from the specimen bank and database of the Ohio SLE Study to understand the vitamin D seasonal variation levels and their correlation with flares. The major finding was that in non–African American SLE patients there was a highly significant decrease in 25(OH)D serum levels at the time of flare, both nonrenal and renal flares, for those flares occurring during low daytime sun exposure season [132]. Later, Schoindre et al. prospectively studied the relationship between 25(OH)D levels and SLEDAI score in 170 SLE patients and assessed the role of vitamin D in predicting SLE flare-ups, finding no association between baseline 25(OH)D levels and relapse-free survival rate [133]. Finally, Susmita Roy et al. published a complex paper, developing a general kinetic model in an attempt to capture the role of vitamin D in immunomodulatory responses. The authors found that although vitamin D plays a negligible role in the initial immune response, it exerts a profound influence in the long term, especially in helping the system to achieve a new, stable steady state. They also observed that the optimal vitamin D level lies in the 50–100 nmol/L range, where both pathogen and effector T cell levels remain at reasonably low-risk range [134].

Despite the general idea that low vitamin D levels are related to higher disease activity, proofs are needed in randomized clinical trials. It seems that large variations of vitamin D can be related to SLE flares, but vitamin D levels themselves cannot predict flares. This statement thus not excludes that vitamin D basal therapy, at least in stable SLE patients, cannot prevent flares. Finally, theoretically, immunomodulation can be achieved with levels between 75 and 100 nmol/L; however, it is shown that optimal individual levels have to be tailored.

This important medical problem leads to the question, whether an insight into the genome- and transcriptome-wide actions of VDR and $1,25(OH)_2D_3$ is a help to a more accurate evaluation of the human individual's responsiveness to, and needs for, vitamin D. Interestingly, only for a subset of individuals, significant correlations between the upregulation of both genes and the intervention-induced raise in serum 25(OH)D concentrations were obtained. This suggests that, on a molecular level, not all study participants benefited from the vitamin D3 supplementation because they had already reached their individual optimal vitamin D status before the start of the intervention, or they carry a genetic polymorphism making them less responsive to vitamin D3 or other undefined reasons.

After 6 months of vitamin D supplementation, FoxP3$^+$/IL-17A ratio in patients with stable SLE was higher than that at baseline ($P < .001$), even in patients with normal 25(OH)D levels at baseline (≥ 75 nmol/L) ($P = .043$) [135]. Considering the same effects before and after a high dose Vitamin D supplementation in patients with severely active disease, no enhancement of Tregs or Tregs/IL-17A was observed (not published, in preparation). Finally, at the epigenetic level, no significant differences were found in miR-146a expression when comparing controls and SLE active patients, before and after Vitamin D supplementation (not published, in preparation). In RA, the documentation of relationship between low levels of vitamin D and lower percentage of disease remission suggest its immunomodulatory action and should be considered an additional option in the management of early RA patients [136]. In a case-control study with early RA, the authors found that a single dose of cholecalciferol (300,000 IU) combined with standard treatment (methotrexate and steroids) significantly ameliorates patients' general health as evaluated on a numeric scale (0–100: 0 worst; 100: best status), but had no effect on DAS28, CRP, ESR, and VAS, already improved with the standard treatment [137].

A study in patients with Hashimoto's thyroiditis and vitamin D deficiency did not find any significant effect on thyroid function and autoimmunity with vitamin D supplementation [138].

REFERENCES

[1] Wimalawansa SJ. Non-musculoskeletal benefits of vitamin D. J Steroid Biochem Mol Biol 2018 Jan;175:60–81. https://doi.org/10.1016/j.jsbmb.2016.09.016. Epub 2016 Sep 2.

[2] Lips P. Relative value of 25(OH)D and 1,25(OH)2D measurements. J Bone Miner Res 2007;22(11):1668–71.

[3] Bikle DD. Vitamin D metabolism, mechanism of action, and clinical applications. Chem Biol 2014;21(3):319–29.

[4] Holick MF. Vitamin D status: measurement, interpretation, and clinical application. Ann Epidemiol 2009;19(2):73–8.

[5] Obi Y, Hamano T, Isaka Y. Prevalence and prognostic implications of vitamin D deficiency in chronic kidney disease. Dis Markers 2015;2015:868961.

[6] Kostner K, Denzer N, Muller CS, Klein R, Tilgen W, Reichrath J. The relevance of vitamin D receptor (VDR) gene polymorphisms for cancer: a review of the literature. Anticancer Res 2009;29(9):3511–36.

[7] Issa LL, Leong GM, Eisman JA. Molecular mechanism of vitamin D receptor action. Inflamm Res 1998;47(12):451–75.

[8] Kongsbak M, Levring TB, Geisler C, von Essen MR. The vitamin d receptor and T cell function. Front Immunol 2013;4:148.

[9] Carlberg C, Quack M, Herdick M, Bury Y, Polly P, Toell A. Central role of VDR conformations for understanding selective actions of vitamin D(3) analogues. Steroids 2001;66(3–5):213–21.

[10] Smolders J, Damoiseaux J, Menheere P, Hupperts R. Vitamin D as an immune modulator in multiple sclerosis, a review. J Neuroimmunol 2008;194(1–2):7–17.

[11] Haussler MR, Jurutka PW, Hsieh JC, Thompson PD, Selznick SH, Haussler CA, et al. New understanding of the molecular mechanism of receptor-mediated genomic actions of the vitamin D hormone. Bone 1995;17(2 Suppl.):33S–8S.

[12] de Azevedo Silva J, Monteiro Fernandes K, Tres Pancotto JA, Sotero Fragoso T, Donadi EA, Crovella S, et al. Vitamin D receptor (VDR) gene polymorphisms and susceptibility to systemic lupus erythematosus clinical manifestations. Lupus 2013;22(11):1110–7.

[13] Whitfield GK, Remus LS, Jurutka PW, Zitzer H, Oza AK, Dang HT, et al. Functionally relevant polymorphisms in the human nuclear vitamin D receptor gene. Mol Cell Endocrinol 2001;177(1–2):145–59.

[14] Yang CY, Leung PS, Adamopoulos IE, Gershwin ME. The implication of vitamin D and autoimmunity: a comprehensive review. Clin Rev Allergy Immunol 2013;45(2):217–26.

[15] Smolders J, Peelen E, Thewissen M, Menheere P, Tervaert JW, Hupperts R, et al. The relevance of vitamin D receptor gene polymorphisms for vitamin D research in multiple sclerosis. Autoimmun Rev 2009;8(7):621–6.

[16] Arai H, Miyamoto K, Taketani Y, Yamamoto H, Iemori Y, Morita K, et al. A vitamin D receptor gene polymorphism in the translation initiation codon: effect on protein activity and relation to bone mineral density in Japanese women. J Bone Miner Res 1997;12(6):915–21.

[17] Jurutka PW, Remus LS, Whitfield GK, Thompson PD, Hsieh JC, Zitzer H, et al. The polymorphic N terminus in human vitamin D receptor isoforms influences transcriptional activity by modulating interaction with transcription factor IIB. Mol Endocrinol 2000;14(3):401–20.

[18] Gross C, Krishnan AV, Malloy PJ, Eccleshall TR, Zhao XY, Feldman D. The vitamin D receptor gene start codon polymorphism: a functional analysis of FokI variants. J Bone Miner Res 1998;13(11):1691–9.

[19] Ingles SA, Haile RW, Henderson BE, Kolonel LN, Nakaichi G, Shi CY, et al. Strength of linkage disequilibrium between two vitamin D receptor markers in five ethnic groups: implications for association studies. Cancer Epidemiol Biomarkers Prev 1997;6(2):93–8. A Publication of the American Association for Cancer Research, Cosponsored by the American Society of Preventive Oncology.

[20] Fukazawa T, Yabe I, Kikuchi S, Sasaki H, Hamada T, Miyasaka K, et al. Association of vitamin D receptor gene polymorphism with multiple sclerosis in Japanese. J Neurol Sci 1999;166(1):47–52.

[21] Niino M, Fukazawa T, Yabe I, Kikuchi S, Sasaki H, Tashiro K. Vitamin D receptor gene polymorphism in multiple sclerosis and the association with HLA class II alleles. J Neurol Sci 2000;177(1):65–71.

[22] Tajouri L, Ovcaric M, Curtain R, Johnson MP, Griffiths LR, Csurhes P, et al. Variation in the vitamin D receptor gene is associated with multiple sclerosis in an Australian population. J Neurogenet 2005;19(1):25–38.

[23] Partridge JM, Weatherby SJ, Woolmore JA, Highland DJ, Fryer AA, Mann CL, et al. Susceptibility and outcome in MS: associations with polymorphisms in pigmentation-related genes. Neurology 2004;62(12):2323–5.

[24] Orton SM, Ramagopalan SV, Para AE, Lincoln MR, Handunnetthi L, Chao MJ, et al. Vitamin D metabolic pathway genes and risk of multiple sclerosis in Canadians. J Neurol Sci 2011;305(1–2):116–20.

[25] Simon KC, Munger KL, Xing Y, Ascherio A. Polymorphisms in vitamin D metabolism related genes and risk of multiple sclerosis. Mult Scler 2010;16(2):133–8.

[26] Sioka C, Papakonstantinou S, Markoula S, Gkartziou F, Georgiou A, Georgiou I, et al. Vitamin D receptor gene polymorphisms in multiple sclerosis patients in northwest Greece. J Negat Results Biomed 2011;10:3.

[27] Smolders J, Damoiseaux J, Menheere P, Tervaert JW, Hupperts R. Fok-I vitamin D receptor gene polymorphism (rs10735810) and vitamin D metabolism in multiple sclerosis. J Neuroimmunol 2009;207(1–2):117–21.

[28] Smolders J, Damoiseaux J, Menheere P, Tervaert JW, Hupperts R. Association study on two vitamin D receptor gene polymorphisms and vitamin D metabolites in multiple sclerosis. Ann NY Acad Sci 2009;1173:515–20.

[29] Steckley JL, Dyment DA, Sadovnick AD, Risch N, Hayes C, Ebers GC. Genetic analysis of vitamin D related genes in Canadian multiple sclerosis patients. Canadian Collaborative Study Group. Neurology 2000;54(3):729–32.

[30] Yeo TW, Maranian M, Singlehurst S, Gray J, Compston A, Sawcer S. Four single nucleotide polymorphisms from the vitamin D receptor gene in UK multiple sclerosis. J Neurol 2004;251(6):753–4.

[31] Bettencourt A, Boleixa D, Guimaraes AL, Leal B, Carvalho C, Bras S, et al. The vitamin D receptor gene FokI polymorphism and multiple sclerosis in a Northern Portuguese population. J Neuroimmunol 2017;309:34–7.

[32] Ozaki Y, Nomura S, Nagahama M, Yoshimura C, Kagawa H, Fukuhara S. Vitamin-D receptor genotype and renal disorder in Japanese patients with systemic lupus erythematosus. Nephron 2000;85(1):86–91.

[33] Huang CM, Wu MC, Wu JY, Tsai FJ. Association of vitamin D receptor gene BsmI polymorphisms in Chinese patients with systemic lupus erythematosus. Lupus 2002;11(1):31–4.

[34] Luo XY, Wu LJ, Yang MH, Liu NT, Liao T, Tang Z, et al. Relationship of vitamin D receptor gene Fok I polymorphism with systemic lupus erythematosus. Xi bao yu fen zi mian yi xue za zhi = Chin J Mol Cell Immunol 2011;27(8):901–5.

[35] Luo XY, Wu LJ, Chen L, Yang MH, Liao T, Liu NT, et al. The association of vitamin D receptor gene ApaI and BsmI polymorphism with systemic lupus erythematosus. Zhonghua nei ke za zhi 2012;51(2):131–5.

[36] Chen XE, Chen P, Chen SS, Lu J, Ma T, Shi G, et al. A population association study of vitamin D receptor gene polymorphisms and haplotypes with the risk of systemic lupus erythematosus in a Chinese population. Immunol Res 2017;65(3):750–6.

[37] Hu W, Niu G, Lin Y, Chen X, Lin L. Impact of the polymorphism in vitamin D receptor gene BsmI and the risk of systemic lupus erythematosus: an updated meta-analysis. Clin Rheumatol 2016;35(4):927–34.

[38] Emerah AA, El-Shal AS. Role of vitamin D receptor gene polymorphisms and serum 25-hydroxyvitamin D level in Egyptian female patients with systemic lupus erythematosus. Mol Biol Rep 2013;40(11):6151–62.

[39] Luo XY, Yang MH, Wu FX, Wu LJ, Chen L, Tang Z, et al. Vitamin D receptor gene BsmI polymorphism B allele, but not BB genotype, is associated with systemic lupus erythematosus in a Han Chinese population. Lupus 2012;21(1):53–9.

[40] Carvalho C, Marinho A, Leal B, Bettencourt A, Boleixa D, Almeida I, et al. Association between vitamin D receptor (VDR) gene polymorphisms and systemic lupus erythematosus in Portuguese patients. Lupus 2015;24(8):846–53.

[41] Dawson-Hughes B, Heaney RP, Holick MF, Lips P, Meunier PJ, Vieth R. Estimates of optimal vitamin D status. Osteoporos Int 2005;16(7):713–6.

[42] Holick MF. Vitamin D deficiency. N Engl J Med 2007;357(3):266–81.

[43] Souberbielle JC, Body JJ, Lappe JM, Plebani M, Shoenfeld Y, Wang TJ, et al. Vitamin D and musculoskeletal health, cardiovascular disease, auto-immunity and cancer: recommendations for clinical practice. Autoimmun Rev 2010;9(11):709–15.

[44] Cashman KD, Dowling KG, Skrabakova Z, Gonzalez-Gross M, Valtuena J, De Henauw S, et al. Vitamin D deficiency in Europe: pandemic? Am J Clin Nutr 2016;103(4):1033–44.

[45] Pludowski P, Grant WB, Bhattoa HP, Bayer M, Povoroznyuk V, Rudenka E, et al. Vitamin d status in central europe. Int J Pediatr Endocrinol 2014;2014:589587.

[46] Quraishi SA, Camargo Jr CA, Manson JE. Low vitamin D status in Europe: moving from evidence to sound public health policies. Am J Clin Nutr 2016;103(4):957–8.

[47] Aleksova A, Belfiore R, Carriere C, Kassem S, La Carrubba S, Barbati G, et al. Vitamin D deficiency in patients with acute myocardial infarction: an Italian single-center study. Int J Vitam Nutr Res Internationale Zeitschrift fur Vitamin- und Ernahrungsforschung Journal international de vita-minologie et de nutrition 2015;85(1–2):23–30.

[48] Bettencourt A, Boleixa D, Reis J, Oliveira JC, Mendonca D, Costa PP, et al. Serum 25-hydroxyvitamin D levels in a healthy population from the North of Portugal. J Steroid Biochem Mol Biol 2016.

[49] Bettica P, Bevilacqua M, Vago T, Norbiato G. High prevalence of hypovitaminosis D among free-living postmenopausal women referred to an osteoporosis outpatient clinic in northern Italy for initial screening. Osteoporos Int 1999;9(3):226–9.

[50] Challa A, Ntourntoufi A, Cholevas V, Bitsori M, Galanakis E, Andronikou S. Breastfeeding and vitamin D status in Greece during the first 6 months of life. Eur J Pediatr 2005;164(12):724–9.

[51] Isaia G, Giorgino R, Rini GB, Bevilacqua M, Maugeri D, Adami S. Prevalence of hypovitaminosis D in elderly women in Italy: clinical conse-quences and risk factors. Osteoporos Int 2003;14(7):577–82.

[52] Cashman KD, Muldowney S, McNulty B, Nugent A, FitzGerald AP, Kiely M, et al. Vitamin D status of Irish adults: findings from the national adult nutrition survey. Br J Nutr 2013;109(7):1248–56.

[53] Christiansen C, Christensen MS, McNair P, Nielsen B, Madsbad S. Vitamin D metabolites in diabetic patients: decreased serum concentration of 24,25-dihydroxyvitamin D. Scand J Clin Lab Investig 1982;42(6):487–91.

[54] Hill T, Collins A, O'Brien M, Kiely M, Flynn A, Cashman KD. Vitamin D intake and status in Irish postmenopausal women. Eur J Clin Nutr 2005;59(3):404–10.

[55] Lamberg-Allardt CJ, Outila TA, Karkkainen MU, Rita HJ, Valsta LM. Vitamin D deficiency and bone health in healthy adults in Finland: could this be a concern in other parts of Europe? J Bone Miner Res 2001;16(11):2066–73.

[56] Lardner E, Fitzgibbon M, Wilson S, Griffin D, Mulkerrin E. Hypovitaminosis D in a healthy female population, aged from 40 to 85 years, in the west of Ireland. Ir J Med Sci 2011;180(1):115–9.

[57] O'Sullivan M, Nic Suibhne T, Cox G, Healy M, O'Morain C. High prevalence of vitamin D insufficiency in healthy Irish adults. Ir J Med Sci 2008;177(2):131–4.

[58] Savolainen K, Maenpaa PH, Alhava EM, Kettunen K. A seasonal difference in serum 25-hydroxyvitamin D3 in a Finnish population. Med Biol 1980;58(1):49–52.

[59] Vik T, Try K, Stromme JH. The vitamin D status of man at 70 degrees north. Scand J Clin Lab Investig 1980;40(3):227–32.

[60] Shah S, Chiang C, Sikaris K, Lu Z, Bui M, Zebaze R, et al. Serum 25-hydroxyvitamin D insufficiency in search of a bone disease. Journal Clin Endocrinol Metab 2017;102(7):2321–8.

[61] Manson JE, Brannon PM, Rosen CJ, Taylor CL. Vitamin D deficiency - is there really a pandemic? N Engl J Med 2016;375(19):1817–20.

[62] Baeke F, Takiishi T, Korf H, Gysemans C, Mathieu C, Vitamin D. Modulator of the immune system. Curr Opin Pharmacol 2010;10(4):482–96.

[63] Ben-Zvi I, Aranow C, Mackay M, Stanevsky A, Kamen DL, Marinescu LM, et al. The impact of vitamin D on dendritic cell function in patients with systemic lupus erythematosus. PLoS One 2010;5(2):e9193.

[64] Adams JS, Hewison M. Unexpected actions of vitamin D: new perspectives on the regulation of innate and adaptive immunity. Nat Clin Pract Endocrinol Metabol 2008;4(2):80–90.

[65] Fernandes de Abreu DA, Eyles D, Feron F, Vitamin D. A neuro-immunomodulator: implications for neurodegenerative and autoimmune diseases. Psychoneuroendocrinology 2009;34(Suppl. 1):S265–77.

[66] Provvedini DM, Tsoukas CD, Deftos LJ, Manolagas SC. 1,25-dihydroxyvitamin D3 receptors in human leukocytes. Science 1983;221(4616):1181–3.

[67] Takahashi K, Nakayama Y, Horiuchi H, Ohta T, Komoriya K, Ohmori H, et al. Human neutrophils express messenger RNA of vitamin D receptor and respond to 1alpha,25-dihydroxyvitamin D3. Immunopharmacol Immunotoxicol 2002;24(3):335–47.

[68] Smolders J, Moen SM, Damoiseaux J, Huitinga I, Holmoy T. Vitamin D in the healthy and inflamed central nervous system: access and function. J Neurol Sci 2011;311(1–2):37–43.

[69] Kamen D, Aranow C. Vitamin D in systemic lupus erythematosus. Curr Opin Rheumatol 2008;20(5):532–7.

[70] Fritsche J, Mondal K, Ehrnsperger A, Andreesen R, Kreutz M. Regulation of 25-hydroxyvitamin D3-1 alpha-hydroxylase and production of 1 alpha,25-dihydroxyvitamin D3 by human dendritic cells. Blood 2003;102(9):3314–6.

[71] Penna G, Adorini L. 1 Alpha,25-dihydroxyvitamin D3 inhibits differentiation, maturation, activation, and survival of dendritic cells leading to impaired alloreactive T cell activation. J Immunol 2000;164(5):2405–11.

[72] van Etten E, Mathieu C. Immunoregulation by 1,25-dihydroxyvitamin D3: basic concepts. J Steroid Biochem Mol Biol 2005;97(1–2):93–101.

[73] D'Ambrosio D, Cippitelli M, Cocciolo MG, Mazzeo D, Di Lucia P, Lang R, et al. Inhibition of IL-12 production by 1,25-dihydroxyvitamin D3. Involvement of NF-kappaB downregulation in transcriptional repression of the p40 gene. J Clin Invest 1998;101(1):252–62.

[74] Ohta M, Okabe T, Ozawa K, Urabe A, Takaku F. 1 alpha,25-Dihydroxyvitamin D3 (calcitriol) stimulates proliferation of human circulating monocytes in vitro. FEBS Lett 1985;185(1):9–13.

[75] Baeke F, Korf H, Overbergh L, van Etten E, Verstuyf A, Gysemans C, et al. Human T lymphocytes are direct targets of 1,25-dihydroxyvitamin D3 in the immune system. J Steroid Biochem Mol Biol 2010;121(1–2):221–7.

[76] Bansal AS, Henriquez F, Sumar N, Patel S. T helper cell subsets in arthritis and the benefits of immunomodulation by 1,25(OH)(2) vitamin D. Rheumatol Int 2012;32(4):845–52.

[77] Guillot X, Semerano L, Saidenberg-Kermanac'h N, Falgarone G, Boissier MC. Vitamin D and inflammation. Joint Bone Spine 2010;77(6):552–7.

[78] Gorman S, Kuritzky LA, Judge MA, Dixon KM, McGlade JP, Mason RS, et al. Topically applied 1,25-dihydroxyvitamin D3 enhances the suppressive activity of CD4+CD25+ cells in the draining lymph nodes. J Immunol 2007;179(9):6273–83.

[79] Penna G, Roncari A, Amuchastegui S, Daniel KC, Berti E, Colonna M, et al. Expression of the inhibitory receptor ILT3 on dendritic cells is dispensable for induction of CD4+Foxp3+ regulatory T cells by 1,25-dihydroxyvitamin D3. Blood 2005;106(10):3490–7.

[80] Brunkow ME, Jeffery EW, Hjerrild KA, Paeper B, Clark LB, Yasayko SA, et al. Disruption of a new forkhead/winged-helix protein, scurfin, results in the fatal lymphoproliferative disorder of the scurfy mouse. Nat Genet 2001;27(1):68–73.

[81] Fontenot JD, Gavin MA, Rudensky AY. Foxp3 programs the development and function of CD4+CD25+ regulatory T cells. Nat Immunol 2003;4(4):330–6.

[82] Fontenot JD, Rasmussen JP, Williams LM, Dooley JL, Farr AG, Rudensky AY. Regulatory T cell lineage specification by the forkhead transcription factor foxp3. Immunity 2005;22(3):329–41.

[83] Hori S, Nomura T, Sakaguchi S. Control of regulatory T cell development by the transcription factor Foxp3. Science 2003;299(5609):1057–61.

[84] Josefowicz SZ, Lu LF, Rudensky AY. Regulatory T cells: mechanisms of differentiation and function. Annu Rev Immunol 2012;30:531–64.

[85] Zhang L, Zhao Y. The regulation of Foxp3 expression in regulatory CD4(+)CD25(+) T cells: multiple pathways on the road. J Cell Physiol 2007;211(3):590–7.

[86] Kang SW, Kim SH, Lee N, Lee WW, Hwang KA, Shin MS, et al. 1,25-Dihyroxyvitamin D3 promotes FOXP3 expression via binding to vitamin D response elements in its conserved noncoding sequence region. J Immunol 2012;188(11):5276–82.

[87] Antico A, Tampoia M, Tozzoli R, Bizzaro N. Can supplementation with vitamin D reduce the risk or modify the course of autoimmune diseases? A systematic review of the literature. Autoimmun Rev 2012;12(2):127–36.

[88] Chen S, Sims GP, Chen XX, Gu YY, Chen S, Lipsky PE. Modulatory effects of 1,25-dihydroxyvitamin D3 on human B cell differentiation. J Immunol 2007;179(3):1634–47.

[89] Muller K, Heilmann C, Poulsen LK, Barington T, Bendtzen K. The role of monocytes and T cells in 1,25-dihydroxyvitamin D3 mediated inhibition of B cell function in vitro. Immunopharmacology 1991;21(2):121–8.

[90] Shirakawa AK, Nagakubo D, Hieshima K, Nakayama T, Jin Z, Yoshie O. 1,25-dihydroxyvitamin D3 induces CCR10 expression in terminally differentiating human B cells. J Immunol 2008;180(5):2786–95.

[91] Veldman CM, Cantorna MT, DeLuca HF. Expression of 1,25-dihydroxyvitamin D(3) receptor in the immune system. Arch Biochem Biophys 2000;374(2):334–8.

[92] Verstuyf A, Carmeliet G, Bouillon R, Mathieu C. Vitamin D: a pleiotropic hormone. Kidney Int 2010;78(2):140–5.

[93] Cocco E, Meloni A, Murru MR, Corongiu D, Tranquilli S, Fadda E, et al. Vitamin D responsive elements within the HLA-DRB1 promoter region in Sardinian multiple sclerosis associated alleles. PLoS One 2012;7(7):e41678.

[94] Ramagopalan SV, Maugeri NJ, Handunnetthi L, Lincoln MR, Orton SM, Dyment DA, et al. Expression of the multiple sclerosis-associated MHC class II Allele HLA-DRB1*1501 is regulated by vitamin D. PLoS Genet 2009;5(2):e1000369.

[95] Fetahu IS, Hobaus J, Kallay E. Vitamin D and the epigenome. Front Physiol 2014;5:164.

[96] Chen Y, Liu W, Sun T, Huang Y, Wang Y, Deb DK, et al. 1,25-Dihydroxyvitamin D promotes negative feedback regulation of TLR signaling via targeting microRNA-155-SOCS1 in macrophages. J Immunol 2013;190(7):3687–95.

[97] Campbell MJ. Vitamin D and the RNA transcriptome: more than mRNA regulation. Front Physiol 2014;5:181.

[98] Giangreco AA, Nonn L. The sum of many small changes: microRNAs are specifically and potentially globally altered by vitamin D3 metabolites. J Steroid Biochem Mol Biol 2013;136:86–93.

[99] Ma Y, Trump DL, Johnson CS. Vitamin D and miRNAs in cancer. Curr Gene Ther 2014;14(4):269–75.

[100] Cutolo M. Vitamin D and autoimmune rheumatic diseases. Rheumatology 2009;48(3):210–2.

[101] Skaaby T, Husemoen LL, Thuesen BH, Linneberg A. Prospective population-based study of the association between vitamin D status and incidence of autoimmune disease. Endocrine 2015;50(1):231–8.

[102] Bizzaro G, Antico A, Fortunato A, Bizzaro N. Vitamin D and autoimmune diseases: is vitamin D receptor (VDR) polymorphism the culprit? Isr Med Assoc J 2017;19(7):438–43.

[103] Agmon-Levin N, Theodor E, Segal RM, Shoenfeld Y. Vitamin D in systemic and organ-specific autoimmune diseases. Clin Rev Allergy Immunol 2013;45(2):256–66.

[104] Adeeb F, Khan MU, Li X, Stack AG, Devlin J, Fraser AD. High vitamin D levels may downregulate inflammation in patients with Behcet's disease. Int J Inflamm 2017;2017:8608716.

[105] Mao S, Huang S. Association between vitamin D receptor gene BsmI, FokI, ApaI and TaqI polymorphisms and the risk of systemic lupus erythematosus: a meta-analysis. Rheumatol Int 2014;34(3):381–8.

[106] Xiong J, He Z, Zeng X, Zhang Y, Hu Z. Association of vitamin D receptor gene polymorphisms with systemic lupus erythematosus: a meta-analysis. Clin Exp Rheumatol 2014;32(2):174–81.

[107] Mandal M, Tripathy R, Panda AK, Pattanaik SS, Dakua S, Pradhan AK, et al. Vitamin D levels in Indian systemic lupus erythematosus patients: association with disease activity index and interferon alpha. Arthritis Res Ther 2014;16(1):R49.

[108] Holick MF. Vitamin D: extraskeletal health. Rheum Dis Clin N Am 2012;38(1):141–60.

[109] Kemp MG, Lindsey-Boltz LA, Sancar A. UV light potentiates STING (stimulator of interferon genes)-dependent innate immune signaling through deregulation of ULK1 (Unc51-like kinase 1). J Biol Chem 2015;290(19):12184–94.

[110] Wion D, MacGrogan D, Neveu I, Jehan F, Houlgatte R, Brachet P. 1,25-Dihydroxyvitamin D3 is a potent inducer of nerve growth factor synthesis. J Neurosci Res 1991;28(1):110–4.

[111] Garcion E, Wion-Barbot N, Montero-Menei CN, Berger F, Wion D. New clues about vitamin D functions in the nervous system. Trends Endocrinol Metab 2002;13(3):100–5.

[112] Cosman F, Nieves J, Komar L, Ferrer G, Herbert J, Formica C, et al. Fracture history and bone loss in patients with MS. Neurology 1998;51(4):1161–5.

[113] Kragt J, van Amerongen B, Killestein J, Dijkstra C, Uitdehaag B, Polman C, et al. Higher levels of 25-hydroxyvitamin D are associated with a lower incidence of multiple sclerosis only in women. Mult Scler 2009;15(1):9–15.

[114] Nieves J, Cosman F, Herbert J, Shen V, Lindsay R. High prevalence of vitamin D deficiency and reduced bone mass in multiple sclerosis. Neurology 1994;44(9):1687–92.

[115] Soilu-Hanninen M, Airas L, Mononen I, Heikkila A, Viljanen M, Hanninen A. 25-Hydroxyvitamin D levels in serum at the onset of multiple sclerosis. Mult Scler 2005;11(3):266–71.

[116] Munger KL, Levin LI, Hollis BW, Howard NS, Ascherio A. Serum 25-hydroxyvitamin D levels and risk of multiple sclerosis. JAMA 2006;296(23):2832–8.

[117] Soilu-Hanninen M, Laaksonen M, Laitinen I, Eralinna JP, Lilius EM, Mononen I. A longitudinal study of serum 25-hydroxyvitamin D and intact parathyroid hormone levels indicate the importance of vitamin D and calcium homeostasis regulation in multiple sclerosis. J Neurol Neurosurg Psychiatry 2008;79(2):152–7.

[118] van der Mei IA, Ponsonby AL, Dwyer T, Blizzard L, Taylor BV, Kilpatrick T, et al. Vitamin D levels in people with multiple sclerosis and community controls in Tasmania, Australia. J Neurol 2007;254(5):581–90.

[119] Bettencourt A, Boleixa D, Reguengo H, Samoes R, Santos E, Oliveira JC, et al. Serum 25-hydroxyvitamin D levels in multiple sclerosis patients from the north of Portugal. J Steroid Biochem Mol Biol 2017.

[120] Bier G, Bongers MN, Ditt H, Bender B, Ernemann U, Horger M. Accuracy of non-enhanced CT in detecting early ischemic edema using frequency selective non-linear blending. PLoS One 2016;11(1):e0147378.

[121] Vojinovic J, Tincani A, Sulli A, Soldano S, Andreoli L, Dall'Ara F, et al. European multicentre pilot survey to assess vitamin D status in rheumatoid arthritis patients and early development of a new Patient Reported Outcome questionnaire (D-PRO). Autoimmun Rev 2017;16(5):548–54.

[122] Urruticoechea-Arana A, Martin-Martinez MA, Castaneda S, Piedra CA, Gonzalez-Juanatey C, Llorca J, et al. Vitamin D deficiency in chronic inflammatory rheumatic diseases: results of the cardiovascular in rheumatology [CARMA] study. Arthritis Res Ther 2015;17:211.

[123] Quintana-Duque MA, Caminos JE, Varela-Narino A, Calvo-Paramo E, Yunis JJ, Iglesias-Gamarra A. The role of 25-hydroxyvitamin D as a predictor of clinical and radiological outcomes in early onset rheumatoid arthritis. J Clin Rheumatol 2017;23(1):33–9.

[124] Cecchetti S, Tatar Z, Galan P, Pereira B, Lambert C, Mouterde G, et al. Prevalence of vitamin D deficiency in rheumatoid arthritis and association with disease activity and cardiovascular risk factors: data from the COMEDRA study. Clin Exp Rheumatol 2016;34(6):984–90.

[125] Hambly R, Kirby B. The relevance of serum vitamin D in psoriasis: a review. Arch Dermatol Res 2017.

[126] Sag MS, Sag S, Tekeoglu I, Solak B, Kamanli A, Nas K, et al. Comparison of 25-hidroksi Vitamin D serum concentrations in patients with psoriasis and psoriatic arthritis. J Back Musculoskelet Rehabil 2017.

[127] Giuggioli D, Colaci M, Cassone G, Fallahi P, Lumetti F, Spinella A, et al. Serum 25-OH vitamin D levels in systemic sclerosis: analysis of 140 patients and review of the literature. Clin Rheumatol 2017;36(3):583–90.

[128] Garcia-Carrasco M, Jimenez-Herrera EA, Galvez-Romero JL, de Lara LV, Mendoza-Pinto C, Etchegaray-Morales I, et al. Vitamin D and Sjogren syndrome. Autoimmun Rev 2017;16(6):587–93.

[129] Grotting LA, Davoudi S, Palenzuela D, Papaliodis GN, Sobrin L. Association of low vitamin D levels with noninfectious anterior uveitis. JAMA Ophthalmol 2016.

[130] Colaris MJL, van der Hulst RR, Tervaert JWC. Vitamin D deficiency as a risk factor for the development of autoantibodies in patients with ASIA and silicone breast implants: a cohort study and review of the literature. Clin Rheumatol 2017;36(5):981–93.

[131] Colotta F, Jansson B, Bonelli F. Modulation of inflammatory and immune responses by vitamin D. J Autoimmun 2017;85:78–97.

[132] Birmingham DJ, Hebert LA, Song H, Noonan WT, Rovin BH, Nagaraja HN, et al. Evidence that abnormally large seasonal declines in vitamin D status may trigger SLE flare in non-African Americans. Lupus 2012;21(8):855–64.

[133] Schoindre Y, Jallouli M, Tanguy ML, Ghillani P, Galicier L, Aumaitre O, et al. Lower vitamin D levels are associated with higher systemic lupus erythematosus activity, but not predictive of disease flare-up. Lupus Sci Med 2014;1(1):e000027.

[134] Roy S, Shrinivas K, Bagchi B. A stochastic chemical dynamic approach to correlate autoimmunity and optimal vitamin-D range. PLoS One 2014;9(6):e100635.

[135] Marinho A, Carvalho C, Boleixa D, Bettencourt A, Leal B, Guimaraes J, et al. Vitamin D supplementation effects on FoxP3 expression in T cells and FoxP3(+)/IL-17A ratio and clinical course in systemic lupus erythematosus patients: a study in a Portuguese cohort. Immunol Res 2017;65(1):197–206.

[136] Di Franco M, Barchetta I, Iannuccelli C, Gerardi MC, Frisenda S, Ceccarelli F, et al. Hypovitaminosis D in recent onset rheumatoid arthritis is predictive of reduced response to treatment and increased disease activity: a 12 month follow-up study. BMC Musculoskeletal Disord 2015;16:53.

[137] Buondonno I, Rovera G, Sassi F, Rigoni MM, Lomater C, Parisi S, et al. Vitamin D and immunomodulation in early rheumatoid arthritis: a randomized double-blind placebo-controlled study. PLoS One 2017;12(6):e0178463.

[138] Vahabi Anaraki P, Aminorroaya A, Amini M, Momeni F, Feizi A, Iraj B, et al. Effect of Vitamin D deficiency treatment on thyroid function and autoimmunity markers in Hashimoto's thyroiditis: a double-blind randomized placebo-controlled clinical trial. J Res Med Sci 2017;vol. 22:103.

Chapter 26

Vitamin D, Pregnancy, and Autoimmunity: An Ongoing Mystery

Xian Chen[1], Shu-Gui He[1], Yehuda Shoenfeld[2,3], Yong Zeng[1]

[1]Shenzhen Key Laboratory of Reproductive Immunology for Peri-implantation, Shenzhen Zhongshan Institute for Reproduction and Genetics, Fertility Center, Shenzhen Zhongshan Urology Hospital, Shenzhen, People's Republic of China; [2]Zabludowicz Center for Autoimmune Diseases, Sheba Medical Center, affiliated to Sackler Faculty of Medicine, Tel Aviv University, Tel Aviv, Israel; [3]Laboratory of the Mosaics of Autoimmunity, Saint-Petersburg University, Saint-Petersburg, Russian Federation

INTRODUCTION

Epidemiological and experimental data demonstrate that a poor vitamin D status is associated with a higher risk of numerous diseases. Vitamin D plays several roles in the human body. It influences the bone health, immune functions, and cell proliferation [1]. Vitamin D levels have been associated with numerous health outcomes such as cancer [2], cardiovascular diseases [3], and some autoimmune diseases [4,5].

Pregnancy is a period where profound immune modulatory changes take place [6]. The profound immunologic adaptations during and after pregnancy have an influence on maternal autoimmune diseases in several ways [7,8]. This typically leads to amelioration of Th1-type autoimmune disease, such as multiple sclerosis (MS) and rheumatoid arthritis, but after the delivery the disease activity often returns [6]. Thus, it can be seen that the relationships between pregnancy and autoimmunity are represented by a bidirectional model. Interestingly, vitamin D levels have been shown to follow a similar pattern, where high vitamin D levels are measured during late pregnancy, and markedly reduced levels are found after the delivery [9].

Vitamin D insufficiency and deficiency are quite common among healthy pregnant women around the world, and it relates to the latitude, season, sunlight exposure behavior, skin color, and vitamin D intake, with lowest values being measured at high latitudes and with low sunlight exposure [10]. Nevertheless, the effects of vitamin D status and its supplementation on pregnancy outcomes and autoimmune disease are not well understood. Therefore, we present recent evidence to discuss that the pregnancy outcome and autoimmunity are influenced by vitamin D status during pregnancy as to gain information on potential vitamin D deficiency in women during pregnancy and in autoimmune diseases patients.

VITAMIN D METABOLISM AND BIOLOGICAL FUNCTIONS

Vitamin D is an essential steroid hormone classically known for its role in maintenance of calcium and phosphate homeostasis. It is mainly synthesized in the skin on exposure to sunlight, while only a small fraction is obtained through dietary intake of dairy products and dark fish [11]. In areas with less sun exposure, the requirements need to be met by external supplementation and fortified foods. Two different forms of vitamin D from dietary sources are vitamin D_2 (ergocalciferol) derived from plants and vitamin D_3 (cholecalciferol) derived from animals [12].

The cutaneous precursor of vitamin D, 7-dehydrocholesterol, is derived from cholesterol in food. After exposure to shortwave UVB radiation, the B ring of 7-dehydrocholesterol is transformed into previtamin D_3 (cholecalciferol) or converted into two inactive products luminosterol and tachysterol [13]. These two products prevent excessive vitamin D production. Vitamin D is transported in blood mostly in a protein-bound form. More than 80% is bound to vitamin D binding protein. It undergoes two hydroxylation steps by P450 mixed function monooxidases. In the liver, vitamin D first hydroxylation into 25-hydroxyvitamin D (25(OH)D) is modulated by the CYP27A1 or CYP2R1. 25(OH)D is the major circulating form of the vitamin [14]. Further hydroxylation takes place in the kidney to its active form, $1\alpha,25$-dihydroxyvitamin D3 $[1,25(OH)_2D_3]$, by CYP27B1, which regulates calcium and phosphate absorption and bone synthesis and metabolism (Fig. 26.1).

The biological activity of vitamin D occurs mainly through the active form of $1,25(OH)_2D_3$ interacting with its receptor, vitamin D receptor (VDR), a member of the superfamily of nuclear receptors for steroid hormones [15]. It occurs through two pathways, a rapid nongenomic response and a slow genomic response [16]. In the nongenomic response pathway,

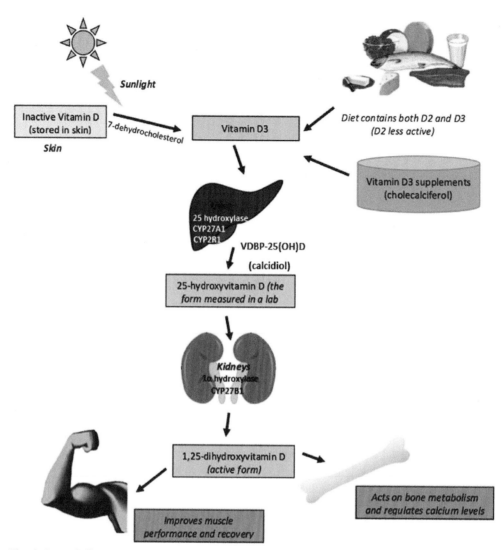

FIGURE 26.1 Vitamin D metabolism overview. The major source of vitamin D is the skin. Here the precursor of vitamin D (7-dehydrocholesterol) is transformed into vitamin D3. A small fraction of active vitamin D precursor is obtained from food and supplements. In the liver, CYP27A1 and CYP2R1 regulate the conversion of vitamin D into 25-hydroxyvitamin D. Bound to vitamin D binding protein (VDBP), it undergoes 1α-hydroxylation by CYP27B1 in the kidney into 1α,25-dihydroxyvitamin D3 (1,25(OH)$_2$D$_3$). 1,25(OH)$_2$D$_3$ improves muscle performance and recovery, as well as acts on bone metabolism and regulates calcium levels. *(Figure reprinted from Bridge Athetic, 2017.)*

1,25(OH)$_2$D$_3$ can bind to VDR of plasma membrane and the ligand-bound VDR then activates one or more signaling cascades, such as protein kinase C, mitogen-activated protein kinases, and phospholipase [16,17]. In the genomic response pathway, ligand-bound VDR then binds the retinoid X receptor, and the heterodimer further regulates the transcription of vitamin D target genes by binding with high affinity to vitamin D response elements in the promoter region of the gene [18], which plays a role in regulating calcium absorption, immune function, cell proliferation, cellular differentiation, and pregnancy [19].

VITAMIN D DEFICIENCY

Vitamin D deficiency has been variably defined. There is still controversy regarding adequate or optimal levels of serum 25(OH)D for overall health. In 2010 year, the United States Institute of Medicine has defined levels of serum 25(OH)D greater than 20 ng/mL (equivalent to 50 nmol/L) as adequate [20]. However, other researchers argue that optimal levels should be set higher (>30 ng/mL or 75 nmol/L) [21,22]. Recently, an accepted definition for vitamin D deficiency is a serum level of 25(OH)D (the form that is measured in the blood) less than 30–40 ng/mL [23]. Lower levels lead to activation of the parathyroid glands, which results in bone damage [24,25], and increased risk for pregnancy complications [26,27] and autoimmune diseases [28,29]. Recently, some literature further divide deficiencies into insufficiency (21–29 ng/mL) and

TABLE 26.1 Definitions of Vitamin D Deficiency and Supplementation Recommendations in Pregnancy [10,70,104,105]

Organization (Country)	Recommended 25(OH)D Levels (nmol/L)	Daily Recommended Supplementation Dose (IU)
WHO	>50	200[a]
IOM (US)	≥30	600[a] 600–1000[b]
Endocrine Society (US)	≥75	1500–2000[a]
ACOG (US)	≥50	600[a]
NICE (UK)	>30	400[a] 800[b,c]
NIH (US)	>50	600[a]
RANZCOG (Australia/NZ)	>50	400[a] 1000[b] 2000[c]

ACOG, American College of Obstetricians and Gynecologists; *IOM*, Institute of Medicine; *NICE*, National Institute of Clinical Excellence; *NIH*, National Institutes of Health; *RANZCOG*, Royal Australia New Zealand College of Obstetricians and Gynecologists; *WHO*, World Health Organization.
[a]*For all pregnant women (or women > 50 nmol/L).*
[b]*For deficient (or at-risk) women (<50 nmol/L).*
[c]*For very deficient women (<30 nmol/L).*

deficiency (under 20 ng/mL) [30,31], while some define an even lower level [32]. An optimal level for the functioning of the immune system, within the normal range of serum vitamin D level, is yet to be determined [25]. Vitamin D deficiency is more common in reproductive failure women or autoimmune disease patients than in healthy individuals [33,34], in women more than men, irrespective of systemic lupus erythematosus (SLE) [32]. Similar findings were indicated in teenagers and young adults diagnosed with juvenile-onset SLE [35,36].

VITAMIN D AND PREGNANCY

Pregnancy is a specific condition characterized with a transient tolerance for the foreign fetal body. It has been widely accepted that immune regulation plays a key role in successful pregnancy. Fetal and maternal factors influence the local mucosal immune system so that the fetus is not rejected by the mother [37]. Vitamin D is a well-recognized immune modulator and has been shown to have an unexpected and crucial effect on the immune response [38]. Human pregnancy is associated with important changes in vitamin D physiology. Reports from across the world have found that between 40% and 98% of pregnancy women have vitamin D levels <50 nmol/L and 15%–84% have levels <25 nmol/L, which are considered insufficient or deficient by most health institutions (Table 26.1). Global vitamin D deficiency in pregnancy has been a major concern. Thus, vitamin D deficiency during pregnancy is hypothesized to influence disease development in female reproduction [39].

Preeclampsia

Preeclampsia (PE) affects 3%–8% of pregnancies in Western countries and remains a remarkable risk factor for mortality and morbidity during pregnancy [40]. PE is characterized by maternal hypertension and proteinuria, and its precise pathophysiology is very complex and poorly understood. Nevertheless, recent evidence strongly supports a therapeutic role for calcium in PE risk, and thus the effect of vitamin D is worth exploring [41]. It has been described that maternal vitamin D status may influence PE via immunomodulatory, inflammatory, and/or angiogenic functions [42]. However, polymorphisms in 1α-hydroxylase have been associated with PE, where trophoblastic cells from preeclamptic mothers had only one-tenth the 1α-hydroxylase activity compared with cells from uncomplicated pregnancies [42].

In recent years, human observational studies find an association between vitamin D deficiency and PE, which women who develop PE tend to have lower 25(OH)D levels [41]. Systematic reviews and metaanalyses have concluded that low serum 25(OH)D levels in pregnancy are associated with a higher risk of PE and suggest a preventive role of vitamin D supplementation [43–45]. However, a recent metaanalysis of three randomized controlled trials (RCTs) on pregnancy outcomes found no association between increased serum vitamin D levels and PE risk [46]. Despite these studies varying in the dose of vitamin D supplementation (400–4000 IU/day) and in the baseline and attained vitamin D levels, it is most important to note that all of the RCTs started the intervention after 20 weeks of gestation. A metaanalysis of the abnormal maternal biomarkers shown during the first trimester of pregnancy in women who developed PE and the findings of previous studies on the association of PE and low vitamin D levels in early pregnancy suggest the necessity of early serum vitamin D level surveillance and modification in pregnancy [43,47]. Because of these limitations, trials to date have not been able to establish a role for vitamin D in prevention of PE, and RCTs designed specifically for this outcome are needed.

Recurrent Miscarriage

Recurrent miscarriage (RM) is the most common adverse outcome of pregnancy and is classically defined as the loss of three or more consecutive pregnancies before 20 week of gestation, with a reported prevalence of 1%–3% [48]. The cause of RM is multifactorial. Known risk factors for RM include genetic abnormalities, endocrine disorders, infectious diseases, and uterine anatomical malformations [49]. It is now widely accepted that immunological dysfunction may play a crucial role in the pathogenesis of RM [50]. A significant proportion of women with RM and autoimmunity have cellular immune abnormalities, including increased percentage of natural killer (NK) cells, NK cytotoxicities, and Th1/Th2 cell ratios [51]. Vitamin D has immune regulatory effects on T and B cell immunity and NK cell cytotoxicity. Therefore, it has been speculated that vitamin D could act as an immune regulator playing an important role in reproductive capacity. Some investigators have reported that a high proportion of women with RM have vitamin D deficiency as compared with women with normal vitamin D levels, which is associated with increased cellular immunity and autoimmunity [26,27,52]. In women with low vitamin D, the prevalence of autoantibodies is higher, which is supported by increased CD19+ B cell population and dysregulated B cell subsets [26]. Vitamin D suppresses NK cytotoxicity through reduction of conjugation with target cells, polarization of perforin, and proinflammatory cytokine secretion [53]. In addition, our findings demonstrate a potential beneficial role of 1,25(OH)$_2$D supplementation as adjuvant therapy in RM patients. The percentage of B cells, the percentage of TNF-α–producing Th cells, and NK cytotoxicity were significantly reduced under 1,25(OH)$_2$D supplementation (0.5 μg/day for 2 months) [26]. Hence, it is possible that appropriate levels of vitamin D and vitamin D supplementation may have a pivotal role to maintain and succeed in early pregnancy. However, further study is needed to elucidate whether vitamin D supplementation can prevent the onset of pregnancy loss.

Gestational Diabetes Mellitus

It has been reported that vitamin D deficiency was associated with impaired glucose tolerance, insulin resistance, and risk of developing type 2 diabetes [54]. Likewise, gestational diabetes mellitus (GDM) is a condition of glucose intolerance with onset or first recognition in pregnancy, characterized by insulin resistance and impaired β-cell function [55], and high risk of progression to type 2 diabetes [56]. In vitro studies have revealed that polymorphisms of the VDR and 1α-hydroxylase result in suboptimal insulin action [57], and these polymorphisms have been proposed as potential biomarkers for GDM susceptibility [58]. However, despite increased knowledge of the links between vitamin D and insulin action and secretion, the potential of vitamin D in mitigating GDM risk remains largely unknown [55].

The metaanalyses of observational studies have concluded that women with GDM had lower mean 25(OH)D levels compared with normoglycemic women and that GDM risk increased by 40%–60% in women with vitamin D deficiency, which persisted after adjusting for multiple confounders [45,59,60]. This is supported by a recent metaanalysis of 20 observational studies including 9209 participants, which showed that the risk of developing GDM was significantly higher among women with vitamin D deficiency (25(OH)D < 50 nmol/L) [61]. However, no association between vitamin D deficiency (<25 or <37.5 nmol/L) and GDM risk was observed in a study included 5109 women in Australia of whom 7.4% developed GDM, after adjusting for age, parity, smoking status, previous illness, maternal weight, and socioeconomic status [62]. Based on the above studies, vitamin D may improve metabolic parameters in women with GDM, but there is insufficient evidence with regard to reducing GDM incidence.

Caesarean Section

A caesarean section (CS) is a life-saving surgical procedure when certain complications arise during pregnancy and labor. However, it is a major surgery and is associated with immediate maternal and prenatal risks and may have implications for future pregnancies and long-term effects that are still being investigated [63,64]. Worldwide, CS rates increased from 6.7% in 1990 to 19.1% in 2014, which represents a 12.4% absolute increase [65]. Risk factors for CS include older maternal age, obesity, parity, ethnicity, and, more recently, nutritional deficiencies including vitamin D deficiency [66].

A systematic review identified six observational studies examining vitamin D deficiency and CS [67]. Only one cross-sectional study of 1153 women [66] and one prospective study of 344 women [68] found significant inverse relationships between maternal 25(OH)D < 37.5 nmol/L and risk of CS after adjusting for age, ethnicity, parity, season, BMI, and gestation at study entry. The remaining four studies found no associations, although two indicated a nonsignificant inverse trend [67]. Additionally, a metaanalysis of RCTs found no effect for vitamin D supplementation on rates of CS [46]. Importantly, none of these trials had assessed or controlled for influential aspects such as having had a previous CS or maternal preference. However, results from a recent trial by Karamali et al. [69] enrolling 60 women with existing GDM found that those supplemented with 50,000 IU vitamin D and 1000 mg calcium at baseline and at 21 days had decreased rates of CS compared with placebo (63.3% vs. 23.3%); however, these effects cannot be attributed to vitamin D because it was combined with calcium. Thus, based on the observational and intervention studies, the preventive potential of vitamin D on CS cannot be derived from existing studies, and the contextual variations driving CS rate should be considered in the design and execution of future trials [70].

VITAMIN D AND AUTOIMMUNE DISEASES

As above mentioned, vitamin D plays a pivotal role in human reproduction, and vitamin D deficiency and insufficiency have been associated with a variety of adverse maternal outcomes. Vitamin D plays a major role in regulating B cell proliferation and function during successful pregnancy. Can vitamin D deficiency during pregnancy impact autoimmune disease? There are some compelling data that suggest an association. Ota et al. [33] reported that 45% of RM patients had vitamin D deficiency and women with vitamin D deficiency had an increased incidence of autoantibodies including antiphospholipid antibody, antithyroperoxidase antibody antinuclear antibody (ANA), and anti-ssDNA antibody when compared with those of recurrent pregnancy loss (RPL) patients with normal vitamin D levels. Vitamin D deficiency is common among antiphospholipid syndrome (APS) patients and it is often associated with clinically defined thrombotic events in APS patients [71]. Vitamin D is a potent inhibitor of tissue factor expression in endothelial cells, activated by anti-β2 glycoprotein I antibody (aβ2GPI) [71]. Vitamin D deficiency is also associated with the prevalence of ANA, and in SLE patient vitamin D supplementation significantly decreased ANA titers [72]. Terrier et al. [73] found the multifaceted immunomodulatory effects of vitamin D, notably, the expansion of Tregs, and the decrease of Th1 and Th17 cells in SLE patients. Moreover, a severe vitamin D deficiency has been demonstrated in patients with Hashimoto's thyroiditis (HT) and in Graves' disease (GD) [74]. The duration of HT was correlated with the severity of 25(OH)D deficiency, which led to an increase in thyroid volume and in ATA levels [75]. In female patients with newly onset GD, serum 25(OH)D concentrations were significantly lower when compared with control group, with a direct correlation between vitamin D deficiency and the increase in thyroid volume [76]. Another condition in which vitamin D is likely to be involved is adverse pregnancy outcome. Vitamin D deficiency is linked with infertility and pregnancy loss, which are consequences of many thyroid autoimmune diseases (AITD) [77,78], suggesting that an even stronger connection between vitamin D deficiency and AITD may exist [79]. Noteworthy, it has long been thought that the development of MS is a result of a complex interaction between genes and environment with an important environmental factor being vitamin D deficiency [80]. It is not yet understood how and when vitamin D acts to modulate MS risk, although there is increasing evidence that this occurs through genetic alterations [81]. For now, it is strongly suggesting vitamin D deficiency during pregnancy as a strong causative agent in the development of MS in later life [82]. Thus, it can be seen that low vitamin D appears to be important for autoimmune disease susceptibility, and vitamin D deficiency was associated with an increased presence of autoantibodies.

Vitamin D deficiency might increase the risk of autoimmune diseases. As a result, vitamin D intervention has been implemented in several studies [83–85]. Agmon-Levin et al. [86] revealed that in patients with systemic and organ-specific autoimmune diseases, vitamin D levels were found to be lower when compared with healthy subjects and that vitamin D supplementation had beneficial effects on autoimmune diseases. In a previous study, Ruiz-Irastorza et al. [87] evaluated the therapeutic effects of oral vitamin D supplementation on SLE in an observational study. After around 2 years of vitamin D treatment, mean 25(OH)D levels in all treated patients were increased. But the majority (71%) of the SLE patients still had insufficient levels of vitamin D. Although it seems that there was no improvement of SLE severity after vitamin D treatment in this study, the effect of vitamin D supplementation in SLE has not been extensively investigated, probably because of too many confounding factors that could impact vitamin D metabolism in clinical medications used to treat SLE [88]. More recently, a double-blind, placebo-controlled trial suggested that cholecalciferol supplementation for 24 weeks is effective in decreasing disease activity and improving fatigue in juvenile-onset SLE patients [89]. Nonetheless, in addition to clinical effectiveness, the current recommendations on the optimal dose and duration of vitamin D supplementation are not well defined and many vary between patients. Hence, a well-designed study needed further to confirm whether vitamin D supplementation has a favorable impact on the development or clinical course of autoimmune diseases.

CURRENT RECOMMENDATION FOR VITAMIN D SUPPLEMENTATION

Based on the current data on the effect of vitamin D supplementation, it is still a matter of debate in what required level, form, and dosage should vitamin D be supplemented [90]. Based on the requirements for calcium homeostasis, current guidelines indicate that a level under 50 nmol/L is considered to be deficient, between 50 and 74 nmol/L as insufficiency, and above 75 nmol/L as a sufficient 25(OH)D level [91,92]. However, in the context of autoimmunity, it is not known whether it is enough to correct deficiency or whether we should strive for an even higher serum 25 (OH)D level. Recently, Wagner et al. [93] suggested that all pregnant women maintain a circulating 25(OH)D concentration of at least 40 ng/mL during the earliest time points of pregnancy. To achieve this, intakes of at least 4000 IU/day vitamin D will be required because of variable individual abilities to convert vitamin D to 25(OH)D [94]. These supplements have proven to be safe in thousands of patients over the past 15 years, as not a single adverse event due to supplementation lies within the safe intake level as defined by the Endocrine Society [91]. Moreover, most clinical trials use cholecalciferol as the form of choice, although some use 1,25(OH)D or less-calcemic analogs such as alfacalcidol. However, the effects of alfacalcidol do not seem better than calcitriol, and at the same dosage, there were no severe side effects from either alfacalcidol or calcitriol [95–97]. Currently, cholecalciferol is the most used supplementation form in clinical practice. Vitamin D supplementation guidelines indicate a maximum safe dose of 4000 IU cholecalciferol/day for healthy adults [91]. But no adverse effects were found with dosages of up to 50,000 IU cholecalciferol weekly for 12 weeks or 100,000 IU weekly for 1 month followed by 100,000 IU monthly for 5 months [98–100]. Interestingly, the dose escalation regime used by Burton et al. [101] and 20,000 IU weekly by Smolders et al. [98] did not elicit hypercalcemia despite reaching a serum 25(OH)D level of 400 and 380 nmol/L, respectively. Altogether, these data indicate that it may be worthwhile to provide more insight into the answers on these remaining questions, and to firmly establish the added value of vitamin D supplementation, large multicenter trials are still required.

CONCLUSION

Vitamin D plays an important role in immunomodulation. This occurs through different possible mechanisms including modification of cytokines and alteration in immune cells activation, proliferation, and destruction [102]. Studies have identified decreased serum vitamin D levels in pregnant women and in patients with autoimmune disease, and inverse association between vitamin D levels and pregnancy outcome and autoimmune diseases [27,103]. However, the potential role of vitamin D supplementation in preventing adverse pregnancy outcome and in preventing autoimmune diseases manifestation and its beneficial role as component of such population treatment remain controversial. Because of the high prevalence of vitamin D insufficiency/deficiency in women during pregnancy and in patients with autoimmune diseases, vitamin D supplementation might be considered a prospective candidate for the treatment of such population. Besides, it is a relatively cheap compound, easy to administer, with no need for a physician's prescription, and without known major side effects. Clearly, further research is needed to confirm the involvement of vitamin D in pregnancy and autoimmunity and to evaluate if vitamin D supplementation should be introduced in clinical practice.

REFERENCES

[1] Vanherwegen AS, Gysemans C, Mathieu C. Regulation of immune function by Vitamin D and its use in diseases of immunity. Endocrinol Metab Clin North Am 2017;46:1061–94.

[2] Yin L, Raum E, Haug U, et al. Meta-analysis of longitudinal studies: serum vitamin D and prostate cancer risk. Cancer Epidemiol 2009;33:435–45.

[3] Pilz S, Tomaschitz A, Ritz E, et al. Vitamin D status and arterial hypertension: a systematic review. Nat Rev Cardiol 2009;6:621–30.

[4] Ascherio A, Munger KL, Simon KC. Vitamin D and multiple sclerosis. Lancet Neurol 2010;9:599–612.

[5] Cutolo M, Otsa K, Paolino S, et al. Vitamin D involvement in rheumatoid arthritis and systemic lupus erythaematosus. Ann Rheum Dis 2009;68:446–7.

[6] Patas K, Engler JB, Friese MA, et al. Pregnancy and multiple sclerosis: feto-maternal immune cross talk and its implications for disease activity. J Reprod Immunol 2013;97:140–6.

[7] Buyon JP. The effects of pregnancy on autoimmune diseases. J Leukoc Biol 1998;63:281–7.

[8] Gordon C. Pregnancy and autoimmune diseases. Best Pract Res Clin Rheumatol 2004;18:359–79.

[9] Brannon PM, Picciano MF. Vitamin D in pregnancy and lactation in humans. Annu Rev Nutr 2011;31:89–115.

[10] Dawodu A, Akinbi H. Vitamin D nutrition in pregnancy: current opinion. Int J Womens Health 2013;5:333–43.

[11] Hollis BW, Wagner CL, Drezner MK, et al. Circulating vitamin D3 and 25-hydroxyvitamin D in humans: an important tool to define adequate nutritional vitamin D status. J Steroid Biochem 2007;103:631–4.

[12] Hollis BW, Wagner CL. New insights into the vitamin D requirements during pregnancy. Bone Res 2017;5:17030.

[13] Nandi A, Sinha N, Ong E, et al. Is there a role for vitamin D in human reproduction. Horm Mol Biol Clin Investig 2016;25:15–28.

[14] Hollis BW, Wagner CL. The role of the parent compound vitamin D with respect to metabolism and function: why clinical dose intervals can affect clinical outcomes. J Clin Endocrinol Metab 2013;98:4619–28.

[15] Deeb KK, Trump DL, Johnson CS. Vitamin D signalling pathways in cancer: potential for anticancer therapeutics. Nat Rev Cancer 2007;7:684–700.

[16] Mizwicki MT, Norman AW. The vitamin D sterol vitamin D receptor ensemble model offers unique insights into both genomic and rapid-response signaling. Sci Signal 2009;2:re4.

[17] Huhtakangas JA, Olivera CJ, Bishop JE, et al. The vitamin D receptor is present in caveolae-enriched plasma membranes and binds 1 alpha,25(OH)2-vitamin D3 in vivo and in vitro. Mol Endocrinol 2004;18:2660–71.

[18] Dusso AS, Brown AJ, Slatopolsky E. Vitamin D. Am J Physiol Renal Physiol 2005;289:F8–28.

[19] Shin JS, Choi MY, Longtine MS, et al. Vitamin D effects on pregnancy and the placenta. Placenta 2010;31:1027–34.

[20] Food and Nutrition Board IOM. Dietary reference intakes for calcium and vitamin D. Washington, DC: National Academy Press; 2010.

[21] Dawson-Hughes B, Heaney RP, Holick MF, et al. Estimates of optimal vitamin D status. Osteoporos Int 2005;16:713–6.

[22] Holick MF. Vitamin D status: measurement, interpretation, and clinical application. Ann Epidemiol 2009;19:73–8.

[23] Azrielant S, Shoenfeld Y. Eppur Si Muove: vitamin D is essential in preventing and modulating SLE. Lupus 2016;0:1–10.

[24] Holick MF. Vitamin D deficiency. N Engl J Med 2007;357:266–81.

[25] Schneider L, Dos Santos AS, Santos M, et al. Vitamin D and systemic lupus erythematosus: state of the art. Clin Rheumatol 2014;33:1033–8.

[26] Chen X, Yin B, Lian RC, et al. Modulatory effects of vitamin D on peripheral cellular immunity in patients with recurrent miscarriage. Am J Reprod Immunol 2016;76:432–8.

[27] Triggianese P, Watad A, Cedola F, et al. Vitamin D deficiency in an Italian cohort of infertile women. Am J Reprod Immunol 2017;78.

[28] Agmon-Levin N, Kivity S, Tzioufas AG, et al. Low levels of vitamin-D are associated with neuropathy and lymphoma among patients with Sjögren's syndrome. J Autoimmun 2012;39:234–9.

[29] Bizzaro G, Shoenfeld Y. Vitamin D and autoimmune thyroid diseases: facts and unresolved questions. Immunol Res 2015;61:46–52.

[30] Mcghie TK, Deceulaer K, Walters CA, et al. Vitamin D levels in Jamaican patients with systemic lupus erythematosus. Lupus 2014;23:1092–6.

[31] Yap KS, Morand EF. Vitamin D and systemic lupus erythematosus: continued evolution. Int J Rheum Dis 2015;18:242–9.

[32] Schoindre Y, Jallouli M, Tanguy ML, et al. Lower vitamin D levels are associated with higher systemic lupus erythematosus activity, but not predictive of disease flare-up. Lupus Sci Med 2014;1:e000027.

[33] Ota K, Dambaeva S, Han AR, et al. Vitamin D deficiency may be a risk factor for recurrent pregnancy losses by increasing cellular immunity and autoimmunity. Hum Reprod 2014;29:208–19.

[34] Sabio JM, Vargas-Hitos JA, Martinez-Bordonado J, et al. Association between low 25-hydroxyvitamin D, insulin resistance and arterial stiffness in nondiabetic women with systemic lupus erythematosus. Lupus 2014;24:155–63.

[35] Stagi S, Cavalli L, Bertini F, et al. Vitamin D levels in children, adolescents, and young adults with juvenile-onset systemic lupus erythematosus: a cross-sectional study. Lupus 2014;23:1059–65.

[36] Garf KE, Marzouk H, Farag Y, et al. Vitamin D status in Egyptian patients with juvenile-onset systemic lupus erythematosus. Rheumatol Int 2015;35:1535–40.

[37] Thellin O, Heinen E. Pregnancy and the immune system: between tolerance and rejection. Toxicology 2003;185:179–84.

[38] Bordon Y. Asthma and allergy: vitamin D primes neonatal immune system. Nat Rev Immunol 2017;17:467.

[39] Shahrokhi SZ, Ghaffari F, Kazerouni F. Role of vitamin D in female reproduction. Clin Chim Acta 2016;455:33–8.

[40] Arain N, Mirza WA, Aslam M. Review-Vitamin D and the prevention of preeclampsia: a systematic review. Pak J Pharm Sci 2015;28:1015–21.

[41] Moon RJ, Harvey NC, Cooper C. Endocrinology in pregnancy: influence of maternal vitamin D status on obstetric outcomes nd the fetal skeleton. Eur J Endocrinol 2015;173:R69–83.

[42] Liu NQ, Hewison M. Vitamin D, the placenta and pregnancy. Arch Biochem Biophys 2012;523:37–47.

[43] Hypponen E, Cavadino A, Williams D, et al. Vitamin D and pre-eclampsia: original data, systematic review and meta-analysis. Ann Nutr Metab 2013;63:331–40.

[44] Tabesh M, Salehi-Abargouei A, Tabesh M, et al. Maternal vitamin D status and risk of pre-eclampsia: a systematic review and meta-analysis. J Clin Endocrinol Metab 2013;98:3165–73.

[45] Wei SQ, Qi HP, Luo ZC, et al. Maternal vitamin D status and adverse pregnancy outcomes: a systematic review and meta-analysis. J Matern Fetal Neonatal Med 2013;26:889–99.

[46] Perez-Lopez FR, Pasupuleti V, Mezones-Holguin E, et al. Effect of vitamin D supplementation during pregnancy on maternal and neonatal outcomes: a systematic review and meta-analysis of randomized controlled trials. Fertil Steril 2015;103:1278–88 e1274.

[47] Allen RE, Rogozinska E, Cleverly K, et al. Abnormal blood biomarkers in early pregnancy are associated with preeclampsia: a meta-analysis. Eur J Obstet Gynecol Reprod Biol 2014;182:194–201.

[48] Alijotas-Reig J, Garrido-Gimenez C. Current concepts and new trends in the diagnosis and management of recurrent miscarriage. Obstet Gynecol Surv 2013;68:445–66.

[49] Rai R, Regan L. Recurrent miscarriage. Lancet 2006;368:601–11.

[50] Souza SS, Ferriani RA, Santos CM, et al. Immunological evaluation of patients with recurrent abortion. J Reprod Immunol 2002;56:111–21.

[51] Kwak-Kim J, Skariah A, Wu L, et al. Humoral and cellular autoimmunity in women with recurrent pregnancy losses and repeated implantation failures: a possible role of vitamin D. Autoimmun Rev 2016;15:943–7.

[52] Ota K, Dambaeva S, Han AR, et al. Vitamin D deficiency may be a risk factor for recurrent pregnancy losses by increasing cellular immunity and autoimmunity. Hum Reprod 2014;29:208–19.

[53] Ota K, Dambaeva S, Kim MW, et al. 1,25-Dihydroxyvitamin D3 regulates NK-cell cytotoxicity, cytokine secretion, and degranulation in women with recurrent pregnancy losses. Eur J Immunol 2015;45:3188–99.

[54] Joham AE, Teede HJ, Cassar S, et al. Vitamin D in polycystic ovary syndrome: relationship to obesity and insulin resistance. Mol Nutr Food Res 2016;60:110–8.

[55] Yeow TP, Lim SL, Hor CP, et al. Impact of vitamin D replacement on markers of glucose metabolism and cardio-metabolic risk in women with former gesta-tional Diabetes-A double-blind, randomized controlled trial. PLoS One 2015;10:e0129017.

[56] Abell SK, De Courten B, Boyle JA, et al. Inflammatory and other biomarkers: role in pathophysiology and prediction of gestational diabetes mel-litus. Int J Mol Sci 2015;16:13442–73.

[57] Mahmoudi T. Genetic variation in the vitamin D receptor and polycystic ovary syndrome risk. Fertil Steril 2009;92:1381–3.

[58] Ramos-Lopez E, Kahles H, Weber S, et al. Gestational diabetes mellitus and vitamin D deficiency: genetic contribution of CYP27B1 and CYP2R1 polymorphisms. Diabetes Obes Metab 2008;10:683–5.

[59] Poel YH, Hummel P, Lips P, et al. Vitamin D and gestational diabetes: a systematic review and meta-analysis. Eur J Intern Med 2012;23:465–9.

[60] Aghajafari F, Nagulesapillai T, Ronksley PE, et al. Association between maternal serum 25-hydroxyvitamin D level and pregnancy and neonatal outcomes: systematic review and meta-analysis of observational studies. BMJ 2013;346.

[61] Zhang MX, Pan GT, Guo JF, et al. Vitamin D deficiency increases the risk of gestational diabetes mellitus: a meta-analysis of observational studies. Nutrients 2015;7:8366–75.

[62] Schneuer FJ, Roberts CL, Guilbert C, et al. Effects of maternal serum 25-hydroxyvitamin D concentrations in the first trimester on subsequent pregnancy outcomes in an Australian population. Am J Clin Nutr 2014;99:287–95.

[63] Marshall NE, Fu R, Guise JM. Impact of multiple cesarean deliveries on maternal morbidity: a systematic review. Am J Obstet Gynecol 2011;205(262):e261–268.

[64] Gregory KD, Jackson S, Korst L, et al. Cesarean versus vaginal delivery: whose risks? Whose benefits? Am J Perinatol 2012;29:7–18.

[65] Betran AP, Ye J, Moller AB, et al. The increasing trend in caesarean section rates: global, regional and national estimates: 1990-2014. PLoS One 2016;11:e0148343.

[66] Scholl TO, Chen X, Stein P. Maternal vitamin D status and delivery by cesarean. Nutrients 2012;4:319–30.

[67] Harvey NC, Holroyd C, Ntani G, et al. Vitamin D supplementation in pregnancy: a systematic review. Health Technol Assess 2014;18:1–190.

[68] Merewood A, Mehta SD, Chen TC, et al. Association between vitamin D deficiency and primary cesarean section. J Clin Endocrinol Metab 2009;94:940–5.

[69] Karamali M, Asemi Z, Ahmadi-Dastjerdi M, et al. Calcium plus vitamin D supplementation affects pregnancy outcomes in gestational diabetes: randomized, double-blind, placebo-controlled trial. Public Health Nutr 2016;19:156–63.

[70] Mousa A, Abell S, Scragg R, et al. Vitamin D in reproductive health and pregnancy. Semin Reprod Med 2016;34:e1–13.

[71] Agmon-Levin N, Blank M, Zandman-Goddard G, et al. Vitamin D: an instrumental factor in the anti-phospholipid syndrome by inhibition of tissue factor expression. Ann Rheum Dis 2011;70:145–50.

[72] Ritterhouse LL, Crowe SR, Niewold TB, et al. Vitamin D deficiency is associated with an increased autoimmune response in healthy individuals and in patients with systemic lupus erythematosus. Ann Rheum Dis 2011;70:1569–74.

[73] Terrier B, Derian N, Schoindre Y, et al. Restoration of regulatory and effector T cell balance and B cell homeostasis in systemic lupus erythemato-sus patients through vitamin D supplementation. Arthritis Res Ther 2012;14:R221.

[74] Bizzaro G, Shoenfeld Y. Vitamin D and thyroid autoimmune diseases: the known and the obscure. Immunol Res 2015;61:107–9.

[75] Bozkurt NC, Karbek B, Ucan B, et al. The association between severity of vitamin D deficiency and Hashimoto's thyroiditis. Endocr Pract 2013;19:479–84.

[76] Yasuda T, Okamoto Y, Hamada N, et al. Serum vitamin D levels are decreased and associated with thyroid volume in female patients with newly onset Graves' disease. Endocrine 2012;42:739–41.

[77] Matalon ST, Blank M, Ornoy A, et al. The association between antithyroid antibodies and pregnancy loss. Am J Reprod Immunol 2001;45:72–7.

[78] Poppe K, Velkeniers B, Glinoer D. Thyroid disease and female reproduction. Clin Endocrinol (Oxf) 2007;66:309–21.

[79] Twig G, Shina A, Amital H, et al. Pathogenesis of infertility and recurrent pregnancy loss in thyroid autoimmunity. J Autoimmun 2012;38:J275–81.

[80] Ebers G. Interactions of environment and genes in multiple sclerosis. J Neurol Sci 2013;334:161–3.

[81] Berlanga-Taylor AJ, Disanto G, Ebers GC, et al. Vitamin D-gene interactions in multiple sclerosis. J Neurol Sci 2011;311:32–6.

[82] Garabédian M, Jacqz E, Guillozo H, et al. Elevated plasma 1,25-dihydroxyvitamin D concentrations in infants with hypercalcemia and an elfin facies. N Engl J Med 1985;312:948–52.

[83] Simsek Y, Cakir I, Yetmis M, et al. Effects of Vitamin D treatment on thyroid autoimmunity. J Res Med Sci 2016;21:85.

[84] Garcia-Carrasco M, Jiménez-Herrera EA, Gálvez-Romero JL, et al. Vitamin D and Sjögren syndrome. Autoimmun Rev 2017;4:1–7.

[85] Holmøy T, Lindstrøm JC, Eriksen EF, et al. High dose vitamin D supplementation does not affect biochemical bone markers in multiple sclerosis-a randomized controlled trial. BMC Neurol 2017;17:67.

[86] Agmon-Levin N, Theodor E, Segal RM, et al. Vitamin D in systemic and organ-specific autoimmune diseases. Clin Rev Allergy Immunol 2013;45:256–66.

[87] Ruiz-Irastorza G, Gordo S, Olivares N, et al. Changes in vitamin D levels in patients with systemic lupus erythematosus: effects on fatigue, disease activity, and damage. Arthritis Care Res (Hoboken) 2010;62:1160–5.

[88] Breslin LC, Magee PJ, Wallace JM, et al. An evaluation of vitamin D status in individuals with systemic lupus erythematosus. Proc Nutr Soc 2011;70:399–407.

[89] Lima GL, Paupitz J, Aikawa NE, et al. Vitamin D supplementation in adolescents and young adults with juvenile systemic lupus erythematosus for improvement in disease activity and fatigue scores: a randomized, double-blind, placebo-controlled Trial. Arthritis Care Res (Hoboken) 2016;68:91–8.

[90] Dankers W, Colin EM, Van Hamburg JP, et al. Vitamin D in autoimmunity: molecular mechanisms and therapeutic potential. Front Immunol 2016;7:697.

[91] Holick M, Binkley N, Ha B-F, et al. Evaluation, treatment, and prevention of vitamin D deficiency: an endocrine society clinical practice guideline. J Clin Endocrinol Metab 2011;96:1911–30.

[92] Aspray TJ, Bowring C, Fraser W, et al. National osteoporosis society vitamin D guideline summary. Age Ageing 2014;43:592–5.

[93] Wagner CL, Baggerly C, Mcdonnell S, et al. Post-hoc analysis of vitamin D status and reduced risk of preterm birth in two vitamin D pregnancy cohorts compared with South Carolina March of Dimes 2009-2011 rates. J Steroid Biochem Mol Biol 2016;155:245–51.

[94] Heaney RP, Davies KM, Chen TC, et al. Human serum 25-hydroxycholecalciferol response to extended oral dosing with cholecalciferol. Am J Clin Nutr 2003;77:204–10.

[95] Bizzarri C, Pitocco D, Napoli N, et al. No protective effect of calcitriol on beta-cell function in recent-onset type 1 diabetes: the IMDIAB XIII trial. Diabetes Care 2010;33:1962–3.

[96] Walter M, Kaupper T, Adler K, et al. No effect of the 1alpha,25-dihydroxyvitamin D3 on beta-cell residual function and insulin requirement in adults with new-onset type 1 diabetes. Diabetes Care 2010;33:1443–8.

[97] Ataie-Jafari A, Loke SC, Rahmat AB, et al. A randomized placebo-controlled trial of alphacalcidol on the preservation of beta cell function in children with recent onset type 1 diabetes. Clin Nutr 2013;32:911–7.

[98] Smolders J, Peelen E, Thewissen M, et al. Safety and T cell modulating effects of high dose vitamin D3 supplementation in multiple sclerosis. PLoS One 2010;5:e15235.

[99] Salesi M, Farajzadegan Z. Efficacy of vitamin D in patients with active rheumatoid arthritis receiving methotrexate therapy. Rheumatol Int 2012;32:2129–33.

[100] Terrier B, Derian N, Schoindre Y, et al. Restoration of regulatory and effector T cell balance and B cell homeostasis in systemic lupus erythematosus patients through vitamin D supplementation. Arthritis Res Ther 2012;14:R221.

[101] Burton JM, Kimball S, Vieth R, et al. A phase I/II dose-escalation trial of vitamin D3 and calcium in multiple sclerosis. Neurology 2010;74:1852–9.

[102] Watad A, Neumann SG, Soriano A, et al. Vitamin D and systemic lupus erythematosus: myth or reality? Isr Med Assoc J 2016;18:177–82.

[103] Bragazzi NL, Watad A, Neumann SG, et al. Vitamin D and rheumatoid arthritis: an ongoing mystery. Curr Opin 2017;29:1–11.

[104] Gallagher JC, Sai AJ. Vitamin D insufficiency, deficiency, and bone health. J Clin Endocrinol Metab 2010;95:2630–3.

[105] Van Schoor NM, Lips P. Worldwide vitamin D status. Best Pract Res Clin Endocrinol Metab 2011;25:671–80.

Chapter 27

Smell and Autoimmunity—State of the Art

Vânia Vieira Borba[1,2,3], Netta Shoenfeld[4], Carlo Perricone[5], Yehuda Shoenfeld[6,7]

[1]Department 'A' of Internal Medicine, Coimbra University Hospital Centre, Coimbra, Portugal; [2]Faculty of Medicine, University of Coimbra, Coimbra, Portugal; [3]Zabludowicz Center for Autoimmune Diseases, Sheba Medical Center, Tel-Hashomer, Israel; [4]Sheba Medical Center, Tel-Hashomer, Israel; [5]Rheumatology, Department of Internal Medicine, Sapienza University of Rome, Rome, Italy; [6]Zabludowicz Center for Autoimmune Diseases, Sheba Medical Center, affiliated to Sackler Faculty of Medicine, Tel Aviv University, Tel Aviv, Israel; [7]Laboratory of the Mosaics of Autoimmunity, Saint-Petersburg University, Saint-Petersburg, Russian Federation

INTRODUCTION

Evolutionarily, the olfactory bulb is the most primitive of brain structures and gives rise to the ancient limbic system that refers to the network of neural structures responsible for emotional processing. Animals survive in harsh and fluctuating environments using sensory neurons to detect and respond to changes in their surroundings. The olfactory system is essential for detecting food, identifying danger, and sensing pheromones [1]. Humans have a superb olfactory sense, capable of discriminating at least 1 trillion different stimuli. Each odorant appears to activate a unique set of olfactory receptors which are known as its "signature" [2]. Considering the great variety among the olfactory receptor genome, it is hypothesized that each person carries a unique nose. Secundo et al. [3] performed a large study to characterize the "olfactory fingerprint" of each individual and described a highly specific olfactory perception that was shown to be variable across individuals. Olfaction involves complex biochemical and electrophysiological processes, which convert the molecular information into sensations. The perception of odor is dominated by the pleasantness–unpleasantness dimension, which dictates the hedonic aspects of aroma. These features influence mood because of the anatomical overlap of the olfactory and limbic systems in the brain. Furthermore, information regarding smell is readily stored in long-term memory and has strong connection with motivation, emotion, and memory. Moreover, the olfactory receptor repertoire represents the largest gene superfamily between mammals, including 1000–1400 coding regions distributed in clusters over most chromosomes [4]. Interestingly, the olfactory receptor genome is linked to HLA genetic makeup, which influences immunological discrimination. Similar to the olfactory system, the immune system allows animals to relate to the external environment and to differentiate threatening from innocuous agents. Only recently has the olfactory capability been tested in autoimmune diseases. Shoenfeld and colleagues discovered this new connection by showing that patients affected with systemic lupus erythematosus have disturbances in their olfactory functions, which are associated with neuropsychiatric manifestations of the disease [5]. Since then, several intricate interactions have been exposed between the olfactory and immune systems and autoimmunity.

OLFACTORY SYSTEM ANATOMY

Nearly 10–20 million olfactory neurons are located within the olfactory epithelium among a variety of supportive cells [6]. The olfactory mucosa has the unique capability of achieving an almost continuous and lifelong neurogenesis in response to external injuries because of the presence of olfactory stem cells that guarantee the maintenance of the olfactory function [7]. Humans can smell between 4000 and 10,000 different odors, which activate a combination of receptor cells, producing unique spatial maps within both the epithelium and the olfactory bulbs, known as the "olfactory code." Olfactory neurons are known to be bipolar cells that project a single dendrite that extends to the epithelial surface and contains cilia where odor molecules bind to their receptor and an axon that transmits signals to the brain without synapsing within the thalamus. In the olfactory bulb, a complex process of signal transduction and coding occurs before signals travel to the olfactory cortex [8]. The great extension of the olfactory regions, both primary and secondary, may account for the close connection between memory, pleasure, and mood. In accordance, the ipsilateral nature and the abundant limbic overlap of the olfactory anatomy might explain the unique ability of odor to affect emotional processing [9]. Recently, An and Liggett [10] were able to identify olfactory receptors expressed deep in the lung, on the human airway smooth muscle cells, and on other cell types in different organs as well. Those olfactory receptors have been

Mosaic of Autoimmunity. https://doi.org/10.1016/B978-0-12-814307-0.00027-X

shown to regulate sperm chemotaxis, respiratory rate, myogenesis, blood pressure regulation, and airway smooth muscle cytoskeletal remodeling and proliferation [11–13]. In accordance, results from several studies indicate a complex chemosensory network in the body, which responds to endogenous and exogenous ligands, carrying out adaptive functions and predisposing to disease [14].

GENETICS AND OLFACTION

The mosaic of autoimmunity describes a complex interaction between genetics, immune defects, environmental, and hormonal factors [15]. It has been proven that olfaction is connected with the aforementioned aspects of the mosaic. The HLA encodes mostly immune-associated proteins whose main purpose is the presentation of antigens to immune cells, strongly implicated in the development of autoimmune diseases [16]. Hence, HLA is the most polymorphic region of the genome. Polymorphisms might be maintained by a balanced selection, and certain populations show deviations from expected gene frequencies [17]. Interestingly, HLA peptides are accepted as natural odors, influencing behavioral decisions in the context of social recognition. Studies into olfactory preferences have suggested that females favor the scent of males with dissimilar HLA to their own [18]. Linda Buck and Richard Axel, the Nobel Prize awardees in 2004, have discovered that mammals usually have 1000 genes for odor receptors. Approximately 63% of those genes are noncoding (pseudogenes), distributed on all human chromosomes, except 20 and Y. In accordance, a large cluster is placed near to the HLA locus, the denominated "MHC-linked" olfactory receptor genes, which appear to be in strong linkage disequilibrium, suggesting a high recombination frequency and a functional connection with the MHC [19].

OLFACTION AND AUTOIMMUNE DISEASES

Abnormalities of olfactory capabilities might be an important manifestation of autoimmune diseases and sometimes represent a clue for nervous system involvement (Table 27.1).

Olfaction and Psychiatric Disorders

Olfactory impairment has been related with several psychiatric disorders, such as depression, schizophrenia, bipolar, and obsessive-compulsive disorder. Olfactory functions are known to share common anatomical regions with psychiatric disorders, which have been seen altered among these patients [20–22]. A consistently decreased sense of smell was reported within the early stages of disease and seems to be correlated with the clinical course [23,24].

Olfaction and Depression

Despite the development of the neocortex, olfactory projections to core limbic structures, such as the hippocampus, insula, amygdala, anterior cingulate cortex, and orbitofrontal cortex, remain. These shared neural connections implicate a bidirectional relationship between olfaction and depression. Patients with depression have been found to show diminished olfactory functioning when compared with nondepressed controls in multiple aspects of olfaction, such as threshold, discrimination, and identification [25]. In patients with primary depression, several pathways emerged to explain the secondary development of olfactory dysfunction, focusing on impaired hippocampal neurogenesis due to increased levels of inflammatory cytokines, which in turn, limit the proliferation of central and peripheral olfactory neurons [26,27]. On the other hand, patients with primary olfactory dysfunction may develop secondary depression because of an abnormal sense of smell, affecting daily life. A recent study performed by Croy et al. [28] explored the olfactory function in 27 female patients with depression at the beginning and at the end of antidepressive therapy, measuring chemosensory event-related potentials and functional magnetic resonance imaging mapping olfactory capabilities. The authors successfully demonstrated an impaired olfactory discrimination, prolonged latencies of the event-related potential, and reduced activation in secondary olfactory structures (thalamus, insula, and left middle orbitofrontal), which normalized after the treatment. Furthermore, depression is associated with a dysfunctional amygdala and subsequent inhibitory projections to the olfactory bulb, disrupting regular olfactory function [21]. Moreover, olfactory loss is thought to decrease the intensity of stimuli going from the olfactory bulb to the limbic system, limiting effective management of emotions and urging feelings of fear and sadness. Recently, it has been proposed that the proinflammatory cytokine dysfunction, which takes part in several conditions causing olfactory loss, can cross the blood–brain barrier to damage the hippocampus, limiting neurogenesis, and amygdala, promoting emotional instability [29].

TABLE 27.1 Relationship Between Smell and Autoimmune Diseases

Disease	Impaired Smell at Diagnosis	Relation With Disease Activity	Relation With Structural Abnormalities	Comments	References
Depression	✓	✓	✓	Proinflammatory cytokine dysfunction limits neurogenesis and promotes emotional instability.	[29]
Schizophrenia	✓	✓	✓	Olfactory impairment precedes the onset of overt psychosis and may be predictive of poor outcome.	[33,34]
Systemic lupus erythematosus	?	✓	✓	Anti-P ribosomal antibodies stained neurons on brain structures consisting with the smell apparatus.	[46]
Sjögren syndrome	?	✗	✓	Olfactory impairment is influenced by mucosal surfaces dryness.	[47,55]
Fibromyalgia	?	✗	✗	Significantly lower threshold for smell when compared with healthy patients.	[58]
Rheumatoid arthritis	?	✓	✓	Might represent a direct effect of inflammation on the nasal mucosa, which is similar to the synovium.	[61]
Behçet disease	?	✗	✓	There is no correlation between nasal lesions and olfaction.	[63]
Systemic sclerosis	?	✓	✗	High degree of depression among systemic sclerosis patients reaching 30% correlated with the severity of their concomitant depression.	[58]
Multiple sclerosis	✓	✓	✓	Olfactory axonal loss correlated with the extent of demyelination in the brain. Both plaque number and distribution of lesions have shown to be relevant to olfactory deficits. Olfactory abilities are inversely correlated with disability status.	[70,72,74]
Psoriasis vulgaris	?	✓	?	Olfactory capabilities worsened with the severity of the disease.	[76]
Autoimmune thyroid disease	✓	✓	✓	High values of thyroid-stimulating hormone have been associated with a longer latency of smell cortex evoked potentials.	[79]
Recurrent spontaneous abortions	✓	✗	✗	Positive correlation between olfaction impairment and number of previous spontaneous abortions.	[82]

✓, yes; ✗, no; ?, unknown.

Olfaction and Schizophrenia

Schizophrenia is a chronic and debilitating mental illness characterized by periods of relapse, which require resource-intensive management. In 1937, Lehmann-Facius suggested that an autoimmune background was involved in the pathogenesis of schizophrenia, based on the presence of autoantibodies in the cerebrospinal fluid of these patients. Subsequently, the autoimmune hypothesis has been reinforced by several studies, which document a wide range of autoantibodies in schizophrenia patients, an inverse association of this disease with rheumatoid arthritis, and a high prevalence of autoimmune diseases among the relatives of schizophrenic patients [30,31]. Interestingly, one-third of the patients have measurable olfactory impairment on their first episode, disproving the bias of a possible adverse effect from psychotropic drugs [32]. Growing evidence indicates that olfactory performance impairment precedes the onset of overt psychosis and that it may be predictive for those who will develop frank psychosis or otherwise progress to a poor functional outcome [33,34]. In accordance, peculiar alterations of the olfactory system have been detected, including a smaller olfactory bulb volume, physiological and molecular anomalies of olfactory receptor neurons in the nose, and reduced gray matter volumes in the primary olfactory cortex [35,36]. Over the course of the disease, the sense of smell progressively declines, with a strong association with the duration of the illness [37].

Olfaction and Systemic Lupus Erythematosus

Systemic lupus erythematosus is a systemic autoimmune disease with high incidence of central nervous system involvement (neuropsychiatric systemic lupus erythematosus) [38]. In 1999, the American College of Rheumatology proposed a standard nomenclature with case definitions for 19 neuropsychiatric syndromes of systemic lupus erythematosus [39]. The pathogenesis of this disorder has been associated with autoantibody-mediated neuronal dysfunction, vasculopathy, and coagulopathy. In accordance, several autoantibodies have been correlated with the neuropsychiatric syndromes of systemic lupus erythematosus, including antineuronal, anti-P ribosomal proteins, antiphospholipids, antiendothelial cell antibodies, antihuman N-methyl-D-aspartate receptor types, and anti-Nedd5 C-ter antibodies [40,41]. Anti-P ribosomal antibodies were firstly reported in association with psychosis and neuropsychiatric lupus, although a positive correlation has also been seen with liver and kidney involvement and disease activity [42,43]. A study performed by Katzav et al. intended to evaluate the relationship between neurological impairment, anti-P ribosomal antibodies, and lupus. Purified anti-P ribosomal antibodies were injected directly into the brain ventricles of a murine model of systemic lupus erythematosus, while irrelevant IgG were employed as controls [44,45]. Interestingly, mice presented a depressive-like behavior, characterized by higher immobilization time in enforced swimming tests. Additionally, impaired olfaction was detected utilizing a smell threshold test. Targeting the anti-P ribosomal antibodies with monoclonal antiidiotypic antibodies and treating mice with an antidepressant drug or aromatherapy resulted in improvement of the depressive-like behavior [45]. In accordance, neurons stained for these highly specific systemic lupus erythematosus autoantibodies were found on brain structures related with the olfactory apparatus [46,47]. Because the stained areas include the limbic system, this binding pattern of the brain is highly suggestive of involvement in the pathogenesis of depression. Shoenfeld et al. contributed with extensive investigations relating to systemic lupus erythematosus and the sense of smell [44,48–50]. A trial implementing active immunization of naïve mice with an anti-DNA antibody carrying the 16/6 Id was capable of inducing the production of anti-P ribosomal antibodies and finally contribute to depression. Likewise, the 16/16 antibody was bound to similar areas in the olfactory apparatus as anti-P ribosomal antibodies. Notwithstanding, olfactory impairment and depressive mood were improved by aromatherapy, entailing specifically orange and lemon smell. In human models, a positive correlation between olfaction, male gender, and older age was found in both the lupus and the control groups. However, patients with systemic lupus erythematosus had significantly impaired olfactory abilities. Interestingly, the performance in score tests was correlated with lupus disease activity index and central nervous system manifestations [51]. The exact mechanism of olfactory impairment is yet to be elucidated; however, the possibility of an immune-mediated mechanism or drug adverse effect is intriguing [52]. Based on these observations, targeting anti-P ribosomal antibodies may be a new therapeutic approach in the treatment of neuropsychiatric lupus patients with depression [53].

Olfaction and Sjögren Syndrome

Primary Sjögren syndrome is a systemic autoimmune rheumatic disorder characterized by the inflammation and destruction of exocrine glands as a result of excessive autoantibodies infiltration [54]. Smell and taste alterations are frequently reported symptoms by Sjögren syndrome patients. Studies have found that smell and taste impairment are correlated with each other and are influenced by mucosal surfaces dryness [55]. Several other mechanisms were suggested to explain these deficits among those patients, including decreased mucin (an odorant carrier), recurrent rhinosinusitis, and immunological abnormalities. Interestingly, some patients were able to improve after cyclophosphamide treatment [56].

Olfaction and Fibromyalgia

Fibromyalgia is a common cause of chronic, diffuse, musculoskeletal pain. This condition is not associated with genuine tissue inflammation and its etiology remains poorly understood. However, a few studies have assessed the olfactory sensitivity in fibromyalgia patients. Lotsch et al. [57] reported a slightly reduced odor identification with no significant differences in smell threshold or discrimination among 17 fibromyalgia patients. More recently, Amital et al. [58] performed a study to evaluate the olfactory functions of female patients with fibromyalgia. A significantly lower threshold of smell was reported among these patients, when compared with healthy controls [58]. The decreased sense of smell among patients with fibromyalgia might connect with concomitant depressed mood.

Olfaction and Rheumatoid Arthritis

Rheumatoid arthritis is a chronic autoimmune disorder characterized by nonreversible progressive joint erosions, movement restrictions, functional limitations, and permanent disability [59]. In addition to the manifestations at the musculoskeletal system, patients are reported to complain about problems with gustatory and olfactory function in their everyday life [60]. A study performed by Steinbach et al. [61] aims to investigate the subjective taste and smell function in patients with rheumatoid arthritis. Interestingly, it was found that those patients were hyposmic and hypogeusic, defining a novel clinical characteristic finding in rheumatoid arthritis. The author hypothesized that it could result from direct effect of systemic inflammation on the nasal mucosa, which is a boundary layer similar to the synovium [61]. Previously, no significant studies have investigated the olfactory impairment among rheumatoid arthritis patients.

Olfaction and Behçet Disease

Behçet disease is a chronic relapsing condition that affects small vessels in multiple systems, with a large spectrum of clinical manifestations involving the vascular, ocular, mucocutaneous, gastrointestinal, musculoskeletal, and central nervous systems [62]. A relationship between Behçet disease and sinonasal disorders, such as olfactory dysfunction and chronic rhinosinusitis, has been reported in a few studies. Nasal symptoms are known to be associated with the presence of nasal lesions, but there is no correlation between nasal findings and olfactory function [63]. Interestingly, the nasal mucociliary clearance time was seen to be prolonged in Behçet disease patients and is correlated with the disease duration [64].

Olfaction and Systemic Sclerosis

Systemic sclerosis is an immune-mediated connective tissue disease, characterized by widespread vascular injury and progressive fibrosis of the skin and internal organs. Patients with systemic sclerosis have decreased survival, with pulmonary involvement as the main cause of death [65]. Amital et al. [58] reported a high degree of depression among systemic sclerosis patients reaching 30%, correlated with the severity of their concomitant disease. Surprisingly, olfactory dysfunction had never been investigated before in patients with systemic sclerosis.

Olfaction and Multiple Sclerosis

Multiple sclerosis is a chronic, lifelong neurological condition associated with inflammation and degeneration of the brain and spinal cord. It is considered an immune-mediated disease, resulting from several genetic and early-life environmental triggering exposures, which are believed to disrupt immunological self-tolerance to myelin in the central nervous system [66]. The prevalence of olfactory dysfunction among patients with multiple sclerosis is believed to be in the range of 40% [67–69]. Olfactory system damage has been seen frequently in demyelinating diseases. The highest prevalence of olfactory axonal loss was found in the multiple sclerosis group (around 71%) and its presence correlated with the extent of demyelination in the brain, particularly the inferior frontal cortex [70]. Considering the wide multifocal damage to the central nervous system seen in multiple sclerosis and that olfactory functions may involve distributed neural regions and pathways, it would be reasonable to suppose that an olfactory deficit could represent a marker for widespread dysfunction in the brain [71]. Furthermore, it has been suggested that olfactory dysfunction may correlate with anxiety, depression, disease activity, relapses, and progression [67,72,73]. Likewise, the extent and progression of olfactory dysfunction appears to correlate with frontal and temporal lobe lesion burden over time. In addition, both plaque number and distribution of lesions have been shown of relevance in olfactory deficits [74]. Interestingly, a recent longitudinal study performed by Good et al. [75] demonstrated that in multiple sclerosis, deficits in odor detection sensitivity and odor identification are not lateralized and are correlated with one another across the two sides of the nose. Finally, olfactory abilities seem to be inversely correlated with multiple sclerosis disability status [72].

Olfaction and Psoriasis Vulgaris

Psoriasis is a chronic systemic disorder characterized by lesions due to T cell–mediated hyperproliferation of keratinocytes. With increased understanding of its immunological basis, it is known that psoriasis is not only limited to skin but also with various comorbidities. Activated T cells and proinflammatory cytokines are believed to play a critical role in the pathophysiology. Only one recent study performed by Aydın et al. [76] was able to demonstrate decreased olfactory capabilities in psoriasis vulgaris patients, which worsened with the severity of the disease. Despite the interesting association, there is insufficient information in the literature regarding this topic.

Olfaction and Autoimmune Thyroid Disease

Smell is known to be influenced by changes in thyroid function. These symptoms are typically neglected both by physicians and hypothyroid patients who are unaware of their dysosmia and dysgeusia [59]. More than 40 years ago, McConnell et al. [77] described smell and taste impairment among 39% of untreated primary hypothyroidism patients. Since then, several studies, involving animal and human models, support this association. Likewise, improved smell thresholds were observed following 3 months of thyroxine replacement therapy, suggesting that thyroid hormones play a prominent role in modulating olfactory sensitivity [78]. In accordance, greater values of thyroid-stimulating hormone have been associated with longer latency of smell cortex evoked potentials recorded from both the trigeminal and olfactory nerve [79]. Interestingly, a recent study performed by Aydin et al. [80] with animal models concluded that diminished hormone secretion due to thyroid gland degradation results in both olfaction loss and vagal complex degeneration in animal models of olfactory bulbectomy, in contrast to the common belief that anosmia results from hypothyroidism.

Olfaction and Recurrent Spontaneous Abortions

Recurrent spontaneous abortion is defined as two or more consecutive spontaneous abortions that may occur at any stage of pregnancy. The etiology of this disease involves immune-mediated pathways, including the presence of a predominant T helper 1 type immunity during pregnancy, a decrease in T regulatory cells, and an increase in natural killer cells [81]. An increased sense of smell has been reported in over two-thirds of pregnant women at some point, although it occurs more frequently among the early stages. A fascinating study performed by Perricone et al. [82] among women with recurrent spontaneous abortions, both idiopathic and secondary, reported a higher prevalence of hyposmia when compared with pregnant women who did not experience recurrent abortions with a positive correlation between smell impairment and number of previous spontaneous abortions. The authors suggested a possible immunological underlining autoimmune condition for the olfactory impairment in women with spontaneous abortions [83].

CONCLUSION

Olfactory dysfunction has been commonly reported in a wide range of autoimmune conditions, frequently associated with disease activity and progression. The recognition of these signs may allow not only for an earlier and more effective management of the underlying condition but also an improvement in patients quality of life. Finally, complementary medicine patterns, such as aromatherapy, could become an important adjunctive therapeutic approach.

HIGHLIGHTS

- The olfactory system might be a target for a spectrum of immune-mediated diseases.
- The great extension of olfactory regions in the brain may account for the close connection between memory, emotion, pleasure, and mood.
- The olfactory system serves many purposes in the central nervous system including prominent interactions with the immune system.
- Because the development of olfactory impairment occurs in the early stages of several diseases, olfaction may serve as a predictor for various illness manifestations and may allow for an earlier and more effective management of the underlying condition.
- Considering that olfactory functions contribute to the quality of life, physicians should be aware of these abnormalities when evaluating their patients.

LIST OF ABBREVIATIONS

HLA Human leukocyte antigen
MHC Major histocompatibility complex

REFERENCES

[1] Hsieh YW, Alqadah A, Chuang CF. Mechanisms controlling diversification of olfactory sensory neuron classes. Cell Mol Life Sci 2017;74(18): 3263–74.

[2] Bushdid C, Magnasco MO, Vosshall LB, Keller A. Humans can discriminate more than 1 trillion olfactory stimuli. Sci (New York, NY) 2014;343(6177):1370–2.

[3] Secundo L, Snitz K, Weissler K, Pinchover L, Shoenfeld Y, Loewenthal R, et al. Individual olfactory perception reveals meaningful nonolfactory genetic information. Proc Natl Acad Sci USA 2015;112(28):8750–5.

[4] Glatz R, Bailey-Hill K. Mimicking nature's noses: from receptor deorphaning to olfactory biosensing. Prog Neurobiol 2011;93(2):270–96.

[5] Strous RD, Shoenfeld Y. To smell the immune system: olfaction, autoimmunity and brain involvement. Autoimmun Rev 2006;6(1):54–60.

[6] Patel RM, Pinto JM. Olfaction: anatomy, physiology, and disease. Clin Anat(New York, NY) 2014;27(1):54–60.

[7] Tanos T, Saibene AM, Pipolo C, Battaglia P, Felisati G, Rubio A. Isolation of putative stem cells present in human adult olfactory mucosa. PLoS One 2017;12(7):e0181151.

[8] Johnson BA, Leon M. Chemotopic odorant coding in a mammalian olfactory system. J Comp Neurol 2007;503(1):1–34.

[9] Mombaerts P. Love at first smell–the 2004 Nobel prize in physiology or medicine. N Engl J Med 2004;351(25):2579–80.

[10] An SS, Liggett SB. Taste and smell GPCRs in the lung: evidence for a previously unrecognized widespread chemosensory system. Cell Signal 2018;41:82–8.

[11] Spehr M, Gisselmann G, Poplawski A, Riffell JA, Wetzel CH, Zimmer RK, et al. Identification of a testicular odorant receptor mediating human sperm chemotaxis. Sci (New York, NY) 2003;299(5615):2054–8.

[12] Pluznick JL, Protzko RJ, Gevorgyan H, Peterlin Z, Sipos A, Han J, et al. Olfactory receptor responding to gut microbiota-derived signals plays a role in renin secretion and blood pressure regulation. Proc Natl Acad Sci USA 2013;110(11):4410–5.

[13] Chang AJ, Ortega FE, Riegler J, Madison DV, Krasnow MA. Oxygen regulation of breathing through an olfactory receptor activated by lactate. Nature 2015;527(7577):240–4.

[14] Kalbe B, Knobloch J, Schulz VM, Wecker C, Schlimm M, Scholz P, et al. Olfactory receptors modulate physiological processes in human airway smooth muscle cells. Front Physiol 2016;7:339.

[15] Shoenfeld Y, Isenberg DA. The mosaic of autoimmunity. Immunol Today 1989;10(4):123–6.

[16] Arango MT, Perricone C, Kivity S, Cipriano E, Ceccarelli F, Valesini G, et al. HLA-DRB1 the notorious gene in the mosaic of autoimmunity. Immunol Res 2017;65(1):82–98.

[17] Colafrancesco S, Agmon-Levin N, Perricone C, Shoenfeld Y. Unraveling the soul of autoimmune diseases: pathogenesis, diagnosis and treatment adding dowels to the puzzle. Immunol Res 2013;56(2–3):200–5.

[18] Roberts T, Roiser JP. In the nose of the beholder: are olfactory influences on human mate choice driven by variation in immune system genes or sex hormone levels? Exp Biol Med (Maywood, NJ) 2010;235(11):1277–81.

[19] Perricone C, Agmon-Levin N, Shoenfeld N, de Carolis C, Guarino MD, Gigliucci G, et al. Evidence of impaired sense of smell in hereditary angio-edema. Allergy 2011;66(1):149–54.

[20] Moscavitch SD, Szyper-Kravitz M, Shoenfeld Y. Autoimmune pathology accounts for common manifestations in a wide range of neuro-psychiatric disorders: the olfactory and immune system interrelationship. Clin Immunol(Orlando, Fla) 2009;130(3):235–43.

[21] Negoias S, Croy I, Gerber J, Puschmann S, Petrowski K, Joraschky P, et al. Reduced olfactory bulb volume and olfactory sensitivity in patients with acute major depression. Neuroscience 2010;169(1):415–21.

[22] Hoexter MQ, Dougherty DD, Shavitt RG, D'Alcante CC, Duran FL, Lopes AC, et al. Differential prefrontal gray matter correlates of treatment response to fluoxetine or cognitive-behavioral therapy in obsessive-compulsive disorder. Eur Neuropsychopharmacol 2013;23(7):569–80.

[23] Rolls ET, Cheng W, Gilson M, et al. Effective connectivity in depression. Biological Psychiatry. Cognitive Neuroscience and Neuroimaging 2018;3:187–97.

[24] Ortega-Hernandez OD, Kivity S, Shoenfeld Y. Olfaction, psychiatric disorders and autoimmunity: is there a common genetic association? Autoimmunity 2009;42(1):80–8.

[25] Kohli P, Soler ZM, Nguyen SA, Muus JS, Schlosser RJ. The association between olfaction and depression: a systematic review. Chem Senses 2016;41(6):479–86.

[26] Furtado M, Katzman MA. Examining the role of neuroinflammation in major depression. Psychiatr Res 2015;229(1–2):27–36.

[27] Yuan TF, Hou G, Arias-Carrion O. Chronic stress impacts on olfactory system. CNS Neurol Disord Drug Targets 2015;14(4):486–91.

[28] Croy I, Symmank A, Schellong J, Hummel C, Gerber J, Joraschky P, et al. Olfaction as a marker for depression in humans. J Affect Disord 2014;160:80–6.

[29] Yuan TF, Slotnick BM. Roles of olfactory system dysfunction in depression. Prog Neuro Psychopharmacol Biol Psychiatr 2014;54:26–30.

[30] Gilvarry CM, Sham PC, Jones PB, Cannon M, Wright P, Lewis SW, et al. Family history of autoimmune diseases in psychosis. Schizophr Res 1996;19(1):33–40.

[31] Gorwood P, Pouchot J, Vinceneux P, Puechal X, Flipo RM, De Bandt M, et al. Rheumatoid arthritis and schizophrenia: a negative association at a dimensional level. Schizophr Res 2004;66(1):21–9.

[32] Cascella NG, Takaki M, Lin S, Sawa A. Neurodevelopmental involvement in schizophrenia: the olfactory epithelium as an alternative model for research. J Neurochem 2007;102(3):587–94.

[33] Kamath V, Turetsky BI, Calkins ME, Kohler CG, Conroy CG, Borgmann-Winter K, et al. Olfactory processing in schizophrenia, non-ill first-degree family members, and young people at-risk for psychosis. World J Biol Psychiatry 2014;15(3):209–18.

[34] Lin A, Brewer WJ, Yung AR, Nelson B, Pantelis C, Wood SJ. Olfactory identification deficits at identification as ultra-high risk for psychosis are associated with poor functional outcome. Schizophr Res 2015;161(2–3):156–62.

[35] Borgmann-Winter KE, Wang HY, Ray R, Willis BR, Moberg PJ, Rawson NE, et al. Altered G protein coupling in olfactory neuroepithelial cells from patients with schizophrenia. Schizophr Bull 2016;42(2):377–85.

[36] Takahashi T, Nakamura Y, Nakamura K, Ikeda E, Furuichi A, Kido M, et al. Altered depth of the olfactory sulcus in first-episode schizophrenia. Prog Neuro Psychopharmacol Biol Psychiatry 2013;40:167–72.

[37] Nguyen AD, Shenton ME, Levitt JJ. Olfactory dysfunction in schizophrenia: a review of neuroanatomy and psychophysiological measurements. Harv Rev Psychiatry 2010;18(5):279–92.

[38] Anaya JM, Shoenfeld Y, Cervera R. Systemic lupus erythematosus 2014. Autoimmune Dis 2014;2014:274323.

[39] Sciascia S, Bertolaccini ML, Baldovino S, Roccatello D, Khamashta MA, Sanna G. Central nervous system involvement in systemic lupus erythematosus: overview on classification criteria. Autoimmun Rev 2013;12(3):426–9.

[40] Conti F, Alessandri C, Perricone C, Scrivo R, Rezai S, Ceccarelli F, et al. Neurocognitive dysfunction in systemic lupus erythematosus: association with antiphospholipid antibodies, disease activity and chronic damage. PLoS One 2012;7(3):e33824.

[41] Su D, Liu R, Li X, Sun L. Possible novel biomarkers of organ involvement in systemic lupus erythematosus. Clin Rheumatol 2014;33(8):1025–31.

[42] Ben-Ami Shor D, Blank M, Reuter S, Matthias T, Beiglass I, Volkov A, et al. Anti-ribosomal-P antibodies accelerate lupus glomerulonephritis and induce lupus nephritis in naive mice. J Autoimmun 2014;54:118–26.

[43] Kivity S, Tsarfaty G, Agmon-Levin N, Blank M, Manor D, Konen E, et al. Abnormal olfactory function demonstrated by manganese-enhanced MRI in mice with experimental neuropsychiatric lupus. Ann N Y Acad Sci 2010;1193:70–7.

[44] Katzav A, Solodeev I, Brodsky O, Chapman J, Pick CG, Blank M, et al. Induction of autoimmune depression in mice by anti-ribosomal P antibodies via the limbic system. Arthritis Rheum 2007;56(3):938–48.

[45] Katzav A, Ben-Ziv T, Chapman J, Blank M, Reichlin M, Shoenfeld Y. Anti-P ribosomal antibodies induce defect in smell capability in a model of CNS -SLE (depression). J Autoimmun 2008;31(4):393–8.

[46] Toubi E, Shoenfeld Y. Clinical and biological aspects of anti-P-ribosomal protein autoantibodies. Autoimmun Rev 2007;6(3):119–25.

[47] Shovman O, Zandman-Goddard G, Gilburd B, Blank M, Ehrenfeld M, Bardechevski S, et al. Restricted specificity of anti-ribosomal P antibodies to SLE patients in Israel. Clin Exp Rheumatol 2006;24(6):694–7.

[48] Shoenfeld Y. To smell autoimmunity: anti-P-ribosomal autoantibodies, depression, and the olfactory system. J Autoimmun 2007;28(2–3):165–9.

[49] Kivity S, Shoenfeld Y, Arango MT, Cahill DJ, O'Kane SL, Zusev M, et al. Anti-ribosomal-phosphoprotein autoantibodies penetrate to neuronal cells via neuronal growth associated protein, affecting neuronal cells in vitro. Rheumatology (Oxford). 2016.

[50] Kiss E, Shoenfeld Y. Are anti-ribosomal P protein antibodies relevant in systemic lupus erythematosus? Clin Rev Allergy Immunol 2007;32(1):37–46.

[51] Blank M, Shoenfeld Y. The story of the 16/6 idiotype and systemic lupus erythematosus. Isr Med Assoc J 2008;10(1):37–9.

[52] Shoenfeld N, Agmon-Levin N, Flitman-Katzevman I, Paran D, Katz BS, Kivity S, et al. The sense of smell in systemic lupus erythematosus. Arthritis Rheum 2009;60(5):1484–7.

[53] Blank M, Beinglass I, Shoenfeld Y. The therapeutic potential of targeting anti-Ribosomal-P antibody in treating SLE patients with depression. Expert Opin Biol Ther 2007;7(9):1283–5.

[54] Peri Y, Agmon-Levin N, Theodor E, Shoenfeld Y. Sjogren's syndrome, the old and the new. Best Pract Res Clin Rheumatol 2012;26(1):105–17.

[55] Al-Ezzi MY, Pathak N, Tappuni AR, Khan KS. Primary Sjogren's syndrome impact on smell, taste, sexuality and quality of life in female patients: a systematic review and meta-analysis. Mod Rheumatol 2017;27(4):623–9.

[56] Kamel UF, Maddison P, Whitaker R. Impact of primary Sjogren's syndrome on smell and taste: effect on quality of life. Rheumatology (Oxford) 2009;48(12):1512–4.

[57] Lotsch J, Kraetsch HG, Wendler J, Hummel T. Self-ratings of higher olfactory acuity contrast with reduced olfactory test results of fibromyalgia patients. Int J Psychophysiol 2012;86(2):182–6.

[58] Amital H, Agmon-Levin N, Shoenfeld N, Arnson Y, Amital D, Langevitz P, et al. Olfactory impairment in patients with the fibromyalgia syndrome and systemic sclerosis. Immunol Res 2014;60(2–3):201–7.

[59] Gershwin ME, Shoenfeld Y. Cutting-edge issues in organ-specific autoimmunity. Clin Rev Allergy Immunol 2011;41(2):123–5.

[60] Anaya JM, Shoenfeld Y, Buttgereit F, Gonzalez-Gay MA. Autoimmune rheumatic diseases. BioMed Res Int 2014;2014:952159.

[61] Steinbach S, Proft F, Schulze-Koops H, Hundt W, Heinrich P, Schulz S, et al. Gustatory and olfactory function in rheumatoid arthritis. Scand J Rheumatol 2011;40(3):169–77.

[62] Watad A, Tiosano S, Yahav D, Comaneshter D, Shoenfeld Y, Cohen AD, et al. Behcet's disease and familial Mediterranean fever: two sides of the same coin or just an association? A cross-sectional study. Eur J Intern Med 2017;39:75–8.

[63] Veyseller B, Dogan R, Ozucer B, Aksoy F, Meric A, Su O, et al. Olfactory function and nasal manifestations of Behcet's disease. Auris Nasus Larynx 2014;41(2):185–9.

[64] Ozbay I, Kucur C, TemIzturk F, Ozkan Y, Kahraman C, Oghan F. Assessment of nasal mucociliary activity in patients with Behcet's disease. J Laryngol Otol 2016;130(4):348–51.

[65] Fischer A, Zimovetz E, Ling C, Esser D, Schoof N. Humanistic and cost burden of systemic sclerosis: a review of the literature. Autoimmun Rev 2017;16:1147–54. https://www.ncbi.nlm.nih.gov/pubmed/28899803.

[66] de Carvalho JF, Pereira RM, Shoenfeld Y. Pearls in autoimmunity. Auto Immun Highlights 2011;2(1):1–4.

[67] Dahlslett SB, Goektas O, Schmidt F, Harms L, Olze H, Fleiner F. Psychophysiological and electrophysiological testing of olfactory and gustatory function in patients with multiple sclerosis. Eur Arch Oto-Rhino-Laryngol 2012;269(4):1163–9.

[68] Erb K, Bohner G, Harms L, Goektas O, Fleiner F, Dommes E, et al. Olfactory function in patients with multiple sclerosis: a diffusion tensor imaging study. J Neurol Sci 2012;316(1–2):56–60.

[69] Uecker FC, Olze H, Kunte H, Gerz C, Göktas Ö HL, et al. Longitudinal testing of olfactory and gustatory function in patients with multiple sclerosis. PLoS One 2017;12(1):e0170492.

[70] DeLuca GC, Joseph A, George J, Yates RL, Hamard M, Hofer M, et al. Olfactory pathology in central nervous system demyelinating diseases. Brain Pathology (Zurich, Switzerland) 2015;25(5):543–51.

[71] Lucassen EB, Turel A, Knehans A, Huang X, Eslinger P. Olfactory dysfunction in Multiple Sclerosis: a scoping review of the literature. Mult Scler Relat Disord 2016;6:1–9.

[72] Lutterotti A, Vedovello M, Reindl M, Ehling R, DiPauli F, Kuenz B, et al. Olfactory threshold is impaired in early, active multiple sclerosis. Mult Scler 2011;17(8):964–9.

[73] Barresi M, Ciurleo R, Giacoppo S, Foti Cuzzola V, Celi D, Bramanti P, et al. Evaluation of olfactory dysfunction in neurodegenerative diseases. J Neurol Sci 2012;323(1–2):16–24.

[74] Doty RL, Li C, Mannon LJ, Yousem DM. Olfactory dysfunction in multiple sclerosis: relation to longitudinal changes in plaque numbers in central olfactory structures. Neurology 1999;53(4):880–2.

[75] Good KP, Tourbier IA, Moberg P, Cuzzocreo JL, Geckle RJ, Yousem DM, et al. Unilateral olfactory sensitivity in multiple sclerosis. Physiol Behav 2017;168:24–30.

[76] Aydin E, Tekeli H, Karabacak E, Altunay IK, Aydin C, Cerman AA, et al. Olfactory functions in patients with psoriasis vulgaris: correlations with the severity of the disease. Arch Dermatol Res 2016;308(6):409–14.

[77] McConnell RJ, Menendez CE, Smith FR, Henkin RI, Rivlin RS. Defects of taste and smell in patients with hypothyroidism. Am J Med 1975;59(3):354–64.

[78] Deniz F, Ay SA, Salihoglu M, Kurt O, Baskoy K, Altundag A, et al. Thyroid hormone replacement therapy improves olfaction and taste sensitivity in primary hypothyroid patients: a prospective randomised clinical trial. Exp Clin Endocrinol Diabetes 2016;124(9):562–7.

[79] Swidzinski T, Linkowska-Swidzinska K, Czerniejewska-Wolska H, Wiskirska-Woznica B, Owecki M, Glowacka MD, et al. Hypothyroidism affects olfactory evoked potentials. BioMed Res Int 2016;2016:9583495.

[80] Aydin N, Ramazanoglu L, Onen MR, Yilmaz I, Aydin MD, Altinkaynak K, et al. Rationalisation of the irrational neuropathological basis of hypothyroidism-olfaction disorders paradox: experimental study. World Neurosurg 2017;107:400–8.

[81] De Carolis C, Perricone C, Perricone R. War and peace at the feto-placental front line: recurrent spontaneous abortion. Isr Med Assoc J 2014;16(10):667–8.

[82] Perricone C, de Carolis C, Perricone R. Pregnancy and autoimmunity: a common problem. Best Pract Res Clin Rheumatol 2012;26(1):47–60.

[83] De Carolis C, Perricone C, Perricone R. NK cells, autoantibodies, and immunologic infertility: a complex interplay. Clin Rev Allergy Immunol 2010;39(3):166–75.

Chapter 28

Breastfeeding and Autoimmunity: A Lesson for Life

Vânia Vieira Borba[1,2,4], Kassem Sharif[3,4,5], Yehuda Shoenfeld[6,7]

[1]Department 'A' of Internal Medicine, Coimbra University Hospital Centre, Coimbra, Portugal; [2]Faculty of Medicine, University of Coimbra, Coimbra, Portugal; [3]Department of Medicine 'B', Sheba Medical Center, Tel-Hashomer, Israel; [4]Zabludowicz Center for Autoimmune Diseases, Sheba Medical Center, Tel-Hashomer, Israel; [5]Sackler Faculty of Medicine, Tel Aviv University, Tel Aviv, Israel; [6]Zabludowicz Center for Autoimmune Diseases, Sheba Medical Center, affiliated to Sackler Faculty of Medicine, Tel Aviv University, Tel Aviv, Israel; [7]Laboratory of the Mosaics of Autoimmunity, Saint-Petersburg University, Saint- Petersburg, Russian Federation

INTRODUCTION

Breast milk is the result of 200 million years of Darwinian pressure on mammalian lactation as the source of infant's nourishment [1]. Diet is one of the most important environmental exposures in early life [2]. Currently the World Health Organization recommends that infants should be exclusively breastfed up to 6 months of age and continue with a partial pattern until the infant is at least 2 years old [3]. During the 19th century, antibodies were the first immunological molecules discovered in breast milk, boosting the possibility that human milk could have an influence on the development of children immune system [4]. Indeed, human milk supplies an impressive array of immune-active molecules, metabolites, oligosaccharides, microbial content, vitamins, and other nutrients that provide protection against infections and modulates mucosal immune responses [3,5]. At this time, more than 80 different autoimmune diseases have been described in which the leading role is characterized by an inappropriate immune reaction [6]. The possibility that decisive imprinting events might be modulated during the first months of life, with potential long-term effects, sparks the importance of breastfeeding in the correct development of the immune system, altering disease susceptibility, mainly in immune-mediated conditions [7,8]. Breast milk is not only a completely adapted nutrition source but also a personalized medicine for the infants, programming to some degree their future health [9].

HUMAN MILK AMONG THE STAGES OF LACTATION

Milk is a complex fluid, the composition of which gradually changes according to the stage of lactation, infant feeding, health status (mother and newborn), maternal diet, environment, and genetics [10]. Colostrum is the first milk produced and is characterized for containing over 250 potentially immunologically active proteins, including enzymes (lactoferrin, lysozyme, etc.), hormones, immunoglobulins, cytokines, signaling molecules, soluble receptors, inflammatory mediators, etc.

The high content of bioactive proteins demonstrates that colostrum main role is immunological rather than nutritional [4,11,12]. Antimicrobial factors present in human milk possess resistance to degradation by the newborn's digestive enzymes, protecting the mucosal surfaces and eliminating pathogens without initiating inflammatory reactions, while the immune system matures [13]. Furthermore, the abundance and diversity of indigestible oligosaccharides promotes the optimal microbiota colonization, which will condition future immune homeostasis [14]. A few days after delivery, tight junctions of the mammary epithelium start to close, the rate of sodium/potassium declines, and the lactose concentration rises, indicating the secretory activation and production of transitional milk. Two weeks postpartum the milk is considered fully mature [15]. It is characterized by decreasing relative concentrations of the immunologically active molecules, whereas the volume and nutritional requirements increase to fulfill the growing infant needs [16].

BREAST MILK AND IMMUNE SYSTEM MODULATION

The postnatal period is crucial for the newborn's immune system maturation. This process is characterized by the development of a balance between Th1 and Th2 response [17]. The thymus is the central immune system organ where bone marrow–derived precursors undergo differentiation and selection before they are apt for migration to the periphery [18];

Mosaic of Autoimmunity. https://doi.org/10.1016/B978-0-12-814307-0.00028-1

therefore thymus plays a major role in the establishment of T cell–mediated immunity [18,19]. Hasselbalch and colleagues [20] reported that the thymus is considerably larger in breastfed infants when compared with formula-fed infants. Subsequently, Jeppesne et al. [21] not only corroborated the previous findings but also discovered a correlation between breastfeeding and CD8+ T cells. The mechanism by which breastfeeding may influence thymus size is unclear, although pathways involving interleukin (IL) 7 are considered to play a critical role in thymopoiesis and Tgd lymphocytes output from the intestinal mucosa [22,23]. In addition, breast milk is known to modulate infant intestinal microbiome [24], which is the main source of bacterial metabolites. This has been proved to play a leading role in T cell development and differentiation and may be the missing link between the benefits of breastfeeding in the intestinal microbiome and enhanced thymus size in breastfed infants [25,26].

Immunological Components of Human Milk

Human milk supplies an impressive array of immunological active molecules (Table 28.1) involved in complex interactions and influence outcomes [5,27]. This effect is because of the amazing nature of the interaction between mother and baby. Breast milk will not only nourish the newborn but also provide a complete arsenal of immune components that will contribute as protective factors and as development and maturation factors (Table 28.1). The protective factors are known to contribute against infections by providing direct immunity (passive) and immune regulatory effects based on antiinflammatory capabilities. They ensure the adequate environment in the infant gastrointestinal tract by preventing microbiome dysbiosis, therefore preserving the immune barrier functions of the epithelium [28,29]. The newborn immune system can be looked at as a very complex machine with amazing capabilities, yet it does not know how to use it. In the last few years, analytical advancements have allowed a better characterization of the human milk composition, discovering new structures such as stem cells, microbiome elements, and miRNA, increasing our knowledge every day [30,31].

Breast Milk and Microbiome

Breastfeeding influences the gut microbiome and metagenome. Recent studies revealed that the main imprinting events on the newborn immune system might be mediated through the microbiome, highlighting the early influence of the infant diet nature [32,33]. The capability to regulate host responses depends on the bacterial composition of milk. Abnormal colonization has a long-term effect on the immune system, mainly in respect to metabolic and autoimmune diseases [34]. The microbiome of breastfed infants has copious amounts of bifidobacteria and Lactobacillus species, promoted by the rich bioactive factors present in the human milk, such as human milk oligosaccharides that function as natural prebiotics [35]. Therefore, there is indeed specificity between the infant microbiome and breastfeeding, resulting in different bacterial-induced effects on metabolism and immunity. Curiously this interaction is based on the mother enteromammary axis, with the release of dendritic cells containing live maternal gut microbiome (which select nonpathogenic bacteria from the gut lumen and carry them to the lactating mammary gland), T cells expressing gut-derived β7 integrins, and plasma cells producing specific immunoglobulin into the milk [36,37]. Naturally the cytokines present in breast milk also depend on the mother immunological experience and this heritage will be transmitted to the infant immature immune system, encouraging tolerogenic responses [38]. Bergstom et al. [39] reported that the major factor affecting infant microbiome up to 12 months of age was the cessation of breastfeeding.

Breast Milk and Immune Tolerance

A healthy mucosal immune system is capable of distinguishing nutritional antigens and nonharmful microbes from pathogens, promoting adequate immunological reactions by suppression of cellular and humoral immune responses to ingested antigens. This "controlled responses" are called "oral tolerance" and are influenced by the intestinal microbiota [40]. Diseases due to a defect in immune tolerance, such as celiac disease (CD) or type 1 diabetes (T1D), are less common in children who were breastfed, suggesting a protective effect [41]. Recent data reported that breastfeed-induced protection may be explained by early antigen-specific tolerance induction, both by the transfer of antigens through milk and the presence of factors that affect the newborn immune maturation and responses [42], adjusting for the deficiency of Ig synthesis during the first year of life. Each mother will produce different milk in accordance with her previous antigen exposure [43], as well as immune responses to transferred antigens, permeability of the mammary gland epithelium [44], microbiome influencing factors, gut growth factors in milk, and the presence of tolerogenic molecules [7,45].

TABLE 28.1 Role of Human Milk Immunological Compounds

Components	Role P	D/M	Function
Proteins			
Lactoferrin	•		Antimicrobial, iron carrier
Lactadherin, lysozyme, defensins	•		Antimicrobial
MicroRNAs	•	•	Lymphocyte development, inflammatory mediator
Cells			
Lymphocytes	•	•	(T cells >80%); lymphocyte development, inflammatory mediator
Macrophages	•	•	Phagocytosis, pathogen defense, T cells stimulation
Neutrophils	•		Unknown, may play a role on maternal protection
Breast milk stem cells		•	Secretion of growth factors; tissue homeostasis, repair, and/or regeneration
Immunoglobulins			
sIgA/IgA	•	•	Antimicrobial, pathogen-binding inhibition
IgM/IgG	•	•	Antimicrobial, antibody-mediated cytotoxicity
Cytokines			
IL-1b	•	•	Inflammatory mediator, intestinal and immune system trophic factor
IL-2	•	•	Modulate T cell development
IL-6	•	•	Intestinal trophic factor, inflammatory mediator, B cell activation
IL-8	•	•	Intestinal trophic factor, recruitment of maternal leukocytes
IL-10	•	•	Intestinal trophic factor, antiinflammatory cytokine, tolerance promoter
IFN-γ	•	•	Stimulate Th1 inflammatory response, suppress Th2 allergic response
TNF-α	•	•	Proinflammatory
Chemokines and other soluble factors			
CXCR-1/CXCR-2	•	•	Cytokine receptor
CXCL-9 (MIP)	•	•	Antimicrobial, NK and T cell chemoattractant
sCD14	•		Inflammatory mediator, promoter of lymphocyte differentiation and activation
IP-10	•		Antimicrobial, NK, and T cell chemoattractant
MCP-1	•	•	T cell chemoattractant
TNF-RI	•		Reduce TNF-α activity, mediate inflammation
G-CSF		•	Stimulate neutrophil growth and differentiation, intestinal trophic factor
Growth factors			
TGF-b, TGF-a, EGF	•	•	Intestinal trophic factor, promote tolerance
IGF-1 and IGF-2		•	Development and maturation of gastrointestinal cells
Oligosaccharides			
HMOs	•	•	Promote colonization of commensal bacteria, antimicrobial effects (pathogen binding, change gut's pH)
Gangliosides	•	•	Prebiotic, suppress inflammation
Other immunological compounds			
LCPUFAs	•	•	Promote tolerance, Th1 and Th2 response
Nucleotides		•	Intestinal trophic factor, promote differentiation and activation of lymphocytes and macrophage, NK activity
Osteoprotegerin	•	•	May regulate Th1/Th2 balance
Food antigens		•	Promote tolerance

EGF, epidermal growth factor; *G-CSF*, granulocyte-macrophage colony-stimulating factor; *HMO*, human milk oligosaccharides; *IFN-γ*, interferon gamma; *Ig*, immunoglobulin; *IGF*, insulin-like growth factor; *IL*, interleukin; *IP*, IFN-γ–inducible protein; *LCPUFA*, long-chain polyunsaturated fatty acid; *MCP*, monocyte chemotactic protein 1; *MIP*, monokine induced by IFN-γ; *TGF*, transforming growth factor; *TNF-α*, tumor necrosis factor alpha.

BREASTFEEDING AND AUTOIMMUNE DISEASES

The benefits of breastfeeding are well recognized worldwide. Current scientific evidence supports the beneficial role of breastfeeding in several immune-mediated diseases.

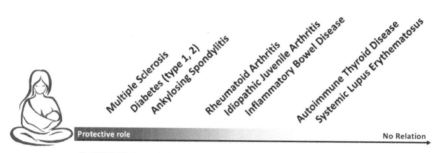

FIGURE 28.1   Relation of breastfeeding and autoimmune diseases.

Breastfeeding and Diabetes

Type 1 Diabetes

T1D is known to be an immune-mediated disease causing destruction of pancreatic B cells, eventually leading to complete and lifelong dependence on exogenous insulin [46]. Although genetic susceptibility variants play a crucial role in the development of T1D, increased incidence over the past 50 years strongly suggests an important role for nongenetic factors [47,48]. The hypothesis that breastfeeding could protect against T1D was proposed more than 30 years ago by Borch-Johnsen et al. [49] and since then several mechanisms have been implied. The reason why human milk might protect against T1D remains uncertain, although numerous theories have been considered for the protective effect of breastfeeding, such as lower incidence of potentially diabetogenic infections, later exposure to dietary antigens, healthier gut microbiota, and correct maturation of the newborn's gut [32,50,51]. Cardwell et al. [52] reported that being breastfed for more than 3 months or exclusively breastfed for more than 2 weeks after birth was associated with 15%–30% lower risk of T1D in childhood. Recently Lund-Blix et al. [53] preformed a large cohort study involving 155 392 children to clarify the relation between the duration of full or any breastfeeding and risk of T1D. The authors concluded that children who were never breastfed had a twofold increased risk for developing T1D. In contrast, the *Diabetes and Autoimmunity Study in the Young (DAISY)* (2015) suggested that the introduction of any solid food before 4 months and after 6 months of age predicted the development of T1D [54]. Likewise, Nucci et al. [55] concluded from the *Type 1 Diabetes Prediction and Prevention Project (DIPP)* study a close link between the risk of islet autoimmunity and early introduction of root vegetables [55]. A recent field of investigation relates microbiome and immune-mediated diseases. Interestingly, recent data suggest that alterations in the proportions of short-chain fatty acids (SCFAs), such as butyrate, might be a potential mechanism contributing to the risk of developing T1D [56,57].

Type 2 Diabetes

Type 2 diabetes (T2D) is an endocrine pathological state affecting young individuals and adults, which has seen a significant increase in the last 30 years, particularly in children worldwide [58]. The etiology is highly heterogeneous, including genetic and environmental factors. These environmental factors, such as diet, may be altered to prevent the onset and the development of the disease [58,59]. The absence of breastfeeding or its improper pattern is recognized as a prime contributive factor in the future development of obesity and metabolic syndrome. Indeed, previous studies related proper breastfeeding with a 24% decreased risk of T2D in childhood [60]. According to earlier data, a systematic review directly correlated the duration of breastfeeding and the risk of development of childhood T2D and obesity in neonates [61]. More recently, Halipchuk et al. [62] preformed a large retrospective case-control study to identify the factors associated with the development of childhood-onset T2D and suggested that exclusive breastfeeding decreases the risk of development of childhood-onset T2D [62].

Breastfeeding and Idiopathic Juvenile Arthritis

Juvenile idiopathic arthritis (JIA) is the most common chronic rheumatic disease of childhood [63]. The pathogenesis and etiology of JIA are unclear, although interactions among genetic factors, immune mechanisms, and environmental exposures are thought to contribute in most cases. Studies relating breastfeeding and JIA have been controversial. A prospective cohort study reported that a longer duration of breastfeeding (both total and exclusive) may protect against development of JIA [64], finding an increased risk of JIA in children who were breastfed for less than 4 months. Recently a cohort study associated breastfeeding with an earlier but milder presentation of JIA and with different patterns of arthritis [65]. The reason why human milk can influence the susceptibility to certain subtypes of JIA is unknown, although studies have related it with differences in microbiome between children with and without enthesitis-related arthritis [65,66]. Indeed, breastfeeding could be indirectly linked to JIA by the gut microbiome because altered microbial profiles have been identified among JIA patients [66]. However, further studies are needed to clarify the role of breastfeeding in JIA disease risk [67].

Breastfeeding and Rheumatoid Arthritis

Rheumatoid arthritis (RA) is the most common autoimmune inflammatory joint disease worldwide, characterized by a distinctive pattern of bone and joint destruction [68]. Several studies have investigated the influence of breastfeeding and the risk of developing RA, but the results were inconsistent [69–71]. An investigation performed by Colebatch et al. [72] reported that in HLA-DR4–negative children, rheumatoid factor–positive infants were less likely to have been breastfed for >3 months when compared with rheumatoid factor–negative children, although this effect was not seen in HLA-DR4–positive infants. A recent metaanalysis *by* Chen et al. [73] included 1672 patients with RA and aimed to estimate the association between breastfeeding and RA risk, and an inverse association was found in the overall study population, relating a decreased risk of RA no matter if breastfeeding was longer or shorter than 12 months.

Breastfeeding and Multiple Sclerosis

Multiple sclerosis (MS) is the most common immune-mediated disease of the central nervous system affecting young adults [74]. Evidence suggests that environmental factors act long before MS becomes symptomatic, suggesting the existence of a prodromal phase for this disease. Conradi et al. [75] recently associated breastfeeding for at least 4 months as a protective factor against the risk of developing MS; however, other studies still debate the impact of breastfeeding duration in determining the risk for MS [76]. Applying data from a large multinational case-control study (EnvIMS), Ragnedda et al. [77] described an increased risk of MS in males who were breastfed for less than 4 months [77]. The protective role of human milk in the pathogenesis of immune-mediated MS could be related with its capacity of promoting the immune system development, safeguarding from toxic agents and pathogens, and modulation of immune responses [78,79], including immunomodulatory effects by IL-10 production and the antiinflammatory properties of transforming growth factor β [80].

Breastfeeding and Celiac Disease

CD is a systemic immune-mediated disorder caused by the ingestion of gluten-containing grains in genetically susceptible individuals [81]. Genetic background plays a crucial role in the predisposition to CD [82], although better long-term health was observed in CD patients who were breastfed [83]. This fact may be due to the delayed introduction of gluten in daily diet and expanding the latency time between the introduction of gluten and the development of the disease [84], lower incidence of gastrointestinal infections in the newborns who are breastfed [85], and the prevention of gut dysbiosis [86]. Metaanalysis and systemic review, including all studies between 1966 and 2004, found that infants who were breastfed had a 52% risk reduction of developing CD when compared with those who were not breastfed at the time of gluten introduction [87]. Recently, a metaanalysis proved that the risk of CD was significantly decreased in infants who were breastfed at the time of gluten introduction [87,88]. Actually, being breastfed at the time of gluten introduction was related with a latter onset of CD [82,87,88]. Interestingly, intestinal dysbiosis may promote an abnormal response to gluten in predisposed individuals [89], a fact that could be due to the role of specific bacteria in the modulation of infant immune responses [90]. However, it is still not clear if human milk truly provides permanent tolerance acquisition or just a symptomatic reduction and delayed diagnosis of CD [91].

Breastfeeding and Inflammatory Bowel Diseases

Inflammatory bowel diseases (IBDs) are known as a chronic inflammatory condition of the gastrointestinal tract, manifesting two major disorders: ulcerative colitis and Crohn's disease [92]. The exact pathogenesis of IBD remains unknown, part of the underlying mechanism is believed to be a deregulated host immune response to intestinal flora, in genetically susceptible individuals [8,93]. The major risk for developing IBD is having a family history of the disease [93]. The greatest incidence of IBD is in early adulthood, bolstering the fact that early exposures might force future susceptibility. Human milk compounds not only protect against infections but also influence the immune tolerance and bacterial colonization of the infant's gut [94]. Considerable investigations found that breastfeeding was protective for IBD [95–97], mainly on early onsets [98].

Breastfeeding and Other Autoimmune Diseases

In 1990, Fort et al. attempted to assess the prevalence of breastfeeding in patients with autoimmune thyroid disease (ATD), which may have a protective role in the development of this disease. Results were unable to document any relationship between the history and duration of breastfeeding and development of ATD; however, a higher prevalence of feedings with soy-containing formulas in early infancy was found [99]. Recently, Simard et al. [100] evaluated the link between breastfeeding and systemic lupus erythematosus (SLE) among two prospective cohort studies, the Nurses' Health Study and the Nurses' Health Study II, but found no statistically significant association between duration and SLE incidence. Further research in this field may lead to novel links and strategies of breastfeeding and immune disorders.

CONCLUSIONS

The benefits of breastfeeding are well recognized worldwide. Current scientific evidence supports the beneficial role of breastfeeding in several immune-mediated diseases, although a few exact pathways are yet to be elucidated. Recent technological progresses allowed a better characterization of the human milk composition, opening new horizons to our knowledge for a better understanding of its capabilities, and plausible mechanisms which play a protective role in a heterogeneous pool of diseases with long-term health effects.

LIST OF ABBREVIATIONS

CD Celiac disease
EGF Epidermal growth factor
G-CSF Granulocyte-macrophage colony-stimulating factor
HMOs Human milk oligosaccharides
IBDs Inflammatory bowel diseases
IFN-γ Interferon gamma
Ig Immunoglobulin
IGF Insulin-like growth factor
IL Interleukin
IP IFN-γ–inducible protein
JIA Juvenile idiopathic arthritis
LCPUFA Long-chain polyunsaturated fatty acid
MCP Monocyte chemotactic protein 1
MIP Monokine induced by IFN-γ
MiRNA micro-RNA
MS Multiple sclerosis
RA Rheumatoid arthritis
sCD14 Soluble CD14
SLE Systemic lupus erythematosus
Tgd Gamma-delta T cells
TGF Transforming growth factor
TNF-α Tumor necrosis factor alpha

REFERENCES

[1] Capuco AV, Akers RM. The origin and evolution of lactation. J Biol 2009;8(4):37.
[2] Dahan S, Segal Y, Shoenfeld Y. Dietary factors in rheumatic autoimmune diseases: a recipe for therapy? Nat Rev Rheumatol 2017;13(6):348–58.
[3] Mosca F, Gianni ML. Human milk: composition and health benefits. La Pediatria medica e chirurgica. Med Surg Pediatr 2017;39(2):155.
[4] Arnold RR, Brewer M, Gauthier JJ. Bactericidal activity of human lactoferrin: sensitivity of a variety of microorganisms. Infect Immun 1980;28(3):893–8.
[5] Andreas NJ, Kampmann B, Mehring Le-Doare K. Human breast milk: a review on its composition and bioactivity. Early Hum Dev 2015;91(11):629–35.
[6] Watad A, Amital H, Aljadeff G, Zandman-Goddard G, Orbach H, Shoenfeld Y. Prolactin: another important player in the mosaic of autoimmunity. Isr Med Assoc J 2016;18(9):542–3.

[7] Hosea Blewett HJ, Cicalo MC, Holland CD, Field CJ. The immunological components of human milk. Adv Food Nutr Res 2008;54:45–80.

[8] Rautava S. Early microbial contact, the breast milk microbiome and child health. J Dev Orig Health Dis 2016;7(1):5–14.

[9] Schack-Nielsen L, Michaelsen KF. Breast feeding and future health. Curr Opin Clin Nutr Metab Care 2006;9(3):289–96.

[10] Lis J, Orczyk-Pawilowicz M, Katnik-Prastowska I. Proteins of human milk involved in immunological processes. Postepy higieny i medycyny doswiadczalnej (Online) 2013;67:529–47.

[11] Donovan SM. The role of lactoferrin in gastrointestinal and immune development and function: a preclinical perspective. J Pediatr 2016;173(Suppl.):S16–28.

[12] Castellote C, Casillas R, Ramirez-Santana C, Perez-Cano FJ, Castell M, Moretones MG, et al. Premature delivery influences the immunological composition of colostrum and transitional and mature human milk. J Nutr 2011;141(6):1181–7.

[13] Palmeira P, Carneiro-Sampaio M. Immunology of breast milk. Revista da Associacao Medica Brasileira 1992;62(6):584–93. 2016.

[14] Zivkovic AM, German JB, Lebrilla CB, Mills DA. Human milk glycobiome and its impact on the infant gastrointestinal microbiota. Proc Natl Acad Sci USA 2011;108(Suppl. 1):4653–8.

[15] Ballard O, Morrow AL. Human milk composition: nutrients and bioactive factors. Pediatr Clin 2013;60(1):49–74.

[16] Munblit D, Treneva M, Peroni DG, Colicino S, Chow L, Dissanayeke S, et al. Colostrum and mature human milk of women from London, Moscow, and Verona: determinants of immune composition. Nutrients 2016;8(11).

[17] Bjorksten B. The intrauterine and postnatal environments. J Allergy Clin Immunol 1999;104(6):1119–27.

[18] Klein L, Kyewski B, Allen PM, Hogquist KA. Positive and negative selection of the T cell repertoire: what thymocytes see (and don't see). Nat Rev Immunol 2014;14(6):377–91.

[19] Garly ML, Trautner SL, Marx C, Danebod K, Nielsen J, Ravn H, et al. Thymus size at 6 months of age and subsequent child mortality. J Pediatr 2008;153(5):683–8. 8.e1-3.

[20] Hasselbalch H, Jeppesen DL, Engelmann MD, Michaelsen KF, Nielsen MB. Decreased thymus size in formula-fed infants compared with breastfed infants. Acta Paediatr (Oslo, Norway: 1992) 1996;85(9):1029–32.

[21] Jeppesen DL, Hasselbalch H, Lisse IM, Ersboll AK, Engelmann MD. T-lymphocyte subsets, thymic size and breastfeeding in infancy. Pediatr Allergy Immunol 2004;15(2):127–32.

[22] Candeias S, Muegge K, Durum SK. IL-7 receptor and VDJ recombination: trophic versus mechanistic actions. Immunity 1997;6(5):501–8.

[23] Ngom PT, Collinson AC, Pido-Lopez J, Henson SM, Prentice AM, Aspinall R. Improved thymic function in exclusively breastfed infants is associated with higher interleukin 7 concentrations in their mothers' breast milk. Am J Clin Nutr 2004;80(3):722–8.

[24] Pannaraj PS, Li F, Cerini C, Bender JM, Yang S, Rollie A, et al. Association between breast milk bacterial communities and establishment and development of the infant gut microbiome. JAMA Pediatr 2017;171(7):647–54.

[25] Munblit D, Peroni DG, Boix-Amoros A, Hsu PS, Land BV, Gay MCL, et al. Human milk and allergic diseases: an unsolved puzzle. Nutrients 2017;9(8).

[26] Rooks MG, Garrett WS. Gut microbiota, metabolites and host immunity. Nat Rev Immunol 2016;16(6):341–52.

[27] Lonnerdal B. Human milk: bioactive proteins/peptides and functional properties. Nestle Nutr Inst Workshop Ser 2016;86:97–107.

[28] Cacho NT, Lawrence RM. Innate immunity and breast milk. Front Immunol 2017;8:584.

[29] Lawrence RM, Lawrence RA. Breast milk and infection. Clin Perinatol 2004;31(3):501–28.

[30] Hassiotou F, Geddes DT, Hartmann PE. Cells in human milk: state of the science. J Hum Lactation 2013;29(2):171–82.

[31] Indumathi S, Dhanasekaran M, Rajkumar JS, Sudarsanam D. Exploring the stem cell and non-stem cell constituents of human breast milk. Cytotechnology 2013;65(3):385–93.

[32] Victora CG, Bahl R, Barros AJD, França GVA, Horton S, Krasevec J, et al. Breastfeeding in the 21st century: epidemiology, mechanisms, and lifelong effect. Lancet 2016;387(10017):475–90.

[33] Schei K, Avershina E, Oien T, Rudi K, Follestad T, Salamati S, et al. Early gut mycobiota and mother-offspring transfer. Microbiome 2017;5(1):107.

[34] Macpherson AJ, de Aguero MG, Ganal-Vonarburg SC. How nutrition and the maternal microbiota shape the neonatal immune system. Nat Rev Immunol 2017;17(8):508–17.

[35] David LA, Maurice CF, Carmody RN, Gootenberg DB, Button JE, Wolfe BE, et al. Diet rapidly and reproducibly alters the human gut microbiome. Nature 2014;505(7484):559–63.

[36] Perez PF, Dore J, Leclerc M, Levenez F, Benyacoub J, Serrant P, et al. Bacterial imprinting of the neonatal immune system: lessons from maternal cells? Pediatrics 2007;119(3):e724–32.

[37] Langa S, Maldonado-Barragan A, Delgado S, Martin R, Martin V, Jimenez E, et al. Characterization of Lactobacillus salivarius CECT 5713, a strain isolated from human milk: from genotype to phenotype. Appl Microbiol Biotechnol 2012;94(5):1279–87.

[38] Rosser EC, Mauri C. A clinical update on the significance of the gut microbiota in systemic autoimmunity. J Autoimmun 2016;74:85–93.

[39] Bergstrom A, Skov TH, Bahl MI, Roager HM, Christensen LB, Ejlerskov KT, et al. Establishment of intestinal microbiota during early life: a longitudinal, explorative study of a large cohort of Danish infants. Appl Environ Microbiol 2014;80(9):2889–900.

[40] Peters RL, Dang TD, Allen KJ. Specific oral tolerance induction in childhood. Pediatr Allergy Immunol 2016;27(8):784–94.

[41] Holmberg H, Wahlberg J, Vaarala O, Ludvigsson J. Short duration of breast-feeding as a risk-factor for beta-cell autoantibodies in 5-year-old children from the general population. Br J Nutr 2007;97(1):111–6.

[42] Breastfeeding OWH. Childhood asthma, and allergic disease. Ann Nutr Metab 2017;70(Suppl. 2):26–36.

[43] Palmer DJ, Gold MS, Makrides M. Effect of cooked and raw egg consumption on ovalbumin content of human milk: a randomized, double-blind, cross-over trial. Clin Exp Allergy 2005;35(2):173–8.

[44] Benn CS, Bottcher MF, Pedersen BV, Filteau SM, Duchen K. Mammary epithelial paracellular permeability in atopic and non-atopic mothers versus childhood atopy. Pediatr Allergy Immunol 2004;15(2):123–6.

[45] Verhasselt V. Neonatal tolerance under breastfeeding influence. Curr Opin Immunol 2010;22(5):623–30.

[46] Atkinson MA, Eisenbarth GS, Michels AW. Type 1 diabetes. Lancet (Lond Engl) 2014;383(9911):69–82.

[47] Patterson CC, Gyurus E, Rosenbauer J, Cinek O, Neu A, Schober E, et al. Trends in childhood type 1 diabetes incidence in Europe during 1989-2008: evidence of non-uniformity over time in rates of increase. Diabetologia 2012;55(8):2142–7.

[48] Skrivarhaug T, Stene LC, Drivvoll AK, Strom H, Joner G. Incidence of type 1 diabetes in Norway among children aged 0-14 years between 1989 and 2012: has the incidence stopped rising? results from the Norwegian childhood diabetes registry. Diabetologia 2014;57(1):57–62.

[49] Borch-Johnsen K, Joner G, Mandrup-Poulsen T, Christy M, Zachau-Christiansen B, Kastrup K, et al. Relation between breast-feeding and incidence rates of insulin-dependent diabetes mellitus. A hypothesis. Lancet (Lond Engl) 1984;2(8411):1083–6.

[50] Chia JSJ, McRae JL, Kukuljan S, Woodford K, Elliott RB, Swinburn B, et al. A1 beta-casein milk protein and other environmental pre-disposing factors for type 1 diabetes. Nutr Diabetes 2017;7(5):e274.

[51] Patelarou E, Girvalaki C, Brokalaki H, Patelarou A, Androulaki Z, Vardavas C. Current evidence on the associations of breastfeeding, infant formula, and cow's milk introduction with type 1 diabetes mellitus: a systematic review. Nutr Rev 2012;70(9):509–19.

[52] Cardwell CR, Stene LC, Ludvigsson J, Rosenbauer J, Cinek O, Svensson J, et al. Breast-feeding and childhood-onset type 1 diabetes: a pooled analysis of individual participant data from 43 observational studies. Diabetes Care 2012;35(11):2215–25.

[53] Lund-Blix NA, Dydensborg Sander S, Stordal K, Nybo Andersen AM, Ronningen KS, Joner G, et al. Infant feeding and risk of type 1 diabetes in two large scandinavian birth cohorts. Diabetes Care 2017;40(7):920–7.

[54] Smithers LG, Kramer MS, Lynch JW. Effects of breastfeeding on obesity and intelligence: causal insights from different study designs. JAMA Pediatr 2015;169(8):707–8.

[55] Nucci AM, Virtanen SM, Becker DJ. Infant feeding and timing of complementary foods in the development of type 1 diabetes. Curr Diabetes Rep 2015;15(9). 62-.

[56] Brown CT, Davis-Richardson AG, Giongo A, Gano KA, Crabb DB, Mukherjee N, et al. Gut microbiome metagenomics analysis suggests a functional model for the development of autoimmunity for type 1 diabetes. PLoS One 2011;6(10):e25792.

[57] Endesfelder D, Engel M, Davis-Richardson AG, Ardissone AN, Achenbach P, Hummel S, et al. Towards a functional hypothesis relating anti-islet cell autoimmunity to the dietary impact on microbial communities and butyrate production. Microbiome 2016;4:17.

[58] Xue Y, Gao M, Gao Y. Childhood type 2 diabetes: risks and complications. Exp Ther Med 2016;12(4):2367–70.

[59] Knip M, Akerblom HK. Early nutrition and later diabetes risk. Adv Exp Med Biol 2005;569:142 50.

[60] Bartz S, Freemark M. Pathogenesis and prevention of type 2 diabetes: parental determinants, breastfeeding, and early childhood nutrition. Curr Diabetes Rep 2012;12(1):82–7.

[61] Rabbitt A, Coyne I. Childhood obesity: nurses' role in addressing the epidemic. Br J Nurs(Mark Allen Pub) 2012;21(12):731–5.

[62] Halipchuk J, Temple B, Dart A, Martin D, Sellers EAC. Prenatal, obstetric and perinatal factors associated with the development of childhood-onset type 2 diabetes. Can J Diabetes 2018;42(1):71–7.

[63] Petty RE, Southwood TR, Manners P, Baum J, Glass DN, Goldenberg J, et al. International League of Associations for Rheumatology classification of juvenile idiopathic arthritis: second revision, Edmonton, 2001. J Rheumatol 2004;31(2):390–2.

[64] Kindgren E, Fredrikson M, Ludvigsson J. Early feeding and risk of Juvenile idiopathic arthritis: a case control study in a prospective birth cohort. Pediatr Rheumatol Online J 2017;15(1):46.

[65] Hyrich KL, Baildam E, Pickford H, Chieng A, Davidson JE, Foster H, et al. Influence of past breast feeding on pattern and severity of presentation of juvenile idiopathic arthritis. Arch Dis Child 2016;101(4):348–51.

[66] Stoll ML, Kumar R, Morrow CD, Lefkowitz EJ, Cui X, Genin A, et al. Altered microbiota associated with abnormal humoral immune responses to commensal organisms in enthesitis-related arthritis. Arthritis Res Ther 2014;16(6):486.

[67] Ellis JA, Munro JE, Ponsonby AL. Possible environmental determinants of juvenile idiopathic arthritis. Rheumatology (Oxford) 2010;49(3):411–25.

[68] Tobon GJ, Youinou P, Saraux A. The environment, geo-epidemiology, and autoimmune disease: rheumatoid arthritis. J Autoimmun 2010;35(1):10–4.

[69] Karlson EW, Mandl LA, Hankinson SE, Grodstein F. Do breast-feeding and other reproductive factors influence future risk of rheumatoid arthritis? Results from the Nurses' Health Study. Arthritis Rheum 2004;50(11):3458–67.

[70] Brennan P, Silman A. Breast-feeding and the onset of rheumatoid arthritis. Arthritis Rheum 1994;37(6):808–13.

[71] Pikwer M, Bergstrom U, Nilsson JA, Jacobsson L, Berglund G, Turesson C. Breast feeding, but not use of oral contraceptives, is associated with a reduced risk of rheumatoid arthritis. Ann Rheum Dis 2009;68(4):526–30.

[72] Colebatch AN, Edwards CJ. The influence of early life factors on the risk of developing rheumatoid arthritis. Clin Exp Immunol 2011;163(1):11–6.

[73] Chen H, Wang J, Zhou W, Yin H, Wang M. Breastfeeding and risk of rheumatoid arthritis: a systematic review and metaanalysis. J Rheumatol 2015;42(9):1563–9.

[74] Ramagopalan SV, Dobson R, Meier UC, Giovannoni G. Multiple sclerosis: risk factors, prodromes, and potential causal pathways. Lancet Neurol 2010;9(7):727–39.

[75] Conradi S, Malzahn U, Paul F, Quill S, Harms L, Then Bergh F, et al. Breastfeeding is associated with lower risk for multiple sclerosis. Mult Scler 2013;19(5):553–8.

[76] Dick G. Breast feeding and multiple sclerosis. Research could have been reviewed. BMJ 1994;309(6954):610–1.

[77] Ragnedda G, Leoni S, Parpinel M, Casetta I, Riise T, Myhr KM, et al. Reduced duration of breastfeeding is associated with a higher risk of multiple sclerosis in both Italian and Norwegian adult males: the EnvIMS study. J Neurol 2015;262(5):1271–7.

[78] Jeong K, Nguyen V, Kim J. Human milk oligosaccharides: the novel modulator of intestinal microbiota. BMB Rep 2012;45(8):433–41.

[79] Fernandez L, Langa S, Martin V, Maldonado A, Jimenez E, Martin R, et al. The human milk microbiota: origin and potential roles in health and disease. Pharmacol Res 2013;69(1):1–10.

[80] Prioult G, Pecquet S, Fliss I. Stimulation of interleukin-10 production by acidic beta-lactoglobulin-derived peptides hydrolyzed with Lactobacillus paracasei NCC2461 peptidases. Clin Diagn Lab Immunol 2004;11(2):266–71.

[81] Husby S, Koletzko S, Korponay-Szabo IR, Mearin ML, Phillips A, Shamir R, et al. European society for pediatric gastroenterology, hepatology, and nutrition guidelines for the diagnosis of coeliac disease. J Pediatr Gastroenterol Nutr 2012;54(1):136–60.

[82] Lionetti E, Castellaneta S, Francavilla R, Pulvirenti A, Tonutti E, Amarri S, et al. Introduction of gluten, HLA status, and the risk of celiac disease in children. N Engl J Med 2014;371(14):1295–303.

[83] Cunningham AS, Jelliffe DB, Jelliffe EF. Breast-feeding and health in the 1980s: a global epidemiologic review. J Pediatr 1991;118(5):659–66.

[84] Diamanti A, Capriati T, Bizzarri C, Ferretti F, Ancinelli M, Romano F, et al. Autoimmune diseases and celiac disease which came first: genotype or gluten? Expert Rev Clin Immunol 2016;12(1):67–77.

[85] Kemppainen KM, Lynch KF, Liu E, Lonnrot M, Simell V, Briese T, et al. Factors that increase risk of celiac disease autoimmunity after a gastrointestinal infection in early life. Clin Gastroenterol Hepatol 2017;15(5):694–702. e5.

[86] Sanz Y, De Pama G, Laparra M. Unraveling the ties between celiac disease and intestinal microbiota. Int Rev Immunol 2011;30(4):207–18.

[87] Akobeng AK, Ramanan AV, Buchan I, Heller RF. Effect of breast feeding on risk of coeliac disease: a systematic review and meta-analysis of observational studies. Arch Dis Child 2006;91(1):39–43.

[88] Guandalini S. The influence of gluten: weaning recommendations for healthy children and children at risk for celiac disease. Nestle Nutr Workshop Ser Pediatr Progr 2007;60:139–51. discussion 51–55.

[89] Cenit MC, Olivares M, Codoner-Franch P, Sanz Y. Intestinal microbiota and celiac disease: cause, consequence or co-evolution? Nutrients 2015;7(8):6900–23.

[90] Pozo-Rubio T, Olivares M, Nova E, De Palma G, Mujico JR, Ferrer MD, et al. Immune development and intestinal microbiota in celiac disease. Clin Dev Immunol 2012;2012:654143.

[91] Nova E, Pozo T, Sanz Y, Marcos A. Dietary strategies of immunomodulation in infants at risk for celiac disease. Proc Nutr Soc 2010;69(3):347–53.

[92] Ek WE, D'Amato M, Halfvarson J. The history of genetics in inflammatory bowel disease. Ann Gastroenterol 2014;27(4):294–303.

[93] Russell RK, Satsangi J. Does IBD run in families? Inflamm Bowel Dis 2008;14(Suppl. 2):S20–1.

[94] Mezoff EA, Aly H. The winding road to understanding the neonatal origins of inflammatory gastrointestinal disorders. J Pediatr Gastroenterol Nutr 2013;57(5):543–9.

[95] Renz H, Brandtzaeg P, Hornef M. The impact of perinatal immune development on mucosal homeostasis and chronic inflammation. Nat Rev Immunol 2011;12(1):9–23.

[96] van der Sloot KWJ, Amini M, Peters V, Dijkstra G, Alizadeh BZ. Inflammatory bowel diseases: review of known environmental protective and risk factors involved. Inflamm Bowel Dis 2017;23(9):1499–509.

[97] Klement E, Cohen RV, Boxman J, Joseph A, Reif S. Breastfeeding and risk of inflammatory bowel disease: a systematic review with meta-analysis. Am J Clin Nutr 2004;80(5):1342–52.

[98] Barclay AR, Russell RK, Wilson ML, Gilmour WH, Satsangi J, Wilson DC. Systematic review: the role of breastfeeding in the development of pediatric inflammatory bowel disease. J Pediatr 2009;155(3):421–6.

[99] Fort P, Moses N, Fasano M, Goldberg T, Lifshitz F. Breast and soy-formula feedings in early infancy and the prevalence of autoimmune thyroid disease in children. J Am Coll Nutr 1990;9(2):164–7.

[100] Simard JF, Karlson EW, Costenbader KH, Hernan MA, Stampfer MJ, Liang MH, et al. Perinatal factors and adult-onset lupus. Arthritis Rheum 2008;59(8):1155–61.

Chapter 29

Vaccines, Adjuvants, and the Mosaic of Autoimmunity

Abdulla Watad[1,2,3], Nicola Luigi Bragazzi[4]

[1]Department of Medicine 'B', Sheba Medical Center, Tel-Hashomer, Israel; [2]Zabludowicz Center for Autoimmune Diseases, Sheba Medical Center, Tel-Hashomer, Israel; [3]Sackler Faculty of Medicine, Tel Aviv University, Tel Aviv, Israel; [4]Postgraduate School of Public Health, Department of Health Sciences (DISSAL), University of Genoa, Genoa, Italy

INTRODUCTION

The immune system is able to carefully distinguish between self- and non–self-components. Therefore, any small deviation of this balanced function may result in an autoimmune activity and harm against self-antigens (autoantigens). Various environmental factors have been described as possible triggers of autoimmune diseases, including drugs, infectious agents [1], smoking [2], vaccination, and adjuvants [3]. Genome-wide association studies have led to the discovery of more than 300 susceptibility loci for autoimmune diseases [4]. However, for almost all loci, understanding of the mechanisms leading to autoimmunity remains limited, and most variants that are likely to be causal are in noncoding regions of the genome.

In the last century science donated humanity the gift of vaccines that have represented a Copernican Revolution by significantly reducing morbidity and virtually eliminating mortality due to infectious diseases [5].

The evidence that vaccines are fundamental for patients with autoimmune diseases has been recently addressed by a committee of experts of the European League Against Rheumatism (EULAR) [6]. These recommendations state that the initial evaluation of a patient with an autoimmune disease should include the assessment of the vaccination status. Other major recommendations include that vaccination should ideally be administered during stable disease, that influenza vaccination and pneumococcal vaccination should be strongly considered for patients with autoimmune rheumatic diseases, that vaccination can be administered during the use of DMARDs and anti-TNF agents but preferably before starting B cell–depleting therapy, and that attenuated live vaccines and BCG vaccination should be avoided whenever possible especially in immunosuppressed patients [7]. Because infections can trigger autoimmunity and may elicit a flare of an autoimmune disease, their prevention can reduce the incidence of the diseases as well as diseases flare-ups.

In some instance, vaccine effect differs because of the genetic background of the recipient individual. Thus, the vaccination schedule would be better if personalized. Thomas et al. have revised this issue gathering a number of examples of genotype/gene polymorphisms mainly in the human leukocyte antigen (HLA) gene family, related to interindividual variation to vaccination [8].

Thus, we will discuss that vaccines and adjuvants may possibly act as triggers of autoimmune diseases in uniquely predisposed and susceptible individuals and report examples of autoimmune diseases induced by diverse vaccines either in clinical reports or experimental animal models. Our hope is that this information would help in advancing the research in the field, which, if properly implemented from a practical standpoint, could pave the way for the introduction of personalized medicine within the context of vaccination practices, considering individual-specific susceptibility factors (the so-called "personalized vaccinology").

The development of autoimmune diseases is a conundrum. In the book authored by Shoenfeld et al., in 1989 [9], entitled "The Mosaic of Autoimmunity," the factors that may contribute to the development of a specific autoimmune disease in an individual were classified into four categories, namely, genetic factors, immune system dysregulation (complement system disorders, T cells dysfunction, etc.), hormonal factors (estrogen, progesterone, prolactin, vitamin D), and environmental factors [10,11], including viral and bacterial infections, UV exposure, and stress, among others. Furthermore, to develop an autoimmune disease, there needs to be an interplay or combination of these four categories of factors. For example, a single environmental trigger is unlikely to precipitate the development of autoimmunity in the absence of genetic predispositions. The wide diversity of these factors may also explain the presence of a large and heterogeneous group of 81 autoimmune diseases [12]. Additionally, the complexity and wide spectrum of possible interactions between susceptibility

Mosaic of Autoimmunity. https://doi.org/10.1016/B978-0-12-814307-0.00029-3

factors also explains why an individual may have more than one autoimmune disease. Thirty years' after "The Mosaic of Autoimmunity," additional important environmental factors were described, including dietary factors (salt, spicy food-protective factor) [13] and obesity [14]. The genetic predisposition plays a pivotal role in all autoimmune diseases, as genetically predisposed individuals possess a very active immune system. It is possible to identify such individuals with a genetic predisposition to autoimmune diseases by the recognition of specific haplotypes of the HLA system [15]. Diverse HLA haplotypes have been described to be linked to the development of autoimmune diseases including (HLA-DRB1) [15], (HLA-DQB1) [16], (HLA-DRB1*07) [4], and several others. Female subjects are also at a higher risk for developing an autoimmune disease, sex hormones having a crucial role in this, with estrogens being a potent stimulators of autoimmunity and androgens playing a protective role [17]. Accumulating evidence further indicates that genetic, epigenetic, and environmental factors may also contribute to sex-related differences both in the risk and clinical course of autoimmune disease [17–20].

Moreover, pregnancy and postpartum periods are linked to autoimmune diseases, characterized by immune–endocrine imbalances, which occur to achieve immunosuppression and tolerance by the immune system to paternal and fetal antigens. These conditions may exacerbate some autoimmune disease and ameliorate others [21,22]. The impact of estrogens on the immune system is highly significant. Not only natural hormones but also endocrine disruptors, such as environmental estrogens, can act in conjunction with other factors to override immune tolerance to self-antigens [23,24].

Of all, probably the most important environmental factors are infections by microbial and viral agents [25–27]. There are five main mechanisms by which infections can lead to an autoimmune disease [10]. These mechanisms are as follows: (1) molecular mimicry, (2) "epitope spreading," (3) polyclonal activation, (4) viral, and (5) bacterial superantigens that possess the ability to bind to the variable domain of the T cell receptor beta chain. Furthermore, environmental factors that possess an immune adjuvant or immune-potentiating activity such as infectious agents, aluminum, and other adjuvants have been associated with both clinically well-defined and nonspecific immune-mediated manifestations, both in animal models and in humans. These agents with immune adjuvant properties may affect diverse components of the immune system through the innate immune response by the activation of diverse toll-like receptors, the production of uric acid, and other molecules [28].

Adjuvants can be found in most vaccines and are added for the purpose of enhancing the host's immune response to target antigens, and, therefore, genetically predisposed individuals may be at risk for developing an autoimmune disease because of vaccination. Altogether, these factors form the core basis underlying the description of the ASIA syndrome "autoimmune/inflammatory syndrome induced by adjuvants" [29–31], which will be discussed in a specific chapter.

AUTOIMMUNE DISEASES INDUCED BY VACCINATION: CASE REPORTS AND SERIES

The main limits discussing the association between vaccine and autoimmune conditions are that most of the data are case reports or case series, that large epidemiological data tend to exclude a causal association, and that most of the associations are reported within a short time from exposure, while the development of an autoimmune response may require a longer exposure. The first cue of possible insurgence of autoimmune events after vaccination dates to 1979, when a large, high-quality epidemiological survey showed a link between influenza vaccination and the emergence of the Guillain-Barré syndrome (GBS). Although disputed, this link has been replicated in further studies. Since then, the emergence of autoimmune disorders related to immunization practices has been described in many recent case reports and series (Table 29.1).

Zafrir et al. [32] reported a case of a 4-month-old female patient who presented with bullous skin rash, 2 months following her second inoculation with the hepatitis B (HBV) vaccine. In addition, during the appearance of the rash she received a second dose of the hexavalent vaccine (containing diphtheria, tetanus, acellular pertussis-DTaP, HBV, inactivated polio, and *Haemophilus influenzae* b), which was followed by irritability and fever. According to the clinical picture, biopsy result, direct immune fluorescent, and indirect immune fluorescent, a diagnosis of infantile bullous pemphigoid was determined. The patient was resistant to most conventional therapies.

Bizjak et al. [33] reported a case of pancreatitis after vaccination in a 20-year-old man. One week after being vaccinated with the first dose of quadrivalent human papillomavirus (HPV) vaccine, he developed severe abdominal pain. Despite ongoing symptoms of nausea and pain, he received the second dose of the vaccine. Only 10 days later, laboratory results revealed significantly elevated pancreatic enzymes, and, with a concomitant abdominal pain and vomiting, he was diagnosed with acute pancreatitis. This case of acute pancreatitis after HPV vaccination is not a novel entity. Although confirming the relationship between pancreatitis and vaccine is challenging, some factors suggest a possible link, including the positive rechallenge on repeated exposure to the vaccine, HPV vaccine relationship to other autoimmune diseases [34–39], and a probable mechanism of molecular mimicry. With regard to the latter, in conjunction with the aluminum adjuvant, the

TABLE 29.1 Selected Recent Reports of Diverse Autoimmune Diseases Induced by Vaccines

References	Vaccine	Autoimmune Disease	Description
Zafrir et al.	Hepatitis B vaccine (HBV)	Bullous pemphigoid	Case report of a 4-month-old child who developed bullous skin rash, 2 months following her second inoculation with HBV vaccine.
Bizjak et al.	Quadrivalent human papillomavirus (HPV)	Pancreatitis	Case report of a 20-year-old male, who developed nausea and pain 1 week after his first vaccine dose. Despite continuing symptoms he received the second dose and 10 days later, laboratory results revealed significantly elevated pancreatic enzymes and with concomitant abdominal pain and vomiting, he was diagnosed with acute pancreatitis.
Agmon-Levin et al.	HBV	Fibromyalgia, chronic fatigue syndrome	Observational study, 19 patients, all patients fulfilled the ASIA criteria.
Zafrir et al.	HBV	Immuno-mediated diseases	Retrospective 93 patients with neuropsychiatric (70%), fatigue (42%) mucocutaneous (30%), musculoskeletal (59%) and gastrointestinal (50%) complaints, elevated titers of autoantibodies were documented in 80%.
Cheng et al.	Influenza vaccine, which contains the MF59 adjuvant	Myositis and myocarditis	Case report of a 65-year-old previously healthy male who 5 days after the vaccination developed severe rhabdomyolysis. Elevated troponin-I and extensive cardiac investigations enabled the diagnosis of myocarditis.
Dansingani et al.	Quadrivalent HPV	Panuveitis	Case report of a 20-year-old woman, who developed panuveitis and exudative retinal detachments 3 weeks after her second dose of the quadrivalent HPV vaccine.
Anaya et al.	Quadrivalent HPV	ASIA syndrome (enthesitis-related arthritis, and systemic lupus erythematosus [SLE])	Three cases of HLA-B27 enthesitis-related arthritis, rheumatoid arthritis, and SLE. Fulfilled the criteria of ASIA.
Lai et al.	Varicella-zoster	Arthritis, alopecia	A case–control study, patients with zoster vaccination had 2.2 and 2.7 times the odds of developing arthritis and alopecia.
Becker et al.	H1N1	Acute disseminated encephalomyelitis	A case report of an 8-year-old boy, who had fever, headache, and somnolence 12 days after the first dose of vaccine against H1N1 influenza, followed by seizures and coma.
Ruhrman-Shahar et al.	Antitetanus	Dermatomyositis, SLE, type 1 diabetes mellitus, antiphospholipid syndrome	Temporal correlation between vaccination and the induction of the diseases. Other causes were excluded.

induction of immunity through molecular mimicry may potentially culminate in production of cytotoxic autoantibodies with a particular affinity for pancreatic acinar cells. We have reported the association between fibromyalgia, chronic fatigue syndrome (CFS), and HBV vaccination [40]. Nineteen patients with CFS and/or fibromyalgia following HBV vaccine immunization were analyzed. The mean age of the patients was 28.6 ± 11 years, of which 68.4% were female and 21.5% had either personal or familial background of autoimmune disease. The mean latency period from the last dose of HBV vaccine to the onset of the symptoms was 38.6 ± 79.4 days, ranging from days to a year. Eight (42.1%) patients continued with the immunization program despite experiencing adverse events. Manifestations that were commonly reported included neurological manifestations (84.2%), musculoskeletal (78.9%), psychiatric (63.1%), fatigue (63.1%), gastrointestinal complains (58%), and mucocutaneous manifestations (36.8%). Autoantibodies were detected in 71% of patients tested. All patients fulfilled the ASIA syndrome criteria [40].

The link between HBV vaccine and autoimmune disease was also reported by analyzing medical records of 114 patients, from different centers in the United States, diagnosed with immune-mediated diseases following immunization with HBV vaccine [41]. The mean age of 93 patients was 26.5 ± 15 years; 69.2% were female and 21% were considered autoimmune-susceptible. The mean latency period from the last dose of HBV vaccine and onset of symptoms was 43.2 days. Of note, 47% of patients continued with the immunization program despite experiencing adverse events. Manifestations that were commonly reported included neuropsychiatric (70%), fatigue (42%) mucocutaneous (30%), musculoskeletal (59%), and gastrointestinal (50%) complaints. Elevated titers of autoantibodies were documented in 80% of sera tested. In this cohort, 80/93 patients (86%), comprising 57/59 (96%) adults and 23/34 (68%) children, fulfilled the required criteria for ASIA.

Recently, a case report of ASIA syndrome was described in a previously healthy patient who received the seasonal influenza vaccine, which contains the MF59 adjuvant [42]. The patient was presented to the hospital with a profound weakness and was diagnosed with severe rhabdomyolysis. He had elevated troponin-I and extensive cardiac investigations enabled the diagnosis of myocarditis. His infectious and rheumatologic workups were negative. He responded well to conservative management and did not require immune suppressive therapy. He had received the influenza vaccine 5 days prior to the onset of symptoms and fulfilled the criteria of ASIA syndrome. A case of a panuveitis with exudative retinal detachments after vaccination against HPV in a 20-year-old white woman was reported recently [43]. The patient presented with a bilateral acute visual loss (visual acuity: 20/60), panuveitis, and exudative retinal detachments 3 weeks after a second dose of quadrivalent HPV vaccine. She was treated with oral prednisolone for 6 weeks and responded rapidly. By week four, the vision had normalized and the clinical signs have resolved. The association between uveitis and the HPV vaccination has been also reported by Holt et al. [44].

Anaya et al. [45] detailed three cases of patients with ASIA syndrome after quadrivalent HPV vaccination. All the patients were women. Diagnosis consisted of HLA-B27 enthesitis-related arthritis, rheumatoid arthritis (RA), and systemic lupus erythematosus (SLE), respectively. These results highlight the risk of developing ASIA after HPV vaccination and may serve to increase the awareness of such complications.

A case-control study has been performed and reported the association between Zoster vaccine and autoimmunity [46]. Compared with the unexposed subjects, patients with zoster vaccination had 2.2 and 2.7 times the odds of developing arthritis and alopecia, respectively ($P < .001$ and $P = .015$, respectively). A case of an acute disseminated encephalomyelitis was reported in a healthy 8-year-old boy, who had fever, headache, and somnolence 12 days after the first dose of vaccine against influenza H1N1 [47]. Ruhrman-Shahar et al. [48] described four cases with a temporal relation between antitetanus vaccination and the appearance of dermatomyositis, SLE, type 1 diabetes mellitus, and antiphospholipid syndrome. The first case was a 38-year-old man, previously healthy, with no known familial autoimmune disease, who was bitten by a black scorpion and received a booster dose of DTaP.

According to the multicenter, international ASIA Web-based registry, up to December 2016, 300 cases of ASIA syndrome have been described, with a mean age at disease onset of 37 years and a mean duration of time latency between exposure to adjuvant and development of autoimmune conditions of 16.8 months (from 3 days to 5 years). Arthralgia, myalgia, and chronic fatigue were the most frequently reported symptoms. Eighty-nine percent of patients were also diagnosed with another defined and with the most frequent autoimmune disease related to ASIA syndrome being connective tissue disease [49].

AUTOIMMUNE DISEASES INDUCED BY VACCINATION: EPIDEMIOLOGICAL SURVEYS

The emergence of autoimmune disorders after vaccination has been observed in several large, high-quality trials. Dodd and coauthors [50] have computed a relative incidence of GBS of 2.42 (95% confidence interval [CI] or CI 1.58–3.72) in the 42 days following exposure to pH1N1 influenza vaccine in an analysis of pooled data and 2.09 (95% CI 1.28–3.42) when carrying out a metaanalytic approach. Similarly, other collaborative groups have replicated this finding: in Italy by Galeotti and collaborators [51], in the United States by Souayah and coworkers [52], in South Korea by Park and collaborators [53], and in Canada by Juurlink and coauthors [54].

Narcolepsy is another autoimmune disorder documented after 2009 Pandemic H1N1 vaccine. Sarkanen and coauthors [55] recently performed a systematic review and metaanalysis and found a relative risk of narcolepsy related to administration increased 5–14-fold in children and adolescents and 2–7-fold in adults during the first year after vaccination. They computed a vaccine-attributable risk in children and adolescents of 1 per 18,400 vaccine doses.

Donahue and coworkers [56] have computed an overall adjusted odds ratio of 2.0 (95% CI 1.1–3.6) in women who spontaneously aborted and received influenza-containing vaccine in the 28-day exposure window. Chambers and colleagues [57] analyzing data of a study from the cohort arm of the Vaccines and Medications in Pregnancy Surveillance System (VAMPSS) found a moderately elevated relative risk for major birth defects.

ANIMAL MODELS OF AUTOIMMUNE DISEASES INDUCED BY ADJUVANTS

A vaccine-related autoimmune reaction should meet a series of requirements to be actually considered vaccine-induced, including consistency, strength, specificity, and temporal relation [58]. In humans, adjuvants can induce nonspecific constitutional, musculoskeletal, or neurological clinical manifestations and, in certain cases, can lead to the appearance or acceleration of an autoimmune disease in a subject with genetic susceptibility. The link between vaccination and pathogenic immune reactions has been reported in animal models. Inbar et al. [59] assessed the behavioral and inflammatory parameters in female mice after the injection of aluminum and quadrivalent HPV vaccine. The C57BL/6 female mice were injected with qHPV, qHPV + pertussis toxin, aluminum hydroxide, or vehicle control in amounts equivalent to human exposure. The qHPV and aluminum-injected mice spent significantly more time floating in the forced swimming test in comparison to vehicle-injected mice (aluminum, $P=.009$; qHPV, $P=.025$; qHPV + pertussis toxin, $P=.005$). No significant differences were observed in the number of stairs climbed in the staircase test, which measures locomotor activity. This suggests that the abnormality observed in the forced swimming test was unlikely because of locomotor dysfunction, but rather because of depression.

Other research in animal models showing toxicity of adjuvant compounds includes the work of Favoino et al. [60], who assessed the effect of diverse adjuvants (incomplete Freund's adjuvant, complete Freund's adjuvant, squalene, or aluminum hydroxide) in lupus-prone New Zealand black/New Zealand white (BW)F1 mice. In the aluminum group, weight decreased by almost half between weeks 29 and 31, indicating some toxic effect of aluminum in the late postimmunization period. Squalene was the least toxic adjuvant as it did not accelerate proteinuria onset compared with incomplete Freund's adjuvant. Similarly, squalene did not induce toxicity compared with aluminum or elicit anti-RNP/Sm autoantibody as observed in the complete Freund's adjuvant group. Quiroz-Rothe et al. [61] described a case of postvaccination polyneuropathy resembling human GBS in a Rottweiler dog. The dog suffered of two separated episodes of acute polyneuropathy after receiving two vaccines (both adjuvanted). Inactivated rabies vaccine was administered 15 days before clinical signs were first noted. Clinical remission was achieved with steroid therapy; however, 3 months later the dog had recurrence of polyneuropathy, following another vaccination administered 12 days earlier. The presence of antibodies against peripheral nerve myelin was demonstrated.

Agmon-Levin et al. [62] examined the effects of immunization with HBV vaccine and aluminum on SLE-like disease in a murine model. NZBWF1 mice were immunized with HBV vaccine or aluminum hydroxide or phosphate-buffered saline (PBS) at 8 and 12 weeks of age. Mice were followed for weight, autoantibodies titers, blood counts, proteinuria, kidney histology, neurocognitive functions (novel object recognition, staircase, Y-maze, and the forced swimming tests), and brain histology. Immunization with HBV vaccine induced acceleration of kidney disease manifested by high anti-dsDNA antibodies ($P<.01$), early onset of proteinuria ($P<.05$), histological damage, and deposition of HBs antigen in the kidney. Mice immunized with HBV vaccine and/or aluminum had decreased cells counts mainly of the red cell lineage ($P<.001$), memory deficits ($P<.01$), and increased activated microglia in different areas of the brain in comparison with mice immunized with PBS. Anxiety-like behavior was more pronounced among mice immunized with aluminum.

Aratani and collaborators [63], in a model of mice vaccinated with HPV and pertussis toxin, reported low responsiveness of the tail reflex and locomotive mobility because of apoptotic damage affecting the hypothalamus and circumventricular regions around the third ventricle.

In summary, animal models are often used to study the relation between autoimmune, inflammatory diseases, and diverse triggers [28]. These are broadly classified as either spontaneous, where an animal's genetic background results in a defined prevalence of disease, or induced, where disease is precipitated by exposure to defined antigens, adjuvants, or other experimental reagents [28]. Experimentally animal models of autoimmune diseases induced by adjuvants are currently widely used to understand the mechanisms and etiology and pathogenesis of these diseases and might thus promote the development of new diagnostic, predictive, and therapeutic methods.

THE CONCEPT OF PERSONALIZED VACCINOLOGY

Vaccination is a pivotal tool to prevent serious infections. In some cases vaccination may lead to adverse events. These are classified in local and systemic events such as allergy, fever, and possibly autoimmune diseases in genetically predisposed individuals [64]. It is important to highlight the fact that a temporal relationship between the induction of an autoimmune phenomenon and a specific vaccine is not always notable. Moreover, a specific vaccine may cause more than one autoimmune disease [65]; likewise, a particular immune process may be induced by diverse vaccines [3]. It is essential to recognize individuals with high risk and prone to develop autoimmunity before the exposure to diverse adjuvants through routine vaccinations. Soriano et al. [66] classified four groups of individuals in which vaccination may represent a risk factor for the induction of autoimmune phenomena. These groups include the following: (1) individuals with prior postvaccination autoimmune phenomena; (2) persons with a medical history of autoimmunity; (3) individuals with a history of allergic reactions (especially vaccination-related reactions); and (4) individuals who are prone to develop autoimmunity (having a family history of autoimmune diseases and presence of specific autoimmune disease markers such as elevated autoantibodies, certain genetic profiles, etc.). The HLA genes encode mostly immune-associated proteins whose main effect is the presentation of antigens to the immune cells. As such, HLA-related protein products are essential for the proper function of the immune response against pathogens; however, their variants are also strongly implicated in the development of autoimmune diseases [66], likewise, the positive correlation between SLE and the allotypes DR2 and DR3 of HLA class II [67], RA and HLA-DRB1 [68], and several others.

In conclusion, physicians should be aware of the rare but possible adverse events to vaccinations, especially not only in cases with previous postvaccination phenomena and those with allergies but also in individuals who might be more prone to develop autoimmune diseases, due to a family history of autoimmune diseases, presence of specific HLA haplotypes and/ or autoantibodies, and other risk factors for autoimmunity (smoking, obesity, etc.).

Factors that are predictive of developing autoimmune diseases should be examined at the population level to establish preventive measures in at-risk individuals for whom health care should be personalized.

We do not stress enough that nowadays the benefits of vaccination overweight its potential risks.

Surely, big data–based epidemiological surveys, metaanalytical approaches, and omics-based studies (exploiting, for instance, new cutting edge high-throughput technologies, such as "adversomics," that is to say the systematic, holistic, data-driven "study of vaccine adverse reactions using immunogenomics and systems biology approaches") [69] can pave the way toward personalized vaccinology.

REFERENCES

[1] Doria A, Canova M, Tonon M, Zen M, Rampudda E, Bassi N, et al. Infections as triggers and complications of systemic lupus erythematosus. Autoimmun Rev 2008;8:24–8.

[2] Perricone C, Versini M, Ben-Ami D, Gertel S, Watad A, Segel MJ, et al. Smoke and autoimmunity: the fire behind the disease. Autoimmun Rev 2016;15:354–74.

[3] Perricone C, Colafrancesco S, Mazor RD, Soriano A, Agmon-Levin N, Shoenfeld Y. Autoimmune/inflammatory syndrome induced by adjuvants (ASIA) 2013: unveiling the pathogenic, clinical and diagnostic aspects. J Autoimmun 2013;47:1–16.

[4] Gutierrez-Arcelus M, Rich SS, Raychaudhuri S. Autoimmune diseases — connecting risk alleles with molecular traits of the immune system. Nat Rev Genet 2016;17:160–74.

[5] Meroni PL, Zavaglia D, Girmenia C. Vaccinations in adults with rheumatoid arthritis in an era of new disease-modifying anti-rheumatic drugs. Clin Exp Rheumatol 2018 Mar-Apr;36(2):317–28.

[6] van Assen S, Agmon-Levin N, Elkayam O, Cervera R, Doran MF, Dougados M, et al. EULAR recommendations for vaccination in adult patients with autoimmune inflammatory rheumatic diseases. Ann Rheum Dis 2011;70:414–22.

[7] Lopez A, Mariette X, Bachelez H, Belot A, Bonnotte B, Hachulla E, Lahfa M, Lortholary O, Loulergue P, Paul S, Roblin X, Sibilia J, Blum M, Danese S, Bonovas S, Peyrin-Biroulet L. Vaccination recommendations for the adult immunosuppressed patient: a systematic review and comprehensive field synopsis. J Autoimmun June 2017;80:10–27. https://doi.org/10.1016/j.jaut.2017.03.011.

[8] Thomas C, Moridani M. Interindividual variations in the efficacy and toxicity of vaccines. Toxicology 2010;278:204–10.

[9] Shoenfeld Y, Isenberg DA. The mosaic of autoimmunity. (English). Holland: Elsevier; 1989. p. 523.

[10] Shoenfeld Y, Zandman-Goddard G, Stojanovich L, Cutolo M, Amital H, Levy Y, et al. The mosaic of autoimmunity: hormonal and environmental factors involved in autoimmune diseases - 2008. Isr Med Assoc J 2008;10:8–12.

[11] Shoenfeld Y, Blank M, Abu-Shakra M, Amital H, Barzilai O, Berkun Y, et al. The mosaic of autoimmunity: prediction, autoantibodies, and therapy in autoimmune diseases - 2008. Isr Med Assoc J 2008;10:13–9.

[12] Hayter SM, Cook MC. Updated assessment of the prevalence, spectrum and case definition of autoimmune disease. Autoimmun Rev 2012;11:754–65.

[13] Deng Y, Huang X, Wu H, Zhao M, Lu Q, Israeli E, et al. Some like it hot: the emerging role of spicy food (capsaicin) in autoimmune diseases. Autoimmun Rev 2016;1–6.

[14] Versini M, Jeandel PY, Rosenthal E, Shoenfeld Y. Obesity in autoimmune diseases: not a passive bystander. Autoimmun Rev 2014;13:981–1000.

[15] Arango M-T, Perricone C, Kivity S, Cipriano E, Ceccarelli F, Valesini G, et al. HLA-DRB1 the notorious gene in the mosaic of autoimmunity. Immunol Res 2016;1–17.

[16] Singh AK, Mahlios J, Mignot E. Genetic association, seasonal infections and autoimmune basis of narcolepsy. J Autoimmun 2013;43:26–31.

[17] Dinesh RK, Hahn BH, Singh RP. PD-1, gender, and autoimmunity. Autoimmun Rev 2010;9:583–7.

[18] Bozzuto G, Paola Ruggieri AM. Molecular aspects of tumor cell migration and invasion. Ann Ist Super Sanita 2010;46:66–80.

[19] Whitacre CC. Sex differences in autoimmune disease. Nat Immunol 2001;2:777–80.

[20] Watad A, Versini M, Jeandel PY, Amital H, Shoenfeld Y. Treating prolactinoma can prevent autoimmune diseases. Cell Immunol 2015;294:84–6.

[21] Borchers AT, Naguwa SM, Keen CL, Gershwin ME. The implications of autoimmunity and pregnancy. J Autoimmun 2010;34.

[22] Pludowski P, Holick MF, Pilz S, Wagner CL, Hollis BW, Grant WB, et al. Vitamin D effects on musculoskeletal health, immunity, autoimmunity, cardiovascular disease, cancer, fertility, pregnancy, dementia and mortality—a review of recent evidence. Autoimmun Rev 2013;12:976–89.

[23] Orbach H, Shoenfeld Y. Hyperprolactinemia and autoimmune diseases. Autoimmun Rev 2007;6:537–42.

[24] Lateef A, Petri M. Hormone replacement and contraceptive therapy in autoimmune diseases. J Autoimmun 2012;38.

[25] Dreyfus DH. Autoimmune disease: a role for new anti-viral therapies? Autoimmun Rev 2011;11:88–97.

[26] Kallenberg CGM, Tadema H. Vasculitis and infections: contribution to the issue of autoimmunity reviews devoted to "autoimmunity and infection". Autoimmun Rev 2008;8:29–32.

[27] Kivity S, Arango MT, Ehrenfeld M, Tehori O, Shoenfeld Y, Anaya JM, et al. Infection and autoimmunity in Sjogren's syndrome: a clinical study and comprehensive review. J Autoimmun 2014;51:17–22.

[28] Shoenfeld Y, Agmon-Levin N. "ASIA" - autoimmune/inflammatory syndrome induced by adjuvants. J Autoimmun 2011;36:4–8.

[29] Colafrancesco S, Perricone C, Shoenfeld Y. Autoimmune/inflammatory syndrome induced by adjuvants and sjögren's syndrome. Isr Med Assoc J 2016;18:150–3.

[30] Meroni PL. Autoimmune or auto-inflammatory syndrome induced by adjuvants (ASIA): old truths and a new syndrome? J Autoimmun 2011;36:1–3.

[31] Luján L, Pérez M, Salazar E, Álvarez N, Gimeno M, Pinczowski P, et al. Autoimmune/autoinflammatory syndrome induced by adjuvants (ASIA syndrome) in commercial sheep. Immunol Res 2013;56:317–24.

[32] Zafrir Y, Zvulunov A, Shoenfeld Y. Infantile bullous pemphigoid following hepatitis B vaccinations. Immunome Res 2014;10.

[33] Bizjak M, Bruck O, Praprotnik S, Dahan S, Shoenfeld Y. Pancreatitis after human papillomavirus vaccination: a matter of molecular mimicry. Immunol Res 2016 [Epub ahead of print].

[34] Pellegrino P, Carnovale C, Pozzi M, Antoniazzi S, Perrone V, Salvati D, et al. On the relationship between human papilloma virus vaccine and autoimmune diseases. Autoimmun Rev 2014;13:736–41.

[35] Baker B, Eça Guimarães L, Tomljenovic L, Agmon-Levin N, Shoenfeld Y. The safety of human papilloma virus-blockers and the risk of triggering autoimmune diseases. Expert Opin Drug Saf 2015;14:1387–94.

[36] Sutton I, Lahoria R, Tan I, Clouston P, Barnett M. CNS demyelination and quadrivalent HPV vaccination. Mult Scler 2009;15:116–9.

[37] Palmieri B, Poddighe D, Vadalà M, Laurino C, Carnovale C, Clementi E. Severe somatoform and dysautonomic syndromes after HPV vaccination: case series and review of literature. Immunol Res 2016:1–11.

[38] Chang J, Campagnolo D, Vollmer L, Bomprezzi R. Demyelinating disease and polyvalent human papilloma virus vaccination. J Neurol Neurosurg Psychiatry 2011;82:1296–8.

[39] Colafrancesco S, Perricone C, Tomljenovic L, Shoenfeld Y. Human papilloma virus vaccine and primary ovarian failure: another facet of the autoimmune/inflammatory syndrome induced by adjuvants. Am J Reprod Immunol 2013;70:309–16.

[40] Agmon-Levin N, Zafrir Y, Kivity S, Balofsky A, Amital H, Shoenfeld Y. Chronic fatigue syndrome and fibromyalgia following immunization with the hepatitis B vaccine: another angle of the autoimmune (auto-inflammatory) syndrome induced by adjuvants (ASIA). Immunol Res 2014;60:376–83.

[41] Zafrir Y, Agmon-Levin N, Paz Z, Shilton T, Shoenfeld Y. Autoimmunity following Hepatitis B vaccine as part of the spectrum of "Autoimmune (Auto-inflammatory) Syndrome induced by Adjuvants" (ASIA): analysis of 93 cases. Lupus 2012;21:146–52.

[42] Cheng MP, Kozoriz MG, Ahmadi AA, Kelsall J, Paquette K, Onrot JM. Post-vaccination myositis and myocarditis in a previously healthy male. Allergy Asthma Clin Immunol 2016;12:6.

[43] Dansingani KK, Suzuki M, Naysan J, Samson CM, Spaide RF, Fisher YL. Panuveitis with exudative retinal detachments after vaccination against human papilloma virus. Ophthalmic Surg Lasers Imaging Retin 2015;46:967–70.

[44] Holt HD, Hinkle DM, Falk NS, Fraunfelder FT, Fraunfelder FW. Human papilloma virus vaccine associated uveitis. Curr Drug Saf 2014;9:65–8.

[45] Anaya JM, Reyes B, Perdomo-Arciniegas AM, Camacho-Rodríguez B, Rojas-Villarraga A. Autoimmune/autoinflammatory syndrome induced by adjuvants (ASIA) after quadrivalent human papillomavirus vaccination in Colombians: a call for personalised medicine. Clin Exp Rheumatol 2015;33:545–8.

[46] Lai YC, Yew YW. Severe autoimmune adverse events post herpes zoster vaccine: a case-control study of adverse events in a national database. J Drugs Dermatol 2015;14:681–4.

[47] Becker MM, Ranzan J, Magalhães LV, Ohlweiler L, Winckler MI, Ramos MS, et al. Post-H1N1 vaccine acute disseminated encephalomyelitis. Pediatr Int 2014;56:437–8.

[48] Ruhrman-Shahar N, Torres-Ruiz J, Rotman-Pikielny P, Levy Y. Autoimmune reaction after anti-tetanus vaccination---description of four cases and review of the literature. Immunol Res 2016;1–7.

[49] Watad A, Quaresma M, Bragazzi NL, Cervera R, Tervaert JWC, Amital H, et al. The autoimmune/inflammatory syndrome induced by adjuvants (ASIA)/Shoenfeld's syndrome: descriptive analysis of 300 patients from the international ASIA syndrome registry. Clin Rheumatol Feb 2018;37(2):483–93.

[50] Dodd CN, Romio SA, Black S, Vellozzi C, Andrews N, Sturkenboom M, et al. International collaboration to assess the risk of Guillain Barré Syndrome following Influenza A (H1N1) 2009 monovalent vaccines. Vaccine 2013;31(40):4448–58. 6.

[51] Galeotti F, Massari M, D'Alessandro R, Beghi E, Chiò A, Logroscino G, et al. Risk of Guillain-Barré syndrome after 2010–2011 influenza vaccination. Eur J Epidemiol 2013;28(5):433–44.

[52] Souayah N, Michas-Martin PA, Nasar A, Krivitskaya N, Yacoub HA, Khan H, et al. Guillain-barre syndrome after gardasil vaccination: data from vaccine adverse event reporting system 2006-2009. Vaccine 2011;29(5):886–9.

[53] Park Y-S, Lee K-J, Kim SW, Kim KM, Suh BC. Clinical features of post-vaccination Guillain-Barré syndrome (GBS) in Korea. J Kor Med Sci 2017;32(7):1154.

[54] Juurlink DN, Stukel TA, Kwong J, Kopp A, McGeer A, Upshur RE, et al. Guillain-Barre syndrome after influenza vaccination in adults: a population-based study. Arch Intern Med 2006;166(20):2217–21.

[55] Sarkanen TO, Alakuijala APE, Dauvilliers YA, Partinen MM. Incidence of narcolepsy after H1N1 influenza and vaccinations: systematic review and meta-analysis. Sleep Med Rev Apr 2018;38:177–86.

[56] Donahue JG, Kieke BA, King JP, DeStefano F, Mascola MA, Irving SA, et al. Association of spontaneous abortion with receipt of inactivated influenza vaccine containing H1N1pdm09 in 2010-11 and 2011-12. Vaccine 2017;35(40):5314–22.

[57] Chambers CD, Johnson D, Xu R, Luo Y, Louik C, Mitchell AA, et al. Risks and safety of pandemic h1n1 influenza vaccine in pregnancy: birth defects, spontaneous abortion, preterm delivery, and small for gestational age infants. Vaccine 2013;31(44):5026–32.

[58] Salemi S, D'Amelio R. Could autoimmunity be induced by vaccination? Int Rev Immunol 2010;29:247–69.

[59] Inbar R, Weiss R, Tomljenovic L, Arango M-T, Deri Y, Shaw CA, et al. Behavioral abnormalities in female mice following administration of aluminum adjuvants and the human papillomavirus (HPV) vaccine Gardasil. Immunol Res 2016;1–14.

[60] Favoino E, Favia EI, Digiglio L, Racanelli V, Shoenfeld Y, Perosa F. Effects of adjuvants for human use in systemic lupus erythematosus (SLE)-prone (New Zealand black/New Zealand white) F(1) mice. Clin Exp Immunol 2014;175:32–40.

[61] Quiroz-Rothe E, Ginel PJ, Perez J, Lucena R, Rivero JLL. Vaccine-associated acute polyneuropathy resembling Guillain-Barré syndrome in a dog. Eur J Companion Anim Pr 2005;15(2):155–9.

[62] Agmon-Levin N, Arango MT, Kivity S, Katzav A, Gilburd B, Blank M, et al. Immunization with hepatitis B vaccine accelerates SLE-like disease in a murine model. J Autoimmun 2014;54:21–32.

[63] Aratani S, Fujita H, Kuroiwa Y, Usui C, Yokota S, Nakamura I, et al. Murine hypothalamic destruction with vascular cell apoptosis subsequent to combined administration of human papilloma virus vaccine and pertussis toxin. Sci Rep November 11, 2016;6:36943.

[64] Cruz-Tapias P, Agmon-Levin N, Israeli E, Anaya J-M, Shoenfeld Y. Autoimmune (auto-inflammatory) syndrome induced by adjuvants (ASIA)--animal models as a proof of concept. Curr Med Chem 2013;20:4030–6.

[65] Soriano A, Nesher G, Shoenfeld Y. Predicting post-vaccination autoimmunity: who might be at risk? Pharmacol Res 2015;92:18–22.

[66] Shoenfeld Y, Agmon-Levin N, Tomljenovic L. Vaccines and autoimmunity. 1st ed. New Jersey: Wiley-Blackwell; 2015.

[67] Relle M, Weinmann-Menke J, Scorletti E, Cavagna L, Schwarting A. Genetics and novel aspects of therapies in systemic lupus erythematosus. Autoimmun Rev 2015;14:1005–18.

[68] Perricone C, Ceccarelli F, Valesini G. An overview on the genetic of rheumatoid arthritis: a never-ending story. Autoimmun Rev 2011;10:599–608.

[69] Whitaker JA, Ovsyannikova IG, Poland GA. Adversomics: a new paradigm for vaccine safety and design. Expert Rev Vaccines July 2015;14(7):935–47.

Chapter 30

Silicone

Jan Willem Cohen Tervaert[1,2]
[1]Division of Rheumatology, University of Alberta, Edmonton, Canada; [2]Maastricht University, Maastricht, The Netherlands

INTRODUCTION

A genetic predisposition has been found to be a prerequisite to develop immune-mediated diseases. Importantly, environmental factors have been shown to play a pivotal role in the pathogenesis of these diseases and various environmental factors have been linked to these immune-mediated diseases. Well-studied examples are infections, smoking, vaccines, silica, and silicones.

Silicones are used in a variety of medical applications such as breast implants, hydrocephalus shunts, catheter lines, intraocular implants, rhinoplasty, hearing aids, laryngotracheal stenosis and various other stents, joint implants, testicular prosthesis, and others. Silicones were introduced in the 60s and were thought to be biologically inert. However, during the last 50 years it became clear that silicones can induce various immunological effects.

Silicone-related complications may occur with all silicone-containing medical devices. During the last 50 years, however, the safety of silicones caused a polarized debate especially in the field of plastic surgery. In this chapter, silicone-induced immune-mediated effects will be reviewed with a focus on silicone breast implants (SBIs).

SILICONE BREAST IMPLANTS

The first SBIs were performed by Cronin and Gerow in 1962 [1]. Silicone gel was wrapped in an impermeable silicone envelope developed by Dow Corning. The SBI implantation procedure was considered a success and since then millions of women received SBI either as a cosmetic procedure or because of postmastectomy reconstruction. Silicon is the basic element of silicones, a family of synthetic polymers with a backbone of repeated Si–O units. Silicones vary in their composition. The longer the side chain and the more cross-links between the side chains, the more solid is the resulting silicone. Therefore, silicones can have the consistency of fluid, oil, gel, or rubber. Polydimethylsiloxane is the polymer used for the mammary prosthetic devices.

In the year 2018, more than one million breast augmentation procedures are performed worldwide. Back in the 1960s, local and distant complications of the SBI procedure were reported. Local complications of SBI are pain, swelling, redness, infections, capsular contracture, implant rupture, and gel bleeding through the intact capsule. Furthermore, general complications occur. In the first case reports, women were described as having developed arthralgias, fatigue, and sometimes an autoimmune disease [2–5]. During the last 50 years, hundreds of patients are reported with similar symptoms and signs [6]. Both patients and doctors suspect that these complaints are caused by the implants. Indeed, removal of the SBI results in an amelioration of symptoms in 60%–80% of the patients [7].

SYMPTOMS AND SIGNS OF SILICONE-MEDIATED DISEASE

Typically, patients with general symptoms that might be related to SBI present with chronic fatigue. Patients are already tired when they wake up, whereas the fatigue is not alleviated by rest. Patients have a substantial reduction in the ability to engage preillness levels of occupational, educational, social, and/or personal activities. Importantly, most patients report postexertional malaise, also referred to as a symptom flare or "crash," which occurs following physical or cognitive exertion and can last from days to weeks. Sleep disturbances such as problems falling asleep and/or staying asleep are often present. Poor sleep quality is linked to greater fatigue. Probably also related to poor sleep quality are the symptoms of cognitive impairment resulting in memory deficits ("Alzheimer-light"), absent-mindedness, word finding difficulties, and difficulty paying attention.

Mosaic of Autoimmunity. https://doi.org/10.1016/B978-0-12-814307-0.00030-X

TABLE 30.1 Fibromyalgia 2016 Criteria

Criteria

A patient satisfies modified 2016 fibromyalgia criteria if the following conditions are met:
1. Widespread pain index (WPI)≥7 and symptom severity scale (SSS) score≥5 OR WPI of 4–6 and SSS score≥9
2. Generalized pain, defined as pain in at least 4 of 5 regions, must be present. Jaw, chest, and abdominal pain are not included in generalized pain definition
3. Symptoms must have been present for at least 3 months
4. A diagnosis of fibromyalgia is valid irrespective of other diagnoses. A diagnosis of fibromyalgia does not exclude the presence of other clinically important illnesses

Notes
1. WPI: note the number of areas in which the patient has had pain over the last week. In how many areas has the patient had pain? Score will be between 0 and 19
2. SSS score
   Fatigue
   Waking unrefreshed
   Cognitive symptoms

For the each of the three symptoms above, the level of severity over the past week using the following scale is indicated:
   0=No problem
   1=Slight or mild problems: generally mild or intermittent
   2=Moderate: considerable problems, often present, and/or at a moderate level
   3=Severe: pervasive, continuous, life-disturbing problems

The SSS score is the sum of the severity scores of the three symptoms (fatigue, waking unrefreshed, and cognitive symptoms) (0–9) plus the sum (0–3) of the number of the following symptoms the patient has been bothered by that occurred during the previous 6 months:
1. Headaches (0–1)
2. Pain or cramps in lower abdomen (0–1)
3. Depression (0–1)

The final SSS is between 0 and 12.

Another early symptom is the occurrence of arthralgia or arthritis, which is present in more than 90% of the patients. Most patients fulfill the 2016 criteria for fibromyalgia (see Table 30.1) [8]. Patients suffer from morning stiffness, which sometimes may last more than an hour. Occasionally, however, patients present with (symmetric) polyarthritis compatible with a diagnosis of rheumatoid arthritis [9,10].

In addition, up to 90% of the patients have myalgia and/or muscle weakness. Weakness can be severe and may render the patient to be bedridden. In one study, an EMG was performed in 93 patients. The EMG was abnormal in 53% of the patients [11]. Most often, a "myopathic" pattern was found in these patients [11].

Furthermore, two-third of the patients report pyrexia, whereas night sweats are common. Some patients additionally have strongly elevated ferritin levels and fulfill the diagnostic criteria for (silicone-induced) Still's disease [12].

Importantly, 75% of patients have dry eyes and/or a dry mouth. Symptoms of the dry eyes are often severe and may result in blurred vision and/or keratitis sicca if left untreated. Anti-Sjögren's-syndrome-related *antigen* A (SSA)/Anti-Sjögren's-syndrome-related *antigen* B (SSB) antibodies are only present in a minority of patients [5], whereas salivary gland biopsies disclose mononuclear cell infiltrates different from what can be found in Sjogren's syndrome [13,14].

30%–50% of the patients develop new-onset Raynaud's phenomenon sometimes with nailfold abnormalities as demonstrated by capillaroscopy suggestive of systemic sclerosis [15].

Another important manifestation that is present in 30%–40% of patients is the occurrence of severe neurological manifestations such as ischemic cerebral disease, multiple sclerosis-like syndrome, or amyotrophic lateral sclerosis-like disease [5,11,16]. In patients with ischemic cerebral disease, anticardiolipin antibodies and/or lupus anticoagulant is detected in only a minority of the patients, whereas traditional risk factors for cerebrovascular accident (CVA) are often lacking as well.

Allergies are reported in 50%–80% of the patients [17]. In most patients, these allergies are preexistent. In many cases, however, the patients report that allergic complaints had disappeared before the SBI operation and returned thereafter. Allergic complaints include sneezing, itching of the nose and eyes, red eyes, rhinorrhea, nasal congestion, and postnasal drip. Furthermore, asthmatic patients may suffer from cough, wheeze, and shortness of breath. Food allergies also occur and about 10%–20% of the patients develop new-onset urticaria and/or Quincke's edema. A remarkable frequent finding (about 50% of patients) is metal allergy with nickel-induced dermatitis. Furthermore, some patients present with episodic symptoms suggesting a diagnosis of mast cell activation syndrome [18,19]. Finally, some patients present with a multiple chemical sensitivity syndrome [20]. Dyspnea in SBI patients can be a result of severe asthma, pulmonary nodules, interstitial lung disease, and/or pulmonary silicone embolism [21–23]. Furthermore, 20%–40% of patients suffer from severe and/or recurrent (upper respiratory tract) infections.

Breast pain, tenderness, and burning sensations are occasionally present. In addition, changes in breast shape, breast asymmetry, firmness of the breasts, and breast enlargement may be noticed. Lymph nodes (axillary, cervical, and inguinal) are often enlarged and tender (70%–80% of patients).

Cardiovascular complaints include signs of orthostatic intolerance such as dizziness, disturbed balance, irregular heartbeat, and sometimes chest pain. A mitral valve prolapse and/or joint hypermobility is found in about half of the patients [24].

20%–40% of patients suffer from gastrointestinal symptoms such as abdominal pain with changes in bowel movement patterns such as found in irritable bowel syndrome. Swallowing difficulties and/or dysphagia are in most cases related to the sicca complaints.

A substantial amount of patients (10%–20%) have interstitial cystitis. These patients suffer from chronic pain localized to the pelvic organs, pelvic floor myofascial support, or external genitalia often accompanied by urinary symptoms, such as urgency or frequency.

The skin may be painful and burning sensations ("pins and needles") suggest that (atypical) small fiber neuropathy is present [25]. A prominent livedo reticularis can be found in about 20%–30% of patients, whereas mild livedo reticularis is present in another 30%–40% of patients. Occasionally, tender subcutaneous nodules can be observed in the arms, legs, abdominal wall, and/or elsewhere in the body. Histologically, these nodules demonstrate granulomatous inflammation (i.e., migratory silicone granulomas) [22,26]. Finally, 20%–40% of patients have ill-defined skin rashes, unexplained (sometimes severe) pruritus, and/or alopecia.

LABORATORY AND RADIOLOGICAL FINDINGS AND OTHER DIAGNOSTIC PROCEDURES IN SILICONE-INDUCED DISEASE

Laboratory findings are often nonspecific. Generally, C-reactive protein (CRP) levels are normal. Angiotensin-converting enzyme and soluble interleukin-2 receptor levels are, however, in up to 50% of patients elevated. Antinuclear antibodies are present in 20% of patients, whereas various other antibodies such as SSA/SSB, anti-dsDNA, anti-Scl-70, anticardiolipin, anti-CCP, IgM-rheumatoid factor, antineutrophil cytoplasmic antibodies, and/or cryoglobulins may be found [5,6]. Furthermore, antipolymer antibodies have been described, but their diagnostic value is at present uncertain [27]. Vitamin D insufficiency and/or deficiency is a frequent finding and 20%–50% of patients have decreased levels of IgG and/or IgG subclasses [5,6].

Magnetic resonance is the examination of choice for evaluating breast implants to detect ruptures. The risk of an SBI rupture increases with implant age. While in the past about 50% of SBIs ruptured after a mean follow-up of 10 years, the risk of modern implants to rupture has been estimated to be 15% after a follow-up of 3–10 years [15]. Rupture rates of SBI made by the French manufacturer Poly Implant Protheses (PIP) are, however, much higher than that of SBIs made by other manufacturers. Mammograms are relatively contraindicated in patients with SBI because compression may induce and/or exacerbate (intracapsular) ruptures [15]. Apart from ruptures, also capsular contractures, seromas, anaplastic large cell lymphoma (ALCL), and silicone-induced granuloma of the breast can be detected by MRI [28]. Furthermore, silicone-containing granulomas in lymph nodes can be detected by MRI. The method of choice to detect this silicone lymphadenopathy is, however, ultrasonographic examination which shows a typical "snowstorm sign" [29].

There are several other diagnostic procedures to objectify the complaints of the patients. These other procedures are, however, nonspecific. Examples are a cardiopulmonary exercise test by cycling till maximal exertion, which is repeated after 24 h to objectify the postexertional malaise [30], overnight polysomnography to ascertain objectively poor sleep quality, capillaroscopy to detect nailfold abnormalities [15], a skin biopsy showing reduced intraepidermal nerve fiber density and/or abnormal temperature threshold testing to confirm small fiber neuropathy [25], and/or ocular surface evaluation including Schirmer testing, tear breakup time, and staining of the cornea and conjunctiva to confirm the impaired tear production. Furthermore, histological examinations of explanted SBI and lymph nodes may confirm granulomatous silicone inflammation and labial salivary gland biopsies may confirm mild lymphocytic infiltration differentiating silicone-induced sicca symptoms from Sjogren's syndrome [14]. Finally, to confirm a diagnosis of ALCL, ultrasonography with fluid aspiration can be used.

ASIA, AUTOIMMUNE DISEASES, AND ALCL

The symptoms described above received during the last 50 years several different names: human adjuvant disease, siliconosis, silicone incompatibility syndrome, silicone-induced toxicity, and, more recently, autoimmune/inflammatory syndrome induced by adjuvants (ASIA) [6,31,32] (Table 30.2). Others, however, state that these patients do not suffer from a separate disease but are merely suffering from idiopathic chronic fatigue syndrome (CFS/ME), fibromyalgia, or mass somatization [33–35].

We hypothesize that as a consequence of the immune activation, ASIA, allergies, autoantibodies, autoimmune diseases, IgG, and/or IgG subclass deficiencies and finally lymphomas may develop.

ASIA was firstly described by Shoenfeld and Agmon-Levin is 2011. This syndrome assembles a spectrum of immune-mediated diseases triggered by adjuvants in persons who are genetically predisposed to it [31]. Potential triggers are silicones, injection of mineral oil or other foreign substances, and/or vaccines.

In 2013, we reported 32 patients with ASIA due to silicone incompatibility syndrome [5]. Median time between start of complaints and time of breast implant was 10 years (2–24 years). 53% of the ASIA patients had an established systemic autoimmune disease, 22% had an organ-specific autoimmune disease, and 47% had a humoral immunodeficiency (either hypogammaglobulinemia or a IgG subclass deficiency). Subsequently, many patients with self-reported symptoms were evaluated in the Netherlands [6,17]. From these, about 95% fulfilled the criteria for ASIA (Table 30.2). These patients all had (1) fatigue and/or cognitive symptoms, (2) arthralgias and/or myalgias, and (3) sicca complaints and/or pyrexia. 70%–80% of these ASIA patients had cosmetic breast augmentation, whereas 20%–30% of these patients had breast reconstruction after mastectomy for breast cancer. More than 99% of the patients were women, the remaining being (transgender) males.

At present, there are no epidemiologic studies performed to calculate the risk of ASIA in SBI patients. In the Netherlands, more than 4700 women with SBI and health issues registered themselves at a Dutch foundation for women with illness because of breast implants. Unfortunately, it is not known how many Dutch women have SBI. Clearly, more epidemiological studies on the association between ASIA and SBI are needed.

Many patients with silicone-related disease fulfill the criteria for CFS/ME [36], fibromyalgia [9], undifferentiated connective tissue disease, and/or sarcoid-like disease [5,37]. Sarcoid-like disease is due to infiltration of silicones in lymph nodes, lungs, and various other tissues. Histopathologically findings are, however, very difficult to differentiate from "idiopathic" sarcoidosis.

Furthermore, a substantial number of patients have well-defined systemic autoimmune diseases such as Sjogren syndrome, rheumatoid arthritis, systemic sclerosis, systemic lupus erythematosus, antiphospholipid syndrome, eosinophilic granulomatosis with polyangiitis, and different other forms of vasculitis [5,6,15,21].

Epidemiologic evidence for an increased occurrence of these autoimmune diseases is, however, sparse [10]. In a recent metaanalysis, increased risks for rheumatoid arthritis and Sjögren syndrome were found. Importantly, the systematic review

---

TABLE 30.2 Criteria for the Diagnosis of Autoimmune/Inflammatory Syndrome Induced by Adjuvants (ASIA)

Major criteria
- Exposure to an external stimulus (infection, vaccine, silicone, adjuvant) prior to clinical manifestations
- The appearance of "typical" clinical manifestations:
  - Myalgia, myositis, or muscle weakness
  - Arthralgia and/or arthritis
  - Chronic fatigue, unrefreshing sleep, or sleep disturbances
  - Neurological manifestations (especially associated with demyelination)
  - Cognitive impairment, memory loss
  - Pyrexia, dry mouth
- Removal of inciting agent induces improvement
- Typical biopsy of involved organs

Minor criteria
- The appearance of autoantibodies or antibodies directed at the suspected adjuvant
- Other clinical manifestations (i.e., irritable bowel syndrome)
- Specific HLA (i.e., HLA DRB1, HLA DQB1)
- Evolvement of an autoimmune disease (i.e., multiple sclerosis, systemic sclerosis)

Patient are considered to have ASIA when either two major or one major and two minor criteria are present.

concluded that studies still do not provide conclusive evidence regarding safety of SBI. Further investigations are required to determine whether increased occurrences exist between silicone gel implants and autoimmune diseases [10].

SBI patients, however, clearly have an increased risk to develop lymphomas [38–40]. Especially, the risk to develop an ALCL of the breast negative for anaplastic lymphoma kinase-1 but positive for CD30 is strongly increased. This lymphoma occurs mainly but not exclusively in SBIs with a textured device.

PATHOPHYSIOLOGY OF SILICONE BREAST IMPLANTS–RELATED DISEASE(S)

In the late 1940s and in the 1950s silicones were directly injected in the breast for augmentation purposes. Injected silicones, however, did not remain at the injection site and spread through the body and induced a foreign body reaction resulting in granulomatous inflammation [41]. Furthermore, autoimmune/inflammatory phenomena may occur. Silicone gel can migrate outside the outer shell after SBI rupture. Migration through an intact shell has also been demonstrated (so-called "gel bleed"). Recently, silicone material was found in multiple organs, nervous tissue, and the brain in a 56-year-old woman at autopsy [42]. The patient had been exposed during a period of 17 years to gel bleed from her silicone breast implants. Two types of silicone material were found in multiple tissue and brain samples of this patient. The first is a droplet-like form composed of elemental Si. The second type was a plaque-like form comprised of elemental Si and Ti (titanium).

The association between SBI and ASIA may result in the following scenario [43–45]: Silicon-containing particles are captured by macrophages, resulting in entrapment within lysosomes. Subsequently, inflammasomes are activated, resulting in the production of cytokines such as interleukin-1β. In addition, reactive oxygen species (ROS) and reactive nitrogen species are produced. Subsequently, apoptosis of macrophages occurs resulting in the release of silicon-containing particles that can be taken up once again by other macrophages. Exposure to silicon-containing particles also leads to a massive production of interleukin-17, resulting in an influx of neutrophils that are activated and produce ROS and release enzymes such as myeloperoxidase. Additionally, silicon-containing particles are transported to the regional lymph nodes, resulting in a pronounced adjuvant effect.

In animal models, it has been shown that SBI induces an adjuvant effect [46–48] and increases the susceptibility to and/or exacerbate autoimmune diseases [49–51]. In nonsusceptible animals, however, autoimmunity could not be induced [49].

Other mechanisms that may be operative in silicone-related disease, however, have been postulated as well [32,52]. Maharaj postulates that platinum and platinum salts—used in the manufacturing of SBI—cause sensitization and may be responsible for (some of the) health problems [52]. In contrast, Brawer postulates that silicone bound to carbon (i.e., organosilicones) is directly toxic for the human body and responsible for the disease [32].

At present it is unknown which women are susceptible for development of SBI-related disease. Several factors, however, have been postulated [53]. Firstly, patients who are known to have (a history of) allergy and/or an established autoimmune disease are at risk. Furthermore, those who have a familial predisposition for autoimmune disease are also prone to develop symptoms after SBI. It is important to realize that not only immunogenetic (i.e., HLA) factors play a role in the development of SBI induced ASIA but also environmental factors such as smoking and obesity [53–55].

Finally, in women with SBI it is found that the capsule around these SBIs contain inflammatory cells that are predominantly Th1/Th17 cells, whereas regulatory T cells in the capsules are defective in suppressing these intracapsular T cells [56]. These findings suggest that the Th17/Treg balance is disturbed, which may result in the development of inflammatory/autoimmune diseases [57]. Importantly, many patients with ASIA due to SBI have a humoral immune deficiency [5] and a vitamin D deficiency [58,59]. These two factors also increase the risk to develop an autoimmune disease in susceptible patients [5,59]. Furthermore, the chronic inflammation by the SBI in the capsule may result in progression from polyclonal lymphocyte stimulation to monoclonal lymphocyte stimulation, which in turn will result in lymphoma formation such as ALCL [39].

DISEASE MANAGEMENT

Unfortunately, there are no randomized clinical trials performed on the management of women with SBI related diseases. In addition, there are no (inter)national guidelines formulated. However, based on our personal experience some therapeutic considerations should be considered [58].

Firstly, vitamin D deficiency and/or insufficiency should be corrected. Because vitamin D may act as a regulatory agent of the immune system [59–61], we prescribe vitamin D supplementation to our patients [61,62]. Importantly, vitamin D also has been demonstrated to decrease chronic widespread pain [63]. Secondly, triggers of immune activation should be avoided and/or treated. The patient should try to quit smoking. Furthermore, antiallergic medication should be prescribed to patients with allergic rhinosinusitis, whereas bacterial (respiratory) infections should be treated with antibiotics, especially

FIGURE 30.1 Explantation of a McGhan breast implant in a 38-year-old woman with ASIA. The implant is clearly not anymore intact. After explantation, the patient recovered nearly completely.

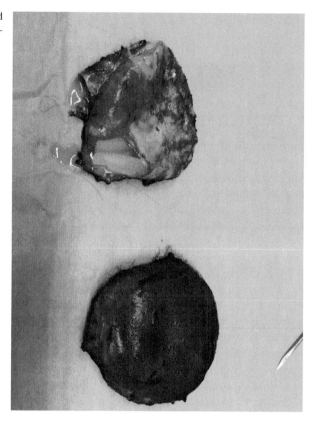

when IgG levels and/or IgG subclasses are deficient [64]. For eye symptoms, preservative-free tear supplements should be prescribed, whereas occasionally plugs should be inserted. Furthermore, sleeping quality should be improved with melatonin, bright light therapy in the morning, cognitive therapy, and/or other approaches.

There is ample evidence that explantation of the SBI is an important first step in the management of women with SBI-related disorders [7,17] (Fig. 30.1). In our recent review, we found that 469 of 622 reported patients (75%) improved after explantation. The shorter the period is that the SBI were in place, the better the amelioration of systemic symptoms and signs following removal [65]. In patients who had already developed an established autoimmune disease, only 16% improved without additional immunosuppressive therapy [7].

Unfortunately, several women still suffer from ASIA after explantation possibly because silicones are present throughout the body [42]. There are no medications that can cure ASIA, but therapy can help reduce symptoms. Suggested medications include minocycline or doxycycline [66–68], hydroxychloroquine, or corticosteroids to dampen inflammation. In severe cases, 2 mg/kg IVIg may be used. In addition, medication may be prescribed for symptoms due to central sensitization [69], gastrointestinal involvement [70], and/or cardiovascular involvement [71]. Finally, as in patients with fibromyalgia, a combination of drug, cognitive behavioral, and exercise treatment should be considered [72,73]. Also, some patients need psychiatric consultation [74].

CONCLUSION

Silicones are associated in a proportion of patients with complaints such as fatigue, cognitive impairment, arthralgias, myalgias, pyrexia, dry eyes, and dry mouth. During the last few years, it has been postulated that these symptoms in patients with SBI are because of an adjuvant effect of migrated silicones. Due to either SBI rupture or gel bleed, silicones can migrate through the body into tissues and the central nervous system. Furthermore, these silicones can induce a chronic inflammatory process that may ultimately result in (an increase of) allergies, autoimmune diseases, immune deficiency, and/or lymphomas. Explantation of SBI results in the majority of patients in an amelioration of the symptoms. There is an urgent need to start adequately adjusted epidemiological studies to obtain better evidence as to which percentage of patients develops symptoms and/or diseases such as ASIA, immune deficiency, autoimmune diseases, and/or ALCL.

REFERENCES

[1] Cronin TD, Gerow FG. Augmentation mammaplasty: a new "natural feel" prostheses. In: Transactions of the third international congress of plastic surgery. Amsterdam: Experta Medical Foundation; 1963. p. 41–4.

[2] Miyoshi K, Miyamura T, Kobayashi Y, Itakura T, Nishijo K. Hyper-gammaglobulinemia by prolonged adjuvanticity in man: disorders developed after augmentation mammaplasty. Jpn Med J 1964;2122:9–14.

[3] Ashley FL, Braley S, Rees TD, Goulian D, Ballantyne DL. The present status of silicone fluid in soft tissue augmentation. Plast Reconstr Surg 1967;39:411–8.

[4] van Nunen SA, Gatenby PA, Basten A. Post-mammoplasty connective tissue disease. Arthritis Rheum 1982;25:694–7.

[5] Cohen Tervaert JW, Kappel RM. Silicone implant incompatibility syndrome (SIIS): a frequent cause of ASIA (Shoenfeld's syndrome). Immunol Res 2013;56:293–8.

[6] Colaris MJ, de Boer M, van der Hulst RR, Cohen Tervaert JW. Two hundreds cases of ASIA syndrome following silicone implants: a comparative study of 30 years and a review of current literature. Immunol Res 2017;65(1):120–8.

[7] de Boer M, Colaris M, van der Hulst RR, Cohen Tervaert JW. Is explantation of silicone breast implants useful in patients with complaints? Immunol Res February 2017;65(1):25–36.

[8] Wolfe F, Clauw DJ, Fitzcharles MA, Goldenberg DL, Häuser W, Katz RL, Mease PJ, Russell AS, Russell IJ, Walitt B. 2016 Revisions to the 2010/2011 fibromyalgia diagnostic criteria. Semin Arthritis Rheum December 2016;46(3):319–29.

[9] Meier LG, Barthel HR, Seidl C. Development of polyarthritis after insertion of silicone breast implants followed by remission after implant removal in 2 HLA-identical sisters bearing rheumatoid arthritis susceptibility genes. J Rheumatol September 1997;24(9):1838–41.

[10] Balk EM, Earley A, Avendano EA, Raman G. Long-Term health outcomes in women with silicone gel breast implants: a systematic review. Ann Intern Med 2016;164(3):164–75.

[11] Shoaib BO, Patten BM, Calkins DS. Adjuvant breast disease: an evaluation of 100 symptomatic women with breast implants or silicone fluid injections. Keio J Med 1994;43:79–87.

[12] Dagan A, Kogan M, Shoenfeld Y, Segal G. When uncommon and common coalesce: adult onset Still's disease associated with breast augmentation as part of autoimmune syndrome induced by adjuvants (ASIA). Clin Rheumatol 2016;35(6):1643–8.

[13] Freundlich B, Altman C, Snadorfi N, Greenberg M, Tomaszewski J. A profile of symptomatic patients with silicone breast implants: a Sjögrens-like syndrome. Semin Arthritis Rheum August 1994;24(1 Suppl. 1):44–53.

[14] Mavromatis BH, Tzioufas AG, Moutsopoulos HM. Sjögren-like disease and silicone implants a Greek experience. J Clin Rheumatol June 1998;4(3):147–50.

[15] Meijs J, de Vries-Bouwstra J, Cohen Tervaert JW, Hoogenberg K. A case of late-onset systemic sclerosis with ruptured silicone breast implants. Neth J Med Jul 2018;76(5):243–8.

[16] Ericsson AD. Syndromes associated with silicone breast implants: a clinical study and review. J Nutr Environ Med 1998;8:35–51.

[17] Maijers MC, de Blok CJ, Niessen FB, van der Veldt AA, Ritt MJ, Winters HA, et al. Women with silicone breast implants and unexplained systemic symptoms: a descriptive cohort study. Neth J Med 2013;71:534–40.

[18] Frieri M, Patel R, Celestin J. Mast cell activation syndrome: a review. Curr Allergy Asthma Rep 2013;13:27–32.

[19] Maharaj S. An atypical immune-inflammatory disorder secondary to breast implant exposure. J Long Term Eff Med Implants 2012;22:33–48.

[20] Spencer TR, Schur PM. The challenge of multiple chemical sensitivity. J Environ Health 2008;70:24–7.

[21] David PR, Dagan A, Colaris M, de Boer M, Cohen Tervaert JW, Shoenfeld Y. Churg-strauss syndrome: singulair or silicone (or both?). Isr Med Assoc J 2016;18:168–70.

[22] Dragu A, Theegarten D, Bach AD, Polykandriotis E, Arkudas A, Kneser U, Horch RE, Ingianni G. Intrapulmonary and cutaneous siliconomas after silent silicone breast implant failure. Breast J 2009;15:496–9.

[23] Gopinath PP, Ali A, Van Tornout F, Kamath A, Crawford M, Nicholson AG. Chronic silicone embolism syndrome due to PIP breast implant leakage: a new entity? Histopathology 2015;66:904–6.

[24] Grahame R, Bird HA, Child A. The revised (Brighton 1998) criteria for the diagnosis of benign joint hypermobility syndrome (BJHS). J Rheumatol 2000;27:1777–9.

[25] Clauw DJ. What is the meaning of "small fiber neuropathy" in fibromyalgia? Pain 2015;156:2115–6.

[26] Teuber SS, Reilly DA, Howell L, Oide C, Gershwin ME. Severe migratory granulomatous reactions to silicone gel in 3 patients. J Rheumatol 1999;26:699–704.

[27] Wolfram D, Oberreiter B, Mayerl C, Soelder E, Ulmer H, Piza-Katzer H, Wick G, Backovic A. Altered systemic serologic parameters in patients with silicone mammary implants. Immunol Lett 2008;118:96–100.

[28] Fleury EF, Rêgo MM, Ramalho LC, Ayres VJ, Seleti RO, Ferreira CA, Roveda Jr D. Silicone-induced granuloma of breast implant capsule (SIGBIC): similarities and differences with anaplastic large cell lymphoma (ALCL) and their differential diagnosis. Breast Cancer (Dove Med Press) 2017;9:133–40.

[29] Klang E, Yosepovich A, Krosser A, Soffer S, Halshtok Neiman O, Shalmon A, Gotlieb M, Sklair-Levy M. Detection of pathologically proven silicone lymphadenopathy: ultrasonography versus magnetic resonance imaging. J Ultrasound Med September 29, 2017. https://doi.org/10.1002/jum.14434. [Epub ahead of print].

[30] Vermeulen RC, Kurk RM, Visser FC, Sluiter W, Scholte HR. Patients with chronic fatigue syndrome performed worse than controls in a controlled repeated exercise study despite a normal oxidative phosphorylation capacity. J Transl Med October 11, 2010;8:93.

[31] Shoenfeld Y, Agmon-Levin N. 'ASIA'-autoimmune/inflammatory syndrome induced by adjuvants. J Autoimmun 2011;36:4–8.

[32] Brawer AE. Mechanisms of breast implant toxicity: will the real ringmaster please stand up. Int Ann Med 2017;1(8).

[33] Fenske TK, Davis P, Aaron SL. Human adjuvant disease revisited: a review of eleven post-augmentation mammoplasty patients. Clin Exp Rheumatol 1994;12:477–81.

[34] Wolfe F. "Silicone related symptoms" are common in patients with fibromyalgia: no evidence for a new disease. J Rheumatol 1999;26:1172–5.

[35] Dush DM. Breast implants and illness: a model of psychological factors. Ann Rheum Dis 2001;60:653–7.

[36] Clayton EW. Beyond myalgic encephalomyelitis/chronic fatigue syndrome: an IOM report on redefining an illness. J Am Med Assoc 2015;313:1101–2.

[37] Teuber SS, Howell LP, Yoshida SH, Gershwin ME. Remission of sarcoidosis following removal of silicone gel breast implants. Int Arch Allergy Immunol 1994;105:404–7.

[38] de Jong D, Vasmel WL, de Boer JP, Verhave G, Barbé E, Casparie MK, van Leeuwen FE. Anaplastic large-cell lymphoma in women with breast implants. J Am Med Assoc 2008;300:2030–5.

[39] Bizjak M, Selmi C, Praprotnik S, Bruck O, Perricone C, Ehrenfeld M, Shoenfeld Y. Silicone implants and lymphoma: the role of inflammation. J Autoimmun 2015;65:64–73.

[40] Clemens MW, Miranda RN, Butler CE. Breast implant informed consent should include the risk of anaplastic large cell lymphoma. Plast Reconstr Surg 2016;137:1117–22.

[41] Barilaro G, Spaziani Testa C, Cacciani A, Donato G, Dimko M, Mariotti A. ASIA syndrome, calcinosis cutis and chronic kidney disease following silicone injections. A case-based review. Immunol Res 2016;64:1142–9.

[42] Kappel RM, Boer LL, Dijkman H. Gel bleed and rupture of silicone breast implants investigated by light-, electron microscopy and energy dispersive X-ray analysis of internal organs and nervous tissue. Clin Med Rev Case Rep 2016;3:087.

[43] Cohen Tervaert JW. Silicon exposure and vasculitis. In: Uversky VN, Kretsinger RH, Permyakov EA, editors. Encyclopedia of metalloproteins. Berlin: Springer Science + Business Media, LLC; 2012. https://doi.org/10.1007/978-1-4614-1533-6.

[44] Lee S, et al. Environmental factors producing autoimmune dysregulation—chronic activation of T cells caused by silica exposure. Immunobiology 2012;217:743–8.

[45] Yoshida SH, Chang CC, Teuber SS, Gershwin ME. Silicon and silicone: theoretical and clinical implications of breast implants. Regul Toxicol Pharmacol 1993;17:3–18.

[46] Narins RS, Beer K. Liquid injectable silicone: a review of its history, immunology, technical considerations, complications, and potential. Plast Reconstr Surg 2006;118(3 Suppl.):77S–84S.

[47] Naim JO, Lanzafame RJ, van Oss CJ. The adjuvant effect of silicone-gel on antibody formation in rats. Immunol Investig 1993;22:151–61.

[48] Nicholson 3rd JJ, Hill SL, Frondoza CG, Rose NR. Silicone gel and octamethylcyclotetrasiloxane (D4) enhances antibody production to bovine serum albumin in mice. J Biomed Mater Res 1996;31:345–53.

[49] McDonald AH, Weir K, Schneider M, Gudenkauf L, Sanger JR. Silicone gel enhances the development of autoimmune disease in New Zealand black mice but fails to induce it in BALB/cAnPt mice. Clin Immunol Immunopathol 1998;87:248–55.

[50] Schaefer CJ, Lawrence WD, Wooley PH. Influence of long term silicone implantation on type II collagen induced arthritis in mice. Ann Rheum Dis 1999;58:503–9.

[51] Schaefer CJ, Wooley PH. The influence of silicone implantation on murine lupus in MRL lpr/lpr mice. J Rheumatol October 1999;26(10):2215–21.

[52] Maharaj SV. Exposure dose and significance of platinum and platinum salts in breast implants. Arch Environ Occup Health 2007;62(3):139–46.

[53] Goren I, Segal G, Shoenfeld Y. Autoimmune/inflammatory syndrome induced by adjuvant (ASIA) evolution after silicone implants. Who is at risk? Clin Rheumatol 2015;34:1661–6.

[54] Kappel RM, Cohen Tervaert JW, Pruijn GJ. Autoimmune/inflammatory syndrome induced by adjuvants (ASIA) due to silicone implant incompatibility syndrome in three sisters. Clin Exp Rheumatol 2014;32:256–8.

[55] Watad A, Quaresma M, Brown S, Cohen Tervaert JW, Rodríguez-Pint I, Cervera R, Perricone C, Shoenfeld Y. Autoimmune/inflammatory syndrome induced by adjuvants (Shoenfeld's syndrome) - An update. Lupus 2017; Jun;26(7):675–81.

[56] Wolfram D, Rabensteiner E, Grundtman C, Böck G, Mayerl C, Parson W, Almanzar G, Hasenöhrl C, Piza-Katzer H, Wick G. T regulatory cells and TH17 cells in peri-silicone implant capsular fibrosis. Plast Reconstr Surg 2012;129:327e–37e.

[57] Noack M, Miossec P. Th17 and regulatory T cell balance in autoimmune and inflammatory diseases. Autoimmun Rev 2014;13:668–77.

[58] Cohen Tervaert JW, Colaris MJ, van der Hulst RR. Silicone breast implants and autoimmune rheumatic diseases: myth or reality. Curr Opin Rheumatol 2017;29(4):348–54.

[59] Colaris MJL, van der Hulst RR, Cohen Tervaert JW. Vitamin D deficiency as a risk factor for the development of autoantibodies in patients with ASIA and silicone breast implants: a cohort study and review of the literature. Clin Rheumatol 2017;36(5):981–93.

[60] Peelen E, Knippenberg S, Muris AH, Thewissen M, Smolders J, Tervaert JW, Hupperts R, Damoiseaux J. Effects of vitamin D on the peripheral adaptive immune system: a review. Autoimmun Rev 2011;10:733–43.

[61] Smolders J, Peelen E, Thewissen M, Cohen Tervaert JW, Menheere P, Hupperts R, Damoiseaux J. Safety and T cell modulating effects of high dose vitamin D3 supplementation in multiple sclerosis. PLoS One 2010;5(12):e15235.

[62] Vieth R. Implications for 25-hydroxyvitamin D testing of public health policies about the benefits and risks of vitamin D fortification and supplementation. Scand J Clin Lab Invest Suppl 2012;243:144–53.

[63] Yong WC, Sanguankeo A, Upala S. Effect of vitamin D supplementation in chronic widespread pain: a systematic review and meta-analysis. Clin Rheumatol 2017;36(12):2825–33.

[64] Jolles S, Chapel H, Litzman J. When to initiate immunoglobulin replacement therapy (IGRT) in antibody deficiency: a practical approach. Clin Exp Immunol June 2017;188(3):333–41.

[65] Brawer AE. Ameloration of systemic disease after removal of silicone gel-filled breast implants. J Nutr Environ Med 2000;10:125–32.

[66] Crocco E, Pascini M, Suzuki N, Alves R, Proença T, Lellis R. Minocycline for the treatment of cutaneous silicone granulomas: a case report. J Cosmet Laser Ther 2016;18:48–9.

[67] Rieger UM, Mesina J, Kalbermatten DF, Haug M, Frey HP, Pico R, Frei R, Pierer G, Lüscher NJ, Trampuz A. Bacterial biofilms and capsular contracture in patients with breast implants. Br J Surg 2013;100:768–74.

[68] Cohen JB, Carroll C, Tenenbaum MM, Myckatyn TM. Breast implant-associated infections: the role of the national surgical quality improvement program and the local microbiome. Plast Reconstr Surg 2015;36:921–9.

[69] Clauw DJ. Fbromyalgia and related conditions. Mayo Clin Proc 2015;90:680–92.

[70] Schoenfeld PS. Advances in IBS 2016: a review of current and emerging data. Gastroenterol Hepatol (NY) 2016;12(8 Suppl. 3):1–11.

[71] Arnold AC, Okamoto LE, Diedrich A, Paranjape SY, Raj SR, Biaggioni I, Gamboa A. Low-dose propranolol and exercise capacity in postural tachycardia syndrome: a randomized study. Neurology 2013;80:1927–33.

[72] Sarzi-Puttini P, Atzeni F, Salaffi F, Cazzola M, Benucci M, Mease PJ. Multidisciplinary approach to fibromyalgia: what is the teaching? Best Pract Res Clin Rheumatol 2011;25:311–9.

[73] Borchers AT, Gershwin ME. Fibromyalgia: a critical and comprehensive review. Clin Rev Allergy Immunol 2015;49:100–51.

[74] Manoloudakis N, Labiris G, Karakitsou N, Kim JB, Sheena Y, Niakas D. Characteristics of women who have had cosmetic breast implants that could be associated with increased suicide risk: a systematic review, proposing a suicide prevention model. Arch Plast Surg 2015;42:131–42.

Chapter 31

Nutritional Aspects of the Mosaic of Rheumatic Autoimmune Diseases a Recipe for Therapy?

Shani Dahan[1,2,*], Yahel Segal[2], Yehuda Shoenfeld[2,3]

[1]*Department of medicine "B", Assuta Ashdod Medical Center, Ashdod, Israel;* [2]*Zabludowicz Center for Autoimmune Diseases, Sheba Medical Center, affiliated to Sackler Faculty of Medicine, Tel Aviv University, Tel Aviv, Israel;* [3]*Laboratory of the Mosaics of Autoimmunity, Saint-Petersburg University, Saint-Petersburg, Russian Federation*

INTRODUCTION

The concept of the "mosaic of autoimmunity" was initially coined in 1989 by Shoenfeld and Isenberg [1], referring to the complex interaction of genetic, hormonal, immunological, and environmental factors in the pathogenesis of autoimmune diseases. This multifaceted pathogenic process contributes to the variety of expressions of autoimmune diseases, much as the reassembling of the pieces of a mosaic in different patterns might result in a new picture.

During the past decades, much progress has been made in illustrating the genetic factors involved in autoimmunity. Strong familial associations reported in autoimmune diseases and significant disease concordance in monozygotic twins all indicated a major role of genetics in disease evolvement [2]. Although there is yet much to explore, revelations such as the unveiling of HLA-DRB1 polymorphism as a determinant in predisposition to autoimmunity [3] shed valuable light in this field. However, when examining the incidence and prevalence of autoimmune diseases, interesting findings arise, suggesting factors other than genetic predisposition to be crucial for autoimmunity development. First, one must address the fact that though there is a disease concordance in monozygotic twins, it does not express a full correlation between genetic information and disease expression. Second, the incidence of autoimmune diseases has increased over the last years [4,5], whereas human genetics have not experienced much turmoil. Third, there is a clear geographical distribution pattern for many autoimmune diseases with a higher prevalence in North America and northern Europe, as well as a latitudinal gradient with lower prevalence around the equator [6,7]. These findings emphasize the significant role of environmental factors, as opposed to genetic factors, in autoimmunity expression.

In an attempt to elucidate this unique geoepidemiology, many environmental factors have been explored in relation to their correlation with autoimmune diseases. A prominent example is vitamin D deficiency, which has long been studied as one of the environmental factors in the development of autoimmune diseases such as multiple sclerosis (MS), type 1 diabetes, and systemic lupus erythematosus (SLE) [8–13]. Considering the pivotal role of vitamin D in regulating the immune system [14,15], it may explain the latitudinal distribution of these diseases as correlated with UV light strength, which affects vitamin D availability [16].

In this article, we aim to review a key group of novel environmental factors that may attenuate autoimmunity—our diet. Dietary habits have long been known to have a crucial influence on human health, affecting the risk for hypertension, heart diseases, and stroke, as well as influencing the development of cancer [17–20]. Therefore, when considering the complex web of factors compiling the mosaic of autoimmunity, it is not surprising that various novel dietary elements were recently found to play a role in disease development and prevention. In fact, there is no question to *we are what we eat,* and it is probably safe to assume every ingredient we consume has some effect on our health and specifically on our immune system. There are several common components of our everyday diet, for which there are relevant evidence as to their effect on rheumatic autoimmune diseases, with each component exerting its effects on the immune system through different complex molecular pathways (Fig. 31.1).

---

*The first two authors share equal contribution

Mosaic of Autoimmunity. https://doi.org/10.1016/B978-0-12-814307-0.00031-1

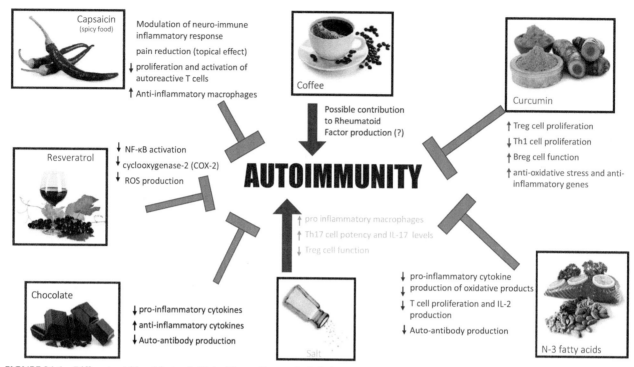

FIGURE 31.1 Different nutritional factors hold significant effects on both the innate and the adaptive immune system via different molecular pathways.

THE GOOD KIND OF FAT (N-3 FATTY ACIDS)

A common folk remedy mentioned in children tales as the terror of every sick child is a generous spoonful of castor oil, which has since been demonstrated to have valid immunological benefits. However, the interaction of fatty acids (FAs) with the human immune system appears to be complex, as they possess qualities of immune augmentation and immunomodulation.

On the one hand, essential FAs are required as membrane constitutes in immune cells and as substrates for the production of arachidonic acid, a precursor for synthesis of important proinflammatory metabolites. These FAs promote immune response and inflammation, as demonstrated in a study in which synovial fibroblasts from rheumatoid arthritis (RA) patients were cultured with different doses of various free FAs. The fibroblasts showed a dose-dependent enhanced secretion of proinflammatory cytokines and chemokines [21].

On the other hand, long-chain n-3 polyunsaturated fatty acids (PUFA) might compete with essential FAs for the enzymes that process them into proinflammatory metabolites, thus creating a contrary effect [22]. Therefore, it is not surprising that recent studies demonstrate a beneficial effect of n-3 PUFA in the settings of an overactive immune system. One noteworthy publication reviews the immunomodulatory effects of marine n-3 PUFA on immune function, among them inhibition of proinflammatory cytokine production; decreased production of reactive oxygen species (ROS) by neutrophils and monocytes; inhibition of T cell proliferation and IL-2 production, and decreased MHC-II expression and antigen presentation [23].

Similar findings of inhibition of proinflammatory cytokine production were found in a study conducted on circulating mononuclear cells of patients with Crohn's disease (CD) [24].

In addition to an in vitro immunomodulatory effect, evidence in vivo points to the effect of an n-3 FA-rich diet in inhibitions of Th1-type cytokines in mice, with little effect on Th2-type cytokines [25]. Supplementation with n-3 FA was found to be associated with lower prevalence of rheumatoid factor positivity among individuals carrying the shared haplotype HLA-DR, a known genetic factor associated with many autoimmune diseases, including RA [26]. Furthermore, in a prospective cohort study performed in Sweden, long-term n-3 FA intake consistently higher than 0.21 g/day was associated with a 52% decreased risk for development of RA [27]. When reviewing the effects of n-3 FA on RA patients in clinical trials, many trials demonstrate a beneficial effect expressed in reduced number of swollen joints, reduced joint pain, and morning stiffness duration, as well as decreased use of nonsteroidal antiinflammatory drugs (NSAIDs) [23]. Although many of these trials report improvement as compared to the baseline status of the patients rather than a significant benefit as compared to a placebo group, it is worth mentioning that when examining trials administering higher doses, significant results comparing to placebo are more common [28–32]. A thorough metaanalysis published in 2012 reviews the effect of n-3 FAs on RA patients in 10 randomized controlled trials and summarized the various doses tested and their effect. The authors conclude that use of n-3 FAs at dosages >2.7 g/day for >3 months reduces NSAID consumption by RA patients [33].

RUBBING SALT IN THE WOUND

Salt has had a major role in human history dating as far back as ancient Egypt where it was used for mummification, cleaning, and even as an antiseptic. It has been used for food preservation and, perhaps most remarkably, it was considered for centuries a valuable currency [34]. However, it is only in the past few decades that the effects of salt on human health have been properly explored. Recent studies bring to light a new aspect in this field as it appears that salt exerts an effect on the human immune system via several mechanisms.

First, salt was demonstrated to influence Th17 cells, which are known to play an integral part in several autoimmune diseases such as RA, SLE, MS, and psoriasis [35]. In 2013, two separate research groups simultaneously published their results of elaborate studies conducted to evaluate the effect of sodium chloride (NaCl) on Th17 differentiation and IL-17 expression.

Both groups examined naïve CD4 cells differentiation into TH17 cells in the presence or absence of additional 40 mM NaCl. IL-17A expression (a cytokine secreted chiefly by Th17 cells) and the expression of several transcription factors related to Th17 lineage differentiation and maturation were found to be significantly elevated in the presence of NaCl. Furthermore, T cells differentiated in the presence of NaCl were found to express factors characteristic of a highly pathogenic Th17 cell type.

When examining the effect of high-salt diet on mice with experimental autoimmune encephalitis, a murine model for MS, both groups found the disease to be aggravated by high salt intake [18,19].

However, the effects of salt on the immune system are mediated by its influence on Th17 cells. A recent study [36] demonstrated the effect of high-salt diet on regulatory T cells (Tregs). Tregs play an integral part in mediating immune tolerance, exerting their effect through various mechanisms. Nevertheless, Tregs are known to possess functional plasticity and under certain conditions may secret proinflammatory cytokines such as IFNγ and IL-17 [37]. By examining the effect of elevated NaCl levels on the suppressive capacity of human and murine Treg cells in vitro and in vivo, it has been found that high salt conditions induced a sixfold increase in IFNγ secreted by Tregs. This resulted in a loss of the suppressive function of these cells, as measured by the amount of T effector cells inhibited by Treg cells. In addition, it has been demonstrated that adding a human IFNγ neutralizing antibody to the culture led to a recovery of the suppressive functions, proving that suppression is mediated by IFNγ.

Significant clinical trials assessing the effect of limited salt intake on autoimmune diseases have yet to be completed; however, there are observational retrospective studies linking salt consumption to autoimmune diseases. One of these is a study performed on a cohort of 18,555 participants in Spain [38]. Daily sodium intake was assessed using a validated food frequency questionnaire and explored for its correlation with self-reported cases of RA. In the fourth quartile of total sodium daily intake, a significant association with RA was found (OR 1.5, CI 1.1–2.1, $P = .02$). Interestingly, the association between increased sodium intake and RA was higher among never smokers as compared with ever smokers, perhaps suggesting that smoking is a significantly stronger determinant of RA than salt intake. However, a similar study conducted in Sweden, harnessing the database of a well-established community intervention program for the prevention of cardiovascular diseases, presented somewhat contradictory results. The study included 386 individuals who had stated their dietary habits as part of the program, a median of 7.7 years before the onset of symptoms of RA, and 1886 matched healthy controls. In this study, sodium intake more than doubled the risk for RA among smokers [39], an association which was not demonstrated among nonsmokers. Furthermore, the authors describe conducting an additive interaction analysis which suggested that approximately half of the risk for the development of RA among smokers may be attributed to interaction with sodium intake. In fact, several more studies addressed the relationship between high sodium intake, smoking, and RA. One of them, evaluating 1285 subjects from the Epidemiological Investigation of Rheumatoid Arthritis study performed in Sweden, showed an increased risk of anticitrullinated peptide antibodies (ACPA) positivity among high sodium intake heavy smokers [40]. Nonetheless, when examining a possible correlation of SGK1 polymorphisms and high sodium intake with ACPA positivity, the researchers found no significant association. SGK1 polymorphisms have been explored and implicated in influencing physiological response to sodium intake and cellular stress response [41,42], yet current evidence as to their part in the development of RA is still lacking. Even so, the relationship between sodium intake and smoking with regard to the risk for development of RA is an intriguing demonstration of the complex interplay of genetic and environmental factors in the development of autoimmunity. This example of the intricate web of factors involved in the development of autoimmunity serves as a potential pathway for designing personalized medical recommendations for the treatment of rheumatic patients in the future. These should take into account the genetic features, such as SGK1 polymorphisms, along with environmental factors, such as smoking history.

These data, though relatively preliminary, along with the described effects of salt observed in vitro and in animal models, raise the need for more extensive clinical trials assessing the therapeutic potential of a low-salt diet in various autoimmune diseases.

SOME LIKE IT HOT—SPICY FOOD (CAPSAICIN)

Spices have been a cardinal part of culinary cultures around the world, with chili peppers being the most widely used seasoning, especially in China, Mexico, and Italy [43]. The increased use of spices as flavorings in foods is a major trend worldwide. In fact, it is estimated that today, as many as three-quarters of the entire world population include peppers in their diet on a daily basis [44].

The beneficial effects of spices are related to their bioactive ingredients such as capsaicin. Capsaicin, the main active ingredient of chili peppers, is a phytochemical (8-methyl-N-vanillyl-6-nonenamide), which is responsible for the characteristic hot taste of these plants [45]. Capsaicin was found to exert multiple pharmacological and physiological effects, documented in experimental or small-sized population studies. Capsaicin has shown mild to moderate efficacy in randomized trials in hand and knee osteoarthritis (OA) in comparison with placebo, with lack of systemic effects [46,47]. It is suggested today as an adjunct or sole therapy for OA patients who are unresponsive to, or intolerant of, other treatments [48].

The chilli spiciness is not technically a taste, but rather a sensation of burning, mediated by nociceptive sensory neuronal fibers [49]. This pathway is initiated by the target receptor of capsaicin, transient receptor potential vanilloid subfamily member 1 (TRPV1), a $Ca^{(2+)}$ permeable ion channel [50]. Considering the close interplay between the peripheral nervous system and autoimmunity, it is not surprising that TRPV1 has also been found to play a role in the immune system. Several studies have demonstrated both proinflammatory and antiinflammatory properties of the TRPV1 receptors, showing them to be widely expressed in innate and adaptive immune cells [51]. This includes modulation and upregulation the function of dendritic cells [52], induction of neurogenic inflammation through the activation of mast cells [53], and T cell–mediated tumorigenesis suppressive effects [54].

Consequently, recent studies have focused on investigating the influence of capsaicin in the pathogenesis of some autoimmune rheumatic diseases, with the most extensive data available in RA. Capsaicin-sensitive peptidergic sensory nerves innervate the synovium and the joint capsule, playing an important role in mediating the classical afferent pain pathway. In addition, on activation of TRPV1 receptors widely expressed on these fibers, sensory neuropeptides are released, including the proinflammatory substance P, neurokinin A, and calcitonin gene-related peptide (CGRP), as well as the potent antiinflammatory somatostatin [55]. All these are crucial mediators in neurogenic inflammation, the relevance of which in the pathophysiology of human RA has been demonstrated beyond doubt. For example, proinflammatory and antiinflammatory neuropeptide levels have been shown to be increased and decreased, respectively, in the serum and synovial fluid of RA patients [56–58]. In an early study [59], arthritic rats pretreated with capsaicin had significantly lower concentrations of substance P and CGRP in the dorsal root ganglia compared with the arthritic controls. This was accompanied by a 40% reduction in the development of ankle joint inflammation.

Based on these data, a recent study [60] analyzed the involvement of capsaicin-sensitive sensory nerves in a murine model of autoimmune arthritis. Inactivation of these fibers resulted in significantly more severe characteristics of arthritis, such as increased swelling, matrix metalloproteinase and neutrophil-derived myeloperoxidase activities, ROS production, and inflammatory cell accumulation, as well as histopathological alterations and decreased late hyperalgesia. In another model of adjuvant-induced arthritis in Lewis rats, capsaicin-induced loss of small, unmyelinated, afferent fibers in the joint draining lymph vessels resulted in markedly reduced limb inflammation [61]. These studies raise the important and complex regulatory role of capsaicin in modulating inflammation in the development and the progression of autoimmune arthritis.

Capsaicin exerts its immunomodulatory effects via neuroimmune mechanisms. E. Nevius et al. showed that oral administration of capsaicin protected mice from development of type 1 diabetes, through enhancement of a discrete population of macrophages and attenuation of the proliferation and activation of autoreactive T cells in pancreatic lymph nodes [49].

In terms of human studies, capsaicin was demonstrated to exert a beneficial effect in a clinical randomized controlled trial involving 31 RA patients [46]. Topical capsaicin administration (0.025%), applied on painful knees four times a day, for a period of 4 weeks, was demonstrated to induce a 57% reduction in pain assessment as compared with the placebo group. The most common side effects were local irritation which occurred in approximately 40% of patients.

There is a lack of human trials evaluating the oral administration of capsaicin, compared with placebo or with other agents, in autoimmune rheumatic diseases. As mentioned above, capsaicin has been found to induce to local irritation when administered topically to humans. One might wonder whether it is really feasible to carry out clinical trials with oral capsaicin with these results. To address this issue, the exact concentration of capsaicin administered should be determined. The pungency of chili peppers has been traditionally measured using the Scoville scale, first developed in 1912 by Wilbur Scoville [62]. There are five levels of pungency classified using Scoville heat units (SHU), a function of capsaicin concentration, from nonpungent (0–700 SHU) to very highly pungent (>80,000 SHU) [63]. However, this method is inaccurate as it is a subjective measurement, depended on the taste buds of the human tasters and the number of their TRPV1 receptors. Therefore, since the 1980s, the chilli spiciness has been more precisely and reliably measured by a method using high-performance liquid chromatography [64,65]. We believe that when performing a clinical trial with oral administration of capsaicin, its concentrations can be tittered to the different doses using a chromatographic method, thus comparing the distinct doses and their corresponding efficacy, as well as possible oropharyngeal or gastro-intestinal irritability.

To conclude, further studies are needed to explore spicy food as a novel modulator, a possible risk factor or a potential therapy of autoimmune diseases.

THE ANCIENT INDIAN GOLD—CURCUMIN

Curcumin is a principal active component of the common spice turmeric, and its use dates back nearly 4000 years to India, where it has been used as a culinary spice and had religious significance. Recently, the scientific community began exploring this substance for its effects on the human immune system and immune pathologies. The described mechanisms for the effect induced by curcumin included elevated expression of antioxidative stress and antiinflammatory-related genes; increased Treg cells expression along with decreased Th1 expression; and a shift toward regulatory B cells, with a rise in protective antiinflammatory antibody production [21].

A clinical trial that assessed the effect of turmeric supplementation on lupus nephritis patients showed a significant decrease in proteinuria, systolic blood pressure, and hematuria in the turmeric group, whereas the control group presented no significant effect [66].

SUMMARY

The mosaic of autoimmunity has been a well-established concept for more than two decades; however, various pieces of the mosaic continue to unravel as research progresses. Today, we are facing a new era of digitization of the health-care system [67]. With the widespread availability and accessibility of quality health data and information, there is a growing demand for safe, cost-effective, and simple way to administer therapies [68]. Moreover, autoimmune rheumatic diseases are chronic diseases, which accompany patients through their lives and are greatly influenced by the life style of their carrier. In light of this, it stands to reason that the search for additional therapies to attenuate these diseases would lead to investigating life style modifications. In this respect, nutritional agents represent an attractive alternative to conventional therapeutics and require further investigation.

Current data suggest that these ingredients hold significant effects on both the innate and the adaptive immune system. While salt appears to promote inflammation in various mechanisms, it seems that consumption of curcumin and spicy food may attenuate immune hyperactivity, whereas consumption of FAs appears to have an ambivalent effect on immunity (Fig. 31.1).

These data should raise the question whether there is a common denominator to the strong influence of these dietary bioactive compounds on the immune system. And indeed, the human microbiome is emerging as a key contributor. Several studies [69–71] have revealed the cardinal role of the worldwide, daily consumed set of dietary components presented in this review in shaping and regulating our gut microbiota population and its diverse functions, thereby affecting autoimmune rheumatic diseases (Box 31.1, Fig. 31.2).

There is still much research to be done to elucidate the various mechanisms of action of these ingredients and determine proper recommendations for doses and frequency of consumption. However, the data present to date are suffice to determine that these factors compile a novel, unexplored mosaic of autoimmunity, leaving some piquant taste for more.

BOX 31.1 Trust Your Gut Feeling

Since the invention of microscopy back in the 17th century, it has become evident that humans are mostly microbes. Humans are actually a home to a complex microbial community, most notable in the gastrointestinal tract that harbors up to 100 trillion of microbial cells, reaching levels as high as 10^{12} cells per gram.

The physician Arthur Kendall was the first to notice that diet changes the bacterial content in the stools of primates. He stated in his article that *"the predominating types of bacteria which take part in the decomposition are determined largely by the nature of the diet".*

And indeed, extensive research in the last few years has revealed the important role of the diet in shaping our microbiome community. Ley et al. analyzed the fecal microbiota of humans and 59 other mammalian species, showing that the host diet influences bacterial diversity, which increased from carnivory to omnivory to herbivory. In another study, consumption of a high-fat, high-sugar diet reproducibly altered the gut microbiota in genetically different mice strains. These findings strongly emphasize that diet plays a more important role than the host genetics in driving the microbiota community structure. Another example is capsaicin, which has recently gained considerable interest because of its bactericidal and antivirulence activity against different types of bacteria, including *Helicobacter pylori*, *Staphylococcus aureus*, and *Porphyromonas gingivalis*. The antimicrobial properties of spicy food may have important effects on the human gut microbiota population, its composition, and its diverse functions, but this is yet to be further investigated.

The microbiome has been studied and implicated in a variety of autoimmune diseases, including rheumatoid arthritis, multiple sclerosis, type 1 diabetes, and inflammatory bowel disease. The interaction between the microbiome and the immune system is complex, with different potential molecular mechanisms. These include, for example, suppression of antiinflammatory Treg cells and induction of Th17 cell differentiation in mice, leading to susceptibility toward autoimmunity.

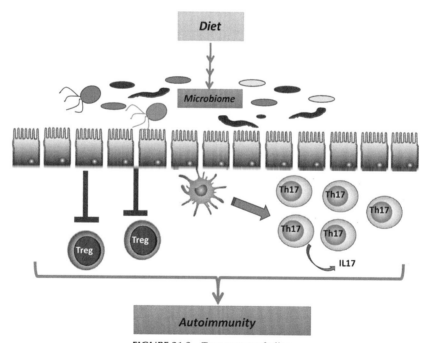

FIGURE 31.2 Trust your gut feeling.

REFERENCES

[1] Shoenfeld Y, Isenberg DA. The mosaic of autoimmunity. Immunol Today 1989;10(4):123–6.

[2] Cooper GS, Miller FW, Pandey JP. The role of genetic factors in autoimmune disease: implications for environmental research. Environ Health Perspect 1999;107(Suppl. 5):693.

[3] Cruz-Tapias P, Pérez-Fernández OM, Rojas-Villarraga A, Rodríguez-Rodríguez A, Arango M-T, Anaya J-M. Shared HLA Class II in six autoimmune diseases in Latin America: a meta-analysis. Autoimmune Dis 2012;2012:569728.

[4] Versini M, Jeandel P-Y, Bashi T, Bizzaro G, Blank M, Shoenfeld Y. Unraveling the Hygiene Hypothesis of helminthes and autoimmunity: origins, pathophysiology, and clinical applications. BMC Med 2015;13:81.

[5] Lerner A, Matthias T. Changes in intestinal tight junction permeability associated with industrial food additives explain the rising incidence of autoimmune disease. Autoimmun Rev 2015;14(6):479–89.

[6] Yinon L, Shapira NAJ. Defining and analyzing geoepidemiology and human autoimmunity. J Autoimmun 2010;34(3):J168–77. SRC - GoogleScholar.

[7] Ramos-Casals M, Brito-Zerón P, Kostov B, Sisó-Almirall A, Bosch X, Buss D, et al. Google-driven search for big data in autoimmune geoepidemiology: analysis of 394,827 patients with systemic autoimmune diseases. Autoimmun Rev 2015;14(8):670–9.

[8] Agmon-Levin N, Theodor E, Segal RM, Shoenfeld Y. Vitamin D in systemic and organ-specific autoimmune diseases. Clin Rev Allergy Immunol 2013;45(2):256–66.

[9] Azrielant S, Shoenfeld Y. Eppur Si Muove: vitamin D is essential in preventing and modulating SLE. Lupus 2016;25(6):563–72.

[10] Amital H, Szekanecz Z, Szucs G, Danko K, Nagy E, Csepany T, et al. Serum concentrations of 25-OH vitamin D in patients with systemic lupus erythematosus (SLE) are inversely related to disease activity: is it time to routinely supplement patients with SLE with vitamin D? Annals Rheum Dis 2010;69(6):1155–7.

[11] Carvalho JF, Blank M, Kiss E, Tarr T, Amital H, Shoenfeld Y, Anti-vitamin D. Vitamin D in SLE: preliminary results. Ann NY Acad Sci 2007;1109:550–7.

[12] Orbach H, Zandman-Goddard G, Amital H, Barak V, Szekanecz Z, Szucs G, et al. Novel biomarkers in autoimmune diseases: prolactin, ferritin, vitamin D, and TPA levels in autoimmune diseases. Ann NY Acad Sci 2007;1109:385–400.

[13] Oren Y, Shapira Y, Agmon-Levin N, Kivity S, Zafrir Y, Altman A, et al. Vitamin D insufficiency in a sunny environment: a demographic and seasonal analysis. Isr Med Assoc J 2010;12(12):751–6.

[14] Bizzaro G, Shoenfeld Y. Vitamin D: a panacea for autoimmune diseases? Can J Physiol Pharmacol 2015;93(5):395–7.

[15] Rosen Y, Daich J, Soliman I, Brathwaite E, Shoenfeld Y. Vitamin D and autoimmunity. Scand J Rheumatol 2016:1–9.

[16] Lindqvist PG, Epstein E, Nielsen K, Landin-Olsson M, Ingvar C, Olsson H. Avoidance of sun exposure as a risk factor for major causes of death: a competing risk analysis of the Melanoma in Southern Sweden cohort. J Intern Med 2016;280:375–87.

[17] Abnet CC, Corley DA, Freedman ND, Kamangar F. Diet and upper gastrointestinal malignancies. Gastroenterology 2015;148(6):1234–43.e4.

[18] Del Gobbo LC, Falk MC, Feldman R, Lewis K, Mozaffarian D. Effects of tree nuts on blood lipids, apolipoproteins, and blood pressure: systematic review, meta-analysis, and dose-response of 61 controlled intervention trials. Am J Clin Nutr 2015;102(6):1347–56.

[19] Jayalath VH, de Souza RJ, Ha V, Mirrahimi A, Blanco-Mejia S, Di Buono M, et al. Sugar-sweetened beverage consumption and incident hypertension: a systematic review and meta-analysis of prospective cohorts. Am J Clin Nutr 2015;102(4):914–21.

[20] Widmer RJ, Flammer AJ, Lerman LO, Lerman A. The Mediterranean diet, its components, and cardiovascular disease. Am J Med 2015;128(3):229–38.

[21] Frommer KW, Schäffler A, Rehart S, Lehr A, Müller-Ladner U, Neumann E. Free fatty acids: potential proinflammatory mediators in rheumatic diseases. Ann Rheum Dis 2015;74(1):303–10.

[22] Hsieh C-C, Lin B-F. Dietary factors regulate cytokines in murine models of systemic lupus erythematosus. Autoimmun Rev 2011;11(1):22–7.

[23] Miles EA, Calder PC. Influence of marine n-3 polyunsaturated fatty acids on immune function and a systematic review of their effects on clinical outcomes in rheumatoid arthritis. Br J Nutr 2012;107(Suppl. 2):S171–84.

[24] Trebble TM, Arden NK, Wootton SA, Calder PC, Mullee MA, Fine DR, et al. Fish oil and antioxidants alter the composition and function of circulating mononuclear cells in Crohn disease. Am J Clin Nutr 2004;80(5):1137–44.

[25] Wallace FA, Miles EA, Evans C, Stock TE, Yaqoob P, Calder PC. Dietary fatty acids influence the production of Th1- but not Th2-type cytokines. J Leukoc Biol 2001;69(3):449–57.

[26] Gan RW, Demoruelle MK, Deane KD, Weisman MH, Buckner JH, Gregersen PK, et al. Omega-3 fatty acids are associated with a lower prevalence of autoantibodies in shared epitope-positive subjects at risk for rheumatoid arthritis. Ann Rheum Dis 2016.

[27] Di Giuseppe D, Wallin A, Bottai M, Askling J, Wolk A. Long-term intake of dietary long-chain n-3 polyunsaturated fatty acids and risk of rheumatoid arthritis: a prospective cohort study of women. Ann Rheum Dis 2014;73(11):1949–53.

[28] Galarraga B, Ho M, Youssef HM, Hill A, McMahon H, Hall C, et al. Cod liver oil (n-3 fatty acids) as an non-steroidal anti-inflammatory drug sparing agent in rheumatoid arthritis. Rheumatology (Oxf Engl) 2008;47(5):665–9.

[29] Kremer JM, Jubiz W, Michalek A, Rynes RI, Bartholomew LE, Bigaouette J, et al. Fish-oil fatty acid supplementation in active rheumatoid arthritis. A double-blinded, controlled, crossover study. Ann Intern Med 1987;106(4):497–503.

[30] Lau CS, Morley KD, Belch JJ. Effects of fish oil supplementation on non-steroidal anti-inflammatory drug requirement in patients with mild rheumatoid arthritis–a double-blind placebo controlled study. Br J Rheumatol 1993;32(11):982–9.

[31] Volker D, Fitzgerald P, Major G, Garg M. Efficacy of fish oil concentrate in the treatment of rheumatoid arthritis. J Rheumatol 2000;27(10):2343–6.

[32] James MJ, Cleland LG. Dietary n-3 fatty acids and therapy for rheumatoid arthritis. Semin Arthritis Rheum 1997;27(2):85–97.

[33] Lee YH, Bae SC, Song GG. Omega-3 polyunsaturated fatty acids and the treatment of rheumatoid arthritis: a meta-analysis. Arch Med Res 2012;43(5):356–62.

[34] Cirillo M, Capasso G, Di Leo VA, De Santo NG. A history of salt. Am J Nephrol 1994;14(4–6):426–31.

[35] Zhu S, Qian Y. IL-17/IL-17 receptor system in autoimmune disease: mechanisms and therapeutic potential. Clin Sci (Lond Engl 1979) 2012;122(11):487–511.

[36] Hernandez AL, Kitz A, Wu C, Lowther DE, Rodriguez DM, Vudattu N, et al. Sodium chloride inhibits the suppressive function of FOXP3+ regulatory T cells. J Clin Investig 2015;125(11):4212–22. SRC - GoogleScholar.

[37] Kleinewietfeld M, Hafler DA. The plasticity of human Treg and Th17 cells and its role in autoimmunity. Semin Immunol 2013;25(4):305–12.

[38] Salgado E, Bes-Rastrollo M, de Irala J, Carmona L, Gomez-Reino JJ. High sodium intake is associated with self-reported rheumatoid arthritis: a cross sectional and case control analysis within the SUN cohort. Medicine 2015;94(37):e924.

[39] Sundström B, Johansson I, Rantapää-Dahlqvist S. Interaction between dietary sodium and smoking increases the risk for rheumatoid arthritis: results from a nested case-control study. Rheumatology (Oxf Engl) 2015;54(3):487–93.

[40] Jiang X, Sundström B, Alfredsson L, Klareskog L, Rantapää-Dahlqvist S, Bengtsson C. High sodium chloride consumption enhances the effects of smoking but does not interact with SGK1 polymorphisms in the development of ACPA-positive status in patients with RA. Ann Rheum Dis 2016;75(5):943–6.

[41] Li C, Yang X, He J, Hixson JE, Gu D, Rao DC, et al. A gene-based analysis of variants in the serum/glucocorticoid regulated kinase (SGK) genes with blood pressure responses to sodium intake: the GenSalt Study. PLoS One 2014;9(5):e98432.

[42] Luca F, Kashyap S, Southard C, Zou M, Witonsky D, Di Rienzo A, et al. Adaptive variation regulates the expression of the human SGK1 gene in response to stress. PLoS Genet 2009;5(5):e1000489.

[43] Deng Y, Huang X, Wu H, Zhao M, Lu Q, Israeli E, et al. Some like it hot: the emerging role of spicy food (capsaicin) in autoimmune diseases. Autoimmun Rev 2016;15(5):451–6.

[44] Mortensen JM, Mortensen JE. The power of capsaicin. Top Issues 2009;9:8.

[45] Cichewicz RH, Thorpe PA. The antimicrobial properties of Chile peppers (Capsicum species) and their uses in Mayan medicine. J Ethnopharmacol 1996;52(2):61–70.

[46] Deal CL, Schnitzer TJ, Lipstein E, Seibold JR, Stevens RM, Levy MD, et al. Treatment of arthritis with topical capsaicin: a double-blind trial. Clin Therapeut 1991;13(3):383–95.

[47] McCarthy GM, McCarty DJ. Effect of topical capsaicin in the therapy of painful osteoarthritis of the hands. J Rheumatol 1992;19(4):604–7.

[48] Mason L, Moore RA, Derry S, Edwards JE, McQuay HJ. Systematic review of topical capsaicin for the treatment of chronic pain. BMJ 2004;328(7446):991.

[49] Nevius E, Srivastava PK, Basu S. Oral ingestion of Capsaicin, the pungent component of chili pepper, enhances a discreet population of macrophages and confers protection from autoimmune diabetes. Mucosal Immunol 2012;5(1):76–86.

[50] Sharma SK, Vij AS, Sharma M. Mechanisms and clinical uses of capsaicin. Eur J Pharmacol 2013;720(1–3):55–62.

[51] Majhi RK, Sahoo SS, Yadav M, Pratheek BM, Chattopadhyay S, Goswami C. Functional expression of TRPV channels in T cells and their implications in immune regulation. FEBS J 2015;282(14):2661–81.

[52] Basu S, Srivastava P. Immunological role of neuronal receptor vanilloid receptor 1 expressed on dendritic cells. Proc Natl Acad Sci USA 2005;102(14):5120–5.

[53] Biro T, Maurer M, Modarres S, Lewin NE, Brodie C, Acs G, et al. Characterization of functional vanilloid receptors expressed by mast cells. Blood 1998;91(4):1332–40.

[54] Aggarwal BB, Van Kuiken ME, Iyer LH, Harikumar KB, Sung B. Molecular targets of nutraceuticals derived from dietary spices: potential role in suppression of inflammation and tumorigenesis. Exp Biol Med (Maywood NJ) 2009;234(8):825–49.

[55] Yoo S, Lim JY, Hwang SW. Sensory TRP channel interactions with endogenous lipids and their biological outcomes. Molecules 2014;19(4):4708–44.

[56] Anichini M, Cesaretti S, Lepori M, Maddali Bongi S, Maresca M, Zoppi M. Substance P in the serum of patients with rheumatoid arthritis. Revue du rhumatisme (English ed) 1997;64(1):18–21.

[57] Larsson J, Ekblom A, Henriksson K, Lundeberg T, Theodorsson E. Concentration of substance P, neurokinin A, calcitonin gene-related peptide, neuropeptide Y and vasoactive intestinal polypeptide in synovial fluid from knee joints in patients suffering from rheumatoid arthritis. Scand J Rheumatol 1991;20(5):326–35.

[58] Denko C, Malemud C. The serum growth hormone to somatostatin ratio is skewed upward in rheumatoid arthritis patients. Front Biosci J Virtual Libr 2004;9:1660–4.

[59] Ahmed M, Bjurholm A, Srinivasan GR, Lundeberg T, Theodorsson E, Schultzberg M, et al. Capsaicin effects on substance P and CGRP in rat adjuvant arthritis. Regul Pept 1995;55(1):85–102.

[60] Borbely E, Botz B, Bolcskei K, Kenyer T, Kereskai L, Kiss T, et al. Capsaicin-sensitive sensory nerves exert complex regulatory functions in the serum-transfer mouse model of autoimmune arthritis. Brain Behav Immun 2015;45:50–9.

[61] Lorton D, Lubahn C, Engan C, Schaller J, Felten DL, Bellinger DL. Local application of capsaicin into the draining lymph nodes attenuates expression of adjuvant-induced arthritis. Neuroimmunomodulation 2000;7(3):115–25.

[62] Scoville WL. Note on capsicums. J Am Pharm Assoc 1912;1(5):453–4.

[63] Weiss EA. Spice crops. CABI; 2002.

[64] Nwokem C, Agbaji E, Kagbu J, Ekanem E. Determination of capsaicin content and pungency level of five different peppers grown in Nigeria. NY Sci J 2010;3(9):17–21.

[65] Othman ZAA, Ahmed YBH, Habila MA, Ghafar AA. Determination of capsaicin and dihydrocapsaicin in Capsicum fruit samples using high performance liquid chromatography. Molecules 2011;16(10):8919–29.

[66] Khajehdehi P, Zanjaninejad B, Aflaki E, Nazarinia M, Azad F, Malekmakan L, et al. Oral supplementation of turmeric decreases proteinuria, hematuria, and systolic blood pressure in patients suffering from relapsing or refractory lupus nephritis: a randomized and placebo-controlled study. J Ren Nutr 2012;22(1):50–7.

[67] Shoenfeld Y, Caspi D. The digital doctor. Harefuah 2015;154(3):148.

[68] Omolo MA, Wong Z-Z, Mergen AK, Hastings JC, Le NC, Reiland HA, et al. Antimicrobial properties of chili peppers. J Infect Dis Ther 2014:2014.

[69] Carmody RN, Gerber GK, Luevano Jr JM, Gatti DM, Somes L, Svenson KL, et al. Diet dominates host genotype in shaping the murine gut microbiota. Cell Host Microbe 2015;17(1):72–84.

[70] Nayak RR, Turnbaugh PJ. Mirror, mirror on the wall: which microbiomes will help heal them all? BMC Med 2016;14:72.

[71] Chu DM, Antony KM, Ma J, Prince AL, Showalter L, Moller M, et al. The early infant gut microbiome varies in association with a maternal high-fat diet. Genome Med 2016;8(1):77.

Chapter 32

Gluten and Autoimmunogenesis

Aaron Lerner[1,2], Torsten Matthias[2]

[1]B. Rappaport School of Medicine, Technion-Israel Institute of Technology, Haifa, Israel; [2]AESKU.KIPP Institute, Wendelsheim, Germany

INTRODUCTION

According to the Food and Agriculture Organization of the United Nations official report, worldwide production of wheat increased from 711.4 in 2013 to 750.1 million tons in 2017 (October 5, 2017) [1].

On the other hand, however, since the early 1990s, strong economic growth in many Asian countries, particularly in China and India, halted the upward trend in global per capita rice consumption as consumers diversified their diet from rice to high-value products such as meat, dairy products, fruits, and vegetables. For the past two decades, global per capita consumption has been flat at around 65 kg, with a dip between 2001 and 2004 due to severe drought in China and India [2]. The ratio of wheat/rice consumption seems to decrease following the westernization process that Asia and Africa are experiencing. This trend has a major implication on gluten consumption, being the most prevalent protein in wheat and also because rice, contrary to wheat, is a gluten-free staple. The present chapter will highlight the gluten status in modern wheat and its potential impact on human health, mainly on autoimmune diseases (ADs) development.

Increased Consumption of Gluten

Gluten is an important component in wheat, representing around 80% of the proteins. Wheat is cultured in larger surfaces than for any other crop and its global trade is greater than that for all other crops combined. Notably, more wheat flour is produced than any other flour. In addition to its agronomic adaptability and improved yield, in contrast to rice, wheat offers convenient grain storage and easiness of grinding grain into flour to produce eatable, palatable, tastier, and satisfying foods. In the last century, global wheat output expanded by about fivefold; however, since 1955, there has been a dramatic tenfold increase in the rate of wheat yield improvement per year, and this has become the major factor associated with increases in global wheat production. Average 2.5 tons wheat was produced on 1 ha of cropland in the world in the first half of 1990s, but this was increased to about 3 tons in 2009. According to a recent survey, the global wheat yield is increasing at 0.9% per year but, unfortunately, is less than the rate required to double global production by 2050, to meet global population needs [3]. It is not only that wheat production surge is directly related to contemporary increase in gluten consumption but also that, in many developing countries, the frequency of gluten-dependent conditions is likely to increase in the near future, given the diffuse tendency to adopt Western, gluten-rich dietary patterns [4].

Evolution Drove the Abundance, Toxicity, and Immunogenicity of Gluten

The ancient wheat originated in the "Fertile Crescent" in Southeast Asia and was discovered around 10,000–15,000 years ago. Triticum monococcum is the oldest and most primitive cultivated wheat. It was genetically diploid, very fragile, low yield, difficult to harvest, and with low survival. Following plant domestication of the Near Eastern crops and the beginning of farming, improved irrigation and multiple interwheat artificial/natural crossbreeding, the polyploid plants improved, had better survival rate and expanded globally. Genetic adaptability and diversity was essential for the wheat species to survive the changing environmental conditions, a process that continues till today [5,6]. During the last centuries of our modern age, extensive genetic natural selection occurred because of changing environment and breeding manipulations, selective advantage of wheat toward improved grains number, and wheat survival and adaptation [7]. The process was accompanied by enrichment of gluten content in wheat. In fact, multiple old and less recent studies documented the increased celiac disease epitopes along the process of gluten gene enrichment in the passage of ancient diploid to modern tetraploid and hexaploid wheat species [8–12]. It should be emphasized that lately, several groups opposed those studies and concluded that the ancient strains contained immunogenic and toxic gluten peptides and recommended the celiac patients to avoid ancient wheat strains consumption [13–17]. Moreover, Kasarda D.D. results do not support the likelihood that wheat breeding has increased the protein content of wheat, at least, in the United States [18]. The author allocated the increased incidence of celiac disease (CD) to changes in the per capita consumption of wheat flour and the use of vital gluten as a processed food additive. Finally, a more neutral conclusion is that toxicity of wheat exists not only in the modern varieties but also in wheat strains grown up around a century ago [8]. In summary, as aforementioned, it seems that the strategy to recultivate the ancient wheat as a new gluten-free diet nutritional therapy is not only very complicated but also not going along the newer observations [19].

Increased Incidence of Autoimmune Diseases

ADs are the third most common category of disease in the United States after cancer and cardiovascular disease, affecting ~5%–8% of the population [20]. Conservative estimates indicate that ~78% of the people affected with ADs are women [21]. One of the major arguments that the modern increase in incidence and prevalence of ADs is environmentally and not genetically mediated is at surge in the last decades. In fact, multiple studies documented this trend in a large repertoire of ADs [22–27]. Multiple sclerosis, type 1 diabetes, inflammatory bowel diseases (mainly Crohn's disease), systemic lupus erythematosus, primary biliary cirrhosis, myasthenia gravis, autoimmune thyroiditis, hepatitis and rheumatic diseases, bullous pemphigoid, and CD are several examples [27–30]. In their seminal papers, Bach JF et al. correlated the rise in ADs to the surge in allergic and cancer conditions while infections are less frequent in the Western societies, creating the basis for the hygiene hypothesis [31–34]. More recently, screening long-term, follow-up, national or local epidemiological studies, comparing incidences and prevalences of ADs, in the last three decades, the mean ± s.d. of the net percentage increased per year worldwide were 19.1 ± 43.1 and 12.5 ± 7.9, respectively. Rheumatic, endocrinological, gastrointestinal, and neurological ADs revealed the following annual percentage increases per year: 7.1, 6.3, 6.2, and 3.7, respectively. In all of these, differences between old versus new frequencies were highly significant [28]. Based on the above information, one can see the longitudinal trend that can be traced between the worldwide increased gluten consumption, the higher content and potential toxicity of gluten in the modern wheat, and the recent increased frequency of gluten-dependent and nonceliac ADs.

GUT ECOEVENTS THAT MIGHT DRIVE SYSTEMIC AUTOIMMUNITY

When dealing with gluten ingestion, it is interesting and challenging to unravel the potential interactions that may be initiated or driven by gluten in the human enteric luminal and mucosal compartments. Several pathophysiologic pathways can be affected by gluten:

Gluten Effects on the Microbiome

The effects of gluten and the dysbiotic changes that occur in untreated CD compared with gluten-free patients were extensively studied. In general, changes in diversity of the following microbial species were detected: an increase in Lachnoanaerobaculum, Prevotella, Actinomycetes, Lachnoanaerobaculum umeaense, a decrease in Bifidobacterium spp., Bacteroides, Parabacteroides, and an increase in Candida albicans, Escherichia, and Helicobacter [35–37]. It is generally accepted that reduced abundance of bifidobacteria and lactobacilli is linked to CD [38,39]. However, it should be emphasized that exploration of the microbiome/dysbiome in CD is complex and, comparing studies results between them, is much more. The enteric bacterial composition and diversity depends on gluten consumption, dietary composition of the meals, fiber amount and origin, topographical sampling (duodenal lumen/biopsy, colonic/rectal lumen, stools or saliva), age, recent antibiotic consumption, or probiotic intake [39]. The last point brings an additional factor that might affect the gluten–microbiome interrelationship. Recent studies reported on the capacity of certain strains of bacteria to hydrolyze gluten, thus affecting its breakdown, immunogenicity, and microbiota composition [40–42]. At the end of the day, at least for now, the gluten–CD–microbiota axis is far from being elucidated. Is it the cause, consequence, or coevolution? It is still unknown [43]. The human enteric immunoecology: how the microbiome regulates tolerance and autoimmunity is still an enigma [44].

Gluten as a Processed Food Additive

The industrial food processing additives affect enteric ecoevents. We recently listed seven heavily used industrial food additives that alter luminal and mucosal behaviors [30,45]. Glucose, salt, emulsifiers, organic solvents, gluten, microbial transglutaminase (mTg), and nanoparticles impact microbiota composition, can breach tight junction integrity impact microbiota composition can breach tight junction integrity and potentially induce a leaky gut, setting the stage for autoimmunogenesis [30,45–47].

Evidence exists that intestinal barrier defects have a role in initiating celiac disease [48–50]. Gluten is a well-characterized enhancer of intestinal permeability [51,52]. Interestingly, when gliadin was applied on intestinal biopsies, an increased intestinal permeability was noticed in active and treated CD, not only in nonceliac gluten sensitivity but also in nonceliac controls [51]. This is only one aspect of gluten side effects in normal population, as will be described below.

Luminal Posttranslational Modification of Gluten

The luminal fate of the ingested gluten is constantly unraveled. After microbial and endogenous enzymatic digestion, several gluten peptides are created, the most characterized one is the 33mer gluten peptide, considered to be the supramolecule playing an important role in CD induction in susceptible patients [19]. Gluten is an ideal substrate for deamidation and cross-linking by the enzymatic autoantigen of CD, namely, tissue transglutaminase (tTg). This essential step occurs below the epithelium, following the passage of the toxic/immunogenic gluten peptides through the enteric epithelium. But, there is another member of the Tgase family, mTg, which, despite very low sequence homology, imitates functionally the endogenous tTg. mTg is essential for microbial survival and it is heavily used as a peptide linker in the processed food industries [52–54]. More so, gluten being rich in glutamine, lysine is an attractive substrate for cross-linking of gliadin, representing luminal posttranslational modification (PTM) of it by the mTg [37,55]. Based on those luminal events, we investigated the immunogenicity of celiac patient's sera/controls and found high activity of IgG anti–neo-epitope mTg antibodies (against the neo-complex created when gliadin is docked on the mTg) in celiac affected children [56,57]. Based on the gluten-induced intestinal permeability, the mTg-induced PTM of gliadin, and the increased immunogenicity of the mTg-gliadin neo-complex, we forwarded the hypothesis that mTg might represent a new environmental factor in CD initiation and progression [37,52–57]. Its place in nonceliac gluten sensitivity is currently under investigations.

Gluten and the Leaky Gut

Disruption of epithelial tight junctions leads to intestinal hyperpermeability, which is the basis for the leaky gut syndrome [58]. The leaky gut is an important step in connecting luminal ecoevents to intestinal and remote organ ADs [59]. Several avenues can be suggested for the role of the luminal gluten/gliadin peptides in the leaky gut induction (Table 32.1). It should be stressed that the side effects of gluten mentioned in Table 32.1 were shown mainly on animal models, human-originated cell lines, and ex vivo and not on human subjects. No doubt that gluten peptides are essential in the leaky gut progression. One of the operating pathway is the induction of zonulin, a major enhancer of gut permeability [63,64].

Luminal Microbial Horizontal Gene Transfer of Virulent Factors

Horizontal gene transfer (HGT) is a genetic conserved mechanism in prokaryotes enabling them to exchange genetic material, including virulent genes between them [65]. This foreign environmental genetic cargo carried by ingested microbes, when entering the human gut, can impact the microbiome/dysbiome balance. Several mechanistic pathways can be envisioned. Microbes used to improve food, microbiota of engineered plants, fruits and vegetables or transformed livestock,

TABLE 32.1 Potential Mechanisms of Gluten Involvement in the Leaky Gut Syndrome

Pathophysiological Pathway	References
Decreased microbiota/dysbiota ratio	[35–39]
Enzymatic post translational modification of protein (PTMP) creating toxic/immunogenic peptides	[55–57]
Breaching tight junction integrity	[48–51]
Side effects of gluten: immunogenic, cytotoxic, proinflammatory, proapoptotic, and activates the immune systems	[60]
Side effects of gluten: decreasing cellular viability and differentiation, enhancer of oxidative stress, and impacts epigenetic processes	[60]
Potential pathobiont or dysbiotic degradation/remodeling of gluten, enhancing its toxicity/immunogenicity/pathogenicity	[61,62]

TABLE 32.2 Gut-Remote Organs' Axes Involvement in Autoimmunity and Chronic Diseases

Axis Name	Organ Involved	Autoimmune Disease (AD)	References
Gut–joint	Articulations	Rheumatoid arthritis	[68,69]
Gut–bone	Skeleton	ADs associated osteoporosis/penia	[70]
Gut–gut	Intestine	Celiac, Crohn's diseases, *Helicobacter pylori* gastritis	[71,72]
Gut–thyroid	Thyroid	Hashimoto thyroiditis, Graves' disease	[73,74]
Gut–kidney	Kidney	IgA nephropathy	[75]
Gut–brain	Brain	Neurodegenerative/inflammatory conditions	[76]
Gut–liver	Liver	Autoimmune hepatitis	[77]
Gut–skin	Skin	Psoriasis	[78]
Gut–lung	Lung	Chronic lung diseases	[79]
Gut–heart	Heart	Chronic heart diseases and failure	[80,81]
Gut–bone	Bone	Osteopenia, osteoporosis	[82]

ingested probiotics, and bioengineered microbes in the processed food industries are some of them [30,35,37,45–47,52–57]. Those prokaryotes are potential carriers of virulent genes (e.g., antibiotics resistant genes), which are important for bacterial survival but might be detrimental for human health, including ADs induction [66]. The significant magnitude of HGT in the human intestine may induce multiple neo-proteins' or neo-peptides' formations that, by imitating self-ones, result in autoantigen creation. Following molecular mimicry or epitope spreading, antigen-directed autoantibodies are formed, thus establishing the basis for autoimmunity progression. Adding the leaky gut to the autoimmune puzzle, the resultant autoantibodies may enhance the snowball effect, exenterating the tissue damage and amplifying the inflammatory cascades. Notably, it was Robinson and others that in 2013 forwarded the hypothesis of the role of the bacteria–animal HGT in carcinogenesis [67]. It should be stressed here that the magnitude of human gut HGT in ADs induction is far from being unraveled, and nowadays, it is a mere hypothesis that should be investigated thoroughly.

The Gut as the Trojan Horse of Remote Organ Autoimmunity

As shown above, multiple nutritional, chemical, biochemical, pathophysiological, genetic, and bacteriological events are taking place in the human enteric compartment, where gluten can be involved and impact the enteric homeostasis. In fact, multiple autoimmune axes originate in the intestinal domain, resulting in intestinal and peripheral specific ADs. Table 32.2 summarizes some of them. Classic examples of gluten-dependent remote organs' pathologies, starting from the intestine, are the numerous extraintestinal manifestations of CD [45].

GLUTEN MIGHT BE BENEFICIAL IN NONCELIAC AUTOIMMUNE DISEASES

In view of the major place played by gut ecoevents in autoimmunogenesis, the toxic, immunogenic, and pathophysiologic features of gluten, the parallel surge in ADs incidence and the surge in gluten consumption in the recent decades, and the heavy usage of gluten by the processed food industries, its withdrawal might be beneficial in certain ADs. Most recently, we have summarized the topic, reviewing the literature on nonceliac ADs that were treated, in certain circumstances, and responded to gluten-free diet [60]. Type 1 diabetes mellitus, rheumatoid arthritis, autoimmune thyroiditis, autoimmune hepatitis, psoriasis, multiple sclerosis, IgA nephropathy, mainly when associated with CD or positive for antigluten antibodies or other CD-associated autoantibodies, can benefit from gluten withdrawal [60].

CONCLUSIONS

Gluten is a major constituent in modern human food. Its increasing consumption, evolutionary increased toxicity and immunogenicity, and heavy usage in food and other industries make it a prime candidate as a modern environmental factor that might impact autoimmunogenesis. Its capacity to change microbiome, being a good substrate for PTMP, enhancer of

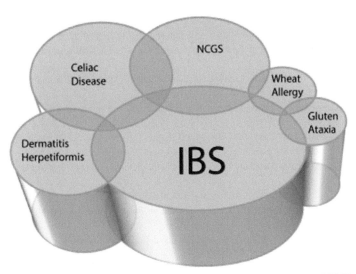

FIGURE 32.1 Classic gluten-dependent conditions in relation to irritable bowel syndrome (IBS). *NCGS,* Nonceliac gluten sensitivity.

intestinal permeability resulting in a leaky gut and its multiple detrimental effects represent pathophysiological pathways that might drive ADs' initiation, maintenance, and progression. Its beneficial effects, when withdrawn in multiple ADs, further reinforce its place in impacting ADs. As gluten-dependent (Fig. 32.1) and non–gluten-related various ADs cohabit in the same affected individual and their closed relatives and since gluten withdrawal might attenuate some of them, the medical and the scientific communities should be aware of such a combination. The present chapter aims to increase the awareness of the treating teams for the potential place of gluten ingestion in autoimmune development. It is suggested that not only gluten-dependent or functional abdominal conditions (Fig. 32.1) but also non–gluten-related ADs should be checked for CD-associated antibodies.

ACKNOWLEDGMENTS

The authors acknowledge Mr. Alf Neu for the figure design.

REFERENCES

[1] Food and Agriculture Organization of the United Nations report. FAO Cereal Supply and Demand Brief, World food Situation, Summary tables, World wheat production market. 2017. Available at: http://www.fao.org/worldfoodsituation/csdb/en/.

[2] Rice today. IRRI -Trends in global rice consumption. Written by Samarendu Mohanty. October 6, 2017. Available at: www.irri.org/rice-today/trends-in-global-rice-consumption.

[3] Ray DK, Mueller ND, West PC, Foley JA. Yield trends are insufficient to double global crop production by 2050. PLoS One 2013;8:e66428.

[4] Catassi C, Gatti S, Lionetti E. World perspective and celiac disease epidemiology. Dig Dis 2015;33:141–6.

[5] Lerner A. The last two millennias eco-catastrophes are the driving forces for the potential genetic advantage mechanisms in celiac disease. Med Hypothesis 2011;77:773–6.

[6] Zhao C, Liu B, Piao S, Wang X, Lobell DB, Huang Y, et al. Temperature increase reduces global yields of major crops in four independent estimates. Proc Natl Acad Sci USA 2017;114:9326–31.

[7] Greco L. From the Neolithic revolution to gluten intolerance: benefits and problems associated with the cultivation of wheat. J Pediatr Gastroenterol Nutr 1997;24s:14–7.

[8] Van den Broeck HC, de Jong HC, Salentijn EMJ, et al. Presence of celiac disease epitopes in modern and old hexaploid wheat varieties: wheat breeding may have contributed to increased prevalence of celiac disease. Theor Appl Genet 2010;121:1527–39.

[9] Molberg O, Uhlen AK, Flaete NS, et al. Mapping of gluten T-cell epitopes in the bread wheat ancestors: implications for celiac disease. Gastroenterology 2005;128:393–401.

[10] Spaenij-Dekking L, Kooy-Winkelaar Y, van Veelen P, et al. Nature variation in toxicity of wheat: potential for selection of nontoxic varieties for celiac disease patients. Gastroenterology 2005;129:797–806.

[11] Yan Y, Hsam SL, Yu JZ, Jiang Y, Ohtsuka I, Zeller FJ. HMW and LMW glutenin alleles among putative tetraploid and hexaploid European splet wheat (Triticum spelta L.) progenitors. Theor Appl Genet 2003;107:1321–30.

[12] de Lorgeril M, Salen P. Gluten and wheat intolerance today: are modern wheat strains involved? Int J Food Sci Nutr 2014;65:577–81.

[13] Šuligoj T, Gregorini A, Colomba M, Ellis HJ, Ciclitira PJ. Evaluation of the safety of ancient strains of wheat in coeliac disease reveals heterogeneous small intestinal T cell responses suggestive of coeliac toxicity. Clin Nutr 2013;32:1043–9.

[14] Gregorini A, Colomba M, Ellis HJ, Ciclitira PJ. Immunogenicity characterization of two ancient wheat α-gliadin peptides related to coeliac disease. Nutrients 2009;1:276–90.

[15] Colomba MS, Gregorini A. Are ancient durum wheats less toxic to celiac patients? A study of α-gliadin from Graziella Ra and Kamut. Sci World J 2012;2012:837416.

[16] Prandi B, Tedeschi T, Folloni S, Galaverna G, Sforza S. Peptides from gluten digestion: a comparison between old and modern wheat varieties. Food Res Int 2017;91:92–102.

[17] Ribeiro M, Rodriguez-Quijano M, Nunes FM, Carrillo JM, Branlard G, Igrejas G. New insights into wheat toxicity: breeding did not seem to contribute to a prevalence of potential celiac disease's immunostimulatory epitopes. Food Chem 2016;213:8–18.

[18] Kasarda DD. Can an increase in celiac disease be attributed to an increase in the gluten content of wheat as a consequence of wheat breeding? J Agric Food Chem 2013;61:1155–9.

[19] Lerner A. New therapeutic strategies for celiac disease. Autoimmun Rev 2010;9:144–7.

[20] Progress in Autoimmune Diseases Research. Report to congress, National Institutes of health, the autoimmune diseases coordinating committee. March 2005.

[21] Fairweather D, Frisancho-Kiss S, Rose NR. Sex differences in autoimmune disease from a pathological perspective. Am J Pathol 2008;173:600–9.

[22] Kondrashova A, Seiskari T, Ilonen J, Knip M, Hyöty H. The 'Hygiene hypothesis' and the sharp gradient in the incidence of autoimmune and allergic diseases between Russian Karelia and Finland. APMIS 2013;121:478–93.

[23] Zenouzi R, Hartl J, Lohse AW. Autoimmune hepatitis: news about a disease on the rise. Dtsch Med Wochenschr 2014;139:2020–2.

[24] Brick KE, Weaver CH, Lohse CM, Pittelkow MR, Lehman JS, Camilleri MJ, Al-Hashimi M, Wieland CN. Incidence of bullous pemphigoid and mortality of patients with bullous pemphigoid in Olmsted County, Minnesota, 1960 through 2009. J Am Acad Dermatol 2014;71:92–9.

[25] Rees F, Doherty M, Grainge M, Davenport G, Lanyon P, Zhang W. The incidence and prevalence of systemic lupus erythematosus in the UK, 1999-2012. Ann Rheum Dis 2016;75:136–41.

[26] Sipetic S, Maksimovic J, Vlajinac H, Ratkov I, Sajic S, Zdravkovic D, Sipetic T. Rising incidence of type 1 diabetes in Belgrade children aged 0-14 years in the period from 1982 to 2005. J Endocrinol Investig 2013;36:307–12.

[27] Lerner A, Jermias P, Matthias T. The world incidence of celiac disease is increasing: a review. Internat J Recent Sci Res 2015;7:5491–6.

[28] Lerner A, Jeremias P, Matthias T. The world incidence and prevalence of autoimmune diseases is increasing: a review. Int J Celiac Dis 2015;3:151–5.

[29] Lohi S, Mustalahti K, Kaukinen K, Laurila K, Collin P, Rissanen H, et al. Increasing prevalence of coeliac disease over time. Aliment Pharmacol Ther 2007;26:1217–25.

[30] Lerner A, Matthias T. Changes in intestinal tight junction permeability associated with industrial food additives explain the rising incidence of autoimmune disease. Autoimmun Rev 2015;14:479–89.

[31] Bach JF. The effect of infections on susceptibility to autoimmune and allergic diseases. N Engl J Med 2002;347:911–20.

[32] Bach JF, Chatenoud L. The hygiene hypothesis: an explanation for the increased frequency of insulin-dependent diabetes. Cold Spring Harb Perspect Med 2012;2:a007799.

[33] Okada H, Kuhn C, Feillet H, Bach JF. The 'hygiene hypothesis' for autoimmune and allergic diseases: an update. Clin Exp Immunol 2010;160:1–9.

[34] León K, Faro J, Lage A, Carneiro J. Inverse correlation between the incidences of autoimmune disease and infection predicted by a model of T cell mediated tolerance. J Autoimmun 2004;22:31–42.

[35] Lerner A, Neidhöfer S, Matthias T. The gut microbiome feelings of the brain: perspective for Non-Microbiologists. Microorganisms 2017;5:66–90.

[36] Lerner A, Jeremias P, Matthias T. Nutrients, bugs and us: the short-chain fatty acids story in celiac disease. Int J Celiac Dis 2016;4:92–4.

[37] Lerner A, Aminov R, Matthias T. Intestinal dysbiotic transglutaminases are potential environmental drivers of systemic autoimmunogenesis. Front Microbiol 2017;8. article 66.

[38] Sanz Y. Microbiome and gluten. Ann Nutr Metab 2015;67(Suppl. 2):28–41.

[39] de Sousa Moraes LF, Grzeskowiak LM, de Sales Teixeira TF, Gouveia Peluzio Mdo C. Intestinal microbiota and probiotics in celiac disease. Clin Microbiol Rev 2014;27:482–9.

[40] Caminero A, Galipeau HJ, McCarville JL, Johnston CW, Bernier SP, Russell AK, et al. Duodenal bacteria from patients with celiac disease and healthy subjects distinctly affect gluten breakdown and immunogenicity. Gastroenterology 2016;151:670–83.

[41] Gutiérrez S, Pérez-Andrés J, Martínez-Blanco H, Ferrero MA, Vaquero L, Vivas S, et al. The human digestive tract has proteases capable of gluten hydrolysis. Mol Metab 2017;6:693–702.

[42] Wagh SK, Gadge PP, Padul MV. Significant hydrolysis of wheat gliadin by Bacillus tequilensis (10bT/HQ223107): a pilot study. Probiotics Antimicrob Proteins September 25, 2017. https://doi.org/10.1007/s12602-017-9331-5. [Epub ahead of print].

[43] Cenit MC, Olivares M, Codoñer-Franch P, Sanz Y. Intestinal microbiota and celiac disease: cause, consequence or Co-Evolution? Nutrients 2015;7:6900–23.

[44] Paun A, Danska JS. Immuno-ecology: how the microbiome Regulates tolerance and autoimmunity. Curr Opin Immunol 2015;37:34–9.

[45] Lerner A, Matthias T. Extraintestinal manifestations of CD: common pathways in the gut-remote organs' axes. Int J Celiac Dis 2017;5:24–7.

[46] Lerner A, Matthias T. Comment to Nature publication: chassaing B et al. Dietary emulsifiers impact the mouse gut microbiota promoting colitis and metabolic syndrome. Nature 2015;519:92–6. [e-correspondance].

[47] Lerner A, Matthias T. Multiple food additives enhance human chronic diseases. SOJ Microbiol Infect Dis 2016;4:1–2.

[48] Heyman M, Abed J, Lebreton C, Cerf-Bensussan N. Intestinal permeability in coeliac disease: insight into mechanisms and relevance to pathogenesis. Gut 2012;61:1355–64.

[49] Sapone A, Lammers KM, Casolaro V, Cammarota M, Giuliano MT, De Rosa M, et al. Divergence of gut permeability and mucosal immune gene expression in two gluten-associated conditions: celiac disease and gluten sensitivity. BMC Med 2011;9:23.

[50] Jauregi-Miguel A, Fernandez-Jimenez N, Irastorza I, Plaza-Izurieta L, Vitoria JC, Bilbao JR. Alteration of tight junction gene expression in celiac disease. J Pediatr Gastroenterol Nutr 2014;58:762–7.

[51] Hollon J, Puppa EL, Greenwald B, Goldberg E, Guerrerio A, Fasano A. Effect of gliadin on permeability of intestinal biopsy explants from celiac disease patients and patients with non-celiac gluten sensitivity. Nutrients 2015;7:1565–76.

[52] Lerner A, Matthias T. Possible association between celiac disease and bacterial transglutaminase in food processing: a hypothesis. Nutr Rev 2015;73:544–52.

[53] Lerner A, Matthias T. Food industrial microbial transglutaminase in celiac disease: treat or trick. Int J Celiac Dis 2015;3:1–6.

[54] Lerner A, Matthias T. Are microbial enzymes used safe in the processed food industries? Food Bioprocess Technol 2016;9:2125–6. https://doi.org/10.1007/s11947-016-1795-x.

[55] Lerner A, Aminov R, Matthias T. Dysbiosis may trigger autoimmune diseases via inappropriate posttranslational modification of host proteins. Front Microbiol 2016;7. Article 84.

[56] Matthias T, Jeremias P, Neidhöfer S, Lerner A. The industrial food additive microbial transglutaminase, mimics the tissue transglutaminase and is immunogenic in celiac disease patients. Autoimmun Rev 2016;15:1111–9.

[57] Lerner A, Matthias T. Don't forget the exogenous microbial transglutaminases: it is immunogenic and potentially pathogenic. AIMS Biophys 2016;3:546–52.

[58] Liu Z, Li N, Neu J. Tight junctions, leaky intestines, and pediatric diseases. Acta Paediatr 2005;94:386–93.

[59] Lerner A, Matthias T. GUT-the Trojan horse in remote organs' autoimmunity. J Clin Cell Immunol 2016;7:401.

[60] Lerner A, Shoenfeld Y, Matthias T. Gluten ingestion side effects and withdrawal advantages in non-celiac autoimmune diseases. Nutr Rev 2017;75:1046–58. https://doi.org/10.1093/nutrit/nux054.

[61] Lerner A, Arleevskaya M, Schmiedl A, Matthias T. Microbes and viruses are bugging the gut in celiac disease. Are they friends or foes? Front Microbiol 2017;8:1392. https://doi.org/10.3389/fmicb.2017.01392.

[62] Rostami Nejad M, Ishaq S, Al Dulaimi D, Zali MR, Rostami K. The role of infectious mediators and gut microbiome in the pathogenesis of celiac disease. Arch Iran Med 2015;18:244–9.

[63] Fasano A. Zonulin, regulation of tight junctions, and autoimmune diseases. Ann NY Acad Sci 2012;1258:25–33.

[64] Fasano A. Zonulin and its regulation of intestinal barrier function: the biological door to inflammation, autoimmunity, and cancer. Physiol Rev 2011;91:151–75.

[65] Aminov RI. The extent and regulation of lateral gene transfer in natural microbial ecosystems. In: Francino MP, editor. Horizontal gene transfer in microorganisms. Norwich NR9 3DB, UK: Horizon Scientific Press; 2012. p. 93–100. [Chapter 6].

[66] Lerner A, Aminov R, Matthias T. Horizontal gene transfer in the gut. Front Immunol 2017, 8:article 1630.

[67] Robinson KM, Sieber KB, Hotopp JCD. A review of bacteria-animal lateral gene transfer may inform our understanding of diseases like cancer. PLoS Genet 2013;9:e1003877.

[68] Lerner A, Matthias T. Rheumatoid arthritis-celiac disease relationship: joints get that gut feeling. Autoimm Rev 2015;14:1038–47.

[69] Lerner A, Neidhöfer S, Matthias T. Beyond the joint: what's happening in the gut. Int J Celiac Dis 2016;4:127–9.

[70] Lerner A, Matthias T. Gut- bone cross talks and implications in celiac disease. Int J Celiac Dis 2016;4:19–23.

[71] Lerner A, Neidhöfer S, Matthias T. The gut-gut axis: cohabitation of celiac, Crohn's disease and IgA deficiency. Int J Celiac Dis 2016;4:68–70.

[72] Lerner A, Matthias T. The gut-stomach axis: *Helicobacter pylori* and celiac disease. Int J Celiac Dis 2016;4(3):77–9.

[73] Lerner A, Matthias T. Autoimmune thyroid diseases in celiac disease: if and when to screen? Int J Celiac Dis 2016;4:124–6.

[74] Lerner A, Jeremias P, Matthias T. The gut-thyroid axis and celiac disease. Endocrinol Cennections 2017;6:R52–8.

[75] Lerner A, Berthelot L, Jeremias P, Abbad L, Matthias T, Monteiro RC. Gut-kidney axis: gluten, transglutaminase, celiac disease and IgA nephropathy. J Clin Cell Immunol 2017;8:499–503.

[76] Lerner A, Neidhöfer S, Matthias T. The gut microbiome feelings of the brain: perspective for Non-Microbiologists. Microorganisms 2017;5:66.

[77] Lin R, Zhou L, Zhang J, Wang B. Abnormal intestinal permeability and microbiota in patients with autoimmune hepatitis. Int J Clin Exp Pathol 2015;8:5153–60.

[78] Yan D, Issa N, Afifi L, Jeon C, Chang HW, Liao W. The role of the skin and gut microbiome in psoriatic disease. Curr Dermatol Rep 2017;6:94–103.

[79] Marsland BJ, Trompette A, Gollwitzer ES. The gut-lung Axis in respiratory disease. Ann Am Thorac Soc 2015;12(Suppl. 2):S150–6.

[80] Kamo T, Akazawa H, Suzuki JI, Komuro I. Novel concept of a heart-gut axis in the pathophysiology of heart failure. Korean Circ J 2017;47:663–9.

[81] Brown JM, Hazen SL. The gut microbial endocrine organ: bacterially derived signals driving cardiometabolic diseases. Annu Rev Med 2015;66:343–59.

[82] Villa CR, Ward WE, Comelli EM. Gut microbiota-bone axis. Crit Rev Food Sci Nutr 2017;57:1664–72.

Chapter 33

Psychological Stress and the Kaleidoscope of Autoimmune Diseases

Kassem Sharif[1,2,3], Abdulla Watad[1,2,3], Alec Krosser[3], Louis Coplan[3], Howard Amital[1,2,3], Arnon Afek[2,3], Yehuda Shoenfeld[4,5]

[1]Department of Medicine 'B', Sheba Medical Center, Tel-Hashomer, Israel; [2]Zabludowicz Center for Autoimmune Diseases, Sheba Medical Center, Tel-Hashomer, Israel; [3]Sackler Faculty of Medicine, Tel Aviv University, Tel Aviv, Israel; [4]Zabludowicz Center for Autoimmune Diseases, Sheba Medical Center, affiliated to Sackler Faculty of Medicine, Tel Aviv University, Tel Aviv, Israel; [5]Laboratory of the Mosaics of Autoimmunity, Saint-Petersburg University, Saint-Petersburg, Russian Federation

INTRODUCTION

Stress is defined as the complex pshycophysiological reaction of the body in which normal homeostasis is disturbed or threatened [1]. Stress is considered negative when it results in detrimental behavioral and physical symptoms [2,3]. In contrast, eustress, or positive stress, results in an action-enhancing effect. The role of stress in the clinical course of autoimmune diseases is oftentimes overlooked [4]. The association between stress and autoimmunity is elusive, and the downstream effects are thought to occur in parallel to immunologic perturbations. Hormones, neurotransmitters, and other factors are shown to influence these phenomena. The role of stress in inducing or directing the clinical course of autoimmune diseases is oftentimes overlooked. In this review, we inspect the clinical evidence regarding the role of stress on various aspects of disease entities (Fig. 33.1).

RHEUMATOID ARTHRITIS AND STRESS

Rheumatoid arthritis (RA) is a chronic autoimmune disease marked by joint swelling with destruction of the synovial membrane in diarthrodial joints [5]. RA is influenced by genetic and environmental factors [6], and various factors, including stress, may contribute its pathogenesis.

Many studies support the notion that stress may precede RA by years. In one retrospective study (N = 18,309), researchers showed that two or more childhood stressful events increased a person's risk of developing RA, confirming that more stress in childhood is related to RA incidence [7]. In another large prospective study (N = 9159), researchers found an increased risk in self-reported arthritis in people with >2 traumatic childhood experiences [8].

Even with the genetic association [9], a study of 3143 twin pairs found that RA is more prevalent in those with more combat exposure. The same study found that those with RA had significantly more Posttraumatic stress disorder (PTSD) symptoms [10]. In a separate study of 54,224 female nurses, participants with >4 PTSD symptoms had an increased risk of developing RA in the next 2 years [11].

Stress and RA activity have been studied during stressful life events (i.e., divorce, bereavement) [12–15]; a literature review involving over 3000 patients found that minor and major stressors are related to an increase in disease activity [16]. Another prospective study found that worrying preceded overall disease activity. One study of 41 women with RA saw a positive association between interpersonal stress and disease activity for the same and following week [30]. No association between daily stressors and any of the immune or Hypothalamic–pituitary–adrenal axis (HPA) axis variables was found [17].

Self-reported daily stress events were correlated with pain in one study of 35 RA patients [18]. Another study found that daily job stress was related to increased pain [19]. Stressful spousal relationships were associated with increased pain scores in RA as well [20].

Researchers found that RA patients in well-adjusted marriages had reduced pain compared with distressed marriages and unmarried patients, suggesting that nonstressful marriages are protective against pain in RA [21]. Another study also found that those with well-adjusted spousal relationships did not have any changes in these variables during stressful times [22].

Mosaic of Autoimmunity. https://doi.org/10.1016/B978-0-12-814307-0.00033-5

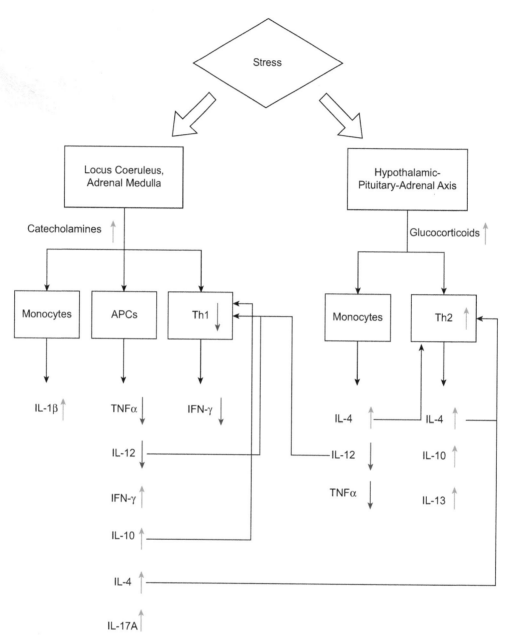

FIGURE 33.1 **The role of stress on the various aspects of the immune system.** During the stress response, catecholamines and glucocorticoids are released from their respective origins. These biomolecules exert control over various immune cells, thereby causing them to alter the production of various cytokines. The increase of IL-4 promotes T_h2 cell differentiation, whereas the decrease in IL-12 and the increased IL-10 production reduce the number of T_h1 cells. These changes favor a shift toward a humoral immune response. *APCs*, antigen-presenting cells.

Different coping styles impacted future RA activity, pain, and functional disability in newly diagnosed RA patients as well. A passive coping style (i.e., feeling of hopelessness and relying on others to resolve the situation) predicted functional disability at 3 years follow-up [23]. Disease activity 3 and 5 years postdiagnosis was worse in with stress avoidance coping mechanisms [24] and greater perceived stress without active coping strategies increased the risk of developing psychological comorbidities [25].

STRESS AND MULTIPLE SCLEROSIS

Multiple sclerosis (MS) is characterized by inflammation and demyelination of the central nervous system [26] and affects over 2.3 million people worldwide [27]. Past studies have shown that stress may play a role in the inflammatory and autoimmune processes [28].

When MS patients were compared with hospital controls, it was found that MS patients had more adverse life events in the 2 years prior to the onset of disease [29–32]. Using MRI technology, psychological stress was correlated with the appearance of new brain lesions [33].

High levels of anxiety were strongly related to severity and number of stressful life events and were found to increase the likelihood of exacerbations [34]. Similarly, after rocket attacks on civilian centers in northern Israel during the 2006 war between Hezbollah and Israel, 18 relapses were observed in the 156 patients, compared with only 1–6 relapses in similar time periods in the previous 12 months [35]. Ackerman et al. also found that exacerbations more likely followed stressful life events [36].

Alleviating stress has shown many benefits in MS patients. A recent study found that patients who received stress management therapies developed fewer new lesions compared with controls [37]. Likewise, many studies concluded that physical exercise and mindfulness-based interventions can benefit patients with MS [38–40]. Pharmacological treatments used for depression and anxiety have shown efficacy in the treatment of MS [41–43].

Regions displaying high levels of oxidative damage in oligodendrocytes correlated with increased presence of T cells and microglia [44] cells responsible for maintaining the integrity of the Blood–brain barrier (BBB) [45]. When microglial activation was inhibited or NADPH oxidase was blocked, the BBB constituents were preserved in vitro and BBB disruption was reduced in vivo [46].

Mast cells are thought to exacerbate MS by facilitating vascular permeability and allowing extravasation of lymphocytes [47]. Acute stress induced by immobilization or forced swimming was caused to cause BBB disruption in mice [48,49].

The HPA axis has also been studied in relation to MS pathogenesis. Increased levels of glucocorticoids inhibit NF-κB activity, leading to downregulation of the inflammatory cascade. Normally, cortisol exerts an inhibitory effect on corticotropin-releasing hormone (CRH) secretion. Under chronic stress, the negative feedback loop can be disrupted, leading to increased levels of cortisol [50]. With sustained stress, hypocortisolemia may occur [51]. In response to CRH stimulation, patients with secondary progressive MS exhibit less cortisol production [52]. The decreased cortisol levels suggest an impaired ability to control inflammation.

STRESS AND INFLAMMATORY BOWEL DISEASES

Crohn's disease (CD) and ulcerative colitis (UC), the two most prevalent inflammatory bowel diseases (IBDs), involve chronic gastrointestinal inflammation [53]. Stress is thought to influence physiological functions of inflammation and normal responses to inflammatory conditions [54].

In a prospective cohort study of 62 patients with UC, Levenstein et al. [55] found a positive association of long-term perceived stress on disease exacerbation. The authors did not find this same association for stressful life events or short-term stress. Bitton et al. [56] also found a positive association between perceived stress and IBD severity. Patients who scored lower on avoidance coping and those with lower perceived stress were less likely to relapse ($P = .003$).

A recent study found no association between the perceived stress level and markers of active intestinal inflammation, though it did find a relationship between perceived stress levels and reported GI symptoms [57]. In a later prospective study, the authors found that among CD and UC patients, higher symptom activity predicted higher perceived stress levels after 3 months [58].

Although the majority of studies on the effects of stress on IBD suggest that stress worsens IBD, not all studies came to the same conclusion and not everyone is in agreement.

Bitton et al. [59] found that patients with UC and stressful events had an earlier time until relapse of the disease. Langhorst et al. [60] found that short-term stress was predictive of relapse in UC and that baseline long-term stress was not. Bernstein et al. [61] monitored patients with IBD and found that perceived stress and major life events significantly correlated with disease flares. Vidal et al. [62] showed that stressful life events were not associated with relapses in UC or CD. A consensus has not been reached regarding the role of psychiatric treatment in IBD. A study by Wahed et al. [63] found that counseling improved the psychological well-being of IBD patients and also improved the course of IBD. Another study by Boye et al. [64] found that stress management psychotherapy did not improve the disease course or reduce replaces, though it may impact quality of life. A study assessing mindfulness-based stress reduction found that it did not reduce the number of flares or the severity of the flares but, however, did prevent a change in the quality of life questionnaire during flares [65]. A multicenter trial examining 488 CD patients found that after 1 year of standard treatment and psychotherapy, patients used fewer sick days and had fewer hospital days, compared with control subjects using only standard therapy [66].

STRESS AND SYSTEMIC LUPUS ERYTHEMATOSUS

Systemic lupus erythematosus (SLE) is an autoimmune disease that results in attacks on multiple body systems, including the joints, skin, lungs, kidneys, and nervous system [67,68]. Environmental factors, including stressors, may act as to induce and exacerbate SLE.

Roberts et al. [69] conducted a longitudinal cohort study of 54,753 women and found that trauma exposure and PTSD were associated with increased incidence of SLE, with a stronger incidence if there was concomitant trauma with PTSD. Stress, and its association with SLE and lupus flares, is a well-studied phenomenon [70–75]. Patients carrying the serotonin receptor 1A–1019 G allele, which has been linked to stress-related behaviors, were more susceptible to self-perceived stress and thus had an increased risk for lupus flares [70]. Kozora et al. [73] found that patients with SLE had more major life stresses ($P < .002$) than controls. Dobkin et al. [74] found that the global physical health scale scores in SF-36 were significantly lower in SLE patients than in healthy women.

Lupus patients with higher Perceived Stress Scale scores have also been found to show cognitive impairment and experience a higher prevalence of forgetfulness and difficulty concentrating [76].

Greco et al. [77] found improvement in pain, psychological functioning, and perceived physical functioning using biofeedback-assisted cognitive behavioral treatment compared with symptom monitoring or usual medical care [77]. Williams et al. [78] found that by using workshops to reduce stress, the perceived stress levels and quality of life increased among patients. Although no significant differences were found for biological indicators of stress (cortisol or Dehydroepiandrosterone (DHEA) levels), stress-reduction interventions improved depression, fatigue, and pain [78].

STRESS AND AUTOIMMUNE THYROID DISEASE

Loss of self-tolerance and subsequent production of autoantibodies against self-thyroid antigens result in varied production of thyroid hormones.

Stress and Graves' Disease

Winsa et al. [79] found that patients with Graves' disease (GD) had more negative life events compared with matched controls in the 12 months preceding diagnosis (OR 6.3). Similarly, Kung et al. [80] demonstrated that more negative events were experienced by GD patients than controls. Yoshiuchi et al. [81] inspected the role of stress in GD for men and women and found that stressful events in the last 12 months increased risk of disease development exclusively in women.

Radosavljevic et al. [82] evaluated 100 GD patients and found that subjects had significantly higher stressful life events in the last 12 months as compared with the healthy controls. Matos-Santos et al. [83] investigated three groups of 31 patients: GD, toxic goiter, and healthy controls. Patients with GD had a significantly higher number of stressful life events compared with toxic goiter and healthy controls. The addition of another control group was aimed to account for thyrotoxicosis.

In a study of patients treated with iodine-131, patients with stressful events reached a hypothyroid status significantly earlier than controls. Thus, stress has been shown to potentiate the development of hypothyroidism in patients receiving a standard dose of radioiodine [84].

Fukao et al. [85] examined the effect of emotional stress and patients' personality traits on hyperthyroid status in antithyroid-treated GD patients who are currently at euthyroid levels. They found that higher stress scores were associated with higher levels of Thyroid-stimulating hormone (TSH) receptor antibodies and larger thyroid volume after treatment termination.

Stress and Hashimoto's Disease

Martin au Pan et al. aimed to investigate whether stress and pregnancy could induce Hashimoto's disease [86]. The authors enrolled 95 patients with Hashimoto's thyroiditis (HT) and 97 with benign thyroid nodules as controls, and no significant differences were noted between the two groups [86]. The evaluation of the role of stress remains a challenge because HT is slow in onset and patients are usually discovered only when they develop overt hypothyroidism [87].

STRESS AND TYPE 1 DIABETES MELLITUS

Type 1 diabetes mellitus (T1DM) is a chronic disease characterized by insulin deficiency as a consequence of autoimmune destruction of pancreatic β-cells. Genetic susceptibility and environmental factors have been shown to precipitate T1DM [88]. Stressful events have been suggested to play a role in the onset of both type 1 and type 2 diabetes. From as early as the 17th century, Thomas Willis, an English physician, linked the disease onset to prolonged sorrow [89].

A Swedish case control study set to investigate the role of psychological stress on the emergence of diabetes. New onset T1DM children, aged 0–14, were enrolled in the investigation and the findings suggested that stressful events in the vulnerable age group 5–9 may be associated with disease development [90]. In another report, 67 T1DM patients 0–14 years of age were compared to 61 matched healthy control subjects. When compared with controls, T1DM patients showed more statistically significant negative stressful events during the first 2 years of life ($P=.039$). This indicates that negative events may be a risk factor for T1DM [91].

The influence of stressful life events and glycemic control has been the focus of various reports. Lloyd et al. [92] examined the occurrence of stressful experiences in 55 adult patients with T1DM, mean age 27.6 ± 8.9 years old, average duration of diabetes 12.7 ± 8.0 years. Subjects with poor glycemic control (HbA1c > 7.7%) were significantly more likely to report severe personal stressors 1 month before HbA1c measurements compared with patients whose glycemic control remained fair or improved (43% and 25% vs. 7% and 0%, $P=.000$).

A metaanalysis of randomized controlled trials on the effectiveness of psychological therapies in improving glycemic control in patients with T1DM was performed [93], totaling 543 participants (children and adolescents). The mean standardized effect sizes were -0.35, 95% CI -0.66 -0.04, $P=.03$, translating to a reduction in glycosylated hemoglobin of 0.48%, a level sufficient to decrease the microvascular complications of diabetes [94]. This demonstrates that psychological treatment can help improve glycemic control in children and adolescents.

SYSTEMIC SCLEROSIS AND STRESS

Systemic sclerosis (SSc) is a chronic multisystemic connective tissue disease. Scleroderma is divided into diffuse and limited cutaneous forms based on the extent of skin involvement [95]. Stress has been proposed to play a factor in disease pathogenesis, progression, and exacerbation.

Chen et al. [96] investigated the occurrence of stressful events prior to SSc onset in 40 patients and found that SSc subjects reported a higher number of stressful life events in all measured categories than controls ($P<.05$), highlighting the association between stress and SSc onset.

Another report found that prior to disease onset, 72% of the SSc respondents reported increased psychological stress, 50% reported emotional and personal problems, and 40% had a history of anger and anxiety [97]. Few studies discuss the association between stress and SSc. Further investigations of the association between stress and SSc are needed.

STRESS AND PEMPHIGUS

Pemphigus entails a collection of various autoimmune conditions characterized by blistering. Robust reports have implicated the role of certain environmental causes, including infections, dietary factors, and emotional stress, in pemphigus disease onset and propagation [98].

Several case reports highlight the role of stress in modulating various aspects of disease onset and exacerbation [99–101]. *Brenner* et al. [100] report two cases of pemphigus developing after war-related stress. *Tamir* et al. [101] documented a 68-year-old woman who did not improve with standard treatment; however, the addition of anxiolytics resulted in gradual healing.

Additionally, one prospective epidemiological study showed stressful events graded as "important" life events occurred in numerous patients 1–6 months prior to first signs or worsening of pemphigus, highlighting the role of stressful events in the disease course [102].

The exact pathomechanism of stress and pemphigus remains obscure. However, during stress, the skin is a prominent target for CRH, cortisol, catecholamines, and substance P [103]. Exposure of animals to stress has shown increased cutaneous inflammation, perifollicular accumulation of antigen-presenting cells, and mastocyte degranulation [104].

Taken together, these observations underscore the putative role of stressful events in inducing and worsening disease activity.

CONCLUSION

The relationship between stress and autoimmune diseases appears to be complex and intricate. A formidable amount of evidence supports the association and role of stress in influencing various aspects of autoimmune diseases including disease onset, severity of disease, and exacerbations. Active management of stress through various psychological techniques demonstrates significant benefits on disease outcomes and quality of life. Given the interrelation between these two factors, clinical physicians should encourage patients with autoimmune disease to seek stress management practices as part of their daily routines.

REFERENCES

[1] Schneiderman N, Ironson G, Siegel SD. Stress and health: psychological, behavioral, and biological determinants. Annu Rev Clin Psychol 2005;1:607–28. https://doi.org/10.1146/annurev.clinpsy.1.102803.144141.

[2] Selye H. The stress of life. New York: McGraw Hill; 1956.

[3] Salleh MR. Life event, stress and illness. Malays J Med Sci 2008;15(4):9–18.

[4] Davidson A, Diamond B. Autoimmune diseases. N Engl J Med 2001;345(5):340–50. https://doi.org/10.1056/nejm200108023450506.

[5] Aletaha D, Neogi T, Silman AJ, Funovits J, Felson DT, Bingham CO, Birnbaum NS, Burmester GR, Bykerk VP, Cohen MD. 2010 rheumatoid arthritis classification criteria: an American College of Rheumatology/European League against Rheumatism collaborative initiative. Arthritis Rheumatol 2010;62(9):2569–81.

[6] Angelotti F, Parma A, Cafaro G, Capecchi R, Alunno A, Puxeddu I. One year in review 2017: pathogenesis of rheumatoid arthritis. Clin Exp Rheumatol 2017;35(3):368–78.

[7] Von Korff M, Alonso J, Ormel J, Angermeyer M, Bruffaerts R, Fleiz C, De Girolamo G, Kessler RC, Kovess-Masfety V, Posada-Villa J. Childhood psychosocial stressors and adult onset arthritis: broad spectrum risk factors and allostatic load. Pain 2009;143(1):76–83.

[8] Kopec JA, Sayre EC. Traumatic experiences in childhood and the risk of arthritis: a prospective cohort study. Can J Public Health (Revue Canadienne de Sante'e Publique) 2004:361–5.

[9] MacGregor AJ, Snieder H, Rigby AS, Koskenvuo M, Kaprio J, Aho K, Silman AJ. Characterizing the quantitative genetic contribution to rheumatoid arthritis using data from twins. Arthritis Rheum 2000;43(1):30–7. https://doi.org/10.1002/1529-0131(200001)43:1<30::aid-anr5>3.0.co;2-b.

[10] Boscarino JA, Forsberg CW, Goldberg J. A twin study of the association between PTSD symptoms and rheumatoid arthritis. Psychosom Med 2010;72(5):481–6.

[11] Lee YC, Agnew-Blais J, Malspeis S, Keyes K, Costenbader K, Kubzansky LD, Roberts AL, Koenen KC, Karlson EW. Post-traumatic stress disorder and risk for incident rheumatoid arthritis. Arthritis Care Res 2016;68(3):292–8.

[12] Leymarie F, Jolly D, Sanderman R, Briancon S, Marchand A, Guillemin F, Eschard J, Suurmeijer T, Poitrinal P, Blanchard F. Life events and disability in rheumatoid arthritis: a European cohort. Br J Rheumatol 1997;36(10):1106–12.

[13] Dekkers JC, Geenen R, Evers AW, Kraaimaat FW, Bijlsma JW, Godaert GL. Biopsychosocial mediators and moderators of stress–health relationships in patients with recently diagnosed rheumatoid arthritis. Arthritis Care Res 2001;45(4):307–16.

[14] Haller C, Holzner B, Mur E, Günther V. The impact of life events on patients with rheumatoid arthritis: a psychological myth? Clin Exp Rheumatol 1996;15(2):175–9.

[15] Conway SC, Creed FH, Symmons DP. Life events and the onset of rheumatoid arthritis. J Psychosom Res 1994;38(8):837–47.

[16] Herrmann M, Schölmerich J, Straub RH. Stress and rheumatic diseases. Rheum Dis Clin N Am 2000;26(4):737–63.

[17] Evers AW, Zautra A, Thieme K. Stress and resilience in rheumatic diseases: a review and glimpse into the future. Nat Rev Rheumatol 2011;7(7):409–15. https://doi.org/10.1038/nrrheum.2011.80.

[18] Stone AA, Broderick JE, Porter LS, Kaell AT. The experience of rheumatoid arthritis pain and fatigue: examining momentary reports and correlates over one week. Arthritis Rheumatol 1997;10(3):185–93.

[19] Fifield J, Mcquillan J, Armeli S, Tennen H, Reisine S, Affleck G. Chronic strain, daily work stress and pain among workers with rheumatoid arthritis: does job stress make a bad day worse? Work Stress 2004;18(4):275–91.

[20] Waltz M, Kriegel W, Bosch PVT. The social environment and health in rheumatoid arthritis: marital quality predicts individual variability in pain severity. Arthritis Rheumatol 1998;11(5):356–74.

[21] Reese JB, Somers TJ, Keefe FJ, Mosley-Williams A, Lumley MA. Pain and functioning of rheumatoid arthritis patients based on marital status: is a distressed marriage preferable to no marriage? J Pain 2010;11(10):958–64.

[22] Zautra AJ, Hoffman JM, Matt KS, Yocum D, Potter PT, Castro WL, Roth S. An examination of individual differences in the relationship between interpersonal stress and disease activity among women with rheumatoid arthritis. Arthritis Rheumatol 1998;11(4):271–9.

[23] Evers AW, Kraaimaat FW, Geenen R, Jacobs JW, Bijlsma JW. Pain coping and social support as predictors of long-term functional disability and pain in early rheumatoid arthritis. Behav Res Ther 2003;41(11):1295–310.

[24] Evers AW, Kraaimaat FW, Geenen R, Jacobs JW, Bijlsma JW. Stress–vulnerability factors as long-term predictors of disease activity in early rheumatoid arthritis. J Psychosom Res 2003;55(4):293–302.

[25] Treharne GJ, Lyons AC, Booth DA, Kitas GD. Psychological well-being across 1 year with rheumatoid arthritis: coping resources as buffers of perceived stress. Br J Health Psychol 2007;12(3):323–45. https://doi.org/10.1348/135910706X109288.

[26] Types of MS: National Multiple Sclerosis Society. 2017. https://www.nationalmssociety.org/What-is-MS/Types-of-MS.

[27] Rogers KA, MacDonald M. Therapeutic yoga: symptom management for multiple sclerosis. J Alternative Compl Med 2015;21(11):655–9.

[28] Stojanovich L, Marisavljevich D. Stress as a trigger of autoimmune disease. Autoimmun Rev 2008;7(3):209–13. https://doi.org/10.1016/j.autrev.2007.11.007.

[29] Warren S, Greenhill S, Warren K. Emotional stress and the development of multiple sclerosis: case-control evidence of a relationship. J Chronic Dis 1982;35(11):821–31.

[30] Grant I, Brown GW, Harris T, McDonald WI, Patterson T, Trimble MR. Severely threatening events and marked life difficulties preceding onset or exacerbation of multiple sclerosis. J Neurol Neurosurg Psychiatry 1989;52(1):8–13.

[31] Li J, Johansen C, Brønnum–Hansen H, Stenager E, Koch–Henriksen N, Olsen J. The risk of multiple sclerosis in bereaved parents a nationwide cohort study in Denmark. Neurology 2004;62(5):726–9.

[32] Mohr DC, Hart SL, Julian L, Cox D, Pelletier D. Association between stressful life events and exacerbation in multiple sclerosis: a meta-analysis. BMJ 2004;328(7442):731.

[33] Mohr D, Goodkin D, Bacchetti P, Boudewyn A, Huang L, Marrietta P, Cheuk W, Dee B. Psychological stress and the subsequent appearance of new brain MRI lesions in MS. Neurology 2000;55(1):55–61.

[34] Potagas C, Mitsonis C, Watier L, Dellatolas G, Retziou A, Mitropoulos P, Sfagos C, Vassilopoulos D. Influence of anxiety and reported stressful life events on relapses in multiple sclerosis: a prospective study. Mult Scler J 2008;14(9):1262–8.

[35] Golan D, Somer E, Dishon S, Cuzin Disegni L, Miller A. Impact of exposure to war stress on exacerbations of multiple sclerosis. Ann Neurol 2008;64(2):143–8.

[36] Ackerman KD, Stover A, Heyman R, Anderson BP, Houck PR, Frank E, Rabin BS, Baum A. Relationship of cardiovascular reactivity, stressful life events, and multiple sclerosis disease activity. Brain Behav Immun 2003;17(3):141–51.

[37] Mohr DC, Lovera J, Brown T, Cohen B, Neylan T, Henry R, Siddique J, Jin L, Daikh D, Pelletier D. A randomized trial of stress management for the prevention of new brain lesions in MS. Neurology 2012;79(5):412–9.

[38] Filipi ML, Kucera DL, Filipi EO, Ridpath AC, Leuschen MP. Improvement in strength following resistance training in MS patients despite varied disability levels. NeuroRehabilitation 2011;28(4):373–82.

[39] Leavitt V, Cirnigliaro C, Cohen A, Farag A, Brooks M, Wecht J, Wylie G, Chiaravalloti N, DeLuca J, Sumowski J. Aerobic exercise increases hippocampal volume and improves memory in multiple sclerosis: preliminary findings. Neurocase 2014;20(6):695–7.

[40] Simpson R, Booth J, Lawrence M, Byrne S, Mair F, Mercer S. Mindfulness based interventions in multiple sclerosis-a systematic review. BMC Neurol 2014;14(1):15.

[41] Mitsonis CI, Zervas IM, Potagas CM, Mitropoulos PA, Dimopoulos NP, Sfagos CA, Papadimitriou GN, Vassilopoulos DC. Effects of escitalopram on stress-related relapses in women with multiple sclerosis: an open-label, randomized, controlled, one-year follow-up study. Eur Neuropsychopharmacol 2010;20(2):123–31.

[42] Bibolini M, Chanaday N, Báez N, Degano A, Monferran C, Roth G. Inhibitory role of diazepam on autoimmune inflammation in rats with experimental autoimmune encephalomyelitis. Neuroscience 2011;199:421–8.

[43] Núñez-Iglesias MJ, Novío S, Almeida-Dias A, Freire-Garabal M. Inhibitory effects of alprazolam on the development of acute experimental autoimmune encephalomyelitis in stressed rats. Pharmacol Biochem Behav 2010;97(2):350–6.

[44] Haider L, Fischer MT, Frischer JM, Bauer J, Höftberger R, Botond G, Esterbauer H, Binder CJ, Witztum JL, Lassmann H. Oxidative damage in multiple sclerosis lesions. Brain 2011;134(7):1914–24.

[45] da Fonseca ACC, Matias D, Garcia C, Amaral R, Geraldo LH, Freitas C, Lima FRS. The impact of microglial activation on blood-brain barrier in brain diseases. Front Cell Neurosci 2014;8.

[46] Yenari MA, Xu L, Tang XN, Qiao Y, Giffard RG. Microglia potentiate damage to blood–brain barrier constituents. Stroke 2006;37(4):1087–93.

[47] Theoharides TC. Mast cells and stress—a psychoneuroimmunological perspective. J Clin Psychopharmacol 2002;22(2):103–8.

[48] Esposito P, Gheorghe D, Kandere K, Pang X, Connolly R, Jacobson S, Theoharides TC. Acute stress increases permeability of the blood–brain-barrier through activation of brain mast cells. Brain Res 2001;888(1):117–27.

[49] Sharma HS, Cervós-Navarro J, Dey PK. Increased blood-brain barrier permeability following acute short-term swimming exercise in conscious normotensive young rats. Neurosci Res 1991;10(3):211–21.

[50] Chrousos GP. The hypothalamic–pituitary–adrenal axis and immune-mediated inflammation. N Engl J Med 1995;332(20):1351–63.

[51] Heim C, Ehlert U, Hellhammer DH. The potential role of hypocortisolism in the pathophysiology of stress-related bodily disorders. Psychoneuroendocrinology 2000;25(1):1–35.

[52] Wei T, Lightman SL. The neuroendocrine axis in patients with multiple sclerosis. Brain 1997;120(6):1067–76.

[53] Fakhoury M, Negrulj R, Mooranian A, Al-Salami H. Inflammatory bowel disease: clinical aspects and treatments. J Inflamm Res 2014;7:113–20. https://doi.org/10.2147/JIR.S65979.

[54] Collins SM. Stress and the Gastrointestinal Tract IV. Modulation of intestinal inflammation by stress: basic mechanisms and clinical relevance. Am J Physiol Gastrointest Liver Physiol 2001;280(3):G315–8.

[55] Levenstein S, Prantera C, Varvo V, Scribano ML, Andreoli A, Luzi C, Arca M, Berto E, Milite G, Marcheggiano A. Stress and exacerbation in ulcerative colitis: a prospective study of patients enrolled in remission. Am J Gastroenterol 2000;95(5):1213–20. https://doi.org/10.1111/j.1572-0241.2000.02012.x.

[56] Bitton A, Dobkin PL, Edwardes MD, Sewitch MJ, Meddings JB, Rawal S, Cohen A, Vermeire S, Dufresne L, Franchimont D, Wild GE. Predicting relapse in Crohn's disease: a biopsychosocial model. Gut 2008;57(10):1386–92. https://doi.org/10.1136/gut.2007.134817.

[57] Targownik LE, Sexton KA, Bernstein MT, Beatie B, Sargent M, Walker JR, Graff LA. The relationship among perceived stress, symptoms, and inflammation in persons with inflammatory bowel disease. Am J Gastroenterol 2015;110(7):1001–12. https://doi.org/10.1038/ajg.2015.147. quiz 1013.

[58] Sexton KA, Walker JR, Graff LA, Bernstein MT, Beatie B, Miller N, Sargent M, Targownik LE. Evidence of bidirectional associations between perceived stress and symptom activity: a prospective longitudinal investigation in inflammatory bowel disease. Inflamm Bowel Dis 2017;23(3):473–83. https://doi.org/10.1097/MIB.0000000000001040.

[59] Bitton A, Sewitch MJ, Peppercorn MA, deB Edwardes MD, Shah S, Ransil B, Locke SE. Psychosocial determinants of relapse in ulcerative colitis: a longitudinal study. Am J Gastroenterol 2003;98(10):2203–8. https://doi.org/10.1111/j.1572-0241.2003.07717.x.

[60] Langhorst J, Hofstetter A, Wolfe F, Hauser W. Short-term stress, but not mucosal healing nor depression was predictive for the risk of relapse in patients with ulcerative colitis: a prospective 12-month follow-up study. Inflamm Bowel Dis 2013;19(11):2380–6. https://doi.org/10.1097/MIB.0b013e3182a192ba.

[61] Bernstein CN, Singh S, Graff LA, Walker JR, Miller N, Cheang M. A prospective population-based study of triggers of symptomatic flares in IBD. Am J Gastroenterol 2010;105(9):1994–2002. https://doi.org/10.1038/ajg.2010.140.

[62] Vidal A, Gomez-Gil E, Sans M, Portella MJ, Salamero M, Pique JM, Panes J. Life events and inflammatory bowel disease relapse: a prospective study of patients enrolled in remission. Am J Gastroenterol 2006;101(4):775–81. https://doi.org/10.1111/j.1572-0241.2006.00476.x.

[63] Wahed M, Corser M, Goodhand JR, Rampton DS. Does psychological counseling alter the natural history of inflammatory bowel disease? Inflamm Bowel Dis 2010;16(4):664–9. https://doi.org/10.1002/ibd.21098.

[64] Boye B, Lundin KE, Jantschek G, Leganger S, Mokleby K, Tangen T, Jantschek I, Pripp AH, Wojniusz S, Dahlstroem A, Rivenes AC, Benninghoven D, Hausken T, Roseth A, Kunzendorf S, Wilhelmsen I, Sharpe M, Blomhoff S, Malt UF, Jahnsen J. INSPIRE study: does stress management improve the course of inflammatory bowel disease and disease-specific quality of life in distressed patients with ulcerative colitis or Crohn's disease? A randomized controlled trial. Inflamm Bowel Dis 2011;17(9):1863–73. https://doi.org/10.1002/ibd.21575.

[65] Jedel S, Hoffman A, Merriman P, Swanson B, Voigt R, Rajan KB, Shaikh M, Li H, Keshavarzian A. A randomized controlled trial of mindfulness-based stress reduction to prevent flare-up in patients with inactive ulcerative colitis. Digestion 2014;89(2):142–55. https://doi.org/10.1159/000356316.

[66] Deter HC, Keller W, von Wietersheim J, Jantschek G, Duchmann R, Zeitz M, German Study Group on Psychosocial Intervention in Crohn's Disease. Psychological treatment may reduce the need for healthcare in patients with Crohn's disease. Inflamm Bowel Dis 2007;13(6):745–52. https://doi.org/10.1002/ibd.20068.

[67] Watad A, Neumann SG, Soriano A, Amital H, Shoenfeld Y. Vitamin D and systemic lupus erythematosus: myth or reality? Isr Med Assoc J 2016;18(3–4):177–82.

[68] Gurevitz SL, Snyder JA, Wessel EK, Frey J, Williamson BA. Systemic lupus erythematosus: a review of the disease and treatment options. Consult Pharm 2013;28(2):110–21. https://doi.org/10.4140/TCP.n.2013.110.

[69] Roberts AL, Malspeis S, Kubzansky LD, Feldman CH, Chang SC, Koenen KC, Costenbader KH. Association of trauma and posttraumatic stress disorder with incident systemic lupus erythematosus in a longitudinal cohort of women. Arthritis Rheumatol 2017. https://doi.org/10.1002/art.40222.

[70] Birmingham DJ, Nagaraja HN, Rovin BH, Spetie L, Zhao Y, Li X, Hackshaw KV, Yu CY, Malarkey WB, Hebert LA. Fluctuation in self-perceived stress and increased risk of flare in patients with lupus nephritis carrying the serotonin receptor 1A -1019 G allele. Arthritis Rheum 2006;54(10):3291–9. https://doi.org/10.1002/art.22135.

[71] Mills SD, Azizoddin D, Racaza GZ, Wallace DJ, Weisman MH, Nicassio PM. The psychometric properties of the perceived stress scale-10 among patients with systemic lupus erythematosus. Lupus 2017;26(11):1218–23. https://doi.org/10.1177/0961203317701844.

[72] Pawlak CR, Witte T, Heiken H, Hundt M, Schubert J, Wiese B, Bischoff-Renken A, Gerber K, Licht B, Goebel MU, Heijnen CJ, Schmidt RE, Schedlowski M. Flares in patients with systemic lupus erythematosus are associated with daily psychological stress. Psychother Psychosom 2003;72(3):159–65. https://doi.org/10.1159/000069735.

[73] Kozora E, Ellison MC, Waxmonsky JA, Wamboldt FS, Patterson TL. Major life stress, coping styles, and social support in relation to psychological distress in patients with systemic lupus erythematosus. Lupus 2005;14(5):363–72. https://doi.org/10.1191/0961203305lu2094oa.

[74] Dobkin PL, Fortin PR, Joseph L, Esdaile JM, Danoff DS, Clarke AE. Psychosocial contributors to mental and physical health in patients with systemic lupus erythematosus. Arthritis Care Res 1998;11(1):23–31.

[75] Bultink IE, Turkstra F, Dijkmans BA, Voskuyl AE. High prevalence of unemployment in patients with systemic lupus erythematosus: association with organ damage and health-related quality of life. J Rheumatol 2008;35(6):1053–7.

[76] Plantinga L, Lim SS, Bowling CB, Drenkard C. Perceived stress and reported cognitive symptoms among Georgia patients with systemic lupus erythematosus. Lupus 2017;26(10):1064–71. https://doi.org/10.1177/0961203317693095.

[77] Greco CM, Rudy TE, Manzi S. Effects of a stress-reduction program on psychological function, pain, and physical function of systemic lupus erythematosus patients: a randomized controlled trial. Arthritis Rheum 2004;51(4):625–34. https://doi.org/10.1002/art.20533.

[78] Williams EM, Penfield M, Kamen D, Oates JC. An intervention to reduce psychosocial and biological indicators of stress in African American lupus patients: the balancing lupus experiences with stress strategies study. Open J Prev Med 2014;4(1):22–31. https://doi.org/10.4236/ojpm.2014.41005.

[79] Winsa B., Karlsson A., Bergstrom R., Adami H.O., Gamstedt A., Jansson R., Adamson U., Dahlberg P.A. Stressful life events and Graves' disease. Lancet 338(8781):1475–1479. doi:10.1016/0140-6736(91)92298-G.

[80] Kung AW. Life events, daily stresses and coping in patients with Graves' disease. Clin Endocrinol 1995;42(3):303–8.

[81] Yoshiuchi K, Kumano H, Nomura S, Yoshimura H, Ito K, Kanaji Y, Ohashi Y, Kuboki T, Suematsu H. Stressful life events and smoking were associated with Graves' disease in women, but not in men. Psychosom Med 1998;60(2):182–5.

[82] Radosavljevic VR, Jankovic SM, Marinkovic JM. Stressful life events in the pathogenesis of Graves' disease. Eur J Endocrinol 1996;134(6):699–701.

[83] Matos-Santos A, Nobre EL, Costa JG, Nogueira PJ, Macedo A, Galvao-Teles A, de Castro JJ. Relationship between the number and impact of stressful life events and the onset of Graves' disease and toxic nodular goitre. Clinical Endocrinol 2001;55(1):15–9.

[84] Stewart T, Rochon J, Lenfestey R, Wise P. Correlation of stress with outcome of radioiodine therapy for Graves' disease. Journal Nucl Med 1985;26(6):592–9.

[85] Fukao A, Takamatsu J, Murakami Y, Sakane S, Miyauchi A, Kuma K, Hayashi S, Hanafusa T. The relationship of psychological factors to the prognosis of hyperthyroidism in antithyroid drug-treated patients with Graves' disease. Clin Endocrinol 2003;58(5):550–5.

[86] Martin-du Pan RC. [Triggering role of emotional stress and childbirth. Unexpected occurrence of Graves' disease compared to 96 cases of Hashimoto thyroiditis and 97 cases of thyroid nodules]. Ann Endocrinol 1998;59(2):107–12.

[87] Mizokami T, Wu Li A, El-Kaissi S, Wall JR. Stress and thyroid autoimmunity. Thyroid 2004;14(12):1047–55. https://doi.org/10.1089/thy.2004.14.1047.

[88] van Belle TL, Coppieters KT, von Herrath MG. Type 1 diabetes: etiology, immunology, and therapeutic strategies. Physiol Rev 2011;91(1):79–118. https://doi.org/10.1152/physrev.00003.2010.

[89] Willis T, Pharmaceutice Rationalis, or, an Exercitation of the Operations of Medicines in Humane Bodies: Shewing the Signs, Causes, and Cures of Most Distempers Incident Thereunto. In: Dring T, Harper C, Leigh J, editors. Two Parts: as Also a Treatise of the Scurvy, and the Several Sorts Thereof, with Their Symptoms, Causes, and Cure, 1679.

[90] Hagglof B, Blom L, Dahlquist G, Lonnberg G, Sahlin B. The Swedish childhood diabetes study: indications of severe psychological stress as a risk factor for type 1 (insulin-dependent) diabetes mellitus in childhood. Diabetologia 1991;34(8):579–83.

[91] Thernlund GM, Dahlquist G, Hansson K, Ivarsson SA, Ludvigsson J, Sjöblad S, Hägglöf B. Psychological stress and the onset of IDDM in children: a case-control study. Diabetes Care 1995;18(10):1323–9. https://doi.org/10.2337/diacare.18.10.1323.

[92] Lloyd CE, Dyer PH, Lancashire RJ, Harris T, Daniels JE, Barnett AH. Association between stress and glycemic control in adults with type 1 (insulin-dependent) diabetes. Diabetes Care 1999;22(8):1278–83.

[93] Winkley K, Landau S, Eisler I, Ismail K. Psychological interventions to improve glycaemic control in patients with type 1 diabetes: systematic review and meta-analysis of randomised controlled trials. BMJ 2006;333(7558):65. https://doi.org/10.1136/bmj.38874.652569.55.

[94] Control D, Group CTR. The effect of intensive treatment of diabetes on the development and progression of long-term complications in insulin-dependent diabetes mellitus. N Engl J Med 1993;1993(329):977–86.

[95] Viswanath V, Phiske MM, Gopalani VV. Systemic sclerosis: current concepts in pathogenesis and therapeutic aspects of dermatological manifestations. Indian J Dermatol 2013;58(4):255–68. https://doi.org/10.4103/0019-5154.113930.

[96] Chen Y, Huang J-Z, Qiang Y, Wang J, Han M-M. Investigation of stressful life events in patients with systemic sclerosis. J Zhejiang Univ Sci B 2008;9(11):853–6. https://doi.org/10.1631/jzus.B0820069.

[97] Hui K-K, Johnston MF, Brodsky M, Tafur J, Kim Ho M. Scleroderma, stress and CAM utilization. Evid Base Compl Alternative Med 2009;6(4):503–6. https://doi.org/10.1093/ecam/nem142.

[98] Brenner S, Tur E, Shapiro J, Ruocco V, D'Avino M, Ruocco E, Tsankov N, Vassileva S, Drenovska K, Brezoev P, Barnadas MA, Gonzalez MJ, Anhalt G, Nousari H, Ramos-e-Silva M, Pinto KT, Miranda MF. Pemphigus vulgaris: environmental factors. Occupational, behavioral, medical, and qualitative food frequency questionnaire. Int J Dermatol 2001;40(9):562–9.

[99] Perry HO, Brunsting LA. Pemphigus foliaceus. Further observations. Arch Dermatol 1965;91:10–23.

[100] Brenner S, Bar-Nathan EA. Pemphigus vulgaris triggered by emotional stress. J Am Acad Dermatol 1984;11(3):524–5. https://doi.org/10.1016/S0190-9622(84)80380-1.

[101] Tamir A, Ophir J, Brenner S. Pemphigus vulgaris triggered by emotional stress. Dermatology (Basel Switz) 1994;189(2):210.

[102] Morell-Dubois S, Carpentier O, Cottencin O, Queyrel V, Hachulla E, Hatron PY, Delaporte E. Stressful life events and pemphigus. Dermatology (Basel Switz) 2008;216(2):104–8. https://doi.org/10.1159/000111506.

[103] Misery L. Skin, immunity and the nervous system. Br J Dermatol 1997;137(6):843–50. https://doi.org/10.1046/j.1365-2133.1997.19762090.x.

[104] Arck PC, Slominski A, Theoharides TC, Peters EMJ, Paus R. Neuroimmunology of stress: skin takes center stage. J Investig Dermatol 2006;126(8):1697–704. https://doi.org/10.1038/sj.jid.5700104.

Chapter 34

Coffee and Autoimmunity: More Than a Mere Hot Beverage!

Kassem Sharif[1,2,3], Alec Krosser[3], Abdulla Watad[1,2,3], Howard Amital[1,2,3], Yehuda Shoenfeld[4,5]

[1]Department of Medicine 'B', Sheba Medical Center, Tel-Hashomer, Israel; [2]Zabludowicz Center for Autoimmune Diseases, Sheba Medical Center, Tel-Hashomer, Israel; [3]Sackler Faculty of Medicine, Tel Aviv University, Tel Aviv, Israel; [4]Zabludowicz Center for Autoimmune Diseases, Sheba Medical Center, affiliated to Sackler Faculty of Medicine, Tel Aviv University, Tel Aviv, Israel; [5]Laboratory of the Mosaics of Autoimmunity, Saint-Petersburg University, Saint- Petersburg, Russian Federation

INTRODUCTION

Coffee is one of the most commonly consumed beverages, and as a complex blend of bioactive compounds, coffee has attracted a huge body of research. Caffeine, the most frequently ingested psychoactive molecule [1], has important anti-apoptotic effects. Moreover, coffee contains the lipid molecules, such as cafestol and kahweol, and antioxidant substances, such as polyphenols [2]. In addition, coffee has antimutagens that lead to a decreased risk of developing colorectal cancer, liver, renal, pancreatic cancer, and other solid tumors [3–5].

However, the beneficial effect of coffee remains debatable. Coffee contains some carcinogens, such as glyoxal, methyl-glyoxal, ethylglyoxal, propylglyoxal, diacetyl, acetol, and other dicarbonyls, and tannin, which may counteract the effects of antimutagens. Additionally, in large population-based studies, coffee is inversely associated with total mortality in a dose-dependent manner [3].

Autoimmune diseases occur as a consequence of immune system attack on self-tissues due to intrinsic tolerance loss [6]. Genetic predisposition and environmental factors such as dietary intake impact the development and progression of various autoimmune diseases [7]. Dietary habits may induce changes in the gut microbiota, influencing both innate and adaptive immunity [8].

Evidence regarding the impact of coffee intake and the development, as well as progression of autoimmune disease, is conflicting. Caffeine and other molecules present in coffee appear to have a role that goes beyond a mere neurostimulatory function. The purpose of this chapter is to describe the relationship between coffee and autoimmune disease as reported in the literature (Table 34.1).

THE ROLE OF COFFEE INTAKE IN IMMUNE SYSTEM MODULATION

Molecules present in coffee, particularly caffeine, act in an antiinflammatory manner on multiple components of the immune system [9] (Fig. 34.1). Although numerous studies have been conducted on caffeine's impact, most did not use physiological ranges [10].

Caffeine Impact on Innate Immunity

Impaired natural killer (NK) cells can contribute to the initiation of autoimmune processes [11]. The effect of caffeine on NK cells was investigated in vitro, and changes in NK cell activity were not observed with coffee dose changes [12]. Caffeine intake decreases chemotaxis of neutrophils and monocytes, which play a substantial role in mediating inflammation and contributing to autoimmune disease pathogenesis by influencing adaptive immune system activation [13,14].

Caffeine Intake and Cytokine Release

Caffeine has been linked to modified production of cell signaling molecules, including increased release of antiinflammatory cytokines, such as interleukin (IL)-10. In general, IL-10 promotes immune regulation and downregulation of

Mosaic of Autoimmunity. https://doi.org/10.1016/B978-0-12-814307-0.00034-7

TABLE 34.1 Summary of the Relationship Between Coffee Intake on Autoimmune Disease Aspects

Autoimmune Disease	Disease Occurrence	Other Disease Aspect
Rheumatoid arthritis	⬆	Influence methotrexate efficacy
Thyroid disease	No effect.	Influence levothyroxine gut absorption
Type 1 diabetes mellitus	⬆	Lowers insulin sensitivity, and elevate epic. levels
Systemic lupus erythematosus	No effect.	
Psoriasis	No effect.	Does not influence methotrexate activity
Multiple sclerosis	⬇	Coffee decreases clinical severity and progression
Primary sclerosing cholangitis	⬇	Decreases proctocolectomy in UC concomittant with PSC
Primary biliary cirrhosis	No effect.	
Inflammatory bowel disease	No effect.	
Celiac disease.	No effect.	23% anti-gliadin cross reactivity with instant preparation, as compared to pure preparations

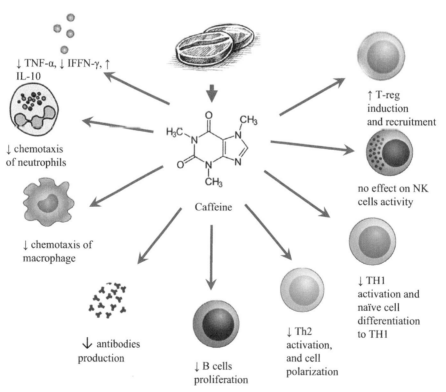

FIGURE 34.1 Effects of caffeine on immune system.

proinflammatory cell signaling pathways [15,16]. Furthermore, caffeine mediates immunosuppression of proinflammatory cytokine release, such as tumor necrosis factor alpha (TNF-α), IL-2, and interferon-gamma (IFN-γ) [17–19].

The Role of Caffeine on Adaptive Immune System

Both B and T cells play an integral part in autoimmune diseases [20,21]. Caffeine intake suppresses proliferation of Th1 and Th2 cells [19]. Both lineages, when activated in an uncontrolled manner, can lead to overt cytokine release damaging self-tissue [21]. Moreover, caffeine intake can lead to alterations of B cell function, suppressing antibody production [22–24].

The molecular mechanism by which caffeine induces its immunosuppressive effects is postulated to be based on its phosphodiesterase action, which leads to cyclic adenosine monophosphate (cAMP) accumulation. cAMP, an immunomodulator, promotes antiinflammatory cytokine production and inhibits proinflammatory cytokine release [25–27]. Other coffee constituents, including the antioxidant polyphenols, have an important role in scavenging reactive oxygen species, which have been implicated in autoimmune disease processes [28,29].

COFFEE AND RHEUMATOID ARTHRITIS

The exact pathogenesis of rheumatoid arthritis (RA) is largely unclear, but an interplay of genetics and the environment influence the onset and activity of the disease [30], with dietary habits proposed as one possible etiological factor [31,32]. Many studies support an increased RA risk in coffee consumers.

In a metaanalysis of 1279 RA cases, people consuming more than four cups of coffee were more at risk of developing RA (relative risk (RR) 2.426 [95% CI 1.060–5.554], $P=.036$). Limiting the analysis to cohort studies, an RR of 4.145 for RA was documented in those with high coffee consumption. Similarly, an association between RA and coffee intake was found in case-control studies (RR 2.01 [95% CI 1.058–1.361], $P=.005$). After stratifying based on the presence of autoimmune antibodies, a significant association between coffee intake and RA existed only in seropositive subjects [33].

In a cohort study, Mikuls et al. [34] found that decaffeinated coffee consumers showed a higher association of RA development compared with noncoffee consumers (RR 2.58, 95% CI 1.63–4.06). Dissimilarly, consumption of caffeinated coffee was not associated with increased development of RA [34]; however, other studies could not replicate these findings [35].

Furthermore, coffee may influence management of RA. Methotrexate (MTX), a disease-modifying agent [36], inhibits a series of enzymes resulting in adenosine accumulation [37]. Caffeine, a methylxanthine (adenosine receptor antagonist) [38], may decrease MTX efficacy [39]. Nesher et al. [39] reported a worse outcome and a slower improvement, indicated by the number of tender joint ($P=.086$) and swollen joints ($P=.072$), in patients with higher caffeine intake treated with MTX. Joint pain and morning stiffness showed significant differences only when comparing the highest caffeine versus lowest caffeine consumers ($P-.028$ and $P-.013$, respectively).

On the contrary, Benito-Garcia et al. did not find a significant difference in MTX efficacy in RA patients as assessed by disease activity score 28 (DAS-28), multidimensional health assessment questionnaire, and morning stiffness duration [40].

COFFEE AND THYROID AUTOIMMUNE DISEASE

The etiopathogenesis of autoimmune thyroid diseases has been linked to dietary habits [41–44], but no studies examine the relationship between coffee consumption and thyroid disease onset in humans. In rat models, intraperitoneal caffeine administration led to decreased thyroid-stimulating hormone levels and subsequently decreased thyroid hormone (T3, T4) [45]. By contrast, chronic caffeine administration stimulated the release of both thyroglobulin and thyroxine [46].

Hashimoto's thyroiditis is usually managed by supplementation of levothyroxine [47]. Benvenga et al. showed that coffee could interfere with levothyroxine intestinal absorption [48]. Compared with water, coffee lowered average and peak incremental rise of thyroxine by 36% and 30%, respectively, and delayed the time to reach peak serum level by 38 min.

COFFEE AND TYPE 1 DIABETES MELLITUS

The incidence of type 1 diabetes mellitus (T1DM) has increased substantially during the last two decades, even in patients not possessing high-risk genetic haplotypes [49,50].

In a case-control study of 600 children (<15-year-old) with T1DM, consuming more than two cups of coffee was associated with development of T1DM (OR 1.94 [95% CI 1.08–3.47]) [51]. On the contrary, a case-control Swedish study showed no association between coffee intake and latent autoimmune diabetes in adults (OR 1.04 [95% CI 0.96–1.13]). A significant association was found when stratifying according to the levels of autoantibody (glutamic acid decarboxylase); levels were proportional with additional coffee consumption (OR 1.11 [95% CI 1.00–1.23] per 1 cup per day) [52].

Watson et al. found that T1DM patients had an increased number of daytime hypoglycemic episodes with higher consumption of caffeine (1.3 vs. 0.9 per week, $P<.003$). Patients with higher coffee consumption had more severe warning symptoms (29 vs. 26 on symptoms scoring, $P<.05$) [53]. In a placebo-controlled study using continuous glucose monitoring, caffeine reduced the number of nighttime hypoglycemic episodes ($P=.04$) and was associated with a decrease in the mean duration of nocturnal hypoglycemia (29 vs. 132 min $P=.035$) [54].

In a double-blinded placebo-controlled study, caffeine decreased tissue sensitivity to insulin by 15% ($P<.05$), with concurrent increases in plasma epinephrine ($P<.0005$) and norepinephrine ($P<.02$) [55]. In another study, glucose ingestion following caffeinated coffee intake showed a 40% decrease in insulin sensitivity and elevated glucose levels ($P<.001$) when compared with decaffeinated coffee [56]. Both studies support a negative influence of caffeine on glycemic profile with a putative role of epinephrine, a known insulin counterregulatory hormone [57].

COFFEE AND MULTIPLE SCLEROSIS

The progression of multiple sclerosis (MS) is unpredictable [58]; however, both genetic and environmental factors, such as diet, may contribute to the etiology of this disease [59,60]. In MS animal models, caffeine administration exerted a neuroprotective role, putatively upregulating the adenosine receptor A1R [61], which is known to prevent neurotoxic injury caused by excessive glutamate secretion [62].

In a case-control study of 210 MS cases, coffee consumption was associated with MS development (OR 1.7, $P=.047$) [63]. In a Swedish study, coffee intake was associated with a reduced risk of developing MS (OR 0.7 [95% CI 0.49–0.99], $P=.04$). A similar association was reported in a US study (adjusted OR 0.69 [95% CI 0.5–0.96], $P=.05$).

In a case-control study conducted in Belgium, higher coffee consumption was associated with decreased disease progression in a dose-dependent manner, as measured by Expanded Disability Status Scale (EDSS) score (HR 0.60 [95% CI 0.44–0.81]) [64]. Relapsing MS patients who consumed coffee daily had a 5 years latency to reaching an EDSS score of 6 compared with patients who did not drink coffee ($P=.09$) [64].

By contrast, a cohort study with 258 MS patients failed to show a significant association between coffee and MS (RR 0.98 [95% CI 0.66–1.44], $P=.95$) [65].

COFFEE AND PSORIASIS

Psoriasis is a common disease, with approximately 2% of the general population being affected [66]. Susceptibility to psoriasis is determined by interactions between genetic and environmental factors [67], including ultraviolet light, smoking, obesity, and dietary intake [67], among others.

The role of coffee and caffeine on psoriasis development was studied in a large cohort study, which showed no association in psoriasis development or proportional increase in RR with increased coffee intake (p_{trend} 0.56) [68]. A case-control study of Australian twins with discordant occurrence of psoriasis also did not show coffee consumption to affect disease development ($P=.65$) [69].

The impact of coffee on treating psoriasis was also investigated, and no correlation between the required MTX dose and levels of coffee consumption was found (r=.03, $P=.22$) [70]. Topical application of caffeine on plaque psoriasis demonstrated a significant improvement in psoriasis area and severity index in psoriatic patients ($P<.05$) [71].

COFFEE AND SYSTEMIC LUPUS ERYTHEMATOSUS

In patients with systemic lupus erythematosus (SLE), interplay between genetic and environmental factors, such as dietary factors, may contribute to the disease etiopathogenesis and progression [72,73]. Kiyohara et al. [74] found coffee intake was marginally associated with development of SLE (crude OR 2.01 [95% CI 1.33–3.03]); however, after adjusting for confounding factors, the strength of association decreased to nonsignificant values (OR 1.57 [95% CI 0.95–2.61]).

Specific polymorphisms of N-acetyltransferase 2 (NAT2), an enzyme that helps to metabolize xenobiotics (including coffee), may be linked to SLE development. Polymorphisms that lead to slower acetylation increase the risk of SLE [75]. Coffee consumption in fast acetylators is not associated with SLE (OR 0.71 [95% CI 0.25–2.03]) [74]. Additionally, coffee intake was not associated with an increased risk of SLE development in SLE slow acetylators versus healthy slow acetylators (OR 2.05 [95% CI 0.86–4.95]) [74]. An increase was noticed in SLE slow acetylators versus SLE fast acetylators (*P*=.094) [74]. Increased association of SLE in fast acetylators supports the possible role of NAT2 polymorphism and slow acetylation in SLE development [74].

COFFEE AND AUTOIMMUNE LIVER DISEASES

Autoimmune liver disease predominantly includes three diseases: autoimmune hepatitis, primary sclerosing cholangitis (PSC), and primary biliary cirrhosis (PBC) [76,77]. Each disease has a different target of attack, but in all three cirrhosis it is inevitably present [78,79]. Environmental factors, such as smoking, infectious agents, chemical toxins, and dietary intake, have been linked to disease onset and activity [80,81]. Coffee is associated with decreased progression to cirrhosis, lower rates of hepatocellular carcinoma, and decreased mortality in cirrhotic patients [82–84].

Concerning liver autoimmune diseases, in a case-control study, 24% of PSC patients and 16% of healthy controls did not consume coffee (*P*<.05). Among coffee consumers, PSC patients were found to consume less than healthy controls (45% vs. 47%, *P*<.05) [85]. Additionally, PSC patients had a smaller duration of coffee consumption compared with healthy adults (46.6% vs. 66.7%, *P*<.05) [85]. These results highlight a protective role of coffee on PSC onset. Furthermore, patients drinking more than 20 cups of coffee per month had an inverse relationship with PSC onset (OR 0.89 [95% CI 0.83–0.94], *P*<.001).

Other research also found PSC patients consume less coffee than controls (76% vs. 86%, OR 0.52 [95% CI 0.32–0.82], *P*=.006), and drinking coffee was found to be inversely associated with PSC onset (*P*=.048) [86].

To date, no significant association was found between coffee consumption and PBC onset [85].

COFFEE AND INFLAMMATORY BOWEL DISEASES

Progression of Crohn's disease and ulcerative colitis (UC), the two major inflammatory bowel diseases (IBDs), is unpredictable and occasionally life-threatening [87]. While increased susceptibility to IBD has been linked to genetic predisposition, environmental factors play a key role in disease onset and activity [88].

In a case-control study conducted in Stockholm, coffee consumption significantly reduced the risk of Crohn's disease and UC development [89]. In a prospective cohort conducted in Australia, caffeine consumption showed a protective effect on UC (OR 0.51 [95% CI 0.30–0.87], *P*=.002), and a marginal inverse association between disease onset and caffeine consumption was noticed in Crohn's patients (R 0.59 [95% CI 0.34–1.03], *P*=.031) [90].

Boyko et al. did not document a significant association between coffee consumption or cumulative coffee intake and the risk of UC development [91].

COFFEE AND CELIAC DISEASE

Around 1% of the population is affected by celiac disease [92], but its etiology remains unclear. Although associations between haplotypes and disease development are well documented [93] and high rates of celiac disease concordance are found in monozygotic twins [94], environmental triggers were shown to play a role in disease susceptibility and etiopathogenesis [95].

Strict adherence to a gluten-free diet prevents colonic inflammation and complications [96]. Intriguingly, around one-third of celiac disease patients have persistent symptoms with adherence to a gluten-free diet [97], and one-quarter of patients did not report any histological improvement on intestinal biopsies [98]. These phenomena raise suspicion for cross-reactivity between gluten-free food and gliadin peptide. Vojdani et al. found that antigliadin antibody did cross-react with two instant coffee preparations at a rate of 23% [99]. Espresso preparation and Turkish and Israeli coffee did not show any reaction with antigliadin [99]. Therefore, it appears that pure coffee is safer than instant coffee preparations for patient with celiac disease.

CONCLUSIONS AND FINAL RECOMMENDATIONS

Although the relationship between coffee intake and the previously mentioned autoimmune disease remains controversial, data on certain autoimmune diseases such as systemic sclerosis, Sjögren's syndrome, and Behçet's disease, among others, are lacking in the extant literature.

From a clinical standpoint, the association between coffee and autoimmune diseases appears to be disease-specific. In a number of diseases, coffee and caffeine intake seem to not affect the risk of disease development, while influencing other aspects of the disease including medication absorption and antigen cross-reactivity.

Taking into mind that most data presented here have been collected from case-control studies, whose experimental design makes them prone to selection and recall biases, the following measures may be taken to prevent or, at least, to diminish the risk of adverse outcomes:

- MS patients could benefit from coffee because of its role in mitigating disease progression.
- Hashimoto's thyroiditis patients on levothyroxine supplementation therapy should avoid concomitant coffee consumption because of its possible impact on drug absorption.
- Due to its postulated impact on drug efficacy, it might be advantageous for patients treated with MTX to avoid coffee.
- Celiac patients adhering to a gluten-free diet with clinical symptoms may improve after switching to a coffee blend characterized by lower reactivity with antigliadin peptide.
- T1DM patients should decrease their coffee consumption because of their lowered insulin sensitivity and impaired glycemic control.

REFERENCES

[1] Belay A, Ture K, Redi M, Asfaw A. Measurement of caffeine in coffee beans with UV/vis spectrometer. Food Chem 2008;108:310–5.

[2] Yashin A, Yashin Y, Wang JY, Nemzer B. Antioxidant and antiradical activity of coffee. Antioxidants 2013;2:230–45.

[3] Butt MS, Sultan MT. Coffee and its consumption: benefits and risks. Crit Rev Food Sci Nutr 2011;51:363–73.

[4] Dong J, Zou J, Yu XF. Coffee drinking and pancreatic cancer risk: a meta-analysis of cohort studies. World J Gastroenterol 2011;17:1204–10.

[5] Schmit SL, Rennert HS, Rennert G, Gruber SB. Coffee consumption and the risk of colorectal cancer. Cancer Epidemiol Biomarkers Prev 2016;25:634–9.

[6] Smith DA, Germolec DR. Introduction to immunology and autoimmunity. Environ Health Perspect 1999;107:661–5.

[7] Wang L, Wang FS, Gershwin ME. Human autoimmune diseases: a comprehensive update. J Intern Med 2015;278:369–95.

[8] Vieira SM, Pagovich OE, Kriegel MA. Diet, microbiota and autoimmune diseases. Lupus 2014;23:518–26.

[9] Koroglu OA, MacFarlane PM, Balan KV, Zenebe WJ, Jafri A, Martin RJ, Kc P. Anti-inflammatory effect of caffeine is associated with improved lung function after lipopolysaccharide-induced amnionitis. Neonatology 2014;106:235–40.

[10] Horrigan LA, Kelly JP, Connor TJ. Immunomodulatory effects of caffeine: friend or foe? Pharmacol Ther 2006;111:877–92.

[11] Vivier E, Tomasello E, Baratin M, Walzer T, Ugolini S. Functions of natural killer cells. Nat Immunol 2008;9:503–10.

[12] Kantamala D, Vongsakul M, Satayavivad J. The in vivo and in vitro effects of caffeine on rat immune cells activities: B, T and NK cells. Asian Pac J Allergy Immunol 1990;8:77–82.

[13] Horrigan LA, Diamond M, Connor TJ, Kelly JP. Caffeine inhibits monocyte and neutrophil chemotaxis at concentrations relevant to normal human consumption. In: Proceedings of the International Cytokine Society Annual Meeting, Trinity College Dublin, Ireland. 2013.

[14] Tse RL, Phelps P, Urban D. Polymorphonuclear leukocyte motility in vitro. VI. Effect of purine and pyrimidine analogues: possible role of cyclic AMP. J Lab Clin Med 1972;80:264–74.

[15] Tauler P, Martinez S, Martinez P, Lozano L, Moreno C, Aguilo A. Effects of caffeine supplementation on plasma and blood mononuclear cell Interleukin-10 levels after exercise. Int J Sport Nutr Exerc Metab 2016;26:8–16.

[16] Ouyang W, Rutz S, Crellin NK, Valdez PA, Hymowitz SG. Regulation and functions of the IL-10 family of cytokines in inflammation and disease. Annu Rev Immunol 2011;29:71–109.

[17] Ritter M, Hohenberger K, Alter P, Herzum M, Tebbe J, Maisch M. Caffeine inhibits cytokine expression in lymphocytes. Cytokine 2005;30:177–81.

[18] Horrigan LA, Kelly JP, Connor TJ. Caffeine suppresses TNF-alpha production via activation of the cyclic AMP/protein kinase A pathway. Int Immunopharm 2004;4:1409–17.

[19] Rosenthal LA, Taub DD, Moors MA, Blank KJ. Methylxanthine-induced inhibition of the antigen- and superantigen-specific activation of T and B lymphocytes. Immunopharmacology 1992;24:203–17.

[20] Hampe CS. B cells in autoimmune diseases. Scientifica 2012;2012:18.

[21] Jäger A. Effector and regulatory T cell subsets in autoimmunity and tissue inflammation. Scand J Immunol 2010;72:173–84.

[22] Laux DC, Klesius PH. Suppressive effects of caffeine on the immune response of the mouse to sheep erythrocytes. Proc Soc Exp Biol Med 1973;144:633–8.

[23] Saxena AK, Singh KP, Srivastava SN, Khanna S, Shukla LJ, Shanker R. Immunomodulating effects of caffeine (1,3,7-trimethylxanthine) in rodents. Indian J Exp Biol 1984;22:298–301.

[24] Lau CE, Falk JL. Dose-dependent surmountability of locomotor activity in caffeine tolerance. Pharmacol Biochem Behav 1995;52:139–43.

[25] Wells JN, Wu YJ, Baird CE, Hardman JG. Phosphodiesterases from porcine coronary arteries: inhibition of separated forms by xanthines, papaverine, and cyclic nucleotides. Mol Pharmacol 1975;11:775–83.

[26] Kammer GM. The adenylate cyclase-cAMP-protein kinase A pathway and regulation of the immune response. Immunol Today 1988;9:222–9.

[27] Procopio DO, Teixeira MM, Camargo MM, Travassos LR, Ferguson MA, Almeida IC, Gazzinelli RT. Differential inhibitory mechanism of cyclic AMP on TNF-alpha and IL-12 synthesis by macrophages exposed to microbial stimuli. Br J Pharmacol 1999;127:1195–205.

[28] Di Dalmazi G, Hirshberg J, Lyle D, Freij JB, Caturegli P. Reactive oxygen species in organ-specific autoimmunity. Auto Immun Highlights 2016;7.

[29] Priftis A, Stagos D, Konstantinopoulos K, Tsitsimpikou C, Spandidos DA, Tsatsakis AM, Tzatzarakis MN, Kouretas D. Comparison of antioxidant activity between green and roasted coffee beans using molecular methods. Mol Med Rep 2015;12:7293–302.

[30] McInnes IB, Schett G. The pathogenesis of rheumatoid arthritis. N Engl J Med 2011;365:2205–19.

[31] Pattison DJ, Symmons DP, Young A. Does diet have a role in the aetiology of rheumatoid arthritis? Proc Nutr Soc 2004;63:137–43.

[32] Watad A, Agmon-Levin N, Gilburd B, Lidar M, Amital H, Shoenfeld Y. Predictive value of anti-citrullinated peptide antibodies: a real life experience. Immunol Res 2014;60:348–55.

[33] Lee YH, Bae S-C, Song GG. Coffee or tea consumption and the risk of rheumatoid arthritis: a meta-analysis. Clin Rheumatol 2014;33:1575–83.

[34] Mikuls TR, Cerhan JR, Criswell LA, Merlino L, Mudano AS, Burma M, Folsom AR, Saag KG. Coffee, tea, and caffeine consumption and risk of rheumatoid arthritis: results from the Iowa Women's Health Study. Arthritis Rheum 2002;46:83–91.

[35] Pedersen M, Stripp C, Klarlund M, Olsen SF, Tjonneland AM, Frisch M. Diet and risk of rheumatoid arthritis in a prospective cohort. J Rheumatol 2005;32:1249–52.

[36] Braun J. Methotrexate: optimizing the efficacy in rheumatoid arthritis. Ther Adv Musculoskelet Dis 2011;3:151–8.

[37] Cutolo M, Sulli A, Pizzorni C, Seriolo B, Straub R. Anti-inflammatory mechanisms of methotrexate in rheumatoid arthritis. Ann Rheum Dis 2001;60:729–35.

[38] Chen JF, Chern Y. Impacts of methylxanthines and adenosine receptors on neurodegeneration: human and experimental studies. Handb Exp Pharmacol 2011:267–310.

[39] Nesher G, Mates M, Zevin S. Effect of caffeine consumption on efficacy of methotrexate in rheumatoid arthritis. Arthritis Rheum 2003;48:571–2.

[40] Benito-Garcia E, Heller JE, Chibnik LB, Maher NE, Matthews HM, Bilics JA, Weinblatt ME, Shadick NA. Dietary caffeine intake does not affect methotrexate efficacy in patients with rheumatoid arthritis. J Rheumatol 2006;33:1275–81.

[41] Brent GA. Environmental exposures and autoimmune thyroid disease. Thyroid 2010;20:755–61.

[42] Prummel MF, Strieder T, Wiersinga WM. The environment and autoimmune thyroid diseases. Eur J Endocrinol 2004;150:605–18.

[43] Gaitan E. Goitrogens. Bailliere Clin Endocrinol Metab 1988;2:683–702.

[44] Porcelli B, Pozza A, Bizzaro N, Fagiolini A, Costantini M-C, Terzuoli L, Ferretti F. Association between stressful life events and autoimmune diseases: a systematic review and meta-analysis of retrospective case–control studies. Autoimmun Rev 2016;15:325–34.

[45] Spindel E, Arnold M, Cusack B, Wurtman RJ. Effects of caffeine on anterior pituitary and thyroid function in the rat. J Pharmacol Exp Therapeut 1980;214:58.

[46] Clozel M, Branchaud CL, Tannenbaum GS, Dussault JH, Aranda JV. Effect of caffeine on thyroid and pituitary function in newborn rats. Pediatr Res 1983;17:592–5.

[47] Ellerbroek V, Warncke K, Kohle J, Bonfig W. A levothyroxine dose recommendation for the treatment of children and adolescents with autoimmune thyroiditis induced hypothyroidism. J Pediatr Endocrinol Metab 2013;26:1023–8.

[48] Benvenga S, Bartolone L, Pappalardo MA, Russo A, Lapa D, Giorgianni G, Saraceno G, Trimarchi F. Altered intestinal absorption of L-thyroxine caused by coffee. Thyroid 2008;18:293–301.

[49] Hermann R, Knip M, Veijola R, Simell O, Laine AP, Akerblom HK, Groop PH, Forsblom C, Pettersson-Fernholm K, Ilonen J. Temporal changes in the frequencies of HLA genotypes in patients with Type 1 diabetes–indication of an increased environmental pressure? Diabetologia 2003;46:420–5.

[50] Ferretti C, La Cava A. Adaptive immune regulation in autoimmune diabetes. Autoimmun Rev 2016;15:236–41.

[51] Virtanen SM, Rasanen L, Aro A, Ylonen K, Lounamaa R, Akerblom HK, Tuomilehto J. Is children's or parents' coffee or tea consumption associated with the risk for type 1 diabetes mellitus in children? Childhood Diabetes in Finland Study Group. Eur J Clin Nutr 1994;48:279–85.

[52] Lofvenborg JE, Andersson T, Carlsson PO, Dorkhan M, Groop L, Martinell M, Rasouli B, Storm P, Tuomi T, Carlsson S. Coffee consumption and the risk of latent autoimmune diabetes in adults–results from a Swedish case-control study. Diabet Med 2014;31:799–805.

[53] Watson JM, Jenkins EJ, Hamilton P, Lunt MJ, Kerr D. Influence of caffeine on the frequency and perception of hypoglycemia in free-living patients with type 1 diabetes. Diabetes Care 2000;23:455–9.

[54] Richardson T, Thomas P, Ryder J, Kerr D. Influence of caffeine on frequency of hypoglycemia detected by continuous interstitial glucose monitoring system in patients with long-standing type 1 diabetes. Diabetes Care 2005;28:1316.

[55] Keijzers GB, De Galan BE, Tack CJ, Smits P. Caffeine can decrease insulin sensitivity in humans. Diabetes Care 2002;25:364–9.

[56] Moisey LL, Kacker S, Bickerton AC, Robinson LE, Graham TE. Caffeinated coffee consumption impairs blood glucose homeostasis in response to high and low glycemic index meals in healthy men. Am J Clin Nutr 2008;87:1254–61.

[57] Capaldo B, Napoli R, Di Marino L, Sacca L. Epinephrine directly antagonizes insulin-mediated activation of glucose uptake and inhibition of free fatty acid release in forearm tissues. Metabolism 1992;41:1146–9.

[58] Goldenberg MM. Multiple sclerosis review. Pharm Ther 2012;37:175–84.

[59] Lauer K. Notes on the epidemiology of multiple sclerosis, with special reference to dietary habits. Int J Mol Sci 2014;15:3533–45.

[60] Watad A, Azrielant S, Soriano A, Bracco D, Abu Much A, Amital H. Association between seasonal factors and multiple sclerosis. Eur J Epidemiol 2016;31:1081–9.

[61] Wang T, Xi NN, Chen Y, Shang XF, Hu Q, Chen JF, Zheng RY. Chronic caffeine treatment protects against experimental autoimmune encephalomyelitis in mice: therapeutic window and receptor subtype mechanism. Neuropharmacology 2014;86:203–11.

[62] Cunha RA. Neuroprotection by adenosine in the brain: from A(1) receptor activation to A(2A) receptor blockade. Purinergic Signal 2005;1:111–34.

[63] Pekmezovic T, Drulovic J, Milenkovic M, Jarebinski M, Stojsavljevic N, Mesaros S, Kisic D, Kostic J. Lifestyle factors and multiple sclerosis: a case-control study in Belgrade. Neuroepidemiology 2006;27:212–6.

[64] D'hooghe MB, Haentjens P, Nagels G, De Keyser J. Alcohol, coffee, fish, smoking and disease progression in multiple sclerosis. Eur J Neurol 2012;19:616–24.

[65] Massa J, O'Reilly E, Munger K, Ascherio A. Caffeine and alcohol intakes have no association with risk of multiple sclerosis in a prospective study of women. Mult Scler (Houndmills Basingstoke Engl) 2013;19:53–8.

[66] Mahil SK, Capon F, Barker JN. Update on psoriasis immunopathogenesis and targeted immunotherapy. Semin Immunopathol 2016;38:11–27.

[67] Smith CH, Barker J. Psoriasis and its management. BMJ 2006;333:380–4.

[68] Li W, Han J, Qureshi AA. No association between coffee and caffeine intake and risk of psoriasis in us women. Arch Dermatol 2012;148:395–7.

[69] Duffy DL, Spelman LS, Martin NG. Psoriasis in Australian twins. J Am Acad Dermatol 1993;29:428–34.

[70] Swanson DL, Barnes SA, Mengden Koon SJ, El-Azhary RA. Caffeine consumption and methotrexate dosing requirement in psoriasis and psoriatic arthritis. Int J Dermatol 2007;46:157–9.

[71] Vali A, Asilian A, Khalesi E, Khoddami L, Shahtalebi M, Mohammady M. Evaluation of the efficacy of topical caffeine in the treatment of psoriasis vulgaris. J Dermatol Treat 2005;16:234–7.

[72] Kamen DL. Environmental influences on systemic lupus erythematosus expression. Rheum Dis Clin N Am 2014;40:401–12. vii.

[73] Watad A, Tiosano S, Azrielant S, Whitby A, Comaneshter D, Cohen AD, Shoenfeld Y, Amital H. Low levels of calcium or vitamin D - which is more important in systemic lupus erythematosus patients? An extensive data analysis. Clin Exp Rheumatol 2017;35:108–12.

[74] Kiyohara C, Washio M, Horiuchi T, Asami T, Ide S, Atsumi T, Kobashi G, Takahashi H, Tada Y, Kyushu Sapporo SLE (KYSS) Study Group. Modifying effect of N-Acetyltransferase 2 genotype on the association between systemic lupus erythematosus and consumption of alcohol and caffeine-rich beverages. Arthritis Care Res 2014;66:1048–56.

[75] Hein DW. Acetylator genotype and arylamine-induced carcinogenesis. Biochim Biophys Acta 1988;948:37–66.

[76] Liberal R, Grant CR. Cirrhosis and autoimmune liver disease: current understanding. World J Hepatol 2016;8:1157–68.

[77] Chapman RW, Williamson KD. Chapter 7-primary sclerosing cholangitis. In: Ramos-Casals M, Khamashta M, Brito-Zeron P, Atzeni F, Rodés TJ, editors. Handbook of systemic autoimmune diseases. Elsevier; 2017. p. 119–39.

[78] Trivedi PJ, Hirschfield GM. Treatment of autoimmune liver disease: current and future therapeutic options. Ther Adv Chronic Dis 2013;4:119–41.

[79] Chung BK, Guevel BT, Reynolds GM, Gupta Udatha DBRK, Henriksen EKK, Stamataki Z, Hirschfield GM, Karlsen TH, Liaskou E. Phenotyping and auto-antibody production by liver-infiltrating B cells in primary sclerosing cholangitis and primary biliary cholangitis. J Autoimmun 2017;77:45–54.

[80] Juran BD, Lazaridis KN. Environmental factors in primary biliary cirrhosis. Semin Liver Dis 2014;34:265–72.

[81] Perricone C, Versini M, Ben-Ami D, Gertel S, Watad A, Segel MJ, Ceccarelli F, Conti F, Cantarini L, Bogdanos DP, Antonelli A, Amital H, Valesini G, Shoenfeld Y. Smoke and autoimmunity: the fire behind the disease. Autoimmun Rev 2016;15:354–74.

[82] Saab S, Mallam D, Cox 2nd GA, Tong MJ. Impact of coffee on liver diseases: a systematic review. Liver Int 2014;34:495–504.

[83] Kuper H, Tzonou A, Kaklamani E, Hsieh CC, Lagiou P, Adami HO, Trichopoulos D, Stuver SO. Tobacco smoking, alcohol consumption and their interaction in the causation of hepatocellular carcinoma. Int J Cancer 2000;85:498–502.

[84] Anty R, Marjoux S, Iannelli A, Patouraux S, Schneck AS, Bonnafous S, Gire C, Amzolini A, Ben-Amor I, Saint-Paul MC, Marine-Barjoan E, Pariente A, Gugenheim J, Gual P, Tran A. Regular coffee but not espresso drinking is protective against fibrosis in a cohort mainly composed of morbidly obese European women with NAFLD undergoing bariatric surgery. J Hepatol 2012;57:1090–6.

[85] Lammert C, Juran BD, Schlicht E, Xie X, Atkinson EJ, de Andrade M, Lazaridis KN. Reduced coffee consumption among individuals with primary sclerosing cholangitis but not primary biliary cirrhosis. Clin Gastroenterol Hepatol 2014;12:1562–8.

[86] Andersen IM, Tengesdal G, Lie BA, Boberg KM, Karlsen TH, Hov JR. Effects of coffee consumption, smoking, and hormones on risk for primary sclerosing cholangitis. Clin Gastroenterol Hepatol 2014;12:1019–28.

[87] Kaser A. Inflammatory bowel disease. Annu Rev Immunol 2010;28:573–621.

[88] Ponder A, Long MD. A clinical review of recent findings in the epidemiology of inflammatory bowel disease. Clin Epidemiol 2013;5:237–47.

[89] Persson PG, Ahlbom A, Hellers G. Diet and inflammatory bowel disease: a case-control study. Epidemiology (Camb Mass) 1992;3:47–52.

[90] Niewiadomski O, Studd C, Wilson J, Williams J, Hair C, Knight R, Prewett E, Dabkowski P, Alexander S, Allen B, Dowling D, Connell W, Desmond P, Bell S. Influence of food and lifestyle on the risk of developing inflammatory bowel disease. Intern Med J 2016;46:669–76.

[91] Boyko EJ, Perera DR, Koepsell TD, Keane EM, Inui TS. Coffee and alcohol use and the risk of ulcerative colitis. Am J Gastroenterol 1989;84:530–4.

[92] Lebwohl B, Ludvigsson JF, Green PHR. Celiac disease and non-celiac gluten sensitivity. BMJ 2015;351.

[93] Kagnoff MF. Celiac disease: pathogenesis of a model immunogenetic disease. J Clin Investig 2007;117:41–9.

[94] Greco L, Romino R, Coto I, Di Cosmo N, Percopo S, Maglio M, Paparo F, Gasperi V, Limongelli MG, Cotichini R, D'Agate C, Tinto N, Sacchetti L, Tosi R, Stazi MA. The first large population based twin study of coeliac disease. Gut 2002;50:624–8.

[95] Sarno M, Discepolo V, Troncone R, Auricchio R. Risk factors for celiac disease. Ital J Pediatr 2015;41.

[96] Francavilla R, Cristofori F, Stella M, Borrelli G, Naspi G, Castellaneta S. Treatment of celiac disease: from gluten-free diet to novel therapies. Minerva Pediatr 2014;66:501–16.

[97] Green PHR, Cellier Celiac C. Disease. N Engl J Med 2007;357:1731–43.

[98] Lanzini A, Lanzarotto F, Villanacci V, Mora A, Bertolazzi S, Turini D, Carella G, Malagoli A, Ferrante G, Cesana BM, Ricci C. Complete recovery of intestinal mucosa occurs very rarely in adult coeliac patients despite adherence to gluten-free diet. Aliment Pharmacol Ther 2009;29:1299–308.

[99] Vojdani A, Tarash I. Cross-reaction between gliadin and different food and tissue antigens. Food Nutr Sci 2013;4:20–32.

Chapter 35

Obesity in Autoimmune Diseases: Not a Passive Bystander

Mathilde Versini[1], Pierre-Yves Jeandel[2], Eric Rosenthal[2], Yehuda Shoenfeld[3,4]

[1]Institut Arnault Tzanck, Saint Laurent du Var, France; [2]Department of Internal Medicine, Archet-1 Hospital, University of Nice-Sophia-Antipolis, Nice, France; [3]Zabludowicz Center for Autoimmune Diseases, Sheba Medical Center, affiliated to Sackler Faculty of Medicine, Tel Aviv University, Tel Aviv, Israel; [4]Laboratory of the Mosaics of Autoimmunity, Saint-Petersburg University, Saint-Petersburg, Russian Federation

INTRODUCTION

For several decades, industrialized countries face an increased prevalence of immune-mediated diseases [1,2]. Most of these inflammatory conditions result from a complex interaction between genetic background and multiple environmental factors [3–8]. Because genetic basis has remained constant over time, there is increasing recognition that environmental factors, especially the Western lifestyle, have a preponderant role in this growing prevalence [9]. Westernization is accompanied by profound changes in dietary habits, promoting high-fat, high-sugar, and high-salt foods [10] with excess calorie intake, leading to obesity outbreak over the past 20 years [11,12]. Therefore, the links between obesity and autoimmunity were questioned and the involvement of obesity in the rise of autoimmune conditions was strongly suggested. This link became even more fascinating in recent years since the discovery of the remarkable properties of adipose tissue. Indeed, the white adipose tissue (WAT), long regarded as an inert energy storage tissue, has been recognized to be an essential endocrine organ, secreting a wide variety of soluble mediators termed "adipokines" or "adipocytokines" [13]. Initially identified for their metabolic and appetite regulation activities, adipokines are known to be involved in various processes including immunity and inflammation [14]. By their proinflammatory action, these molecules contribute to the so-called "low-grade inflammatory state" in obese subjects, resulting in a cluster of comorbidities such as metabolic syndrome, diabetes, or cardiovascular complications [13]. On this basis, it is now of major interest to clarify the relationship between obesity and autoimmune/inflammatory diseases. In this review, following a short overview of the main mechanisms highlighted so far to link obesity and autoimmunity, we will detail metabolic and immunological activities of the main adipokines. Then, we shall focus on obesity and more precisely adipokines involvement in the development and prognosis of several immune-mediated conditions.

CONNECTING OBESITY AND AUTOIMMUNITY

Obesity corresponds to an abnormal accumulation of adipose tissue within the body. According to World Health Organization (WHO), approximately 35% of the world population is estimated to be overweight (body mass index, BMI 25–30 kg/m^2) or obese (BMI > 30 kg/m^2) [12]. As mentioned above, it is widely known that obese persons exhibit a subclinical chronic state of inflammation leading to multiple metabolic disorders [13]. Moreover, as will be discussed further below, a large number of studies found a significant correlation between obesity and a higher prevalence or a worse prognosis of many immune-mediated conditions. Therefore, understanding the underlying immune disorders in obesity, which promote inflammatory autoimmune diseases, is a major topic of research. Thus, to date, several mechanisms have been postulated. These mechanisms are schematically illustrated in Fig. 35.1.

First, numerous studies have documented the properties of WAT as a crucial site in the generation of soluble mediators named "adipokines," most of which carry a proinflammatory activity. These include classical cytokines such as interleukin (IL)-6 and tumor necrosis factor alpha (TNFα) and specific molecules such as leptin and adiponectin [13]. These mediators are secreted by adipocytes and by a diverse set of immune cells found to abundantly infiltrate adipose tissue under obese conditions [15,16]. As will be discussed later in this review, adipokines appear to be key players in the interactions between adipose tissue and the immune system.

Mosaic of Autoimmunity. https://doi.org/10.1016/B978-0-12-814307-0.00035-9

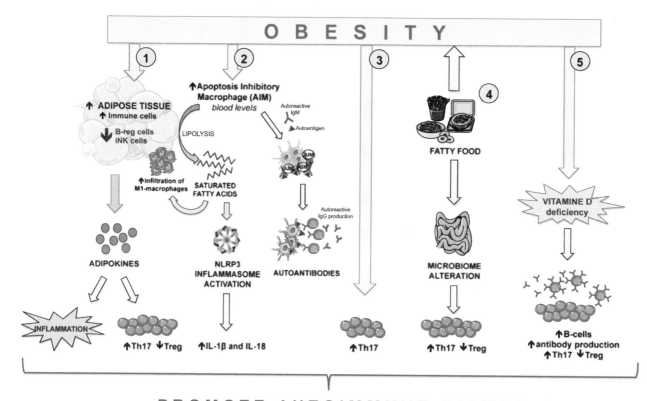

FIGURE 35.1 Representation of the main mechanisms suggested to promote autoimmune diseases in obesity. (1) In obesity, fat mass increases. Both adipocytes and immune cells massively infiltrating adipose tissue secrete high levels of adipokines, responsible for a proinflammatory state and deregulation of Th17/Treg balance. Furthermore, obesity is associated with lower B regulatory and iNK cells within the adipose tissue. (2) AIM blood levels increase under obese conditions. First, AIM induces lipolysis, thereby producing saturated fatty acids. The latter will in turn act on adipose tissue by promoting proinflammatory M1-macrophage infiltration; moreover, saturated fatty acids can activate the NLRP3-inflammasome, which secretes IL-1β and IL-18, both being involved in the pathogenesis of autoimmune diseases. Second, AIM forms immune complexes with natural autoreactive IgM associated with autoantigens, promoting their retention on follicular dendritic cells. Subsequent autoantigens presentation to follicular B cells leads to the production of IgG autoantibodies. (3) Obesity has been found to promote a Th17 profile, a subset implicated in the pathogenesis of immune-mediated conditions. (4) The Western diet, partially responsible for obesity, may also cause dysbiosis, an alteration of gut microbiota, resulting in a modulation of extraintestinal immune responses and subsequent deregulation of the Th17/Treg balance. (5) Obese subjects exhibit a higher prevalence of vitamin D deficiency. Lower vitamin D levels have been associated with increased Th17 cells, B cells, and secretion of antibodies as well as reduced Treg cells. *AIM*, apoptosis inhibitor of macrophage; *Breg cells*, B regulatory cells; *iNK cells*, invariant natural killer T cells; *IL*, interleukin; *NLRP3-inflammasome*, NOD-like receptor protein 3 inflammasome; *Th17*, T helper 17 cells; *Treg*, regulatory T cells.

Recently, several authors have also highlighted the role of the apoptosis inhibitor of macrophage (AIM) in the pathogenesis of obesity-associated autoimmune diseases [17,18]. AIM is produced by tissue macrophages and was initially found to promote the survival of macrophages against various apoptosis-inducing stimuli [19]. Briefly, it was demonstrated that lipolysis induced by increased blood AIM under obese conditions releases large amounts of saturated fatty acids from adipocytes. The latter stimulate chemokine production in adipocytes via TLR4 activation, which results in increased M1-macrophage infiltration in adipose tissue. Moreover, AIM forms immune complexes with natural autoreactive IgM associated with autoantigens. Thus, AIM promotes their retention on follicular dendritic cells and autoantigens presentation to follicular B lymphocytes, leading to production of IgG autoantibodies.

The T helper 17 cells (Th17) are a recently discovered subset of CD4 effector T lymphocytes. Th17 cells secrete IL-17 and are now recognized for their involvement in the pathogenesis of autoimmune diseases [20]. Recently it has been reported that obesity may predispose induction of Th17 cells, at least in part in an IL-6-dependent process, which exacerbates autoinflammatory diseases such as multiple sclerosis and colitis in several mouse models [21]. Paradoxically, IL-17 has also been shown to inhibit adipogenesis [22,23]. The precise role of Th17 cells and IL-17 in obesity-associated inflammatory conditions needs to be clarified.

Another exciting field of investigation is the contribution of nutrients, especially the influence of a high-salt, high-fat diet on immune-mediated conditions [10,24]. Indeed, recent studies suggest that Western diet may cause dysbiosis, an alteration of intestinal microbiome. This modification induces profound modulation of extraintestinal immune responses, including Th17/T regulatory cells (Treg) imbalance [25]. However, it is not yet clear if dysbiosis contributes to or is a consequence of autoimmune diseases. In the same area, another possibility involves the higher prevalence of vitamin D deficiency among obese subjects [26]. Vitamin D regulates many processes, including immune response. Thus, it has been shown to increase Treg cells and inhibits Th1 and Th17 differentiation [27]. Hence, some studies report an association between vitamin D deficiency and the development of autoimmune diseases, although these observations are still controversial [28,29].

Some areas still require further investigations. It has been demonstrated that the NLRP3 (NOD-like receptor protein 3) inflammasome, a highly regulated protein complex involved via its secretion of IL-1β and IL-18 in the pathogenesis of many autoimmune diseases, can be activated in macrophages by numerous factors associated with obesity, including ceramides, saturated fatty acids, and reactive oxygen species [30]. Additionally, Nishimura et al. [31] recently showed that B regulatory lymphocytes, a subset of B lymphocytes known to hamper inflammation by their secretion of IL-10 and TGF-β, are constitutively present in the adipose tissue. B regulatory cells and subsequent antiinflammatory cytokines are progressively diminished in obese adipose tissue, promoting the development of inflammation. Likewise, the role of invariant natural killer T cells (iNK cells) also remains unclear. iNK cells are a subset of natural killer (NK) cells abundantly present in adipose tissue (10%–20% of resident T lymphocytes). They seem to contribute to the maintenance of adipose tissue homeostasis, and their number decreases significantly in obese patients [32].

Although these mechanisms require further investigations to be specified, one of the most documented areas to date is the role of adipokines in the pathophysiology of obesity-associated immune-mediated diseases. WAT has been found to produce more than 50 adipokines. Herein, we will consider four of those—leptin, adiponectin, resistin, and visfatin—whose involvement in autoimmune and inflammatory conditions has been reported. The main metabolic, vascular, and immunological effects of these four adipokines are summarized in Table 35.1 and Fig. 35.2.

ADIPOKINES: METABOLIC AND IMMUNOLOGICAL PROPERTIES

Leptin

Leptin [33–37] (from the Greek word leptos = thin) was the first adipokine identified in 1994 by positional cloning of a single gene mutation in the *ob/ob* mouse. It is a 16 kDa nonglycosylated polypeptide hormone, classified as a member of the long-chain helical cytokine family, such as IL-6, IL-11, IL-12, and leukemia inhibitory factor. It is encoded by the obese (*ob*) gene, which is the murine homolog of human Lep gene. Leptin exerts its biological actions through the activation of its OB-Rb long-isoform receptor, encoded by the diabetes (*db*) gene. OB-Rb receptors are expressed in different tissues including the central nervous and the cardiovascular systems, as well as in immune system cells. Leptin is predominantly produced by WAT, and circulating levels of leptin directly correlate with the body adipose mass and adipocyte size. Starvation and hormones such as testosterone and glucocorticoids inhibit its synthesis. It is upregulated by inflammatory mediators (TNFα, IL-1β) insulin and ovarian sex steroids, the latter likely explaining the higher levels of leptin found in women.

Leptin is a major regulator of body weight by promoting satiety and stimulating energy expenditure. It acts on specific hypothalamic nuclei, inducing anorexigenic factors and suppressing orexigenic neuropeptides. Leptin has antidiabetic effects and inhibits hepatic lipogenesis. Either *ob*- or *db*-deficient mice develops severe obese phenotype. This is due to the lack of perception of satiety, together with deregulation of glucose and lipid metabolisms. In addition to its metabolic effects, leptin exerts pleiotropic actions on physiological functions, including fertility, bone metabolism, angiogenesis, inflammation, and immunity.

Leptin is a potent modulator of immune responses. Thus, congenital leptin-deficient patients have a higher incidence of infection-related death because of dysfunctional immune response. Similarly, starvation causes a dramatic decrease in leptin levels, causing immunosuppression. In both cases, the effects can be reversed by leptin replacement therapy. Leptin affects both innate and acquired immunity. In innate immunity, leptin activates proliferation of monocytes, enhances macrophages phagocytosis activity, and induces them to produce leukotriene B4, eicosanoids, and proinflammatory cytokines such as TNFα, IL-6, and IL-12. In neutrophils, it increases chemotaxis and release of oxygen radicals. It promotes proliferation, differentiation, activation, and cytotoxicity of NK cells. Finally, leptin is involved in dendritic cell maturation and survival by activating signaling pathways such as Akt and nuclear factor kappa beta. Leptin is also an important regulator of the acquired response. Indeed, leptin-deficient mice have defective cellular immunity and exhibit thymic and lymphoid atrophy. These effects are reversed by exogenous leptin administration. Leptin stimulates proliferation of naive T cells and promotes memory T cells differentiation toward Th1, producing proinflammatory cytokines such as interferon gamma (IFN-γ) and IL-2 and suppressing the production of the Th2 cytokines IL-4 and IL-10. Furthermore, it inhibits

TABLE 35.1 Major Metabolic, Vascular, and Immune Actions of Adipokines

	Metabolic Effects	Vascular Effects	Innate Immune System Effects	Acquired Immune System Effects
Leptin ↑ in obesity	Anorexigen ↑Resting energy expenditure (REE) Antidiabetic effect ↑Lipolytic activity Hepatic ↓lipogenesis	Proatherogenic: Causes endothelial dysfunction ↑Platelets aggregation	Proinflammatory: Monocytes: ↑ proliferation, ↑ production of IL-1 RA, ↑ CD25, CD71 Macrophages: ↑phagocytosis, ↑ production of IL-6, IL-12, LTB4, NO, eicosanoids, COX2 PMNLs: ↑ chemotaxis, ↑ release of oxygen radicals NK cells: ↑ differentiation ↑ proliferation, activation ↑cytotoxicity, survival Dendritic cells: ↑ maturation, ↑ production of IL-1, IL-6, IL-12, TNF$_\alpha$, ↑survival	Proinflammatory: T cells: ↑ thymocytes maturation, ↑ naive T cells proliferation and activation, ↑ differentiation of memory T cells toward Th1 phenotype ↑ production of IFN-γ, IL-2, ↓ production of IL-4, IL-10 ↓T cells apoptosis B cells: ↑ lymphopoiesis, ↓ IgG2-switch Treg cells, ↓ proliferation, ↑ anergy
Adiponectin ↓ in obesity	↑Appetite ↑Insulin sensitivity, ↑insulin gene expression, ↑ glucose uptake in adipose tissue and skeletal muscle, ↓hepatic glycogenesis ↑Free-fatty acid oxidation in liver and skeletal muscle	Antiatherogenic: ↓Endothelial adhesion molecules (ICAM-1, VCAM-1, E-selectin) ↓Macrophage transformation into foam cells	Antiinflammatory: Monocytes: ↓ Secretion of TNFα, IFN-γ IL-6 and ↑IL-10, IL-1 RA Macrophages: ↓ maturation, proliferation, phagocytosis activity, if ↑ phagocytosis of apoptotic cells,↓ production of TNFα, IFN-γ, ↑ M2-profile NK cells: ↓ cytotoxicity Dendritic cells: ↑ maturation, activation	Antiinflammatory: T cells: ↓ activation ↓ proliferation B cells: ↓lymphopoiesis Treg cells: ↑ proliferation Proinflammatory effects suspected in autoimmune diseases
Resistin ↑ in obesity	Anorexigen ↑Insulin resistance ↑Free-fatty release from adipose tissue	Proatherogenic: ↑Endothelial adhesion molecules (ICAM-1, VCAM-1, E-selectin)	Proinflammatory: Monocytes: ↑ production of 1L1β, IL-6, IL-12, TNFα Macrophages: ↑ production of IL-12, TNFα	Proinflammatory: Lymphocytes: ↑ production of IL-1β, IL-6, IL-12, TNFα
Visfatin ↑ in obesity	Insulin-like effects suggested	Proatherogenic: ↑Endothelial adhesion molecules (ICAM-1, VCAM-1, E-selectin) ↑Atherosclerotic plaque instability	Proinflammatory: Monocytes: ↑ chemotaxis, ↑ activation, ↑ production of IL-1β, IL-6, IL-12, TNFα PMNLs: ↓ apoptosis	Proinflammatory: Lymphocytes: ↑ maturation, ↑ activation, ↑ production of IL-1β, IL-6, IL-12, TNFα

COX2, cyclooxygenase-2; *ICAM-1*, intercellular adhesion molecule-1; *IL*, interleukin; *IL-1 RA*, interleukin-1 receptor antagonist; *LTB4*, leukotriene B4; *NK cells*, natural killer cells; *PMNL*, polymorphonuclear leukocytes; *Treg cells*, regulatory T cells; *VCAM-1*, vascular cell adhesion molecule-1.

the proliferation of Treg cells, known as critical mediators of immune tolerance. In summary, leptin modulates immune response toward a proinflammatory profile, being critical in infection control. As it is at the crossroad between inflammation and autoimmunity, upsetting the balance may result in immunosuppressed condition or conversely proinflammatory state facilitating the development of autoimmune diseases.

Adiponectin

Adiponectin [33,35–38] was independently characterized by four research groups as a 244-amino acid protein with various names: Acrp30 (adipocyte complement-related protein of 30 kDa), apM1 (adipose most abundant gene transcript 1), adipoQ, or GBP28 (gelatin-binding protein of 28 kDa). The human adiponectin gene is located on 3q27 chromosome. It structurally belongs to the collagen superfamily, sharing homologies with collagens VIII and X and complement factor C1q. The primary structure of adiponectin contains an N-terminal signal sequence, a variable domain, a collagen-like domain, and a C-terminal domain, known as globular adiponectin. The monomeric 30 kDa form of adiponectin seems to be confined to the adipocyte, whereas oligomeric complexes circulate in plasma as low-, middle-, and high molecular weight multimers. Adiponectin can also be found in the plasma as a 16 kDa proteolytic globular form.

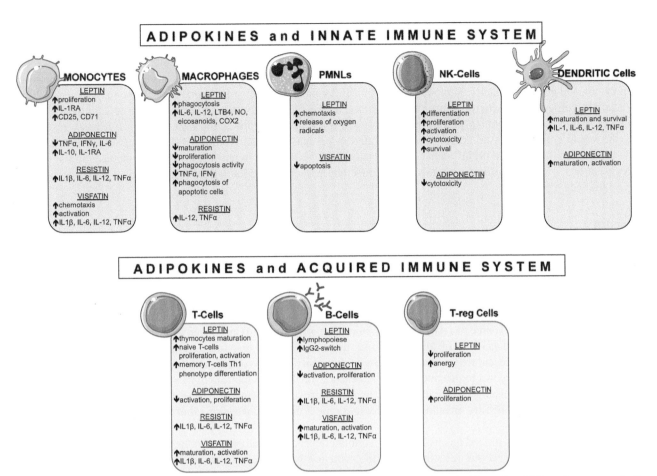

FIGURE 35.2 Main effects of leptin, adiponectin, resistin, and visfatin on cells of the innate and acquired immunity. *COX2*, cyclooxygenase-2; *IL*, interleukin; *IL-1 RA*, interleukin-1 receptor antagonist; *LTB4*, leukotriene B4; *NK cells*, natural killer cells; *PMNLs*, polymorphonuclear leukocytes; *Treg cells*, regulatory T cells.

Three receptors mediate adiponectin signaling: AdipoR1, found predominantly in skeletal muscle; AdipoR2, expressed more abundantly in the liver; and T-cadherin, mainly expressed in the cardiovascular system. It is important to note that adiponectin isoforms differ in their biological function, possibly depending on tissue and receptor subtype. Adiponectin is mainly secreted by WAT. Of all adipokines, it has the highest serum levels, ranging from 0.5 to 30 mg/mL in human, which accounts for about 0.01% of all plasma proteins in humans [39]. Unlike most adipokines, plasma levels of adiponectin are decreased in obese individuals and increase with weight loss. Adiponectin exerts important effects on metabolic modulation and energy homeostasis. Adiponectin is, together with leptin, an insulin-sensitizing adipokine. Besides enhancing insulin sensitivity, it decreases hepatic glycogenesis and promotes insulin gene expression and glucose uptake in skeletal muscle and in adipose tissue. Furthermore, adiponectin increases free fatty acid oxidation in the liver and in the skeletal muscle.

While leptin has proinflammatory activity, adiponectin has been consistently shown to be an antiinflammatory adipokine, especially with regard to protective effects on the vascular wall. Indeed, adiponectin acts on endothelial cells by inhibiting the expression of TNFα-induced adhesion molecules, such as vascular cell adhesion molecule-1, endothelial–leukocyte adhesion molecule-1, and intracellular adhesion molecule-1. It results in reduced monocyte adhesion to endothelial cells. Furthermore, adiponectin can modulate transformation of macrophages into foam cells. Thus, low circulating adiponectin levels are closely associated with obesity-linked metabolic and cardiovascular disorders, including insulin resistance, type 2 diabetes, hypertension, and coronary artery disease.

Besides acting as a metabolic and antiatherogenic factor, adiponectin also exhibits its antiinflammatory effects on immune system cells. Adiponectin inhibits maturation, proliferation, and phagocytic activity of macrophages, as well as their TNFα and IFN-γ production in response to lipopolysaccharide stimulation. Moreover, adiponectin promotes phagocytosis of apoptotic cells by macrophages, whose accumulation can trigger inflammation or immune system dysfunction.

It reduces the secretion and activity of TNFα and IL-6 and induces production of antiinflammatory mediators, such as IL-10 and IL-1 receptor antagonist, in monocytes, macrophages, and dendritic cells. Adiponectin also increases the number of Treg cells. Conversely, it promotes the maturation and activation of dendritic cells. Interestingly, both TNFα and IL-6 are potent inhibitors of adiponectin secretion, which suggests the existence of a negative feedback between adiponectin and proinflammatory cytokines. Further antiinflammatory effects of adiponectin involve suppression of IL-2-induced NK cell cytotoxic activity. In acquired immunity, it inhibits the activation and proliferation of T lymphocytes and B cell lymphopoiesis. Surprisingly, some reports suggest a proinflammatory action of adiponectin. It has been proven that the serum concentration of adiponectin is elevated in patients with autoimmune inflammatory conditions [38,40]. This bidirectional, anti-, and proinflammatory effects of adiponectin may in part result from the changes in the relative proportion of its various isoforms, as much as the different molecular weight and truncated forms of adiponectin exert differential activities.

Resistin

Resistin [35,37,41], also known as ADSF (adipocyte-secreted factor) or FIZZ3 (found in inflammatory zone 3), was discovered in 2001. It is a 12.5 kDa polypeptide that belongs to a family of cysteine-rich proteins called "resistin-like molecules." The term "resistin" was originally proposed for its role as a mediator of insulin resistance. To date, resistin receptor and its signaling pathways have not been identified. The study of resistin in human disease is complicated by the fact that there are marked interspecies differences in the source of production and structure of this protein. Indeed, while in rodents the major source of resistin is WAT, human resistin is mainly produced by circulating and WAT-resident peripheral blood mononuclear cells (PBMC). Moreover, human and rodent resistins only share 59% identity at the amino acid level. Serum resistin levels are known to increase with obesity in both rodents and humans. In animal models, resistin has consistently been shown to promote insulin resistance. Yet, data on the role of this adipokine in the regulation of glucose homeostasis and insulin sensitivity in humans are controversial. Some authors report that high serum levels are associated with increased obesity, insulin resistance, and type 2 diabetes, whereas other groups failed to observe such correlations.

In humans, resistin may instead be involved in inflammatory processes rather than in the modulation of glucose homeostasis. Recent studies showed that resistin induces the secretion by PBMC and is induced by several proinflammatory cytokines, such as TNFα, IL-1β, and IL-6, indicating that resistin can increase its own activity by a positive feedback mechanism. Resistin also increases the expression of cytokines and adhesion molecules in vascular endothelial cells, thereby contributing to atherogenesis. Metabolic syndrome by itself is associated with inflammation. Some authors suggest that resistin may be associated with inflammatory markers of metabolic syndrome, its correlation with metabolic parameters such as glucose or blood lipids being just an indirect effect.

Visfatin

Visfatin [36,37,41] corresponds to a 52 kDa-protein previously identified as pre-B cell colony-enhancing factor as well as identified to act as an enzyme, nicotinamide phosphoribosyl transferase. It was originally discovered in liver, skeletal muscle, and bone marrow as a growth factor for B lymphocyte precursors. Adipose tissue and leucocytes also secrete visfatin. The role of this adipokine on glucose metabolism remains unclear, although most studies indicate insulin-like effects. Visfatin appears to be increased in obese subjects, even if these data are also controversial. Certainly, it is a potent mediator of inflammation. Visfatin increases the production of inflammatory cytokines (IL-6, TNFα, and IL-1β) by leucocytes. Additionally, it promotes activation of T cells by enhancing the expression of co-stimulatory molecules, such as CD40, CD54, and CD80, on monocytes. Visfatin acts as a chemotactic factor on monocytes and lymphocytes. It strongly affects the development of both T and B lymphocytes. Moreover, its proinflammatory effects might contribute to the process of atherosclerosis. As resistin, visfatin is upregulated by inflammatory mediators.

OBESITY AND IMMUNE-MEDIATED DISEASES

An association between obesity and various inflammatory/autoimmune conditions has been suggested in many observational studies. Recently, the discovery of adipokines and better knowledge of their pleiotropic role, particularly on the immune system, has led to major advances in the understanding of the relationships between obesity and autoimmune diseases. Below, we summarize and discuss the data in this field in several immune-mediated conditions. An overview of experimental and clinical data from the literature is presented in Table 35.2 and Fig. 35.3.

TABLE 35.2 Synthesis of Clinical and Experimental Data Regarding the Effects of Obesity and Adipokines in Several Autoimmune Diseases

	Obesity as a Risk Factor	Obesity as a Worsening Factor	Experimental Data
Rheumatoid arthritis (RA)	Obesity ↑ risk (OR=1.2–3.4) of ACPA->ACPA+RA in women>men [50–57], weight loss ↓ risk of RA [58]	Obesity ↑ severity, comorbidities [67–72] and ↓ treatment efficacy [114–119] Paradoxical protective role on radiographic damage [67,73,98–100]	Patients: ↑ leptin, adiponectin, resistin, and visfatin levels in RA correlated with severity [79–94] Mice: Leptin-KO mice and inhibition of visfatin ↓ severity [95–97]
Systemic lupus erythematosus (SLE)	Insufficient data; one negative study but several bias [126]	Obesity correlated with renal and cognitive involvement,↓quality of life [134,145,146,151,152] and ↑CVD [134,156] No correlation with disease activity [133–135]	Patients: ↑ leptin levels in SLE not correlated with disease activity [138–140] Mice: leptin ↑ lupus autoimmunity, Th17 and ↓Treg. Leptin deficiency ↓ severity, Th17 and,↑ Treg [127–130] ↑ Leptin, resistin and ↓adiponectin levels correlated with ↑ renal damage and CVD [128,136,137,141,142,144,147–149,160,161]
Inflammatory bowel disease	Conflicting results [126,167–169]; overall data suggesting obesity as a risk factor	Obesity correlated with an unfavorable course of the disease and ↓ treatment efficacy [174,175,194–197]	Patients: ↑ leptin, resistin and visfatin levels in plasma, visceral adipose tissue, or gut lumen [176–180,183–186] Mice: Leptin-KO mice ↓colitis [181,182] High-fat diet ↑ intestinal inflammation [172,173]
Multiple sclerosis (MS)	Childhood and adolescent obesity ↑ risk (OR≈2) of MS in women>men [204–207]; risk potentiated by genetic predisposition [208]	No clinical data Experimental data suggesting a harmful role	Patients: ↑ leptin, resistin, visfatin and ↓adiponectin levels correlated with ↑ inflammation and ↓Treg Mice: Inhibition of visfatin ↓ severity [219] Adiponectin-KO mice ↑ severity and ↓Treg [217] Strong data for a key role of leptin in induction and progression of the disease [220–223]
Type 1 diabetes (T1D)	High birthweight, early weight gain, childhood, and adult obesity ↑ risk of T1D (OR≈2) [126,236,237,241]; earlier onset rather than ↑ risk?	No clinical data	Mice: High birthweight ↑ risk of T1D [238] Pregnancy calorie restriction ↓birthweight and subsequent T1D [239] ↑ leptin, resistin and ↓adiponectin levels: ↑ βcell autoimmunity [258–261]
Psoriasis and psoriatic arthritis (PsA)	Obesity ↑ risk of psoriasis and PsA (OR=1.48–6.46) [126,271,273–275]; risk potentiated by genetic predisposition [286,287]	Obesity ↑ severity, CVD, metabolic syndrome and ↓ biologic therapies efficacy [277,288–290,322,326,328–330] Weight loss ↓ severity, CVD and ↑ treatment efficacy [296–302,332]	Patients: ↑ leptin and resistin levels in psoriasis and PsA correlated with severity [305–309,315] ↑ leptin levels in skin lesions [313,314]
Hashimoto thyroiditis (HT)	Childhood obesity ↑ risk of HT (OR=1.21) [357] Obesity ↑TAI [356]	No clinical data	Patients: ↑ leptin levels correlated with Th17 [356,358]

ACPA, anticitrullinated protein antibodies; *CVD*, cardiovascular diseases; *KO*, knockout; *OR*, odds ratio; *TAI*, thyroid autoimmunity; *Th17*, T helper 17 cells; *Treg*, regulatory T cells.

Obesity and Rheumatoid Arthritis

RA is an inflammatory autoimmune disease characterized by chronic synovial inflammation. If left untreated, RA ultimately leads to irreversible erosive joint destruction, responsible for disability and impaired quality of life. Extra-articular manifestations may include cutaneous, pulmonary, cardiac, ocular, renal, and hematological involvement [42]. It is the most common inflammatory joint disease, affecting almost 1% of the population, and it has experienced an increase over the last decades. RA has a higher prevalence in women than in men [43,44]. Most RA patients are recognized to have altered

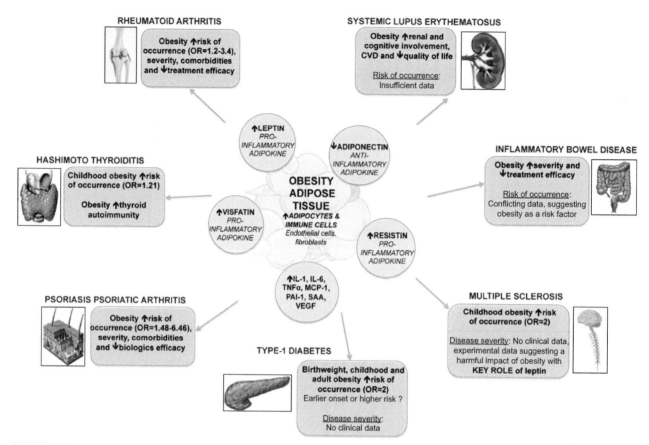

FIGURE 35.3 Schematic overview of the actions of adipose tissue on several immune-mediated diseases during obesity. Adipose tissue consists primarily of adipocytes and many other cell types. In obesity, there is an increase in the number of adipocytes and a major infiltration of adipose tissue by a variety of immune cells. Both adipocytes and immune cells are responsible for the secretion of multiple inflammatory mediators called "adipokines" including conventional molecules (IL-1, IL-6, TNF, MCP-1, PAI-1, SAA, VEGF) and specific hormones, such as leptin, adiponectin, resistin, and visfatin. In obesity, the levels of leptin, resistin, and visfatin, three proinflammatory molecules, increase proportionally to fat mass. Conversely adiponectin, a mostly antiinflammatory adipokine, decreases. The boxes present the major effects of obesity on the onset and progression of several autoimmune diseases. This partially results from the harmful action of adipokines. *CVD*, cardiovascular diseases; *IL*, interleukin; *MCP-1*, monocyte chemotactic protein-1; *OR*, odds ratio; *PAI-1*, plasminogen activator inhibitor-1; *SAA*, serum amyloid A; *VEGF*, vascular endothelial growth factor.

body composition. This change is characterized by reduced lean tissue and preserved or increased fat mass with stable or increased body weight, a condition known as "rheumatoid cachexia" [45], believed to accelerate morbidity and mortality [46]. This state has received significant scientific attention, but less is known about the relation between obesity and RA. However, both conditions—obesity and RA—share several common features. Indeed, RA is characterized by chronic inflammation, with reduced life expectancy compared with the general population mainly because of increased prevalence of cardiovascular diseases [47]. Similarly, obese patients exhibit a chronic subclinical inflammatory state, resulting in an increased incidence of various comorbidities, especially cardiovascular diseases [48,49].

First, concerning obesity as a risk factor for RA onset, several studies associated obesity with a higher risk for the occurrence of RA [50–55]. In a large retrospective case–control study, Crowon et al. [53] found that a history of obesity more than obesity at incidence date was modestly correlated (OR = 1.24; CI 1.01–1.53) with the likelihood of developing RA. Interestingly, their findings indicate that obesity could explain 52% of the recent rise in incidence of RA in Minnesota. Two additional large case–control studies [51,55] brought out an increased risk in obese individuals (BMI $\geq 30\,kg/m^2$) to develop an ACPA (anticitrullinated protein antibodies)–negative RA (OR ranging 1.6–3.45), this rise affecting only women in one of these studies [55]. There is no biologic explanation for this specific association. It should be noted that, in both studies, patients fulfilled old 1987 American College of Rheumatology criteria for RA diagnosis, and the authors cannot exclude misdiagnosed osteoarthritis, which is positively correlated with BMI. The association between obesity and risk of seronegative RA was recently found again in a population-based study from the European Prospective Investigation of Cancer Norfolk and Norfolk Arthritis Register (EPIC-2-NOAR Study) with an hazard ratio (HR) = 2.75 for BMI $\geq 30\,kg/m^2$ [56]. Recently, a large prospective study [57] using two cohort of women, Nurses' Health Study (NHS, 109,896 women) and

Nurses' Health Study II (NHS II, 108,727 women), observed a significant association between being overweight and obese and developing seropositive and seronegative RA, which appeared to be stronger among women diagnosed at younger ages (≤55 years) with an HR = 1.45–1.65. They also observed that a BMI ≥25 kg/m² at 18 years of age was associated with a 35% increased risk of developing RA, and an almost 50% increased risk of developing seropositive RA in adulthood. Finally, they reported a "dose effect" of obesity years on risk of RA at age 55 years or younger with a 37% increased risk of RA associated with a history of 10 years of being obese. Interestingly, an intensive prevention program in Finland reported a decline in the incidence of RA accompanying weight reduction [58]. Conversely, many studies failed to show obesity as being a predisposing factor for RA [59–65]. Several reasons have been discussed to account for this discrepancy, including the lack of power of some studies (insufficient number of patients) to detect a modest risk (OR b1.5), methodological variability across studies, many biases or confounding factors, particularly in case–control studies, and the relevance of BMI as a measuring tool of obesity especially in RA patients [66]. Indeed, BMI is not a good marker of body fat content because it neither distinguishes between the tissues that comprise it or consider abdominal obesity, which is a key prognostic factor.

Regarding the impact of obesity on RA activity, available data suggest a correlation between obesity and disease severity. In 2013, Ajeganovic et al. [67] followed a cohort of 1596 patients with early RA for a mean duration of 9.5 years. They found that a BMI ≥30 kg/m² was directly correlated with higher disease activity, indicated by higher HAQ (Health Assessment Questionnaire) score, DAS28, visual analog scale pain, CRP (C-reactive protein), and ESR (erythrocyte sedimentation rate) levels. BMI was also correlated with worse global health scores, decreased probability of remission, and higher prevalence of comorbidities, such as type 2 diabetes, cardiovascular disease, and chronic pulmonary disease. These results are consistent with previous studies [68–72]. In contrast, several authors do not correlate obesity with increased disease activity [73–75] or with cardiovascular disease [76,77]. However, some results may be biased by a well-described phenomenon. Indeed, all studies report a paradoxical association between a low BMI (<18–20 kg/m²) and a higher morbidity and mortality of RA [46,78]. Actually, this is more likely related to a state of rheumatoid cachexia, mentioned above, which is the result of a more active disease. This association may distort the results, finding a more severe disease in lean subjects and ignoring the deleterious effect of fat.

In addition, a correlation between the increase in fat mass and disease activity seems consistent in the light of recently acquired knowledge on adipokines. Indeed, despite some conflicting results, most studies report higher levels of serum leptin [79–83], adiponectin [79,84,85], resistin [81,86–92], and visfatin [79,93,94] in patients with RA when compared with control subjects. This rise is commonly correlated with severity parameters, such as DAS28, HAQ score, radiographic damage, and with inflammation markers ESR and CRP. These data are supported by different mouse models, including leptin-deficient mice [95] or mice treated by pharmacological inhibition of visfatin [96,97], exhibiting a milder form of experimental arthritis. It is important to note that the proinflammatory action of adiponectin and visfatin in RA is widely recognized, but conflicting data are reported regarding leptin and resistin effects. It may be because of various biases, including differences in race, age, sex, BMI, body fat distribution, and medication used between the studies. However, the overall findings and the experimental data are in favor of higher levels and proinflammatory effects of adipokines in RA. Thus, considering that the rate of three of these adipokines (leptin, resistin, and visfatin) is correlated with fat mass in obese subjects, these data argue for a more severe RA activity in obese patients.

Furthermore, data unanimously show a surprising protective action of obesity for radiographic joint damage in RA [67,73,98–100]. Possible explanations for these phenomena include stimulation of bone synthesis because of the increased mechanical loading [101], the higher levels of estrogens in obese individuals [102], known to exhibit bone protective effects, and the involvement of adiponectin. Indeed, regarding the role of adipokines in erosive joint damage, studies report increased rates of four previously cited adipokines—that is, leptin, adiponectin, resistin, and visfatin—in the synovial fluid of patients compared with healthy controls or osteoarthritis patients [82,84,87,103,104]. High synovial rates were most frequently correlated with joint damage [94,105–107]. Moreover, in vitro data demonstrate proinflammatory effects of these adipokines on synovial fibroblasts and chondrocytes by enhancing the secretion of numerous chemokines (IL-2, IL-8), proinflammatory cytokines (IL-1β, IL-6), and matrix metalloproteinases (MMP-1, MMP-3, MMP-9) [85,93,108–113]. Adiponectin, the most abundant adipokines in human, is inversely correlated with body fat. We can therefore assume that the decreased levels of adiponectin in obese individuals are partly responsible for the paradoxical relationship between obesity and protection against radiographic damage.

Finally, all the studies investigating the consequences of obesity on treatment efficacy in RA suggest a poorer remission rate in obese conditions [114–119]. Thus, in a cohort of 495 patients with early RA, Sandberg et al. [119] showed that there were significantly lower odds of remission at 6 months (OR = 0.49) among overweight or obese patients (BMI ≥25 kg/m²). This effect appears to be even more pronounced with infliximab, which is consistent with previous studies [114,115,118]. It is postulated that the adipose tissue leads to an inflammatory and therapy-resistant state. In this regard, however, studies investigating the effect of TNF blockade on adipokine plasma levels in patients with RA are not conclusive, most of these failing to demonstrate an impact of anti-TNFα therapy on the levels of adipokines [120–122]. Further clarification is needed regarding the reason why obesity mostly affects RA outcome in patients treated with infliximab.

In conclusion, data suggest that obesity may modestly predispose RA, especially ACPA-negative RA, and is associated with higher severity of the disease and lower response rate to treatment. These effects seem to be partially related to the proinflammatory action of adipokines, most of which increase their circulating levels along with the fat mass. However, further studies are needed to confirm these observations.

Obesity and Systemic Lupus Erythematosus

Systemic lupus erythematosus (SLE) is a chronic autoimmune disorder characterized by multisystem organ involvement, ranging from relatively mild manifestations (skin rash or nonerosive arthritis) to severe or life-threatening complications, such as lupus nephritis, neuropsychiatric disorders, cardiac involvement, and a wide profile of autoantibodies [123]. SLE affects people worldwide, though the incidence and prevalence may diverge across different countries. Young women are predominantly affected, representing about 80%–90% of patients [124]. Although the pathogenesis of SLE is still poorly understood, various genetic and environmental factors appear to be involved in the onset as in disease activity.

To date, no study has demonstrated an epidemiological link between obesity and the risk of developing lupus. However, while other environmental factors such as hormones or chemical exposures have been widely investigated [125], it is important to specify that data on the role of obesity in the onset of lupus are extremely rare. Only one large prospective cohort study recently investigated the association between BMI and the risk of 43 autoimmune diseases [126]. In a cohort of 75,008 Danish women followed for a mean duration of 11 years, the authors found no correlation between obesity and the risk of developing SLE. However, despite the power of this study, no definite conclusion can be made from these data because of several methodological limitations that may bias the results. Moreover, several recent studies [127–130] demonstrated that leptin, commonly elevated in obese subjects, could promote the survival and proliferation of autoreactive T lymphocytes, as well as the expansion of Th17 cells, while decreasing Treg cells in lupus-prone mice. Conversely, fasting-induced hypoleptinemia [130] or leptin-deficient mice [128,129] exhibit decreased Th17 cells and higher Treg cells.

Several studies have examined the impact of obesity on various parameters of SLE. This is even more important considering that the prevalence of obesity in patients with SLE is very high, ranging from 28% to 50% depending on the measurement methods [131,132]. None found an association between high BMI and disease activity, generally defined by the SLE disease activity index [133–135]. Similarly, many [136–141], but not all studies [142,143], have demonstrated that leptin rates were enhanced in SLE patients, as in obese individuals, and this was not correlated with disease activity [138–140]. However, in a lupus-prone murine model [128], leptin deficiency was shown to ameliorate lupus severity and was associated with decreased concentrations of anti-dsDNA antibodies. Regarding other adipokines, less data are available, but none showed a direct correlation between circulating levels and lupus activity in SLE patients. Only one experiment in a strain of lupus-prone mice suggests that adiponectin deficiency is correlated with a more severe disease [144].

Nevertheless, some studies associated obesity with a higher risk of renal impairment (lupus nephritis), as measured by increased proteinuria [134], and a significant increase in inflammatory markers (TNFα, CRP, IL-6) [133,145]. This corroborates experimental data on mouse models of SLE, reporting that high-fat diet [146], as well as increased levels of leptin [128], resistin [147,148], and reduced levels of adiponectin [144,149] as found in obese subjects are associated with more severe renal impairment. However, observations on adiponectin are contradictory because another study [150] found that plasma levels and urinary adiponectin levels were higher in patients with lupus renal disease. Furthermore, several studies have clearly linked obesity with worsened functional and cognitive capacities, decreased physical activity, more fatigue, and altered quality of life [134,145,151,152]. Even more interesting are the findings that high inflammation markers and leptin levels appear to be related to cognitive impairment in the general population [153–155]. Finally, obesity appears to predispose cardiovascular risk factors (hypertension, dyslipidemia) and atherosclerosis [134,156]. This is a key observation considering the increased prevalence of atherosclerosis and metabolic syndrome in SLE [157] and that cardiovascular disease is a major cause of mortality in SLE patients [158,159]. Here again, high levels of leptin [136,137,141,160] and resistin [161] and low levels of adiponectin [136,137,141,142] were correlated with an increased risk of cardiovascular disease and metabolic syndrome.

In summary, despite suggestive experimental data, the relationship between obesity and the likelihood of developing SLE has not been really investigated to date. However, it appears that a high BMI is associated with more severe cognitive and renal involvement, alteration of the quality of life, and contributes to the enhanced cardiovascular risk in SLE patients. Indeed, pathophysiological data provide evidence on the involvement of adipokines in the pathogenesis of SLE through their proinflammatory and proatherosclerotic effects.

Obesity and Inflammatory Bowel Disease

Crohn's disease (CD) and ulcerative colitis (UC) are the main forms of IBD, a group of chronic, idiopathic, pathological conditions affecting the gut, characterized by a relapsing-remitting course and the frequent development of various intestinal and extraintestinal complications. Despite some shared characteristics, these forms can be distinguished by differences in genetic predisposition, risk factors, and clinical, endoscopic, and histological features. The precise cause of inflammatory bowel disease (IBD) is unknown; however, genetically susceptible individuals seem to have a dysregulated mucosal immune response to commensal gut flora, which results in bowel inflammation [162–165]. The prevalence of IBD has increased mainly in Western countries in the past 50 years up to 120–200/100,000 and 50–200/100,000 for UC and CD, respectively [166]. The reasons for this rise are unknown, but environmental factors are likely to have a preponderant role. Similar to IBD, obesity has followed the same upward curve in industrialized countries, which seems obvious to discuss its involvement in the recent outbreak of IBD.

A single very large international prospective study, including 300,724 participants, investigated the link between BMI and the risk of developing IBD [167]. The findings revealed no association of obesity measured by BMI and the risk of incident UC or CD. Yet, a previous retrospective study suggested a link between BMI and CD in subjects aged 50–70 years [168]. This correlation between obesity and an increased risk of CD was also found in a recent large study (OR = 1.02–3.47) [126]. Moreover, a recent systematic literature review of epidemiological data from 19 studies comprising 1269 CD and 1340 UC patients concluded that a high dietary intake of fat increases the risk of IBD development [169]. Several deficiencies in the first-mentioned cohort study should be pointed out [167]. First, BMI alone is a poor measuring tool of adiposity fat, especially to assess visceral adipose tissue. Secondly, only one measurement of BMI was performed when participants were recruited, sometimes several years before diagnosis. Lastly, the population was predominantly middle to elderly aged (median age of recruitment: 50–53 years), although classically IBD presents in younger patients. Thus, this study, although major, does not enable us to have a formal conclusion regarding the relationship between obesity and the risk of developing IBD, given the conflicting data from other studies.

Obesity has previously been considered to be uncommon in IBD. As the prevalence of obesity has increased worldwide, this epidemic has also influenced the IBD patients population [170]. Moreover, mesenteric adipose depots, so-called "creeping fat," have long been recognized as hallmarks of CD, its extent being correlated with the severity of intestinal inflammation [171]. Due to the proinflammatory state induced by the adipose tissue, it is necessary to clarify its impact on disease progression. Studies on this topic are unfortunately rare. Some experiments in murine models of IBD have shown that high-fat diet-induced obesity aggravates intestinal and systemic inflammation [172,173]. Furthermore, only two clinical studies have correlated a high BMI with an unfavorable course of IBD, including a higher risk of relapses, abscesses, surgical complications, and therefore hospitalizations [174,175]. These findings seem consistent with several studies reporting a link between the level of some adipokines and the severity of inflammation in IBD. Indeed, higher leptin levels are found in the plasma [176], the mesenteric visceral adipose tissue [177,178], and the gut lumen [179,180] of IBD subjects. Moreover, leptin-deficient mice are protected from inflammation in experimental colitis [181,182]. Similarly, the plasma [183,184] and adipose tissue levels [185] of resistin, as visfatin serum levels [183,186], are elevated in patients with IBD. Regarding adiponectin, results are contradictory on mouse models [187–190], as well as with serum [183,184,191] and tissue levels [178,192]. These discrepancies may be related to methodological variations and the various actions of adiponectin isoforms. Conversely, Suibhne et al. [193] recently failed to correlate obesity with disease activity score in CD. Only CRP concentration was increased in obese IBD patients. Finally, several studies found worse responses to treatment with adalimumab [194,195], infliximab [196], and azathioprine [197] in obese patients, respectively, for both diseases, CD and UD.

To summarize, data are still too sparse to conclude regarding the involvement of obesity in the risk of IBD. Nevertheless, in our opinion, despite a negative large cohort study [167] affected by some noteworthy bias, much evidence argues for obesity as a risk factor of IBD: it includes several positive studies [126,168,169], including a broad review reporting a promoting effect of a high-fat diet on the risk of IBD [169], knowledge acquired on the involvement of adipokines in this disease, and, last but not the least, the troubling outbreak of IBD concomitantly with increase in obesity worldwide, particularly with the dramatic rise in prevalence of obesity in IBD patients. Moreover, experimental and pathophysiological data prove that adipose tissue, particularly visceral mesenteric adipose tissue, plays an important role in the pathogenesis of IBD and could result in more severe presentations. However, clinical studies are lacking on this topic and further studies will likely clarify its involvement.

Obesity and Multiple Sclerosis

Multiple sclerosis (MS) is the most common chronic inflammatory demyelinating disease of the central nervous system. It is characterized by localized areas of inflammation, demyelination, axonal loss, and gliosis in the brain and spinal cord, resulting in a variety of neurological symptoms disseminated in time and space. MS mainly affects young people with onset usually at the age of 20–50 and a mean age of onset of 30, although the disease may develop also in childhood and after the age of 60 [198]. The total number of people living with MS worldwide is estimated to be 2.3 million in 2013, with increasing prevalence in recent decades. In many countries, it is the leading cause of nontraumatic disability in young adults [199]. The cause of MS is still unknown. However, genetic, environmental, and immunological factors have been implicated in the etiology of the disease [200,201]. Childhood and adolescence are thought to be a critical period of susceptibility to promoting factors. Concomitant with the rise of MS is the increased prevalence of overweight and obese children over the past decades; thus, in some countries the number of overweight children has tripled since 1980. Globally, 170 million children (aged <18 years) are estimated to be overweight [202,203].

Therefore, several studies investigated obesity during childhood and late adolescence as a risk factor of developing MS [204–208]. Thereby, two large studies, one using two cohorts of over 200,000 American women [204] and the other based on a Swedish population case–control study [205], reported a twofold increased risk of developing MS among subjects with a BMI $\geq 30\,kg/m^2$ at age 18 and 20, respectively, compared with normal weight subjects in both men and women in the second study (the first including only women). Although these studies are limited by several biases, including retrospective self-report of body size, this trend was confirmed in subsequent studies [206,207] with a more pronounced risk in women than in men. Indeed, in a prospective cohort study, Munger et al. [206] found that a higher BMI at ages 7–13 was associated with a significant 1.61–1.95-fold increased risk of MS only among girls. Similarly, another study [207] identified a higher risk of pediatric MS and clinically isolated syndrome (encompassing optic neuritis and transverse myelitis) in extremely obese adolescent girls (BMI $\geq 35\,kg/m^2$) with an OR = 2.57.

The explanation for the higher female-to-male risk observed in MS is still unknown. However, it is likely that an interaction between childhood obesity and estrogens or the X chromosome may contribute to this phenomenon [207].

Interestingly, one study [208] investigated the interactions between human leukocyte antigen (HLA) genotype and BMI status. Many genes have been identified for predisposition to MS [201], HLA-DRB1*15 allele conferring a threefold higher risk and HLA-A*02 being protective with a twofold lower risk. Using two case–control studies, the authors showed that subjects with a BMI <27 kg/m² and the two risk genotypes (carriage of DRB1*15 and absence of A*02) displayed an OR = 5.1–5.7, whereas the same genotype for subjects with BMI $\geq 27\,kg/m^2$ rendered an OR = 13.8–16.2 in the two cohorts.

Different hypotheses were suggested attempting to explain this association. First, vitamin D has been found to reduce the incidence and progression of an animal model of MS [209]. Moreover, high levels of circulating 25-hydroxyvitamin D have been associated with lower risk of MS [210]. It is well established that obese people, including obese children, have decreased serum levels of vitamin D metabolites [26,211,212], which may offer a partial explanation for the increased risk of MS in this population. Furthermore, adipose tissue macrophages infiltrating adipose tissue during obesity under high-fat feeding switch from an antiinflammatory M2 polarization state to a proinflammatory M1 polarization [213]. A recent study [214] demonstrated that imbalance toward M1 monocytes promotes relapsing experimental autoimmune encephalomyelitis (EAE), whereas administration of ex vivo activated M2 monocytes suppressed ongoing severe EAE.

The most exciting field of investigation is the role of adipokines in the pathogenesis of MS. Indeed, several studies [215,216] reported increased levels of leptin, resistin, and visfatin and decreased levels of adiponectin, a profile also observed among obese subjects, in MS patients. This profile was correlated with higher levels of inflammatory mediators (CRP, TNFα, IL-1β) [216] and lower Foxp3 Treg cells [215,216]. Using an EAE mice model, the most commonly used animal model for MS, Piccio et al. [217] showed that adiponectin-deficient mice developed worse clinical and histological disease, with higher amounts of IFN-γ, IL-17, TNFα, and IL-6, and fewer Treg cells than wild-type mice. Treatment with globular adiponectin almost completely suppressed the development of EAE and increased Treg cells. Moreover, prior study [218] found that calorie restriction ameliorated murine EAE and was associated with higher adiponectin plasma levels and lower concentrations of leptin and IL-6. In the same way, pharmacological inhibition of visfatin decreased the clinical manifestations of EAE by reducing T lymphocytes IFN-γ and TNFα production [219].

However, the stronger body of evidence has been shown with leptin. Indeed, Matarese et al. investigated the role of leptin in several experimental studies in murine models of MS [220–223] (reviewed in Refs. [224,225]). First, using a leptin-deficient *ob/ob* mice [220], they showed that leptin is required in the induction and progression of EAE; leptin replacement converted disease resistance to susceptibility by shifting the Th2 to a Th1 response and by inducing production of myelin-specific antibodies. Additionally, [221], they demonstrated in C57BL/6J and SJL/J mice, two EAE-susceptible strains of mice, that a marked surge in serum leptin levels, starting after immunization with myelin antigens, anticipates the onset of the acute phase of EAE; interestingly, this increase was accompanied by in situ production of leptin by pathogenic T cells and macrophages in demyelinating lesions in the brain and the spinal cord. A 48-h starvation at this time prevented rise in serum leptin along with EAE onset and clinical symptoms by inducing a Th2 cytokine switch. The effects of starvation could be reversed by administration of recombinant leptin. Finally [222,223], leptin neutralization with either antileptin antibodies or leptin receptor-Fc fusion protein reduced EAE onset, severity, and mortality by promoting a Th2 and Treg profile. Moreover, in patients with MS, leptin levels were found enhanced in both the serum and the cerebrospinal fluid (CSF), correlating with IFN-γ production in CSF [222].

To summarize, there is strong evidence linking obesity with the risk of developing MS. The pathophysiological mechanisms are likely to be complex but clearly involve adipokines by promoting a proinflammatory Th1 profile and reducing Treg cells. Although to date there is no clinical study investigating the involvement of obesity on the course and prognosis of MS, experimental data detailed above suggest a harmful impact. This issue needs to be investigated in subsequent studies.

Obesity and Type 1 Diabetes

Diabetes mellitus refers to a group of diseases characterized by dysregulation of glucose metabolism, resulting from defects in insulin secretion, decreased insulin sensitivity, or a combination of both; it leads to chronic hyperglycemia and subsequent acute and chronic complications. It has traditionally been subdivided into type 1 diabetes (T1D, previously named insulin-dependent or juvenile-onset diabetes), a childhood acute disorder characterized by autoimmune destruction of insulin-secreting β-cells, and type 2 diabetes (T2D, formerly known as non–insulin-dependent diabetes), a slow-onset, middle-life disorder presenting with insulin resistance and features of metabolic syndrome, including overweightness [226,227]. Autoantibodies associated with T1D include islet cell autoantibodies, glutamic acid decarboxylase autoantibodies, insulinoma-associated 2 autoantibodies, insulin autoantibodies, and zinc transporter-8 autoantibodies.

However, distinctions between type 1 and type 2 diabetes are becoming increasingly blurred both clinically and etiologically. Indeed, the last decades have been marked by profound changes in epidemiological and clinical features of "diabetic diseases," giving rise to an intense debate on the underlying pathophysiological mechanisms. First, incidence and prevalence of both T1D and T2D are dramatically increasing worldwide. Thus, the number of people with diabetes rose from 153 million in 1980 to 347 million in 2008 [228]. T1D is the most common (90%) type of diabetes in children and adolescent. Its incidence is increasing by approximately 4% per year [2]. As genetic changes cannot cause such a rapid rise, environmental factors are strongly suspected to be involved in this outbreak. Second, clinical presentations are becoming more complex and overlapping. In addition to the "classical" type 1 and type 2 diabetes, the following are described: overweight or obese T1D, T2D in adolescents, latent autoimmune diabetes in adults, enclosing a group of patients over 35 years with features of T2D but with T1D autoimmunity markers, and conversely "double diabetes" or "1.5 diabetes," characterized by the presence of overlapping T1D and T2D symptoms in children or adolescents [227]. One common point is noted: obesity has experienced the same dramatic increase as diabetes in recent decades [11,12] and is found as a common characteristic in the overlapping forms of diabetes mentioned above.

These findings led Wilkin to propose a provocative and controversial theory in 2001, the "Accelerator Hypothesis" [229]. It postulates that T1D and T2D are the same disorder of insulin resistance set against different genetic background. Both diseases are distinguishable only by their rate of β-cell loss and the "accelerators" responsible; at the end, all diabetes progress to a final insulin-dependent state. Thus, the difference between T1D and T2D would only rely on the tempo of disease progression, depending on the presence of the various accelerators. Three accelerators are described: genetic susceptibility, insulin resistance, and β-cell autoimmunity. Insulin resistance would be a common accelerator, resulting from weight gain, and is widely believed to explain the epidemic rise of both T1D and T2D.

To focus on T1D, the question of the relationship between obesity and the risk of developing T1D has long been raised [230]. The Accelerator Hypothesis puts overweightness at the heart of the pathogenesis of T1D in a continuum with T2D [229]. It has sparked renewed interest in this topic and has been investigated in subsequent studies. Several questions are raised: does obesity influence the occurrence of T1D, partly driving its recent outbreak? If so, what are the mechanisms involved? The literature on this subject is not uniform, this issue being addressed at different levels. According to the studies, authors analyze the influence of maternal weight and weight gain during pregnancy, birthweight, weight gain in the early years of life, or childhood obesity, on the occurrence of T1D.

Prenatal factors (including maternal obesity and weight gain during pregnancy) will not be discussed herein. Briefly, studies are scarce and contradictory [231], some correlating maternal obesity and weight gain during pregnancy with increased islet autoimmunity and higher risk of T1D in offspring [232,233] and others failing to evidence an association [234,235]. Two large metaanalyses [236,237] were made regarding the role of birthweight and early weight gain during the first years of life, one of these investigating 29 studies [237]. A significant positive relation was found between higher birthweight or increased early weight gain and the risk of developing subsequent T1D. Children with birthweight >4000 g exhibit an increased risk of T1D ranging from 10% [237] to 43% [236]. The observed association is supported by several studies in non-obese diabetic mice, an animal model spontaneously developing T1D. A higher risk of diabetes was seen with increased birthweight [238], whereas calorie restriction during pregnancy leads to reduced birthweight and lower risk of diabetes in mice at 24 weeks [239]. However, it is worth mentioning that despite the adjustment for potential confounders in these large metaanalyses, it is impossible to exclude all exposure factors that may affect both birthweight and risk of T1D, such as maternal diseases, weight, and nutrition, or some HLA predisposing both conditions [240]. Similarly, childhood obesity has been investigated as a potential risk factor for T1D and reviewed in a recent metaanalysis [241]. Despite heterogeneous data, there is overall evidence for a positive association between childhood obesity and increased risk of T1D, with a calculated pooled OR=2.03.

Interestingly, only one study [126] examining the association between obesity and certain autoimmune diseases in a cohort of 75,000 adult women (mean age 30 years) followed during a median time of 11 years reported a twofold increased risk of T1D among obese women (BMI ≥30 kg/m²). Unfortunately, BMI was only measured once at the start of the follow-up, and no data were available on eventual childhood obesity and weight change throughout the duration of the follow-up.

Yet, it remains unclear if increased birthweight and childhood obesity are acting as real risk factors or simply as accelerators, leading to an earlier presentation of T1D in genetically susceptible subjects. Although a number of studies demonstrated that among heavier children T1D occurs at a younger age [242–244], several authors argue that this is balanced by a decreased incidence among older age groups, resulting in a stable overall risk [245,246]. Thus, obesity may decrease the age at onset of T1D without necessarily changing lifetime risk. According to the Accelerator Hypothesis, overweightness would be a precipitating factor rather than an etiological factor.

Nevertheless, the mechanisms underlying this effect are still poorly understood. Increased body weight may promote T1D in a number of ways. Overload Hypothesis [247] suggests that overload of the β-cell, mediated by a variety of mechanisms, may sensitize them to immune damage and apoptosis and accelerate ongoing autoimmune processes leading to their destruction. Thus, obesity-induced insulin resistance, by increased insulin demand on β-cells at a critical period in early life, leads to β-cell overload by making them work harder metabolically. Both glucotoxicity and β-cell stress may accelerate their apoptosis, rendering β-cells more immunogenic. Therefore, individuals with susceptible genotypes will subsequently mount an autoimmune response, further accelerating β-cell loss.

Adipokines may also have a crucial role in the relationship between T1D and obesity, their action being at the crossroads of metabolism, immunity, and obesity. Leptin and adiponectin are two major insulin-sensitizing mediators and regulate glucose metabolism through various mechanisms, including promotion of insulin secretion and storage of glucose and inhibition of glucagon secretion and hepatic gluconeogenesis [33]. According to the studies, leptin is found to be increased [248], reduced [249], or unchanged [250] among T1D patients, possibly because of variations in insulin levels that regulate leptin. Concerning adiponectin, most studies report high levels [251,252], suggesting that increased adiponectin is a compensatory mechanism secondary to hyperglycemia and loss of endogenous insulin secretion in T1D patients [253]. Paradoxically, although adiponectin has antiinflammatory and vascular protective properties, high adiponectin levels appear to be associated with microvascular and macrovascular complications [254,255] and increased cardiovascular and overall mortality in diabetes [256]. Several explanations have been proposed to this observation. Hyperadiponectimenia may reflect poorly controlled diabetes, thus at high risk of complications, or it may be a compensatory mechanism, the adiponectin exhibiting cardioprotective effects. Conversely, resistin, known to promote insulin resistance, is found at increased levels in T1D [257], suggesting a pathophysiological involvement.

The most exciting point concerns the action of adipokines on the autoimmune destruction of β-cells. Indeed, adiponectin has been shown to protect β-cells from apoptosis and islet immunoreactivity [258,259]; inversely, leptin, by its proinflammatory effects, accelerates autoimmune destruction of β-cells in murine models [260], and resistin decreases β-cell viability [261]. Considering now the adipokine profile observed among obese patients, low adiponectin and high leptin and resistin promote both insulin resistance via decreased adiponectin and elevated resistin; it also leads to the immune-mediated destruction of β-cell through the joint action of the three mediators.

Thus, an extensive literature suggests that childhood and adolescence obesity leads to an overall twofold increase in the risk of subsequent T1D. However, it remains unclear whether this trend reflects an earlier onset of T1D in obese subjects or an enhanced risk of developing the disease. In all cases, prevention of obesity may have substantial benefits on preventing late complications of T1D by delaying or preventing its occurrence. Even more, the "adipokine profile" observed in obese subjects has been shown to aggravate both metabolic and autoimmune processes involved in T1D.

Obesity, Psoriasis, and Psoriatic Arthritis

Psoriasis is a highly common chronic inflammatory skin disease, its prevalence ranging from 1% to 8.5% of the population according to the countries [262]. Psoriasis is associated with a wide range of comorbid conditions [263] and responsible for significant impairment of the quality of life [264]. Its common variant, termed psoriasis vulgaris, affects 90% of all patients and is characterized by papulosquamous well-delineated plaques [265]. However, the disease is not necessarily restricted to skin and nails; notably, about 30% of patients may develop a chronic inflammatory arthritis, included in the group of spondyloarthritis, namely psoriatic arthritis (PsA) [266]. The pathogenesis of both psoriasis and PsA is thought to result from the interplay between a strong genetic background, environmental factors, and immune dysfunction [267].

The existence of an association between obesity and both psoriasis and PsA has long been suggested [268] and has been strongly confirmed in many studies since [269,270]. Indeed, a recent metaanalysis [269] of 16 observational studies with a total of 2.1 million subjects (including 201,831 psoriasis patients) analyzed the epidemiological association between psoriasis and obesity; the findings conclude that compared with the general population, psoriasis patients are at significantly higher odds of obesity, with a pooled OR=1.46 for mild-psoriasis and an OR=2.23 for severe-psoriasis patients. However, the direction of this relationship is still a matter of debate. Several authors suggest that obesity may be a risk factor predisposing the development of psoriasis [271–273] and PsA [274–276], whereas others argue that overweightness is a consequence of these conditions rather than a predisposing factor [277,278]. To date, available data suggest that both phenomena are intricate in a bidirectional relationship [279].

First, psoriasis and PsA are thought to promote weight gain, which may partly explain the high prevalence of obesity among these patients. Thus, Herron et al. [277] reported in a retrospective study of 557 psoriatic patients that obesity at 18 years did not increase the risk of subsequent psoriasis; conversely, patients who developed psoriasis were more likely to become obese compared with Utah population (OR=2.39). This study was based on a recall method and despite the controversy of this design, the observation seems consistent as numerous studies have demonstrated that psoriasis and PsA promote increased social isolation, depression [280], overeating and high-fat diets [281], alcohol consumption [282], and physical inactivity [283], all of which may lead to excess weight gain. Moreover, some studies have suggested that anti-TNFα treatments could result in a significant increase in body weight in psoriasis patients [284,285].

Furthermore, strong evidence suggests that obesity is an independent risk factor for both psoriasis and PsA [271–276]. In support of this hypothesis are two large prospective cohort studies [271,273] of American female nurses including 67,300 and 76,626 women (with 809 and 892 incident cases of psoriasis) followed, respectively, for 12 and 14 years in NHS [273] and NHS II [271] The studies report that higher BMI and weight gain since the age of 18 years are strong risk factors for incident psoriasis in both young [271] and old [273] women (mean age of 36 and 62 years). The relative risks (RR) of psoriasis are 1.48–1.63 for a BMI of 30–34.9 and 2.03–2.68 for a BMI of 35 or greater. BMI is also suggested as a risk factor for psoriasis in a recently published Danish cohort of over 75,000 women [126]. Similarly, two simultaneous large prospective studies [274,275], one from a UK population database (about 2 million individuals, 75,395 psoriasis patients, 976 incident PsA) [274] and the other from the NHS II (89,049 women, 146 incident PsA) [275], provide evidence linking obesity with the risk of incident PsA, with an RR among all individuals (regardless of psoriasis) of 1.57–3.12 for BMI 30–34.9 and 1.96–6.46 for BMI over 35. Interestingly, the influence of BMI on the risk of developing psoriasis could partially depend on the genetic background as suggested by two studies which demonstrated that the risk of subsequent psoriasis was influenced by the interaction between BMI and several genetic risk factors [286,287].

Moreover, the potential pathogenic role of obesity in psoriasis is strengthened by several studies [277,288–290] reporting a positive correlation between obesity measured by various parameters (BMI, waist circumference, bioelectrical impedance analysis) and psoriasis severity determined by the Psoriasis Area and Severity Index (PASI) score. Furthermore, besides its potential direct pathogenic role in psoriasis and PsA, obesity is also known to aggravate cardiovascular risk and increase the prevalence of metabolic syndrome features [48,49,291]. These comorbidities are more commonly seen in subjects with inflammatory diseases, especially psoriasis and PsA [292–294].

Supporting this hypothesis, a recent review [295] examining the impact of weight loss intervention found that losing weight through decreased calorie intake [296,297] or gastric bypass [298,299], alone or in conjunction with other treatments [300,301], significantly improved psoriasis or PsA severity, as well as the cardiovascular risk profile in both diseases [302]. Naldi et al. [296] recently conducted a randomized controlled trial including overweight or obese patients with moderate-to-severe psoriasis, randomized to receive either a dietary plan associated with physical exercise or simple information counseling. At 20 weeks, a significant improvement of psoriasis severity was shown in the dietary intervention arm when compared with the information-only arm, with a PASI score reduction of 48% versus 25.5%.

Thus, there is strong evidence suggesting a pathogenic role of obesity on both the occurrence and the severity of psoriasis and PsA. This is supported by extensive data acquired on the proinflammatory role of adipocytes. First, we must remember that psoriasis and PsA are characterized by the expansion of Th1, Th17, and Th22 cells, resulting in the production of large amounts of proinflammatory mediators, including IFN-γ, TNFα, IL-6, IL-17, and IL-22 [303,305]. As it is now recognized that fat cells secrete a wide variety of mediators, including TNFα and IL-6 [304], it might contribute to the inflammatory state in psoriasis. Moreover, many studies have demonstrated that high levels of both leptin and resistin, two adipokines enhanced in obese subjects, were found in psoriasis and PsA patients [305–309] and were correlated to the severity of the disease. Furthermore, resistin plasma levels have been shown to decrease under treatment [309–311].

Regarding leptin, a recent metaanalysis of 11 studies [305] confirmed that psoriasis patients exhibit increased levels of leptin compared with controls. Both leptin and resistin are known to promote the production of proinflammatory mediators involved in the pathogenesis of psoriasis, such as TNFα and CXCL8 [307,312]. Interestingly, tissue levels of leptin are also enhanced in the skin of psoriasis patients [313,314] and induce secretion of proinflammatory cytokines by human keratinocytes in vitro [314]. Moreover, leptin is increased in PsA patients and correlates with both the severity score of PsA and soluble mediators of osteoclastogenesis [315]. Studies investigating the role of visfatin in psoriasis are sparse. However, some data [316,317] suggest that high levels of visfatin are associated with more severe psoriasis and, considering its pro-atherogenic role, visfatin may contribute to the cardiovascular morbidity in psoriasis.

Finally, on adiponectin, its role is still uncertain. Indeed, despite several studies [318–320] suggesting that psoriasis patients exhibit lower rates inversely correlated to the severity, a recent metaanalysis [321] found no difference between serum adiponectin levels in patients and controls. However, the authors state that most studies have a case–control design and small sample sizes. In addition, as mentioned above, the action of adiponectin is different depending on the isoform considered, and studies may not all measure the same isoform. Larger studies are needed to clarify the role of adiponectin.

Equally important, obesity has also been shown to significantly affect the efficacy and safety of psoriasis and PsA treatments; several reviews summarize literature data on this topic [279,322]. First, conventional systemic drugs, especially methotrexate and cyclosporine, exhibit a higher risk of toxicity in overweight patients. Indeed, nonalcoholic steatohepatitis, usually associated with obesity, may potentiate the hepatotoxicity of methotrexate, requiring closer hepatic monitoring in obese individuals [323]. Alternatively, the distribution volume of cyclosporine, a highly lipophilic drug, seems to be influenced by increased fat mass, leading to higher concentrations and subsequent nephrotoxicity in psoriasis patients [324]. Thus, it is recommended to adjust the dose of cyclosporine to the ideal weight instead of the actual weight of the patient to reduce the risk of toxicity [325].

Regarding biologic therapies, non–weight-adjusted drugs may be less effective in overweight patients [322,326]. Thus, infliximab weight-adjusted regimen provides constant results in psoriasis according to the weight [327]. Conversely, in most studies, response to etanercept and adalimumab, two fixed dose anti-TNFα treatments, was lower in heavier psoriasis patients, with an inverse correlation between BMI or weight and response rate [328,329]. Moreover, a prospective trial [330] concluded that obesity is a negative predictor of achieving and maintaining minimal disease activity in PsA patients treated by anti-TNFα blockers. Similarly, large trials found that in psoriasis patients, a weight N100 kg was associated with decreased serum levels and efficacy of ustekinumab, an anti–IL-12 and IL-23 inhibitor. The switch for a double dose of ustekinumab restored its efficacy [331]. The lower efficiency is likely related to the modification of the drug distribution, as well as the secretion of proinflammatory factors, including TNFα, by adipose tissue.

In support of this hypothesis, Mutairi et al. [332] carried out a randomized controlled prospective trial including 262 psoriasis patients under biologic therapies and demonstrated the beneficial effects of weight reduction on the efficacy of biologics. They reported that PASI-75 (a 75% reduction in PASI score) was achieved by 85.9% in the diet group and 59.3% in the control group. These results are consistent with previous studies reporting a positive effect of weight loss on the response to treatment, both in psoriasis and PsA [300,301]. Therefore, the treatment of obese patients with psoriasis and PsA is associated with decreased effectiveness and higher risk of adverse events, which may lead to drug discontinuation [333,334]. Consequently, it clearly appears that the type and the dose of treatment should be considered and adapted according to the patient's weight.

In conclusion, there is strong evidence suggesting that obesity, through its proinflammatory action, predisposes the development of psoriasis and PsA, aggravates the evolution of both diseases, increases the risk of cardiovascular and metabolic comorbidities, and decreases biologic therapy efficacy. This should make nutritional care a central part of the management of psoriasis and PsA patient, particularly as the beneficial effects of weight loss have been demonstrated.

Obesity and Thyroid Autoimmunity

Autoimmune thyroid diseases encompass a spectrum of disorders characterized by an autoimmune attack on the thyroid gland, including Hashimoto thyroiditis (HT), Grave's disease, and postpartum thyroiditis. Herein, we will focus on HT, as there are no sufficient data on the relationship between obesity and the other autoimmune thyroid diseases. HT (also named chronic autoimmune thyroiditis and autoimmune hypothyroidism) is the most common autoimmune disease [335], the most common endocrine disorder [336], and the most common cause of hypothyroidism [337]. Its incidence ranges from 27 to 448/100,000 per year according to the studies and the geographic areas, and women show to be at least 8 times more affected than men [335]. It is an organ-specific autoimmune disease characterized by the presence of a goiter with lymphocytic infiltration, associated with serum thyroid antibodies—including anti–thyroid peroxidase (anti-TPO) and antithyroglobulin (anti-Tg) antibodies – and systemic manifestation related to hypothyroidism [338]. The etiopathogenesis of HT has not been fully elucidated; however, it is clearly a multifactorial disease, resulting from a complex interaction between genetic and environmental factors, such as excess iodine, synthetic chemicals, or infections [339,340].

Thyroid function was extensively investigated in obese subjects. Relationship between obesity and thyroid is complex and several processes seem to be intricate [341]. On the one hand, an elevated serum thyroid-stimulating hormone (thyrotropin, TSH) concentration is frequently reported in obese individuals and positively correlated with BMI [342,343]. However, this elevation is not always indicative of hypothyroidism, as peripheral thyroid hormones (T3 and T4) might be increased, decreased, or in the normal range [344–346]. Moreover, in most studies, these hormonal changes do not appear to be related to an autoimmune process in the thyroid, insofar as these patients with raised serum TSH exhibit low prevalence of HT-related autoantibodies [344–346]. Some authors initially postulated that thyroid dysfunction was responsible for obesity [347]. However, it seems unlikely, as the treatment of severe hypothyroidism was found to result only in a minimal improvement in weight [348]. Conversely, weight loss by hypocaloric diet or by bariatric surgery led to a significant reduction in TSH levels [349,350]. Thus, this hyperthyrotropinemia appears to be the consequence rather than the cause of excess weight. Several mechanisms have been suggested. It might correspond to an adaptive process of the hypothalamus–pituitary–thyroid axis in obese individuals, elevated thyroid hormones promoting the resting energy expenditure [351]. Furthermore, there is increased evidence that leptin is contributing to TSH elevation [352], as it has been shown that leptin regulates, at least partially, TSH secretion in humans [353,354] and is correlated both with BMI and TSH [355].

Besides these hormonal changes associated with obesity, some studies have suggested that obese people could also be more prone to develop HT [356,357]. Ong et al. [357] reported on a cohort study including almost 2500 subjects that childhood weight gain and childhood overweightness conferred a slightly increased risk (OR = 1.21) of HT at the age of 60–64 years particularly in women. Similarly, Marzullo et al. [356] recently showed a greater prevalence of hypothyroidism and HT-related autoantibodies among obese individuals, correlated with increased leptin levels. In support of this concept is a recently published study [358] describing higher leptin levels in HT patients, positively correlating with the percentage of Th17 cells, which are suggested to be involved in the pathogenesis of HT [359,360].

In conclusion, it is now recognized that variations in thyroid hormones during obesity are mostly related to a deregulation of the hypothalamic–pituitary axis, without underlying autoimmune process. This does not exclude that overweightness might also lead to an excess risk of autoimmune thyroiditis, with leptin playing a major role in this process. Given the frequency of HT, future studies will probably help clarify this relationship.

CONCLUSION

Currently, many efforts are underway to attempt to explain the recent outbreak of autoimmune diseases, which is a hot topic today. The combination of variety of environmental factors is highly suspected to promote this phenomenon. Of these environmental factors, available data provide strong evidence for the deleterious impact of obesity on several immune-mediated conditions. Thus, obesity clearly appears to increase the risk of developing RA, MS, psoriasis, and PsA and could also promote the occurrence of IBD, T1D, and TAI. Furthermore, obese patients are prone to experience a more severe course of RA, SLE, IBD, psoriasis, and PsA and reduced therapeutic response in RA, IBD, psoriasis, and PsA.

Multiple and complex pathophysiological processes are likely to be engaged and result in these harmful effects. In this review, we focused on the key role of adipokines. Indeed, extensive clinical and pathophysiological studies have demonstrated their pathogenic action in various diseases, including immune-mediated diseases, mostly through their pro-inflammatory properties. More than a passive storage area, adipose tissue is an active endocrine organ responsible for the promotion and the worsening of pathological conditions in obese subjects. When considering globally all of the pathogenic mechanisms suggested to affect the immune system under obese conditions, it provides pathophysiological arguments, in addition to clinical data, to answer two major issues: do obese individuals have more autoimmune disorders? And is obesity aggravating these conditions? Schematically, on the one hand, obesity has been associated with decreased Treg and B regulatory subsets, expansion of Th17 cells, and promotion of autoantibodies. Altogether, these mechanisms may lead to a breakdown of self-tolerance, promoting the development of autoimmunity and subsequent autoimmune disease. On the other hand, obesity is recognized to result in a strong proinflammatory environment, which once the autoimmune disease has occurred may worsen its progression and its treatment.

Despite abundant literature, this review also highlights several limitations and gaps in this topic. Thus, studies are often heterogeneous, and their interpretation may be limited by numerous biases, related to an insufficient number of patients, retrospective methodology, inadequate measure of body fat, and variations in considering potential confounders.

In conclusion, in the light of recent advances, obesity appears to be a new component of the complex mosaic of autoimmunity. Although some trends are emerging, further studies are needed to confirm these observations and specify the effects and pathogenic mechanisms involved. Furthermore, the impact of obesity should be investigated in a wide range of autoimmune diseases, such as antiphospholipid syndrome, inflammatory myopathies, and juvenile idiopathic arthritis, in which a few data [361–364] already suggest the involvement of obesity and adipokines.

TAKE-HOME MESSAGES

- WAT is an active endocrine organ secreting soluble mediators called "adipokines."
- Adipokines are responsible for a proinflammatory state in obese subjects promoting and worsening various pathological conditions.
- Obesity promotes autoimmunity through variety of mechanisms including the secretion of adipokines.
- Obesity may increase the risk of several autoimmune diseases, especially RA, MS, psoriasis, PsA, IBD, T1D, and HT.
- Obesity may aggravate the course of RA, SLE, IBD, psoriasis, and PsA.
- Obesity would affect the treatment response of RA, IBD, psoriasis, and PsA.

LIST OF ABBREVIATIONS

ACPA Anticitrullinated protein antibodies
ACR American College of Rheumatology
AIM Apoptosis inhibitor of macrophage
Anti-Tg Antithyroglobulin antibodies
Anti-TPO Antithyroperoxidase antibodies
BMI Body mass index
CCL Chemokine ligand
CD Crohn's disease
CSF Cerebrospinal fluid
CRP C-reactive protein
EAE Experimental autoimmune encephalomyelitis
ESR Erythrocyte sedimentation rate
Foxp3 Forkhead box protein 3
HAQ Health Assessment Questionnaire
HLA Human leukocyte antigen
HT Hashimoto thyroiditis
HR Hazard ratio
IBD Inflammatory bowel disease
IFN-γ Interferon gamma
IL Interleukin
iNK cells Invariant natural killer T cells
MS Multiple sclerosis
NLRP3-inflammasome NOD-like receptor protein 3 inflammasome
OR Odds ratio
PASI Psoriasis Area and Severity Index
PBMC Peripheral blood mononuclear cell
PsA Psoriatic arthritis
RA Rheumatoid arthritis
RR Relative risk
SLE Systemic lupus erythematosus
T1D Type 1 diabetes
T2D Type 2 diabetes
TAI Thyroid autoimmunity
Th17 cells T helper 17 cells
TNFα Tumor necrosis factor alpha
Treg cells T regulatory cells
TSH Thyroid-stimulating hormone
UC Ulcerative colitis
WAT White adipose tissue

REFERENCES

[1] Pedersen JK, Svendsen AJ, Hørslev-Petersen K. Incidence of rheumatoid arthritis in the southern part of Denmark from 1995 to 2001. Open Rheumatol J January 2007;1:18–23.

[2] Patterson CC, Dahlquist GG, Gyürüs E, Green A, Soltész G. Incidence trends for childhood type 1 diabetes in Europe during 1989–2003 and predicted new cases 2005–20: a multicentre prospective registration study. Lancet July 13, 2009;373(9680):2027–33.

[3] Zandman-Goddard G, Shoenfeld Y. Parasitic infection and autoimmunity. Lupus November 2009;18(13):1144–8.

[4] De Carvalho JF, Pereira RMR, Shoenfeld Y. The mosaic of autoimmunity: the role of environmental factors. Front Biosci (Elite Ed) January 2009;1:501–9.

[5] Bogdanos DP, Smyk DS, Invernizzi P, Rigopoulou EI, Blank M, Pouria S, et al. Infectome: a platform to trace infectious triggers of autoimmunity. Autoimmun Rev May 2013;12(7):726–40.

[6] Agmon-Levin N, Theodor E, Segal RM, Shoenfeld Y. Vitamin D in systemic and organ-specific autoimmune diseases. Clin Rev Allergy Immunol October 2013;45(2):256–66.

[7] Doria A, Sarzi-Puttini P, Shoenfeld Y. Infections, rheumatism and autoimmunity: the conflicting relationship between humans and their environment. Autoimmun Rev October 2008;8(1):1–4.

[8] Kivity S, Agmon-Levin N, Blank M, Shoenfeld Y. Infections and autoimmunity—friends or foes? Trends Immunol August 2009;30(8):409–14.

[9] Moroni L, Bianchi I, Lleo A. Geoepidemiology, gender and autoimmune disease. Autoimmun Rev May 2012;11(6–7):A386–92.

[10] Van der Meer JW, Netea MG. A salty taste to autoimmunity. N Engl J Med June 27, 2013;368(26):2520–1.

[11] Flegal KM, Carroll MD, Ogden CL, Curtin LR. Prevalence and trends in obesity among US adults, 1999–2008. JAMA January 20, 2010;303(3):235–41.

[12] World Health Organization. Overweight/obesity: overweight by country. In: Global Health Observatory Data Repository 2008. 2013.

[13] Cao H. Adipocytokines in obesity and metabolic disease. J Endocrinol 2014;220(2):T47–59.

[14] Gómez R, Conde J, Scotece M, Gómez-Reino JJ, Lago F, Gualillo O. What's new in our understanding of the role of adipokines in rheumatic diseases?. Nat Rev Rheumatol September 2011;7(9):528–36. Nature Publishing Group.

[15] Weisberg SP, McCann D, Desai M, Rosenbaum M, Leibel RL, Ferrante AW. Obesity is associated with macrophage accumulation in adipose tissue. J Clin Investig December 2003;112(12):1796–808.

[16] Nishimura S, Manabe I, Nagasaki M, Eto K, Yamashita H, Ohsugi M, et al. CD8+ effector T cells contribute to macrophage recruitment and adipose tissue inflammation in obesity. Nat Med August 2009;15(8):914–20.

[17] Arai S, Maehara N, Iwamura Y, Honda S, Nakashima K, Kai T, et al. Obesityassociated autoantibody production requires AIM to retain the immunoglobulin M immune complex on follicular dendritic cells. Cell Rep 2013;3(4):1187–98. The Authors.

[18] Arai S, Miyazaki T. Impacts of the apoptosis inhibitor of macrophage (AIM) on obesityassociated inflammatory diseases. Semin Immunopathol January 2013;36(1):3–12.

[19] Miyazaki T, Hirokami Y, Matsuhashi N, Takatsuka H, Naito M. Increased susceptibility of thymocytes to apoptosis in mice lacking AIM, a novel murine macrophage-derived soluble factor belonging to the scavenger receptor cysteine-rich domain superfamily. J Exp Med January 18, 1999;189(2):413–22.

[20] Noack M, Miossec P. Th17 and regulatory T cell balance in autoimmune and inflammatory diseases. Autoimmun Rev June 2014;13(6):668–77.

[21] Winer S, Paltser G, Chan Y, Tsui H, Engleman E, Winer D, et al. Obesity predisposes to Th17 bias. Eur J Immunol October 2009;39(9):2629–35.

[22] Ahmed M, Gaffen S. IL-17 inhibits adipogenesis in part bia C/EBP-alpha, PPAR-gamma and Krüppel-like factors. Cytokine 2014;61(3):898–905.

[23] Ahmed M, Gaffen S. IL-17 in obesity and adipogenesis. Cytokine Growth Factor Rev 2012;21(6):449–53.

[24] Manzel A, Muller DN, Hafler DA, Kleinewietfeld M. Role of "western diet" in inflammatory autoimmune diseases. Curr Allergy Asthma Rep 2014;14(1):404.

[25] Brown K, DeCoffe D, Molcan E, Gibson DL. Diet-induced dysbiosis of the intestinal microbiota and the effects on immunity and disease. Nutrients August 2012;4(11):1552–3.

[26] Soskić S, Stokić E, Isenović ER. The relationship between vitamin D and obesity. Curr Med Res Opin July 2014;30(6):1197–9.

[27] Schoindre Y, Terrier B, Kahn J-E, Saadoun D, Souberbielle J-C, Benveniste O, et al. Vitamin D and autoimmunity. First part: fundamental aspects. La Rev Méd Interne March 2012;33(2):80–6.

[28] Yang C-Y, Leung PSC, Adamopoulos IE, Gershwin ME. The implication of vitamin D and autoimmunity: a comprehensive review. Clin Rev Allergy Immunol October 2013;45(2):217–26.

[29] Pludowski P, Holick MF, Pilz S, Wagner CL, Hollis BW, Grant WB, et al. Vitamin D effects on musculoskeletal health, immunity, autoimmunity, cardiovascular disease, cancer, fertility, pregnancy, dementia and mortality—a review of recent evidence. Autoimmun Rev August 2013;12(10):976–89.

[30] Lukens JR, Dixit VD, Kanneganti T-D. Inflammasome activation in obesity-related inflammatory diseases and autoimmunity. Discov Med July 2011;12(62):65–74.

[31] Nishimura S, Manabe I, Takaki S, Nagasaki M, Otsu M, Yamashita H, et al. Adipose natural regulatory B cells negatively control adipose tissue inflammation. Cell Metab October 22, 2013;18(5):759–66. Elsevier Inc.

[32] Rakhshandehroo M, Kalkhoven E, Boes M. Invariant natural killer T cells in adipose tissue: novel regulators of immune–mediated metabolic disease. Cell Mol Life Sci 2013;70(24):4711–27.

[33] Stofkova A. Leptin and adiponectin: from energy and metabolic dysbalance to inflammation and autoimmunity. Endocr Regul 2009;43(4):157–68.

[34] Iikuni N, Lam Q, Lu L, Matarese G, La Cava A. Leptin and inflammation. Curr Immunol Rev 2010;4(2):70–9.

[35] Krysiak R, Handzlik-Orlik G, Okopien B. The role of adipokines in connective tissue diseases. Eur J Nutr August 2012;51(5):513–28.

[36] Derdemezis CS, Voulgari PV, Drosos AA, Kiortsis DN. Obesity, adipose tissue and rheumatoid arthritis: coincidence or more complex relationship? Clin Exp Rheumatol 2011;29(4):712–27.

[37] Stavropoulos-kalinoglou A, Metsios GS, Koutedakis Y, Kitas GD. Obesity in rheumatoid arthritis. Rheumatology (Oxford) 2011;50(3):450–62.

[38] Li L, Wu L-L. Adiponectin and interleukin-6 in inflammation-associated disease. Vitam Horm January 2012;90:375–95.

[39] Sun Y, Xun K, Wang C, Zhao H, Bi H, Chen X, et al. Adiponectin, an unlocking adipocytokine. Cardiovasc Ther January 2009;27(1):59–75.

[40] Toussirot E, Gaugler B, Bouhaddi M, Nguyen NU, Saas P, Dumoulin G. Elevated adiponectin serum levels in women with systemic autoimmune diseases. Mediators Inflamm January 2010, E-pub.

[41] Stofkova A. Resistin and Visfatin: regulators of insulin sensitivity inflammation and immunity. Endocr Regul 2010;44(1):25–36.

[42] Kourilovitch M, Galarza-Maldonado C, Ortiz-Prado E. Diagnosis and classification of rheumatoid arthritis. J Autoimmun 2014;48–49:26–30.

[43] Myasoedova E, Crowson CS, Kremers HM, Therneau TM, Gabriel SE. Is the incidence of rheumatoid arthritis rising? Results from Olmsted County, Minnesota, 1955–2007. Arthritis Rheum July 2010;62(6):1576–82.

[44] Neovius M, Simard JF, Askling J. Nationwide prevalence of rheumatoid arthritis and penetration of disease-modifying drugs in Sweden. Ann Rheum Dis May 2011;70(4):624–9.

[45] Roubenoff R, Roubenoff RA, Cannon JG, Kehayias JJ, Zhuang H, Dawson-Hughes B, et al. Rheumatoid cachexia: cytokine-driven hypermetabolism accompanying reduced body cell mass in chronic inflammation. J Clin Investig June 1994;93(6):2379–86.

[46] Kremers HM, Nicola PJ, Crowson CS, Ballman KV, Gabriel SE. Prognostic importance of low body mass index in relation to cardiovascular mortality in rheumatoid arthritis. Arthritis Rheum November 2004;50(11):3450–7.

[47] Crowson CS, Liao KP, Davis JM, Solomon DH, Matteson EL, Knutson KL, et al. Rheumatoid arthritis and cardiovascular disease. Am Heart J October 2013;166(4):622–8 [e1].

[48] Landsberg L, Aronne LJ, Beilin LJ, Burke V, Igel LI, Lloyd-Jones D, et al. Obesityrelated hypertension: pathogenesis, cardiovascular risk, and treatment—a position paper of the the Obesity Society and the American Society of Hypertension. Obesity (Silver Spring) January 2013;21(1):8–24.

[49] Chen Y, Copeland WK, Vedanthan R, Grant E, Lee JE, Gu D, et al. Association between body mass index and cardiovascular disease mortality in east Asians and south Asians: pooled analysis of prospective data from the Asia Cohort Consortium. BMJ January 2013;347:f5446.

[50] Symmons DP, Bankhead CR, Harrison BJ, Brennan P, Barrett EM, Scott DG, et al. Blood transfusion, smoking, and obesity as risk factors for the development of rheumatoid arthritis: results from a primary care-based incident case–control study in Norfolk. Engl Arthritis Rheum December 1997;40(11):1955–61.

[51] Pedersen M, Jacobsen S, Klarlund M, Pedersen BV, Wiik A, Wohlfahrt J, et al. Environmental risk factors differ between rheumatoid arthritis with and without auto-antibodies against cyclic citrullinated peptides. Arthritis Res Ther January 2006;8(4):R133.

[52] Lahiri M, Morgan C, Symmons DPM, Bruce IN. Modifiable risk factors for RA: prevention, better than cure? Rheumatology (Oxford) 2012;51(3):499–512.

[53] Crowson CS, Matteson EL, Davis JMGS. Contribution of obesity to the rise in incidence of rheumatoid arthritis. Arthritis Care Res (Hoboken) 2014;65(1):71–7.

[54] De Hair MJ, Landewé RB, Van De Sande MG, Van Schaardenburg D, Van Baarsen LGM, Gerlag DM, et al. Smoking and overweight determine the likelihood of developing rheumatoid arthritis. Ann Rheum Dis 2013;72(10):1654–8.

[55] Wesley A, Bengtsson C, Elkan A, Klareskog L, Alfredsson L, Wedre S. Association between body mass index and anti-citrullinated protein antibody-positive and anti-citrullinated protein antibody-negative rheumatoid arthritis: results from a population-based case–control study. Arthritis Care Res (Hoboken) 2013;65(1):107–12.

[56] Lahiri M, Luben RN, Morgan C, Bunn DK, Marshall T, Lunt M, et al. Using lifestyle factors to identify individuals at higher risk of inflammatory polyarthritis (results from the European Prospective Investigation of Cancer-Norfolk and the Norfolk Arthritis Register—the EPIC-2-NOAR Study). Ann Rheum Dis January 2014;73(1):219–26.

[57] Lu B, Hiraki L, Sparks JA, Malspeis S, Chen C-Y, Awosogba JA, et al. Being overweight or obese and risk of developing rheumatoid arthritis among women: a prospective cohort study. Ann Rheum Dis July 23, 2014. [Online First] https://doi.org/10.1136/annrheumdis-2014-205459.

[58] Kaipiainen-Seppanen O, Kautiainen H. Declining trend in the incidence of rheumatoid factor-positive rheumatoid arthritis in Finland 1980–2000. J Rheumatol December 2006;33(11):2132–8.

[59] Vessey MP, Villard-Mackintosh L, Yeates D. Oral contraceptives, cigarette smoking and other factors in relation to arthritis. Contraception May 1987;35(5):457–64.

[60] Hernández Avila M, Liang MH, Willett WC, Stampfer MJ, Colditz GA, Rosner B, et al. Reproductive factors, smoking, and the risk for rheumatoid arthritis. Epidemiology July 1990;1(4):285–91.

[61] Voigt LF, Koepsell TD, Nelson JL, Dugowson CE, Daling JR. Smoking, obesity, alcohol consumption, and the risk of rheumatoid arthritis. Epidemiology October 1994;5(5):525–32.

[62] Uhlig T, Hagen KB, Kvien TK. Current tobacco smoking, formal education, and the risk of rheumatoid arthritis. J Rheumatol January 1999;26(1):47–54.

[63] Cerhan JR, Saag KG, Criswell LA, Merlino LA, Mikuls TR. Blood transfusion, alcohol use, and anthropometric risk factors for rheumatoid arthritis in older women. J Rheumatol March 2002;29(2):246–54.

[64] Bartfai T, Waalen J, Buxbaum JN. Adipose tissue as a modulator of clinical inflammation: does obesity reduce the prevalence of rheumatoid arthritis? J Rheumatol March 2007;34(3):488–92.

[65] Rodríguez LAG, Tolosa LB, Ruigómez A, Johansson S, Wallander M-A. Rheumatoid arthritis in UK primary care: incidence and prior morbidity. Scand J Rheumatol 2009;38(3):173–7.

[66] Stavropoulos-Kalinoglou A, Metsios GS, Koutedakis Y, Nevill AM, Douglas KM, Jamurtas A, et al. Redefining overweight and obesity in rheumatoid arthritis patients. Ann Rheum Dis October 2007;66(10):1316–21.

[67] Ajeganova S, Andersson ML, Hafström I. Association of obesity with worse disease severity in rheumatoid arthritis as well as with comorbidities: a long-term followup from disease onset. Arthritis Care Res (Hoboken) January 2013;65(1):78–87.

[68] Hollingworth P, Melsom RD, Scott JT. Measurement of radiographic joint space in the rheumatoid knee: correlation with obesity, disease duration, and other factors. Rheumatol Rehabil March 1982;21(1):9–14.

[69] García-Poma A, Segami MI, Mora CS, Ugarte MF, Terrazas HN, Rhor EA, et al. Obesity is independently associated with impaired quality of life in patients with rheumatoid arthritis. Clin Rheumatol November 2007;26(11):1831–5.

[70] Kremers HM, Crowson CS, Therneau TM, Roger VL, Gabriel SE. High ten-year risk of cardiovascular disease in newly diagnosed rheumatoid arthritis patients: a population-based cohort study. Arthritis Rheum August 2008;58(8):2268–74.

[71] Stavropoulos-Kalinoglou A, Metsios GS, Panoulas VF, Nevill AM, Jamurtas AZ, Koutedakis Y, et al. Underweight and obese states both associate with worse disease activity and physical function in patients with established rheumatoid arthritis. Clin Rheumatol April 2009;28(4):439–44.

[72] Jawaheer D, Olsen J, Lahiff M, Forsberg S, Lähteenmäki J, da Silveira IG, et al. Gender, body mass index and rheumatoid arthritis disease activity: results from the QUEST-RA Study. Clin Exp Rheumatol 2010;28(4):454–61.

[73] Westhoff G, Rau R, Zink A. Radiographic joint damage in early rheumatoid arthritis is highly dependent on body mass index. Arthritis Rheum November 2007;56(11):3575–82.

[74] Caplan L, Davis LA, Bright CM, Kerr GS, Lazaro DM, Khan NA, et al. Body mass index and the rheumatoid arthritis swollen joint count: an observational study. Arthritis Care Res (Hoboken) January 2013;65(1):101–6.

[75] Choe JY, Bae J, Lee H, Park S, Kim S. Lack association of body mass index with disease activity composites of rheumatoid arthritis in Korean population: cross-sectional observation. Clin Rheumatol 2014;33(4):485–92.

[76] Wolfe F, Michaud K. Effect of body mass index on mortality and clinical status in rheumatoid arthritis. Arthritis Care Res (Hoboken) 2012;64(10):1471–9.

[77] Naranjo A, Sokka T, Descalzo MA, Calvo-Alén J, Hørslev-Petersen K, Luukkainen RK, et al. Cardiovascular disease in patients with rheumatoid arthritis: results from the QUEST-RA study. Arthritis Res Ther January 2008;10(2):R30.

[78] Escalante A, Haas RW, del Rincón I. Paradoxical effect of body mass index on survival in rheumatoid arthritis: role of comorbidity and systemic inflammation. Arch Intern Med July 25, 2005;165(14):1624–9.

[79] Otero M, Lago R, Gomez R, Lago F, Dieguez C, Gómez-Reino JJ, et al. Changes in plasma levels of fat-derived hormones adiponectin, leptin, resistin and visfatin in patients with rheumatoid arthritis. Ann Rheum Dis October 2006;65(9):1198–201.

[80] Lee S-W, Park M-C, Park Y-B, Lee S-K. Measurement of the serum leptin level could assist disease activity monitoring in rheumatoid arthritis. Rheumatol Int May 2007;27(6):537–40.

[81] Yoshino T, Kusunoki N, Tanaka N, Kaneko K, Kusunoki Y, Endo H, et al. Elevated serum levels of resistin, leptin, and adiponectin are associated with C-reactive protein and also other clinical conditions in rheumatoid arthritis. Intern Med January 2011;50(4):269–75.

[82] Olama SM, Senna MK, Elarman M. Synovial/serum leptin ratio in rheumatoid arthritis: the association with activity and erosion. Rheumatol Int March 2012;32(3):683–90.

[83] Xibillé-Friedmann D, Bustos-Bahena C, Hernàndez-Gongora S, Burgos-Vargas R, Montiel-Hernàndez J. Two-year follow-up of plasma leptin and other cytokines in patients with rheumatoid arthritis. Ann Rheum Dis 2010;69(5):9–11.

[84] Schäffler A, Ehling A, Neumann E, Herfarth H, Tarner I, Schölmerich J, et al. Adipocytokines in synovial fluid. JAMA October 1, 2003;290(13):1709–10.

[85] Chen X, Lu J, Bao J, Guo J, Shi J, Wang Y. Adiponectin: a biomarker for rheumatoid arthritis? Cytokine Growth Factor Rev March 2013;24(1):83–9.

[86] Fadda SMH, Gamal SM, Elsaid NY, Mohy AM. Resistin in inflammatory and degenerative rheumatologic diseases. Relationship between resistin and rheumatoid arthritis disease progression. Z Rheumatol August 2013;72(6):594–600.

[87] Senolt L, Housa D, Vernerová Z, Jirásek T, Svobodová R, Veigl D, et al. Resistin in rheumatoid arthritis synovial tissue, synovial fluid and serum. Ann Rheum Dis April 2007;66(4):458–63.

[88] Migita K, Maeda Y, Miyashita T, Kimura H, Nakamura M, Ishibashi H, et al. The serum levels of resistin in rheumatoid arthritis patients. Clin Exp Rheumatol 2006;24(6):698–701.

[89] Forsblad d'Elia H, Pullerits R, Carlsten H, Bokarewa M. Resistin in serum is associated with higher levels of IL-1Ra in post-menopausal women with rheumatoid arthritis. Rheumatology (Oxford) July 2008;47(7):1082–7.

[90] Kontunen P, Vuolteenaho K, Nieminen R, Lehtimäki L, Kautiainen H, Kesäniemi Y, et al. Resistin is linked to inflammation, and leptin to metabolic syndrome, in women with inflammatory arthritis. Scand J Rheumatol January 2011;40(4):256–62.

[91] Straburzyńska-Lupa A, Nowak A, Pilaczyńska-Szcześniak Ł, Straburzyńska-Migaj E, Romanowski W, Karolkiewicz J, et al. Visfatin, resistin, hsCRP and insulin resistance in relation to abdominal obesity in women with rheumatoid arthritis. Clin Exp Rheumatol 2010;28(1):19–24.

[92] Alkady EAM, Ahmed HM, Tag L, Abdou MA. Serum and synovial adiponectin, resistin, and visfatin levels in rheumatoid arthritis patients. Relation to disease activity. Z Rheumatol October 2011;70(7):602–8.

[93] Brentano F, Schorr O, Ospelt C, Stanczyk J, Gay RE, Gay S, et al. Pre-B cell colony-enhancing factor/visfatin, a new marker of inflammation in rheumatoid arthritis with proinflammatory and matrix-degrading activities. Arthritis Rheum October 2007;56(9):2829–39.

[94] Rho YH, Solus J, Sokka T, Oeser A, Chung CP, Gebretsadik T, et al. Adipocytokines are associated with radiographic joint damage in rheumatoid arthritis. Arthritis Rheum July 2009;60(7):1906–14.

[95] Busso N, So A, Chobaz-Péclat V, Morard C, Martinez-Soria E, Talabot-Ayer D, et al. Leptin signaling deficiency impairs humoral and cellular immune responses and attenuates experimental arthritis. J Immunol January 15, 2002;168(2):875–82.

[96] Busso N, Karababa M, Nobile M, Rolaz A, Van Gool F, Galli M, et al. Pharmacological inhibition of nicotinamide phosphoribosyltransferase/visfatin enzymatic activity identifies a new inflammatory pathway linked to NAD. PLoS One January 2008;3(5):e2267.

[97] Evans L, Williams AS, Hayes AJ, Jones SA, Nowell M. Suppression of leukocyte infiltration and cartilage degradation by selective inhibition of pre-B cell colonyenhancing factor/visfatin/nicotinamide phosphoribosyltransferase: Apo866-mediated therapy in human fibroblasts and murine collagen-induced arthrit. Arthritis Rheum July 2011;63(7):1866–77.

[98] Kaufmann J, Kielstein V, Kilian S, Stein G, Hein G. Relation between body mass index and radiological progression in patients with rheumatoid arthritis. J Rheumatol December 2003;30(11):2350–5.

[99] Van der Helm-van Mil A, van der Kooij S, Allaart C, Toes R, Huizinga T. A high body mass index has a protective effect on the amount of joint destruction in small joints in early rheumatoid arthritis. Ann Rheum Dis June 2008;67(6):769–74.

[100] De Rooy D, van der Linden MP, Knevel R, Huizinga TW. van der Helm-van Mil AH. Predicting arthritis outcomes—what can be learned from the Leiden Early Arthritis Clinic? Rheumatology (Oxford) January 2011;50(1):93–100.

[101] Tremollieres FA, Pouilles JM, Ribot C. Vertebral postmenopausal bone loss is reduced in overweight women: a longitudinal study in 155 early postmenopausal women. J Clin Endocrinol Metab October 1993;77(3):683–6.

[102] Rohrmann S, Shiels MS, Lopez DS, Rifai N, Nelson WG, Kanarek N, et al. Body fatness and sex steroid hormone concentrations in US men: results from NHANES III. Cancer Causes Control August 2011;22(8):1141–51.

[103] Tan W, Wang F, Zhang M, Guo D, Zhang Q, He S. High adiponectin and adiponectin receptor 1 expression in synovial fluids and synovial tissues of patients with rheumatoid arthritis. Semin Arthritis Rheum July 2009;38(6):420–7.

[104] Matsui H, Tsutsumi A, Sugihara M, Suzuki T, Iwanami K, Kohno M, et al. Visfatin (pre-B cell colony-enhancing factor) gene expression in patients with rheumatoid arthritis. Ann Rheum Dis May 2008;67(4):571–2.

[105] Klein-wieringa IR, Van Der Linden MPM, Knevel R, Kwekkeboom JC, Van Beelen E, Huizinga TWJ, et al. Baseline serum adipokine levels predict radiographic progression in early rheumatoid arthritis. Arthritis Rheum 2011;63(9):2567–74.

[106] Giles J, van der Heijde D, Bathon J. Association of circulating adiponectin levels with progression of radiographic joint destruction in rheumatoid arthritis. Ann Rheum Dis 2013;70(9):1562–8.

[107] Bokarewa M, Nagaev I, Dahlberg L, Smith U, Tarkowski A. Resistin, an adipokine with potent proinflammatory properties. J Immunol May 1, 2005;174(9):5789–95.

[108] Gómez R, Scotece M, Conde J, Gómez-Reino JJ, Lago F, Gualillo O. Adiponectin and leptin increase IL-8 production in human chondrocytes. Ann Rheum Dis December 2011;70(11):2052–4.

[109] Bao J, Chen W, Feng J, Hu P, Shi Z, Wu L. Leptin plays a catabolic role on articular cartilage. Mol Biol Rep October 2010;37(7):3265–72.

[110] Tong K-M, Chen C-P, Huang K-C, Shieh D-C, Cheng H-C, Tzeng C-Y, et al. Adiponectin increases MMP-3 expression in human chondrocytes through AdipoR1 signaling pathway. J Cell Biochem May 2011;112(5):1431–40.

[111] Lago R, Gomez R, Otero M, Lago F, Gallego R, Dieguez C, et al. A new player in cartilage homeostasis: adiponectin induces nitric oxide synthase type II and pro-inflammatory cytokines in chondrocytes. Osteoarthritis Cartilage October 2008;16(9):1101–9.

[112] Kusunoki N, Kitahara K, Kojima F, Tanaka N, Kaneko K, Endo H, et al. Adiponectin stimulates prostaglandin E(2) production in rheumatoid arthritis synovial fibroblasts. Arthritis Rheum July 2010;62(6):1641–9.

[113] Frommer KW, Schäffler A, Büchler C, Steinmeyer J, Rickert M, Rehart S, et al. Adiponectin isoforms: a potential therapeutic target in rheumatoid arthritis? Ann Rheum Dis October 2012;71(10):1724–32.

[114] Heimans L, van den Broek M, le Cessie S, Siegerink B, Riyazi N, Han KH, et al. Association of high body mass index with decreased treatment response to combination therapy in recent-onset rheumatoid arthritis patients. Arthritis Care Res (Hoboken) August 2013;65(8):1235–42.

[115] Klaasen R, Wijbrandts CA, Gerlag DM, Tak PP. Body mass index and clinical response to infliximab in rheumatoid arthritis. Arthritis Rheum March 2011;63(2):359–64.

[116] Smolen J, Szumski A, Koening A, Jones T. Impact of body mass index on response to etanercept therapy in subjects with moderate active rheumatoid arthritis in the PRESERVE trial. Arthritis Rheum 2011;63:S156–7. [Abstract Supplement].

[117] Gonzálezgay MA, González-juanatey C. Rheumatoid arthritis: obesity impairs efficacy of anti-TNF therapy in patients with RA. Nat Rev Rheumatol 2012;8(11):641–2. Nature Publishing Group.

[118] Gremese E, Carletto A, Padovan M, Atzeni F, Raffeiner B, Giardina AR, et al. Obesity and reduction of the response rate to anti-tumor necrosis factor alpha in rheumatoid arthritis: an approach to a personalized medicine. Arthritis Care Res (Hoboken) 2013;65(1):94–100.

[119] Sandberg MEC, Bengtsson C, Källberg H, Wesley A, Klareskog L, Alfredsson L, et al. Overweight decreases the chance of achieving good response and low disease activity in early rheumatoid arthritis. Ann Rheum Dis May 2014;12.

[120] Derdemezis CS, Filippatos TD, Voulgari PV, Tselepis AD, Drosos AA, Kiortsis DN. Effects of a 6-month infliximab treatment on plasma levels of leptin and adiponectin in patients with rheumatoid arthritis. Fundam Clin Pharmacol October 2009;23(5):595–600.

[121] Gonzalez-Gay MA, Vazquez-Rodriguez TR, Garcia-Unzueta MT, Berja A, Miranda-Filloy JA, de Matias JM, et al. Visfatin is not associated with inflammation or metabolic syndrome in patients with severe rheumatoid arthritis undergoing anti-TNF-alpha therapy. Clin Exp Rheumatol 2010;28(1):56–62.

[122] Gonzalez-Gay MA, Garcia-Unzueta MT, Berja A, Gonzalez-Juanatey C, Miranda-Filloy JA, Vazquez-Rodriguez TR, et al. Anti-TNF-alpha therapy does not modulate leptin in patients with severe rheumatoid arthritis. Clin Exp Rheumatol 2009;27(2):222–8.

[123] Agmon-Levin N, Mosca M, Petri M, Shoenfeld Y. Systemic lupus erythematosus one disease or many? Autoimmun Rev June 2012;11(8):593–5.

[124] Gatto M, Zen M, Ghirardello A, Bettio S, Bassi N, Iaccarino L, et al. Emerging and critical issues in the pathogenesis of lupus. Autoimmun Rev February 2013;12(4):523–36.

[125] Oliver JE, Silman AJ. What epidemiology has told us about risk factors and aetiopathogenesis in rheumatic diseases. Arthritis Res Ther January 2009;11(3):223.

[126] Harpsøe MC, Basit S, Andersson M, Nielsen NM, Frisch M, Wohlfahrt J, et al. Body mass index and risk of autoimmune diseases: a study within the Danish National Birth Cohort. Int J Epidemiol 2014:1–13.

[127] Amarilyo G, Iikuni N, Shi F, Liu A, Matarese G, La A. Leptin promotes lupus T-cell autoimmunity. Clin Immunol 2013;149(3):530–3. Elsevier Inc.

[128] Fujita Y, Fujii T, Mimori T, Sato T, Nakamura T, Iwao H, et al. Deficient leptin signaling ameliorates systemic lupus erythematosus lesions in MRL/Mp- Fas lpr mice. J Immunol 2014;192(3):979–84.

[129] Yu Y, Liu Y, Shi F-D, Zou H, Matarese G, La Cava A. Leptin-induced ROR-gamma-t expression in CD4+ T cells promotes Th17 responses in systemic lupus erythematosus. J Immunol 2014;190(7):3054–8.

[130] Liu Y, Yu Y, Matarese G, La Cava A. Fasting-induced hypoletinemia expands functional regulatory T cells in systemic lupus erythematosus. J Immunol 2013;188(5):2070–3.

[131] Katz P, Gregorich S, Yazdany J, Trupin L, Julian L, Yelin E, et al. Obesity and its measurement in a community-based sample of women with systemic lupus erythematosus. Arthritis Care Res (Hoboken) March 2011;63(2):261–8.

[132] Borges MC, dos Santos F de MM, Telles RW, Lanna CCD, Correia MITD. Nutritional status and food intake in patients with systemic lupus erythematosus. Nutrition 2012;28(11–12):1098–103.

[133] Sinicato NA, Postal M, Peres FA, Peliçari KDO, Marini R, De Oliveira A, et al. Obesity and cytokines in childhood-onset systemic lupus erythematosus. J Immunol Res 2014;2014:162047.

[134] Rizk A, Gheita TA, Nassef S, Abdallah A. The impact of obesity in systemic lupus erythematosus on disease parameters, quality of life, functional capacity and the risk of atherosclerosis. Int J Rheum Dis July 2012;15(3):261–7.

[135] Chaiamnuay S, Bertoli AM, Fernández M, Apte M, Vilá LM, Reveille JD, et al. The impact of increased body mass index on systemic lupus erythematosus: data from LUMINA, a multiethnic cohort (LUMINA XLVI) [corrected]. J Clin Rheumatol July 2007;13(3):128–33.

[136] Sada K-E, Yamasaki Y, Maruyama M, Sugiyama H, Yamamura M, Maeshima Y, et al. Altered levels of adipocytokines in association with insulin resistance in patients with systemic lupus erythematosus. J Rheumatol August 2006;33(8):1545–52.

[137] Vadacca M, Margiotta D, Rigon A, Cacciapaglia F, Coppolino G, Amoroso A, et al. Adipokines and systemic lupus erythematosus: relationship with metabolic syndrome and cardiovascular disease risk factors. J Rheumatol February 2009;36(2):295–7.

[138] Kim H, Choi G, Jeon J, Yoon J, Sung J, Suh C. Leptin and ghrelin in Korean systemic lupus erythematosus. Lupus 2010;19(2):170–4.

[139] Al M, Ng L, Tyrrell P, Bargman J, Bradley T, Silverman E. Adipokines as novel biomarkers in paediatric systemic lupus erythematosus. Rheumatology (Oxford) May 2009;48(5):497–501.

[140] Garcia-Gonzalez A, Gonzalez-Lopez L, Valera-Gonzalez IC, Cardona-Muñoz EG, Salazar-Paramo M, González-Ortiz M, et al. Serum leptin levels in women with systemic lupus erythematosus. Rheumatol Int August 2002;22(4):138–41.

[141] Chung CP, Long AG, Solus JF, Rho YH, Oeser A, Raggi P, et al. Adipocytokines in systemic lupus erythematosus: relationship to inflammation, insulin resistance and coronary atherosclerosis. Lupus August 2009;18(9):799–806.

[142] De Sanctis JB, Zabaleta M, Bianco NE, Garmendia JV, Rivas L. Serum adipokine levels in patients with systemic lupus erythematosus. Autoimmunity May 2009;42(4):272–4.

[143] Wisłowska M, Rok M, Stepień K, Kuklo-Kowalska A. Serum leptin in systemic lupus erythematosus. Rheumatol Int March 2008;28(5):467–73.

[144] Parker J, Menn-Josephy H, Laskow B, Takemura Y, Aprahamian T. Modulation of lupus phenotype by adiponectin deficiency in autoimmune mouse models. J Clin Immunol 2012;31(2):167–73.

[145] Oeser A, Chung CP, Asanuma Y, Avalos I, Stein CM. Obesity is an independent contributor to functional capacity and inflammation in systemic lupus erythematosus. Arthritis Rheum December 2005;52(11):3651–9.

[146] Gilbert EL, Ryan MJ. High dietary fat promotes visceral obesity and impaired endothelial function in female mice with systemic lupus erythematosus. Gend Med 2012;8(2):150–5.

[147] Boström E, Ekstedt M, Kechagias S, Sjöwall C, Bokarewa MI, Almer S. Resistin is associated with breach of tolerance and anti-nuclear antibodies in patients with hepatobiliary inflammation. Clin Immunol 2011;74(5):463–70.

[148] Baker JF, Morales M, Qatanani M, Nackos E, Lazar MA, Teff K, et al. Resistin levels in lupus and associations with disease-specific measures, insulin resistance, and coronary calcification. J Rheumatol 2011;38(11):2369–75.

[149] Aprahamian T, Bonegio RG, Richez C, Yasuda K, Chiang L-K, Sato K, et al. The peroxisome proliferator-activated receptor gamma agonist rosiglitazone ameliorates murine lupus by induction of adiponectin. J Immunol January 1, 2009;182(1):340–6.

[150] Rovin BH, Song H, Hebert LA, Nadasdy T, Nadasdy G, Birmingham DJ, et al. Plasma, urine, and renal expression of adiponectin in human systemic lupus erythematosus. Kidney Int October 2005;68(4):1825–33.

[151] Katz P, Julian L, Tonner MC, Yazdany J, Trupin L, Yelin E, et al. Physical activity, obesity, and cognitive impairment among women with systemic lupus erythematosus. Arthritis Care Res (Hoboken) 2013;64(4):502–10.

[152] Katz P, Yazdany J, Julian L, Trupin L, Margaretten M, Yelin E, et al. The impact of obesity on functioning among women with SLE. Arthritis Care Res (Hoboken) 2011;63(10):1357–64.

[153] Yaffe K, Lindquist K, Penninx BW, Simonsick EM, Pahor M, Kritchevsky S, et al. Inflammatory markers and cognition in well-functioning African–American and white elders. Neurology July 8, 2003;61(1):76–80.

[154] Gunstad J, Spitznagel MB, Keary TA, Glickman E, Alexander T, Karrer J, et al. Serum leptin levels are associated with cognitive function in older adults. Brain Res September 16, 2008;1230:233–6.

[155] Holden KF, Lindquist K, Tylavsky FA, Rosano C, Harris TB, Yaffe K. Serum leptin level and cognition in the elderly: findings from the Health ABC Study. Neurobiol Aging September 2009;30(9):1483–9.

[156] Chaiamnuay S, Bertoli AM, Roseman JM, McGwin G, Apte M, Durán S, et al. African– American and Hispanic ethnicities, renal involvement and obesity predispose to hypertension in systemic lupus erythematosus: results from LUMINA, a multiethnic cohort (LUMINAXLV). Ann Rheum Dis May 2007;66(5):618–22.

[157] Nikpour M, Urowitz MB, Gladman DD. Epidemiology of atherosclerosis in systemic lupus erythematosus. Curr Rheumatol Rep August 2009;11(4):248–54.

[158] Knight JS, Kaplan MJ. Cardiovascular disease in lupus: insights and updates. Curr Opin Rheumatol September 2013;25(5):597–605.

[159] Chung CP, Avalos I, Oeser A, Gebretsadik T, Shintani A, Raggi P, et al. High prevalence of the metabolic syndrome in patients with systemic lupus erythematosus: association with disease characteristics and cardiovascular risk factors. Ann Rheum Dis February 2007;66(2):208–14.

[160] McMahon M, Skaggs BJ, Sahakian L, Grossman J, FitzGerald J, Ragavendra N, et al. High plasma leptin levels confer increased risk of atherosclerosis in women with systemic lupus erythematosus, and are associated with inflammatory oxidised lipids. Ann Rheum Dis September 2011;70(9):1619–24.

[161] Almehed K, d'Elia HF, Bokarewa M, Carlsten H. Role of resistin as a marker of in-flammation in systemic lupus erythematosus. Arthritis Res Ther January 2008;10(1):R15.

[162] Cassinotti A, Sarzi-Puttini P, Fichera M, Shoenfeld Y, de Franchis R, Ardizzone S. Immunity, autoimmunity and inflammatory bowel disease. Autoimmun Rev January 2014;13(1):1–2.

[163] Baumgart DC, Sandborn WJ. Crohn's disease. Lancet November 3, 2012;380(9853):1590–605.

[164] Ordás I, Eckmann L, Talamini M, Baumgart DC, Sandborn WJ. Ulcerative colitis. Lancet November 3, 2012;380(9853):1606–19.

[165] Abraham C, Cho JH. Inflammatory bowel disease. N Engl J Med November 19, 2009;361(21):2066–78.

[166] Cosnes J, Gower-Rousseau C, Seksik P, Cortot A. Epidemiology and natural history of inflammatory bowel diseases. Gastroenterology May 2011;140(6):1785–94.

[167] Chan SSM, Luben R, Olsen A, Tjonneland A, Kaaks R, Teucher B, et al. Body mass index and the risk for Crohn's disease and ulcerative colitis: data from a European Prospective Cohort Study (The IBD in EPIC study). Am J Gastroenterol April 2013;108(4):575–82.

[168] Mendall MA, Gunasekera AV, John BJ, Kumar D. Is obesity a risk factor for Crohn's disease? Dig Dis Sci March 2011;56(3):837–44.

[169] Hou JK, Abraham B, El-Serag H. Dietary intake and risk of developing inflammatory bowel disease: a systematic review of the literature. Am J Gastroenterol April 2011;106(4):563–73.

[170] Steed H, Walsh S, Reynolds N. A brief report of the epidemiology of obesity in the inflammatory bowel disease population of Tayside, Scotland. Obes Facts January 2009;2(6):370–2.

[171] Sheehan AL, Warren BF, Gear MW, Shepherd NA. Fat-wrapping in Crohn's disease: pathological basis and relevance to surgical practice. Br J Surg September 1992;79(9):955–8.

[172] Paik J, Fierce Y, Treuting PM, Brabb T, Maggio-price L. High-fat diet-induced obesity exacerbates inflammatory bowel disease in genetically susceptible Mdr1a–/– male mice. J Nutr 2013;143(8):1240–7.

[173] Teixeira LG, Leonel AJ, Aguilar EC, Batista NV, Alves AC, Coimbra CC, et al. The combination of high-fat diet-induced obesity and chronic ulcerative colitis reciprocally exacerbates adipose tissue and colon inflammation. Lipids Health Dis 2011 Jan.;10(1):204. BioMed Central Ltd.

[174] Blain A, Cattan S, Beaugerie L, Carbonnel F, Gendre JP, Cosnes J. Crohn's disease clinical course and severity in obese patients. Clin Nutr February 2002;21(1):51–7.

[175] Hass DJ, Brensinger CM, Lewis JD, Lichtenstein GR. The impact of increased body mass index on the clinical course of Crohn's disease. Clin Gastroenterol Hepatol April 2006;4(4):482–8.

[176] Tuzun A, Uygun A, Yesilova Z, Ozel AM, Erdil A, Yaman H, et al. Leptin levels in the acute stage of ulcerative colitis. J Gastroenterol Hepatol April 2004;19(4):429–32.

[177] Barbier M, Vidal H, Desreumaux P, Dubuquoy L, Bourreille A, Colombel J-F, et al. Overexpression of leptin mRNA in mesenteric adipose tissue in inflammatory bowel diseases. Gastroentérol Clin Biol November 2003;27(11):987–91.

[178] Ponemone V, Keshavarzian A, Brand MI, Saclarides T, Abcarian H, Cabay RJ, et al. Apoptosis and inflammation: role of adipokines in inflammatory bowel disease. Clin Transl Gastroenterol January 2010;1:e1. Nature Publishing Group.

[179] Sitaraman S, Liu X, Charrier L, Gu LH, Ziegler TR, Gewirtz A, et al. Colonic leptin: source of a novel proinflammatory cytokine involved in IBD. FASEB J April 2004;18(6):696–8.

[180] Hoda MR, Scharl M, Keely SJ, McCole DF, Barrett KE. Apical leptin induces chloride secretion by intestinal epithelial cells and in a rat model of acute chemotherapy-induced colitis. Am J Physiol Gastrointest Liver Physiol May 2010;298(5):G714–21.

[181] Siegmund B, Lear-Kaul KC, Faggioni R, Fantuzzi G. Leptin deficiency, not obesity, protects mice from Con A-induced hepatitis. Eur J Immunol February 2002;32(2):552–60.

[182] Siegmund B, Sennello JA, Jones-Carson J, Gamboni-Robertson F, Lehr HA, Batra A, et al. Leptin receptor expression on T lymphocytes modulates chronic intestinal inflammation in mice. Gut July 2004;53(7):965–72.

[183] Valentini L, Wirth EK, Schweizer U, Hengstermann S, Schaper L, Koernicke T, et al. Circulating adipokines and the protective effects of hyperinsulinemia in inflammatory bowel disease. Nutrition February 2009;25(2):172–81.

[184] Karmiris K, Koutroubakis IE, Xidakis C, Polychronaki M, Voudouri T, Kouroumalis EA. Circulating levels of leptin, adiponectin, resistin, and ghrelin in inflammatory bowel disease. Inflamm Bowel Dis February 2006;12(2):100–5.

[185] Paul G, Schäffler A, Neumeier M, Fürst A, Bataillle F, Buechler C, et al. Profiling adipocytokine secretion from creeping fat in Crohn's disease. Inflamm Bowel Dis June 2006;12(6):471–7.

[186] Moschen AR, Kaser A, Enrich B, Mosheimer B, Theurl M, Niederegger H, et al. Visfatin, an adipocytokine with proinflammatory and immuno-modulating properties. J Immunol March 1, 2007;178(3):1748–58.

[187] Nishihara T, Matsuda M, Araki H, Oshima K, Kihara S, Funahashi T, et al. Effect of adiponectin on murine colitis induced by dextran sulfate sodium. Gastroenterology September 2006;131(3):853–61.

[188] Fayad R, Pini M, Sennello JA, Cabay RJ, Chan L, Xu A, et al. Adiponectin deficiency protects mice from chemically induced colonic inflammation. Gastroenterology February 2007;132(2):601–14.

[189] Pini M, Gove ME, Fayad R, Cabay RJ, Fantuzzi G. Adiponectin deficiency does not affect development and progression of spontaneous colitis in IL-10 knockout mice. Am J Physiol Gastrointest Liver Physiol February 2009;296(2):G382–7.

[190] Gove ME, Pini M, Fayad R, Cabay RJ, Fantuzzi G. Adiponectin deficiency modulates adhesion molecules expression and cytokine production but does not affect disease severity in the transfer model of colitis. Cytokine August 2009;47(2):119–25. Elsevier Ltd.

[191] Rodrigues VS, Milanski M, Fagundes JJ, Torsoni AS, Ayrizono ML, Nunez CE, et al. Serum levels and mesenteric fat tissue expression of adiponectin and leptin in patients with Crohn's disease. Clin Exp Immunol December 2012;170(3):358–64.

[192] Yamamoto K, Kiyohara T, Murayama Y, Kihara S, Okamoto Y, Funahashi T, et al. Production of adiponectin, an anti-inflammatory protein, in mesenteric adipose tissue in Crohn's disease. Gut June 2005;54(6):789–96.

[193] Nic Suibhne T, Raftery TC, McMahon O, Walsh C, O'Morain C, O'Sullivan M. High prevalence of overweight and obesity in adults with Crohn's disease: associations with disease and lifestyle factors. J Crohns Colitis August 2013;7(7):e241–8.

[194] Billioud V, Sandborn WJ, Peyrin-Biroulet L. Loss of response and need for adalimumab dose intensification in Crohn's disease: a systematic review. Am J Gastroenterol April 2011;106(4):674–84.

[195] Bultman E, de Haar C, van Liere-Baron A, Verhoog H, West RL, Kuipers EJ, et al. Predictors of dose escalation of adalimumab in a prospective cohort of Crohn's disease patients. Aliment Pharmacol Ther February 2012;35(3):335–41.

[196] Harper JW, Sinanan MN, Zisman TL. Increased body mass index is associated with earlier time to loss of response to infliximab in patients with inflammatory bowel disease. Inflamm Bowel Dis September 2013;19(10):2118–24.

[197] Holtmann MH, Krummenauer F, Claas C, Kremeyer K, Lorenz D, Rainer O, et al. Significant differences between Crohn's disease and ulcerative colitis regarding the impact of body mass index and initial disease activity on responsiveness to azathioprine: results from a European multicenter study in 1176 patients. Dig Dis Sci April 2010;55(4):1066–78.

[198] Milo R, Miller A. Revised diagnostic criteria of multiple sclerosis. Autoimmun Rev 2014;13(4–5):518–24.

[199] World Health Organization. Altas of multiple sclerosis. 2013.

[200] Milo R, Kahana E. Multiple sclerosis: geoepidemiology, genetics and the environment. Autoimmun Rev March 2010;9(5):A387–94.

[201] Sawcer S, Franklin RJM, Ban M. Multiple sclerosis genetics. Lancet Neurol July 2014;13(7):700–9.

[202] Lobstein T, Baur L, Uauy R. Obesity in children and young people: a crisis in public health. Obes Rev May 2004;5(Suppl. 1):4–104.

[203] World Health Organization. Global strategy on diet. Physical activity and health: a framework to monitor and evaluate implementation. 2006. [Geneva].

[204] Munger KL, Chitnis T, Ascherio A. Body size and risk of MS in two cohorts of US women. Neurology November 10, 2009;73(19):1543–50.

[205] Hedström AK, Olsson T, Alfredsson L. High body index before age 20 is associated with increased risk for multiple sclerosis men and women. Mult Scler J 2012;18(9):1334–6.

[206] Munger KL, Bentzen J, Laursen B, Stenager E, Koch-henriksen N, Sørensen TIA. Childhood body mass index and multiple sclerosis risk: a long-term cohort study. Mult Scler J 2013;19(10):1323–9.

[207] Langer-gould A, Beaber BE. Childhood obesity and risk of pediatric multiple sclerosis and clinically isolated syndrome. Neurology 2013;80(6):548–52.

[208] Hedström AK, Lima Bomfim I, Barcellos L, Gianfrancesco M, Schaefer C, Kockum I, et al. Interaction between adolescent obesity and HLA risk genes in the etiology of multiple sclerosis. Neurology March 11, 2014;82(10):865–72.

[209] Pedersen LB, Nashold FE, Spach KM, Hayes CE. 1,25-dihydroxyvitamin D3 reverses experimental autoimmune encephalomyelitis by inhibiting chemokine synthesis and monocyte trafficking. J Neurosci Res August 15, 2007;85(11):2480–90.

[210] Munger KL, Levin LI, Hollis BW, Howard NS, Ascherio A. Serum 25-hydroxyvitamin D levels and risk of multiple sclerosis. JAMA December 20, 2006;296(23):2832–8.

[211] Wortsman J, Matsuoka LY, Chen TC, Lu Z, Holick MF. Decreased bioavailability of vitamin D in obesity. Am J Clin Nutr September 2000;72(3):690–3.

[212] Alemzadeh R, Kichler J, Babar G, Calhoun M. Hypovitaminosis D in obese children and adolescents: relationship with adiposity, insulin sensitivity, ethnicity, and season. Metabolism February 2008;57(2):183–91.

[213] Lumeng CN, Bodzin JL, Saltiel AR. Obesity induces a phenotypic switch in adipose tissue macrophage polarization. J Clin Investig January 2007;117(1):175–84.

[214] Mikita J, Dubourdieu-Cassagno N, Deloire MS, Vekris A, Biran M, Raffard G, et al. Altered M1/M2 activation patterns of monocytes in severe relapsing experimental rat model of multiple sclerosis. Amelioration of clinical status by M2 activated monocyte administration. Mult Scler January 2011;17(1):2–15.

[215] Kraszula L, Jasińska A, Eusebio M-O, Kuna P, Głąbiński A, Pietruczuk M. Evaluation of the relationship between leptin, resistin, adiponectin and natural regulatory T cells in relapsing-remitting multiple sclerosis. Neurol Neurochir Pol 2012;46(1):22–8.

[216] Emamgholipour S, Eshaghi SM, Hossein-nezhad A, Mirzaei K. Adipocytokine profile, cytokine levels and Foxp3 expression in multiple sclerosis: a possible link to susceptibility and clinical course of disease. PLoS One 2013;8(10):6–8.

[217] Piccio L, Cantoni C, Henderson JG, Hawiger D, Ramsbottom M, Mikesell R, et al. Lack of adiponectin leads to increased lymphocyte activation and increased disease severity in a mouse model of multiple sclerosis. Eur J Immunol 2013;43(8):2089–100.

[218] Piccio L, Stark JL, Cross AH. Chronic calorie restriction attenuates experimental autoimmune encephalomyelitis. J Leukoc Biol October 2008;84(4):940–8.

[219] Bruzzone S, Fruscione F, Morando S, Ferrando T, Poggi A, Garuti A, et al. Catastrophic NAD+ depletion in activated T lymphocytes through Nampt inhibition reduces demyelination and disability in EAE. PLoS One January 2009;4(11):e7897.

[220] Matarese G, Di Giacomo A, Sanna V, Lord GM, Howard JK, Di Tuoro A, et al. Requirement for leptin in the induction and progression of autoimmune encephalomyelitis. J Immunol May 15, 2001;166(10):5909–16.

[221] Sanna V, Di Giacomo A, La Cava A, Lechler RI, Fontana S, Zappacosta S, et al. Leptin surge precedes onset of autoimmune encephalomyelitis and correlates with development of pathogenic T cell responses. J Clin Investig January 2003;111(2):241–50.

[222] Matarese G, Carrieri PB, La Cava A, Perna F, Sanna V, De Rosa V, et al. Leptin increase in multiple sclerosis associates with reduced number of CD4(+)CD25+ regulatory T cells. Proc Natl Acad Sci USA April 5, 2005;102(14):5150–5.

[223] De Rosa V, Procaccini C, La Cava A, Chieffi P, Nicoletti GF, Fontana S, et al. Leptin neutralization interferes with pathogenic T cell autoreactivity in autoimmune encephalomyelitis. J Clin Investig February 2006;116(2):447–55.

[224] Matarese G, Procaccini C, De Rosa V. The intricate interface between immune and metabolic regulation: a role for leptin in the pathogenesis of multiple sclerosis? J Leukoc Biol 2008;84(4):893–9.

[225] Matarese G, Carrieri PB, Montella S, De Rosa V, La Cava A. Leptin as a metabolic link to multiple sclerosis. Nat Rev Neurol 2010;6(8):455–61. Nature Publishing Group.

[226] Tuomi T, Santoro N, Caprio S, Cai M, Weng J, Groop L. The many faces of diabetes: a disease with increasing heterogeneity. Lancet March 22, 2014;383(9922):1084–94.

[227] Canivell S, Gomis R. Diagnosis and classification of autoimmune diabetes mellitus. Autoimmun Rev 2014;13(4–5):403–7.

[228] Danaei G, Finucane MM, Lu Y, Singh GM, Cowan MJ, Paciorek CJ, et al. National, regional, and global trends in fasting plasma glucose and diabetes prevalence since 1980: systematic analysis of health examination surveys and epidemiological studies with 370 country-years and 2·7 million participants. Lancet July 2, 2011;378(9785):31–40.

[229] Wilkin TJ. The accelerator hypothesis: weight gain as the missing link between Type I and Type II diabetes. Diabetologia July 2001;44(7):914–22.

[230] Baum JD, Ounsted M, Smith MA. Weight gain in infancy and subsequent development of diabetes mellitus in childhood. Lancet November 1, 1975;2(7940):866.

[231] Islam ST, Srinivasan S, Craig ME. Environmental determinants of type 1 diabetes: a role for overweight and insulin resistance. J Paediatr Child Health Nov 2014;50(11):874–9.

[232] Rasmussen T, Stene LC, Samuelsen SO, Cinek O, Wetlesen T, Torjesen PA, et al. Maternal BMI before pregnancy, maternal weight gain during pregnancy, and risk of persistent positivity for multiple diabetes-associated autoantibodies in children with the high-risk HLA genotype: the MIDIA study. Diabetes Care October 2009;32(10):1904–6.

[233] McKinney PA, Parslow R, Gurney K, Law G, Bodansky HJ, Williams DR. Antenatal risk factors for childhood diabetes mellitus; a case–control study of medical record data in Yorkshire, UK. Diabetologia August 1997;40(8):933–9.

[234] Arkkola T, Kautiainen S, Takkinen H-M, Kenward MG, Nevalainen J, Uusitalo U, et al. Relationship of maternal weight status and weight gain rate during pregnancy to the development of advanced beta cell autoimmunity in the offspring: a prospective birth cohort study. Pediatr Diabetes August 2011;12(5):478–84.

[235] Robertson L, Harrild K. Maternal and neonatal risk factors for childhood type 1 diabetes: a matched case–control study. BMC Publ Health January 2010;10:281.

[236] Harder T, Roepke K, Diller N, Stechling Y, Dudenhausen JW, Plagemann A. Birth weight, early weight gain, and subsequent risk of type 1 diabetes: systematic review and meta-analysis. Am J Epidemiol June 15, 2009;169(12):1428–36.

[237] Cardwell CR, Stene LC, Joner G, Davis EA, Cinek O, Rosenbauer J, et al. Birthweight and the risk of childhood-onset type 1 diabetes: a meta-analysis of observational studies using individual patient data. Diabetologia April 2010;53(4):641–51.

[238] Pedersen CR, Bock T, Hansen SV, Hansen MW, Buschard K. High juvenile body weight and low insulin levels as markers preceding early diabetes in the BB rat. Autoimmunity January 1994;17(4):261–9.

[239] Oge A, Isganaitis E, Jimenez-Chillaron J, Reamer C, Faucette R, Barry K, et al. In utero undernutrition reduces diabetes incidence in non-obese diabetic mice. Diabetologia May 2007;50(5):1099–108.

[240] Larsson HE, Lynch K, Lernmark B, Nilsson A, Hansson G, Almgren P, et al. Diabetes-associated HLA genotypes affect birthweight in the general population. Diabetologia August 2005;48(8):1484–91.

[241] Verbeeten KC, Elks CE, Daneman D, Ong KK. Association between childhood obesity and subsequent Type 1 diabetes: a systematic review and meta-analysis. Diabet Med January 2011;28(1):10–8.

[242] Kibirige M, Metcalf B, Renuka R, Wilkin TJ. Testing the accelerator hypothesis: the relationship between body mass and age at diagnosis of type 1 diabetes. Diabetes Care October 2003;26(10):2865–70.

[243] Knerr I, Wolf J, Reinehr T, Stachow R, Grabert M, Schober E, et al. The "accelerator hypothesis": relationship between weight, height, body mass index and age at diagnosis in a large cohort of 9248 German and Austrian children with type 1 diabetes mellitus. Diabetologia December 2005;48(12):2501–4.

[244] Dabelea D, D'Agostino RB, Mayer-Davis EJ, Pettitt DJ, Imperatore G, Dolan LM, et al. Testing the accelerator hypothesis: body size, beta-cell function, and age at onset of type 1 (autoimmune) diabetes. Diabetes Care February 2006;29(2):290–4.

[245] Weets I, De Leeuw IH, Du Caju MVL, Rooman R, Keymeulen B, Mathieu C, et al. The incidence of type 1 diabetes in the age group 0–39 years has not increased in Antwerp (Belgium) between 1989 and 2000: evidence for earlier disease manifestation. Diabetes Care May 2002;25(5):840–6.

[246] Pundziute-Lyckå A, Dahlquist G, Nyström L, Arnqvist H, Björk E, Blohmé G, et al. The incidence of Type I diabetes has not increased but shifted to a younger age at diagnosis in the 0–34 years group in Sweden 1983–1998. Diabetologia June 2002;45(6):783–91.

[247] Dahlquist G. Can we slow the rising incidence of childhood-onset autoimmune diabetes? The overload hypothesis. Diabetologia January 2006;49(1):20–4.

[248] Luna R, Garcia-Mayor RV, Lage M, Andrade MA, Barreiro J, Pombo M, et al. High serum leptin levels in children with type 1 diabetes mellitus: contribution of age, BMI, pubertal development and metabolic status. Clin Endocrinol (Oxf) November 1999;51(5):603–10.

[249] Kirel B, Doğruel N, Korkmaz U, Kiliç FS, Ozdamar K, Uçar B. Serum leptin levels in type 1 diabetic and obese children: relation to insulin levels. Clin Biochem August 2000;33(6):475–80.

[250] Verrotti A, Basciani F, Morgese G, Chiarelli F. Leptin levels in non-obese and obese children and young adults with type 1 diabetes mellitus. Eur J Endocrinol July 1998;139(1):49–53.

[251] Imagawa A, Funahashi T, Nakamura T, Moriwaki M, Tanaka S, Nishizawa H, et al. Elevated serum concentration of adipose-derived factor, adiponectin, in patients with type 1 diabetes. Diabetes Care September 2002;25(9):1665–6.

[252] Leth H, Andersen KK, Frystyk J, Tarnow L, Rossing P, Parving H-H, et al. Elevated levels of high-molecular-weight adiponectin in type 1 diabetes. J Clin Endocrinol Metab August 2008;93(8):3186–91.

[253] Pham MN, Kolb H, Mandrup-Poulsen T, Battelino T, Ludvigsson J, Pozzilli P, et al. Serum adipokines as biomarkers of beta-cell function in patients with type 1 diabetes: positive association with leptin and resistin and negative association with adiponectin. Diabetes Metab Res Rev February 2013;29(2):166–70.

[254] Habeeb NMM, Youssef OI, Saab AAR, El Hadidi ES. Adiponectin as a marker of complications in type I diabetes. Indian Pediatr April 2012;49(4):277–80.

[255] Saraheimo M, Forsblom C, Thorn L, Wadén J, Rosengård-Bärlund M, Heikkilä O, et al. Serum adiponectin and progression of diabetic nephropathy in patients with type 1 diabetes. Diabetes Care June 2008;31(6):1165–9.

[256] Forsblom C, Thomas MC, Moran J, Saraheimo M, Thorn L, Wadén J, et al. Serum adiponectin concentration is a positive predictor of all-cause and cardiovascular mortality in type 1 diabetes. J Intern Med October 2011;270(4):346–55.

[257] Geyikli İ KM, Kör Y, Akan M. Increased resistin serum concentrations in patients with type 1 diabetes mellitus. J Clin Res Pediatr Endocrinol 2013;5(3):189–93.

[258] Pang TTL, Chimen M, Goble E, Dixon N, Benbow A, Eldershaw SE, et al. Inhibition of islet immunoreactivity by adiponectin is attenuated in human type 1 diabetes. J Clin Endocrinol Metab March 2013;98(3):E418–28.

[259] Wijesekara N, Krishnamurthy M, Bhattacharjee A, Suhail A, Sweeney G, Wheeler MB. Adiponectin-induced ERK and Akt phosphorylation protects against pancreatic beta cell apoptosis and increases insulin gene expression and secretion. J Biol Chem October 29, 2010;285(44):33623–31.

[260] Matarese G, Sanna V, Lechler RI, Sarvetnick N, Fontana S, Zappacosta S, et al. Leptin accelerates autoimmune diabetes in female NOD mice. Diabetes May 2002;51(5):1356–61.

[261] Brown JEP, Onyango DJ, Dunmore SJ. Resistin down-regulates insulin receptor expression, and modulates cell viability in rodent pancreatic beta-cells. FEBS Lett July 10, 2007;581(17):3273–6.

[262] Parisi R, Symmons DPM, Griffiths CEM, Ashcroft DM. Global epidemiology of psoriasis: a systematic review of incidence and prevalence. J Invest Dermatol February 2013;133(2):377–85.

[263] Ni C, Chiu MW. Psoriasis and comorbidities: links and risks. Clin Cosmet Investig Dermatol January 2014;7:119–32.

[264] Gelfand JM, Feldman SR, Stern RS, Thomas J, Rolstad T, Margolis DJ. Determinants of quality of life in patients with psoriasis: a study from the US population. J Am Acad Dermatol November 2004;51(5):704–8.

[265] Nestle FO, Kaplan DH, Barker J. Psoriasis. N Engl J Med July 30, 2009;361(5):496–509.

[266] Raychaudhuri SK, Maverakis E, Raychaudhuri SP. Diagnosis and classification of psoriasis. Autoimmun Rev 2014;13(4–5):490–5.

[267] Griffiths CEM, Barker JNWN. Pathogenesis and clinical features of psoriasis. Lancet July 21, 2007;370(9583):263–71.

[268] Lindegård B. Diseases associated with psoriasis in a general population of 159,200 middle-aged, urban, native Swedes. Dermatologica January 1986;172(6):298–304.

[269] Armstrong AW, Harskamp CT, Armstrong EJ. The association between psoriasis and obesity: a systematic review and meta-analysis of observational studies. Nutr Diabetes January 2012;2:e54.

[270] Russolillo A, Iervolino S, Peluso R, Lupoli R, Di Minno A, Pappone N, et al. Obesity and psoriatic arthritis: from pathogenesis to clinical outcome and management. Rheumatology (Oxford) January 2013;52(1):62–7.

[271] Setty AR, Curhan G, Choi HK. Obesity, waist circumference, weight change, and the risk of psoriasis in women: nurses' Health Study II. Arch Intern Med 2007;167(15):1670–5.

[272] Naldi L, Chatenoud L, Linder D, Belloni Fortina A, Peserico A, Virgili AR, et al. Cigarette smoking, body mass index, and stressful life events as risk factors for psoriasis: results from an Italian case–control study. J Investig Dermatol July 2005;125(1):61–7.

[273] Kumar S, Han J, Li T, Qureshi AA. Obesity, waist circumference, weight change and the risk of psoriasis in US women. J Eur Acad Dermatol Venereol October 2013;27(10):1293–8.

[274] Love TJ, Zhu Y, Zhang Y, Wall-Burns L, Ogdie A, Gelfand JM, et al. Obesity and the risk of psoriatic arthritis: a population-based study. Ann Rheum Dis August 2012;71(8):1273–7.

[275] Li W, Han J, Qureshi AA. Obesity and risk of incident psoriatic arthritis in US women. Ann Rheum Dis August 2012;71(8):1267–72.

[276] Soltani-Arabshahi R, Wong B, Feng B-J, Goldgar DE, Duffin KC, Krueger GG. Obesity in early adulthood as a risk factor for psoriatic arthritis. Arch Dermatol July 2010;146(7):721–6.

[277] Herron MD, Hinckley M, Hoffman MS, Papenfuss J, Hansen CB, Callis KP, et al. Impact of obesity and smoking on psoriasis presentation and management. Arch Dermatol December 2005;141(12):1527–34.

[278] Kaye JA, Li L, Jick SS. Incidence of risk factors for myocardial infarction and other vascular diseases in patients with psoriasis. Br J Dermatol September 2008;159(4):895–902.

[279] Carrascosa JM, Rocamora V, Fernandez-Torres RM, Jimenez-Puya R, Moreno JC, Coll-Puigserver N, et al. Obesity and psoriasis: inflammatory nature of obesity, relationship between psoriasis and obesity, and therapeutic implications. Actas Dermosifiliogr 2014;105(1):31–44.

[280] McDonough E, Ayearst R, Eder L, Chandran V, Rosen CF, Thavaneswaran A, et al. Depression and anxiety in psoriatic disease: prevalence and associated factors. J Rheumatol May 2014;41(5):887–96.

[281] Solis MY, de Melo NS, Macedo MEM, Carneiro FP, Sabbag CY, Lancha Júnior AH, et al. Nutritional status and food intake of patients with systemic psoriasis and psoriatic arthritis associated. Einstein (Sao Paulo) 2012;10(1):44–52.

[282] Brenaut E, Horreau C, Pouplard C, Barnetche T, Paul C, Richard M-A, et al. Alcohol consumption and psoriasis: a systematic literature review. J Eur Acad Dermatol Venereol August 2013;27(Suppl. 3):30–5.

[283] Torres T, Alexandre JM, Mendonça D, Vasconcelos C, Silva BM, Selores M. Levels of physical activity in patients with severe psoriasis: a cross-sectional questionnaire study. Am J Clin Dermatol April 2014;15(2):129–35.

[284] Florin V, Cottencin AC, Delaporte E, Staumont-Sallé D. Body weight increment in patients treated with infliximab for plaque psoriasis. J Eur Acad Dermatol Venereol February 2013;27(2):e186–90.

[285] Renzo LDI, Saraceno R, Schipani C, Rizzo M, Bianchi A, Noce A, et al. Prospective assessment of body weight and body composition changes in patients with psoriasis receiving anti-TNF-α treatment. Dermatol Ther 2011;24(4):446–51.

[286] Jin Y, Zhang F, Yang S, Kong Y, Xiao F, Hou Y, et al. Combined effects of HLA-Cw6, body mass index and waist–hip ratio on psoriasis vulgaris in Chinese Han population. J Dermatol Sci November 2008;52(2):123–9.

[287] Li W-Q, Han J-L, Zhang M-F, Qureshi AA. Interactions between adiposity and genetic polymorphisms on the risk of psoriasis. Br J Dermatol March 2013;168(3):639–42.

[288] Takahashi H, Tsuji H, Takahashi I, Hashimoto Y, Ishida-Yamamoto A, Iizuka H. Prevalence of obesity/adiposity in Japanese psoriasis patients: adiposity is correlated with the severity of psoriasis. J Dermatol Sci July 2009;55(1):74–6.

[289] Duarte GV, de FSP Oliveira M, Cardoso TM, Follador I, Silva TS, Cavalheiro CMA, et al. Association between obesity measured by different parameters and severity of psoriasis. Int J Dermatol February 2013;52(2):177–81.

[290] Tobin AM, Hackett CB, Rogers S, Collins P, Richards HL, O'Shea D, et al. Body mass index, waist circumference and HOMA-IR correlate with PASI in psoriasis patients receiving phototherapy. Br J Dermatol Feb 2014;23.

[291] Nikolopoulou A, Kadoglou NPE. Obesity and metabolic syndrome as related to cardiovascular disease. Expert Rev Cardiovasc Ther July 2012;10(7):933–9.

[292] Horreau C, Pouplard C, Brenaut E, Barnetche T, Misery L, Cribier B, et al. Cardiovascular morbidity and mortality in psoriasis and psoriatic arthritis: a systematic literature review. J Eur Acad Dermatol Venereol August 2013;27(Suppl. 3):12–29.

[293] Miller IM, Ellervik C, Yazdanyar S, Jemec GBE. Meta-analysis of psoriasis, cardiovascular disease, and associated risk factors. J Am Acad Dermatol December 2013;69(6):1014–24.

[294] Armstrong AW, Harskamp CT, Armstrong EJ. Psoriasis and metabolic syndrome: a systematic review and meta-analysis of observational studies. J Am Acad Dermatol April 2013;68(4):654–62.

[295] Debbaneh M, Millsop JW, Bhatia BK, Koo J, Liao W. Diet and psoriasis, part I: impact of weight loss interventions. J Am Acad Dermatol July 2014;71(1):133–40.

[296] Naldi L, Conti A, Cazzaniga S, Patrizi A, Pazzaglia M, Lanzoni A, et al. Diet and physical exercise in psoriasis: a randomized controlled trial. Br J Dermatol 2014;170(3):634–42.

[297] Jensen P, Zachariae C, Christensen R, Geiker NRW, Schaadt BK, Stender S, et al. Effect of weight loss on the severity of psoriasis: a randomized clinical study. JAMA Dermatol July 2013;149(7):795–801.

[298] Farias MM, Achurra P, Boza C, Vega A, de la Cruz C. Psoriasis following bariatric surgery: clinical evolution and impact on quality of life on 10 patients. Obes Surg June 2012;22(6):877–80.

[299] Hossler EW, Wood GC, Still CD, Mowad CM, Maroon MS. The effect of weight loss surgery on the severity of psoriasis. Br J Dermatol March 2013;168(3):660–1.

[300] Gisondi P, Del Giglio M, Di Francesco V, Zamboni M, Girolomoni G. Weight loss improves the response of obese patients with moderate-to-severe chronic plaque psoriasis to low-dose cyclosporine therapy: a randomized, controlled, investigator-blinded clinical trial. Am J Clin Nutr November 2008;88(5):1242–7.

[301] Di Minno MND, Peluso R, Iervolino S, Russolillo A, Lupoli R, Scarpa R. Weight loss and achievement of minimal disease activity in patients with psoriatic arthritis starting treatment with tumour necrosis factor α blockers. Ann Rheum Dis June 1, 2014;73(6):1157–62.

[302] Jensen P, Zachariae C, Christensen R, Geiker NRW, Schaadt BK, Stender S, et al. Effect of weight loss on the cardiovascular risk profile of obese patients with psoriasis. Acta Derm Venereol Feb 2014;20.

[303] Michalak-Stoma A, Pietrzak A, Szepietowski JC, Zalewska-Janowska A, Paszkowski T, Chodorowska G. Cytokine network in psoriasis revisited. Eur Cytokine Netw December 2011;22(4):160–8.

[304] Bulló M, García-Lorda P, Megias I, Salas-Salvadó J. Systemic inflammation, adipose tissue tumor necrosis factor, and leptin expression. Obes Res April 2003;11(4):525–31.

[305] Zhu K-J, Zhang C, Li M, Zhu C-Y, Shi G, Fan Y-M. Leptin levels in patients with psoriasis: a meta-analysis. Clin Exp Dermatol July 2013;38(5):478–83.

[306] Wang Y, Chen J, Zhao Y, Geng L, Song F, Chen H-D. Psoriasis is associated with increased levels of serum leptin. Br J Dermatol May 2008;158(5):1134–5.

[307] Johnston A, Arnadottir S, Gudjonsson JE, Aphale A, Sigmarsdottir AA, Gunnarsson SI, et al. Obesity in psoriasis: leptin and resistin as mediators of cutaneous inflammation. Br J Dermatol August 2008;159(2):342–50.

[308] Coimbra S, Oliveira H, Reis F, Belo L, Rocha S, Quintanilha A, et al. Circulating adipokine levels in Portuguese patients with psoriasis vulgaris according to body mass index, severity and therapy. J Eur Acad Dermatol Venereol December 2010;24(12):1386–94.

[309] Takahashi H, Tsuji H, Honma M, Ishida-Yamamoto A, Iizuka H. Increased plasma resistin and decreased omentin levels in Japanese patients with psoriasis. Arch Dermatol Res March 2013;305(2):113–6.

[310] Ozdemir M, Yüksel M, Gökbel H, Okudan N, Mevlitoğlu I. Serum leptin, adiponectin, resistin and ghrelin levels in psoriatic patients treated with cyclosporin. J Dermatol May 2012;39(5):443–8.

[311] Kawashima K, Torii K, Furuhashi T, Saito C, Nishio E, Nishida E, et al. Phototherapy reduces serum resistin levels in psoriasis patients. Photodermatol Photoimmunol Photomed June 2011;27(3):152–5.

[312] Nakajima H, Nakajima K, Tarutani M, Sano S. Clear association between serum levels of adipokines and T-helper 17-related cytokines in patients with psoriasis. Clin Exp Dermatol 2012;38(1):66–70.

[313] Cerman AA, Bozkurt S, Sav A, Tulunay A, Elbaşi MO, Ergun T. Serum leptin levels, skin leptin and leptin receptor expression in psoriasis. Br J Dermatol September 2008;159(4):820–6.

[314] Xue K, Liu H, Jian Q, Liu B, Zhu D, Zhang M, et al. Leptin induces secretion of pro-inflammatory cytokines by human keratinocytes in vitro—a possible reason for increased severity of psoriasis in patients with a high body mass index. Exp Dermatol June 2013;22(6):406–10.

[315] Xue Y, Jiang L, Cheng Q, Chen H, Yu Y, Lin Y, et al. Adipokines in psoriatic arthritis patients: the correlations with osteoclast precursors and bone erosions. PLoS One 2012;7(10):1–11.

[316] Gerdes S, Osadtschy S, Rostami-Yazdi M, Buhles N, Weichenthal M, Mrowietz U. Leptin, adiponectin, visfatin and retinol-binding protein-4—mediators of comorbidities in patients with psoriasis? Exp Dermatol January 2012;21(1):43–7.

[317] Ismail SA, Mohamed SA. Serum levels of visfatin and omentin-1 in patients with pso-riasis and their relation to disease severity. Br J Dermatol August 2012;167(2):436–9.

[318] Shibata S, Tada Y, Hau C, Tatsuta A, Yamamoto M, Kamata M, et al. Adiponectin as an anti-inflammatory factor in the pathogenesis of psoriasis: induction of elevated serum adiponectin levels following therapy. Br J Dermatol March 2011;164(3):667–70.

[319] Shibata S, Saeki H, Tada Y, Karakawa M, Komine M, Tamaki K. Serum high molecular weight adiponectin levels are decreased in psoriasis patients. J Dermatol Sci July 2009;55(1):62–3.

[320] Takahashi H, Tsuji H, Takahashi I, Hashimoto Y, Ishida-Yamamoto A, Iizuka H. Plasma adiponectin and leptin levels in Japanese patients with psoriasis. Br J Dermatol November 2008;159(5):1207–8.

[321] Zhu K-J, Shi G, Zhang C, Li M, Zhu C-Y, Fan Y-M. Adiponectin levels in patients with psoriasis: a meta-analysis. J Dermatol June 2013;40(6):438–42.

[322] Puig L. Obesity and psoriasis: body weight and body mass index influence the response to biological treatment. J Eur Acad Dermatol Venereol September 2011;25(9):1007–11.

[323] Montaudié H, Sbidian E, Paul C, Maza A, Gallini A, Aractingi S, et al. Methotrexate in psoriasis: a systematic review of treatment modalities, incidence, risk factors and monitoring of liver toxicity. J Eur Acad Dermatol Venereol May 2011;25(Suppl. 2):12–8.

[324] Shibata N, Hayakawa T, Hoshino N, Minouchi T, Yamaji A, Uehara M. Effect of obesity on cyclosporine trough concentrations in psoriasis patients. Am J Health Syst Pharm August 1, 1998;55(15):1598–602.

[325] Maza A, Montaudié H, Sbidian E, Gallini A, Aractingi S, Aubin F, et al. Oral cyclosporin in psoriasis: a systematic review on treatment modalities, risk of kidney toxicity and evidence for use in non-plaque psoriasis. J Eur Acad Dermatol Venereol May 2011;25(Suppl. 2):19–27.

[326] Clark L, Lebwohl M. The effect of weight on the efficacy of biologic therapy in patients with psoriasis. J Am Acad Dermatol March 2008;58(3):443–6.

[327] Reich K, Gottlieb A, Kimaball A, Li S. Consistency of infliximab response across subgroups of patients with psoriasis: integrated results from randomized controlled clinical trials. J Am Acad Dermatol 2006;54:AB215.

[328] Gordon K, Korman N, Frankel E, Wang H, Jahreis A, Zitnik R, et al. Efficacy of etanercept in an integrated multistudy database of patients with psoriasis. J Am Acad Dermatol March 2006;54(3 Suppl. 2):S101–11.

[329] Menter A, Gordon KB, Leonardi CL, Gu Y, Goldblum OM. Efficacy and safety of adalimumab across subgroups of patients with moderate to severe psoriasis. J Am Acad Dermatol September 2010;63(3):448–56.

[330] Di Minno MND, Peluso R, Iervolino S, Lupoli R, Russolillo A, Scarpa R, et al. Obesity and the prediction of minimal disease activity: a prospective study in psoriatic arthritis. Arthritis Care Res (Hoboken) January 2013;65(1):141–7.

[331] Lebwohl M, Yeilding N, Szapary P, Wang Y, Li S, Zhu Y, et al. Impact of weight on the efficacy and safety of ustekinumab in patients with moderate to severe psoriasis: rationale for dosing recommendations. J Am Acad Dermatol October 2010;63(4):571–9.

[332] Al-mutairi N, Nour T. The effect of weight reduction on treatment outcomes in obese patients with psoriasis on biologic therapy: a randomized controlled prospective trial. Expert Opin Biol Ther 2014;14(6):749–56.

[333] Di Lernia V, Tasin L, Pellicano R, Zumiani G, Albertini G. Impact of body mass index on retention rates of anti-TNF-alfa drugs in daily practice for psoriasis. J Dermatolog Treat December 2012;23(6):404–9.

[334] Carrascosa JM, Vilavella M, Garcia-Doval I, Carretero G, Vanaclocha F, Daudén E, et al. Body mass index in patients with moderate-to-severe psoriasis in Spain and its impact as an independent risk factor for therapy withdrawal: results of the Biobadaderm Registry. J Eur Acad Dermatol Venereol July 2014;28(7):907–14.

[335] McLeod DSA, Cooper DS. The incidence and prevalence of thyroid autoimmunity. Endocrine October 2012;42(2):252–65.

[336] Golden SH, Robinson KA, Saldanha I, Anton B, Ladenson PW. Clinical review: prevalence and incidence of endocrine and metabolic disorders in the United States: a comprehensive review. J Clin Endocrinol Metab July 2009;94(6):1853–78.

[337] Vanderpump MPJ. The epidemiology of thyroid disease. Br Med Bull January 2011;99:39–51.

[338] Caturegli P, De Remigis A, Rose NR. Hashimoto thyroiditis: clinical and diagnostic criteria. Autoimmun Rev 2014;13(4–5):391–7.

[339] Burek CL, Talor MV. Environmental triggers of autoimmune thyroiditis. J Autoimmun 2009;33(3–4):183–9.

[340] Cogni G, Chiovato L. An overview of the pathogenesis of thyroid autoimmunity. Hormones (Athens) 2013;12(1):19–29.

[341] Rotondi M, Magri F, Chiovato L. Thyroid and obesity: not a one-way interaction. J Clin Endocrinol Metab February 2011;96(2):344–6.

[342] Fox CS, Pencina MJ, D'Agostino RB, Murabito JM, Seely EW, Pearce EN, et al. Relations of thyroid function to body weight: cross-sectional and longitudinal observations in a community-based sample. Arch Intern Med March 24, 2008;168(6):587–92.

[343] Nyrnes A, Jorde R, Sundsfjord J. Serum TSH is positively associated with BMI. Int J Obes (Lond) January 2006;30(1):100–5.

[344] Michalaki MA, Vagenakis AG, Leonardou AS, Argentou MN, Habeos IG, Makri MG, et al. Thyroid function in humans with morbid obesity. Thyroid January 2006;16(1):73–8.

[345] Rotondi M, Leporati P, La Manna A, Pirali B, Mondello T, Fonte R, et al. Raised serum TSH levels in patients with morbid obesity: is it enough to diagnose subclinical hypothyroidism? Eur J Endocrinol March 2009;160(3):403–8.

[346] Radetti G, Kleon W, Buzi F, Crivellaro C, Pappalardo L, Iorgi N. Thyroid function and structure are affected in childhood obesity. J Clin Endocrinol Metab 2014;93(12):4749–54.

[347] Knudsen N, Laurberg P, Rasmussen LB, Bülow I, Perrild H, Ovesen L, et al. Small differences in thyroid function may be important for body mass index and the occurrence of obesity in the population. J Clin Endocrinol Metab July 2005;90(7):4019–24.

[348] Portmann L, Giusti V. Obesity and hypothyroidism: myth or reality? Rev Med Suisse April 4, 2007;3(105):859–62.

[349] de Moraes CMM, Mancini MC, de Melo ME, Figueiredo DA, Villares SMF, Rascovski A, et al. Prevalence of subclinical hypothyroidism in a morbidly obese population and improvement after weight loss induced by Roux-en-Y gastric by-pass. Obes Surg October 2005;15(9):1287–91.

[350] Kok P, Roelfsema F, Langendonk JG, Frölich M, Burggraaf J, Meinders AE, et al. High circulating thyrotropin levels in obese women are reduced after body weight loss induced by caloric restriction. J Clin Endocrinol Metab August 2005;90(8):4659–63.

[351] Danforth E, Burger A. The role of thyroid hormones in the control of energy expenditure. Clin Endocrinol Metab November 1984;13(3):581–95.

[352] Duntas LH, Biondi B. The interconnections between obesity, thyroid function, and autoimmunity: the multifold role of leptin. Thyroid 2013;23(6):646–53.

[353] Feldt-Rasmussen U. Thyroid and leptin. Thyroid May 2007;17(5):413–9.

[354] Seoane LM, Carro E, Tovar S, Casanueva FF, Dieguez C. Regulation of in vivo TSH secretion by leptin. Regul Pept August 25, 2000;92(1–3):25–9.

[355] Oge A, Bayraktar F, Saygili F, Guney E, Demir S. TSH influences serum leptin levels independent of thyroid hormones in hypothyroid and hyperthyroid patients. Endocr J April 2005;52(2):213–7.

[356] Marzullo P, Minocci A, Tagliaferri MA, Guzzaloni G, Di Blasio A, De Medici C, et al. Investigations of thyroid hormones and antibodies in obesity: leptin levels are associated with thyroid. J Clin Endocrinol Metab 2014;95(8):3965–72.

[357] Ong KK, Kuh D, Pierce M, Franklyn JA. Childhood weight gain and thyroid autoimmunity at age 60–64 years: the 1946 British Birth Cohort Study. J Clin Endocrinol Metab 2014;98(4):1435–42.

[358] Wang S, Baidoo SE, Liu Y, Zhu C, Tian J, Ma J, et al. T cell-derived leptin contributes to increased frequency of T helper type 17 cells in female patients with Hashimoto's thyroiditis. Clin Exp Immunol 2012;171(1):63–8.

[359] Figueroa-Vega N, Alfonso-Pérez M, Benedicto I, Sánchez-Madrid F, González-Amaro R, Marazuela M. Increased circulating pro-inflammatory cytokines and Th17 lymphocytes in Hashimoto's thyroiditis. J Clin Endocrinol Metab February 2010;95(2):953–62.

[360] Shi Y, Wang H, Su Z, Chen J, Xue Y, Wang S, et al. Differentiation imbalance of Th1/Th17 in peripheral blood mononuclear cells might contribute to pathogenesis of Hashimoto's thyroiditis. Scand J Immunol September 2010;72(3):250–5.

[361] Rodrigues CEM, Vendramini MB, Bueno C, Bonfá E, De Carvalho JF, Paulo-sp S, et al. Adipocytokines in primary antiphospholipid syndrome : potential markers of low-grade inflammation, insulin resistance and metabolic syndrome. Clin Exp Rheumatol 2012;30(6):871–8.

[362] Gary T, Belaj K, Bruckenberger R, Hackl G, Hafner F, Froehlich H, et al. Primary antiphospholipid antibody syndrome — one further aspect of thrombophilia in overweight and obese patients with venous thromboembolism. Obesity 2013;21(9):463–6.

[363] Gheita T, El-Gazzar I, El Shazly R, El-Din A, Abdel-Rasheed E, Bassyouni R. Elevated serum resistin in juvenile idiopathic arthritis: relation to categories and disease activity. J Clin Immunol 2013;33(1):297–301.

[364] Filkovà M, Senolt L, Vencovsky J. The role of resistin in inflammatory myopathies. Curr Rheumatol Rep 2013;15(6):336.

Chapter 36

Physical Activity and the Mosaic of Autoimmunity. Get Moving to Manage the Disease

Kassem Sharif[1,2,3], Michael Lichtbroun[2,3], Abdulla Watad[1,2,3], Vânia Vieira Borba[2,4,5], Yehuda Shoenfeld[6,7]

[1]Department of Medicine 'B', Sheba Medical Center, Tel-Hashomer, Israel; [2]Zabludowicz Center for Autoimmune Diseases, Sheba Medical Center, Tel-Hashomer, Israel; [3]Sackler Faculty of Medicine, Tel Aviv University, Tel Aviv, Israel; [4]Department 'A' of Internal Medicine, Coimbra University Hospital Centre, Coimbra, Portugal; [5]Faculty of Medicine, University of Coimbra, Coimbra, Portugal; [6]Zabludowicz Center for Autoimmune Diseases, Sheba Medical Center, affiliated to Sackler Faculty of Medicine, Tel Aviv University, Tel Aviv, Israel; [7]Laboratory of the Mosaics of Autoimmunity, Saint-Petersburg University, Saint-Petersburg, Russian Federation

INTRODUCTION

Physical inactivity is one of the most prevalent modifiable risk factors for acquiring disease worldwide [1]. It is the fourth leading risk factor for global mortality and is responsible for an estimated 13.4 million disability-adjusted life years worldwide [1]. Physical activity levels have been shown to correlate with many chronic diseases including type 2 diabetes mellitus, cardiovascular disease (CVD), and metabolic syndrome [2].

In the past, research on physical activity primarily focused on various health determinants such as the all-cause mortality risk. Eventually, due to the growing evidence that physical activity is beneficial in such a diverse list of diseases, researcher explored its effect on immunomodulation. This chapter will review how this modifiable risk factor influences the prevalence and symptomology of the many different autoimmune diseases (Table 36.1).

PHYSICAL ACTIVITY AND RHEUMATOID ARTHRITIS

Rheumatoid Arthritis Risk of Occurrence and Future Disease Severity

In a large prospective study of rheumatoid arthritis (RA) women, Di Giuseppe et al. [3] found that physical activity habits were associated with a reduced risk of developing RA. The strongest association was seen in those who bicycled or walked more than 20 min/day, and those who exercised more than 1 h/week [3]. In another study, researchers found that high physical activity levels 5 years leading up to a formal diagnosis of RA reduced an individuals risk of having a disease activity score (DAS)-28 above the median [4].

Impact of Physical Activity on Cardiovascular Risk in Rheumatoid Arthritis Patients

CVD is considered a leading cause of mortality in patients with RA [5,6]. The increased susceptibility has been postulated to result from the continuous inflammatory process seen in RA patients [5].

Metsios et al. [7] investigated the effect that 6 months of aerobic and resistance exercises had on microvascular and macrovascular function in RA patients in a matched controlled design study. At the end of the 6 months, the experimental group had an increased aerobic capacity, a reduced DAS-28 score, and an improvement in microvascular function [7]. Based on the modest results available, physical activity should be advised in RA patients due to its antiinflammatory and antiatherogenic effects.

The Impact of Physical Activity on Joint Mobility

It was initially believed that exercise might cause an exacerbation of joint damage, and thus RA patients were advised to refrain from engaging in physical activity [8]. Over the years, a considerable amount of study results contradict this notion [9]. The underlying mechanism is believed to occur through enhanced muscle coordination and muscle hypertrophy.

Mosaic of Autoimmunity. https://doi.org/10.1016/B978-0-12-814307-0.00036-0

TABLE 36.1 The Effect of Physical Activity on the Various Aspects of Selected Autoimmune Conditions

Disease	Incidence	Other Effects
Rheumatoid arthritis	↓	↓ Disease severity, ↑ motility, ↑ strength.
Multiple sclerosis	↓	↓ Fatigue, ↓ depression, ↓ spasticity, ↑ balance, ↑ motility.
Systemic lupus erythematosus		↓ Fatigue, ↓ heart dysautonomia.
Fibromyalgia		↑ Pain, ↑ stiffness, ↑ physical function, ↓ tenderness.
Type 1 diabetes mellitus		↑ HbA1c, ↓ nephropathy, ↓ retinopathy, ↓ cardiovascular disease.
Inflammatory bowel disease	↓	↓ Episodes of colitis, ↑ antiinflammatory mediators.
Psoriasis	↓	

Van den Ende et al. [10] investigated the influence that an intensive exercise regimen has on physical function in RA patients. The intensive exercise regimen consisted of range of motion, isometric, and isokinetic exercises involving the joints of the feet, hand, and knee. During the observation period, joint motility, strength, and functional ability significantly improved.

PHYSICAL ACTIVITY AND MULTIPLE SCLEROSIS

Physical Activity and Multiple Sclerosis Risk of Occurrence

Dorans et al. [11] studied the association between multiple sclerosis (MS) and physical activity in two prospective cohort studies, termed the Nurses' Health Study. Of the subjects who developed MS after the baseline physical activity assessment, there was significantly higher proportion of MS cases in the group of women reporting lower physical activity (RR = 0.73, 95% CI [0.55–0.98], $P = .08$).

It has been suggested that exercise reduces MS occurrence by increasing the release of neuroprotective molecules including, for example, IGF-1, as well as other molecules which are important in maintaining neuroplasticity [12].

Impact of Physical Activity on Cognition

The ability to process new information, memory, and executive function has been shown to be reduced in roughly 40%–60% of patients with MS [13]. The studies investigating cognition and MS are scarce. In a *post hoc* correlational pilot study of MS patients with an Expanded disability status scale (EDSS) of less than 5.5, researchers found that those who exercised had significant improvement in executive functioning. In another randomized controlled pilot study, 42 secondary progressive MS patients with EDSS of 4–6 and who did not have a physical disability were randomized into exercise interventions. Patients engaging in bicycle ergometry over 8–10 weeks demonstrated an improvement in verbal learning, delayed memory, alertness, and shift of attention.

Impact of Physical Activity on Mobility

The prevalence of impaired mobility in MS varies depending on the definitions used and population studied from 50% to as high as 90% [14,15]. Snook et al. [16] metaanalyzed 22 studies that pooled 600 MS patients investigating the influence of various types of exercises on physical strength in patients with MS. Of the 22 studies, 20 of them enrolled patients with an EDSS score less than 4.5. Recruited MS patients were not exclusive to RRMS and instead included the various forms of the disease. Exercise was shown to significantly improve physical strength. The beneficial effect of exercise on muscular strength was replicated with different exercise interventions including aquatic fitness [17], aerobic activity [18], and treadmill training [19]. Of note, most of these studies were conducted in patients with RRMS and moderate disability. Further studies are needed to include MS patients with different subtypes and variable levels of disability.

In addition to muscle strength, balance and spasticity are essential components to mobility that may be dysfunctional in MS patients. One study (N = 110) found that patients undergoing 12 weeks of a supervised exercise program had a significant improvement in balance, spasticity, fatigue, and quality of life when compared to a control group [68]. In the study, the mean EDSS score was 4.2 and included RRMS primary and secondary progressive subtypes. Exercise interventions were devised and conducted by physical therapists that focused on lower extremity, core stability, and coordination exercises [20]. In a separate study, improvements in spasticity scores were also observed in leg cycling and locomotor exercises [21,22].

Impact of Physical Activity on Fatigue

In MS, fatigue has been associated with higher disability scores including depression, cognitive impairment, and pain [23]. The influence of exercise on fatigue was assessed in a large metaanalysis which revealed a reduction in fatigue levels in MS patients engaging in physical activity (correlation coefficient r=0.22) [24,25].

Impact of Physical Activity on Mood

Roughly 50% of people affected by MS will develop a clinically diagnosed depression over the course of the disease [26]. Depression in MS patients affects cognition, decision-making, compliance to medication, and increases the ideation of suicide [27,28].

Ensari et al. [29] compared the effect of exercise versus control on depression in patients with MS by pooling 477 patients from 13 RCTs. EDSS of MS patients ranged from 2.2 to 6.0. Physical activity was shown to have a beneficial effect on depression (r=0.18).

PHYSICAL ACTIVITY AND SYSTEMIC LUPUS ERYTHEMATOSUS

Traditionally, physical activity was infrequently incorporated as a behavioral modality in the care for patients with SLE. The European League Against Rheumatism highlighted the proposed benefit of physical exercise as adjuvant therapy in patients with SLE in general, and in SLE patients with increased risk of CVD in particular [30]. Physical activity has been shown to be effective in influencing multiple aspects of the disease process including cardiovascular risk, psychological symptoms, physical fitness, quality of life, and fatigue.

Impact of Physical Activity on Cardiovascular Disease Risk

SLE patients are at a higher risk of developing CVD due to medications employed (i.e., glucocorticoids) and systemic inflammation [31–34]. In response to exercise, SLE patients have been shown to possess an abnormal cardiovascular response characterized by chronotropic incompetence and a delayed postexercise heart rate recovery. The dysautonomia associated with SLE consequently results in an elevated risk for cardiovascular events [35,36]. Miossi et al. [37] investigated the impact of treadmill exercise for 12 weeks on SLE patients with mild disease (SLEDAI <4) and without a cardiovascular or conduction disturbance to sedentary SLE patients and healthy controls. The exercise training program was shown to be effective in increasing the chronotropic reserve and improving heart rate recovery. The results of this study highlight the safety of exercise training as well as its efficacy in reducing the dysautonomia that results from the disease itself.

Dos Reis-Neto et al. [38] evaluated the impact of walking exercise three times per week for 16 weeks on SLE patients. Endothelial function measured by brachial artery flow–mediated dilation showed a significant improvement in the exercise group versus control. Exercise tolerance and threshold speed also demonstrated similar effects. These findings underlined the role of physical exercise in improving endothelial function and aerobic capacity in patients with SLE without causing a deterioration in SLE disease clinical severity.

Impact of Physical Activity on Fatigue

Fatigue is considered to be one of the most common symptoms in patients with SLE, affecting roughly 80% of patients. Wu et al. [39] conducted a metaanalysis that focused on the effectiveness of physical activity in ameliorating fatigue in patients with SLE. 163 adults were pooled with a mean SLE-disease activity index (SLEDAI) score of 2–5.6 and a median duration of SLE ranging from 2.5 to 14.4. Aerobic exercise was shown to significantly decrease fatigue severity as assessed by the Fatigue Severity Scale (MD=−0.52, 95% CI [−0.92 to −0.13], P<.009).

PHYSICAL ACTIVITY AND TYPE 1 DIABETES MELLITUS

Impact of Physical Activity on Glycemic Indices

A primary goal in disease management revolves around maintaining glucose levels within normal range while minimizing hypoglycemic episodes [40]. Tonoli et al. [41] carried out a metaanalysis that investigated the effect of a wide variety of exercise interventions on glycemic control. Although all exercise forms had a statistically significant influence on both glucose and HbA1c levels, regular aerobic exercise was shown to significantly decrease HbA1c the most. One major limitation in both metaanalyses was that dietary intake, a factor that influences glycemic markers, was not strictly reported [42].

Impact of Physical Activity and T1DM Chronic Complications

T1DM patients engaging in physical activity require less insulin dosages due to an increase in peripheral insulin sensitivity and other mechanisms. This ultimately leads to a reduction in chronic complications [43]. In the cross-sectional Finnish diabetic nephropathy study (FinnDianne), increased leisure time physical activity was associated with a lower risk of renal dysfunction, proteinuria, retinopathy, and cerebrovascular disease [44]. In the "Pittsburgh Insulin Dependent Diabetes Mellitus Morbidity and Mortality Study," it was demonstrated that T1DM male patients who engaged in sport activities during their teen years showed a significantly decreased risk in CVD and all year mortality 25 years after disease diagnosis. In addition, engagement in physical exercise during teenage years was found to be protective against the development of diabetic nephropathy and neuropathy [45].

Moreover, longstanding type T1DM can lead to autonomic dysfunction. The engagement in physical activity in type 1 diabetes mellitus has been shown to improve spontaneous baroreflex, and heart rate variability, both of which are good measures for autonomic function [46,47].

PHYSICAL ACTIVITY AND INFLAMMATORY BOWEL DISEASE

Physical Activity and Risk of Disease Occurrence

Khalili et al. [48] examined the association between physical activity and the risk of developing IBD by examining two prospective cohort studies (Nurses' Health Study I&II) that included a total of 194,711 women. On follow-up, the risk of developing CD was shown to be inversely associated with increased physical activity ($P<.02$), even after adjusting for confounding variables. The finding of this study was consistent with the results of previous studies that highlighted the inverse relationship between higher physical activity and risk of IBD development [49–52]. This relationship has been more pronounced in CD as compared to UC [53]. It should be noted that Khalili et al. found no association between physical activity and the risk of developing UC [48].

Impact of Physical Activity on Disease Activity in Mouse Models

The effectiveness of physical activity on IBD progression has not been studied in humans and is poorly understood. However, the influence of physical activity on IBD was observed in colitis mouse models. Cook et al. [54] revealed that voluntary running in colitis mouse models decreased colitis symptoms by significantly reducing diarrhea episodes, as well as reducing inflammatory gene expression of proinflammatory markers including IL-17 and IL-1β. Hoffman-Goetz et al. [55] showed that 16 weeks of wheel running led to a significant decrease of TNF-α secretion and enhanced the section of IL-10: a well-known antiinflammatory cytokine [55]. Several other studies supported the positive role of exercise in reducing proinflammatory process and decreasing the intestinal barrier dysfunction [56,57].

PHYSICAL ACTIVITY AND FIBROMYALGIA

Fibromyalgia is treated by the combination of pharmacological and nonpharmacological approaches. The best nonpharmacological approaches include health education, cognitive behavioral therapy, and exercise. To achieve long-term desired effects, adherence to exercise and physical activity should be encouraged.

Accumulating evidence supports the integral role of physical exercise in the management of fibromyalgia. This relationship has been substantiated across a variety of exercise interventions. Bidonde et al. [58] conducted a metaanalysis that involved 839 patients with fibromyalgia examining the effect of aerobic exercise on major fibromyalgia outcomes. The aerobic interventions varied and included walking, cycling, and running. Aerobic exercise was shown to be well tolerated among fibromyalgia patients with a similar withdrawal rate in the exercise group as compared to the control group. Quality of life, physical function, and pain were significantly improved after aerobic exercise engagement. The influence of aerobic activity on fatigue and stiffness was shown to be positive, albeit not reaching significant levels.

In another report, Bidone et al. [59] explored the influence of aquatic exercise on fibromyalgia outcomes. Significant improvements were found in multidimensional function as assessed by fibromyalgia impact questionnaire, self-reported physical function, pain, stiffness, strength, and cardiovascular submaximal function. When compared to land-based exercising activities, aquatic interventions were not shown to confer a statistically significant advantage. It is also important to note that land-based training was superior to aquatic exercise in increasing strength.

Finally, based on another metaanalysis, moderate to high intensity resistance exercise with the intention of improving muscle strength, endurance, and power over 16–21 weeks was shown to significantly improve multidimensional functioning, self-reported physical function, pain, tenderness, and muscles strength. Similar to previous comparisons, engagement in resistance training was not proven to confer statistical significance over aerobic exercises in any reported measure. Withdrawal rates between the resistance and aerobic interventions were shown to be similar [60].

The improvement of fibromyalgia parameters subsequent to various exercise regimens highlights the importance of engagement in physical activity as adjuvant to standard disease management.

PHYSICAL ACTIVITY AND SYSTEMIC SCLEROSIS

Physical activity has been shown to be generally well tolerated among patients with SSc [61–63]. Nevertheless, in the subset of patients with interstitial lung disease, exercise can result in desaturation. Furthermore, SSc patients are at a higher risk of developing exercise-induced pulmonary artery hypertension [64,65].

In one randomized controlled study, researchers investigated how exercise affects the disease course of SSc patients. All patients in the intervention group, regardless of their disability, received muscle strengthening exercises, respiratory exercises, and functional rehabilitation for 1 year. At 1 month, there was a significant reduction in disability score and pain, and an improvement in hand motility. Additionally, microstomia was found to be significantly improved in the intervention group at both one and 12 months [63].

Schouffoer et al. [66] compared the effectiveness individually tailored therapy that consisted of a standardized group of sessions (general exercise and hand/mouth exercises) on a mixed sample of patients of diffuse and limited SSc and revealed a significant improvement in the grip strength, mouth opening, and 6-minute walking distance.

In summary, exercise is proven to be safe and tolerable in patients with SSc and therefore patients should be encouraged to engage in exercise interventions.

PHYSICAL ACTIVITY AND PSORIASIS

Physical Activity and Risk of Disease Occurrence

In the Nurses' Health Study II, a large cohort study involving 86,655 women, Frankel et al. [67] showed that after adjusting for confounding factors, women who engaged in higher levels of physical activity had a lower relative risk of developing psoriasis as compared with women in the least active quintile. Vigorous physical activity, defined as >6 metabolic equivalents, was also shown to be significantly inversely associated with the risk of psoriasis development. The mechanism explaining these findings requires further analysis, but such effects have been postulated to be mediated by the immunomodulatory effect of exercise on proinflammatory cytokine release of TNF-α, IFN-γ, and CRP [68].

CONCLUSION

Patients with autoimmune disease are less active than their healthy counterparts. Physical activity is shown to be safe, and its integration in patients' lifestyle is highly recommended.

Given the interrelation between physical activity and mental health, improving psychological parameters through physical activity could be reflected with higher compliance to medications. Thus, it stands to reason that clinical physicians should encourage patients to include exercise regimens as part of their daily life routines.

REFERENCES

[1] Ding D, Lawson KD, Kolbe-Alexander TL, Finkelstein EA, Katzmarzyk PT, van Mechelen W, et al. The economic burden of physical inactivity: a global analysis of major non-communicable diseases. Lancet 2016;388(10051):1311–24.

[2] Laaksonen DE, Lakka HM, Salonen JT, Niskanen LK, Rauramaa R, Lakka TA. Low levels of leisure-time physical activity and cardiorespiratory fitness predict development of the metabolic syndrome. Diabetes Care 2002;25(9):1612–8.

[3] Di Giuseppe D, Bottai M, Askling J, Wolk A. Physical activity and risk of rheumatoid arthritis in women: a population-based prospective study. Arthritis Res Ther 2015;17(1)).

[4] Sandberg ME, Wedren S, Klareskog L, Lundberg IE, Opava CH, Alfredsson L, et al. Patients with regular physical activity before onset of rheumatoid arthritis present with milder disease. Ann Rheum Dis 2014;73(8):1541–4.

[5] Crowson CS, Liao KP, Davis JM, Solomon DH, Matteson EL, Knutson KL, et al. Rheumatoid arthritis and cardiovascular disease. Am Heart J 2013;166(4):622–8.e1.

[6] Dhawan SS, Quyyumi AA. Rheumatoid arthritis and cardiovascular disease. Curr Atherosclerosis Rep 2008;10(2):128–33.

[7] Metsios GS, Stavropoulos-Kalinoglou A, Veldhuijzen van Zanten JJ, Nightingale P, Sandoo A, Dimitroulas T, et al. Individualised exercise improves endothelial function in patients with rheumatoid arthritis. Ann Rheum Dis 2013;73(4):748–51.

[8] de Jong Z, Munneke M, Zwinderman AH, Kroon HM, Jansen A, Ronday KH, et al. Is a long-term high-intensity exercise program effective and safe in patients with rheumatoid arthritis? Results of a randomized controlled trial. Arthritis Rheum 2003;48(9):2415–24.

[9] Metsios GS, Stavropoulos-Kalinoglou A, Veldhuijzen van Zanten JJ, Treharne GJ, Panoulas VF, Douglas KM, et al. Rheumatoid arthritis, cardio-vascular disease and physical exercise: a systematic review. Rheumatology (Oxford England) 2008;47(3):239–48.

[10] van den Ende CHM, Breedveld FC, le Cessie S, Dijkmans BAC, de Mug AW, Hazes JMW. Effect of intensive exercise on patients with active rheumatoid arthritis: a randomised clinical trial. Ann Rheum Dis 2000;59(8):615–21.

[11] Dorans KS, Massa J, Chitnis T, Ascherio A, Munger KL. Physical activity and the incidence of multiple sclerosis. Neurology 2016;87(17):1770–6.

[12] White LJ, Castellano V. Exercise and brain health–implications for multiple sclerosis: part 1–neuronal growth factors. Sports Med (Auckland NZ) 2008;38(2):91–100.

[13] Jongen PJ, Ter Horst AT, Brands AM. Cognitive impairment in multiple sclerosis. Minerva Med 2012;103(2):73–96.

[14] Wu N, Minden SL, Hoaglin DC, Hadden L, Frankel D. Quality of life in people with multiple sclerosis: data from the Sonya Slifka longitudinal multiple sclerosis study. J Health Hum Serv Adm 2007;30(3):233–67.

[15] Hobart J, Lamping D, Fitzpatrick R, Riazi A, Thompson A. The Multiple Sclerosis Impact Scale (MSIS-29): a new patient-based outcome measure. Brain J Neurol 2001;124(Pt 5):962–73.

[16] Snook EM, Motl RW. Effect of exercise training on walking mobility in multiple sclerosis: a meta-analysis. Neurorehabil Neural Repair 2009;23(2):108–16.

[17] Gehlsen GM, Grigsby SA, Winant DM. Effects of an aquatic fitness program on the muscular strength and endurance of patients with multiple sclerosis. Phys Ther 1984;64(5):653–7.

[18] Petajan JH, Gappmaier E, White AT, Spencer MK, Mino L, Hicks RW. Impact of aerobic training on fitness and quality of life in multiple sclerosis. Ann Neurol 1996;39(4):432–41.

[19] Beer S, Aschbacher B, Manoglou D, Gamper E, Kool J, Kesselring J. Robot-assisted gait training in multiple sclerosis: a pilot randomized trial. Mult Scler (Houndmills Basingstoke Engl) 2008;14(2):231–6.

[20] Tarakci E, Yeldan I, Huseyinsinoglu BE, Zenginler Y, Eraksoy M. Group exercise training for balance, functional status, spasticity, fatigue and qual-ity of life in multiple sclerosis: a randomized controlled trial. Clin Rehabil 2013;27(9):813–22.

[21] Sosnoff J, Motl RW, Snook EM, Wynn D. Effect of a 4-week period of unloaded leg cycling exercise on spasticity in multiple sclerosis. NeuroRehabilitation 2009;24(4):327–31.

[22] Giesser B, Beres-Jones J, Budovitch A, Herlihy E, Harkema S. Locomotor training using body weight support on a treadmill improves mobility in persons with multiple sclerosis: a pilot study. Mult Scler (Houndmills Basingstoke Engl) 2007;13(2):224–31.

[23] Larocca NG. Impact of walking impairment in multiple sclerosis: perspectives of patients and care partners. Patient 2011;4(3):189–201.

[24] Pilutti LA, Greenlee TA, Motl RW, Nickrent MS, Petruzzello SJ. Effects of exercise training on fatigue in multiple sclerosis: a meta-analysis. Psychosom Med 2013;75(6):575–80.

[25] Filippini G, Munari L, Incorvaia B, Ebers GC, Polman C, D'Amico R, et al. Interferons in relapsing remitting multiple sclerosis: a systematic review. Lancet (Lond Engl) 2003;361(9357):545–52.

[26] Siegert R, Abernethy D. Depression in multiple sclerosis: a review. J Neurol Neurosurg Psychiatry 2005;76(4):469–75.

[27] Arnett PA, Higginson CI, Voss WD, Wright B, Bender WI, Wurst JM, et al. Depressed mood in multiple sclerosis: relationship to capacity-demand-ing memory and attentional functioning. Neuropsychology 1999;13(3):434–46.

[28] Feinstein A. An examination of suicidal intent in patients with multiple sclerosis. Neurology 2002;59(5):674–8.

[29] Ensari I, Motl RW, Pilutti LA. Exercise training improves depressive symptoms in people with multiple sclerosis: results of a meta-analysis. J Psychosom Res 2014;76(6):465–71.

[30] Bertsias G, Ioannidis JP, Boletis J, Bombardieri S, Cervera R, Dostal C, et al. EULAR recommendations for the management of systemic lupus erythematosus. Report of a task force of the EULAR standing committee for international clinical studies including therapeutics. Ann Rheum Dis 2008;67(2):195–205.

[31] Esdaile JM, Abrahamowicz M, Grodzicky T, Li Y, Panaritis C, Berger RD, et al. Traditional Framingham risk factors fail to fully account for acceler-ated atherosclerosis in systemic lupus erythematosus. Arthritis Rheum 2001;44(10):2331–7.

[32] Chung CP, Avalos I, Oeser A, Gebretsadik T, Shintani A, Raggi P, et al. High prevalence of the metabolic syndrome in patients with systemic lupus erythematosus: association with disease characteristics and cardiovascular risk factors. Ann Rheum Dis 2007;66(2):208–14.

[33] Aydemir M, Yazisiz V, Basarici I, Avci AB, Erbasan F, Belgi A, et al. Cardiac autonomic profile in rheumatoid arthritis and systemic lupus erythe-matosus. Lupus 2010;19(3):255–61.

[34] Robert M, Miossec P. Effects of Interleukin 17 on the cardiovascular system. Autoimmun Rev 2017;16(9):984–99.

[35] do Prado DL, Gualano B, Miossi R, Sa-Pinto A, Lima F, Roschel H, et al. Abnormal chronotropic reserve and heart rate recovery in patients with SLE: a case-control study. Lupus 2011;20(7):717–20.

[36] Dogdu O, Yarlioglues M, Kaya MG, Ardic I, Oguzhan N, Akpek M, et al. Deterioration of heart rate recovery index in patients with systemic lupus erythematosus. J Rheumatol 2010;37(12):2511–5.

[37] Miossi R, Benatti FB, Lúciade de Sá Pinto A, Lima FR, Borba EF, Prado DML, et al. Using exercise training to counterbalance chronotropic incom-petence and delayed heart rate recovery in systemic lupus erythematosus: a randomized trial. Arthritis Care Res 2012;64(8):1159–66.

[38] dos Reis-Neto ET, da Silva AE, Monteiro CM, de Camargo LM, Sato EI. Supervised physical exercise improves endothelial function in patients with systemic lupus erythematosus. Rheumatology (Oxford Engl) 2013;52(12):2187–95.

[39] Wu ML, Yu KH, Tsai JC. The effectiveness of exercise in adults with systemic lupus erythematosus: a systematic review and meta-analysis to guide evidence-based practice. Worldviews Evid Based Nurs 2017;14(4):306–15.

[40] Monnier L, Colette C. Target for Glycemic Control: Concentrating on glucose. Diabetes Care 2009;32:S199–S204.

[41] Tonoli C, Heyman E, Roelands B, Buyse L, Cheung SS, Berthoin S, et al. Effects of different types of acute and chronic (training) exercise on glycaemic control in type 1 diabetes mellitus: a meta-analysis. Sports Med (Auckland NZ) 2012;42(12):1059–80.

[42] Kennedy A, Nirantharakumar K, Chimen M, Pang TT, Hemming K, Andrews RC, et al. Does exercise improve glycaemic control in type 1 diabetes? A systematic review and meta-analysis. PLoS One 2013;8(3).

[43] Langfort J, Viese M, Ploug T, Dela F. Time course of GLUT4 and AMPK protein expression in human skeletal muscle during one month of physical training. Scand J Med Sci Sports 2003;13(3):169–74.

[44] Wadén J, Forsblom C, Thorn LM, Saraheimo M, Rosengård-Bärlund M, Heikkilä O, et al. Physical activity and diabetes complications in patients with type 1 diabetes. Fin Diabet Nephropathy (FinnDiane) Study 2008;31(2):230–2.

[45] LaPorte RE, Dorman JS, Tajima N, Cruickshanks KJ, Orchard TJ, Cavender DE, et al. Pittsburgh insulin-dependent diabetes mellitus morbidity and mortality study: physical activity and diabetic complications. Pediatrics 1986;78(6):1027–33.

[46] Chen SR, Lee YJ, Chiu HW, Jeng C. Impact of physical activity on heart rate variability in children with type 1 diabetes. Child's Nervous Syst 2008;24(6):741–7.

[47] Lucini D, Zuccotti GV, Scaramuzza A, Malacarne M, Gervasi F, Pagani M. Exercise might improve cardiovascular autonomic regulation in adolescents with type 1 diabetes. Acta Diabetol 2013;50(3):341–9.

[48] Khalili H, Ananthakrishnan AN, Konijeti GG, Liao X, Higuchi LM, Fuchs CS, et al. Physical activity and risk of inflammatory bowel disease: prospective study from the Nurses' Health Study cohorts. BMJ 2013;347.

[49] Sonnenberg A. Occupational distribution of inflammatory bowel disease among German employees. Gut 1990;31(9):1037–40.

[50] Persson P-G, Leijonmarck C-E, Bernell O, Hellers G, Ahlbom A. Risk indicators for inflammatory bowel disease. Int J Epidemiol 1993;22(2):268–72.

[51] Klein I, Reif S, Farbstein H, Halak A, Gilat T. Preillness non dietary factors and habits in inflammatory bowel disease. Ital J Gastroenterol Hepatol 1998;30(3):247–51.

[52] Cucino C, Sonnenberg A. Occupational mortality from inflammatory bowel disease in the United States 1991–1996. Am J Gastroenterol 2001;96(4):1101–5.

[53] Bøggild H, Tüchsen F, Ørhede E. Occupation, employment status and chronic inflammatory bowel disease in Denmark. Int J Epidemiol 1996;25(3):630–7.

[54] Cook MD, Martin SA, Williams C, Whitlock K, Wallig MA, Pence BD, et al. Forced treadmill exercise training exacerbates inflammation and causes mortality while voluntary wheel training is protective in a mouse model of colitis. Brain Behav Immun 2013;33:46–56.

[55] Hoffman-Goetz L, Pervaiz N, Packer N, Guan J. Freewheel training decreases pro- and increases anti-inflammatory cytokine expression in mouse intestinal lymphocytes. Brain Behav Immun 2010;24(7):1105–15.

[56] Hoffman-Goetz L, Thorne R, Houston M. Splenic immune responses following treadmill exercise in mice. Can J Physiol Pharmacol 1988;66(11):1415–9.

[57] Hoffman-Goetz L, Spagnuolo P, Guan J. Repeated exercise in mice alters expression of IL-10 and TNF-α in intestinal lymphocytes. Brain Behav Immun 2008;22(2):195–9.

[58] Bidonde JBA, Schachter CL, Overend TJ, Kim SY, Góes SM, Boden C, Foulds HJA. Aerobic exercise training for adults with fibromyalgia. Cochrane Database Syst Rev 2017;CD012700.

[59] Bidonde J, Busch AJ, Webber SC, Schachter CL, Danyliw A, Overend TJ, et al. Aquatic exercise training for fibromyalgia. Cochrane Database Syst Rev 2014;(10).

[60] Busch AJ, Webber SC, Richards RS, Bidonde J, Schachter CL, Schafer LA, et al. Resistance exercise training for fibromyalgia. Cochrane Database Syst Rev 2013;(12):Cd010884.

[61] Alexanderson H, Bergegard J, Bjornadal L, Nordin A. Intensive aerobic and muscle endurance exercise in patients with systemic sclerosis: a pilot study. BMC Res Notes 2014;7:86.

[62] Schouffoer AA, Ninaber MK, Beaart-van de Voorde LJ, van der Giesen FJ, de Jong Z, Stolk J, et al. Randomized comparison of a multidisciplinary team care program with usual care in patients with systemic sclerosis. Arthritis Care Res 2011;63(6):909–17.

[63] Rannou F, Boutron I, Mouthon L, Sanchez K, Tiffreau V, Hachulla E, et al. Personalized physical therapy versus usual care for patients with systemic sclerosis: a randomized controlled trial. Arthritis Care Res 2017;69(7):1050–9.

[64] Someya F, Mugii N, Hasegawa M, Yahata T, Nakagawa T. Predictors of exercise-induced oxygen desaturation in systemic sclerosis patients with interstitial lung disease. Respir Care 2014;59(1):75–80.

[65] Voilliot D, Magne J, Dulgheru R, Kou S, Henri C, Laaraibi S, et al. Determinants of exercise-induced pulmonary arterial hypertension in systemic sclerosis. Int J Cardiol 2014;173(3):373–9.

[66] Schouffoer AA, Ninaber MK, Beaart-van de Voorde LJJ, van der Giesen FJ, de Jong Z, Stolk J, et al. Randomized comparison of a multidisciplinary team care program with usual care in patients with systemic sclerosis. Arthritis Care Res 2011;63(6):909–17.

[67] Frankel HC, Han J, Li T, Qureshi AA. The association between physical activity and the risk of incident psoriasis. Arch Dermatol 2012;148(8):918–24.

[68] Nicklas BJ, Hsu FC, Brinkley TJ, Church T, Goodpaster BH, Kritchevsky SB, et al. Exercise training and plasma C-reactive protein and interleukin-6 in elderly people. J Am Geriatr Soc 2008;56(11):2045–52.

FURTHER READING

[1] Metsios GS, Stavropoulos-Kalinoglou A, Panoulas VF, Wilson M, Nevill AM, Koutedakis Y, et al. Association of physical inactivity with increased cardiovascular risk in patients with rheumatoid arthritis. Eur J Cardiovasc Prev Rehabil 2009;16(2):188–94.

[2] Lemmey AB, Marcora SM, Chester K, Wilson S, Casanova F, Maddison PJ. Effects of high-intensity resistance training in patients with rheumatoid arthritis: a randomized controlled trial. Arthritis Rheum 2009;61(12):1726–34.

[3] Beier M, Bombardier CH, Hartoonian N, Motl RW, Kraft GH. Improved physical fitness correlates with improved cognition in multiple sclerosis. Arch Phys Med Rehabil 2014;95(7):1328–34.

[4] Briken S, Gold SM, Patra S, Vettorazzi E, Harbs D, Tallner A, et al. Effects of exercise on fitness and cognition in progressive MS: a randomized, controlled pilot trial. Mult Scler 2014;20(3):382–90.

[5] Dalgas U, Stenager E, Jakobsen J, Petersen T, Hansen HJ, Knudsen C, et al. Resistance training improves muscle strength and functional capacity in multiple sclerosis. Neurology 2009;73(18):1478–84.

[6] Avaux M, Hoellinger P, Nieuwland-Husson S, Fraselle V, Depresseux G, Houssiau FA. Effects of two different exercise programs on chronic fatigue in lupus patients. Acta Clinica Belgica 2016;71(6):403–6.

[7] Miossi R, Benatti FB, Luciade de Sa Pinto A, Lima FR, Borba EF, Prado DM, et al. Using exercise training to counterbalance chronotropic incompetence and delayed heart rate recovery in systemic lupus erythematosus: a randomized trial. Arthritis Care Res 2012;64(8):1159–66.

[8] Seeger JP, Thijssen DH, Noordam K, Cranen ME, Hopman MT, Nijhuis-van der Sanden MW. Exercise training improves physical fitness and vascular function in children with type 1 diabetes. Diabetes Obes Metab 2011;13(4):382–4.

[9] Strombeck BE, Theander E, Jacobsson LT. Effects of exercise on aerobic capacity and fatigue in women with primary Sjogren's syndrome. Rheumatology (Oxford Engl) 2007;46(5):868–71.

[10] Antonioli CM, Bua G, Frigè A, Prandini K, Radici S, Scarsi M, et al. An individualized rehabilitation program in patients with systemic sclerosis may improve quality of life and hand mobility. Clin Rheumatol 2009;28(2):159–65.

[11] Oliveira NC, dos Santos Sabbag LM, de Sa Pinto AL, Borges CL, Lima FR. Aerobic exercise is safe and effective in systemic sclerosis. Int J Sports Med 2009;30(10):728–32.

Chapter 37

Smoke and Autoimmunity: The Fire Behind the Disease

Carlo Perricone[1], Mathilde Versini[2], Dana Ben-Ami[3], Smadar Gertel[4], Abdulla Watad[3,4,5], Michael J. Segel[5,6], Fulvia Ceccarelli[1], Fabrizio Conti[1], Luca Cantarini[7], Dimitrios P. Bogdanos[8], Alessandro Antonelli[9], Howard Amital[3,4,5], Guido Valesini[1], Yehuda Shoenfeld[10,11]

[1]*Rheumatology, Department of Internal Medicine, Sapienza University of Rome, Rome, Italy;* [2]*Institut Arnault Tzanck, Saint Laurent du Var, France;* [3]*Department of Medicine 'B', Sheba Medical Center, Tel-Hashomer, Israel;* [4]*Zabludowicz Center for Autoimmune Diseases, Sheba Medical Center, Tel-Hashomer, Israel;* [5]*Sackler Faculty of Medicine, Tel Aviv University, Tel Aviv, Israel;* [6]*The Pulmonary Institute, Sheba Medical Center, Tel-Hashomer, Israel;* [7]*Department of Medical Sciences, Surgery and Neurosciences, Research Center of Systemic Autoinflammatory Diseases and Behçet's Disease, Rheumatology Unit, University of Siena, Policlinico Le Scotte, Siena, Italy;* [8]*Department of Rheumatology and Clinical Immunology, Faculty of Medicine, School of Health Sciences, University of Thessaly, Larissa, Greece;* [9]*Department of Clinical and Experimental Medicine, University of Pisa, Pisa, Italy;* [10]*Zabludowicz Center for Autoimmune Diseases, Sheba Medical Center, affiliated to Sackler Faculty of Medicine, Tel Aviv University, Tel Aviv, Israel;* [11]*Laboratory of the Mosaics of Autoimmunity, Saint-Petersburg University, Saint-Petersburg, Russian Federation*

INTRODUCTION

The association between smoke habit and autoimmunity has been hypothesized a long time ago [1]. Indeed, within the milestones achieved in the knowledge of the pathogenesis of autoimmune diseases, the discovery of novel autoantibodies possibly triggered by environmental agents has gained the attention of researchers [2]. Moreover, it is now recognized that autoantibodies often precede the development of an overt autoimmune disorder; however, because their presence does not necessarily lead to a full-blown disease, it is still a matter of debate whether they represent epiphenomena, some result of a genetic predisposition, or true risk factors [3]. Nonetheless, in the last years, the concept of "second hit" has been suggested for instance in antiphospholipid syndrome to explain the occurrence of a full-blown condition in a genetically predisposed individual [4]. Smoke has been found to play a pathogenic role because in certain conditions it may trigger the development of autoantibodies favoring citrullination [5], or acting as the "second hit" responsible for disease manifestation. Indeed, both epidemiological studies and animal models have showed the potential deleterious effect caused by smoke [6,7]. For example, smoke, by provoking oxidative stress, may contribute to lupus disease by dysregulating DNA demethylation, upregulating immune genes thereby leading to autoreactivity [6]. Moreover, it can alter the lung microenvironment, facilitating an exaggerated proinflammatory response to infection [8]. This, in turn, may result in a dysregulation of immune system leading to autoimmune phenomena. Not only cigarette smoke (CS) but also air pollution has been reported as being responsible for the development of autoimmunity. Indeed, it has been recently suggested that air pollution may represent a risk factor for rheumatoid arthritis (RA) [9,10]. Nevertheless, the results are still conflicting for some conditions while more clear in other autoimmune diseases such as RA. Thus, we aimed to review the role of smoke in the some of the most prominent autoimmune diseases.

SMOKE AND RHEUMATOID ARTHRITIS

RA is a common rheumatologic condition affecting approximately 1% of the adult population [11]. The disease has a complex pathogenesis in which both environmental and genetic factors interplay [12]. The synoviocytes are within the major effectors leading to the formation of pannus and production of proinflammatory cytokines and chemokines [13]. The inflammatory response leads to cartilage degradation and bone damage through the production of proteases and reactive oxygen intermediates, proliferation of synovial fibroblasts, recruitment of inflammatory cells, and neoangiogenesis [14]. The complement system is involved in disease pathogenesis possibly influencing serological phenotype and response to therapy [15–17].

The risk factors suggested so far include diet, coffee intake, alcohol, and body mass index [18]. However, cigarette smoking is the only risk factor clearly associated with disease susceptibility [19]. A number of evidences link cigarette smoking and disease development and outcome in patients with RA [20]. Animal models with collagen-induced arthritis suggest that CS can augment the induction and clinical development of arthritis at both young and older mice [21].

In humans, estimations from the Swedish EIRA cohort study indicate that the excess fraction of anticitrullinated peptide antibody (ACPA) positive RA due to smoking (without considering the HLA-SE status) is 35% (95% CI 25–45). This could indicate that over one-third of RA cases would be prevented if people did not smoke [22].

Back to the late 1980s, Vessey et al. [23] found a marked increase in hospital admissions due to RA in smokers. It is not well established whether the association between smoke and RA is more frequent in men or women because there are studies suggesting both scenarios [24,25]. As previously mentioned, there is a correlation between packs smoked in a year and the risk for RA. Indeed, it is more elevated in 10 pack-years or more of smoking and increased linearly with increasing pack-years (HR 1.5e2). Nonetheless, the risk of RA remains substantially elevated even until 10–20 years after smoking ceased [26]. Data from a metaanalysis suggest that the risk for developing RA is about twice for male smokers than nonsmokers, whereas for female smokers, this risk seems to be about 1.3 times higher. This is not valid for heavy smokers (20 pack-years of smoking or more) in which the risk seems equally high for both genders [27].

Smoking seems to influence also the clinical phenotype of patients with RA. Tobacco habit contributes to the occurrence of extraarticular manifestations of RA in European, African American, and Korean populations. The occurrence of rheumatoid nodules is more frequent in seropositive RA smokers [19]. Even the response to therapy is influenced by smoking status [28]. Those patients who smoke more than 20 pack-years are less likely to improve after treatment; moreover, they seem to need a more aggressive treatment with disease-modifying antirheumatic drugs and have a poor response to anti–tumor necrosis factor (TNF) treatment. The most important variable is intensity of previous smoking rather than the smoking status at initiation of TNF antagonists [28]. Smokers are more frequently nonresponders, as it was recently suggested by data from the Swedish Rheumatology Register cohort [29]. Current smokers were less likely than nonsmokers to achieve a good response at 3 months following the start of MTX (27% vs. 36%) and at 3 months following the start of TNF inhibitors (29% vs. 43%; $P = .03$). Such lower likelihood of a good response was still present after at later follow-up visits (6 months, 1 year, and 5 years) with adjusted odds ratios (ORs) of 0.65, 0.78, 0.66, and 0.61, respectively.

Hutchinson and colleagues found that [30] heavy smoking was a risk factor for the disease development especially in patients without a family history of RA. When considering the first 7 years of age, maternal smoking during pregnancy can be responsible for infant RA and other inflammatory polyarthritis [31].

Another question is whether RA smokers also do develop a more severe joint damage. If there are studies suggesting they do not [32,33], or even that smoke may ameliorate disease progression [34,35] in others, tobacco exposure has been associated with a more erosive disease [36–38]. In a recent study from patients with early arthritis, the simple erosion narrowing score was found higher in current smokers and former smokers than in never smokers with a statistically significant difference [39].

The exact mechanisms are still unclarified. Lee and colleagues suggested that benzo[a]pyrene may increase the expression of Slug thus upregulating the invasive function of fibroblast-like synoviocytes [40]. This, in turn, may explain the increased radiological progression observed in RA smokers.

Noteworthy, it has been shown that complement, which has an important pathogenic role in RA, can be activated by smoke in vitro [41]. More recently, polymorphisms in the immune-related genes complement component 5 (C5) and/or TNF receptor-associated factor 1 (TRAF1) have been associated with increased susceptibility and disease progression (as determined by radiographic damage over time) in RA patients [42].

Moreover, polycyclic aromatic hydrocarbons (PAHs) such as 3-methylcholanthrene (3-MC), benzo[a]pyrene (B[a]P), and 2,3,7,8-tetrachlorodibenzo-p-dioxin (TCDD), which are contained in tobacco smoke, can upregulate IL1β mRNA in RA cell line that has the same features of parental synoviocytes [43]. Moreover, CS condensate can induce IL-1α, IL-1β, IL-6, and IL-8 at both mRNA and protein levels in these cells [44].

Ospelt et al. have shown that CS extract can induce changes in gene expressions with a significant upregulation of the heat shock proteins in synovial fibroblasts [45]. Finally, as it will be later discussed, despite that the strongest association with smoke is found in ACPA+ patients displaying the HLA-SE, it has been suggested that the role of smoke in the pathogenesis of RA is so strong to be even independent of the effect of *Porphyromonas gingivalis* [46], the notorious bacterium implicated in citrullination process [47].

SMOKING AND ANTICITRULLINATED PEPTIDE ANTIBODY—THE EVIL DUO

The etiology of RA is not fully understood, yet it is speculated that a complex interplay between genetic and environmental factors is involved in the pathogenesis of the disease [48]. Many of the RA-specific autoantibodies are generated against citrullinated antigens and termed ACPA [49]. ACPA can be detected in almost 80% of RA patients with a diagnosis specificity reaching 98% [50] and were reported to be more specific than rheumatoid factor for diagnosing RA [51]. ACPA are used as diagnostic markers of RA [51,52] in ELISA test that attains a high sensitivity and exhibits remarkable specificity for RA over other autoimmune conditions [53]. The assay has since been optimized, and it is included among the revised 2010 classification criteria for RA [54]. ACPA can be detected years before the onset of symptoms [55] and are associated with a more erosive disease course and poor remission rate [56].

The major targets for ACPA are citrullinated peptides, i.e., peptides, which underwent posttranslation conversion of arginine to citrulline-based residues. Citrullination is mediated by peptidylarginine deiminases (PADs), of which PAD2 and PAD4 are likely to be most important in RA [57]. In RA, many proteins, such as filaggrin, fibrinogen, vimentin, and collagen type II, are subjected to citrullination [58]. Inflamed joints of RA patients contain three times more citrullinated proteins within erosive tissue compared to nonerosive tissue [59]. It is widely acceptable that alterations in protein structure and antigenicity, resulting from the posttranslational modification of arginine to citrulline may break tolerance to citrullinated proteins and drive an autoimmune response, which eventually leads to disease [60]. Autoreactivity toward citrullinated peptides may contribute to the development of RA by giving rise to sets of neo-self-antigens in susceptible individuals.

Citrullinated-specific T cells may contribute to the pathogenesis of RA [61]. The hypothesis that ACPA response is T-cell dependent is supported by the following facts:

1. The PAD enzyme that catalyzes citrullination is not expressed in the thymus [62]; therefore, T cells reactive to citrullinated antigens are not likely to be eliminated, leaving an option of possible future immune reaction against citrullinated antigens.
2. ACPA formation correlates with specific human leukocyte antigen (HLA)-DRB1, DRB4, and DRB10 alleles [63,64]. These alleles encode for a specific peptide-binding pocket, on the antigen presenting cells the so-called shared epitope (SE) [65]. Citrullination increases self-antigen immunogenicity through better binding to SE-containing HLA-DRB molecules. The latter results in loss of tolerance to citrullinated antigens mediated by significant immune response to citrulline-specific autoreactive T cells, activation of immune cells, production of inflammatory cytokines that eventually results in synovial inflammation [63,66–68]. Studies in transgenic mice expressing the human HLA DRB1*0401 demonstrated that citrullination leads to enhanced T-cell activation and increased binding of peptides through the SE [66].

Smoking contributes to citrullination in RA patients who carry HLA-DRB1 SE alleles [69]. Smoking can induce citrullination through upregulation of PAD enzymes [70,71]. Susceptible individuals that possess the SE alleles in their HLA molecules may preferentially present citrullinated peptides to the immune system [72]. Smoking and the SE may therefore act in concert to drive the development of ACPAs and ultimately RA [73].

More genes contribute to RA predisposition such as polymorphisms in the PTPN22 gene. PTPN22 encodes for a tyrosine phosphatase; with a potential function in the regulation of T-cell and B-cell activation, it was found that single-nucleotide polymorphism (SNP) at 1858C/T substitutes the arginine to tryptophan residue in position 620 of mature protein and was found to be associated with ACPA-positive RA [74].

RA is a disorder comprising a complex onset mechanism and many associated complications, in particular, within the spectrum of pulmonary complications [75]. Smoking increases the risk of extraarticular RA occurring in the lung resulting in complications that carry high morbidity and mortality in RA [76]. In addition, smokers without RA have increased ACPA prevalence [77].

CS contains a mixture of over 4000 toxic substances including nicotine, carcinogens (PAHs), organic compounds (unsaturated aldehydes such as acrolein), solvents, gas substances (carbon monoxide), and free radicals [78].

Chronic exposure to CS has an effect on immune cells, such as macrophages, neutrophils, dendritic cells, and CD8+ T lymphocytes [79,80], and induce proinflammatory cytokines IL-6, IL-8, and TNF-α upregulation [81]. CS contains high levels of free radicals and other reactive oxygen species (ROS) that contribute to proinflammatory activation of lung cells via NF-κB and other redox-sensitive transcription factors [82]. Additional ROS, including superoxide, H_2O_2, and hypochlorous acid, are released by inflammatory macrophages and neutrophils via the action of enzymes, including xanthine/xanthine oxidase, myeloperoxidase, and NADPH oxidase, which have been linked to alveolar injury [83].

Other mediators such as elastase, matrix metalloproteases [81,84], somatic mutations, epigenetic mechanisms [85], and apoptosis [86] are enhanced in exposure to CS and play a critical role in the progressive destruction of the lung, leading to emphysema. It is believed that these pathways may also be activated in response to short-term tobacco smoke exposure in humans. CS exposure also augmented PAD expression and enhanced immune responses to citrullinated collagen and vimentin in mice [87].

Early events in the lungs may occur in the course of ACPA-positive individuals and might contribute to the systemic autoimmunity that precedes the onset of RA [71]. Smoking is likely to play a critical role in the onset of RA-associated autoimmunity because in the bronchoalveolar lavage (BAL) of healthy smokers, citrullination and PAD2 expression were increased compared with nonsmokers [71]. In addition, germinal center–like structures were found in rheumatoid lungs [88] and local enrichment of ACPAs in BAL fluids in early stages of ACPA-positive RA [89]. Smoking can also induce different autoantibodies formation; antinuclear autoantibodies were observed in the lungs of CS-exposed mice [90].

Cigarette smoking is the most dominant risk factor for chronic obstructive pulmonary disease (COPD), a common destructive inflammatory lung disease and increasing global health problem that is now the fourth leading cause of death in the western world [91]. The inhalation of toxic particles, mostly tobacco smoke, seems to be a seminal risk factor for COPD.

An increased incidence of COPD was demonstrated in patients diagnosed with RA compared to the non-RA population [92]. Furthermore, our group has shown that RA is associated with an increased risk of COPD independently of smoking [93].

Increasing evidence indicates that chronic inflammatory and autoimmune responses play a key role in the development and progression of COPD [94,95]. However, little is known on the association linking smoking, COPD, and serological markers associated with autoimmunity. Inflammation persists in patients with COPD after they stop smoking, suggesting an ongoing self-perpetuating immune process that continues after the initial stimulus of tobacco smoke has been removed [96].

In COPD, it is possible to hypothesize that the body regulatory system is not effective in preventing the lung damage caused by the effects of CS and subsequent inflammation; therefore, the immune system switches to a T helper 1 (Th1), Th17 response, which is proinflammatory [97].

Increased presence of citrullinated proteins has been demonstrated in the lungs of smokers; for example, elastin is often citrullinated in COPD [98]. Pathogenic features such as significant follicular B-cell hyperplasia has been demonstrated in lungs of RA patients. The follicular B lymphocyte may contribute to the humoral immune response through the production of ACPA. These antibodies complex with citrullinated peptides through Fc receptors might induce production of proinflammatory cytokines, including TNF-α. T lymphocytes are often recruited to the lung, where many displayed an activated phenotype and are essential to support B-cell activation and differentiation following antigen exposure. Fig. 37.1 illustrates as the presence of ACPA could contribute to autoimmune RA and COPD. The mechanisms by which ACPA elicits autoimmunity and the downstream effects on specific immune cells and humoral and cellular ACPA-specific immune responses in RA and COPD remain to be revealed. In wide perspective, treatment against the citrulline-specific immune response that aims to suppress the arthritis disease could putatively be applicable for COPD patients as well.

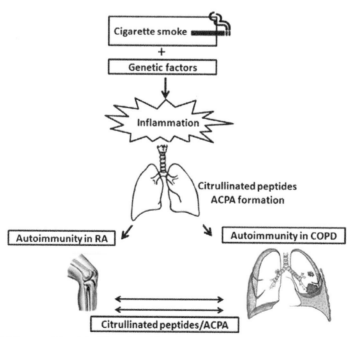

FIGURE 37.1 A schematic model for potential anticitrullinated peptide antibody (ACPA) formation in autoimmune process of rheumatoid arthritis (RA) and chronic obstructive pulmonary disease (COPD).

SMOKING AND INFLAMMATORY BOWEL DISEASE

Smoking was first recognized as a risk factor in the development of inflammatory bowel disease (IBD) more than 30 years ago [99,100]. Studies constantly show that smoking is the most significant environmental risk factor in Crohn's disease (CD) [101–104] while it positively affects the disease course of ulcerative colitis (UC) [104]. The different effects of smoking on cellular and humoral immune function in both diseases, their cytokine profiles, as well as bowel wall motility and permeability are among the potential mechanisms explaining such an opposite influence [105]. Moreover, studies suggest that smoking has diverse effects on the small and large intestine [103] and that the effect of smoking on CD and UC depends on the site of inflammation rather than on the type of disease [106]. Apparently, the influence of smoking is not identical in all clinical settings, and certain populations have not demonstrated any association between smoking and IBD [107–110]. The role of smoking in IBD was assessed in both animal models and clinical trials, but so far no single culprit mediator was identified. Nicotine is considered to be the active moiety in cigarettes and has been the leading focus in most studies [103,111,112]. It was shown that chronic nicotine exposure causes different effect on small and large intestine, a finding that might explain the opposite effect of smoking on CD and UC. For example, in the small intestine, nicotine exposure decreases prostaglandin E2, increases nitric oxide synthetase (NOS) activity, increases interleukin (IL)-6 and IL-10 levels, and has no effect on the circulation of the jejunum, whereas in the large intestine, nicotine exposure increases microcirculation and decreases IL-2 levels but has no effect on IL-6 and IL-10 as well as NOS and PGE2 [113,114]. Other suggested mechanisms include the effects of smoking on antioxidant and oxygen free radicals [115,116]; gut permeability [117]; microbiota changes [118]; and influence on gene expression profile of the colonic mucosa [119]. Further research is needed to understand the biological pathways and/or genetic predispositions, which explain why smoking is correlated with an increased risk for CD and a reduced risk for UC.

SMOKING AND CROHN'S DISEASE

Active smoking increases the risk for CD [102], as was confirmed in a previous metaanalysis (OR, 1.76; 95% confidence interval [CI] 1.40–2.22) [104]. Moreover, smoking may alter the course of CD; active smokers are more likely to suffer from frequent relapses [120,121], as this is involved with an increased probability of hospital admission and intestinal resection among patients with ileal involvement [120]. Current smoking is associated with late-onset CD (≥40 years old) and current smokers are more likely to progress to stricturing or penetrating type CD than nonsmoking patients [122]. Conflicting evidence exists regarding the association between smoking with respect to CD disease location [122]. Smoking seems to negatively affect the clinical course of CD in both females and males, but more so in females [123].

CD patients who start or continue smoking after disease diagnosis are at risk for higher therapeutic requirements, increasing the need for steroids, immunosuppressants, and reoperations [101,124]. Only a few studies investigating the influence of smoking on drug efficacy have been performed to date. Despite initial data [125,126], larger studies found no relation between smoking and infliximab response [127,128]. There is evidence that interventions designed to facilitate smoking cessation may improve the course of the disease [129]. When a CD patient is not able to quit smoking, a close monitoring is recommended and early step-up of more intensive therapeutic strategies should be considered, especially in females with ileal involvement [101].

SMOKING AND ULCERATIVE COLITIS

Current smoking was found to be protective against the development of UC (OR 1.79, 95% CI 1.37–2.34) [104]. After the onset of the disease, smoking might improve its course, decreasing the rate of relapses [130] and hospitalizations [131,132] reducing the need for corticosteroid and immunosuppressant therapy [133,134].

It remains controversial as to whether smoking reduces the rate of surgery required in UC, particularly colectomy [131,134,135]. Also, smoking's effect on pouchitis following colectomy with ileal pouch–anal anastomosis remains diverse. Some reported a reduced rate of pouchitis among current smokers [136], whereas others observed no significant difference [137]. In several studies, male ex-smokers have demonstrated delayed onset of disease compared with lifetime nonsmokers. Interestingly, no difference was detected in disease onset between female ex-smokers and nonsmokers [137,138].

Nicotine has demonstrated variable efficacy in the induction of remission in UC when compared to placebo and conventional therapy, including oral corticosteroids or mesalazine [139–141]. Different application methods have been used, including transdermal nicotine patches, nicotine chewing gum, and a nicotine-based enema [139–141]. However, nicotine's usage as a therapeutic treatment in UC is limited due to a high frequency of adverse events.

SMOKING, ANKYLOSING SPONDYLITIS, AND SPONDYLOARTHRITIS

During the last years, smoking has been largely investigated as a possible risk factor for disease onset and progression in ankylosing spondylitis (AS) and spondyloarthritis (SpA) patients. To date, data regarding this topic are mostly unclear, but the majority of studies highlight that smoking is associated with a higher disease activity, a worsening in functional ability, and a reduced quality of life in such cases [142–158]. In particular, several studies point out that smoking represents an inducing factor for a more rapid progression toward functional disability and a poor long-term outcome in patients diagnosed with AS and SpA [142–144]. In addition, smoking appears among factors associated with increased risk for advanced stages of the disease, a higher activity, and an earlier onset of inflammatory back pain in young axial SpA patients [144,145]. In line with this findings, many studies found that smoking has a dose-dependent relationship with measures of disease severity such as Bath AS Functional Index, a numerical rating scale of pain, the AS quality of life questionnaire, and the evaluation of AS quality of life measures [146–149]. In this regard, current smoking has been proven to have a negative impact on quality of life and activity efficacy of patients affected with AS and SpA [150,151] and has also been listed among variables associated with absenteeism and presenteeism [151,152]. In addition, also physical examination proves a more severe impairment among smoker than nonsmoker patients as finger floor distance, Schober test, cervical rotation, total spinal movement, later lumbar flexion, and chest expansion and occiput-wall distance are worse among smokers [143,144]. In line with these data, cigarette smoking has also been associated with radiographic severity and progression. In this regard, Waard et al. found that smoking status represents a variable able to estimate the likelihood of severe radiographic damage after 20 years of AS duration [153]. Similarly, Poddubnyy et al. demonstrated that smoking status is independently associated with radiographic progression and can be considered as a predictor of radiographic progression in axial SpA [154]. In addition, smoking intensity itself can affect radiographic progression in axial SpA patients [155]. Furthermore, smoking may be related not only to progression but also to development of AS itself. In support of this, a recent Norwegian population-based study including a large cohort of about 396.000 person-years follow-up time identified current smoking as one of the clinical variables significantly associated with incident AS [156]. In addition, smoking status has been found to be associated with the presence of MRI inflammation and structural damage in early axial SpA patients and inflammatory markers have been identified to be higher in smoker than nonsmoker AS patients [144]. Interestingly, a longitudinal study over 2 years highlighted that although Bath Ankylosing Spondylitis Disease Activity Index (BASDAI) evolution was similar between smoker and nonsmoker, the subgroup of SpA nonsmoker patients with increased C-reactive protein showed a better BASDAI decrease than smoker subjects. This finding suggested that smoking influence is driven by inflammatory mechanisms [157].

The different effect between current smoking and cumulative exposure represents a further conflicting issue. According to some studies, current smoking is associated with worse outcomes while cumulative exposure (pack-years of smoking) does not lead to any association with AS progression and functional limitation [156,158]. On the contrary, Mattey et al. also found that an increasing BASDAI score increased along with pack-year history. However, the strongest association was with current smoking, whereas increased levels of pain were primarily identified in current smokers rather than in past smokers. In any case, the authors conceded that distinguishing current and long-term smoking effects was difficult [146].

To date, the role of smoking on AS and SpA progression and severity is still a subject of debate and studies standing out from the crowd are available. Dincer et al., basing on data from 36 patients, found no differences in disease activity between smoking and nonsmoking AS patients. In addition, there was no association between poorer quality of life and smoking [159]. Furthermore, the risk of orthopedic AS-related spinal, root, and peripheral orthopedic surgery has not been found to be associated with smoking history [160]. Noteworthy, a recent study conducted on Australian AS patients showed that smoking did not induce a diminished or modified response to anti-TNF treatment. In fact, although current smokers tended to report poorer scores in some health-related quality of life (HRQoL) measures when compared to nonsmoker patients, active smoking did not affect the improvements in HRQoL from anti-TNF treatment [161].

Finally, although proinflammatory and pro-oxidative effects of smoking could contribute to the evolution toward AS and SpA onset and progression, smoking may partly act as a proxy for other important environmental factors [156]. Nevertheless, ceasing smoking seems an advisable treatment suggestion in AS and SpA patients.

PSORIASIS AND PSORIATIC ARTHRITIS

With regard to psoriasis, a large amount of data proves a significant association of prevalent psoriasis among former and current smokers. Cigarette smoking has been found to be more common in patients with psoriasis than in patients without psoriasis [162–167]. In addition, smoking has been also identified as an inducer factor responsible for a more severe disease course, an earlier disease onset, and a diminished response to treatment [166–169].

A dose–effect relation between smoking and psoriasis has been demonstrated in past cross-sectional and case-control studies with pack-years associated to a graded increase in the risk for psoriasis [170,171]. In particular, some authors found that smoking association with psoriasis was mostly sex-related, with a stronger and more consistent association among women than men [172,173]. However, a recent large study conducted on a United States (US) population of 185,836 people confirmed that smoking increases the risk for psoriasis development among both women and men without showing differences in the association among younger versus older women or between women and men [174]. In the same way, disease severity appears to be correlated with smoking in both genders [175].

To study the association between smoking and psoriasis, a recent systematic review and metaanalysis identified a total of 25 studies assessing the prevalence of psoriasis among smokers and nonsmokers. This metaanalysis revealed a significant association between psoriasis and current smoking. However, studies of higher quality and multivariate adjustment were found to generally report lower ORs for the association between psoriasis and smoking, thus suggesting some residual confounding in studies without multivariate adjustment [167]. Metaanalysis results also pointed out that both former and current smoking patients were more likely to develop incident psoriasis when compared with nonsmokers [167]. In this regard, Li et al. found that 15%–20% of incident psoriasis cases could be attributed to current or past smoking status, with a risk of developing psoriasis higher in current smokers than in past smokers. This finding suggests that quitting smoking could positively affect disease course [174]. Interestingly, the risk of psoriasis seems to monotonically increase with increasing duration of smoking. Specularly, the risk of incident psoriasis among former smokers progressively decreases over time [170,174]. Notably, Li et al. disclosed that both male and female past smokers had an augmented risk after having quit for more than 10 years. However, the risk was still higher for women after having quit for 20–29 years [174]. Similarly, Setty et al. found that the risk of psoriasis became comparable to that of nonsmoker 20 or more years after smoking cessation [170].

A graded association between smoking intensity and the risk of psoriasis has also been found, with current smokers subject to a greater risk than past smokers [170,176]. Likewise, studies generally support an association between psoriasis and the number of cigarette smoked daily with a significantly elevated relative risk of psoriasis in patients currently smoking 15 cigarettes or more per day [173,177,178].

Noteworthy, also prenatal and childhood passive smoke exposure itself has been associated with an increased risk of psoriasis [170,174]. In particular, Setty et al. found that second-hand smoke works as a risk factor in the case of prenatal and childhood exposure, whereas the risk was attenuated with passive smoke exposure after age 18 [170]. Conversely, Li et al. found that a positive association with adulthood passive smoking was observed only among male subjects [174].

Interestingly, the association between smoking and genetic predisposition should be also taken into account [176,179]. In particular, Zhu et al. demonstrated in a Chinese population that a specific *CHRNB3-CHRNA6* region gene polymorphism, encoding for nicotinic acetylcholine receptor subunits, may have impact on psoriasis severity when combined with smoking [179].

With regard to treatment efficacy, smoking was associated with nonresponse to anti–TNF-α treatment in patients with psoriasis [180]. Similarly, a smoking habit over 20 cigarettes/day has been found to likely affect the quality of the response to the anti–IL-12/23 agent ustekinumab [181] and an inverse relationship between smoking intensity and response to narrowband-UVB treatment in patients with early-onset psoriasis has also been described [182]. However, basing on data from 66 psoriatic patients, a recent retrospective review found no statistical difference in terms of clinical improvement in cutaneous psoriasis among nonsmokers and smokers on various systemic treatment regimens. For these reasons, the authors suggested that smoking did not affect response to systemic treatment in such patients. Nevertheless, they advocated further studies to better explore this issue [183].

Interestingly, despite the large amount of data about the correlation between smoking status and psoriasis, nicotine replacement therapy has been recently reported as leading to beneficial effects on psoriasis in one patient [184]. Conversely, the antismoking drug bupropion employed for smoking cessation has been found to aggravate psoriasis in another patient [185].

Psoriatic arthritis (PsA) is an inflammatory joint condition occurring in 6%–42% of psoriasis cases [186]. A relationship between PsA and smoking has been investigated in many association studies [187–194]. However, only sparse evidence on this link has been identified: according to Tey et al., smoking did not lead to a difference in the frequency of PsA in psoriasis patients [187]. In addition, a trend for a less-common smoking status among PsA patients compared with those with psoriasis alone was also reported [188]. In the wake of these data, other authors stated that smoking was associated with a delayed onset of PsA in patients with psoriasis [189], whereas Eder et al. even found an inverse association between smoking and PsA [190,191] although this peculiarity vanished in HLA-Cw6-positive patients [191].

Nevertheless, a large cohort study conducted on a US female population published in 2012 found that smokers showed an increased risk of incident PsA among past or current smokers. In addition, the risk was positively correlated with smoking intensity and duration, in particular among patients currently smoking 15 or more cigarettes daily, those with smoking duration of 25 years or more or smoking at least 20 pack-years. More severe PsA phenotypes by increasing smoking intensity and duration were also found. The authors explained the discrepancy with previous data by indicating that former studies did not take into account the main confounders, did not indicate a dose–response relationship, and could not determine the temporal association between smoking and later PsA onset because of study design [192]. Supporting such evidence, a year later, Tillett et al. suggested that smoking is associated with worse physical function in established PsA [193]. Similarly, recent data from a Swedish population-based cohort confirm that ever smokers report worse health status and more pain and fatigue than never smokers [194]. Notably, a shorter disease duration on start of anti-TNF agents has been found among current compared to never smokers, thus suggesting neither a more aggressive disease course nor a worse disease perception among smokers [195].

With regard to treatment response, according to data from an observational study in 1388 PsA patients initiating their first TNF inhibitor, current smokers reduced response rates, mostly among male smokers. In addition, current smokers had shorter treatment adherence than never smokers. In particular, treatment adherence was poorer for infliximab and etanercept but not for adalimumab. Interestingly, the effect of smoking on drug adherence among previous smokers diminished over time and was equivalent to never smokers after 4 years of smoking cessation [195]. In line with these findings, a single-centered study evaluating 78 PsA patients administered with TNF inhibitors showed that smokers were more likely to achieve a poorer treatment response both at 3- and at 6-month follow-up [196]. Furthermore, an observational study conducted on 440 patients found that current smoking at baseline was a significant predictor of anti-TNF agents termination at 3-year follow-up [197].

Ultimately, the recent National Psoriasis Foundation guidelines recommend quitting smoking in daily practice when treating psoriatic patients [198]. This appears desirable to remove a risk factor strongly suspected to induce a more severe disease course, an earlier disease onset, and a diminished response to psoriasis treatment. Because both psoriasis and PsA are linked to metabolic disorders and increased risk for cardiovascular diseases [199], removing smoking can also represent a useful clinical procedure beyond disease-specific considerations.

SMOKING AND BEHÇET'S DISEASE

During the past years, smoking has been identified as a behavioral factor capable to induce good clinical results in subjects suffering from recurrent oral aphtosis [200]. Although in 1999 a smoking-related worsening of oral aphtosis was reported by 3 out of 12 patients [201], cigarette smoking has been described to induce healing also in oral and genital ulcers related to Behçet disease (BD). Simultaneously, improvements on skin, articular, and subjective neuropsychiatric BD manifestations were also reported [202–204]. At first, the healing action of cigarettes had been considered local in action. However, further evidence suggested also systemic mechanisms [205,206]. In this regard, an increasing number of studies found an aggravation of both oral aphtosis and systemic BD-related features after smoking cessation [203,204,207–209]. Soy et al. found that 31 out of 47 (66%) asymptomatic BD current smokers experienced oral aphtosis after 1 week of smoking discontinuation. Conversely, among nonsmoking BD patients oral ulcers developed in only 25% in the same period [204]. Similarly, this inverse association between smoking and oral aphtosis occurrence has been also corroborated by a retrospective study on 118 BD patients [66]. In line with these findings, according to a small prospective trial by Kaklamani et al., five out of eight BD patients showed an increase in oral and/or genital aphtosis during a smoking discontinuation of at least 3 weeks. Notably, four of these patients started smoking again and no other mucosal lesions occurred. In addition, in the same study, one smoker and two nonsmoker BD patients underwent therapeutic nicotine administration showing no further lesions [208]. Accordingly, a case series describing five ex-smoker BD patients with refractory mucocutaneous manifestations reported that four patients quickly responded to nicotine-patch therapy experiencing a complete regression of all mucocutaneous lesions within 6 months. Nevertheless, nicotine therapy did not prove efficacy in the treatment and/or prevention of arthritis and uveitis [209]. Comparable results had been obtained in a previously reported BD woman suffering from severe oral aphtosis after stopping smoking [210].

The role of nicotine in BD has also been investigated in an in vitro study showing that nicotine inhibited IL-6 and IL-8 release from the keratinocyte and dermal microvascular endothelial cells thus suggesting a specific antiinflammatory effect of nicotine [211]. In addition, the antiinflammatory action of nicotine can be linked to skin nonneural cholinergic system and mediated by specific nicotinic acetylcholine receptors [212].

Toward mucocutaneous BD manifestations, the effect of smoking on other BD-related features remains controversial. In particular, although smoking has been repeatedly related to inflammatory eye diseases, a recent study found neither relations with BD uveitis nor with types of uveitis, time to resolution, and time to recurrences [213]. Similarly, Aramaki et al. found that cigarette smoking is even a risk factor for chronic progressive neuro-BD, especially when associated with

HLA-B51 positivity [205]. Therefore, smoking could affect BD manifestations according to a specific genetic background. In support of this, Özer et al. found that smoking influence on BD features can be augmented in patients carrying glutathione S-transferase (GST) polymorphisms, encoding for enzymes involved in the detoxification of chemicals. In particular, the specific GSTM1 null-polymorphism decreased the risk for papulopustular lesions and chronic arthritis also among smokers. Conversely, the risk for chronic arthritis was increased among nonsmoker patients carrying the same null-polymorphism. Instead, smoking made worse the risk for large-vessel vasculitis and venous insufficiency among male smoking BD patients with the GSTM1 and the GSTT1 null-polymorphisms, respectively [206].

In any case, smoking remains an important risk factor for several life-threatening clinical conditions. In addition, smoking can increase the risk for nonnecessarily BD-related clinical manifestations such as retinal vein occlusion and other vascular complications [214]. Consequently, an indirect unfavorable effect of smoking habit on some BD-related clinical manifestations is very likely and recommending cigarette smoking as a therapeutic approach does not seem advisable.

SMOKING AND SYSTEMIC LUPUS ERYTHEMATOSUS

Systemic lupus erythematosus (SLE) is an autoimmune inflammatory disease in which genetic and environmental factors interplay determining disease susceptibility [215]. Among the environmental factors, the trigger most widely accepted is the exposure to ultraviolet rays, associated with disease development and relapse. Within other environmental factors that intervene in the pathogenesis, similarly for the RA, the role of smoking has been suggested. Several studies evaluated this topic, suggesting an association not only between smoking and the systemic form of lupus, but also with the cutaneous lupus erythematosus (CLE).

Concerning the studies conducted on CLE patients, Miot et al. in 2005 performed a case-control study involving 57 patients with discoid CLE and 215 healthy controls [216]. A higher cigarette smoking prevalence was registered in patients (84.2%) than in controls (33.5%). Moreover, skin involvement at the disease onset was more extensive in smoker than nonsmoker patients [216]. The Finnish multicenter study published in 2008 analyzed three groups of subjects: 178 discoid LE, 55 subacute LE, and 77 SLE. Smoking at the onset of disease was significantly more frequent in all subgroups (57% for discoid CLE, 35% for subacute CLE, and 34% for SLE) compared with the age-/gender-matched healthy subjects [217].

These results were confirmed by the study of Boeckler et al. aiming at evaluating the association between smoking and cutaneous manifestations. The assessment of 108 CLE patients and 216 control subjects demonstrated a significant higher percentage of smokers in the patients compared with control subjects (73.1% vs. 49.5%; p < 0.001) [218].

In a recent retrospective descriptive study, conducted on 405 CLE, it was observed that 45.9% of patients smoked at the time of diagnosis. Moreover, significantly more CLE patients were smokers (45.9%) compared to the general population (33.2%, $P<.0001$). The analysis of the smoking prevalence in different CLE subgroups demonstrated a significantly higher prevalence of smokers in the population with tumidus and chronic LE ($P<.0001$) [219].

The study published by Kuhun et al. in 2014 aimed at investigating the influence of smoking on disease severity and antimalarial treatment in patients with CLE using the Core Set Questionnaire of the European Society of Cutaneous Lupus Erythematosus [220]. The analysis of 1002 patients, the greatest population described so far, demonstrated a higher percentage (87.2%) of patients with CLE already smoking at the time of diagnosis, compared with the 12.4% of the patients still not smoking at the date of their first diagnosis [220]. The Cutaneous Lupus Erythematosus Disease Area and Severity Index activity and damage score was higher in patients who have ever smoked than in nonsmokers [220]. These results were in agreement with previous data obtained by Piett et al. and Turchin et al. suggesting the influence of smoke habit on the severity of CLE [221,222].

Moving on SLE patients, the role of tabagism on the disease development was suggested by Hardy et al. in 1998 and Ghaussy et al. in 2001 [223,224]. These authors identified a higher risk of developing SLE in the current smokers compared with nonsmokers and ex-smokers [223,224]. The metaanalysis conducted by Costenbader et al. in 2004, in which nine studies were evaluated, revealed a small but significantly increased risk of SLE development among current smokers compared with nonsmokers (OR 1.50, 95% CI 1.09–2.08) [225]. More recently, a literature review published by Takvorian et al. in 2014, evaluated the epidemiology on the association between smoking and SLE [226]. Indeed, most of the studies evidenced such relationship, confirming that current smoking could be a stronger risk factor than former smoking [226]. Taken together, the results deriving from this literature review may suggest that smoking status could confer an immediate risk for SLE, with an OR at 1.31 (95% CI 1.02–1.70). On the other hand, the cessation of smoking seems associated with a reduction of the risk, which seems to return to that observed in subjects who have never smoked [226]. Moreover, the risk of developing SLE is also related with the average number of cigarettes smoked per day, cigarette-years of smoking, fraction smoked per cigarette, and degree of smoke inhalation. This result seems to find further confirmation in prospective studies in which a more accurate measure of CS exposure before the onset of disease was possible [226].

The results from the "1000 Canadian Faces of Lupus cohort" were in agreement with previous studies. The evaluation of 1346 SLE patients demonstrated that, according to the smoking use, 41.2% of the patients reported ever smoking, 34.1% of whom were current smokers and 65.9% of whom (27.1% of the entire cohort) were past smokers. Throughout multivariate analysis, an association between the condition of current smoker and the presence of active rash, as recorded by the SLEDAI-2K, was found. Moreover, among current smokers, the number of smoked packs-year seems to have a predictive role on the development of SLE. In addition, an association between past smoking and the ACR criteria of discoid rash and photosensitivity was also observed [227]. The absence of an association between smoking and cutaneous damage could be explained by the small number of patients with cutaneous damage in this cohort or could suggest the need of a longer observation period to demonstrate this possible relationship [227].

Contrasting results have been achieved from the evaluation of the influence of smoking habit on disease activity. The study conducted by Ghaussy et al. showed significantly higher SLEDAI scores over a 6-month period in current smokers compared to former and never smokers [228]. However, more recent studies showed different results. Smoking was not associated with SLE activity, evaluated by using the SLEDAI-2K, in a prospective study including 276 SLE patients conducted by Turchin et al. in 2009 [216]. Similar findings have been identified in a study conducted on 223 SLE patients. No significant differences in the SLEDAI scores between current smokers, ex-smokers, and never smokers have been identified; moreover, current smokers tended to have lower disease activity and anti-dsDNA antibodies levels [229].

Several studies have evaluated the association between smoking and specific SLE-related manifestations. As above-mentioned, an association with skin manifestations has been reported by studies conducted on CLE and SLE populations [216–218,220,237]. The study conducted by Ward et al. on an inception cohort of 160 adults with lupus nephritis identified a strong association between smoking at the onset of nephritis and the development of the end-stage renal disease (ESDR). The median time to ESRD was significantly lower in smokers compared with nonsmoker subjects [230].

As expected, the smoking status may influence the occurrence of thrombotic events. Data from the LUMINA cohort indicated that smoking is a predictor of vascular events and should be strongly discouraged and contributes in the occurrence of thrombotic events (OR = 2.777) [231,232].

Smoking can also affect the response to antimalarial drugs agents. A recent metaanalysis, focusing on this topic, analyzed 10 observational studies evaluating 1398 CLE patients and found that smoke may impair the response to antimalarial drugs. Indeed, an overall twofold decrease in the proportion of smoker versus nonsmoker patients reaching response to antimalarial drugs in CLE has been demonstrated [233]. The association between smoking and poor response to antimalarial drugs was confirmed for both chloroquine and hydroxychloroquine drugs [220,234,235]. Moreover, the study conducted by Jewell et al. suggested a negative correlation between response and the number of packs smoked per day [234]. The mechanisms by which smoking may interfere with antimalarial drugs remain largely unknown. Some hypothesis have been suggested; among these, the role of tobacco smoking on the induction of the cytochrome p450 system could influence the response to antimalarial agents, due to the involvement of this pathway in their metabolism [236].

Smoke has been shown to have a role in the production of anticitrullinated protein antibodies in RA patients. Similarly, some studies attempted to find a correlation between smoke and the production of pathogenic antibodies in SLE patients, with contrasting results [237–239]. The study conducted by Freemer and colleagues in 2006 suggested the mechanism by which smoking could determine the development of anti-dsDNA. The authors suggest that smoking could damage DNA molecules, determining the development of antibodies targeting these molecules. These data seem confirmed by the identification of significant higher frequency of anti-dsDNA in SLE smoker patients [236]. Data from the recent study published by Young et al. are not in agreement with these results. The evaluation of 1242 SLE patients, 981 first-degree relatives, and 946 controls in the Lupus Family Registry and Repository did not identify a clear association between smoking and autoantibodies development in all the three groups evaluated [239]. In particular, no associations were found between ever smoking and being positive for more than one autoantibody in SLE subjects, nor in unaffected first-degree relatives and healthy controls. In addition, a similar lack of association between higher number of pack-years smoked and autoantibody positivity was identified [239].

Despite these contrasting results, several data demonstrated the presence of multiple chemical factors in the cigarettes, able to generate free radicals, with possible modification of both the innate and adaptive immune arms [240]. Smoking seems able to modify the inflammatory cell function: in particular, CS has been associated with the activation of macrophage and dendritic cell and with the increase of autoreactive B cells. Taken together, these modifications could determine an increased production of proinflammatory cytokines (i.e., TNF, IL-1, IL-6, IL-8 GM-CSF) and the reduction of antiinflammatory cytokines levels, such as IL-10. At the same extent, an increased production of autoantibodies could be observed [240]. More recently, a positive association between ever, and above all former, regular cigarette smoking and presence of antiphospholipid (aPL) antibodies has been demonstrated among patients with SLE [241]. In particular, former smoking status was associated with aPL IgG isotype as well as with lupus anticoagulant positivity, widely accepted as the strongest risk factor for thrombotic events. Conversely, current smoking tended to be associated with IgM isotype aPL. This association may suggest that smoking may act triggering an immunological response with initial IgM production and a later persistent "IgG memory," as was the case of infections. This is confirmed by the observation that smoking cessation does not seem to influence the aPL status, with persistent positivity [242].

SMOKING AND MULTIPLE SCLEROSIS

Multiple sclerosis (MS) is the most common chronic inflammatory demyelinating disease of the central nervous system (CNS). It is characterized by localized areas of inflammation, demyelination, axonal loss, and gliosis in the brain and spinal cord, resulting in a variety of neurological symptoms disseminated in time and space. In many countries, it is the leading cause of nontraumatic disability in young adults [243,244].

Understanding the etiology of MS is of increasing importance because a universal rise in the incidence and prevalence of the disease is observed over the last decade [244,245]. However, despite recent advances in the understanding of its pathogenesis, the cause of MS is still unclear. MS is thought to involve both genetic susceptibility and environmental factors [246]. The strongest genetic associations with MS are presence of HLA-DRB1*15 providing a threefold higher risk of developing MS and HLA-A*02 conferring a twofold protective effect [247]. Furthermore, growing evidence indicates that environmental factors, such as previous infection with Epstein–Barr virus, low levels of vitamin D, and obesity contribute to MS susceptibility [248–250].

Alongside other autoimmune conditions, cigarette smoking is now clearly established as a risk factor of MS. The role of smoking in MS was first consistently investigated in 2001 by Hernàn et al. [251] in a large prospective study based on two cohorts of women, Nurses' Health Study (NHS, 121,700 women) and Nurses' Health Study II (NHSII, 116,671 women). Smoking exposure was assessed by biennial questionnaires. During the follow-up, 315 MS cases were documented, with a relative incidence rate of 1.6 among current smokers and 1.2 among past smokers. Remarkably, the relative risk increased proportionally with cumulative exposure to smoking. These observations have subsequently been supported by several studies [252–262] demonstrating that both active and passive smoking were risk factor for MS with an OR ranging from 1.5 to 2.67. Unlike other environmental factors that seem to act only if the exposure takes place early in life (gestation, childhood, or adolescence), smoking appears to affect MS risk irrespective of age at exposure [258].

These data were confirmed in 2015 by Belbasis et al. in a broad metaanalysis [258]. Among 44 metaanalyses regarding environmental risk factors for MS, three meeting all the methodological requirements were included and showed smoking as one of the strongest consistent risk factors of developing MS with an overall OR = 1.52, corresponding to a 50% higher risk.

More interestingly, Hedström et al. provided evidence of gene–environment interactions. In two Swedish population-based case-control studies [263,264], the authors observed a potentiated risk of developing MS when combining passive or active smoke exposure with genetic risk factors (presence of HLA-DRB1*15 and absence of HLA-1*02). Although smokers and passive smoking-exposed subjects with any of the two genetic risk factors displayed an OR = 1.3–1.4 for MS, and nonsmokers genetically susceptible subjects had an OR = 4.5–4.9, surprisingly combination of both genetic risk factors and passive or active smoking rendered an OR = 7.7–13.5.

A number of mechanisms have been proposed to explain the involvement of tobacco in the occurrence of MS. Especially, it has been demonstrated that contrary to smoked tobacco, tobacco snuff use does not increase MS risk [264], suggesting that tobacco does not exert a systemic effect but acts through lung irritation. This hypothesis is supported by experiments conducted in experimental autoimmune encephalomyelitis (EAE) mice, detecting that the lungs constitute a niche for resting autoimmune memory cells; after local stimulation of the lungs, these cells strongly proliferate and after assuming migratory properties, enter the CNS and induce paralytic disease [265].

Besides its role as a risk factor in MS onset, tobacco has also been shown to accelerate disease progression and worsen prognosis. First evidence was provided in 2005 by Hernàn et al. [266], demonstrating in a cohort study including 179 relapsing remitting MS that the risk for transforming to a secondary progressive MS (SPMS) was 3.6 times higher for ever smokers compared with never smokers. Subsequently, despite some negative studies [267–269], most reports have confirmed these observations, while providing new data [270–282]. Thus, it was shown that in addition to promoting acceleration of MS to secondary progressive course, smoking also enhances disease activity as measured by the Expanded Disability Status Scale, increases the number and volume of demyelinating lesions on MRI as well as cerebral atrophy, and alters cognitive functions and quality of life [271–282]. Similarly, smoking is an independent factor associated with a higher risk for early conversion to clinically definite MS after a clinically isolated syndrome(namely a first episode of neurologic symptoms that lasts at least 24h and is caused by inflammation and demyelination in one or more sites in the CNS) [271–282]. In 2015, Ramanuajam et al. [281] provided evidence in an elegant cross-sectional study that each additional year of smoking after diagnosis of MS accelerated the time to conversion to SPMS by 4.7%. Those who continued smoking reached SP disease at 48 versus 56 years of age for those who quit. Consequently, tobacco is a major modifiable factor representing a key target. Furthermore, concerning prognosis, tobacco smoking is associated with MS with greater mortality with hazard ratio ranging from 1.38 to 2.70 [283–285]. Even more surprisingly, current smokers have been found to exhibit an enhanced risk of developing neutralizing antibodies to interferon (IFN)-beta therapy with an OR = 1.9–5.6 [286–288].

Whether the mechanisms underlying this observation are still unknown, several hypotheses have been proposed to explain the deleterious effect of smoking on the overall course of MS [288–290]. In an EAE mice model, Gao et al. [290] found that nicotine in CS prevented disease exacerbation, whereas nonnicotine components, especially acrolein, were responsible for acceleration and increase of clinical symptoms by promoting demyelinization, activating microglia and eventually becoming cytotoxic to the cells. Recently, Correale et al. [289] demonstrated that cigarette smoking conducted to reduced indoleamine 2,3 dioxygenase activity and subsequent higher production of IL-6 and IL-13. Moreover, smoking patients exhibit elevated levels of renin–angiotensin system activity, inducing IL-17 and IL-22 producing cells number, as well as CCL2, CCL3, and CXCL10 production by monocytes. Both pathways lead to a significant decrease in CD4 + CD25 + FoxP3 + regulatory T cells. Exposure to CS has also been found to induce blood–brain barrier oxidative stress [291].

In summary, to date, strong evidence demonstrates that smoking is an independent risk factor for developing MS, in a dose-dependent manner, regardless of the age of exposure. Moreover, many data show a major detrimental effect of tobacco on the course of the disease, promoting a more active disease and an earlier transition to a secondary progressive form. Therefore, smoking is so far the most important modifiable factor involved in the pathogenesis of MS. Further studies are needed to clarify the pathogenic mechanisms.

SMOKING AND AUTOIMMUNE LIVER DISEASE

Autoimmune hepatitis (AIH), primary biliary cirrhosis (PBC), and primary sclerosing cholangitis (PSC) are the tree major forms of autoimmune liver disease, which differ according to the focus of autoimmune injury, the pattern of inflammation, and the clinical phenotype [292]. PBC is an autoimmune liver disease characterized by chronic inflammation and targeted destruction of biliary epithelial cells lining the small to medium-sized interlobular bile ducts [293]. The disease is characterized by circulating antimitochondrial antibodies (AMA) as well as disease-specific antinuclear antibodies, cholestatic liver biochemistry, and characteristic histology. The disease primarily affects middle-aged females, and its incidence is apparently increasing worldwide [294]. As with most other autoimmune diseases, development of PBC is thought to entail the action of environmental stressors in genetically susceptible individuals [295]. Robust genetic associations with specific HLA alleles, a marked female predominance, and the near ubiquity of AMA specific for the E2 subunit of the pyruvate dehydrogenase complex (PDC-E2) in PBC patients indicate that PBC is a prototypical autoimmune disease. Evidence for the role of genetic factors is provided by high disease concordance in monozygotic twins, increased sibling risk of AMA positivity and PBC development, and overlap with other autoimmunity [296]. Epidemiological studies have indicated several risk factors for the development of PBC, with family history of PBC, recurrent urinary tract infection, and smoking being the most widely cited [294]. A questionnaire was developed by the Mayo Clinic Survey Center and collected information regarding demographics, anthropometric features, education, lifestyle, and environmental exposures as well as extensive personal and familial medical history to assess risk factors for PBC [297]. A history of regular cigarette smoking, defined as lifetime smoking of more than 100 cigarettes, was reported by 53% of PBC cases compared to 40% of controls ($P<.001$). The total duration as a regular smoker was slightly longer among PBC cases compared to controls (22.0 years vs. 21.0 years, $P=.04$), with a median of 10.5 pack-years smoked by cases prior to the diagnosis to PBC. Lifetime exposure to second-hand smoke at home (81% vs. 73%, $P=.01$) was significantly higher in PBC cases compared to controls. There was no difference between the groups in regard to exposure at work, although among the exposed, the total number of years of second-hand smoke was higher in the cases ($P<.001$) (6). A study by Gershwin et al. enrolled patients with PBC (n = 1032) from 23 tertiary referral centers for liver diseases in the US and random digit–dialed controls (n = 1041) matched for sex, age, race, and geographical location and reported that a greater proportion of PBC cases reported a past history of cigarette smoking (60% vs. 54%; $P=.0034$), but more controls were active smokers at the time of the interview (32% vs. 16%; $P<.0001$). Compared with controls, patients with PBC reported a lesser time of passive smoke in both the workplace and at home [298]. Parikh-Patel et al. conducted a survey using standardized NHANES (National Health and Nutrition Examination Survey) questions to 241 PBC patients in the US, 261 of their siblings, and 141 friends without PBC and reported the elevated adjusted ORs for smoking (OR 2.04, 95% CI 1.10–3.78) when cases were compared with their siblings and the significance of smoking in the multivariate models supports the findings of previous studies and raises the issue of the influence of smoking on a Th1 response [299]. A study by Corpechot et al. was performed and enrolled 222 patients with PBC and 509 controls matched for age, gender, and residential location with standardized questionnaire data confirming the individual history of active or passive smoking (OR 3.1, 95% CI 2.0–5.0) as a risk factor for PBC [300]. AIH is a complex disease: it is a multifactorial polygenic disorder that is probably caused by the interaction of a trigger and environmental factors in a genetically susceptible individual. Specific genetic variants or polymorphisms increase or decrease the risk of disease, and possession of a potential disease-causing mutation in itself does not cause disease [301–303]. Several environmental agents, such as viruses, have been suggested as putative triggers for AIH [304]. Research has identified several agents that precipitate AIH, such as minocycline, tienilic acid, nitrofurantoin, pemoline, melatonin, ornidazole, diclofenac, propylthiouracil, and statins. Herbal remedies, such as dai-taiko-so (da chai hu tang; commonly used in Japan), have also been associated with the disorder [304]. To the best of our knowledge, smoking was not reported as a risk factor for AIH.

PSC is a challenging illness that is characterized by chronic bile duct destruction and progression to end-stage liver disease. No effective medical treatments are available. Although PSC affects both sexes and all age groups, more than 60% of patients are men and the median age at onset is 30–40 years. Patients are usually nonsmokers, and 60%–80% of cases in northern European populations are clearly associated with IBD (compared with 30%–50% of cases in southern European and Asian populations) [305]. PSC without colitis probably shows the effects of a mosaic of interacting genetic and environmental risks of different strengths. A recent study by Andersen et al. investigated the relationship between environmental risk factors and susceptibility to PSC and the data were analyzed from 240 patients with PSC and 245 control subjects, matched for gender and age. Twenty percent of the patients were ever (current or former) daily smokers compared with 43% of control subjects (OR 0.33, 95% CI 0.22–0.50, $P < .001$), which means that smoking might protect against development of PSC [306]. Another study aiming to examine the risk factors in patients with PSC with and without underlying IBD by Mitchell et al. enrolled 170 patients with PSC, 41 without underlying IBD, 170 patients with UC but normal liver function tests, and 170 age- and sex-matched community controls were obtained by questionnaire and reported that PSC, like UC, is a disease of nonsmokers as the odds of having PSC was significantly decreased among current and former smokers and the OR of having PSC was 0.17 (95% CI 0.08–0.35) among current smokers and 0.33 (95% CI 0.21–0.52) among ever (former + current) smokers [307]. A case-control study by Loftus EV et al. reported OR of having PSC was significantly decreased among current smokers [308].

SMOKING AND SYSTEMIC SCLEROSIS

Systemic sclerosis (SSc) is a multisystem disorder characterized by microvascular disease, a disturbance in fibroblast function, and immune system activation, culminating in fibrosis of skin and internal organs [309]. SSc is very heterogeneous, but skin involvement is nearly universal and two common clinical subsets based on the extent of skin involvement are typically recognized, namely, limited SSc with skin involvement below the elbows and knees and diffuse SSc with skin involvement of the proximal limbs and/or trunk [310]. Although environmental factors have been implicated as contributors to the development of SSc in a genetically susceptible host, the exact role of environmental triggers in the etiology of SSc remains unclear [311]. Few studies have been investigating the role of cigarette exposure in susceptibility to SSc. A review of 1379 patients with SSc enrolled in the SSc family registry was conducted and reported that the majority of patients had never smoked (57%), whereas 43% of patients were classified as ever smokers. The patients with SSc did not differ from control subjects in terms of their smoking behavior (OR 1.020, 95% CI 0.839–1.240, $P = .842$) [311]. A study from Hudson et al. investigated the effects of cigarette smoking on vascular, gastrointestinal, and respiratory outcomes in patients with SSc. This study included 606 patients with SSc; of these patients, 16% were current smokers, 42% were past smokers, and 42% were never smokers. The regression analyses showed that smoking had a significant negative effect on almost all vascular, gastrointestinal, and respiratory outcomes. The effects of smoking were in some cases long-lasting (e.g., persistent respiratory abnormalities), and smoking cessation appeared beneficial with respect to some outcomes (e.g., reduced severity of Raynaud's phenomenon) [312]. Hissaria et al. reported in a cohort consisted of 786 SSc patients that there is no association of smoking history (ever smoked, never smoked, or pack-year history) with any clinical variables (vascular, gastrointestinal, or respiratory). Moreover, the cumulative proportional survival analysis revealed that survival was decreased in past or present smokers (i.e., those designated as ever having smoked) compared with those who had never smoked [313].

SMOKING AND THYROID AUTOIMMUNITY

A dysregulation of the immune system causes an immune attack on the thyroid leading to the onset of autoimmune thyroid diseases (AITDs) that are T-cell mediated organ-specific autoimmune disorders [314,315].

The prevalence of AITD is estimated to be about 5%, whereas the frequency of antithyroid autoantibodies may be even higher [316,317].

Two main clinical presentations are typical of AITD: Graves' disease (GD) and Hashimoto's thyroiditis (HT) (both characterized by lymphocytic infiltration of the thyroid parenchyma), whose clinical hallmarks are, respectively, thyrotoxicosis and hypothyroidism [314,318].

Systemic autoimmune diseases (Sjögren's syndrome, RA, SLE, SSc, cryoglobulinemia, sarcoidosis, PsA) and other organ-specific autoimmune disorders (polyglandular autoimmune syndromes) are associated with AITD.

The determinant role of cytokines and chemokines in the pathogenesis of autoimmune thyroiditis (AT) and GD has been shown by different studies. In the thyroid gland, recruited Th1 lymphocytes may be responsible for an increase in the secretion of IFN-γ and TNF)-α, which in turn stimulates CXCL10 (the prototype of the IFN-γ–inducible Th1 chemokines) secretion from thyrocytes, in this way creating an amplification feedback loop, which attracts other lymphocytes and initiates and perpetuates the autoimmune process [319,320].

The etiology of the autoimmune attack to the thyroid is still unknown, but it is suggested by epidemiological data that an interaction among genetic susceptibility and environmental triggers could be the determinant factor causing the breakdown of tolerance and the development of the disease.

The familial clustering of the disease (20%–30% of AITD in siblings of affected patients; sibling risk ratio of about 17 for AITD), the increased prevalence of thyroid antibodies (50%) in siblings of affected subjects, and the results of twin studies (with a concordance rate for AITD of 0.3–0.6 for monozygotic, compared to 0.00–0.1 for dizygotic twins) demonstrate the importance of genetic susceptibility in AITD. The heritability of GD has been calculated to be about 80%, while that associated with the presence of thyroid antibodies is about 70% [321–323]. Genome-wide association studies and Immunochip have also identified various genes significantly associated with the AITD and the presence of thyroid antibodies [324]. Most of the susceptibility genes whose function is known are involved in T cells function, suggesting the importance of T lymphocytes in the immunopathogenesis of AITD. Environmental factors (as radiation, iodine, smoking, infection, stress, and drugs) contribute to the occurrence of AITD for about 20% [325]. Among environmental factors, cigarette smoking has been associated with GD and Graves' ophthalmopathy (GO) [326,327], whereas it has been suggested that it decreases the risk of overt hypothyroidism as well as the prevalence of thyroid antibodies [328,329].

SMOKING AND THYROIDITIS

Controversial results are reported about the effect of smoking on thyroid autoantibodies (antithyroglobulin [AbTg] and antithyroperoxidase [AbTPO]) and chronic AT [330].

A first study reviewed the smoking habits of 1730 women. The prevalence of smokers in AT was about 30%, not different from that of controls. In addition, other studies confirmed the absence of association between smoking and thyroid autoimmunity [331].

A discordant result was reported in a retrospective study that examined the relationship between smoking history and thyroid function in 387 women patients with HT, suggesting that an increase in serum thiocyanate concentration from smoking may contribute to the development of hypothyroidism in patients with HT [332]. A metaanalysis suggested that HT and postpartum thyroid dysfunction were associated with smoking [333]. However, the results of a large prospective cohort study in subjects at risk of developing AITD, for example, healthy female relatives of AITD patients, showed that smoking was negatively correlated with the presence of AbTPO [334]. The relationship between smoking and thyroid abnormalities was also evaluated in the 1988–94 Third National Health and Nutrition Examination Survey (NHANES III), a cross-sectional study. Smoking appeared to be negatively associated with serological evidence of thyroid autoimmunity and hypothyroidism and positively associated with mild thyroid-stimulating hormone decreases [335].

A study investigated a cohort of 874,507 parous women with self-reported information on smoking during pregnancy, registered in the Swedish Registry, with hospital diagnoses of thyroiditis (n=286) and hypothyroidism (n=690). Smoking was inversely associated with risk of overt thyroiditis, while increased the risk of thyroiditis occurring in the postpartum period [336].

In a cross-sectional comparative population study performed in two areas of Denmark with moderate and mild iodine deficiency, 4649 subjects were examined, and AbTPO and AbTg were determined. There was a negative association between smoking and the presence of thyroid autoantibodies in serum [337].

A prospective cohort study of 521 euthyroid women without thyroid antibodies in serum who were relatives of AITD patients and were followed for 5 years was conducted. Discontinuation of smoking was associated with an increased risk for occurrence of AbTPO and/or AbTg in serum [338].

Subsequently, a nested case-control study was conducted, within the prospective Amsterdam AITD cohort study, in which 790 healthy euthyroid women, with at least one first- or second-degree relative with documented AITD, were followed for 5 years. At the time of event, hypothyroid cases were less common among current smokers than their controls [339].

In a population-based, case-control study, 140 cases of newly diagnosed primary autoimmune overt hypothyroidism were identified prospectively by population monitoring and individually, age-, sex-, and region-matched with euthyroid controls (n=560). The risk of having overt autoimmune hypothyroidism was more than sixfold increased in the first 2 years after cessation of smoking [340].

Even more recently, smoking habit was not associated to an increased risk of HT in an Italian study [341].

Overall, the abovementioned studies suggest that smoking reduces the risk of occurrence of AbTPO and AbTg and autoimmune hypothyroidism by about 40%. The protective effect of smoking on thyroid autoimmunity is dose dependent and disappears a few years after the cessation. It is not clear how smoking could exert these protective effects; however, it has been suggested that this effect might be related to activation of nicotine receptors on immune cells, which leads to a shift of the autoimmune profile away from Th1 and Th17 responses [328,329].

GRAVES' DISEASE, OPHTHALMOPATHY, AND SMOKING

Bartalena et al. first studied the smoking habits of 1730 women. Smokers were 47.9% in GD and 64.2% in GO groups, versus about 30% in controls. The percentage of heavy smokers was higher in patients with more severe ophthalmopathy [330]. Similar results were confirmed in other studies [342–345].

In a consecutive entry case-control study with two age- and sex-matched control subjects, smoking was associated with GD, and it especially increased the risk for the development of more severe ophthalmopathy [326]. Furthermore, in an epidemiological study of thyrotoxicosis in Sweden, the increased incidence of GD in females was partially related to changes in smoking habits [346].

A randomized, single-blind study of smoking and mild ophthalmopathy after radioiodine therapy showed an increased risk for progression of ophthalmopathy after radioiodine therapy and a decreased efficacy of orbital radiation therapy and glucocorticoid therapy [327]. Moreover, in a double-blind prospective randomized study, of levothyroxine administration, both during and after antithyroid drugs (ATD) treatment in GD, showed that two factors, namely positive thyroid stimulating hormone receptor antibodies at the end of ATD treatment, and regular smoking habits may represent clinically useful predictors of the risk of recurrence in patients with Graves' hyperthyroidism treated with ATD [347]. These results were confirmed in other studies [348,349].

A study compared the occurrence of worsening or development of thyroid-associated ophthalmopathy (TAO) in patients who were treated with radioiodine or ATD. Radioiodine treatment was a significant risk factor for the development of TAO in Graves' hyperthyroidism. However, smokers run the highest risk for worsening or development of TAO irrespective of treatment modality [350]. In addition, other studies confirmed these last results [351,352].

In 95 consecutive patients with untreated GO, the ratios of fat volume/orbital volume (FV/OV) and muscle volume/OV (MV/OV) were calculated with validated software. Smoking was associated with an increase in extraocular MV in untreated patients with GO and not with an increase in FV [353]. The abovementioned studies suggest that smoking increases about twofold the risk of Graves' hyperthyroidism and about three- to fourfold the risk of GO. Furthermore, smoking habit is related to a more severe GO, and to worsening or development of GO in GD patients irrespective of treatment modality, or relapse of GD or GO. It is not clear how smoking could increase these effects in GD or GO, even if many studies have addressed this point. In one study, it has been shown that extraocular muscle fibroblasts respond differently from dermal fibroblasts following cytokine stimulation, which may explain in part the anatomical localization of ophthalmopathy. Hypoxia stimulates fibroblasts and this could contribute, as an enhancing factor, to the adverse effects of smoking on thyroid eye disease [354]. Later it has been shown that oxygen-free radicals may contribute to the retroocular fibroblast proliferation observed in patients with GO [355]. Cigarette smoking might also act by enhancing generation of oxygen-reactive species and reducing antioxidant production [356].

Oxidative DNA damage was assessed by determination of the 8-hydroxy-2'-deoxyguanosine (8-OHdG) level in urine in GO patients. The results demonstrated that urinary 8-OHdG was increased in GO patients and was correlated with the disease activity; smoking had a higher impact on the increased 8-OHdG among GO patients [357].

Furthermore, it has been shown that CS extract induced adipogenesis in Graves' orbital fibroblasts, which was inhibited by quercetin via reduction in oxidative stress [358]. More recently, hypoxia has been shown to induce adipogenesis in orbital fibroblasts, suggesting that it may represent a mechanism by which smoking contributes to the deterioration of GO [359]. The expression of HLA (HLA-DR) increased threefold when nicotine (25 ng/mL) in combination with IFN-γ (500 U/mL) was added to cultured orbital fibroblasts, suggesting a further possible molecular mechanism for the more severe ophthalmopathy observed in Graves' patients who smoke cigarettes [360]. Furthermore, smoking was associated with increased sICAM-1 and decreased sVCAM-1 levels in another study in GO patients [361]. Genetic studies were also performed. In a prospective case-control study GSTP1, CYP1A1, and TP53 germline polymorphisms were associated with smoking-related GD susceptibility [362].

A total of 98 SNPs in 12 genes were genotyped in 594 GD patients with (n=267) or without (n=327) GO and 1147 sex- and ethnicity-matched controls from Malmö, Sweden. It was found an association of SNPs in immediate early genes (IEGs) and stearoyl-coenzyme A desaturase with GD and/or GO. Smoking and cysteine-rich, angiogenic inducer 61 (CYR61) rs12756618 interacted to increase the risk of GO [363].

More recently, gene expression in intraorbital fat was studied in smokers and nonsmokers with severe active GO. IEGs, IL-1B, and IL-6 were overexpressed in smokers with severe active GO compared to nonsmokers, suggesting that smoking activates pathways associated with adipogenesis and inflammation [364].

In conclusion, smoking increases about twofold the risk of Graves' hyperthyroidism and about three- to fourfold the risk of GO. Furthermore, smoking habit is related to a more severe GO, and to worsening or development of GO in GD patients irrespective of treatment modality, or relapse of GD or GO, and to a less favorable outcome of GO treatment with steroids or retrobulbar irradiation. These effects of cigarette smoking might be due, at least in part, to enhancing generation of oxygen-reactive species and reducing antioxidant production.

SMOKING AND TYPE 1 DIABETES

Type 1 diabetes (T1D) affects about 36 million individuals worldwide, and the incidence is increasing worldwide by about 3% annually [365]. An antigen-specific assault on the insulin-producing β-cells of the pancreas by T cells is the cause of T1D; this leads to deficient insulin secretion, resulting in dysregulation of blood glucose [366]. ThCD4+ cells and cytotoxic (CD8+) T lymphocyte induce an immune reaction that leads to destroy β-cells and to a deficient insulin secretion [367,368].

A predominance of the Th1 immune response is associated with the development of the autoimmune response in T1D [369]. Th1 cytokines and chemokines (CXCL10) play an important role in this process [370,371].

The production of a number of autoantibodies against β-cell antigens (i.e., insulin, glutamic acid decarboxylase [GAD]65, tyrosine phosphatase autoantibodies [IA–2A], Zinc Transporter 8, CD38, etc.) precedes or accompanies this immune reaction. These autoantibodies are useful in identifying subjects at risk of developing T1D [369,372].

T1D results from interactions between susceptibility genes and environmental triggers. Many progresses have been done in finding T1D susceptibility genes [373,374]. However, the identification and confirmation of environmental risk factors associated with T1D need more efforts [375–378]. Among studies that evaluated a possible association between maternal or paternal smoking during pregnancy and childhood T1D, only two found a significant risk for smoking. In a case-control study, a total of 105 recently onset diabetic and 210 control children, individually matched by age (±1 year), sex, and place of residence, were included. The frequency of maternal smoking during pregnancy was higher in T1D cases (37%) compared to controls (25%) [379].

Wahlberg et al. studied 7208 unselected 2.5-year-old children from the All Babies in Southeast Sweden cohort. Maternal smoking during pregnancy and heavy smoking at home (>10 vs. ≤10 cigarettes) were associated with a significant risk for IA–2A, but not for GAD+ antibody [380]. Other studies failed to find any effect of maternal smoking on islet autoimmunity in newborns [381–383].

Paternal smoking was associated with a decreased prevalence of T1D among offsprings in two national British birth cohort studies [384]. The relation between passive smoking and development of GAD or IA–2A autoantibodies was evaluated in another study with negative results. It was concluded that passive smoking does not seem to influence the development of diabetes-related autoantibodies early in life [385].

Several studies reported that T1D was less prevalent among children whose mothers smoked during pregnancy than among the children of nonsmoking mothers [385–387]. More recently in the study by Svensson et al. in a multiple logistic regression analysis, maternal smoking was associated with a decreased risk of T1D [388].

Other studies have evaluated the possible association of T1D with exposure to smoke during childhood. In the study by Halthot et al., passive smoking was more frequent in children with diabetes (30% vs. 10%) [389]. In the study by Skrodeniene et al., children with islet cell autoantibody positive lived more frequently in a home where family members smoked indoors than children who were islet cell autoantibody negative (54% vs. 27%) [390]. Thus, most of the existing human studies do not provide support for an association between maternal, or paternal, smoking during pregnancy, and T1D in offspring. However, a possible association between smoking exposure during childhood and T1D needs to be further investigated.

SMOKING AND OTHER IMMUNE-MEDIATED DISEASES

To date, studies analyzing the relationship between smoking and other inflammatory conditions are scarce. Considering the large group of vasculitis, with the exception of thromboangiitis obliterans (Buerger's disease) wherein tobacco's involvement is widely recognized [391], data are rare and controversial. Thus regarding giant cell arteritis (GCA), smoking has been found to be associated with an increased risk of developing this disease, in particular in women, with an OR ranging from 2.3 to 6.5 [392–394]. But in a recent population-based study, Jakobsson et al. [395] did not confirm these results with smoking being not a significant risk factor for GCA (OR = 1.36, CI 0.77–2.57), although there was a trend toward a higher risk among female smokers (OR = 2.14, CI = 0.97–4.68). This last study confirmed Kermani's findings, who did not find any differences between GCA patients and controls with respect to smoking history (ever/never) [396].

Similarly, two studies failed to find a correlation between smoking habits and the risk of ANCA vasculitis [397,398]. A third study [399] even suggested a possible protective effect of smoking on the risk of ANCA vasculitis. The authors proposed that nicotine might exert a protective effect on ANCA vasculitis development by impairing T-cell response [399]. However, the limited power of these studies does not allow a firm conclusion.

Unsurprisingly, as other risk factors for atherosclerosis, smoking was unanimously reported as an aggravating factor in the evolution of the GCA and ANCA vasculitis. It was found to increase severe ischemic complications and aortic aneurysm in GCA [400,401]. In ANCA vasculitis, tobacco consumption was associated with more common cutaneous ischemia, amputation, myocardial infarction, and ESDR, whereas ear–nose–throat involvement was less frequent [402–404].

Similarly, tobacco appears to affect negatively myasthenia gravis (MG). Maniaol et al. first investigated the relationship between smoking and MG [405]. They suggested that smokers were 3.6 times more likely to present an early onset subtype of MG compared with nonsmokers. Subsequently, another study addressed the effects of smoking on clinical course of ocular MG [406]. Current smokers had significantly higher activity score than never smokers. However, these observations must be carefully considered and should be verified in larger studies. Conversely, in several studies, tobacco use has been strongly suggested as a protective factor for celiac disease [407–410]. However, the challenge when such an association is highlighted is to prove the causality between smoking and the protective effect. In their study, Suman et al. [409] have worked to support this hypothesis based on causal Bradford Hill criteria. Their conclusions strengthen a causal relationship by showing a strong, temporally appropriate, and dose-dependent effect. The most impressive protective effect was found among heavy smokers with an OR = 0.15 for the risk of celiac disease when compared to nonsmokers. Despite some negative reports [411–414] failing to reach the same outcome, most evidence support these findings. Interestingly, there is an analogy with now recognized protective effect of smoking on the risk of developing UC.

Although the mechanisms of this beneficial action are unclear, some assume that tobacco would act both through its effects on the intestinal barrier and its immunosuppressive action. On a gut scale, smoking has been shown to reduce mucosal intestinal permeability, whereas an abnormal intestinal permeability, with gliadin being an offensive agent, is considered to be an early pathogenic event in the celiac lesion. Smoking could also inhibit tissue transglutaminase activity that is responsible for rendering dietary gliadin immunogenic [408,409]. Pemphigus is a bullous autoimmune disease of complex etiology. Interestingly, it also seems to be positively influenced by smoking. Several series [415–418] have shown a significantly lower proportion of smokers in the pemphigus groups compared to controls, arguing for a protective effect of smoking on the risk of developing the disease. Moreover, few data suggest that remission may be achieved sooner in smokers [418,419]. Acantholysis in pemphigus would notably be the consequence of effects of autoantibodies targeting various keratinocytes cell membrane antigens, including acetylcholine receptors. Human keratinocytes contain an elaborated acetylcholine network. Both nicotinic and muscarinic acetylcholine receptors regulate cell-to-cell adhesion. Interaction of nicotine with nicotinic acetylcholine receptors on keratinocytes would help increase cell-to-cell adherence, stop acantholysis, and stimulate keratinocytes to move laterally to heal erosions [417–420].

CONCLUSIONS

It is evident that the role of smoke, no matter if tobacco, cigarette, or water pipe, is strictly dependent on the autoimmune condition that is taken into consideration [421]. Indeed, as summarized in Table 37.1, smoke habit can have both protective effects as well as it can represent a risk factor for disease exacerbation or worsening. Nonetheless, its effects on the immune system and on the local microbiome are manifold and influence the disease manifestations. As it has been recently reviewed by Hollan et al. [422], there is an enormous need to develop adequate cardiovascular risk stratification tools and to identify the optimal prevention strategies in autoimmune conditions such as RA [422,423]. Smoking relies within those preventable risk factors associated with increased cardiovascular risk. As rheumatologists, and in general, as physicians, we should take responsibility for the education of health care providers and patients [424]. Moreover, the occupational exposure to fumes and other substances should be also taken into account in the evaluation process of each patient to implement preventive measures [425,426]. We should stress also that smoke represents a negative burden on treatment response in several conditions, including RA and IBD [427,428].

It is also evident that the effects of smoke may vary from a person to another because different genetic backgrounds may significantly change the effects of smoke. This is the case for instance of NAT2 polymorphisms in SLE. Indeed, individuals

TABLE 37.1 Summary of the reported main genetic associations between several autoimmune/inflammatory diseases and possible mechanisms of interaction between smoke and diseases pathophysiology

Disease	Genetic Association	Mechanism	Other
Rheumatoid arthritis	HLADRB1, DRB4, DRB10, especially HLA DRB1*0401, PTPN22, NAT2	Proinflammatory on synoviocytes, triggers citrullination, upregulates proinflammatory cytokines, production of radical oxygen species, switch to Th17 response, follicular B hyperplasia	Reduces the response to therapy, both to methotrexate and anti-TNF; patients have a more severe disease and progression of erosive bone damage, association with parodontopathy by *Porphyromonas gingivalis*, association with chronic obstructive pulmonary disease
			Risk factor for a more severe stricturing disease, increases the need for immunosuppressants and steroids, especially in females
Crohn's disease	NOD2/CARD15, IL23R, ATG16L1	Decreases prostaglandin (PG) E2, increases nitric oxide synthetase (tNOS) activity, increases interleukin (IL)-6 and IL-10 levels; no effect on the circulation of the jejunum, whereas in the large intestine, it increases microcirculation and decreases IL-2 levels; no effect on IL-6 and IL-10 as well as NOS and PGE2, influence on gut permeability and microbiome. Possible effect on gut microbiome	*Protective!* Smoking might improve its course, decreasing the rate of relapses [130] and hospitalizations [131, 132], reducing the need for corticosteroid and immunosuppressant therapy [133,134]. It remains controversial as to whether smoking reduces the rate of surgery required in UC, particularly colectomy.
Ulcerative colitis			Higher disease activity, worsening in functional ability, reduced quality of life, more rapid radiographic progression and disability
Ankylosing spondylitis and spondyloarthritis Psoriasis and psoriatic arthritis	CHRNB3–CHRNA6, notably no association with HLA-Cw6	Induces oxidative stress-mediated IL-8 production in human keratinocytes via the aryl-hydrocarbon receptor signaling pathway, upregulation of TNFα mediated by Egr-1 in HaCaT human keratinocytes	Nonresponse to anti–TNF-α treatment and to the anti–IL 12/23 agent ustekinumab in patients with psoriasis
Behçet's Disease	Glutathione S-transferase (GST)	Local action, nicotine inhibits IL-6 and IL-8 release from the keratinocyte and dermal microvascular endothelial cells	Induces healing in oral and genital ulcers and improves skin, articular, and subjective neuro-psychiatric manifestations
Systemic lupus erythematosus	NAT2	Possible development of anti-dsDNA antibodies and antiphospholipid antibodies, epigenetic change of T lymphocytes	More severe skin disease, contrasting data on disease activity, triggers flares
Multiple sclerosis	Presence of HLA-DRB1*15 and absence of HLA-1*02	Lung irritation, change of local lymphocytes genetic expression that acquire the capability of migrating in the CNS, promoting demyelination, activating microglia and eventually becoming cytotoxic to the cells, elevated levels of renin–angiotensin system activity, induction of IL-17 and IL-22 producing cells number, and CCL2, CCL3, and CXCL10 production by monocytes, significant decrease in CD4+CD25+FoxP3+ regulatory T cells Possible trigger of AMA in individuals with HLA predisposing alleles	Accelerates disease progression and worsen prognosis

Autoimmune liver disease			Contrasting results: associated with primary biliary cirrhosis and autoimmune hepatitis, possible reduced odds ratio for primary sclerosing cholangitis
Systemic sclerosis (SSc)		Induction of oxidative stress	Significant negative effect on almost all vascular, gastrointestinal, and respiratory outcomes
Autoimmune thyroid disease (Hashimoto's)	CYP1A1	Recruitment of Th1 lymphocytes with increased secretion of interferon (IFN)-γ and TNF-α, stimulation of CXCL10 secretion from thyrocytes	Controversial results on thyroid autoantibodies (seems to reduce the risk of occurrence of AbTPO and AbTg and autoimmune hypothyroidism)
Graves' disease, ophthalmopathy	HLA-DR, GSTP1, CYP1A1, and TP53	Oxidative DNA damage, increased sICAM-1 and decreased sVCAM-1 levels, overexpression IL-1B, and IL-6	Heavy smokers present more severe ophthalmopathy
Type 1 diabetes (T1D)	CYP1A1, renin–angiotensin–aldosterone	DNA methylation	Significant risk for IA-2A, but not for GAD+ antibody
Vasculitis		Protective effect on ANCA vasculitis development by impairing T cell response	Association with Buerger's disease, controversial on giant cell arteritis. Reported more common cutaneous ischemia, amputation, myocardial infarction, and end-stage renal disease and less frequent ear–nose–throat involvement. Lower proportion of smokers in the pemphigus groups compared to controls
Pemphigus	Both nicotinic and muscarinic acetylcholine receptors regulate cell-to-cell adhesion. Interaction of nicotine with nicotinic acetylcholine receptors on keratinocytes would help increase cell-to-cell adherence, stop acantholysis, and stimulate keratinocytes to move laterally to heal erosions		

who possess homozygous polymorphic alleles have a slower rate of metabolic detoxification of aromatic amines. It was shown that those individuals who possess the slow acetylator genotype of NAT2 had an increased risk of SLE compared with the rapid acetylator genotype in a Japanese population [429]. Thus, the relationship between genetic factors, pathogenic mechanism, microbiome, and smoke needs to be elucidated. Furthermore, all these evidences highlight the need for large epidemiological studies to further explore the accountability of smoking in the pathogenesis of autoimmune disease.

REFERENCES

[1] Shoenfeld Y, Tincani A. Autoantibodies-the smoke and the fire. Autoimmunity February 2005;38(1):1–2.

[2] Colafrancesco S, Agmon-Levin N, Perricone C, Shoenfeld Y. Unraveling the soul of autoimmune diseases: pathogenesis, diagnosis and treatment adding dowels to the puzzle. Immunol Res July 2013;56(2–3):200–5.

[3] Perricone C, Agmon-Levin N, Ceccarelli F, Valesini G, Anaya JM, Shoenfeld Y. Genetics and autoantibodies. Immunol Res July 2013;56(2–3):206–19.

[4] Meroni PL, Chighizola CB, Rovelli F, Gerosa M. Antiphospholipid syndrome in 2014: more clinical manifestations, novel pathogenic players and emerging biomarkers. Arthritis Res Ther 2014;16(2):209.

[5] Valesini G, Gerardi MC, Iannuccelli C, Pacucci VA, Pendolino M, Shoenfeld Y. Citrullination and autoimmunity. Autoimmun Rev June 2015;14(6):490–7.

[6] Strickland FM, Li Y, Johnson K, Sun Z, Richardson BC. J CD4(+) T cells epigenetically modified by oxidative stress cause lupus-like autoimmunity in mice. Autoimmunity August 2015;62:75–80. https://doi.org/10.1016/j.jaut.2015.06.004. Epub 2015 Jul 9.

[7] Costenbader KH, Karlson EW. Cigarette smoking and systemic lupus erythematosus: a smoking gun? Autoimmunity November 2005;38(7):541–7.

[8] Kearley J, Silver JS, Sanden C, Liu Z, Berlin AA, White N, et al. Cigarette smoke silences innate lymphoid cell function and facilitates an exacerbated type I interleukin-33-dependent response to infection. Immunity March 17, 2015;42(3):566–79.

[9] Farhat SC, Silva CA, Orione MA, Campos LM, Sallum AM, Braga AL. Air pollution in autoimmune rheumatic diseases: a review. Autoimmun Rev November 2011;11(1):14–21. https://doi.org/10.1016/j.autrev.2011.06.008. Epub 2011 Jul 6.

[10] Essouma M, Noubiap JJ. Is air pollution a risk factor for rheumatoid arthritis? J Inflamm (Lond) July 30, 2015;12(48). https://doi.org/10.1186/s12950-015-0092-1eCollection 2015.

[11] Astorri E, Nerviani A, Bombardieri M, Pitzalis C. Towards a stratified targeted approach with biologic treatments in rheumatoid arthritis: role of synovial pathobiology. Curr Pharm Des 2015;21(17):2216–24.

[12] Perricone C, Ceccarelli F, Valesini G. An overview on the genetic of rheumatoid arthritis: a never-ending story. Autoimmun Rev August 2011;10(10):599–608. https://doi.org/10.1016/j.autrev.2011.04.021.

[13] Tak PP, Bresnihan B. The pathogenesis and prevention of joint damage in rheumatoid arthritis: advances from synovial biopsy and tissue analysis. Arthritis Rheum 2000;43:2619–33.

[14] Raij L, DeMaster EG, Jaimes EA. Cigarette smoke-induced endothelium dysfunction: role of superoxide anion. J Hypertens May 2001;19(5):891–97.

[15] Ballanti E, Perricone C, Greco E, Ballanti M, Di Muzio G, Chimenti MS, et al. Complement and autoimmunity. Immunol Res July 2013;56(2–3):477–91.

[16] Di Muzio G, Perricone C, Ballanti E, Kroegler B, Greco E, Novelli L, et al. Complement system and rheumatoid arthritis: relationships with autoantibodies, serological, clinical features, and anti-TNF treatment. Int J Immunopathol Pharmacol 2011 Apr-Jun;24(2):357–66.

[17] Ballanti E, Perricone C, di Muzio G, Kroegler B, Chimenti MS, Graceffa D, et al. Role of the complement system in rheumatoid arthritis and psoriatic arthritis: relationship with anti-TNF inhibitors. Autoimmun Rev August 2011;10(10):617–23. https://doi.org/10.1016/j.autrev.2011.04.012.

[18] Symmons DP, Bankhead CR, Harrison BJ, Brennan P, Barrett EM, Scott DG, et al. Blood transfusion, smoking, and obesity as risk factors for the development of rheumatoid arthritis: results from a primary care-based incident case-control study in Norfolk, England. Arthritis Rheum 1997;40:1955e61.

[19] Nyhall-Wahlin BM, Jacobsson LT, Petersson IF, et al. Smoking is a strong risk factor for rheumatoid nodules in early rheumatoid arthritis. Ann Rheum Dis 2006;65:601–6.

[20] Papadopoulos NG, Alamanos Y, Voulgari PV, et al. Does cigarette smoking influence disease expression, activity and severity in early rheumatoid arthritis patients? Clin Exp Rheumatol 2005;23:861–6.

[21] Chujo S, Okamoto S, Sunahara R, Adachi M, Yamada K, Hayashi H, et al. Cigarette smoke condensate extracts augment collagen-induced arthritis in mice. Int Immunopharmacol October 2010;10(10):1194–9. https://doi.org/10.1016/j.intimp. 2010.06.026.

[22] Kallberg H, Ding B, Padyukov L, Bengtsson C, Ronnelid J, Klareskog L, et al. Smoking is a major preventable risk factor for rheumatoid arthritis: estimations of risks after various exposures to cigarette smoke. Ann Rheum Dis 2010;70(3):508–11.

[23] Vessey MP, Villard-Mackintosh L, Yeates D. Oral contraceptives, cigarette smoking and other factors in relation to arthritis. Contraception 1987;35:457e64.

[24] Heliovaara M, Aho K, Aromaa A, Knekt P, Reunanen A. Smoking and risk of rheumatoid arthritis. J Rheumatol 1993;20:1830e5.

[25] Karlson EW, Lee IM, Cook NR, Manson JE, Buring JE, Hennekens CH. A retrospective cohort study of cigarette smoking and risk of rheumatoid arthritis in female health professionals. Arthritis Rheum 1999;42:910e7.

[26] Costenbader KH, Feskanich D, Mandl LA, Karlson EW. Smoking intensity, duration, and cessation, and the risk of rheumatoid arthritis in women. Am J Med 2006;119:503e9.

[27] Sugiyama D, Nishimura K, Tamaki K, Tsuji G, Nakazawa T, Morinobu A, et al. Impact of smoking as a risk factor for developing rheumatoid arthritis: a meta-analysis of observational studies. Ann Rheum Dis January 2010;69(1):70–81.

[28] Mattey DL, Brownfield A, Dawes PT. Relationship between pack-year history of smoking and response to tumor necrosis factor antagonists in patients with rheumatoid arthritis. J Rheumatol 2009;36:1180e7.

[29] Saevarsdottir S, Wedrén S, Seddighzadeh M, Bengtsson C, Wesley A, Lindblad S, et al. Patients with early rheumatoid arthritis who smoke are less likely to respond to treatment with methotrexate and tumor necrosis factor inhibitors: observations from the epidemiological investigation of rheumatoid arthritis and the Swedish Rheumatology Register cohorts. Arthritis Rheum January 2011;63(1):26–36. https://doi.org/10.1002/art.27758.

[30] Hutchinson D, Shepstone L, Moots R, Lear JT, Lynch MP. Heavy cigarette smoking is strongly associated with rheumatoid arthritis (RA), particularly in patients without a family history of RA. Ann Rheum Dis 2001;60:223–7.

[31] Jaakkola JJ, Gissler M. Maternal smoking in pregnancy as a determinant of rheumatoid arthritis and other inflammatory polyarthropathies during the first 7 years of life. Int J Epidemiol 2005;34:664–71.

[32] Westhoff G, Rau R, Zink A. Rheumatoid arthritis patients who smoke have a higher need for DMARDs and feel worse, but they do not have more joint damage than non-smokers of the same serological group. Rheumatology (Oxf) 2008;47:849e54.

[33] Manfredsdottir VF, Vikingsdottir T, Jonsson T, et al. The effects of tobacco smoking and rheumatoid factor seropositivity on disease activity and joint damage in early rheumatoid arthritis. Rheumatology (Oxf) 2006;45:734–40.

[34] Vesperini V, Lukas C, Fautrel B, Le Loet X, Rincheval N, Combe B. Association of tobacco exposure and reduction of radiographic progression in early rheumatoid arthritis: results from a French multicenter cohort. Arthritis Care Res December 2013;65(12):1899–906. https://doi.org/10.1002/acr.22057.

[35] Finckh A, Dehler S, Costenbader KH, et al. Cigarette smoking and radiographic progression in rheumatoid arthritis. Ann Rheum Dis 2007;66:1066–71.

[36] Saag KG, Cerhan JR, Kolluri S, et al. Cigarette smoking and rheumatoid arthritis severity. Ann Rheum Dis 1997;56:463–9.

[37] Wolfe F. The effect of smoking on clinical, laboratory, and radiographic status in rheumatoid arthritis. J Rheumatol 2000;27:630–7.

[38] Ruiz-Esquide V, Gomez-Puerta JA, Canete JD, et al. Effects of smoking on disease activity and radiographic progression in early rheumatoid arthritis. J Rheumatol 2011;38:2536–9.

[39] Haye Salinas MJ, Retamozo S, Alvarez AC, Maldonado Ficco H, Dal Pra F, Citera G, et al. Effects of cigarette smoking on early arthritis: a cross-sectional study-data from the Argentine Consortium for Early Arthritis (CONAART). Rheumatol Int December 2014:16.

[40] Lee J, Jeong H, Park EJ, Hwang JW, Bae EK, Ahn JK, et al. A role for benzo[a]pyrene and slug in invasive properties of fibroblast-like synoviocytes in rheumatoid arthritis: a potential molecular link between smoking and radiographic progression. Joint Bone Spine December 2013;80(6):621–5. https://doi.org/10.1016/j.jbspin. 2013.02.009.

[41] Perricone R, de Carolis C, de Sanctis G, Fontana L. Complement activation by cigarette smoke condensate and tobacco infusion. Arch Environ Health 1983 May-Jun;38(3):176–9.

[42] Kurreeman FA, Padyukov L, Marques RB, Schrodi SJ, Seddighzadeh M, StoekenRijsbergen G, et al. A candidate gene approach identifies the TRAF1/C5 region as a risk factor for rheumatoid arthritis. PLoS Med September 2007;4(9):e278. Erratum in: PLoS Med. 2007 Dec;4(12):e358.

[43] Kobayashi S, Okamoto H, Iwamoto T, Toyama Y, Tomatsu T, Yamanaka H, et al. A role for the aryl hydrocarbon receptor and the dioxin TCDD in rheumatoid arthritis. Rheumatology (Oxf) September 2008;47(9):1317–22. https://doi.org/10.1093/rheu-matology/ken259.

[44] Henley DV, Bellone CJ, Williams DA, et al. Aryl hydrocarbon receptor-mediated posttranscriptional regulation of IL-1beta. Arch Biochem Biophys 2004;422:42–51.

[45] Ospelt C, Camici GG, Engler A, Kolling C, Vogetseder A, Gay RE, et al. Smoking induces transcription of the heat shock protein system in the joints. Ann Rheum Dis July 2014;73(7):1423–6. https://doi.org/10.1136/annrheumdis-2013-204486.

[46] Seror R, Le Gall-David S, Bonnaure-Mallet M, Schaeverbeke T, Cantagrel A, Minet J, et al. Anti-*Porphyromonas gingivalis* antibodies titres are associated with non-smoking status in early rheumatoid arthritis: results from the ESPOIR cohort. Arthritis Rheumatol July 2015;67(7):1729–37. https://doi.org/10.1002/art.39118.

[47] Mikuls TR, Payne JB, Yu F, Thiele GM, Reynolds RJ, Cannon GW, et al. Periodontitis and *Porphyromonas gingivalis* in patients with rheumatoid arthritis. Arthritis Rheumatol May 2014;66(5):1090–100. https://doi.org/10.1002/art.38348.

[48] McInnes IB, Schett G. The pathogenesis of rheumatoid arthritis. N Engl J Med December 8, 2011;365(23):2205–19. PubMed PMID: 22150039.

[49] Vincent C, Nogueira L, Clavel C, Sebbag M, Serre G. Autoantibodies to citrullinated proteins: ACPA. Autoimmunity February 2005;38(1):17–24. PubMed PMID: 15804701.

[50] Vincent C, Nogueira L, Sebbag M, Chapuy-Regaud S, Arnaud M, Letourneur O, et al. Detection of antibodies to deiminated recombinant rat filaggrin by enzyme-linked immunosorbent assay: a highly effective test for the diagnosis of rheumatoid arthritis. Arthritis Rheum August 2002;46(8):2051–8. PubMed PMID: 12209508.

[51] Nishimura K, Sugiyama D, Kogata Y, Tsuji G, Nakazawa T, Kawano S, et al. Meta-analysis: diagnostic accuracy of anti-cyclic citrullinated peptide antibody and rheumatoid factor for rheumatoid arthritis. Ann Intern Med June 5, 2007;146(11):797–808. PubMed PMID: 17548411.

[52] Avouac J, Gossec L, Dougados M. Diagnostic and predictive value of anti-cyclic citrullinated protein antibodies in rheumatoid arthritis: a systematic literature review. Ann Rheum Dis July 2006;65(7):845–51. PubMed PMID: 16606649. Pubmed Central PMCID:1798205.

[53] van Venrooij WJ, van Beers JJ, Pruijn GJ. Anti-CCP antibodies: the past, the present and the future. Nat Rev Rheumatol July 2011;7(7):391–8. PubMed PMID: 21647203.

[54] Aletaha D, Neogi T, Silman AJ, Funovits J, Felson DT, Bingham 3rd CO, et al. Rheumatoid arthritis classification criteria: an American College of Rheumatology/European League Against Rheumatism collaborative initiative. Arthritis Rheum September 2010;62(9):2569–81. PubMed PMID: 20872595.

[55] Nielen MM, van Schaardenburg D, Reesink HW, van de Stadt RJ, van der Horst-Bruinsma IE, de Koning MH, et al. Specific autoantibodies precede the symptoms of rheumatoid arthritis: a study of serial measurements in blood donors. Arthritis Rheum February 2004;50(2):380–6. PubMed PMID: 14872479.

[56] Meyer O, Labarre C, Dougados M, Goupille P, Cantagrel A, Dubois A, et al. Anticitrullinated protein/peptide antibody assays in early rheumatoid arthritis for predicting five year radiographic damage. Ann Rheum Dis February 2003;62(2):120–6. PubMed PMID: 12525380. Pubmed Central PMCID: 1754441.

[57] Foulquier C, Sebbag M, Clavel C, Chapuy-Regaud S, Al Badine R, Mechin MC, et al. Peptidyl arginine deiminase type 2 (PAD-2) and PAD-4 but not PAD-1, PAD-3, and PAD-6 are expressed in rheumatoid arthritis synovium in close association with tissue inflammation. Arthritis Rheum November 2007;56(11):3541–53. PubMed PMID: 17968929.

[58] Simon M, Girbal E, Sebbag M, Gomes-Daudrix V, Vincent C, Salama G, et al. The cytokeratin filament-aggregating protein filaggrin is the target of the so-called "antikeratin antibodies," autoantibodies specific for rheumatoid arthritis. J Clin Investig September 1993;92(3):1387–93. PubMed PMID: 7690781. Pubmed Central PMCID: 288281.

[59] Turunen S, Koivula MK, Melkko J, Alasaarela E, Lehenkari P, Risteli J. Different amounts of protein-bound citrulline and homocitrulline in foot joint tissues of a patient with anti-citrullinated protein antibody positive erosive rheumatoid arthritis. J Transl Med 2013;11:224. PubMed PMID: 24060405. Pubmed Central PMCID: 3848878.

[60] Uysal H, Nandakumar KS, Kessel C, Haag S, Carlsen S, Burkhardt H, et al. Antibodies to citrullinated proteins: molecular interactions and arthritogenicity. Immunol Rev January 2010;233(1):9–33. PubMed PMID: 20192990.

[61] Snir O, Rieck M, Gebe JA, Yue BB, Rawlings CA, Nepom G, et al. Identification and functional characterization of T cells reactive to citrullinated vimentin in HLA-DRB1*0401-positive humanized mice and rheumatoid arthritis patients. Arthritis Rheum October 2011;63(10):2873–83. PubMed PMID: 21567378. Pubmed Central PMCID: 3174345.

[62] Suzuki A, Yamada R, Chang X, Tokuhiro S, Sawada T, Suzuki M, et al. Functional haplotypes of PADI4, encoding citrullinating enzyme peptidyl-larginine deiminase 4, are associated with rheumatoid arthritis. Nat Genet August 2003;34(4):395–402. PubMed PMID: 12833157.

[63] Auger I, Sebbag M, Vincent C, Balandraud N, Guis S, Nogueira L, et al. Influence of HLA-DR genes on the production of rheumatoid arthritis-specific autoantibodies to citrullinated fibrinogen. Arthritis Rheum November 2005;52(11):3424–32. PubMed PMID: 16255019.

[64] Gonzalez-Gay MA, Garcia-Porrua C, Hajeer AH. Influence of human leukocyte antigen-DRB1 on the susceptibility and severity of rheumatoid arthritis. Semin Arthritis Rheum June 2002;31(6):355–60. PubMed PMID: 12077707.

[65] Gregersen PK, Silver J, Winchester RJ. The shared epitope hypothesis. An approach to understanding the molecular genetics of susceptibility to rheumatoid arthritis. Arthritis Rheum November 1987;30(11):1205–13. PubMed PMID: 2446635.

[66] Hill JA, Southwood S, Sette A, Jevnikar AM, Bell DA, Cairns E. Cutting edge: the conversion of arginine to citrulline allows for a high-affinity peptide interaction with the rheumatoid arthritis-associated HLA-DRB1*0401 MHC class II molecule. J Immunol July 15, 2003;171(2):538–41. PubMed PMID: 12847215.

[67] Law SC, Street S, Yu CH, Capini C, Ramnoruth S, Nel HJ, et al. T-cell autoreactivity to citrullinated autoantigenic peptides in rheumatoid arthritis patients carrying HLA-DRB1 shared epitope alleles. Arthritis Res Ther 2012;14(3):R118. PubMed PMID: 22594821. Pubmed Central PMCID: 3446499.

[68] van der Helm-van Mil AH, Verpoort KN, Breedveld FC, Huizinga TW, Toes RE, de Vries RR. The HLA-DRB1 shared epitope alleles are primarily a risk factor for anti-cyclic citrullinated peptide antibodies and are not an independent risk factor for development of rheumatoid arthritis. Arthritis Rheum April 2006;54(4):1117–21. PubMed PMID: 16572446.

[69] Linn-Rasker SP, van der Helm-van Mil AH, van Gaalen FA, Kloppenburg M, de Vries RR, le Cessie S, et al. Smoking is a risk factor for anti-CCP antibodies only in rheumatoid arthritis patients who carry HLA-DRB1 shared epitope alleles. Ann Rheum Dis March 2006;65(3):366–71. PubMed PMID: 16014670. Pubmed Central PMCID: 1798061.

[70] Makrygiannakis D, Af Klint E, Lundberg IE, Lofberg R, Ulfgren AK, Klareskog L, et al. Citrullination is an inflammation-dependent process. Ann Rheum Dis September 2006;65(9):1219–22. PubMed PMID: 16540548. Pubmed Central PMCID: 1798285.

[71] Makrygiannakis D, Hermansson M, Ulfgren AK, Nicholas AP, Zendman AJ, Eklund A, et al. Smoking increases peptidylarginine deiminase 2 enzyme expression in human lungs and increases citrullination in BAL cells. Ann Rheum Dis October 2008;67(10):1488–92. PubMed PMID: 18413445.

[72] Hill JA, Bell DA, Brintnell W, Yue D, Wehrli B, Jevnikar AM, et al. Arthritis induced by posttranslationally modified (citrullinated) fibrinogen in DR4-IE transgenic mice. J Exp Med April 14, 2008;205(4):967–79. PubMed PMID: 18391064. Pubmed Central PMCID: 2292232.

[73] Klareskog L, Stolt P, Lundberg K, Kallberg H, Bengtsson C, Grunewald J, et al. A new model for an etiology of rheumatoid arthritis: smoking may trigger HLA-DR (shared epitope)-restricted immune reactions to autoantigens modified by citrullination. Arthritis Rheum January 2006;54(1):38–46. PubMed PMID: 16385494.

[74] Lee YH, Rho YH, Choi SJ, Ji JD, Song GG, Nath SK, et al. The PTPN22 C1858T functional polymorphism and autoimmune diseases—a meta-analysis. Rheumatology January 2007;46(1):49–56. PubMed PMID: 16760194.

[75] Turesson C, Jacobsson LT. Epidemiology of extra-articular manifestations in rheumatoid arthritis. Scand J Rheumatol 2004;33(2):65–72. PubMed PMID: 15163106.

[76] Harel-Meir M, Sherer Y, Shoenfeld Y. Tobacco smoking and autoimmune rheumatic diseases. Nat Clin Pract Rheumatol December 2007;3(12):707–15. PubMed PMID: 18037930.

[77] Ruiz-Esquide V, Gomara MJ, Peinado VI, Gomez Puerta JA, Barbera JA, Canete Jde D, et al. Anti-citrullinated peptide antibodies in the serum of heavy smokers without rheumatoid arthritis. A differential effect of chronic obstructive pulmonary disease?. Clin Rheumatol July 2012;31(7):1047–50. PubMed PMID: 22466712.

[78] Costenbader KH, Karlson EW. Cigarette smoking and autoimmune disease: what can we learn from epidemiology?. Lupus 2006;15(11):737–45. PubMed PMID: 17153844.

[79] Bracke KR, D'Hulst AI, Maes T, Moerloose KB, Demedts IK, Lebecque S, et al. Cigarette smoke-induced pulmonary inflammation and emphysema are attenuated in CCR6-deficient mice. J Immunol October 1, 2006;177(7):4350–9. PubMed PMID: 16982869.

[80] Sopori M. Effects of cigarette smoke on the immune system. Nat Rev Immunol May 2002;2(5):372–7. PubMed PMID: 12033743.

[81] Churg A, Dai J, Tai H, Xie C, Wright JL. Tumor necrosis factor-alpha is central to acute cigarette smoke-induced inflammation and connective tissue breakdown. Am J Respir Crit Care Med September 15, 2002;166(6):849–54. PubMed PMID: 12231496.

[82] Chung S, Sundar IK, Hwang JW, Yull FE, Blackwell TS, Kinnula VL, et al. NF-kappaB inducing kinase, NIK mediates cigarette smoke/TNFalpha-induced histone acetylation and inflammation through differential activation of IKKs. PLoS One 2011;6(8):e23488. PubMed PMID: 21887257. Pubmed Central PMCID: 3160853.

[83] Heijink IH, Pouwels SD, Leijendekker C, de Bruin HG, Zijlstra GJ, van der Vaart H, et al. Cigarette smoke induced DAMP release from necrotic neutrophils triggers proinflammatory mediator release. Am J Respir Cell Mol Biol September 2014:5. PubMed PMID: 25192219.

[84] Lee J, Taneja V, Vassallo R. Cigarette smoking and inflammation: cellular and molecular mechanisms. J Dent Res February 2012;91(2):142–9. PubMed PMID: 21876032. Pubmed Central PMCID: 3261116.

[85] Pulling LC, Vuillemenot BR, Hutt JA, Devereux TR, Belinsky SA. Aberrant promoter hypermethylation of the death-associated protein kinase gene is early and frequent in murine lung tumors induced by cigarette smoke and tobacco carcinogens. Cancer Res June 1, 2004;64(11):3844–8. PubMed PMID: 15172992.

[86] Hodge S, Hodge G, Holmes M, Reynolds PN. Increased airway epithelial and T-cell apoptosis in COPD remains despite smoking cessation. Eur Respir J March 2005;25(3):447–54. PubMed PMID: 15738287.

[87] Vassallo R, Luckey D, Behrens M, Madden B, Luthra H, David C, et al. Cellular and humoral immunity in arthritis are profoundly influenced by the interaction between cigarette smoke effects and host HLA-DR and DQ genes. Clin Immunol 2014 May-Jun;152(1–2):25–35. PubMed PMID: 24631425. Pubmed Central PMCID: 4004713.

[88] Rangel-Moreno J, Hartson L, Navarro C, Gaxiola M, Selman M, Randall TD. Inducible bronchus-associated lymphoid tissue (iBALT) in patients with pulmonary complications of rheumatoid arthritis. J Clin Invest December 2006;116(12):3183–94. PubMed PMID: 17143328. Pubmed Central PMCID: 1678820.

[89] Reynisdottir G, Karimi R, Joshua V, Olsen H, Hensvold AH, Harju A, et al. Structural changes and antibody enrichment in the lungs are early features of anti-citrullinated protein antibody-positive rheumatoid arthritis. Arthritis Rheumatol January 2014;66(1):31–9. PubMed PMID: 24449573.

[90] Morissette MC, Jobse BN, Thayaparan D, Nikota JK, Shen P, Labiris NR, et al. Persistence of pulmonary tertiary lymphoid tissues and anti-nuclear antibodies following cessation of cigarette smoke exposure. Respir Res 2014;15:49. PubMed PMID: 24754996. Pubmed Central PMCID: 4021094.

[91] Mannino DM, Homa DM, Akinbami LJ, Ford ES, Redd SC. Chronic obstructive pulmonary disease surveillance–United States, 1971–2000. Respir Care October 2002;47(10):1184–99. PubMed PMID: 12354338.

[92] Shen TC, Lin CL, Chen CH, Tu CY, Hsia TC, Shih CM, et al. Increased risk of chronic obstructive pulmonary disease in patients with rheumatoid arthritis: a population-based cohort study. QJM July 2014;107(7):537–43. PubMed PMID: 24497528.

[93] Bieber V, Cohen AD, Freud T, Agmon-Levin N, Gertel S, Amital H. Autoimmune smoke and fire—coexisting rheumatoid arthritis and chronic obstructive pulmonary disease: a cross-sectional analysis. Immunol Res July 2013;56(2–3):261–6. PubMed PMID: 23568054.

[94] Agusti A, MacNee W, Donaldson K, Cosio M. Hypothesis: does COPD have an auto- immune component?. Thorax October 2003;58(10):832–4. PubMed PMID: 14514931. Pubmed Central PMCID: 1746486.

[95] Cosio MG, Saetta M, Agusti A. Immunologic aspects of chronic obstructive pulmonary disease. N Engl J Med June 4, 2009;360(23):2445–54. PubMed PMID: 19494220.

[96] Lane N, Robins RA, Corne J, Fairclough L. Regulation in chronic obstructive pulmonary disease: the role of regulatory T-cells and Th17 cells. Clin Sci July 2010;119(2):75–86. PubMed PMID: 20402669.

[97] Zhang MQ, Wan Y, Jin Y, Xin JB, Zhang JC, Xiong XZ, et al. Cigarette smoking promotes inflammation in patients with COPD by affecting the polarization and survival of Th/Tregs through up-regulation of muscarinic receptor 3 and 5 expression. PLoS One 2014;9(11):e112350. PubMed PMID: 25375131. Pubmed Central PMCID: 4223024.

[98] Karsdal MA, Henriksen K, Leeming DJ, Woodworth T, Vassiliadis E, Bay-Jensen AC. Novel combinations of post-translational modification (PTM) neo-epitopes provide tissue-specific biochemical markers—are they the cause or the consequence of the disease?. Clin Biochem July 2010;43(10–11):793–804. PubMed PMID: 20381482.

[99] Harries AD, Baird A, Rhodes J. Non-smoking: a feature of ulcerative colitis. Br Med J 1982;284:706.

[100] Somerville KW, Logan RF, Edmond M, Langman MJ. Smoking and Crohn's disease. Br Med J 1984;289:954–6.

[101] Nos P, Domenech E. Management of Crohn's disease in smokers: is an alternative approach necessary? World J Gastroenterol 2011;17:3567–74.

[102] Calkins BM. A meta-analysis of the role of smoking in inflammatory bowel disease. Dig Dis Sci 1989;34:1841–54.

[103] Karban A, Eliakim R. Effect of smoking on inflammatory bowel disease: is it disease or organ specific? World J Gastroenterol 2007;13:2150–2.

[104] Mahid SS, Minor KS, Soto RE, Hornung CA, Galandiuk S. Smoking and inflammatory bowel disease: a meta-analysis. Mayo Clin Proc 2006;81:1462–71.

[105] Birrenbach T, Bocker U. Inflammatory bowel disease and smoking: a review of epidemiology, pathophysiology, and therapeutic implications. Inflamm Bowel Dis 2004;10:848–59.

[106] Verschuere S, De Smet R, Allais L, Cuvelier CA. The effect of smoking on intestinal inflammation: what can be learned from animal models? J Crohns Colitis 2012;6:1–12.

[107] Probert CS, Jayanthi V, Hughes AO, Thompson JR, Wicks AC, Mayberry JF. Prevalence and family risk of ulcerative colitis and Crohn's disease: an epidemiological study among Europeans and south Asians in Leicestershire. Gut 1993;34:1547–51.

[108] Reddy SI, Burakoff R. Inflammatory bowel disease in African Americans. Inflamm Bowel Dis 2003;9:380–5.

[109] Reif S, Klein I, Arber N, Gilat T. Lack of association between smoking and inflammatory bowel disease in Jewish patients in Israel. Gastroenterology 1995;108:1683–7.

[110] Ben-Horin S, Avidan B, Yanai H, Lang A, Chowers Y, Bar-Meir S. Familial clustering of Crohn's disease in Israel: prevalence and association with disease severity. Inflamm Bowel Dis 2009;15:171–5.

[111] McGilligan VE, Wallace JM, Heavey PM, Ridley DL, Rowland IR. Hypothesis about mechanisms through which nicotine might exert its effect on the interdependence of inflammation and gut barrier function in ulcerative colitis. Inflamm Bowel Dis 2007;13:108–15.

[112] Galeazzi F, Blennerhassett PA, Qiu B, O'Byrne PM, Collins SM. Cigarette smoke aggravates experimental colitis in rats. Gastroenterology 1999;117:877–83.

[113] Eliakim R, Karmeli F. Divergent effects of nicotine administration on cytokine levels in rat small bowel mucosa, colonic mucosa, and blood. Isr Med Assoc J 2003;5:178–80.

[114] Eliakim R, Karmeli F, Cohen P, Heyman SN, Rachmilewitz D. Dual effect of chronic nicotine administration: augmentation of jejunitis and amelioration of colitis induced by iodoacetamide in rats. Int J Colorectal Dis 2001;16:14–21.

[115] Beltran B, Nos P, Dasi F, Iborra M, Bastida G, Martinez M, et al. Mitochondrial dysfunction, persistent oxidative damage, and catalase inhibition in immune cells of naive and treated Crohn's disease. Inflamm Bowel Dis 2010;16:76–86.

[116] Kalra J, Chaudhary AK, Prasad K. Increased production of oxygen free radicals in cigarette smokers. Int J Exp Pathol 1991;72:1–7.

[117] Prytz H, Benoni C, Tagesson C. Does smoking tighten the gut? Scand J Gastroenterol 1989;24:1084–8.

[118] Wang H, Zhao JX, Hu N, Ren J, Du M, Zhu MJ. Side-stream smoking reduces intestinal inflammation and increases expression of tight junction proteins. World J Gastroenterol 2012;18:2180–7.

[119] Nielsen OH, Bjerrum JT, Csillag C, Nielsen FC, Olsen J. Influence of smoking on colonic gene expression profile in Crohn's disease. PLoS One 2009;4:e6210.

[120] Holdstock G, Savage D, Harman M, Wright R. Should patients with inflammatory bowel disease smoke? Br Med J 1984;288:362.

[121] Timmer A, Sutherland LR, Martin F. Oral contraceptive use and smoking are risk factors for relapse in Crohn's disease. The Canadian Mesalamine for Remission of Crohn's Disease Study Group. Gastroenterology 1998;114:1143–50.

[122] Mahid SS, Minor KS, Stevens PL, Galandiuk S. The role of smoking in Crohn's disease as defined by clinical variables. Dig Dis Sci 2007;52:2897–903.

[123] Ashley MJ. Smoking and diseases of the gastrointestinal system: an epidemiological review with special reference to sex differences. Can J Gastroenterol 1997;11:345–52. Journal canadien de gastroenterologie.

[124] Lakatos PL, Szamosi T, Lakatos L. Smoking in inflammatory bowel diseases: good, bad or ugly? World J Gastroenterol 2007;13:6134–9.

[125] Arnott ID, McNeill G, Satsangi J. An analysis of factors influencing short-term and sustained response to infliximab treatment for Crohn's disease. Aliment Pharmacol Ther 2003;17:1451–7.

[126] Parsi MA, Achkar JP, Richardson S, Katz J, Hammel JP, Lashner BA, et al. Predictors of response to infliximab in patients with Crohn's disease. Gastroenterology 2002;123:707–13.

[127] Orlando A, Colombo E, Kohn A, Biancone L, Rizzello F, Viscido A, et al. Infliximab in the treatment of Crohn's disease: predictors of response in an Italian multicentric open study. Dig Liver Dis 2005;37:577–83.

[128] Fefferman DS, Lodhavia PJ, Alsahli M, Falchuk KR, Peppercorn MA, Shah SA, et al. Smoking and immunomodulators do not influence the response or duration of response to infliximab in Crohn's disease. Inflamm Bowel Dis 2004;10:346–51.

[129] Johnson GJ, Cosnes J, Mansfield JC. Review article: smoking cessation as primary therapy to modify the course of Crohn's disease. Aliment Pharmacol Ther 2005;21:921–31.

[130] Hoie O, Wolters F, Riis L, Aamodt G, Solberg C, Bernklev T, et al. Ulcerative colitis: patient characteristics may predict 10-yr disease recurrence in a European-wide population-based cohort. Am J Gastroenterol 2007;102:1692–701.

[131] Boyko EJ, Perera DR, Koepsell TD, Keane EM, Inui TS. Effects of cigarette smoking on the clinical course of ulcerative colitis. Scand J Gastroenterol 1988;23:1147–52.

[132] van der Heide F, Dijkstra A, Weersma RK, Albersnagel FA, van der Logt EM, Faber KN, et al. Effects of active and passive smoking on disease course of Crohn's disease and ulcerative colitis. Inflamm Bowel Dis 2009;15:1199–207.

[133] Bastida G, Beltran B. Ulcerative colitis in smokers, non-smokers and ex-smokers. World J Gastroenterol 2011;17:2740–7.

[134] Fraga XF, Vergara M, Medina C, Casellas F, Bermejo B, Malagelada JR. Effects of smoking on the presentation and clinical course of inflammatory bowel disease. Eur J Gastroenterol Hepatol 1997;9:683–7.

[135] Aldhous MC, Drummond HE, Anderson N, Baneshi MR, Smith LA, Arnott ID, et al. Smoking habit and load influence age at diagnosis and disease extent in ulcerative colitis. Am J Gastroenterol 2007;102:589–97.

[136] Merrett MN, Mortensen N, Kettlewell M, Jewell DO. Smoking may prevent pouchitis in patients with restorative proctocolectomy for ulcerative colitis. Gut 1996;38:362–4.

[137] Motley RJ, Rhodes J, Kay S, Morris TJ. Late presentation of ulcerative colitis in ex-smokers. Int J Colorectal Dis 1988;3:171–5.

[138] Srivasta ED, Newcombe RG, Rhodes J, Avramidis P, Mayberry JF. Smoking and ulcerative colitis: a community study. Int J Colorectal Dis 1993;8:71–4.

[139] Lunney PC, Leong RW. Review article: ulcerative colitis, smoking and nicotine therapy. Aliment Pharmacol Ther 2012;36:997–1008.

[140] McGrath J, McDonald JW, McDonald JK. Transdermal nicotine for induction of remission in ulcerative colitis. Cochrane Database Syst Rev 2004:CD004722.

[141] Nikfar S, Ehteshami-Ashar S, Rahimi R, Abdollahi M. Systematic review and meta-analysis of the efficacy and tolerability of nicotine preparations in active ulcerative colitis. Clin Ther 2010;32:2304–15.

[142] Ward MM. Predictors of the progression of functional disability in patients with ankylosing spondylitis. J Rheumatol 2002;29:1420–5.

[143] Averns HL, Oxtoby J, Taylor HG, Jones PW, Dziedzic K, Dawes PT. Smoking and outcome in ankylosing spondylitis. Scand J Rheumatol 1996;25:138–42.

[144] Chung HY, Machado P, van der Heijde D, D'Agostino MA, Dougados M. Smokers in early axial spondyloarthritis have earlier disease onset, more disease activity, inflammation and damage, and poorer function and health-related quality of life: results from the DESIR cohort. Ann Rheum Dis 2012;71:809–16.

[145] Koko V, Ndrepepa A, Skënderaj S, Ploumis A, Backa T, Tafaj A. An epidemiological study on ankylosing spondylitis in southern Albania. Mater Sociomed 2014;26:26–9.

[146] Mattey DL, Dawson SR, Healey EL, Packham JC. Relationship between smoking and patient-reported measures of disease outcome in ankylosing spondylitis. J Rheumatol 2011;38:2608–15.

[147] Kaan U, Ferda O. Evaluation of clinical activity and functional impairment in smokers with ankylosing spondylitis. Rheumatol Int 2005;25:357–60.

[148] Doran MF, Brophy S, MacKay K, Taylor G, Calin A. Predictors of longterm outcome in ankylosing spondylitis. J Rheumatol 2003;30:316–20.

[149] Ward MM, Weisman MH, Davis Jr JC, Reveille JD. Risk factors for functional limitations in patients with long-standing ankylosing spondylitis. Arthritis Rheum 2005;53:710–7.

[150] Bodur H, Ataman S, Rezvani A, Buğdaycı DS, Cevik R, Birtane M, et al. Quality of life and related variables in patients with ankylosing spondylitis. Qual Life Res 2011;20:543–9.

[151] Haglund E, Petersson IF, Bremander A, Bergman S. Predictors of presenteeism and activity impairment outside work in patients with spondyloarthritis. J Occup Rehabil June 2015;25(2):288–95. [Epub ahead of print].

[152] Boonen A, Boone C, Albert A, Mielants H. Understanding limitations in at-work productivity in patients with active ankylosing spondylitis: the role of work-related contextual factors. J Rheumatol 2015;42:93–100.

[153] Ward MM, Hendrey MR, Malley JD, Learch TJ, Davis Jr JC, Reveille JD, et al. Clinical and immunogenetic prognostic factors for radiographic severity in ankylosing spondylitis. Arthritis Rheum 2009;61:859–66.

[154] Poddubnyy D, Haibel H, Listing J, Märker-Hermann E, Zeidler H, Braun J, et al. Baseline radiographic damage, elevated acute-phase reactant levels, and cigarette smoking status predict spinal radiographic progression in early axial spondylarthritis. Arthritis Rheum 2012;64:1388–98.

[155] Poddubnyy D, Haibel H, Listing J, Märker-Hermann E, Zeidler H, Braun J, et al. Cigarette smoking has a dose-dependent impact on progression of structural damage in the spine in patients with axial spondyloarthritis: results from the German SPondyloarthritis Inception rohort (GESPIC). Ann Rheum Dis 2013;72:1430–2.

[156] Videm V, Cortes A, Thomas R, Brown MA. Current smoking is associated with incident ankylosing spondylitis - the HUNT population-based Norwegian health study. J Rheumatol 2014;41:2041–8.

[157] Ciurea A, Finckh A. Smoking and spondyloarthritis. Joint Bone Spine 2013;80:234–5.

[158] Reed MD, Dharmage S, Boers A, Martin BJ, Buchanan RR, Schachna L. Ankylosing spondylitis: an Australian experience. Intern Med J 2008;38:321–7.

[159] Dincer U, Cakar E, Kiralp MZ, Bozkanat E, Kilac H, Dursun H. The pulmonary involvement in rheumatic diseases: pulmonary effects of ankylosing spondylitis and its impact on functionality and quality of life. Tohoku J Exp Med 2007;212:423–30.

[160] Jadon D, Shaddick G, Jobling A, Ramanan AV, Sengupta R. Clinical outcomes and progression to orthopedic surgery in juvenile versus adult-onset ankylosing spondylitis. Arthritis Care Res May 2015;67(5):651–7. [Epub ahead of print].

[161] Kydd AS, Chen JS, Makovey J, Chand V, Henderson L, Buchbinder R, et al. Smoking did not modify the effects of anti-TNF treatment on health-related quality of life among Australian ankylosing spondylitis patients. Rheumatology (Oxf) February 2015;54(2):310–7. [Epub ahead of print].

[162] Kimball AB, Leonardi C, Stahle M, Gulliver W, Chevrier M, Fakharzadeh S, et al. Demography, baseline disease characteristics and treatment history of patients with psoriasis enrolled in a multicentre, prospective, disease-based registry (PSOLAR). Br J Dermatol 2014;171:137–47.

[163] Hayes J, Koo J. Psoriasis: depression, anxiety, smoking, and drinking habits. Dermatol Ther 2010;23:174–80.

[164] Guenther L, Gulliver W. Psoriasis comorbidities. J Cutan Med Surg 2009;13:S77–87.

[165] Helmick CG, Lee-Han H, Hirsch SC, Baird TL, Bartlett CL. Prevalence of psoriasis among adults in the U.S.: 2003–2006 and 2009–2010 national health and nutrition examination surveys. Am J Prev Med 2014;47:37–45.

[166] Fortes C, Mastroeni S, Leffondré K, Sampogna F, Melchi F, Mazzotti E, et al. Relationship between smoking and the clinical severity of psoriasis. Arch Dermatol 2005;141:1580–4.

[167] Armstrong AW, Harskamp CT, Dhillon JS, Armstrong EJ. Psoriasis and smoking: a systematic review and meta-analysis. Br J Dermatol 2014;170:304–14.

[168] Asokan N, Prathap P, Rejani P. Severity of psoriasis among adult males is associated with smoking, not with alcohol use. Indian J Dermatol 2014;59:237–40.

[169] Dębniak T, Soczawa E, Boer M, Różewicka-Czabańska M, Wiśniewska J, Serrano-Fernandez P, et al. Common variants of ZNF750, RPTOR and TRAF3IP2 genes and psoriasis risk. Arch Dermatol Res 2014;306:231–8.

[170] Setty AR, Curhan G, Choi HK. Smoking and the risk of psoriasis in women: Nurses' health study II. Am J Med 2007;120:953–9.

[171] Wolkenstein P, Revuz J, Roujeau JC, Bonnelye G, Grob JJ, Bastuji-Garin S, et al. Psoriasis in France and associated risk factors: results of a case-control study based on a large community survey. Dermatology 2009;218:103–9.

[172] Naldi L, Peli L, Parazzini F. Association of early-stage psoriasis with smoking and male alcohol consumption: evidence from an Italian case-control study. Arch Dermatol 1999;135:1479–84.

[173] Poikolainen K, Reunala T, Karvonen J. Smoking, alcohol and life events related to psoriasis among women. Br J Dermatol 1994;130:473–7.

[174] Li W, Han J, Choi HK, Qureshi AA. Smoking and risk of incident psoriasis among women and men in the United States: a combined analysis. Am J Epidemiol 2012;175:402–13.

[175] Gerdes S, Zahl VA, Weichenthal M, Mrowietz U. Smoking and alcohol intake in severely affected patients with psoriasis in Germany. Dermatology 2010;220:38–43.

[176] Jin Y, Yang S, Zhang F, Kong Y, Xiao F, Hou Y, et al. Combined effects of HLA-Cw6 and cigarette smoking in psoriasis vulgaris: a hospital-based case-control study in China. J Eur Acad Dermatol Venereol 2009;23:132–7.

[177] Mills CM, Srivastava ED, Harvey IM, Swift GL, Newcombe RG, Holt PJ, et al. Smoking habits in psoriasis: a case control study. Br J Dermatol 1992;127:18–21.

[178] Naldi L, Parazzini F, Brevi A, Peserico A, Veller Fornasa C, Grosso G, et al. Family history, smoking habits, alcohol consumption and risk of psoriasis. Br J Dermatol 1992;127:212–7.

[179] Zhu KJ, Quan C, Zhang C, Liu Z, Liu H, Li M, et al. Combined effect between CHRNB3-CHRNA6 region gene variant (rs6474412) and smoking in psoriasis vulgaris severity. Gene 2014;544:123–7.

[180] Di Lernia V, Ricci C, Lallas A, Ficarelli E. Clinical predictors of nonresponse to any tumor necrosis factor (TNF) blockers: a retrospective study. J Dermatolog Treat 2014;25:73–4.

[181] Umezawa Y, Saeki H, Nakagawa H. Some clinical factors affecting quality of the response to ustekinumab for psoriasis. J Dermatol 2014;41:690–6.

[182] Serwin AB, Sokolowska M, Chodynicka B. Tumor necrosis factor-alpha-converting enzyme as a potential mediator of the influence of smoking on the response to treatment with narrowband ultraviolet B in psoriasis patients. Photodermatol Photoimmunol Photomed 2010;26:36–40.

[183] Kinahan CE, Mazloom S, Fernandez AP. Impact of smoking on response to systemic treatment in patients with psoriasis: a retrospective case-control study. Br J Dermatol February 2015;172(2):428–36. https://doi.org/10.1111/bjd.13359. [Epub ahead of print].

[184] Staples J, Klein D. Can nicotine use alleviate symptoms of psoriasis? Can Fam Physician 2012;58:404–8.

[185] Gómez-Fernández C, Herranz Pinto P, Casado Verrier B, Sendagorta Cudós E, Beato-Merino MJ, Jiménez MC. Drug eruption and exacerbation of psoriasis related to bupropion. Eur J Dermatol 2011;21:120–1.

[186] Gelfand JM, Gladman DD, Mease PJ, Smith N, Margolis DJ, Nijsten T, et al. Epidemiology of psoriatic arthritis in the population of the United States. J Am Acad Dermatol 2005;53:573.

[187] Tey HL, Ee HL, Tan AS, Theng TS, Wong SN, Khoo SW. Risk factors associated with having psoriatic arthritis in patients with cutaneous psoriasis. J Dermatol 2010;37:426–30.

[188] Pattison E, Harrison BJ, Griffiths CE, Silman AJ, Bruce IN. Environmental risk factors for the development of psoriatic arthritis: results from a case-control study. Ann Rheum Dis 2008;67:672–6.

[189] Duffin KC, Freeny IC, Schrodi SJ, Wong B, Feng BJ, Soltani-Arabshahi R, et al. Association between IL13 polymorphisms and psoriatic arthritis is modified by smoking. J Invest Dermatol 2009;129:2777–83.

[190] Eder L, Law T, Chandran V, Shanmugarajah S, Shen H, Rosen CF, et al. Association between environmental factors and onset of psoriatic arthritis in patients with psoriasis. Arthritis Care Res 2011;63:1091–7.

[191] Eder L, Shanmugarajah S, Thavaneswaran A, Chandran V, Rosen CF, Cook RJ, et al. The association between smoking and the development of psoriatic arthritis among psoriasis patients. Ann Rheum Dis 2012;71:219–24.

[192] Li W, Han J, Qureshi AA. Smoking and risk of incident psoriatic arthritis in US women. Ann Rheum Dis 2012;71:804–8.

[193] Tillett W, Jadon D, Shaddick G, Cavill C, Korendowych E, de Vries CS, et al. Smoking and delay to diagnosis are associated with poorer functional outcome in psoriatic arthritis. Ann Rheum Dis 2013;72:1358–61.

[194] Bremander A, Jacobsson LT, Bergman S, Haglund E, Löfvendahl S, Petersson IF. Smoking is associated with a worse self-reported health status in patients with psoriatic arthritis: data from a Swedish population-based cohort. Clin Rheumatol March 2015;34(3):579–83. [Epub ahead of print].

[195] Højgaard P, Glintborg B, Hetland ML, Hansen TH, Lage-Hansen PR, Petersen MH, et al. Association between tobacco smoking and response to tumour necrosis factor α inhibitor treatment in psoriatic arthritis: results from the DANBIO registry. Ann Rheum Dis December 2015;74(12):2130–6. [Epub ahead of print] https://doi.org/10.1136/annrheumdis-2014-205389.

[196] Miller S, Bawa S. The effect of smoking on treatment response and drug survival in psoriatic arthritis patients treated with their first anti-TNFa drug: a single-Centre restrospective analysis [abstract]. Ann Rheum Dis 2013;72:686.

[197] Fagerli KM, Lie E, van der Heijde D, Heiberg MS, Lexberg AS, Rødevand E, et al. The role of methotrexate co-medication in TNF-inhibitor treatment in patients with psoriatic arthritis: results from 440 patients included in the NOR-DMARD study. Ann Rheum Dis 2014;73:132–7.

[198] Tablazon IL, Al-Dabagh A, Davis SA, Feldman SR. Risk of cardiovascular disorders in psoriasis patients: current and future. Am J Clin Dermatol 2013;14:1–7.

[199] Katsiki N, Anagnostis P, Athyros VG, Karagiannis A, Mikhailidis DP. Psoriasis and vascular risk: an update. Curr Pharmaceut Des 2014;20(39):6114–25. [Epub ahead of print].

[200] Grady D, Ernster VL, Stillman L, Greenspan J. Smokeless tobacco use prevents aphthous stomatitis. Oral Surg Oral Med Oral Pathol 1992;74:463–5.

[201] Krause I, Rosen Y, Kaplan I, Milo G, Guedj D, Molad Y, et al. Recurrent aphthous sto-matitis in Behçet's disease: clinical features and correlation with systemic disease expression and severity. J Oral Pathol Med 1999;28:193–6.

[202] Salonen L, Axéll T, Helldén L. Occurrence of oral mucosal lesions, the influence of tobacco habits and an estimate of treatment time in an adult Swedish population. J Oral Pathol Med 1990;19:170–6.

[203] Rizvi SW, McGrath Jr H. The therapeutic effect of cigarette smoking on oral/genital aphthosis and other manifestations of Behçet's disease. Clin Exp Rheumatol 2001;19:S77–8.

[204] Soy M, Erken E, Konca K, Ozbek S. Smoking and Behçet's disease. Clin Rheumatol 2000;19:508–9.

[205] Aramaki K, Kikuchi H, Hirohata S. HLA-B51 and cigarette smoking as risk factors for chronic progressive neurological manifestations in Behçet's disease. Mod Rheumatol 2007;17:81–2.

[206] Özer HT, Günesaçar R, Dinkçi S, Özbalkan Z, Yildiz F, Erken E. The impact of smoking on clinical features of Behçet's disease patients with glutathione S-transferase polymorphisms. Clin Exp Rheumatol 2012;30:S14–7.

[207] Kaklamani VG, Tzonou A, Markomichelakis N, Papazoglou S, Kaklamanis PG. The effect of smoking on the clinical features of Adamantiades–Behçet's disease. Adv Exp Med Biol 2003;528:323–7.

[208] Kaklamani VG, Markomichelakis N, Kaklamanis PG. Could nicotine be beneficial for behçet's disease? Clin Rheumatol 2002;21:341–2.

[209] Ciancio G, Colina M, La Corte R, Lo Monaco A, De Leonardis F, Trotta F, et al. Nicotine-patch therapy on mucocutaneous lesions of Behçet's disease: a case series. Rheumatology (Oxf) 2010;49:501–4.

[210] Scheid P, Bohadana A, Martinet Y. Nicotine patches for aphthous ulcers due to Behçet's syndrome. N Engl J Med 2000;343:1816–7.

[211] Kalayciyan A, Orawa H, Fimmel S, Perschel FH, González JB, Fitzner RG, et al. Nico-tine and biochanin A, but not cigarette smoke, induce anti-inflammatory effects on keratinocytes and endothelial cells in patients with Behçet's disease. J Invest Dermatol 2007;127:81–9.

[212] Ingram JR. Nicotine: does it have a role in the treatment of skin disease? Postgrad Med J 2009;85:196–201.

[213] Bilgin AB, Turkoglu EB, Ilhan HD, Unal M, Apaydin KC. Is smoking a risk factor in ocular behçet disease?. Ocul Immunol Inflamm August 2015;23(4):283–286. [Epub ahead of print].

[214] Kolar P. Risk factors for central and branch retinal vein occlusion: a meta-analysis of published clinical data. J Ophthalmol 2014;2014:724780.

[215] Tsokos GC. Systemic lupus erythematosus. N Engl J Med 2011;365:2110–21.

[216] Miot HA, Bartoli Miot LD, Haddad GR. Association between discoid lupus erythematosus and cigarette smoking. Dermatology 2005;211:118–22.

[217] Koskenmies S, Jarvinen TM, Onkamo P, Panelius J, Tuovinen U, Hasan T, et al. Clinical and laboratory characteristics of Finnish lupus erythematosus patients with cutaneous manifestations. Lupus 2008;17:337–47.

[218] Boeckler P, Cosnes A, Frances C, Hedelin G, Lipsker D. Association of cigarette smoking but not alcohol consumption with cutaneous lupus erythematosus. Arch Dermatol 2009;145:1012–6.

[219] Böckle BC, Sepp NT. Smoking is highly associated with discoid lupus erythematosus and lupus erythematosus tumidus: analysis of 405 patients. Lupus June 2015;24(7):669–74.

[220] Kuhn A, Sigges J, Biazar C, Ruland V, Patsinakidis N, Landmann A, et al. Influence of smoking on disease severity and antimalarial therapy in cutaneous lupus erythematosus: analysis of 1002 patients from the EUSCLE database. Br J Dermatol 2014;171:571–9.

[221] Piette EW, Foering KP, Chang AY, Okawa J, Ten Have TR, Feng R, et al. Impact of smoking in cutaneous lupus erythematosus. Arch Dermatol 2012;148:317–22.

[222] Turchin I, Bernatsky S, Clarke AE, St-Pierre Y, Pineau CA. Cigarette smoking and cutaneous damage in systemic lupus erythematosus. J Rheumatol 2009;36:2691–3.

[223] Hardy CJ, Palmer BP, Muir KR, Sutton AJ, Powell RJ. Smoking history, alcohol consumption, and systemic lupus erythematosus: a case-control study. Ann Rheum Dis 1998;57:451–5.

[224] Ghaussy NO, Sibbitt Jr WL, Qualls CR. Cigarette smoking, alcohol consumption, and the risk of systemic lupus erythematosus: a case-control study. J Rheumatol 2001;28:2449–53.

[225] Costenbader KH, Kim DJ, Peerzada J, Lockman S, Nobles-Knight D, Petri M, et al. Cigarette smoking and the risk of systemic lupus erythematosus: a meta-analysis. Arthritis Rheum 2004;50:849–57.

[226] Takvorian SU, Merola JF, Costenbader KH. Cigarette smoking, alcohol consumption and risk of systemic lupus erythematosus. Lupus 2014;23:537–44.

[227] Bourré-Tessier J, Peschken CA, Bernatsky S, Joseph L, Clarke AE, Fortin PR, et al. Canadian network for improved outcomes in systemic lupus erythematosus 1000 Canadian faces of lupus investigators, pineau CA. Association of smoking with cutaneous manifestations in systemic lupus erythematosus. Arthritis Care Res 2013;65:1275–80.

[228] Ghaussy NO, Sibbitt Jr W, Bankhurst AD, Qualls CR. Cigarette smoking and disease activity in systemic lupus erythematosus. J Rheumatol 2003;30:1215–21.

[229] Ekblom-Kullberg S, Kautiainen H, Alha P, Leirisalo-Repo M, Miettinen A, Julkunen H. Smoking, disease activity, permanent damage and dsDNA autoantibody production in patients with systemic lupus erythematosus. Rheumatol Int 2014;34:341–5.

[230] Ward MM, Studenski S. Clinical prognostic factors in lupus nephritis. The importance of hypertension and smoking. Arch Intern Med 1992;152:2082–8.

[231] Toloza SM, Uribe AG, McGwin Jr G, Alarcón GS, Fessler BJ, Bastian HM, et al. Systemic lupus erythematosus in a multiethnic US cohort (LUMINA). XXIII. Baseline predictors of vascular events. Arthritis Rheum 2004;50:3947–57.

[232] Ho KT, Ahn CW, Alarcón GS, Baethge BA, Tan FK, Roseman J, et al. Systemic lupus erythematosus in a multiethnic cohort (LUMINA): XXVIII. Factors predictive of thrombotic events. Rheumatology (Oxf) 2005;44:1303–7.

[233] Chasset F, Francès C, Barete S, Amoura Z, Arnaud L. Influence of smoking on the efficacy of antimalarials in cutaneous lupus: a meta-analysis of the literature. J Am Acad Dermatol January 2015;30.

[234] Jewell ML, McCauliffe DP. Patients with cutaneous lupus erythematosus who smoke are less responsive to antimalarial treatment. J Am Acad Dermatol 2000;42:983–7.

[235] Dutz J, Werth VP. Cigarette smoking and response to antimalarials in cutaneous lupus erythematosus patients: evolution of a dogma. J Invest Dermatol 2011;131:1968–70.

[236] Schein JR. Cigarette smoking and clinically significant drug interactions. Ann Pharmacother 1995;29:1139–48.

[237] Rubin RL, Hermanson TM, Bedrick EJ, McDonald JD, Burchiel SW, Reed MD, et al. Effect of cigarette smoke on autoimmunity in murine and human systemic lupus erythematosus. Toxicol Sci 2005;87:86–96.

[238] Freemer MM, King Jr TE, Criswell LA. Association of smoking with dsDNA autoantibody production in systemic lupus erythematosus. Ann Rheum Dis 2006;65:581–4.

[239] Young KA, Terrell DR, Guthridge JM, Kamen DL, Gilkeson GS, Karp DR, et al. Smoking is not associated with autoantibody production in systemic lupus erythematosus patients, unaffected first-degree relatives, nor healthy controls. Lupus 2014;23:360–9.

[240] Arnson Y, Shoenfeld Y, Amital H. Effects of tobacco smoke on immunity, inflammation and autoimmunity. J Autoimmun 2010;34:J258–65.

[241] Gustafsson JT, Gunnarsson I, Källberg H, Pettersson S, Zickert A, Vikerfors A, et al. Cigarette smoking, antiphospholipid antibodies and vascular events in systemic lupus erythematosus. Ann Rheum Dis August 2015;74(8):1537–43.

[242] Vikerfors A, Johansson AB, Gustafsson JT, Jönsen A, Leonard D, Zickert A, et al. Clinical manifestations and anti-phospholipid antibodies in 712 patients with systemic lupus erythematosus: evaluation of two diagnostic assays. Rheumatology (Oxf) 2013;52:501–9.

[243] Milo R, Miller A. Revised diagnostic criteria of multiple sclerosis. Autoimmun Rev 2014;13(4–5):24–518. World Health Organization. Atlas of multiple sclerosis; 2013.

[244] Koch-Henriksen N, Sørensen PS. The changing demographic pattern of multiple sclerosis epidemiology. Lancet Neurol May 2010;9(5):520–32.

[245] Milo R, Kahana E. Multiple sclerosis: geoepidemiology, genetics and the environment. Autoimmun Rev March 2010;9(5):A387–94.

[246] Sawcer S, Franklin RJM, Ban M. Multiple sclerosis genetics. Lancet Neurol May 19, 2014;13(7):700–9.

[247] Belbasis L, Bellou V, Evangelou E, Ioannidis JPA, Tzoulaki I. Environmental risk factors and multiple sclerosis: an umbrella review of systematic reviews and meta-analyses. Lancet Neurol March 2015;14(3):263–73.

[248] Versini M, Jeandel P-Y, Rosenthal E, Shoenfeld Y. Obesity in autoimmune diseases: not a passive bystander. Autoimmun Rev August 2, 2014;13(9):981–1000.

[249] Munger KL, Levin LI, Hollis BW, Howard NS, Ascherio A. Serum 25-hydroxyvitamin D levels and risk of multiple sclerosis. JAMA December 20, 2006;296(23):2832–8.

[250] Hernán MA, Olek MJ, Ascherio A. Cigarette smoking and incidence of multiple sclerosis. Am J Epidemiol July 1, 2001;154(1):69–74.

[251] Riise T, Nortvedt MW, Ascherio A. Smoking is a risk factor for multiple sclerosis. Neurology October 28, 2003;61(8):1122–4.

[252] Mikaeloff Y, Caridade G, Tardieu M, Suissa S. Parental smoking at home and the risk of childhood-onset multiple sclerosis in children. Brain October 1, 2007;130(10):2589–95.

[253] Sundström P, Nyström L, Hallmans G. Smoke exposure increases the risk for multiple sclerosis. Eur J Neurol June 2008;15(6):579–83.

[254] Palacios N, Alonso A, Brønnum-Hansen H, Ascherio A. Smoking and increased risk of multiple sclerosis: parallel trends in the sex ratio reinforce the evidence. Ann Epidemiol July 2011;21(7):536–42.

[255] Maghzi A-H, Etemadifar M, Heshmat-Ghahdarijani K, Moradi V, Nonahal S, Ghorbani A, et al. Cigarette smoking and the risk of multiple sclerosis: a sibling case-control study in Isfahan, Iran. Neuroepidemiology January 2011;37(3–4):238–42.

[256] Ramagopalan SV, Lee JD, Yee IM, Guimond C, Traboulsee AL, Ebers GC, et al. Association of smoking with risk of multiple sclerosis: a population-based study. J Neurol March 2, 2013;260(7):1778–81.

[257] Hedström AK, Hillert J, Olsson T, Alfredsson L. Smoking and multiple sclerosis susceptibility. Eur J Epidemiol November 2013;28(11):867–74.

[258] O'Gorman C, Bukhari W, Todd A, Freeman S, Broadley SA. Smoking increases the risk of multiple sclerosis in Queensland, Australia. J Clin Neurosci October 2014;21(10):1730–3.

[259] Hedström AK, Bäärnhielm M, Olsson T, Alfredsson L. Exposure to environmental tobacco smoke is associated with increased risk for multiple sclerosis. Mult Scler July 2011;17(7):788–93.

[260] Hedstrom A, Olsson T, Alfredsson L. Smoking is a major preventable risk factor for multiple sclerosis. Mult Scler J October 2015;12.

[261] O'Gorman C, Broadley SA. Smoking and multiple sclerosis: evidence for latitudinal and temporal variation. J Neurol September 2014;261(9):1677–83.

[262] Hedström AK, Sundqvist E, Bäärnhielm M, Nordin N, Hillert J, Kockum I, et al. Smoking and two human leukocyte antigen genes interact to increase the risk for multiple sclerosis. Brain March 2011;134(Pt 3):653–64.

[263] Hedström AK, Bomfim IL, Barcellos LF, Briggs F, Schaefer C, Kockum I, et al. Interaction between passive smoking and two HLA genes with regard to multiple sclerosis risk. Int J Epidemiol December 2014;43(6):1791–8.

[264] Hedstrom AK, Baarnhielm M, Olsson T, Alfredsson L. Tobacco smoking, but not Swedish snuff use, increases the risk of multiple sclerosis. Neurology August 31, 2009;73(9):696–701.

[265] Odoardi F, Sie C, Streyl K, Ulaganathan VK, Schläger C, Lodygin D, et al. T cells licensed in the lung to enter the central nervous system. Nature August 30, 2012;488(7413):675–9.

[266] Hernán MA, Jick SS, Logroscino G, Olek MJ, Ascherio A, Jick H. Cigarette smoking and the progression of multiple sclerosis. Brain June 2005;128(Pt 6):1461–5.

[267] Koch M, van Harten A, Uyttenboogaart M, De Keyser J. Cigarette smoking and progression in multiple sclerosis. Neurology October 8, 2007;69(15):1515–20.

[268] Mandia D, Ferraro OE, Nosari G, Montomoli C, Zardini E, Bergamaschi R. Environmental factors and multiple sclerosis severity: a descriptive study. Int J Environ Res Public Health June 2014;11(6):6417–32.

[269] Munger KL, Fitzgerald KC, Freedman MS, Hartung H-P, Miller DH, Montalban X, et al. No association of multiple sclerosis activity and progression with EBV or tobacco use in BENEFIT. Neurology November 10, 2015;85(19):1694–701.

[270] Di Pauli F, Reindl M, Ehling R, Schautzer F, Gneiss C, Lutterotti A, et al. Smoking is a risk factor for early conversion to clinically definite multiple sclerosis. Mult Scler July 16, 2008;14(8):1026–30.

[271] Sundström P, Nyström L. Smoking worsens the prognosis in multiple sclerosis. Mult Scler September 2008;14(8):1031–5.

[272] Pittas F, Ponsonby A-L, Mei IAF, Taylor BV, Blizzard L, Groom P, et al. Smoking is associated with progressive disease course and increased progression in clinical disability in a prospective cohort of people with multiple sclerosis. J Neurol April 9, 2009;256(4):577–85.

[273] Healy BC, Ali EN, Guttmann CRG, Chitnis T, Glanz BI, Buckle G, et al. Smoking and disease progression in multiple sclerosis. Arch Neurol July 1, 2009;66(7):858–64.

[274] Zivadinov R, Weinstock-Guttman B, Hashmi K, Abdelrahman N, Stosic M, Dwyer M, et al. Smoking is associated with increased lesion volumes and brain atrophy in multiple sclerosis. Neurology August 17, 2009;73(7):504–10.

[275] D'hooghe MB, Haentjens P, Nagels G, De Keyser J. Alcohol, coffee, fish, smoking and disease progression in multiple sclerosis. Eur J Neurol April 2012;19(4):616–24.

[276] Roudbari SA, Ansar MM, Yousefzad A. Smoking as a risk factor for development of secondary progressive multiple sclerosis: a study in Iran. Guilan. J Neurol Sci July 15, 2013;330(1–2):52–5.

[277] Arikanoglu A, Shugaiv E, Tüzün E, Eraksoy M. Impact of cigarette smoking on conversion from clinically isolated syndrome to clinically definite multiple sclerosis. Int J Neurosci July 2013;123(7):476–9.

[278] Ozcan ME, Ince B, Bingöl A, Ertürk S, Altınöz MA, Karadeli HH, et al. Association between smoking and cognitive impairment in multiple sclerosis. Neuropsychiatr Dis Treat January 2014;10:1715–9.

[279] Weiland TJ, Hadgkiss EJ, Jelinek GA, Pereira NG, Marck CH, van der Meer DM. The association of alcohol consumption and smoking with quality of life, disability and disease activity in an international sample of people with multiple sclerosis. J Neurol Sci January 15, 2014;336(1–2):211–9.

[280] Durhan G, Diker S, Has AC, Karakaya J, Kurne AT, Karabudak R, et al. Assessment of the effect of cigarette smoking on regional brain volumes and lesion load in patients with clinically isolated syndrome. Int J Neurosci September 2015;3:1–7.

[281] Ramanujam R, Hedström A-K, Manouchehrinia A, Alfredsson L, Olsson T, Bottai M, et al. Effect of smoking cessation on multiple sclerosis prognosis. JAMA Neurol September 8, 2015;72(10):1.

[282] Horakova D, Zivadinov R, Weinstock-Guttman B, Havrdova E, Qu J, Tamaño-Blanco M, et al. Environmental factors associated with disease progression after the first demyelinating event: results from the multi-center SET study. Editor Fujinami R.S PLoS One January 8, 2013;8(1):e53996.

[283] Manouchehrinia A, Weston M, Tench CR, Britton J, Constantinescu CS. Tobacco smoking and excess mortality in multiple sclerosis: a cohort study. J Neurol Neurosurg Psychiatry February 25, 2014;85(10):1091–5.

[284] Turner AP, Hartoonian N, Maynard C, Leipertz SL, Haselkorn JK. Smoking and physical activity: examining health behaviors and 15-year mortality among individuals with multiple sclerosis. Arch Phys Med Rehabil March 2015;96(3):402–9.

[285] Jick SS, Li L, Falcone GJ, Vassilev ZP, Wallander M-A. Epidemiology of multiple sclerosis: results from a large observational study in the UK. J Neurol June 13, 2015;262(9):2033–41.

[286] Sena A, Bendtzen K, Cascais MJ, Pedrosa R, Ferret-Sena V, Campos E. Influence of apolipoprotein E plasma levels and tobacco smoking on the induction of neutralising antibodies to interferon-beta. J Neurol October 2010;257(10):1703–7.

[287] Hedström AK, Ryner M, Fink K, Fogdell-Hahn A, Alfredsson L, Olsson T, et al. Smoking and risk of treatment-induced neutralizing antibodies to interferon β-1a. Mult Scler April 2014;20(4):445–50.

[288] Yadav SK, Mindur JE, Ito K, Dhib-Jalbut S. Advances in the immunopathogenesis of multiple sclerosis. Curr Opin Neurol June 2015;28(3):206–19.

[289] Correale J, Farez MF. Smoking worsens multiple sclerosis prognosis: two different pathways are involved. J Neuroimmunol April 15, 2015;281:23–34.

[290] Gao Z, Nissen JC, Ji K, Tsirka SE. The experimental autoimmune encephalomyelitis disease course is modulated by nicotine and other cigarette smoke components. PLoS One January 2014;9(9):e107979.

[291] Khanna A, Guo M, Mehra M, Royal W. Inflammation and oxidative stress induced by cigarette smoke in Lewis rat brains. J Neuroimmunol January 15, 2013;254(1–2):69–75.

[292] Carbone M, Neuberger JM. Autoimmune liver disease, autoimmunity and liver transplantation. J Hepatol 2014;60:210–23.

[293] Kaplan MM, Gershwin ME. Primary biliary cirrhosis. N Engl J Med 2005;353:1261–73.

[294] Smyk DS, Rigopoulou EI, Muratori L, Burroughs AK, Bogdanos DP. Smoking as a risk factor for autoimmune liver disease: what we can learn from primary biliary cirrhosis. Ann Hepatol 2012;11:7–14.

[295] Hirschfield GM, Chapman RW, Karlsen TH, Lammert F, Lazaridis KN, Mason AL. The genetics of complex cholestatic disorders. Gastroenterology 2013;144:1357–74.

[296] Juran BD, Lazaridis KN. Environmental factors in primary biliary cirrhosis. Semin Liver Dis 2014;34:265–72.

[297] Lammert C, Nguyen DL, Juran BD, Schlicht E, Larson JJ, Atkinson EJ, et al. Questionnaire based assessment of risk factors for primary biliary cirrhosis. Dig Liver Dis 2013;45:589–94.

[298] Gershwin ME, Selmi C, Worman HJ, Gold EB, Watnik M, Utts J, et al. Risk factors and comorbidities in primary biliary cirrhosis: a controlled interview-based study of 1032 patients. Hepatology 2005;42:1194–202.

[299] Parikh-Patel A, Gold EB, Worman H, Krivy KE, Gershwin ME. Risk factors for prima-ry biliary cirrhosis in a cohort of patients from the United States. Hepatology 2001;33:16–21.

[300] Corpechot C, Chrétien Y, Chazouillères O, Poupon R. Demographic, lifestyle, medical and familial factors associated with primary biliary cirrhosis. J Hepatol 2010;53:162–9.

[301] Cookson S, Constantini PK, Clare M, et al. Frequency and nature of cytokine gene polymorphisms in type 1 autoimmune hepatitis. Hepatology 1999;30:851–6.

[302] Czaja AJ, Cookson S, Constantini PK, Clare M, Underhill JA, Donaldson PT. Cytokine polymorphisms associated with clinical features and treatment outcome in type 1 autoimmune hepatitis. Gastroenterology 1999;117:645–52.

[303] Agarwal K, Czaja AJ, Jones DE, Donaldson PT. Cytotoxic T lymphocyte antigen-4 (CTLA-4) gene polymorphisms and susceptibility autoimmune hepatitis. Hepatology 2000;31:49–53.

[304] Heneghan MA, Yeoman AD, Verma S, Smith AD, Longhi MS. Autoimmune hepatitis. Lancet 2013;382:1433–44.

[305] Hirschfield GM, Karlsen TH, Lindor KD, Adams DH. Primary sclerosing cholangitis. Lancet 2013;382:1587–99.

[306] Andersen IM, Tengesdal G, Lie BA, Boberg KM, Karlsen TH, Hov JR. Effects of coffee consumption, smoking, and hormones on risk for primary sclerosing cholangitis. Clin Gastroenterol Hepatol 2014;12:1019–28.

[307] Mitchell SA, Thyssen M, Orchard TR, Jewell DP, Fleming KA, Chapman RW. Cigarette smoking, appendectomy, and tonsillectomy as risk factors for the development of primary sclerosing cholangitis: a case control study. Gut 2002;51:567–73.

[308] Loftus Jr EV, Sandborn WJ, Tremaine WJ, Mahoney DW, Zinsmeister AR, Offord KP, et al. Primary sclerosing cholangitis is associated with nonsmoking: a case-control study. Gastroenterology 1996;110:1496–502.

[309] Siebold J. Scleroderma. In: Harris E, Budd R, Firestein G, Genovese M, Sergent J, Ruddy S, editors. Kelley's textbook of rheumatology. 7th ed. Philadelphia: Elsevier; 2005.

[310] LeRoy EC, Black C, Fleischmajer R, et al. Scleroderma (systemic sclerosis): classification, subsets and pathogenesis. J Rheumatol 1988;15:202–5.

[311] Chaudhary P, Chen X, Assassi S, Gorlova O, Draeger H, Harper BE, et al. Cigarette smoking is not a risk factor for systemic sclerosis. Arthritis Rheum 2011;63:3098–102.

[312] Hudson M, Lo E, Lu Y, Hercz D, Baron M, Steele R. Cigarette smoking in patients with systemic sclerosis. Arthritis Rheum 2011;63:230–8.

[313] Hissaria P, Lester S, Hakendorf P, Woodman R, Patterson K, Hill C, et al. Survival in scleroderma: results from the population-based south Australian Register. Intern Med J 2011;41:381–90.

[314] Orgiazzi J. Thyroid autoimmunity. Presse Med December 2012;41(12 P 2):25–e611.

[315] Antonelli A, Ferrari SM, Corrado A, et al. Autoimmune thyroid disorders. Autoimmun Rev February 2015;14(2):174–80.

[316] Jacobson DL, Gange SJ, Rose NR, Graham NM. Epidemiology and estimated population burden of selected autoimmune diseases in the United States. Clin Immunol Immunopathol September 1997;84(3):223–43.

[317] McLeod DS, Cooper DS. The incidence and prevalence of thyroid autoimmunity. Endocrine October 2012;42(2):252–65.

[318] Tunbridge WM, Evered DC, Hall R, Appleton D, Brewis M, Clark F, et al. The spectrum of thyroid disease in a community: the Whickham survey. Clin Endocrinol (Oxf) 1977;7(6):481–93.

[319] Antonelli A, Ferrari SM, Giuggioli D, Ferrannini E, Ferri C, Fallahi P. Chemokine (C-X-C motif) ligand (CXCL)10 in autoimmune diseases. Autoimmun Rev March 2014;13(3):272–80.

[320] Antonelli A, Ferrari SM, Corrado A, Franceschini SS, Gelmini S, Ferrannini E, et al. Extraocular muscle cells from patients with Graves' ophthalmopathy secrete α (CXCL10) and β (CCL2) chemokines under the influence of cytokines that are modulated by PPARγ. Autoimmun Rev November 2014;13(11):1160–6.

[321] Tomer Y, Davies TF. Searching for the autoimmune thyroid disease susceptibility genes: from gene mapping to gene function. Endocr Rev October 2003;24(5):694–717.

[322] Hansen PS, Brix TH, Iachine I, Kyvik KO, Hegedüs L. The relative importance of genetic and environmental effects for the early stages of thyroid autoimmunity: a study of healthy Danish twins. Eur J Endocrinol January 2006;154(1):29–38.

[323] Brix TH, Hegedus L. Twin studies as a model for exploring the aetiology of autoimmune thyroid disease. Clin Endocrinol (Oxf) April 2012;76(4):457–64.

[324] Simmonds MJ. GWAS in autoimmune thyroid disease: redefining our understanding of pathogenesis. Nat Rev Endocrinol May 2013;9(5):277–87.

[325] Tanda ML, Piantanida E, Lai A, Lombardi V, Dalle Mule I, Liparulo L, et al. Thyroid autoimmunity and environment. Horm Metab Res 2009;41(6):436–42.

[326] Prummel MF, Wiersinga WM. Smoking and risk of Graves' disease. JAMA January 1993;269(4):479–82.

[327] Bartalena L, Marcocci C, Tanda ML, Manetti L, Dell'Unto E, Bartolomei MP, et al. Cigarette smoking and treatment outcomes in graves ophthalmopathy. Ann Intern Med 1998;129(8):632–5.

[328] Wiersinga WM. Smoking and thyroid. Clin Endocrinol (Oxf) August 2013;79(2):145–51.

[329] Nizzi E, Irony-Tur-Sinai M, Lory O, Orr-Urtreger A, Lavi E, Brenner T. Activation of the cholinergic anti-inflammatory system by nicotine attenuates neuroinflammation via suppression of Th1 and Th17 responses. J Immunol November 2009;183(10):6681–8.

[330] Bartalena L, Martino E, Marcocci C, Bogazzi F, Panicucci M, Velluzzi F, et al. More on smoking habits and Graves' ophthalmopathy. J Endocrinol Investig 1989;12(10):733–7.

[331] Ericsson UB, Lindgärde F. Effects of cigarette smoking on thyroid function and the prevalence of goitre, thyrotoxicosis and autoimmune thyroiditis. J Intern Med January 1991;229(1):67–71.

[332] Fukata S, Kuma K, Sugawara M. Relationship between cigarette smoking and hypothyroidism in patients with Hashimoto's thyroiditis. J Endocrinol Investig October 1996;19(9):607–12.

[333] Vestergaard P. Smoking and thyroid disorders—a meta-analysis. Eur J Endocrinol February 2002;146(2):153–61.

[334] Strieder TG, Prummel MF, Tijssen JG, Endert E, Wiersinga WM. Risk factors for and prevalence of thyroid disorders in a cross-sectional study among healthy female relatives of patients with autoimmune thyroid disease. Clin Endocrinol (Oxf) September 2003;59(3):396–401.

[335] Belin RM, Astor BC, Powe NR, Ladenson PW. Smoke exposure is associated with a lower prevalence of serum thyroid autoantibodies and thyrotropin concentration elevation and a higher prevalence of mild thyrotropin concentration suppression in the third national health and nutrition examination survey (NHANES III). J Clin Endocrinol Metab December 2004;89(12):6077–86.

[336] Galanti MR, Cnattingius S, Granath F, Ekbom-Schnell A, Ekbom A. Smoking and environmental iodine as risk factors for thyroiditis among parous women. Eur J Epidemiol 2007;22(7):467–72.

[337] Pedersen IB, Laurberg P, Knudsen N, Jørgensen T, Perrild H, Ovesen L, et al. Smoking is negatively associated with the presence of thyroglobulin autoantibody and to a lesser degree with thyroid peroxidase autoantibody in serum: a population study. Eur J Endocrinol 2008;158(3):367–73.

[338] Effraimidis G, Tijssen JG, Wiersinga WM. Discontinuation of smoking increases the risk for developing thyroid peroxidase antibodies and/or thyroglobulin antibodies: a prospective study. J Clin Endocrinol Metab April 2009;94(4):1324–8.

[339] Effraimidis G, Strieder TG, Tijssen JG, Wiersinga WM. Natural history of the transition from euthyroidism to overt autoimmune hypo- or hyperthyroidism: a prospective study. Eur J Endocrinol January 2011;164(1):107–13.

[340] Carlé A, Bülow Pedersen I, Knudsen N, Perrild H, Ovesen L, Banke Rasmussen L, et al. Smoking cessation is followed by a sharp but transient rise in the incidence of overt autoimmune hypothyroidism - a population-based, case-control study. Clin Endocrinol (Oxf) November 2012;77(5):764–72.

[341] Rendina D, De Palma D, De Filippo G, De Pascale F, Muscariello R, Ippolito R, et al. Prevalence of simple nodular goiter and Hashimoto's thyroiditis in current, previous, and never smokers in a geographical area with mild iodine deficiency. Horm Metab Res March 2015;47(3):214–9.

[342] Balazs C, Stenszky V, Farid NR. Association between Graves' ophthalmopathy and smoking. Lancet September 1990;336(8717):754.

[343] Tellez M, Cooper J, Edmonds C. Graves' ophthalmopathy in relation to cigarette smoking and ethnic origin. Clin Endocrinol (Oxf) March 1992;36(3):291–4.

[344] Vestergaard P, Rejnmark L, Weeke J, Hoeck HC, Nielsen HK, Rungby J, et al. Smoking as a risk factor for Graves' disease, toxic nodular goiter, and autoimmune hypothyroidism. Thyroid 2002;12(1):69–75.

[345] Holm IA, Manson JE, Michels KB, Alexander EK, Willett WC, Utiger RD. Smoking and other lifestyle factors and the risk of Graves' hyperthyroidism. Arch Intern Med July 2005;165(14):1606–11.

[346] Berglund J, Ericsson UB, Hallengren B. Increased incidence of thyrotoxicosis in Malmö during the years 1988–1990 as compared to the years 1970–1974. J Intern Med January 1996;239(1):57–62.

[347] Glinoer D, de Nayer P, Bex M. Belgian collaborative study group on Graves' disease. Effects of L-thyroxine administration, TSH-receptor antibodies and smoking on the risk of recurrence in Graves' hyperthyroidism treated with antithyroid drugs: a double-blind prospective randomized study. Eur J Endocrinol May 2001;144(5):475–83.

[348] Nedrebo BG, Holm PI, Uhlving S, Sorheim JI, Skeie S, Eide GE, et al. Predictors of outcome and comparison of different drug regimens for the prevention of relapse in patients with Graves' disease. Eur J Endocrinol 2002;147(5):583–9.

[349] Orgiazzi J, Madec AM. Reduction of the risk of relapse after withdrawal of medical therapy for Graves' disease. Thyroid October 2002;12(10):849–53.

[350] Träisk F, Tallstedt L, Abraham-Nordling M, Andersson T, Berg G, Calissendorff J, et al. Thyroid-associated ophthalmopathy after treatment for Graves' hyperthyroidism with antithyroid drugs or iodine-131. J Clin Endocrinol Metab 2009;94(10):3700–7.

[351] Hou X, Li Y, Li J, Wang W, Fan C, Wang H, et al. Development of thyroid dysfunction and autoantibodies in Graves' multiplex families: an eight-year follow-up study in Chinese Han pedigrees. Thyroid 2011;21(12):1353–8.

[352] Anagnostis P, Adamidou F, Polyzos SA, Katergari S, Karathanasi E, Zouli C, et al. Predictors of long-term remission in patients with Graves' disease: a single center experience. Endocrine 2013;44(2):448–53.

[353] Regensburg NI, Wiersinga WM, Berendschot TT, Saeed P, Mourits MP. Effect of smoking on orbital fat and muscle volume in Graves' orbitopathy. Thyroid February 2011;21(2):177–81.

[354] Metcalfe RA, Weetman AP. Stimulation of extraocular muscle fibroblasts by cytokines and hypoxia: possible role in thyroid-associated ophthalmopathy. Clin Endocrinol (Oxf) January 1994;40(1):67–72.

[355] Burch HB, Lahiri S, Bahn RS, Barnes S. Superoxide radical production stimulates retroocular fibroblast proliferation in Graves' ophthalmopathy. Exp Eye Res August 1997;65(2):311–6.

[356] Bartalena L, Tanda ML, Piantanida E, Lai A. Oxidative stress and Graves' ophthalmopathy: in vitro studies and therapeutic implications. Biofactors 2003;19(3–4):155–63.

[357] Tsai CC, Cheng CY, Liu CY, Kao SC, Kau HC, Hsu WM, et al. Oxidative stress in patients with Graves' ophthalmopathy: relationship between oxidative DNA damage and clinical evolution. Eye (Lond) 2009;23(8):1725–30.

[358] Yoon JS, Lee HJ, Chae MK, Lee SY, Lee EJ. Cigarette smoke extract-induced adipogenesis in Graves' orbital fibroblasts is inhibited by quercetin via reduction in oxidative stress. J Endocrinol January 2013;216(2):145–56.

[359] Chng CL, OF L, Chew CS, Peh YP, Fook-Chong SM, Seah LL, et al. Hypoxia increases adipogenesis and affects adipocytokine production in orbital fibroblasts-a possible explanation of the link between smoking and Graves' ophthalmopathy. Int J Ophthalmol 2014;7(3):403–7.

[360] Mack WP, Stasior GO, Cao HJ, Stasior OG, Smith TJ. The effect of cigarette smoke constituents on the expression of HLA-DR in orbital fibroblasts derived from patients with Graves ophthalmopathy. Ophthal Plast Reconstr Surg July 1999;15(4):260–71.

[361] Wakelkamp IM, Gerding MN, van der Meer JW, Prummel MF, Wiersinga WM. Smoking and disease severity are independent determinants of serum adhesion molecule levels in Graves' ophthalmopathy. Clin Exp Immunol February 2002;127(2):316–20.

[362] Bufalo NE, Santos RB, Cury AN, Andrade RA, Morari J, Morari EC, et al. Genetic polymorphisms associated with cigarette smoking and the risk of graves' disease. Clin Endocrinol (Oxf) 2008;68(6):982–7.

[363] Planck T, Shahida B, Sjögren M, Groop L, Hallengren B, Lantz M. Association of BTG2, CYR61, ZFP36, and SCD gene polymorphisms with Graves' disease and ophthalmopathy. Thyroid July 2014;24(7):1156–61.

[364] Planck T, Shahida B, Parikh H, Ström K, Asman P, Brorson H, et al. Smoking induces overexpression of immediate early genes in active Graves' ophthalmopathy. Thyroid 2014;24(10):1524–32.

[365] Atkinson MA, Eisenbarth GS, Michels AW. Type 1 diabetes. Lancet January 2014;383(9911):69–82.

[366] Davidson A, Diamond B. Autoimmune diseases. N Engl J Med August 2001;345(5):340–50.

[367] Battaglia M. Experiments by nature: lessons on type 1 diabetes. Tissue Antigens January 2014;83(1):1–9.

[368] Roep BO, Tree TI. Immune modulation in humans: implications for type 1 diabetes mellitus. Nat Rev Endocrinol April 2014;10(4):229–42.

[369] Kawasaki E. Type 1 diabetes and autoimmunity. Clin Pediatr Endocrinol October 2014;23(4):99–105.

[370] Antonelli A, Ferrari SM, Corrado A, Ferrannini E, Fallahi P. CXCR3, CXCL10 and type 1 diabetes. Cytokine Growth Factor Rev February 2014;25(1):57–65.

[371] Antonelli A, Fallahi P, Ferrari SM, Pupilli C, d'Annunzio G, Lorini R, et al. Serum Th1 (CXCL10) and Th2 (CCL2) chemokine levels in children with newly diagnosed type 1 diabetes: a longitudinal study. Diabet Med 2008;25(11):1349–53.

[372] Antonelli A, Baj G, Marchetti P, Fallahi P, Surico N, Pupilli C, et al. Human anti-CD38 autoantibodies raise intracellular calcium and stimulate insulin release in human pancreatic islets. Diabetes 2001;50(5):985–91.

[373] Concannon P, Rich SS, Nepom GT. Genetics of type 1a diabetes. N Engl J Med April 2009;360(16):1646–54.

[374] Stankov K, Benc D, Draskovic D. Genetic and epigenetic factors in etiology of diabetes mellitus type 1. Pediatrics December 2013;132(6):1112–22.

[375] Rønningen KS. Type 1 diabetes: prospective cohort studies for identification of the environmental trigger. Arch Immunol Ther Exp (Warsz) December 2013;61(6):459–68.

[376] Zipris D. The interplay between the gut microbiota and the immune system in the mechanism of type 1 diabetes. Curr Opin Endocrinol Diabetes Obes August 2013;20(4):265–70.

[377] Stene LC, Gale EA. The prenatal environment and type 1 diabetes. Diabetologia September 2013;56(9):1888–97.

[378] Craig ME, Nair S, Stein H, Rawlinson WD. Viruses and type 1 diabetes: a new look at an old story. Pediatr Diabetes May 2013;14(3):149–58.

[379] Sipetic SB, Vlajinac HD, Kocev NI, Marinkovic JM, Radmanovic SZ, Bjekic MD. The Belgrade childhood diabetes study: a multivariate analysis of risk determinants for diabetes. Eur J Public Health April 2005;15(2):117–22.

[380] Wahlberg J, Vaarala O, Ludvigsson J. ABIS study group. Asthma and allergic symptoms and type 1 diabetes-related autoantibodies in 2.5-yr-old children. Pediatr Diabetes November 2011;12(7):604–10.

[381] Stene LC, Barriga K, Norris JM, Hoffman M, Erlich HA, Eisenbarth GS, et al. Perinatal factors and development of islet autoimmunity in early childhood: the diabetes autoimmunity study in the young. Am J Epidemiol 2004;160(1):3–10.

[382] Rosenbauer J, Herzig P, Kaiser P, Giani G. Early nutrition and risk of type 1 diabetes mellitus—a nationwide case-control study in preschool children. Exp Clin Endocrinol Diabetes September 2007;115(8):502–8.

[383] Wadsworth EJ, Shield JP, Hunt LP, Baum JD. A case-control study of environmental factors associated with diabetes in the under 5s. Diabet Med May 1997;14(5):390–6.

[384] Toschke AM, Ehlin A, Koletzko B, Montgomery SM. Paternal smoking is associated with a decreased prevalence of type 1 diabetes mellitus among offspring in two national British birth cohort studies (NCDS and BCS70). J Perinat Med 2007;35(1):43–7.

[385] Johansson A, Hermansson G, Ludvigsson J. ABIS Study Group. Tobacco exposure and diabetes-related autoantibodies in children: results from the ABIS study. Ann N Y Acad Sci December 2008;1150:197–9.

[386] Dahlquist G, Källén B. Maternal-child blood group incompatibility and other perinatal events increase the risk for early-onset type 1 (insulin-dependent) diabetes mellitus. Diabetologia July 1992;35(7):671–5.

[387] Marshall AL, Chetwynd A, Morris JA, Placzek M, Smith C, Olabi A, et al. Type 1 diabetes mellitus in childhood: a matched case control study in Lancashire and Cumbria, UK. Diabet Med 2004;21(9):1035–40.

[388] Svensson J, Carstensen B, Mortensen HB, Borch-johnsen K. Danish study group of childhood diabetes. Early childhood risk factors associated with type 1 diabetes–is gender important? Eur J Epidemiol 2005;20(5):429–34.

[389] Hathout EH, Beeson WL, Ischander M, Rao R, Mace JW. Air pollution and type 1 diabetes in children. Pediatr Diabetes April 2006;7(2):81–7.

[390] Skrodeniene E, Marciulionyte D, Padaiga Z, Jasinskiene E, Sadauskaite-Kuehne V, Ludvigsson J. Environmental risk factors in prediction of childhood prediabetes. Medicina (Kaunas) 2008;44(1):56–63.

[391] Olin JW. Thromboangiitis obliterans (Buerger's disease). N Engl J Med September 21, 2000;343(12):864–9.

[392] Machado EB, Gabriel SE, Beard CM, Michet CJ, O'Fallon WM, Ballard DJ. A population-based case-control study of temporal arteritis: evidence for an associa-tion between temporal arteritis and degenerative vascular disease? Int J Epidemiol December 1989;18(4):836–41.

[393] Duhaut P, Pinede L, Demolombe-Rague S, Loire R, Seydoux D, Ninet J, et al. Giant cell arteritis and cardiovascular risk factors: a multicenter, prospective case-control study. Groupe de recherche sur l'artérite à cellules Géantes. Arthritis Rheum November 1998;41(11):1960–5.

[394] Larsson K, Mellström D, Nordborg E, Nordborg C, Odén A. Early menopause, low body mass index, and smoking are independent risk factors for developing giant cell arteritis. Ann Rheum Dis April 2006;65(4):529–32.

[395] Jakobsson K, Jacobsson L, Warrington K, Matteson EL, Liang K, Melander O, et al. Body mass index and the risk of giant cell arteritis: results from a prospective study. Rheumatology (Oxf) March 2015;54(3):433–40.

[396] Kermani TA, Schäfer VS, Crowson CS, Hunder GG, Ytterberg SR, Matteson EL, et al. Cancer preceding giant cell arteritis: a case-control study. Arthritis Rheum June 2010;62(6):1763–9.

[397] Lane SE, Watts RA, Bentham G, Innes NJ, Scott DGI. Are environmental factors important in primary systemic vasculitis? A case-control study. Arthritis Rheum March 2003;48(3):814–23.

[398] Beaudreuil S, Lasfargues G, Laurière L, El Ghoul Z, Fourquet F, Longuet C, et al. Occupational exposure in ANCA-positive patients: a case-control study. Kidney Int May 2005;67(5):1961–6.

[399] Haubitz M, Woywodt A, de Groot K, Haller H, Goebel U. Smoking habits in patients diagnosed with ANCA associated small vessel vasculitis. Ann Rheum Dis October 2005;64(10):1500–2.

[400] Gonzalez-Gay MA, Piñeiro A, Gomez-Gigirey A, Garcia-Porrua C, Pego-Reigosa R, Dierssen-Sotos T, et al. Influence of traditional risk factors of atherosclerosis in the development of severe ischemic complications in giant cell arteritis. Medicine (Baltim) November 2004;83(6):342–7.

[401] Robson JC, Kiran A, Maskell J, Hutchings A, Arden N, Dasgupta B, et al. The relative risk of aortic aneurysm in patients with giant cell arteritis compared with the general population of the UK. Ann Rheum Dis January 2015;74(1):129–35.

[402] Mohammad AJ, Segelmark M. Association of cigarette smoking with organ damage in primary systemic vasculitis. Scand J Rheumatol January 2011;40(1):51–6.

[403] Lega J-C, Seror R, Fassier T, Aumaître O, Quere I, Pourrat J, et al. Characteristics, prognosis, and outcomes of cutaneous ischemia and gangrene in systemic necrotizing vasculitides: a retrospective multicenter study. Semin Arthritis Rheum April 2014;43(5):681–8.

[404] Benarous L., Terrier B, Puéchal X., Dunogué B, Cohen P., Le Jeunne C., et al. Tobacco differentially affects the clinical-biological phenotypes of ANCA-associated vasculitides. Clin Exp Rheumatol. Jan; 33(2 Suppl 89):S 116–121.

[405] Maniaol AH, Boldingh M, Brunborg C, Harbo HF, Tallaksen CME. Smoking and socio-economic status may affect myasthenia gravis. Eur J Neurol March 2013;20(3):453–60.

[406] Gratton SM, Herro AM, Feuer WJ, Lam BL. Cigarette smoking and activities of daily living in ocular myasthenia gravis. J Neuro Ophthalmol March 2016;36(1):37–40.

[407] Snook JA, Dwyer L, Lee-Elliott C, Khan S, Wheeler DW, Nicholas DS. Adult coeliac disease and cigarette smoking. Gut July 1996;39(1):60–2.

[408] Vazquez H, Smecuol E, Flores D, Mazure R, Pedreira S, Niveloni S, et al. Relation be-tween cigarette smoking and celiac disease: evidence from a case-control study. Am J Gastroenterol March 2001;96(3):798–802.

[409] Suman S, Williams EJ, Thomas PW, Surgenor SL, Snook JA. Is the risk of adult coeliac disease causally related to cigarette exposure? Eur J Gastroenterol Hepatol September 2003;15(9):995–1000.

[410] Austin AS, Logan RFA, Thomason K, Holmes GKT. Cigarette smoking and adult coeliac disease. Scand J Gastroenterol August 2002;37(8):978–82.

[411] Patel AH, Loftus EV, Murray JA, Harmsen WS, Zinsmeister AR, Sandborn WJ. Cigarette smoking and celiac sprue: a case-control study. Am J Gastroenterol August 2001;96(8):2388–91.

[412] Ludvigsson JF, Nordenvall C, Järvholm B. Smoking, use of moist snuff and risk of ce-liac disease: a prospective study. BMC Gastroenterol January 2014;14:120.

[413] Ludvigsson JF, Ludvigsson J. Parental smoking and risk of coeliac disease in off-spring. Scand J Gastroenterol March 2005;40(3):336–42.

[414] Ludvigsson JF, Montgomery SM, Ekbom A. Smoking and celiac disease: a population-based cohort study. Clin Gastroenterol Hepatol September 2005;3(9):869–74.

[415] Brenner S, Tur E, Shapiro J, Ruocco V, D'Avino M, Ruocco E, et al. Pemphigus vulgaris: environmental factors. Occupational, behavioral, medical, and qualitative food frequency questionnaire. Int J Dermatol September 2001;40(9):562–9.

[416] Sullivan TP, Elgart GW, Kirsner RS. Pemphigus and smoking. Int J Dermatol August 2002;41(8):528–30.

[417] Valikhani M, Kavusi S, Chams-Davatchi C, Daneshpazhooh M, Barzegari M, Ghiasi M, et al. Pemphigus and associated environmental factors: a case-control study. Clin Exp Dermatol May 2007;32(3):256–60.

[418] Valikhani M, Kavusi S, Chams-Davatchi C, Hallaji Z, Esmaili N, Ghandi N, et al. Impact of smoking on pemphigus. Int J Dermatol June 2008;47(6):567–70.

[419] Mehta JN, Martin AG. A case of pemphigus vulgaris improved by cigarette smoking. Arch Dermatol January 2000;136(1):15–7.

[420] Grando SA, Dahl MV. Nicotine and pemphigus. Arch Dermatol October 2000;136(10):1269.

[421] Baron-Epel O, Shalata W, Hovell MF. Waterpipe tobacco smoking in three Israeli adult populations. Isr Med Assoc J May 2015;17(5):282–7.

[422] Hollan I, Dessein PH, Ronda N, Wasko MC, Svenungsson E, Agewall S, et al. Prevention of cardiovascular disease in rheumatoid arthritis. Autoimmun Rev October 2015;14(10):952–69.

[423] Selmi C, Cantarini L, Kivity S, Dagaan A, Shovman O, Zandman-Goddard G, et al. The 2014 ACR annual meeting: a bird's eye view of autoim-munity in 2015. Autoimmun Rev July 2015;14(7):622–32.

[424] Sela BA. Time for setting a good example: physicians, quit smoking now. Isr Med Assoc J July 2013;15(7):379–81.

[425] Marie I, Gehanno JF, Bubenheim M, Duval-Modeste AB, Joly P, Dominique S, et al. Prospective study to evaluate the association between systemic sclerosis and occupational exposure and review of the literature. Autoimmun Rev February 2014;13(2):151–6.

[426] Gómez-Puerta JA, Gedmintas L, Costenbader KH. The association between silica exposure and development of ANCA-associated vasculitis: sys-tematic review and metaanalysis. Autoimmun Rev October 2013;12(12):1129–35.

[427] Sakkas LI, Bogdanos DP, Katsiari C, Platsoucas CD. Anti-citrullinated peptides as autoantigens in rheumatoid arthritis-relevance to treatment. Autoimmun Rev November 2014;13(11):1114–20.

[428] Ben-Horin S, Kopylov U, Chowers Y. Optimizing anti-TNF treatments in inflammatory bowel disease. Autoimmun Rev January 2014;13(1):24–30.

[429] Kiyohara C, Washio M, Horiuchi T, Tada Y, Asami T, Ide S, et al. Kobashi G; Kyushu Sapporo SLE (KYSS) study group. Cigarette smoking, N-acetyltransferase 2 polymorphisms and systemic lupus erythematosus in a Japanese population. Lupus June 2009;18(7):630–8.

Chapter 38

Cannabinoids in Autoimmune and Rheumatic Diseases

Luca Navarini, Domenico P. E. Margiotta, Gabriele Gallo Afflitto, Antonella Afeltra

Unit of Allergology, Immunology, Rheumatology, Department of Medicine, Università Campus Bio-Medico di Roma, Rome, Italy

ENDOCANNABINOID SYSTEM AND PHYTOCANNABINOIDS

Cannabis sativa, Cannabis indica, and *Cannabis ruderalis* are three different *Cannabis* species, part of the plant family Cannabaceae. "Marijuana" is a type of cannabis characterized by a high production of the psychoactive cannabinoid delta9-tetrahydrocannabinol (Δ9-THC) and the nonpsychoactive cannabinoid cannabidiol (CBD), and it is considered for recreational and medical use, while "hemp" is another type of cannabis characterized by a high production of CBD and very low production or absence of Δ9-THC and it has mainly industrial applications [1]. The first testimonies of medical use of cannabis date back to 1400–2000 BC in Sanskrit and Hindi literature [2], and different ancient Greek physicians reported medicinal inductions for cannabis [3]. In 1964, a group from Israel isolated the main psychoactive compound of cannabis and the prototypical phytocannabinoid, Δ9-THC [4]. Since then, many of other phytocannabinoids have been identified, such as CBD, cannabinol (CBN), cannabivarin, cannabidivarin, and cannabidiolic acid [5]. Despite the great effort of research in this field, the pharmacodynamics of Δ9-THC remained elusive for many years. Only in the early 90s, Matsuda and coworkers identified a cannabinoid receptor, named cannabinoid type 1 receptor (CB_1), able to bind Δ9-THC [6]; soon after, another cannabinoid receptor, named cannabinoid type 2 receptor (CB_2), has been found and linked to the immunosuppressive features of cannabis [7]. These findings led to hypothesize the existence of one or more molecules able to bind cannabinoid receptors in vivo. In 1992, Devane and coworkers were able to isolate from pig brain the first endogenous ligand for cannabinoid receptor, named *N*-arachidonoylethanolamine (or anandamide, AEA) [8]. At present, it has been well established that many lipid mediators, named endocannabinoids (eCBs), are able to bind CB_1 and/or CB_2. Among them, AEA and 2-arachidonoylglycerol (2-AG) are the most studied (Fig. 38.1). It is widely accepted that eCBs are synthesized "on demand" from membrane lipid precursors by distinct metabolic routes. In particular, AEA is synthesized from the corresponding *N*-acylphosphatidylethanolamines (NAPEs) and the most studied route of its biosynthesis requires a type D phospholipase (PLD) selective for NAPEs (NAPE-PLD) [9,10]. Fatty acid amide hydrolase (FAAH) is the major responsible of AEA [11]. Through the action of two *sn*-2-selective DAG lipases, i.e., DAGL-α and DAGL-β, 1-acyl-2-arachidonoylglycerols (DAGs) can be converted in 2-AG [12], which can be degraded by monoacylglycerol lipase and, to a lesser extent, alpha/beta-hydrolase domain 6 (ABHD6) and 12 (ABHD12) and FAAH itself [11]. For a functional point of view, AEA preferentially activates CB_1 than CB_2, while 2-AG resembles Δ9-THC activating both CB_1 and CB_2. CB_1 is mainly expressed not only in brain (particularly cortex, basal ganglia, hippocampus, and cerebellum) but also to a lesser extent in testes, adrenal glands, pancreas, heart, and lungs, while 2-AG is mainly distributed in peripheral tissue and especially in immune cells [13–15]. Both cannabinoid receptor are G protein–coupled receptors, which electively couple to G proteins of the G_i and G_o classes, and they inhibit certain voltage-dependent calcium channels and adenylyl cyclases, thus reducing cyclic adenosine monophosphate formation, and promote the activation of mitogen-activating protein kinases and inwardly rectifying potassium channels [16]. Of note, eCBs are able to interact also with other receptors, such as the transient receptor potential cation channel subfamily V member 1 (TRPV1) and subfamily A member 1 (TRPA1), as well as the G protein–coupled receptor 55 (GPR55) [13]. eCBs, along with their receptors and the enzymes responsible for their synthesis and degradation, form the eCB system. On the other hand, eCB-like molecules, such as *N*-palmitoylethanolamine (PEA) and *N*-oleoylethanolamine (OEA), are able to modulate the eCB system, mainly competing with eCBs for the degradation through FAAH [11].

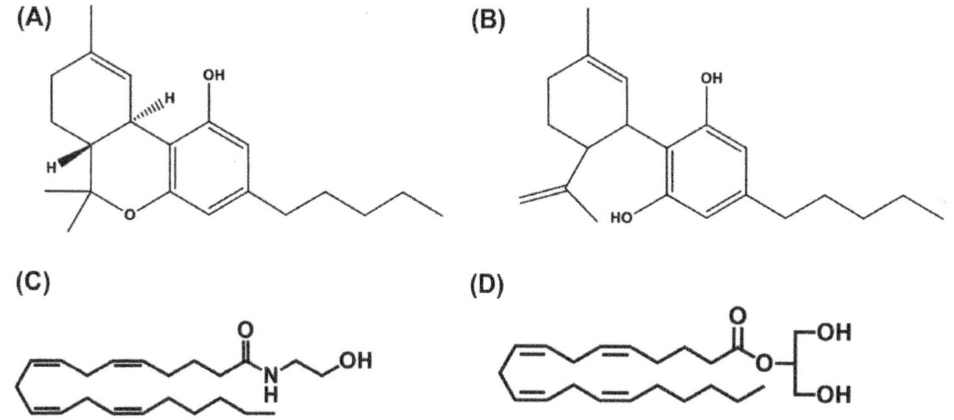

FIGURE 38.1 Structure of (A) tetrahydrocannabinol, (B) cannabidiol, (C) anandamide, and (D) 2-arachidonoylglycerol.

CANNABINOIDS AND IMMUNE SYSTEM

Phytocannabinoids and eCBs exert their immunologic functions through the interaction with CB_2, more expressed in immune cells than CB_1 [17] and present also in neurons and activated microglial cells and astrocytes [18].

Phytocannabinoids have important effects on immune system and exert mainly antiinflammatory effects. Δ9-THC, the main psychoactive phytocannabinoid, plays a pivotal role in immunomodulation and antiinflammation: it reduces the production of many proinflammatory cytokines, such as tumor necrosis factor alpha (TNF-α), interleukin-1 (IL-1), IL-6, and IL-12, and chemokines. Moreover, Δ9-THC deeply affects the migration, proliferation, and apoptosis of inflammatory cells [19–21]. Furthermore, CBD, a nonpsychoactive phytocannabinoid, has proven to be beneficial in inflammatory pain in rats treated with Freund's adjuvant intraplantar injection [22]. CBD is also able to reduce many proinflammatory cytokines, such as IL-2 and interferon-γ (IFN-γ) [23], and its administration seems to be effective in animal models of encephalomyelitis [24], arthritis [25], colitis [26], and diabetes [27]. Recently, a phase II study highlighted the safety and efficacy of CBD in the prevention of graft-versus-host-disease [28].

In recent years, eCB system has been identified as a key modulator of immune system. Both macrophages and monocytes express CB_1 and CB_2 on their membranes [17,29,30]. AEA is able to inhibit alveolar macrophage killing of TNF-sensitive murine L929 fibroblasts [31] in mouse. Similarly, in mouse macrophages AEA is able to reduce the expression of nitric oxide (NO), IL-6, IL-12, and IL-23 and increase the expression of IL-10 mainly through interaction with CB_2 [17,32–36]. The role of 2-AG is still contradictory: on the one hand, 2-AG is able to induce the production of chemokines and promote adhesion and migration of macrophages mainly through CB_2 [37–40]; on the other hand, it has proven to decrease proinflammatory cytokines output and adhesion molecules expression [41].

Only few studies evaluated the role of eCB system on dendritic cells (DCs) in humans [42]. In DCs, the presence of AEA, 2-AG, PEA, and FAAH has been demonstrated and CB_1 and CB_2 expression does not undergo modification during maturation of DCs [43]. Furthermore, AEA is able to reduce the production of TNF-α, IL-12p40, and IL-6 in myeloid DCs and the production of TNF-α and IFN-α from plasmacytoid DCs through CB_2. AEA is also able to reduce the activity of myeloid and plasmacytoid DCs in polarizing naïve CD4+ T cells in T helper lymphocytes 1 (Th1) and Th17 [44].

Other cells of innate immune system are also deeply affected by eCBs. High levels of AEA and 2-AG and expression of CB_1 and CB_2 have been identified in natural killer (NK) cells [29]; particularly, 2-AG could be crucial in inducing the migration of NK cells [45,46].

AEA is able to reduce neutrophil migration [47] and it reduces the production of metalloproteases [48], but its capacity to modulate microbicidal features of neutrophils is highly controversial because AEA is not able to reduce superoxide and hydrogen peroxide release [49–51]. On the other hand, 2-AG is able to not only induce production of myeloperoxidase and leukotriene B_4, thus sustaining neutrophil activity [52], but also control RhoA activation, reducing neutrophil migration [53].

2-AG is also able to promote migration in eosinophils through activation of CB_2 [54]. Furthermore, AEA reduces degranulation and maturation of mast cells mainly through interaction with CB_1 [55,56]. These findings highlight the important role of eCB system in allergy [17].

eCB system exerts a pivotal role also in adaptive immunity. It has been well established that AEA exerts important antiinflammatory features on T lymphocytes and inhibits proliferation of both CD4+ and CD8+ T cells, reducing cytokines output (particularly IL-2, TNF-α, INF-γ, and IL-17) mainly through activation of CB_2 and peroxisome proliferator-activated receptor gamma (PPAR-γ) and inhibition of nuclear factor-κB (NF-κB) [17,42,57]. eCB is also deeply affected by cytokines milieu: particularly, the Th2 cytokines IL-4 and IL-10 are able to enhance FAAH activity, whereas Th1 cytokines IL-12 and INF-γ tend to reduce FAAH activity [58]. In addition, 2-AG seems to be able to reduce the production of IL-2 but mainly through activation of PPAR-γ [59,60]. At present, little is known about the effects of eCB system in human B lymphocytes [42], but data from mouse models highlighted that CB_2 plays a pivotal role in B cells differentiation and immunoglobulin class switching from IgM to IgE [17].

As the immune cells were firstly shown to differentially express both CB_1 and CB_2 receptor on their surface, thus suggesting an immunomodulatory effect of the eCB system, a large amount of studies have been set up in recent years to better understand its exact role in autoimmune and immune-mediated diseases and the effects produced by its exogenous modulation both in in vitro and in vivo models.

RHEUMATOID ARTHRITIS

Rheumatoid arthritis (RA) is a multisystemic chronic inflammatory condition primarily affecting the joint, characterized by synoviocytes dysregulation, proliferation, and migration, along with neoangiogenesis and inflammatory cells synovial invasion, up to the synovial pannus formation, which represents the main histological feature of the disease [61,62]. Even if the major epidemiological studies have been done in Western countries, it is now commonly assumed that RA prevalence is in the range of 0.5%–1.0% worldwide, though geographical (Northern vs. Southern countries), ethnical (Native Americans), and sex-related (female>male) differences exist [61,63].

The cytokine, chemokine, and enzymatic milieu (primarily TNF-α, IL-1b, IL-6, and IL-17, with IL-8 and matrix metalloproteinases [MMPs]) both in RA synovium and synovial fluid have been demonstrated not only to induce but also self-sustain the inflammatory process, responsible for the pannus formation, for the articular cartilage degradation and for the bony erosions, up to the complete joint destruction and ankyloses [64–67].

Data from animal models demonstrated that synthetic and phytocannabinoids could have beneficial effects on inflammatory arthritis [25,68,69]. The first evidence of an altered regulation of the eCB system in human RA came from an in deep analysis of the synovium and the synovial fluid of RA patients, published by Richardson and coworkers in 2008, demonstrating the expression of CB_1 and CB_2 mRNAs and proteins as long as the two main eCBs, AEA and 2-AG, in synovium of patients with end-stage osteoarthritis (OA) and RA. Furthermore, in synovial fluids of patients with RA and OA, a higher expression of both AEA and 2-AG, along with lower levels of PEA, has been demonstrated in comparison with healthy subjects [70].

In the last few years, a better description of the eCB system in RA synovium has been provided, and it could be reasonably summarized, considering the main actors in the pathogenic process of the disease, as follows:

- **Rheumatoid arthritis synovial fibroblasts (RASFs)**: Contributing for a major part in RA pathophysiology, RASFs are nowadays recognized as the potential inducer of the inflammatory process and the engine of joint damage attaching to, invading into, and degrading cartilage and bone [71]. RASFs are able to produce inflammatory cytokines (TNF-α, IL-1β, IL-6), chemokines (RANTES, MCP-1, fractalkine), and metalloproteinases (MMP-1, MMP-3, MMP-10) [72]. RASFs are deeply affected by cannabinoids. Compared with osteoarthritis fibroblasts (OASFs), RASFs have been shown to express more CB_2 mRNA and protein, which may be upregulated by inflammatory stimuli (IL-1β, TNF-α, and lipopolysaccharide); HU-308, a selective CB_2 agonist, is able to reduce RASFs proliferation and MMP-3, MMP-13, and IL-6 production [73,74]. Previously, in a mouse model of collagen-induced arthritis, HU-320, a molecule structurally related to CBD with low affinity to CB_1 and CB_2, ameliorates joint inflammation and destruction [68]. On the other hand, in a first report, Lowin T. and coworkers demonstrated that AEA, PEA, and OEA are able to reduce the production of IL-6, IL-8, and MMP-3 in RASFs and OASFs through activation of TRPV1 and TRPA1 in a COX-2–dependent manner and that AEA reduces the adhesion of synovial fibroblasts to fibronectin through activation of CB_1 [75]. Afterward, Lowin and coworkers highlighted that low concentrations of the synthetic cannabinoid WIN55,212-2 reduce IL-6, IL-8, and MMP-3 production through CB_2, TRPA1, TRPV1, and a still unknown pharmacological target [74]. Ajulemic acid (AJA), another nonpsychoactive cannabinoid, has proven to decrease MMP-1, MMP-3, and MMP-9 in RASFs stimulated by IL-1α and TNF-α [76]; also in vivo, AJA is able to ameliorate adjuvant-induced arthritis [69].

- **Osteoclast and osteoblast:** It is nowadays well known that a dysregulation in osteoblasts/osteoclasts ratio is peculiar in RA, which is responsible for both juxtaarticular osteoporosis and bony erosions, important clinical feature of progressive RA [77]. Even these phenomena are related to the chronic inflammatory process via the TNF-α/RANKL pathway [78]. In addition, it has been shown that, while osteoblasts preferentially express only CB_2 on the cell surface, osteoclasts express CB_1 and TRPV1, too, thus demonstrating a potential role of the eCB system in bone metabolism [79,80]. In fact, according to the most recent data, a reduction in osteoclasts proliferation and a suppression of bone resorption could be obtained by CB_1 inhibition along with a CB_2 agonism [73,81,82].
- **Macrophages:** One of the most abundant cells in RA pannus, macrophages, acting as antigen-presenting cells and mediating the innate and the adaptive branch of the immune response, is likely to firstly trigger off the autoimmune process on the basis of genetic predisposition. Their multipotent inflammatory activity is responsible for most of the nowadays disposable evidence [83,84]; in fact, it has been demonstrated that, in RA patients, the synovial macrophage infiltrate highly correlates with disease activity, joint erosions, and response to treatment with synthetic DMARDs and biologics.

In addition, it has been demonstrated that macrophages express CB_2 on their surface, thus supporting the speculation for a probable role of the eCB system in the regulation of their activity in RA, too [30]. For example, HU-320 is able to reduce the production of TNF-α from murine macrophages and of reactive oxygen intermediates from RAW 264.7 [68].

- **T and B lymphocytes:** It is nowadays extensively accepted the crucial role played by T cells in RA pathogenesis, which is characterized by the particular activation of specific CD4+ T cell subsets, such as T helper 1 (Th1) and T helper 17 (Th17) and the dysregulation of the regulatory T cells (Tregs), mediated by TNF-dependent Foxp3 dephosphorylation [85]. B lymphocytes represent the main source of RF and ACPA and they are one of the most important players in RA pathogenesis, as shown by the formation in some patients' synovium of tertiary lymphoid structures and by the success of therapeutic B cell depletion using, for example, rituximab [86]. Even if few is known about the exact role of the eCBs system in RA pathogenesis, evidences from other diseases have shown an efficacy in reducing T cells proliferation and differentiation, via CB_2 agonism [87]. It was also demonstrated that HU-320 is able to modulate lymphocytes polyclonal responses both in murine and human RA [68].

The immunomodulatory effect and the pain-relieving action expressed by the eCBs system in experimental settings together represent the supporting evidence for a double-blind randomized controlled trial (RCT) observing the effects of nabiximols (a Δ9-THC/CBD oromucosal spray) on 58 patients with RA over a 4 weeks period. In this trial, Nabiximols provided benefit effects on pain on movement, pain at rest, quality of sleep, DAS28, and short-form McGill Pain Questionnaire, while no amelioration on morning stiffness has been proven. Unfortunately, it is not currently possible to recommend this kind of treatments in the clinical approach to the patient with RA because of the reduced sample size, the short observational period, and the lack of other RCTs [88,89].

PSORIASIS

Psoriasis (PSO) is a chronic, immune-mediated disorder, primarily affecting the skin, which can express different phenotypes (plaques or vulgaris PSO, guttate PSO, inverse PSO, pustular PSO, palmoplantar PSO, and erythrodermic PSO), albeit systemic comorbidities, for instance, articular, cardiovascular, and psychiatric, tend to occur [90,91]. Data from a systematic review about the global prevalence of PSO in adults show values ranging from 2.7% in the United States to 8.5% in Norway, with main geographical and age-related differences [92]. PSO can be considered as a multifactorial disease, depending on epigenetic, genetic (PSO susceptibility 1 locus—HLA-C*06—previously known as PSORS1) [93], and environmental factors (infections—bacteria, fungus, and virus; bad habits—smoking, drinking; chemical irritants—UV radiation exposure) concurring to the breach of the self-tolerance [94].

In PSO, keratinocytes, DCs, and T cells take part into the pathogenic process, which is primarily mediated by the IL-23/IL-17 axis, responsible for the main histological features of the disease, comprising, among the others:

- In the epidermis:
  - Acanthosis, parakeratosis, and dyskeratosis, together with abnormal keratinocyte hyperproliferation;
  - Munro microabscesses (an accumulation of neutrophils in the epidermis) and alternating neutrophils.
- In the dermis:
  - Infiltration of mononuclear cells;
  - Dilated, prominent blood vessels [95,96].

In addition, in the last few years, a number of data have shown that the eCBs play a critical role into the pathogenesis of PSO defined as follow:

- **Keratinocytes:** It is now well known that the eCB system is well expressed in the skin, where not only AEA, 2-AG, and all the enzymes responsible for their synthesis and metabolism but also all the receptors linked to the eCB system (CB_1, CB_2, and TRPV1) are expressed [97]. All these are responsible for a variety of effects induced by the eCB system modulation in skin. For example, AEA inhibits keratinocytes proliferation and promotes cell death through CB_1 and TRPV1 activation and subsequent Ca^{++} influx [98]. Furthermore, a CB_1 agonist, arachidonoyl-chloro-ethanolamide, downregulates the expression of keratins K6 and K16, which are overexpressed in a number of skin conditions such as PSO and wound healing [99]. Of note, Δ9-THC, CBD, CBN, and cannabigerol reduce proliferation of keratinocytes, while JWH015 and BML190, which are CB_2 agonists, only partially inhibit their proliferation and their action seems to be not linked with CB_1 and CB_2 activation [97].
- **Endothelium:** Dermal neovascularization, one of the main histological features of PSO, is a process consisting of three main parts: proliferation, migration, and organization in a structured blood vessel of endothelial cells [100]. Each of these mechanisms is regulated by a number of transcription factors (i.e., HIF-1α, NF-κB), cytokines (i.e., TNF-α, IL-8), chemokines (i.e., VCAM-1, ICAM-1), protease (i.e., MMP-2), and growth factors (i.e., VEGF, FGF, Ang2, Tie2), which in turn is at least partly controlled by the eCB system mediators. In fact, the selective agonism to CB_2 has been demonstrated to reduce angiogenesis, in vivo and in vitro, through inhibition of endothelial cells migration and proliferation [101,102].
- **Dendritic cells:** Noteworthy, Δ9-THC pretreatment in *Legionella pneumophila*–infected DCs suppresses IL-12p40 (a pivotal cytokine in PSO immunopathology) and inhibits the expression of maturation markers such as MHC-2, CD86, and CD40 [103].

Altogether, these pieces of evidence demonstrate a possible efficacy of the eCBs in reducing inflammation, angiogenesis, and hyperkeratosis, thus representing a possible, novel, efficacious oral, or topical treatment for PSO.

SYSTEMIC SCLEROSIS

Systemic sclerosis (SSc) is a chronic connective tissue disease, distinctively characterized by the triad microvascular damage, dysregulation of cellular and humoral immunity, and generalized fibrosis in skin and multiple internal organs. It represents just a peculiar manifestation of the diverse scleroderma spectrum, including localized scleroderma and SSc [104].

Pathophysiologically, SSc is considered as a multifactorial disease with a genetic HLA, IRF5, and STAT4, demonstrated by the familiar, ethnic, and geographical distribution of the disease, as well as an environmental component, related to industrial and infectious components according to the molecular mimicry theory [105–107].

Even in SSc, a role for the eCB system has been speculated, and a modest amount of data is now available, especially, on dermal fibroblasts (DFs). Both CB_1 and CB_2 are clearly overexpress by DFs [108], and their agonism has been shown to induce

- Inhibition of the transdifferentiation of DFs in myofibroblasts, specialized fibroblasts, resistant to apoptosis, expressing the cytoskeletal protein α-SMA, and characterized by an intense profibrotic behavior [108];
- Profound reduction in type 1 collagen, TGF-β, and CTGF mRNAs and proteins, thus inhibiting the fibrogenic process, probably through an IL-6-dependent manner;
- Increased apoptosis trend, apparently not mediated by CB1/CB2 activation [108–111].

In fact, recent studies have shown that a number of secondary receptor can mediate the eCBs intracellular cascade; among them PPAR-γ should be considered for its biological relevance in SSc. In fact, the administration of AJA, a nonpsychoactive synthetic analog of THC, is able to bind PPAR-γ, thus reducing dermal and pulmonary fibrosis, acting both as an antifibrotic and as antiinflammatory agent. In fact, it is able to indirectly inhibit NF-κB translocation from cytoplasm to the nucleus, resulting in a reduced production of proinflammatory cytokines, metalloproteases, and acute-phase proteins [111–113].

FIBROMYALGIA

Fibromyalgia, one of the most debated disease, is described in the EULAR revised recommendations for the management of fibromyalgia as a syndrome in which "although pain is the dominant symptom […], other symptoms such as fatigue, non-refreshed sleep, mood disturbance and cognitive impairment are common, but not universal," setting up a heterogeneous and complex condition with a considerable influence on quality of life [114]. A large number of diagnostic criteria has succeeded in the years, till 2016, when the last and most accepted revisions to the 2010/11 fibromyalgia diagnostic criteria was released [115]. Fibromyalgia is a common disease, occurring in all populations worldwide, with prevalence rate ranging from 2% to 4%. A slight difference exists according to sex, being female more affected than man [114,116,117].

The definite etiology of the disease is not today well known, with a probable interaction between biological and psychosocial variables. The former ones would incorporate a wide range of somatic and functional alterations in many systems, with a major involvement of the central nervous system (CNS); on the other hand, depression, obesity, physical and sexual abuse in childhood, sleep problems, and smoking could not only trigger but also worsen symptoms of fibromyalgia. Nowadays, a multidisciplinary approach, with physical and psychological interventions as a first-line treatment, eventually combined with pharmacological therapy, is strongly recommended by evidence-based guidelines. However, just a small proportion of patients (up to 25%) is capable to achieve a noteworthy pain relief, in such a way [114,118].

It has been supposed that eCB system could be deficient in fibromyalgia, thus responsible, among the others, for alterations in nociceptive pathways, low-grade inflammation, and emotional and cognitive impairment; therefore, its modulation was assumed as conceivably effective in fibromyalgia patients [119].

In fact, nabilone, a synthetic cannabinoid available in oral capsule, was proven to be effective and noninferior (if compared with placebo and amitriptyline, respectively) in fibromyalgia in two different RCTs with 72 participants. On the other hand, a higher incidence of not-serious adverse events was reported in nabilone-treated patients, especially dizziness, drowsiness, nausea, and dry mouth. However, the quality of evidence for all outcomes of efficacy, tolerability, and safety was very low in both of the trials beacause of the small size and the short duration of the studies [120]. Two different reviews of the literature about the use of cannabinoids in patients with fibromyalgia reported different results about effectiveness and safety, clearly demonstrating that further studies are requested to better understand the possible role of cannabis-based products in this disease [121,122].

OSTEOARTHRITIS

OA, a chronic degenerative diarthrodial disease, affecting both large and small joints, is the most common rheumatic disorder, with an estimated 27 million affected patients (≥25 yo) in the United States [123]. OA can be described as a multifactorial disease depending on a combination of both endogenous (genetic, structural factors, obesity, physical activity) [124,125] and environmental factors (age, overuse, major trauma) [126] leading to a number of alterations regarding each of the constituents of the diarthrodial joint (articular cartilage, subchondral bone, ligaments, capsule, and synovial membranc) [127], accompanicd by thc dcvclopmcnt of structural damagc and joint pain, till thc complctc joint failurc [128].

In the pathogenesis of OA a large number of different class of cells are involved but a central role is undoubtedly played by articular chondrocytes, which under physiological conditions are responsible for maintaining minimal collagen turnover, while in OA they tend to exhibit an increased synthetic activity (MMP-3, MMP-13, ADAMTS-4, ADAMTS-5, and cathepsins), in turn stimulated by a number of proinflammatory cytokines (TNF-α, IL-1, IL-6, IL-15) responsible for the catabolism of type II collagen, proteoglycans, and aggrecans [127,129,130].

In addition, in 2016, chondrocytes from OA donors were shown to widely express not only the "classical" eCBs receptor (CB$_1$ and CB$_2$) but also GPR55, PPAR-α, and PPAR-γ. On the other hand, the expression of TRPV1 and GPR18 within the deep zone of cartilage was notably decreased [70,131]. The in vitro modulation of these receptors—specifically CB$_2$—mediated by WIN55 resulted efficacious in inhibiting ADAMTS-4 in unstimulated and IL-1β stimulated human OA articular chondrocytes, reducing the mRNA expression and stability of syndecan-1 [129,132].

However, FAAH inhibition has been shown to be ineffective, when compared with naproxen as an active comparator, in pain modulation, as shown by an RCT enrolling 74 patients, which was stopped at the interim analysis for futility [129,133].

SYSTEMIC LUPUS ERYTHEMATOSUS

Less is known about the role played by the eCBs in systemic lupus erythematosus (SLE), the prototypic potentially fatal, chronic, multisystem, and multifactorial autoimmune disorder, commonly affecting women between puberty and menopause. In a mouse model of SLE, an FAAH upregulation has been demonstrated and FAAH inhibition reverted the increase of receptor revision, RAG expression, and polyreactive autoantibodies formation [134]. A first preliminary result demonstrated that SLE patients have higher levels of 2-AG compared with healthy controls [135].

MULTIPLE SCLEROSIS

Multiple sclerosis (MS) is a chronic neurodegenerative disorder which affects 2.3 million people in the world [136]. Many ex vivo studies highlighted that there is an important alteration of CB_1 and CB_2 both in murine models and patients with MS [137]. A first pioneeristic study demonstrated that Δ9-THC, methanandamide (an AEA analog), and CB_1 and CB_2 agonists reduce spasticity and tremor in experimental autoimmune encephalitis (EAE), and administration of CB_1 or CB_2 antagonists reverted these therapeutic effects [138]. It has been also suggested that CB_1 could be able to exert neuroprotective features, reducing neurodegeneration and preventing disability [139], and promote remyelination [140,141]; these effects are probably related to the immunomodulation which leads to reduction of adhesion molecules, T lymphocytes infiltration, and microglial activation [24,142,143] and, to some extent, to recovery to self-tolerance to myelin [144]. CB_2 too has beneficial effects in MS: its activation is able to reduce inflammation in CNS, reducing Th17 differentiation and microglia activation in murine models [145,146] and downregulating T lymphocytes proliferation and activation in MS patients [147]. Overall, recent data demonstrate that CB_1 is more involved in control of spasticity and CB_2 is more involved in immunomodulation in MS [137]. In agreement with these findings, exogenous administration of eCBs is related to reduction of the spasticity and amelioration of CNS inflammation [137]. Of note, in an experimental model of MS, AEA was able to reduce the production of IL-23, IL-12, IL-1β, and IL-6, thus interfering with microglial activation [35,36]. AEA seems to exert specific antiinflammatory features on myeloid DCs [44], but not on plasmacytoid DCs [44]. Furthermore, eCB system through CB_1 activation is able to reduce excitotoxic damage of neurons, another hallmark of neuroinflammation [137]. On the other hand, phytocannabinoids reduce neuroinflammation and neurodegeneration during EAE [148]; in particular, the interaction between Δ9-THC and CB_1 seems to improve neurological deficits in EAE [149], while CBD reduces inflammation and axonal damage in the same mouse model and apoptosis in oligodendrocytes and neurons [24,150]. These findings provided the rationale for the use of Nabiximols in MS, which is now approved for spasticity-related MS [137].

TYPE 1 DIABETES MELLITUS

Type 1 diabetes mellitus T lymphocytes play a pivotal role in destroying insulin pancreatic β-cells [151]. In non–obese diabetes mice, CBD is able to reduce the incidence of diabetes and downregulate Th1 cytokines as well as upregulate Th2 cytokines [27]: these data suggested that CBD could have an important role in preventing the onset of type 1 diabetes mellitus. In macrophages, CBD is also able to reduce the production of IL-12, which is a very important cytokine in the pathogenesis of type 1 diabetes [152]. Further evaluations are required to confirm and/or apply these findings in humans.

INFLAMMATORY BOWEL DISEASES

The term inflammatory bowel diseases (IBDs) comprise two different intestinal diseases differentiated by histology and location. In Crohn's disease, a transmural inflammation which involves any portion of the gastrointestinal tract has been demonstrated, while ulcerative colitis (UC) induces inflammation of the colonic mucosa [153]. In CB_1 and CB_2 knockout mice, an increased susceptibility to chemical colitis has been demonstrated [154,155]. Moreover, AEA is able to promote colonic mucosal healing and both AEA and 2-AG increase intestinal permeability [156]. Particularly, CB_2 is more expressed during inflammatory flares [157], leading to hypothesize that CB_2 could become in the next few years an important therapeutic target in IBDs [158]. eCB-like molecule, PEA, seems to be a fascinating treatment opportunity in IBDs: precisely, it has been demonstrated that PEA could promote mucosal healing in UC [159].

Data about the role of cannabinoids in human autoimmune and rheumatic diseases are summarized in Table 38.1.

CONCLUSIONS

The relationship between cannabinoids and immune system is clearly demonstrated in many studies, both in animal models and humans. eCB system modulation seems to represent a valuable therapeutic strategy in many autoimmune and rheumatic disorders to manage better and better "the fire within" [160].

TABLE 38.1 The Role of Cannabinoids in Human Autoimmune and Rheumatic Diseases: A Summary

Disease	Role of Cannabinoids	References
Rheumatoid arthritis	Higher expression of AEA and 2-AG in synovial fluid	[70]
	Higher expression of CB_2 in RASFs compared with OASFs. CB_2 agonism reduces RASFs proliferation and MMP-3, MMP-13, and IL-6 production	[73,74]
	AEA, PEA, and OEA reduce IL-6, IL-8, and MMP-3 in RASFs and reduce adhesion to fibronectin	[75]
	Nabiximols provided beneficial effects on pain on movement, pain at rest, quality of sleep, DAS28, and short-form McGill Pain Questionnaire	[88]
Psoriasis	AEA inhibits keratinocytes proliferation and promotes cell death through CB_1 and TRPV1 activation	[98]
	Arachidonoyl-chloro-ethanolamide downregulates the expression of keratins K6 and K16	[99]
	Δ9-THC, CBD, CBN, and cannabigerol reduce proliferation of keratinocytes	[97]
Systemic sclerosis	Agonism to CB_1 and CB_2 inhibits the transdifferentiation of DFs in myofibroblasts and reduces type 1 collagen, TGF-β, and CTGF	[108,111]
Fibromyalgia	Hypothesis of an eCB deficiency	[119]
	Controversial results with cannabinoids-based treatments in fibromyalgia	[121,122]
Osteoarthritis (OA)	In OA, chondrocytes express CB_1, CB_2, GPR55, PPAR-α, and PPAR-γ. The expression of TRPV1 and GPR18 within the deep zone of cartilage is decreased	[70,131]
	WIN55 inhibits ADAMTS-4 in chondrocytes, reducing the mRNA expression and stability of syndecan-1	[129]
	FAAH inhibition seems to an ineffective therapeutic strategy	[133]
Systemic lupus erythematosus	Higher levels of 2-AG compared with healthy subjects	[135]
Multiple sclerosis (MS)	Reduction of T lymphocytes proliferation and activation through CB_2 activation	[147]
	AEA exerts antiinflammatory features on myeloid dendritic cells, but not on plasmacytoid dendritic cells	[44]
	Effectiveness of nabiximols in spasticity-related MS	[137]
Inflammatory bowel diseases	CB_2 is more expressed during inflammatory flares	[157]
	PEA promotes mucosal healing in UC	[159]

2-AG, 2-arachidonoylglycerol; *AEA*, anandamide; *CBD*, cannabidiol; *CBN*, cannabinol; *DFs*, dermal fibroblasts; *FAAH*, fatty acid amide hydrolase; *IL*, interleukin; *MMP*, matrix metalloproteinase; *OASFs*, osteoarthritis fibroblasts; *OEA*, oleoylethanolamine; *PEA*, palmitoylethanolamine; *PPAR*, peroxisome proliferator-activated receptor; *RASFs*, rheumatoid arthritis synovial fibroblasts; *UC*, ulcerative colitis.

REFERENCES

[1] Baron EP. Comprehensive review of medicinal marijuana, cannabinoids, and therapeutic implications in medicine and headache: what a long strange trip it's been. Headache 2015;55(6):885–916.

[2] Chopra IC, Chopra RN. The use of cannabis drugs in India. Bull Narc 1957;9:4–29.

[3] Brunner T. Marijuana in ancient Greece and Rome? The literary evidence. Bull Hist Med 1973;47:344–55.

[4] Mechoulam R, Gaoni Y. A total synthesis of dl-delta-1-tetrahydrocannabinol, the active constituent of hashish. J Am Chem Soc 1965;87:3273–5.

[5] ElSohly MA, Radwan MM, Gul W, Chandra S, Galal A. Phytochemistry of *Cannabis sativa* L. Prog Chem Org Nat Prod 2017;103:1–36.

[6] Matsuda LA, Lolait SJ, Brownstein MJ, Young AC, Bonner TI. Structure of a cannabinoid receptor and functional expression of the cloned cDNA. Nature 1990;346(6284):561–4.

[7] Munro S, Thomas KL, Abu-Shaar M. Molecular characterization of a peripheral receptor for cannabinoids. Nature 1993;365(6441):61–5.

[8] Devane WA, Hanus L, Breuer A, Pertwee RG, Stevenson LA, Griffin G, et al. Isolation and structure of a brain constituent that binds to the cannabinoid receptor. Science (New York NY) 1992;258(5090):1946–9.

[9] Ueda N, Tsuboi K, Uyama T. Metabolism of endocannabinoids and related *N*-acylethanolamines: canonical and alternative pathways. FEBS J 2013;280(9):1874–94.

[10] Jin XH, Okamoto Y, Morishita J, Tsuboi K, Tonai T, Ueda N. Discovery and characterization of a Ca^{2+}-independent phosphatidylethanolamine *N*-acyltransferase generating the anandamide precursor and its congeners. J Biol Chem 2007;282(6):3614–23.

[11] Fezza F, Bari M, Florio R, Talamonti E, Feole M, Maccarrone M. Endocannabinoids, related compounds and their metabolic routes. Molecules 2014;19(11):17078–106.

[12] Bisogno T, Howell F, Williams G, Minassi A, Cascio MG, Ligresti A, et al. Cloning of the first sn1-DAG lipases points to the spatial and temporal regulation of endocannabinoid signaling in the brain. J Cell Biol 2003;163(3):463–8.

[13] Pertwee RG. The diverse CB1 and CB2 receptor pharmacology of three plant cannabinoids: delta9-tetrahydrocannabinol, cannabidiol and delta9-tetrahydrocannabivarin. Br J Pharmacol 2008;153(2):199–215.

[14] Lu HC, Mackie K. An introduction to the endogenous cannabinoid system. Biol Psychiatry 2016;79(7):516–25.

[15] Mackie K. Distribution of cannabinoid receptors in the central and peripheral nervous system. Handb Exp Pharmacol 2005;168:299–325.

[16] Howlett AC, Barth F, Bonner TI, Cabral G, Casellas P, Devane WA, et al. International union of pharmacology. XXVII. Classification of cannabinoid receptors. Pharmacol Rev 2002;54(2):161–202.

[17] Chiurchiu V, Battistini L, Maccarrone M. Endocannabinoid signaling in innate and adaptive immunity. Immunology 2015;144:352–4.

[18] Chiurchiu V, Leuti A, Maccarrone M. Cannabinoid signaling and neuroinflammatory diseases: a melting pot for the regulation of brain immune responses. J Neuroimmune Pharmacol 2015;10(2):268–80.

[19] Ligresti A, De Petrocellis L, Di Marzo V. From phytocannabinoids to cannabinoid receptors and endocannabinoids: pleiotropic physiological and pathological roles through complex pharmacology. Physiol Rev 2016;96(4):1593–659.

[20] Klein TW. Cannabinoid-based drugs as anti-inflammatory therapeutics. Nat Rev Immunol 2005;5(5):400–11.

[21] Walter L, Stella N. Cannabinoids and neuroinflammation. Br J Pharmacol 2004;141(5):775–85.

[22] Costa B, Trovato AE, Comelli F, Giagnoni G, Colleoni M. The non-psychoactive cannabis constituent cannabidiol is an orally effective therapeutic agent in rat chronic inflammatory and neuropathic pain. Eur J Pharmacol 2007;556(1–3):75–83.

[23] Kaplan BL, Springs AE, Kaminski NE. The profile of immune modulation by cannabidiol (CBD) involves deregulation of nuclear factor of activated T cells (NFAT). Biochem Pharmacol 2008;76(6):726–37.

[24] Kozela E, Lev N, Kaushansky N, Eilam R, Rimmerman N, Levy R, et al. Cannabidiol inhibits pathogenic T cells, decreases spinal microglial activation and ameliorates multiple sclerosis-like disease in C57BL/6 mice. Br J Pharmacol 2011;163(7):1507–19.

[25] Malfait AM, Gallily R, Sumariwalla PF, Malik AS, Andreakos E, Mechoulam R, et al. The nonpsychoactive cannabis constituent cannabidiol is an oral anti-arthritic therapeutic in murine collagen-induced arthritis. Proc Natl Acad Sci USA 2000;97(17):9561–6.

[26] Borrelli F, Aviello G, Romano B, Orlando P, Capasso R, Maiello F, et al. Cannabidiol, a safe and non-psychotropic ingredient of the marijuana plant *Cannabis sativa*, is protective in a murine model of colitis. J Mol Med (Berl Ger) 2009;87(11):1111–21.

[27] Weiss L, Zeira M, Reich S, Har-Noy M, Mechoulam R, Slavin S, et al. Cannabidiol lowers incidence of diabetes in non-obese diabetic mice. Autoimmunity 2006;39(2):143–51.

[28] Yeshurun M, Shpilberg O, Herscovici C, Shargian L, Dreyer J, Peck A, et al. Cannabidiol for the prevention of graft-versus-host-disease after allogeneic hematopoietic cell transplantation: results of a phase II study. Biol Blood Marrow Transplant 2015;21(10):1770–5.

[29] Maresz K, Carrier EJ, Ponomarev ED, Hillard CJ, Dittel BN. Modulation of the cannabinoid CB2 receptor in microglial cells in response to inflammatory stimuli. J Neurochem 2005;95(2):437–45.

[30] Chiurchiu V, Lanuti M, Catanzaro G, Fezza F, Rapino C, Maccarrone M. Detailed characterization of the endocannabinoid system in human macrophages and foam cells, and anti-inflammatory role of type-2 cannabinoid receptor. Atherosclerosis 2014;233(1):55–63.

[31] Cabral GA, Toney DM, Fischer-Stenger K, Harrison MP, Marciano-Cabral F. Anandamide inhibits macrophage-mediated killing of tumor necrosis factor-sensitive cells. Life Sci 1995;56(23–24):2065–72.

[32] Ross RA, Brockie HC, Pertwee RG. Inhibition of nitric oxide production in RAW264.7 macrophages by cannabinoids and palmitoylethanolamide. Eur J Pharmacol 2000;401(2):121–30.

[33] Correa F, Docagne F, Clemente D, Mestre L, Becker C, Guaza C. Anandamide inhibits IL-12p40 production by acting on the promoter repressor element GA-12: possible involvement of the COX-2 metabolite prostamide E(2). Biochem J 2008;409(3):761–70.

[34] Correa F, Hernangomez M, Mestre L, Loria F, Spagnolo A, Docagne F, et al. Anandamide enhances IL-10 production in activated microglia by targeting CB(2) receptors: roles of ERK1/2, JNK, and NF-kappaB. Glia 2010;58(2):135–47.

[35] Correa F, Hernangomez-Herrero M, Mestre L, Loria F, Docagne F, Guaza C. The endocannabinoid anandamide downregulates IL-23 and IL-12 subunits in a viral model of multiple sclerosis: evidence for a cross-talk between IL-12p70/IL-23 axis and IL-10 in microglial cells. Brain Behav Immun 2011;25(4):736–49.

[36] Hernangomez M, Mestre L, Correa FG, Loria F, Mecha M, Inigo PM, et al. CD200-CD200R1 interaction contributes to neuroprotective effects of anandamide on experimentally induced inflammation. Glia 2012;60(9):1437–50.

[37] Lourbopoulos A, Grigoriadis N, Lagoudaki R, Touloumi O, Polyzoidou E, Mavromatis I, et al. Administration of 2-arachidonoylglycerol ameliorates both acute and chronic experimental autoimmune encephalomyelitis. Brain Res 2011;1390:126–41.

[38] Kishimoto S, Kobayashi Y, Oka S, Gokoh M, Waku K, Sugiura T. 2-Arachidonoylglycerol, an endogenous cannabinoid receptor ligand, induces accelerated production of chemokines in HL-60 cells. J Biochem 2004;135(4):517–24.

[39] Kishimoto S, Gokoh M, Oka S, Muramatsu M, Kajiwara T, Waku K, et al. 2-arachidonoylglycerol induces the migration of HL-60 cells differentiated into macrophage-like cells and human peripheral blood monocytes through the cannabinoid CB2 receptor-dependent mechanism. J Biol Chem 2003;278(27):24469–75.

[40] Gokoh M, Kishimoto S, Oka S, Mori M, Waku K, Ishima Y, et al. 2-arachidonoylglycerol, an endogenous cannabinoid receptor ligand, induces rapid actin polymerization in HL-60 cells differentiated into macrophage-like cells. Biochem J 2005;386(Pt 3):583–9.

[41] Stefano GB, Bilfinger TV, Rialas CM, Deutsch DG. 2-arachidonyl-glycerol stimulates nitric oxide release from human immune and vascular tissues and invertebrate immunocytes by cannabinoid receptor 1. Pharmacol Res 2000;42(4):317–22.

[42] Chiurchiu V. Endocannabinoids and immunity. Cannabis Cannabinoid Res 2016;1(1):59–66.

[43] Matias I, Pochard P, Orlando P, Salzet M, Pestel J, Di Marzo V. Presence and regulation of the endocannabinoid system in human dendritic cells. Eur J Biochem 2002;269(15):3771–8.

[44] Chiurchiu V, Cencioni MT, Bisicchia E, De Bardi M, Gasperini C, Borsellino G, et al. Distinct modulation of human myeloid and plasmacytoid dendritic cells by anandamide in multiple sclerosis. Ann Neurol 2013;73(5):626–36.

[45] Sugiura T, Oka S, Gokoh M, Kishimoto S, Waku K. New perspectives in the studies on endocannabinoid and cannabis: 2-arachidonoylglycerol as a possible novel mediator of inflammation. J Pharmacol Sci 2004;96(4):367–75.

[46] Kishimoto S, Muramatsu M, Gokoh M, Oka S, Waku K, Sugiura T. Endogenous cannabinoid receptor ligand induces the migration of human natural killer cells. J Biochem 2005;137(2):217–23.

[47] McHugh D, Tanner C, Mechoulam R, Pertwee RG, Ross RA. Inhibition of human neutrophil chemotaxis by endogenous cannabinoids and phyto-cannabinoids: evidence for a site distinct from CB1 and CB2. Mol Pharmacol 2008;73(2):441–50.

[48] Montecucco F, Di Marzo V, da Silva RF, Vuilleumier N, Capettini L, Lenglet S, et al. The activation of the cannabinoid receptor type 2 reduces neutrophilic protease-mediated vulnerability in atherosclerotic plaques. Eur Heart J 2012;33(7):846–56.

[49] Kaufmann I, Schelling G, Eisner C, Richter HP, Krauseneck T, Vogeser M, et al. Anandamide and neutrophil function in patients with fibromyalgia. Psychoneuroendocrinology 2008;33(5):676–85.

[50] Kraft B, Wintersberger W, Kress HG. Cannabinoid receptor-independent suppression of the superoxide generation of human neutrophils (PMN) by CP55 940, but not by anandamide. Life Sci 2004;75(8):969–77.

[51] Kraft B, Kress HG. Indirect CB2 receptor and mediator-dependent stimulation of human whole-blood neutrophils by exogenous and endogenous cannabinoids. J Pharmacol Exp Ther 2005;315(2):641–7.

[52] Chouinard F, Lefebvre JS, Navarro P, Bouchard L, Ferland C, Lalancette-Hebert M, et al. The endocannabinoid 2-arachidonoyl-glycerol activates human neutrophils: critical role of its hydrolysis and de novo leukotriene B4 biosynthesis. J Immunol (Baltim Md 1950) 2011;186(5):3188–96.

[53] Kurihara R, Tohyama Y, Matsusaka S, Naruse H, Kinoshita E, Tsujioka T, et al. Effects of peripheral cannabinoid receptor ligands on motility and polarization in neutrophil-like HL60 cells and human neutrophils. J Biol Chem 2006;281(18):12908–18.

[54] Oka S, Ikeda S, Kishimoto S, Gokoh M, Yanagimoto S, Waku K, et al. 2-arachidonoylglycerol, an endogenous cannabinoid receptor ligand, induces the migration of EoL-1 human eosinophilic leukemia cells and human peripheral blood eosinophils. J Leukoc Biol 2004;76(5):1002–9.

[55] Maccarrone M, Bari M, Battista N, Finazzi-Agro A. Endocannabinoid degradation, endotoxic shock and inflammation. Curr Drug Targets Inflamm Allergy 2002;1(1):53–63.

[56] Sugawara K, Biro T, Tsuruta D, Toth BI, Kromminga A, Zakany N, et al. Endocannabinoids limit excessive mast cell maturation and activation in human skin. J Allergy Clin Immunol 2012;129(3):726–38.e8.

[57] Cencioni MT, Chiurchiu V, Catanzaro G, Borsellino G, Bernardi G, Battistini L, et al. Anandamide suppresses proliferation and cytokine release from primary human T-lymphocytes mainly via CB2 receptors. PLoS One 2010;5(1):e8688.

[58] Maccarrone M, Valensise H, Bari M, Lazzarin N, Romanini C, Finazzi-Agro A. Progesterone up-regulates anandamide hydrolase in human lymphocytes: role of cytokines and implications for fertility. J Immunol (Baltim Md 1950) 2001;166(12):7183–9.

[59] Rockwell CE, Raman P, Kaplan BL, Kaminski NE. A COX-2 metabolite of the endogenous cannabinoid, 2-arachidonyl glycerol, mediates suppression of IL-2 secretion in activated Jurkat T cells. Biochem Pharmacol 2008;76(3):353–61.

[60] Rockwell CE, Snider NT, Thompson JT, Vanden Heuvel JP, Kaminski NE. Interleukin-2 suppression by 2-arachidonyl glycerol is mediated through peroxisome proliferator-activated receptor gamma independently of cannabinoid receptors 1 and 2. Mol Pharmacol 2006;70(1):101–11.

[61] Smolen JS, Aletaha D, Barton A, Burmester GR, Emery P, Firestein GS, et al. Rheumatoid arthritis. Nat Rev Dis Primers 2018;4:18001.

[62] Scott DL, Wolfe F, Huizinga TW. Rheumatoid arthritis. Lancet (Lond Engl) 2010;376(9746):1094–108.

[63] Myasoedova E, Crowson CS, Kremers HM, Therneau TM, Gabriel SE. Is the incidence of rheumatoid arthritis rising?: results from Olmsted County, Minnesota, 1955-2007. Arthritis Rheum 2010;62(6):1576–82.

[64] McInnes IB, Schett G. The pathogenesis of rheumatoid arthritis. N Engl J Med 2011;365(23):2205–19.

[65] Ng CT, Biniecka M, Kennedy A, McCormick J, Fitzgerald O, Bresnihan B, et al. Synovial tissue hypoxia and inflammation in vivo. Ann Rheum Dis 2010;69(7):1389–95.

[66] Orr C, Vieira-Sousa E, Boyle DL, Buch MH, Buckley CD, Canete JD, et al. Synovial tissue research: a state-of-the-art review. Nat Rev Rheumatol 2017;13(8):463–75.

[67] McInnes IB, Schett G. Cytokines in the pathogenesis of rheumatoid arthritis. Nat Rev Immunol 2007;7(6):429–42.

[68] Sumariwalla PF, Gallily R, Tchilibon S, Fride E, Mechoulam R, Feldmann M. A novel synthetic, nonpsychoactive cannabinoid acid (HU-320) with antiinflammatory properties in murine collagen-induced arthritis. Arthritis Rheum 2004;50(3):985–98.

[69] Zurier RB, Rossetti RG, Lane JH, Goldberg JM, Hunter SA, Burstein SH. Dimethylheptyl-THC-11 oic acid: a nonpsychoactive antiinflammatory agent with a cannabinoid template structure. Arthritis Rheum 1998;41(1):163–70.

[70] Richardson D, Pearson RG, Kurian N, Latif ML, Garle MJ, Barrett DA, et al. Characterisation of the cannabinoid receptor system in synovial tissue and fluid in patients with osteoarthritis and rheumatoid arthritis. Arthritis Res Ther 2008;10(2):R43.

[71] Bartok B, Firestein GS. Fibroblast-like synoviocytes: key effector cells in rheumatoid arthritis. Immunol Rev 2010;233(1):233–55.

[72] Ospelt C. Synovial fibroblasts in 2017. RMD Open 2017;3(2):e000471.

[73] Gui H, Liu X, Wang ZW, He DY, Su DF, Dai SM. Expression of cannabinoid receptor 2 and its inhibitory effects on synovial fibroblasts in rheumatoid arthritis. Rheumatology (Oxf Engl) 2014;53(5):802–9.

[74] Lowin T, Pongratz G, Straub RH. The synthetic cannabinoid WIN55,212-2 mesylate decreases the production of inflammatory mediators in rheumatoid arthritis synovial fibroblasts by activating CB2, TRPV1, TRPA1 and yet unidentified receptor targets. J Inflamm (Lond Engl) 2016;13:15.

[75] Lowin T, Apitz M, Anders S, Straub RH. Anti-inflammatory effects of N-acylethanolamines in rheumatoid arthritis synovial cells are mediated by TRPV1 and TRPA1 in a COX-2 dependent manner. Arthritis Res Ther 2015;17:321.

[76] Zurier RB, Sun YP, George KL, Stebulis JA, Rossetti RG, Skulas A, et al. Ajulemic acid, a synthetic cannabinoid, increases formation of the endogenous proresolving and anti-inflammatory eicosanoid, lipoxin A4. FASEB J 2009;23(5):1503–9.

[77] Schett G, Gravallese E. Bone erosion in rheumatoid arthritis: mechanisms, diagnosis and treatment. Nat Rev Rheumatol 2012;8(11):656–64.

[78] Redlich K, Smolen JS. Inflammatory bone loss: pathogenesis and therapeutic intervention. Nat Rev Drug Discov 2012;11(3):234–50.

[79] Ofek O, Karsak M, Leclerc N, Fogel M, Frenkel B, Wright K, et al. Peripheral cannabinoid receptor, CB2, regulates bone mass. Proc Natl Acad Sci USA 2006;103(3):696–701.

[80] Rossi F, Siniscalco D, Luongo L, De Petrocellis L, Bellini G, Petrosino S, et al. The endovanilloid/endocannabinoid system in human osteoclasts: possible involvement in bone formation and resorption. Bone 2009;44(3):476–84.

[81] Fukuda S, Kohsaka H, Takayasu A, Yokoyama W, Miyabe C, Miyabe Y, et al. Cannabinoid receptor 2 as a potential therapeutic target in rheumatoid arthritis. BMC Musculoskelet Disord 2014;15:275.

[82] Gui H, Tong Q, Qu W, Mao CM, Dai SM. The endocannabinoid system and its therapeutic implications in rheumatoid arthritis. Int Immunopharmacol 2015;26(1):86–91.

[83] Bresnihan B, Gerlag DM, Rooney T, Smeets TJ, Wijbrandts CA, Boyle D, et al. Synovial macrophages as a biomarker of response to therapeutic intervention in rheumatoid arthritis: standardization and consistency across centers. J Rheumatol 2007;34(3):620–2.

[84] Haringman JJ, Gerlag DM, Zwinderman AH, Smeets TJ, Kraan MC, Baeten D, et al. Synovial tissue macrophages: a sensitive biomarker for response to treatment in patients with rheumatoid arthritis. Ann Rheum Dis 2005;64(6):834–8.

[85] Gao Y, Tang J, Chen W, Li Q, Nie J, Lin F, et al. Inflammation negatively regulates FOXP3 and regulatory T-cell function via DBC1. Proc Natl Acad Sci USA 2015;112(25):E3246–54.

[86] Trouw LA, Huizinga TW, Toes RE. Autoimmunity in rheumatoid arthritis: different antigens–common principles. Ann Rheum Dis 2013;72(Suppl. 2). ii132–6.

[87] Guillot A, Hamdaoui N, Bizy A, Zoltani K, Souktani R, Zafrani ES, et al. Cannabinoid receptor 2 counteracts interleukin-17-induced immune and fibrogenic responses in mouse liver. Hepatology (Baltim Md) 2014;59(1):296–306.

[88] Blake DR, Robson P, Ho M, Jubb RW, McCabe CS. Preliminary assessment of the efficacy, tolerability and safety of a cannabis-based medicine (Sativex) in the treatment of pain caused by rheumatoid arthritis. Rheumatology (Oxf Engl) 2006;45(1):50–2.

[89] Fitzcharles MA, Ste-Marie PA, Hauser W, Clauw DJ, Jamal S, Karsh J, et al. Efficacy, tolerability, and safety of cannabinoid treatments in the rheumatic diseases: a systematic review of randomized controlled trials. Arthritis Care Res (Hoboken) 2016;68(5):681–8.

[90] Griffiths CE, Barker JN. Pathogenesis and clinical features of psoriasis. Lancet (Lond Engl) 2007;370(9583):263–71.

[91] Greb JE, Goldminz AM, Elder JT, Lebwohl MG, Gladman DD, Wu JJ, et al. Psoriasis. Nat Rev Dis Primers 2016;2:16082.

[92] Parisi R, Symmons DP, Griffiths CE, Ashcroft DM. Global epidemiology of psoriasis: a systematic review of incidence and prevalence. J Investig Dermatol 2013;133(2):377–85.

[93] Nair RP, Stuart PE, Nistor I, Hiremagalore R, Chia NV, Jenisch S, et al. Sequence and haplotype analysis supports HLA-C as the psoriasis susceptibility 1 gene. Am J Hum Genet 2006;78(5):827–51.

[94] Zeng J, Luo S, Huang Y, Lu Q. Critical role of environmental factors in the pathogenesis of psoriasis. J Dermatol 2017;44(8):863–72.

[95] Conrad C, Gilliet M. Psoriasis: from pathogenesis to targeted therapies. Clin Rev Allergy Immunol 2018;54(1):102–13.

[96] Raphael I, Nalawade S, Eagar TN, Forsthuber TG. T cell subsets and their signature cytokines in autoimmune and inflammatory diseases. Cytokine 2015;74(1):5–17.

[97] Wilkinson JD, Williamson EM. Cannabinoids inhibit human keratinocyte proliferation through a non-CB1/CB2 mechanism and have a potential therapeutic value in the treatment of psoriasis. J Dermatol Sci 2007;45(2):87–92.

[98] Toth BI, Dobrosi N, Dajnoki A, Czifra G, Olah A, Szollosi AG, et al. Endocannabinoids modulate human epidermal keratinocyte proliferation and survival via the sequential engagement of cannabinoid receptor-1 and transient receptor potential vanilloid-1. J Investig Dermatol 2011;131(5):1095–104.

[99] Ramot Y, Sugawara K, Zakany N, Toth BI, Biro T, Paus R. A novel control of human keratin expression: cannabinoid receptor 1-mediated signaling down-regulates the expression of keratins K6 and K16 in human keratinocytes in vitro and in situ. PeerJ 2013;1:e40.

[100] Folkman J. Angiogenesis. Annu Rev Med 2006;57:1–18.

[101] Vidinsky B, Gal P, Pilatova M, Vidova Z, Solar P, Varinska L, et al. Anti-proliferative and anti-angiogenic effects of CB2R agonist (JWH-133) in non-small lung cancer cells (A549) and human umbilical vein endothelial cells: an in vitro investigation. Folia Biologica 2012;58(2):75–80.

[102] Blazquez C, Gonzalez-Feria L, Alvarez L, Haro A, Casanova ML, Guzman M. Cannabinoids inhibit the vascular endothelial growth factor pathway in gliomas. Canc Res 2004;64(16):5617–23.

[103] Lu T, Newton C, Perkins I, Friedman H, Klein TW. Cannabinoid treatment suppresses the T-helper cell-polarizing function of mouse dendritic cells stimulated with *Legionella pneumophila* infection. J Pharmacol Exp Ther 2006;319(1):269–76.

[104] Allanore Y, Simms R, Distler O, Trojanowska M, Pope J, Denton CP, et al. Systemic sclerosis. Nat Rev Dis Primers 2015;1:15002.

[105] Barsotti S, Bruni C, Orlandi M, Della Rossa A, Marasco E, Codullo V, et al. One year in review 2017: systemic sclerosis. Clin Exp Rheumatol 2017;35(Suppl. 106(4)):3–20.

[106] Andreasson K, Saxne T, Bergknut C, Hesselstrand R, Englund M. Prevalence and incidence of systemic sclerosis in southern Sweden: population-based data with case ascertainment using the 1980 ARA criteria and the proposed ACR-EULAR classification criteria. Ann Rheum Dis 2014;73(10):1788–92.

[107] Stern EP, Denton CP. The pathogenesis of systemic sclerosis. Rheum Dis Clin N Am 2015;41(3):367–82.

[108] Garcia-Gonzalez E, Selvi E, Balistreri E, Lorenzini S, Maggio R, Natale MR, et al. Cannabinoids inhibit fibrogenesis in diffuse systemic sclerosis fibroblasts. Rheumatology (Oxf Engl) 2009;48(9):1050–6.

[109] Servettaz A, Kavian N, Nicco C, Deveaux V, Chereau C, Wang A, et al. Targeting the cannabinoid pathway limits the development of fibrosis and autoimmunity in a mouse model of systemic sclerosis. Am J Pathol 2010;177(1):187–96.

[110] Balistreri E, Garcia-Gonzalez E, Selvi E, Akhmetshina A, Palumbo K, Lorenzini S, et al. The cannabinoid WIN55, 212-2 abrogates dermal fibrosis in scleroderma bleomycin model. Ann Rheum Dis 2011;70(4):695–9.

[111] Garcia-Gonzalez E, Galeazzi M, Selvi E. Can cannabinoids modulate fibrotic progression in systemic sclerosis? Isr Med Assoc J 2016;18(3–4):156–8.

[112] Gonzalez EG, Selvi E, Balistreri E, Akhmetshina A, Palumbo K, Lorenzini S, et al. Synthetic cannabinoid ajulemic acid exerts potent antifibrotic effects in experimental models of systemic sclerosis. Ann Rheum Dis 2012;71(9):1545–51.

[113] Lucattelli M, Fineschi S, Selvi E, Garcia Gonzalez E, Bartalesi B, De Cunto G, et al. Ajulemic acid exerts potent anti-fibrotic effect during the fibrogenic phase of bleomycin lung. Respir Res 2016;17(1):49.

[114] Macfarlane GJ, Kronisch C, Atzeni F, Hauser W, Choy EH, Amris K, et al. EULAR recommendations for management of fibromyalgia. Ann Rheum Dis 2017;76(12):e54.

[115] Wolfe F, Clauw DJ, Fitzcharles MA, Goldenberg DL, Hauser W, Katz RL, et al. 2016 Revisions to the 2010/2011 fibromyalgia diagnostic criteria. Semin Arthritis Rheum 2016;46(3):319–29.

[116] Queiroz LP. Worldwide epidemiology of fibromyalgia. Curr Pain Headache Rep 2013;17(8):356.

[117] Wolfe F, Brahler E, Hinz A, Hauser W. Fibromyalgia prevalence, somatic symptom reporting, and the dimensionality of polysymptomatic distress: results from a survey of the general population. Arthritis Care Res (Hoboken) 2013;65(5):777–85.

[118] Talotta R, Bazzichi L, Di Franco M, Casale R, Batticciotto A, Gerardi MC, et al. One year in review 2017: fibromyalgia. Clin Exp Rheumatol 2017;35(Suppl. 105(3)):6–12.

[119] Russo EB. Clinical endocannabinoid deficiency reconsidered: current research supports the theory in migraine, fibromyalgia, irritable bowel, and other treatment-resistant syndromes. Cannabis Cannabinoid Res 2016;1(1):154–65.

[120] Walitt B, Klose P, Fitzcharles MA, Phillips T, Hauser W. Cannabinoids for fibromyalgia. Cochrane Database Syst Rev 2016;7:Cd011694.

[121] Habib G, Artul S. Medical cannabis for the treatment of fibromyalgia. J Clin Rheumatol 2018;24:255–8.

[122] Rocco M, Rada G. Are cannabinoids effective for fibromyalgia? Medwave 2018;18(1):e7154.

[123] Lawrence RC, Felson DT, Helmick CG, Arnold LM, Choi H, Deyo RA, et al. Estimates of the prevalence of arthritis and other rheumatic conditions in the United States. Part II. Arthritis Rheum 2008;58(1):26–35.

[124] Agricola R, Heijboer MP, Bierma-Zeinstra SM, Verhaar JA, Weinans H, Waarsing JH. Cam impingement causes osteoarthritis of the hip: a nationwide prospective cohort study (CHECK). Ann Rheum Dis 2013;72(6):918–23.

[125] Atukorala I, Makovey J, Lawler L, Messier SP, Bennell K, Hunter DJ. Is there a dose-response relationship between weight loss and symptom improvement in persons with knee osteoarthritis? Arthritis Care Res (Hoboken) 2016;68(8):1106–14.

[126] Dore DA, Winzenberg TM, Ding C, Otahal P, Pelletier JP, Martel-Pelletier J, et al. The association between objectively measured physical activity and knee structural change using MRI. Ann Rheum Dis 2013;72(7):1170–5.

[127] Sandell LJ. Etiology of osteoarthritis: genetics and synovial joint development. Nat Rev Rheumatol 2012;8(2):77–89.

[128] Burr DB, Gallant MA. Bone remodelling in osteoarthritis. Nat Rev Rheumatol 2012;8(11):665–73.

[129] Kong Y, Wang W, Zhang C, Wu Y, Liu Y, Zhou X. Cannabinoid WIN55, 2122 mesylate inhibits ADAMTS4 activity in human osteoarthritic articular chondrocytes by inhibiting expression of syndecan1. Mol Med Rep 2016;13(6):4569–76.

[130] Martel-Pelletier J, Barr AJ, Cicuttini FM, Conaghan PG, Cooper C, Goldring MB, et al. Osteoarthritis. Nat Rev Dis Primers 2016;2:16072.

[131] Dunn SL, Wilkinson JM, Crawford A, Bunning RAD, Le Maitre CL. Expression of cannabinoid receptors in human osteoarthritic cartilage: implications for future therapies. Cannabis Cannabinoid Res 2016;1(1):3–15.

[132] Sophocleous A, Borjesson AE, Salter DM, Ralston SH. The type 2 cannabinoid receptor regulates susceptibility to osteoarthritis in mice. Osteoarthritis Cartilage 2015;23(9):1586–94.

[133] Huggins JP, Smart TS, Langman S, Taylor L, Young T. An efficient randomised, placebo-controlled clinical trial with the irreversible fatty acid amide hydrolase-1 inhibitor PF-04457845, which modulates endocannabinoids but fails to induce effective analgesia in patients with pain due to osteoarthritis of the knee. Pain 2012;153(9):1837–46.

[134] Pathak S, Kumar KR, Kanta H, Carr-Johnson F, Han J, Bashmakov A, et al. Fatty acid amide hydrolase regulates peripheral B cell receptor revision, polyreactivity, and B1 cells in Lupus. J Immunol (Baltim Md 1950) 2016;196(4):1507–16.

[135] Navarini LMP, Margiotta DPE, Basta F, Saracini S, Afeltra A, Maccarrone M, Bisogno T. AB0046 endocannabinoid system and systemic lupus erythematosus. Ann Rheum Dis 2016;75:912–3.

[136] Browne P, Chandraratna D, Angood C, Tremlett H, Baker C, Taylor BV, et al. Atlas of multiple sclerosis 2013: a growing global problem with widespread inequity. Neurology 2014;83(11):1022–4.

[137] Chiurchiu V, van der Stelt M, Centonze D, Maccarrone M. The endocannabinoid system and its therapeutic exploitation in multiple sclerosis: clues for other neuroinflammatory diseases. Prog Neurobiol 2018;160:82–100.

[138] Baker D, Pryce G, Croxford JL, Brown P, Pertwee RG, Huffman JW, et al. Cannabinoids control spasticity and tremor in a multiple sclerosis model. Nature 2000;404(6773):84–7.

[139] Pryce G, Ahmed Z, Hankey DJ, Jackson SJ, Croxford JL, Pocock JM, et al. Cannabinoids inhibit neurodegeneration in models of multiple sclerosis. Brain 2003;126(Pt 10):2191–202.

[140] Croxford JL, Miller SD. Immunoregulation of a viral model of multiple sclerosis using the synthetic cannabinoid R+WIN55, 212. J Clin Investig 2003;111(8):1231–40.

[141] Arevalo-Martin A, Vela JM, Molina-Holgado E, Borrell J, Guaza C. Therapeutic action of cannabinoids in a murine model of multiple sclerosis. J Neurosci 2003;23(7):2511–6.

[142] Mestre L, Docagne F, Correa F, Loria F, Hernangomez M, Borrell J, et al. A cannabinoid agonist interferes with the progression of a chronic model of multiple sclerosis by downregulating adhesion molecules. Mol Cell Neurosci 2009;40(2):258–66.

[143] Zhang M, Martin BR, Adler MW, Razdan RJ, Kong W, Ganea D, et al. Modulation of cannabinoid receptor activation as a neuroprotective strategy for EAE and stroke. J Neuroimmune Pharmacol 2009;4(2):249–59.

[144] Arevalo-Martin A, Molina-Holgado E, Guaza C. A CB(1)/CB(2) receptor agonist, WIN 55,212-2, exerts its therapeutic effect in a viral autoimmune model of multiple sclerosis by restoring self-tolerance to myelin. Neuropharmacology 2012;63(3):385–93.

[145] Maresz K, Pryce G, Ponomarev ED, Marsicano G, Croxford JL, Shriver LP, et al. Direct suppression of CNS autoimmune inflammation via the cannabinoid receptor CB1 on neurons and CB2 on autoreactive T cells. Nat Med 2007;13(4):492–7.

[146] Kong W, Li H, Tuma RF, Ganea D. Selective CB2 receptor activation ameliorates EAE by reducing Th17 differentiation and immune cell accumulation in the CNS. Cell Immunol 2014;287(1):1–17.

[147] Malfitano AM, Laezza C, D'Alessandro A, Procaccini C, Saccomanni G, Tuccinardi T, et al. Effects on immune cells of a new 1,8-naphthyridin-2-one derivative and its analogues as selective CB2 agonists: implications in multiple sclerosis. PLoS One 2013;8(5):e62511.

[148] Pryce G, Riddall DR, Selwood DL, Giovannoni G, Baker D. Neuroprotection in experimental autoimmune encephalomyelitis and progressive multiple sclerosis by cannabis-based cannabinoids. J Neuroimmune Pharmacol 2015;10(2):281–92.

[149] Moreno-Martet M, Feliu A, Espejo-Porras F, Mecha M, Carrillo-Salinas FJ, Fernandez-Ruiz J, et al. The disease-modifying effects of a Sativex-like combination of phytocannabinoids in mice with experimental autoimmune encephalomyelitis are preferentially due to Delta9-tetrahydrocannabinol acting through CB1 receptors. Mult Scler Relat Disord 2015;4(6):505–11.

[150] Giacoppo S, Soundara Rajan T, Galuppo M, Pollastro F, Grassi G, Bramanti P, et al. Purified Cannabidiol, the main non-psychotropic component of Cannabis sativa, alone, counteracts neuronal apoptosis in experimental multiple sclerosis. Eur Rev Med Pharmacol Sci 2015;19(24):4906–19.

[151] Mandrup-Poulsen T. Beta cell death and protection. Ann NY Acad Sci 2003;1005:32–42.

[152] Weiss L, Zeira M, Reich S, Slavin S, Raz I, Mechoulam R, et al. Cannabidiol arrests onset of autoimmune diabetes in NOD mice. Neuropharmacology 2008;54(1):244–9.

[153] Duijvestein M, Battat R, Vande Casteele N, D'Haens GR, Sandborn WJ, Khanna R, et al. Novel therapies and treatment strategies for patients with inflammatory bowel disease. Curr Treat Options Gastroenterol 2018;16:129–6.

[154] Massa F, Marsicano G, Hermann H, Cannich A, Monory K, Cravatt BF, et al. The endogenous cannabinoid system protects against colonic inflammation. J Clin Investig 2004;113(8):1202–9.

[155] Engel MA, Kellermann CA, Burnat G, Hahn EG, Rau T, Konturek PC. Mice lacking cannabinoid CB1-, CB2-receptors or both receptors show increased susceptibility to trinitrobenzene sulfonic acid (TNBS)-induced colitis. J Physiol Pharmacol 2010;61(1):89–97.

[156] Pesce M, D'Alessandro A, Borrelli O, Gigli S, Seguella L, Cuomo R, et al. Endocannabinoid-related compounds in gastrointestinal diseases. J Cell Mol Med 2018;22(2):706–15.

[157] Marquez L, Suarez J, Iglesias M, Bermudez-Silva FJ, Rodriguez de Fonseca F, Andreu M. Ulcerative colitis induces changes on the expression of the endocannabinoid system in the human colonic tissue. PLoS One 2009;4(9):e6893.

[158] Duncan M, Mouihate A, Mackie K, Keenan CM, Buckley NE, Davison JS, et al. Cannabinoid CB2 receptors in the enteric nervous system modulate gastrointestinal contractility in lipopolysaccharide-treated rats. Am J Physiol Gastrointest Liver Physiol 2008;295(1):G78–g87.

[159] Esposito G, Capoccia E, Turco F, Palumbo I, Lu J, Steardo A, et al. Palmitoylethanolamide improves colon inflammation through an enteric glia/toll like receptor 4-dependent PPAR-alpha activation. Gut 2014;63(8):1300–12.

[160] Chiurchiu V, Leuti A, Maccarrone M. Bioactive lipids and chronic inflammation: managing the fire within. Front Immunol 2018;9:38.

Chapter 39

The Role of Plastics in the Spectrum of Autoimmune Disease—Bisphenol A

Kassem Sharif[1,2,3], Benjamin Lichtbroun[2], Chen Rizenbah[2,3], Yehuda Shoenfeld[4,5]

[1]Department of Medicine 'B', Sheba Medical Center, Tel-Hashomer, Israel; [2]Zabludowicz Center for Autoimmune Diseases, Sheba Medical Center, Tel-Hashomer, Israel; [3]Sackler Faculty of Medicine, Tel Aviv University, Tel Aviv, Israel; [4]Zabludowicz Center for Autoimmune Diseases, Sheba Medical Center, affiliated to Sackler Faculty of Medicine, Tel Aviv University, Tel Aviv, Israel; [5]Laboratory of the Mosaics of Autoimmunity, Saint-Petersburg University, Saint-Petersburg, Russian Federation

INTRODUCTION

Bisphenol A (BPA) is a molecule frequently used in the manufacturing of epoxy resins and plastics. BPA is commonly used to make water bottles, dental products, toys, utensils, dental filling sealants, and sports equipment, and it is even found in sales receipts [1,2]. Because of its unique properties, BPA has become increasingly common to the extent that 8 billion pounds of BPA is manufactured annually [3]. Acidic pH of liquids and high temperatures increase the likelihood of BPA leaching out of products [4]. Although this molecule has great promise from a manufacturing standpoint, BPA has recently been shown to exert many negative health effects that warranted the European Chemicals Agency to list BPA as a substance of very high concern as well as the Food and Drug Administration to ban the use of BPA in baby bottles [5,6]. BPA has been extensively studied as an endocrine disruptor. Specifically, it can bind to estrogen receptors and exert various effects on the body. BPA exposure has also been associated with an increased likelihood of developing metabolic syndrome, neurological deficits, atherosclerosis, coronary artery disease, hypertension breast cancer, endometrial cancer, testicular cancer, and prostate cancer [6]. Recently, however, BPA has been heavily studied because of the potential impact on the immune system and the development of autoimmunity. This chapter will discuss the role of BPA in autoimmunity with an emphasis on specific diseases.

IMPACT OF BISPHENOL A ON THE IMMUNE SYSTEM

The role that BPA plays on the immune system is multifaceted. One mechanism by which BPA impacts the immune system is that it acts as an environmental estrogen, specifically a xenoestrogen, because it is not naturally occurring but rather synthesized chemically. An environmental estrogen can either act as an agonist or antagonist at estrogen receptors [7–9]. Estrogen was found to upregulate a Toll-like receptor (TLR) trafficking protein called UNC93B1, which transports TLRs from the endoplasmic reticulum and plays a role in the development of autoimmunity [10]. Likewise, estrogen also stimulates activation-induced deaminase (AID), When there is either an excess or a deficiency in AID, there is an increased propensity to autoimmune processes to occur [11]. Furthermore, estrogen causes macrophages to increase the production of TNF-alpha, which is an acute-phase reactant that upregulates the inflammatory response [12]. Estrogen increases the activity of B-cell activating factor (BAFF), which is primarily expressed by macrophages and dendritic cells and is largely responsible for the expression of genes essential for B cell survival and differentiation [13,14]. When overstimulated, BAFF can lead to autoimmunity [15]. The development and function of dendritic cells are also impacted by estrogen, which can subsequently lead to autoimmunity [16]. Therefore, BPA can act through an estrogen-like mechanism to induce autoimmune processes (Fig. 39.1).

Acting as a xenoestrogen, BPA has also been shown to mimic E2 and subsequently increase serum prolactin levels in women [17]. Hyperprolactinemia has been associated with many systemic autoimmune diseases such as rheumatoid arthritis and systemic lupus erythematosus, as well as organ-specific diseases such as type 1 diabetes mellitus (T1DM) and celiac disease among others. Prolactin causes increased production of IFN-gamma and IL-2 by Th1 lymphocytes. Likewise, prolactin leads to activation of Th2 lymphocytes, which are capable of producing autoantibodies [18]. Prolactin interferes with B cell tolerance and thus increases the likelihood of autoimmune processes [19]. Lastly, prolactin plays a role in autoimmunity in that it aids in the response to MHC complexes presenting self-antigens [20].

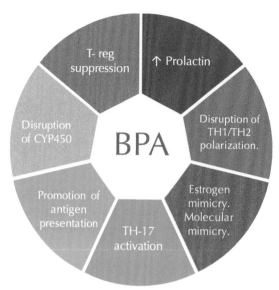

FIGURE 39.1 The mechanism by which bisphenol A is proposed to influence the immune system. *BPA*, bisphenol A; *CYP450*, cytochrome P450; *TH*, T helper; *Treg*, T regulatory cells.

BPA can profoundly disturb the Th1/Th2 homeostatic balance. Researchers found that BPA exposure resulted in a profound increase in IL-4 and IL-10 in mice [21]. On the contrary, in a separate study it was found that when mice were exposed to BPA, there was an increase in IFN-gamma, a Th1-related cytokine, and a decrease in IL-4, a Th2-related cytokine [22]. From this data, it is clear that BPA alters the Th1/Th2 homeostatic balance; however, the literature is still inconclusive with regard to these changes.

Exposure to low doses of BPA has been shown to increase mRNA expression of aryl hydrocarbons, which aid in the development of Th17 cells. Th17 is a key effector cell in the development of autoimmunity and therefore the increased mRNA expression of aryl hydrocarbons is a possible mechanism for the development of autoimmune diseases [23].

B cells are also proposed to play a role in autoimmunity. IgE-producing B cells stimulate the inflammatory response, often in response to allergens. BPA has been impacting immunoglobulin expression into the IgE response and thus increasing the inflammatory response. Likewise, a specific subset of B cells called regulatory B cells (Bregs) produce IL-10 and suppress the inflammatory response [24]. Recent evidence suggests that impairment of Breg activity may play a role in autoimmunity as well [25].

AUTOIMMUNE DISEASES ASSOCIATED WITH BISPHENOL A EXPOSURE

Multiple sclerosis (MS) is a disease with autoimmune destruction of central nervous system (CNS) myelin and oligodendrocytes. It is the most common chronic CNS disease in young adults and is more commonly seen in women [26]. When assessing whether BPA altered susceptibility of autoimmune encephalomyelitis (EAE), an inflammatory model of MS, researchers found that gestational BPA exposure increased the susceptibility in adult male mice but not female mice. The gestational BPA exposure had no effect on female mice even though females have a higher prevalence of MS than males. Of note, the male and female mice that developed EAE had the same severity of their diseases. When attempting to elucidate the mechanism by which gestational BPA exposure increases the susceptibility to EAE in adult male mice, the results did show that stimulated macrophages from gestationally exposed male mice produce significantly more TNF-alpha, Granulocyte-colony stimulating factor (G-CSF), and other cytokines. Polymerase chain reaction (PCR) analysis of spleen RNA samples from these mice showed increased TNF-alpha transcripts and CXCR2, a chemokine receptor important for neutrophil chemotaxis. Therefore, the researchers hypothesized that the activated macrophages release G-CSF and involve the neutrophils as effector cells. This was supported by measurements of blood counts 6 days after a standard EAE protocol that showed male mice gestationally exposed to BPA had increased levels of neutrophils. At this time point, the bone marrow population of neutrophils was also assessed, which showed an increased level of CD11b, an integrin that allows for neutrophil adhesion and migration. Researchers then used a monoclonal antibody to block G-CSF signaling and found that the incidence of EAE in the gestationally exposed mice went down [27]. It is clear that BPA plays a role in the development of MS. These data support the notion that MS development in male mice exposed to BPA occurs through the activity of G-CSF and neutrophils.

T1DM is characterized by autoimmune destruction of beta cells within the islets of Langerhans by T lymphocytes leading to an insulin deficiency and hyperglycemia. Researchers aimed to investigate the effects of BPA exposure on the development of T1DM in a mouse model using streptozotocin to induce T1DM. They exposed the mice to BPA between weeks 4–16 of life and introduced the streptozotocin at week 9. They found that the incidence of T1DM was significantly increased in both low- and high-dose BPA exposure compared with controls. To decipher the mechanism in which BPA causes T1DM, researchers looked at various immunological parameters at days 11 and 50 poststreptozotocin. At day 11, there was a significant decrease in all CD3$^+$ cells including CD4$^+$, CD8$^+$, and natural killer cells and an increase in B cells in the low-dose group compared with the control group. On the contrary, at day 11 there was no difference in cell counts or percentages in the high-dose group compared with the control group. At day 50, there were no differences in the percentages or totals of T cells in either group. Following ConA stimulation of splenocytes, at day 11 there was an increase in TNF-alpha, IL-6, and IFN-gamma and a decrease in IL-2, IL-4, and IL-17 in the low-dose group. On the contrary, in the high-dose group there was a decrease in TNF-alpha and IFN-gamma. At day 50, the cytokine profiles of the BPA-exposed mice were comparable with the controls. One interesting exception though is that in the high-dose group there was a trend toward increasing IL-6 and IFN-gamma at day 50. At day 50, in the low-dose group there was a trend toward decreasing IL-2 and IFN-gamma and a trend toward increasing IL-6. These results indicate that while both doses of BPA are diabetogenic, they seem to have differing mechanisms of exerting their effect [28].

Recent evidence suggests that BPA may play a role in thyroid autoimmunity. In one study, researchers aimed to study the impact of BPA exposure on thyroid autoantibodies to better understand the impact of BPA on thyroid autoimmunity. Researchers analyzed levels of antithyroglobulin, antithyroperoxidase, and antithyrotropin receptor antibodies as well as serum BPA levels from a total of 2700 people. The findings illustrate that as BPA levels increased, there was a trend of increasing levels of antithyroglobulin and antithyroperoxidase antibodies but no relationship between BPA and antithyrotropin receptor antibodies [29].

CONCLUSION

The prevalence of autoimmune diseases has been rising. Environmental factors, such as BPA exposure, are theorized to play a role in this unfortunate reality. Many studies have provided evidence supporting the notion that BPA exposure may play a role in the pathophysiology of autoimmunity. Recent studies have shown that there is a strong association between BPA exposure and the development of specific diseases such as MS, T1DM, and thyroid autoimmunity. With increasing research, it is likely that many more autoimmune diseases impacted by BPA will be discovered. Considering the ubiquity of BPA, further studies need to be performed to better understand the role of BPA in triggering autoimmunity and clarify the mechanisms by which this occurs.

REFERENCES

[1] Pivnenko K, Pedersen GA, Eriksson E, Astrup TF. Bisphenol A and its structural analogues in household waste paper. Waste Manag 2015;44(Suppl. C):39–47.

[2] Kharrazian D. The potential roles of bisphenol A (BPA) pathogenesis in autoimmunity. Autoimmune Dis 2014:2014.

[3] Gardner A. Studies report more harmful effects from BPA U.S. News and World Report. June 10, 2009. Available from: https://health.usnews.com/health-news/family-health/heart/articles/2009/06/10/studies-report-more-harmful-effects-from-bpa.

[4] MSC unanimously agrees that Bisphenol A is an endocrine disruptor European Chemicals Agency. June 6, 2017. Available from: https://echa.europa.eu/-/msc-unanimously-agrees-that-bisphenol-a-is-an-endocrine-disruptor.

[5] Mirmira P, Evans-Molina C. Bisphenol A, obesity, and type 2 diabetes mellitus: genuine concern or unnecessary preoccupation? Transl Res 2014;164(1):13–21.

[6] Jochmanová I, Lazúrová Z, Rudnay M, Baová I, Mareková M, Lazúrová I. Environmental estrogen bisphenol A and autoimmunity. Lupus 2015;24(4–5):392–9.

[7] Alonso-Magdalena P, Ropero AB, Carrera MP, Cederroth CR, Baquie M, Gauthier BR, et al. Pancreatic insulin content regulation by the estrogen receptor ER. PLoS One 2008;3(4):e2069.

[8] Arase S, Ishii K, Igarashi K, Aisaki K, Yoshio Y, Matsushima A, et al. Endocrine disrupter bisphenol A increases in situ estrogen production in the mouse urogenital sinus. Biol Reprod 2011;84(4):734–42.

[9] Zsarnovszky A, Le HH, Wang H-S, Belcher SM. Ontogeny of rapid estrogen-mediated extracellular signal-regulated kinase signaling in the rat cerebellar cortex: potent nongenomic agonist and endocrine disrupting activity of the xenoestrogen bisphenol A. Endocrinology 2005;146(12):5388–96.

[10] Panchanathan R, Liu H, Choubey D. Expression of murine Unc93b1 is up-regulated by interferon and estrogen signaling: implications for sex bias in the development of autoimmunity. Int Immunol 2013;25(9):521–9.

[11] Chen L, Guo L, Tian J, Zheng B, Han S. Deficiency in activation induced cytidine deaminase promotes systemic autoimmunity in lpr mice on a C57BL/6 background. Clin Exp Immunol 2010;159(2):169–75.

[12] Chao T-C, Van Alten PJ, Greager JA, Walter RJ. Steroid sex hormones regulate the release of tumor necrosis factor by macrophages. Cell Immunol 1995;160(1):43–9.

[13] Moore PA, Belvedere O, Orr A, Pieri K, LaFleur DW, Feng P, et al. BLyS: member of the tumor necrosis factor family and B lymphocyte stimulator. Science 1999;285(5425):260–3.

[14] Rickert RC, Jellusova J, Miletic AV. Signaling by the tumor necrosis factor receptor superfamily in B cell biology and disease. Immunol Rev 2011;244(1):115–33.

[15] Panchanathan R, Choubey D. Murine BAFF expression is up-regulated by estrogen and interferons: implications for sex bias in the development of autoimmunity. Mol Immunol 2013;53(1):15–23.

[16] Siracusa MC, Overstreet MG, Housseau F, Scott AL, Klein SL. 17 -estradiol alters the activity of conventional and IFN-producing killer dendritic cells. J Immunol 2008;180(3):1423–31.

[17] Steinmetz R, Brown NG, Allen DL, Bigsby RM, Ben-Jonathan N. The environmental estrogen bisphenol A stimulates prolactin release in vitro and in vivo. Endocrinology 1997;138(5):1780–6.

[18] De Bellis A, Bizzarro A, Pivonello R, Lombardi G, Bellastella A. Prolactin and autoimmunity. Pituitary 2005;8(1):25–30.

[19] Shelly S, Boaz M, Orbach H. Prolactin and autoimmunity. Autoimmun Rev 2012;11(6):A465–70.

[20] Matera L, Mori M, Galetto A. Effect of prolactin on the antigen presenting function of monocyte-derived dendritic cells. Lupus 2001;10(10):728–34.

[21] Lee J, Lim K-T. Plant-originated glycoprotein (36 kDa) suppresses interleukin-4 and-10 in bisphenol A–stimulated primary cultured mouse lymphocytes. Drug Chem Toxicol 2010;33(4):421–9.

[22] Youn J-Y, Park H-Y, Lee J-W, Jung I-O, Choi K-H, Kim K, et al. Evaluation of the immune response following exposure of mice to bisphenol A: induction of Th1 cytokine and prolactin by BPA exposure in the mouse spleen cells. Arch Pharm Res 2002;25(6):946.

[23] Aryl hydrocarbon receptor and experimental autoimmune arthritis. In: Nguyen NT, Nakahama T, Kishimoto T, editors. Seminars in immunopathology. Springer; 2013.

[24] Smits HH. B cells in allergic diseases: bad or better? Autoimmunity 2012;45(5):415–26.

[25] Lee MH, Chung SW, Kang BY, Park J, Lee CH, Hwang SY, et al. Enhanced interleukin 4 production in CD4+ T cells and elevated immunoglobulin E levels in antigen primed mice by bisphenol A and nonylphenol, endocrine disruptors: involvement of nuclear factor AT and Ca2+. Immunology 2003;109(1):76–86.

[26] Orton S-M, Herrera BM, Yee IM, Valdar W, Ramagopalan SV, Sadovnick AD, et al. Sex ratio of multiple sclerosis in Canada: a longitudinal study. Lancet Neurol 2006;5(11):932–6.

[27] Rogers JA, Mishra MK, Hahn J, Greene CJ, Yates RM, Metz LM, et al. Gestational bisphenol-A exposure lowers the threshold for autoimmunity in a model of multiple sclerosis. Proc Natl Acad Sci USA 2017;114(19):4999–5004.

[28] Cetkovic-Cvrlje M, Thinamany S, Bruner KA. Bisphenol A (BPA) aggravates multiple low-dose streptozotocin-induced Type 1 diabetes in C57BL/6 mice. J Immunotoxicol 2017;14(1):160–8.

[29] Chailurkit L-O, Aekplakorn W, Ongphiphadhanakul B. The association of serum bisphenol a with thyroid autoimmunity. Int J Environ Res Public Health 2016;13(11):1153.

Chapter 40

Prolactin and the Mosaic of Autoimmunity

Vânia Vieira Borba[1,2,4], Kassem Sharif[3,4,5], Yehuda Shoenfeld[6,7]

[1]Department 'A' of Internal Medicine, Coimbra University Hospital Centre, Coimbra, Portugal; [2]Faculty of Medicine, University of Coimbra, Coimbra, Portugal; [3]Department of Medicine 'B', Sheba Medical Center, Tel-Hashomer, Israel; [4]Zabludowicz Center for Autoimmune Diseases, Sheba Medical Center, Tel-Hashomer, Israel; [5]Sackler Faculty of Medicine, Tel Aviv University, Tel Aviv, Israel; [6]Zabludowicz Center for Autoimmune Diseases, Sheba Medical Center, affiliated to Sackler Faculty of Medicine, Tel Aviv University, Tel Aviv, Israel; [7]Laboratory of the Mosaics of Autoimmunity, Saint-Petersburg University, Saint-Petersburg, Russian Federation

INTRODUCTION

Nowadays, more than 80 autoimmune disorders are recognized, in which an aberrant immune response against different organs and tissues plays a crucial role [1]. The immune and neuroendocrine systems are intimately connected, partaking of dynamic bidirectional communication. Hormonal homeostasis has great influence in achieving a competent and healthy immune system function [2]. Prolactin is a polypeptide hormone and was firstly described as a pituitary factor stimulating lactation in rabbit models. Since then, a great variety of actions has been attributed to prolactin, although one of the most enigmatic and controversial aspects is related with its capability of regulating immune responses and autoimmune inflammation [3]. Hyperprolactinemia has been detected in many patients with different autoimmune diseases, such as rheumatoid arthritis, systemic lupus erythematosus (SLE), Sjögren syndrome, multiple sclerosis, autoimmune thyroid disease, systemic sclerosis, and others [4]. Although the mechanisms involving this interaction are not completely understood, it has been documented that prolactin can influence the communication and regulation of immune cells [5].

PROLACTIN, THE HORMONE AND THE CYTOKINE

Prolactin is a 23 kDa polypeptide hormone, mainly secreted by the lactotropic cells of the pituitary gland, under tonic inhibition of the hypothalamus via dopamine [6]. This hormone can also be secreted in several extrapituitary locations, including mammary epithelium, ovary, placenta, neurons, endothelium, skin cells, adipose tissue, prostate, spleen, bone marrow, and immune cells, although with a different molecular weight and biologic activity [7]. Serum prolactin levels may be influenced by the circadian rhythm (peak at 2 a.m.) [8], exercise, stress, breast stimulation, and pathologic conditions such as prolactinoma, hypothyroidism, and adrenal insufficiency [9]. Likewise, cytokines interleukin (IL)-1, IL-2, and IL-6 stimulate its secretion, whereas endothelin-3 and interferon-γ play an inhibitory influence [10]. Due to its variations by posttranslational modifications (such as phosphorylation and glycosylation), prolactin exists in several isoforms, each one with different receptor binding and bioactivity [11]. Prolactin is a cytokine which appears to stimulate both cell and humoral immunity [12]. Its receptors are expressed in a great variety of immune cells, including macrophages, monocytes, lymphocytes, granulocytes, natural killer cells, and thymic epithelial cells.

Immune Modulation Properties of Prolactin

The prolactin receptor belongs to the cytokine/hematopoietic receptor superfamily, which also includes receptors from leptin, IL-2, IL-3, IL-4, IL-6, IL-7, growth hormone, erythropoietin, and leukemia-inhibiting factor. The binding of prolactin to its receptor triggers different reaction pathways, namely P13K/Akt, MAPK, and JAK/STAT [13]. The activation of these cascades has the ability to influence immune cells secretion, differentiation, proliferation, and survival (Fig. 40.1) [14]. Prolactin enhances cytokine production and the expression of human T cell markers on mitogen-stimulated normal CD8+ T cells [15]. Recent data support a pleiotropic effect of prolactin in the thymus gland. When thymus dendritic cells were treated with prolactin, there was an increased responsiveness in allogenic mixed leukocyte reactions and enhanced cytokine production was observed [16]. Likewise, prolactin was shown to impair B cell receptor–mediated clonal deletion, deregulate receptor editing, decrease the threshold for activation of anergic B cells, and finally interfere with B cell tolerance induction [17]. In lupus murine models, prolactin decreased

Mosaic of Autoimmunity. https://doi.org/10.1016/B978-0-12-814307-0.00040-2

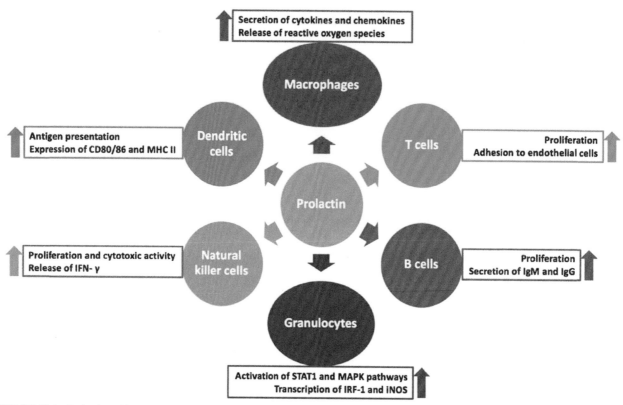

FIGURE 40.1 Prolactin and immune modulation. *IFN*, interferon; *Ig*, immunoglobulin; *IL*, interleukin; *iNOS*, inducible nitric oxide synthase; *MAPK*, phosphoinositide 3-kinase and the mitogen-activated protein kinase; *STAT*, signal transducer and activator of transcription.

apoptosis of transitional B cells and promoted a breakdown of B cell tolerance to self [18]. These antiapoptotic properties activate multiple signaling pathways and lead to a higher expression of survival proteins [19]. Furthermore, prolactin regulates Th1 type cytokines, boosting the production of IL-1, IL-2, IL-6, interferon-γ and enhancing the expression of IL-2 receptor [2,20]. A correlation between prolactin levels and the number of B and CD4+ T lymphocytes was found. Indeed, prolactin was able to influence the maturation of CD4− and CD8− thymocytes, via IL-2 receptor, leading to the enhancement of pro–B cell generation [21]. In addition, its influence on immunoglobulin production, development of antigen-presenting cells, and interaction between B and T cells can also induce autoreactivity [22]. Several studies successfully demonstrated a variety of autoantibodies in patients with hyperprolactinemia, including antibodies against prolactin, cardiolipin, β-2-glycoprotein I, endothelial cells, Ro, and La [23–28]. Induced moderate hyperprolactinemia was shown to break tolerance and induce lupus-like disease in nonspontaneously autoimmune mice with genetic susceptibility [29]. A low dose of prolactin can induce proinflammatory responses and antibody production, whereas high doses suppress these responses. These controversial effects may involve modulation of a key transcription factor directing Th1 inflammatory responses, T-bet [30]. Another strategy to determine the prolactin influence in the immune system was made by reducing its serum levels with a dopamine D2 agonist (bromocriptine).

Prolactin and Genetics

Humans express a single prolactin gene, located on the short arm of chromosome 6, near the HLA-DRB1 region. Its expression is not restricted to the pituitary gland but occurs in a variety of extrapituitary sites. Estrogens are involved in the regulation of the prolactin gene [31]. Adamson et al. [32] successfully demonstrated a novel promoter-specific signaling interaction between estrogen and TNF-α signaling for prolactin regulation. Furthermore, mutations in these genes have been associated with the development of autoimmune diseases. A relationship between HLA-DRB1 alleles and the microsatellite markers alleles near the prolactin gene were seen in women with rheumatoid arthritis and SLE, suggesting the possibility of extended haplotypes encoding for HLA-DRB1 susceptibility and hyperprolactinemia [33]. Recently, a metaanalysis investigated the association between prolactin-1149G/T polymorphism and the susceptibility to develop autoimmune disorders. The authors successfully demonstrated an association for rheumatoid arthritis but not for SLE [34].

In addition, another study examined the prolactin-1149G/T in women with SLE. The findings revealed that prolactin-1149TT genotype was correlated with prolactin gene expression, hyperprolactinemia, and low levels of dehydroepiandrosterone (DHEA), hypothesizing that prolactin-1149TT genotype could represent a risk factor for SLE patients [35].

PROLACTIN AND THE "MOSAIC OF AUTOIMMUNITY"

More than 25 years ago, the concept of the "mosaic of autoimmunity" was introduced to the scientific community by *Shoenfeld and Isenberg* [36]. Since then, new pieces have been regularly added, turning the mosaic into a more complex network each day [37]. Prolactin is an integral member of the immune-neuro-endocrinology chain and has long been related with autoimmune diseases [38]. High levels of serum prolactin have been described in the history of several autoimmune diseases, both organ and non–organ specific (Table 40.1) [39]. The interactions among prolactin, cytokines, antibodies, and organ involvement propose an active influence of prolactin on inflammatory and immune processes, acting as a link between the neuroendocrine and immune systems [40,41].

Systemic Autoimmune Diseases

Prolactin and Systemic Lupus Erythematosus

SLE is a complex and debilitating autoimmune disease, attributed to the development of antinuclear or anti–double-strained DNA antibodies (anti-dsDNA) [42]. The higher incidence of SLE among women at reproductive age when compared with men (ratio 9:1) suggests a crucial role of sex hormones on disease pathogenesis [43]. Notwithstanding, serum levels of prolactin above the normal range have been described in patients with SLE irrespective of gender (15%–45%) [44–47]. In animal models, prolactin receptor was found to be expressed in early bone marrow B cells, emphasizing the influence of this hormone in B cell development [48]. Furthermore, hyperprolactinemia was associated with higher IgG levels, anti-DNA antibodies, immune complexes, glomerulonephritis, and premature death [49]. The prolactin effect appears to be accentuated by estrogen stimulation of prolactin secretion [50]. Peeva et al. [29] proposed that estrogen-induced breakdown in B cell tolerance can be neutralized by bromocriptine, which induces anergy in DNA-reactive B cells. Indeed, both hormones promote the survival and activation of autoreactive B cells in SLE models, offering new targets for novel treatments [21]. In humans, hyperprolactinemia has been largely associated with SLE patients, especially those with active disease. Independent studies were able to find significant correlations between hyperprolactinemia and anti-dsDNA, anticardiolipin, low C3, erythrocyte sedimentation rate, anemia, and all types of serositis [51,52]. Furthermore, clinical observations hypothesize that prolactin might be produced in damaged organs from SLE by accumulation and promotion of lymphocyte infiltration. Patients following an immunosuppressive therapy show lower prolactin levels in relation to disease remission [53]. The link between hyperprolactinemia and SLE activity might be explained by the decreased suppressive function of T regulatory cells, promoting an inflammatory state. Patients with active SLE have an enhanced production of a prolactin-like immune-reactive substance with different molecular weight [54]. Besides low levels of homovanillic acid, a dopamine metabolite was found in SLE, suggesting a dopamine defect among these patients [55]. Despite all, results regarding prolactin and SLE disease severity remain controversial, probably because of altered bioactivity of the prolactin variants, genetic factors, methodologies, and

TABLE 40.1 Hyperprolactinemia and Autoimmune Diseases

Organ-Specific Disease	Non–Organ-Specific Disease
Autoimmune thyroid disease	Systemic lupus erythematosus
Type 1 diabetes	Rheumatoid arthritis
Addison's disease	Psoriatic arthritis
Celiac disease	Antiphospholipid syndrome
Autoimmune uveitis	Sjögren syndrome
Multiple sclerosis	Behçet disease
Myasthenia gravis	Systemic sclerosis
Psoriasis vulgaris	Reactive arthritis
Pemphigus vulgaris	
Peripartum cardiomyopathy	
Rejection of heart transplantation	
Lymphocytic hypophysitis	

others [46,47,51,56]. The exact source of hyperprolactinemia in SLE patients remains unclear, although several studies suggest an extrapituitary production from lymphocytes. Diamond et al. discovered that some anti-DNA antibodies were capable of interaction with the N-methyl-D-aspartate receptor in the brain and promoted the secretion of prolactin, introducing a novel idea for the development of new treatments that could disrupt the vicious cycle of lupus antibodies increasing prolactin levels and promoting disease severity [57,58]. A few controlled studies treating SLE patients with dopamine agonists have been conducted so far. Data strongly support the benefits of bromocriptine on the reduction of flares and disease activity, even when compared with hydroxychloroquine [59]. Interestingly, the injection of CD8 cells from SLE mice treated with bromocriptine abolished disease development in experimental models. These results suggest that bromocriptine might downregulate autoimmune events through the induction of natural nonspecific CD8 suppressor cells [60].

Prolactin and Primary Antiphospholipid Syndrome

Antiphospholipid syndrome is a systemic autoimmune condition, characterized by the presence of antiphospholipid antibodies, recurrent thrombosis, and miscarriages [61,62]. A large cohort performed by Praprotnik et al. [63] unveiled for the first time significantly higher levels of prolactin among 12% of patients with antiphospholipid syndrome (primary and secondary), for both genders, when compared with healthy subjects. Curiously, typical clinical signs of hyperprolactinemia, such as galactorrhea, male gynecomastia, and amenorrhea, were not observed. In contrast, high levels of prolactin were associated with obstetric complications and the presence of lupus anticoagulants, although no significant association was found with thrombosis events. For a long time, prolactin was believed to be a potent coactivator of platelet aggregation and potential promoter of thromboembolic events, although recent studies reported controversial results [64,65]. Interestingly, the presence of hyperprolactinemia was negatively correlated with arthralgia, suggesting a possible protective role and alternative marker for some disease manifestations [63]. In antiphospholipid syndrome experimental models, bromocriptine was shown to downregulate autoimmune phenomena [60,66,67].

Prolactin and Rheumatoid Arthritis

Rheumatoid arthritis is a chronic, autoimmune inflammatory disease affecting the synovial membrane, cartilage, and bone [68]. A large study found a possible correlation between decreased risk of developing rheumatoid arthritis and the prolactin-1149T polymorphism, which has been associated with reduced prolactin production by lymphocytes [69,70]. Studies relating rheumatoid arthritis and hyperprolactinemia have been controversial, although serum prolactin and monomeric prolactin were significantly increased in rheumatoid arthritis patients [71]. Besides, male patients were also proved to have higher titers [72]. Prolactin is thought to play a crucial role in initiating and/or sustaining inflammation in rheumatoid arthritis. It is known that rheumatoid arthritis usually improves during pregnancy and exacerbates during postpartum, probably because of growing levels of prolactin and decreased cortisol and estrogen serum titers [73]. After the corticotropin-releasing hormone test, upregulation of prolactin secretion in women under 40 years old was shown [74,75]. Higher levels of prolactin and prolactin/cortisol ratio at 2 a.m. were demonstrated in postmenopausal women with active disease [76]. Likewise, prolactin was found to be produced by fibroblast-like synovial cells and by T lymphocytes in rheumatoid joints, increasing the synthesis of matrix metalloproteinase-3, IL-6, and IL-8. In addition, serum prolactin has been associated with duration, activity of the disease, severe radiographic damage, and worse functional stage [77].

Prolactin and Sjögren Syndrome

Primary Sjögren syndrome is a chronic autoimmune disease characterized by exocrine glandular insufficiency secondary to lymphocytic and plasma cell infiltration [78]. The spectrum of the disease extends from an organ-specific autoimmune disease to systemic involvement [79,80]. Hyperprolactinemia has been associated with Sjögren syndrome especially in patients diagnosed at a young age with active immunological disease [81]. Studies report levels of prolactin approximately 1.3–2.4 times higher than the healthy population and it was associated with internal organ disease score [81–83]. Despite all, the levels of the hormone were not correlated with disease duration, systemic manifestations, antibodies, or immunoglobulin levels. Prolactin is thought to reflect disease pathology rather than its presence in a subset of patients [84].

Prolactin and Behçet's Disease

Behcet's disease is a chronic relapsing multisystemic inflammatory disorder characterized by orogenital ulcerations, skin lesions, intraocular inflammation, and less commonly arthritic, vascular, gastrointestinal, and neurologic manifestations. The presence of hyperprolactinemia in patients with Behçet disease has been proposed in several studies [85]. Atasoy et al. [86] demonstrated high levels of prolactin in patients with active disease in comparison with inactive Behçet disease patients. The elevated levels of prolactin may contribute to disease activity by augmenting immune processes [87,88].

Prolactin and Psoriatic Arthritis

Psoriatic arthritis is an autoinflammatory disease in which the prolactin receptor is expressed on macrophages [89]. Prolactin was found to be locally expressed in the synovial fluid of patients with psoriatic arthritis by confirmed measuring of synovial micro-RNA expression [90], and it is positively correlated with several clinical disease parameters, including erythrocyte sedimentation rate, swollen joint count of 28 joints, visual analog scale of global disease activity, and disease activity score [91]. Through the years, studies have demonstrated benefits of bromocriptine treatment by modulating the disease [92–94]. Recently, Kokot et al. [95] showed that regardless of serum prolactin levels, administration of bromocriptine improves joint and skin symptoms, which indicates a decrease in disease activity and might be a promising way of alternative therapy for psoriatic arthritis.

Prolactin and Systemic Sclerosis

Systemic sclerosis is a connective tissue disorder characterized by diffuse vascular lesions and fibrotic changes affecting skin and major organs. Its pathogenesis is extremely complex and still poorly understood [96,97]. Systemic sclerosis was found to be five times more common among women at reproductive age when compared with men [98]. Fojtíková et al. [99] described the 1149TT genotype of the extrapituitary prolactin promoter as being specific for systemic sclerosis and that it was also associated with decreased risk of developing the disease in older age. Studies have reported high levels of prolactin among a wide range of patients suffering from systemic sclerosis (3%–81%), probably in relation with an aberrant circadian rhythm [39,44,100–103]. Besides, prolactin levels were also associated with skin sclerosis, peripheral vascular, and lung involvement [104]. Interestingly, almost 80% of the patients with systemic sclerosis were diagnosed with asymptomatic microadenoma. After the metoclopramide test, prolactin levels were found dramatically increased in systemic sclerosis patients, maybe because of a higher dopaminergic tone [105]. Likewise, hyperprolactinemia was correlated with more aggressive skin involvement (mainly in early disease), diastolic dysfunction of the left ventricle, and disease duration [102]. As described in other autoimmune diseases, peripheral blood mononuclear cells were found to contain increased amounts of prolactin and to be more sensitive to prolactin stimulation [103]. These results suggest that the etiology of hyperprolactinemia in systemic sclerosis patients could be due to an increased dopaminergic tone and/or lymphocytic secretion.

Organ-Specific Autoimmune Diseases

Prolactin and Multiple Sclerosis

Multiple sclerosis is a chronic inflammatory disorder of the central nervous system characterized by the presence of multifocal areas of immune cell infiltration, demyelination, and axonal damage mainly located in the white matter [106]. In animal models, this disease is represented by experimental autoimmune encephalomyelitis, believed to be an inflammatory response against oligodendrocytes that form the myelin sheath surrounding neuronal axons driven by myelin-reactive CD4+ Th1/Th17 cells [107]. Almost 35 years ago, Nagy et al. [108] reported a clinical improvement of experimental autoimmune encephalomyelitis following bromocriptine treatment, suggesting a potential negative influence for prolactin. Since then, several studies support the benefits of bromocriptine on animal models [109–111]. In addition, controversial results have been obtained while exploring hyperprolactinemia and multiple sclerosis [112]. Several studies demonstrate a positive correlation between hyperprolactinemia and disease onset, recurrence [113], as well as with the number of antimyelin oligodendrocyte glycoprotein antibody secreting cells [114]. There was no difference in prolactin levels between the relapsing-remitting and the progressive type of multiple sclerosis [115]. Recently, a study documented hyperprolactinemia in 6.7% of patients with multiple sclerosis. Among female patients, prolactin was related to the secondary progressive type of the disease [116]. In accordance, a case report described multiple sclerosis onsets during a developing prolactinoma, followed by disease relapse during adenoma recurrence, suggesting the proinflammatory role of prolactin on the disease [117]. Studies evaluating treatment with bromocriptine showed no efficacy in reducing disease activity [118].

Prolactin and Myasthenia Gravis

Myasthenia gravis is an archetypal autoimmune disease characterized by autoantibodies against the acetylcholine receptor, muscle-specific tyrosine kinase, or against a growing variety of postsynaptic proteins in smaller subsets [119]. Prolactin and its receptor are located on chromosome 6, near the HLA A1-B8 extended haplotype, which is associated with myasthenia gravis in women with thymic hyperplasia [120,121]. Despite the limited data available, few case reports of myasthenia gravis in association with prolactinomas have been published [122]. In accordance with early studies reporting high levels of prolactin among these patients, some of them in relation with prolactinomas, the suggestion that prolactin might be implied in the pathophysiology of the disease is inferred [123,124]. This hormone has been found on thymic epithelial cells and influences T cell function, thymulin production, and thymic epithelial cell growth, which in the other hand can be modulated by antiprolactin receptor antibodies with agonistic function. However, the possible roles of thymus-derived prolactin and the functional involvement in thymic disorders remain unknown.

Prolactin and Celiac Disease

Celiac disease is a gluten-sensitive autoimmune enteropathy where both adaptive and innate immunity are involved in its development [125]. Serum levels of prolactin were shown to have a close relationship with celiac disease activity [126]. Besides, prolactin levels were positively correlated with the degree of mucosal atrophy and with the serum concentration of antiendomysial antibodies. Kapur et al. [127] reported a positive correlation between prolactin levels and disease activity, duration of symptoms, and age at diagnosis. A recent longitudinal study performed by Delvecchio et al. [128] revealed high levels of prolactin among celiac patients when compared with healthy subjects. In addition, levels diminish after 6 months following a gluten-free diet. The evidence of decreasing prolactin simultaneously with the decline of antitransglutaminase antibodies suggests that compliance with a gluten-free diet correlates with prolactin levels.

Prolactin and Autoimmune Thyroid Disease

Autoimmune thyroid diseases comprise mainly two disorders: Grave's disease and Hashimoto thyroiditis. The etiology is multifactorial, involving genetic and environmental factors, with a great preponderance in females [129]. High levels of prolactin were found in 20% of patients with autoimmune thyroid disease and had twice the frequency among autoimmune hypothyroidism. Around 90% of Hashimoto's thyroiditis patients presented significantly higher prolactin levels in association with decreased cortisol titers [130]. The role of dopamine agonists in treatment of autoimmune diseases is yet to be determined.

Prolactin and Pemphigus Vulgaris

Pemphigus vulgaris is an autoimmune bullous disease involving both the skin and mucosal areas, which is characterized by intraepithelial flaccid blisters and erosions [131,132]. It is known that autoantibodies against desmosomal glycoproteins including desmoglein-1 and desmoglein-3 play a role in the pathogenesis of the disease, although the specific molecular steps in initiation and perpetuation of this abnormality remain unknown [133,134]. A cross-sectional study demonstrated that prolactin serum levels were correlated with the extent of body involvement ($P = .01$) [135]. Recently, Yousefi et al. [136] demonstrated that patients with pemphigus had higher total and free prolactin and lower DHEA concentrations. Besides, patients with more severe disease were found to have higher levels of total serum prolactin, suggesting an active role of this hormone in the pathogenesis of the disease. Unfortunately, the available data relating these two entities are remote; therefore, future studies are needed to clarify the influence of prolactin in pemphigus vulgaris.

Prolactin and Psoriasis Vulgaris

Psoriasis vulgaris is an inflammatory, immune-mediated skin disease, characterized by type 1 T cell infiltration. Human skin is also a source of prolactin. Likewise, prolactin acts as a neuroendocrine modulator of both skin epithelial growth and the skin immune system [137]. Rathika et al. [138] found significantly higher levels of prolactin in patients with psoriasis in comparison with healthy subjects, with a positive correlation with disease severity. Besides, levels of prolactin decreased after psoriasis treatment. Hyperprolactinemia might play a role in the proliferation of keratinocytes in psoriasis vulgaris, promoting T cell infiltration via CCL20 [139,140]. Treatment of this disease with bromocriptine has been proposed in the past, displaying evident benefits and mild side effects [141,142].

Prolactin and Autoimmune Uveitis

Autoimmune uveitis is an organ-specific disorder characterized by irreversible lesions to the eye and is among the leading causes of visual deficit and blindness [143]. Hyperprolactinemia has been linked with anterior uveitis, although no significant correlation with disease activity was found. Proença et al. [144] reported high serum levels of prolactin in HLA-B27–related uveitis patients. Likewise, intraocular prolactin was elevated in patients with cataract and anterior uveitis in comparison with patients carrying only cataract [145]. Bromocriptine was found to lower prolactin systemic levels and diminished the inflammatory response in experimental autoimmune uveitis models, in accordance with preliminary trials in humans [146,147].

Prolactin and Peripartum Cardiomyopathy

Peripartum cardiomyopathy is a rare but potentially fatal disease defined by heart failure toward the end of pregnancy or in the months following delivery, affecting previously healthy women [148]. The etiology of this disease remains unclear, although several underlying mechanisms have been proposed, including viral infections, low selenium level, stress-activated cytokines, inflammation and autoimmune reactions, and a pathological response to hemodynamic stress [149]. Prolactin has demonstrated an active role in the pathophysiology of peripartum cardiomyopathy. Increased oxidative stress and subsequent generation of 16 kDa prolactin impairs the cardiac vasculature and its metabolism, finally culminating in systolic heart failure [150–152]. Haghikia et al. [153] identified the presence of autoantibodies against troponin I and sarcomeric myosin in the serum of patients with peripartum cardiomyopathy. Furthermore, the presence of those antibodies was correlated with the severity of left ventricle dysfunction and lower rate of full cardiac recovery on follow-up [153]. In addition to the autoantibodies, these patients demonstrate a heightened level of fetal microchimerism, an abnormal cytokine profile (increased levels of TNF, IL-6, and soluble Fas receptors), decreased levels of CD4+ CD25lo regulatory T cells, and a significant reduction in the plasma levels of progesterone, estradiol, and relaxin, contributing to an aberrant immunologic activity and inflammatory processes [154,155]. Recently, several studies emerged using dopamine agonists in the treatment of this disease, with great results so far [156–159].

Prolactin and Schizophrenia

Schizophrenia is a complex brain disorder characterized by psychotic symptoms, such as hallucinations, as well as cognitive disorganization, withdrawal, and apathy. Interestingly, when analyzing the frequency of the 1149G/T functional polymorphism of the prolactin gene among schizophrenia patients, G allele was found to be significantly more common, particularly in males, similar to autoimmune diseases [160]. Antipsychotic-naive patients with schizophrenia had significantly higher prolactin concentrations when compared with healthy subjects. Serum levels were closely correlated with severity of psychopathology, suicide risk, and negative symptoms [161]. In accordance, pituitary enlargement and/or hyperprolactinemia has also been found in people at high risk for the development of psychosis [162,163]. Recently, Gragnoli et al. [164] hypothesized that activation of dopamine receptor 2 in noncortical areas and functional reduction of dopamine or dopamine receptors in cortical areas may contribute to the development of schizophrenia. The correlation of higher prolactin levels and drug-naive schizophrenia patients might be due to prolactin receptor resistance, which leads to reduced prolactin activity in brain areas, an important aspect for social and cognitive functions.

BROMOCRIPTINE AND AUTOIMMUNITY

Bromocriptine is an ergot alkaloid that binds to the dopamine receptor and inhibits the pituitary synthesis of prolactin. Despite its effects on prolactinemia, it may also directly modulate T and B lymphocytes through the dopamine receptor (Fig. 40.2) [60,165]. Studies in human models suggest an immunosuppressive effect, although its mechanisms are not completely elucidated. Bromocriptine has been shown to decrease autoantibodies production and influence

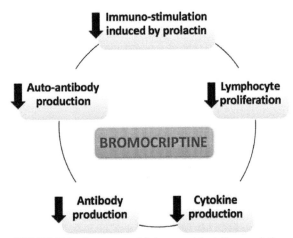

FIGURE 40.2   Immune modulation properties of bromocriptine.

lymphocyte function, quantity modulation, and expression of surface molecules [165]. In contrast, it is inappropriate for downregulating prolactin production in extrapituitary tissues, which can represent an important source in various diseases such as rheumatoid arthritis. Despite all, bromocriptine is considered to have a relatively safe side effect profile and might represent an interesting adjunctive or nonstandard treatment in mild to moderate rheumatic and autoimmune diseases [5,166].

CONCLUSIONS

Prolactin has a bioactive function acting as a hormone and a cytokine. It exerts a great influence in immune system modulation, mainly inhibiting the negative selection of autoreactive B lymphocytes. Hyperprolactinemia has been associated with several autoimmune diseases, and it is believed to play a crucial role in disease pathogenesis. A direct correlation between prolactin levels and disease activity was not found in all disorders. Genetic factors may play a role in humans as in animal models. Dopamine agonists have proven to offer clinical benefits and represent a promising therapy to investigate.

HIGHLIGHTS

- Autoimmune diseases are more common in women, mainly at a reproductive age.
- Prolactin interferes with the negative selection of autoreactive B cells, enhances their proliferation and survival, and increases antibody production.
- Hyperprolactinemia has been associated with several autoimmune disorders and is believed to play a crucial role in disease pathogenesis.
- A consistent correlation between prolactin levels and disease activity is not clear.
- Dopamine agonists have been used in the treatment of many autoimmune diseases with great benefits.

LIST OF ABBREVIATIONS

DHEA Dehydroepiandrosterone
Ig Immunoglobulin
IL Interleukin
JAK/STAT Janus kinase/signal transducer and activator of transcription
MAPK Phosphoinositide 3-kinase and the mitogen-activated protein kinase
NOD Nonobese diabetic
SLE Systemic lupus erythematosus
TNF Tumor necrosis factor

REFERENCES

[1] Shoenfeld Y. Idiotypes and autoimmunity. Curr Opin Immunol 1989;2(4):593–7.
[2] Vera-Lastra O, Jara LJ, Espinoza LR. Prolactin and autoimmunity. Autoimmun Rev 2002;1(6):360–4.
[3] Buskila D, Sukenik S, Shoenfeld Y. The possible role of prolactin in autoimmunity. Am J Reprod Immunol 1991;26(3):118–23.
[4] Watad A, Amital H, Aljadeff G, Zandman-Goddard G, Orbach H, Shoenfeld Y. Prolactin: another important player in the mosaic of autoimmunity. Isr Med Assoc J 2016;18(9):542–3.
[5] Tang MW, Garcia S, Gerlag DM, Tak PP, Reedquist KA. Insight into the endocrine system and the immune system: a review of the inflammatory role of prolactin in rheumatoid arthritis and psoriatic arthritis. Front Immunol 2017;8:720.
[6] Costanza M, Binart N, Steinman L, Pedotti R. Prolactin: a versatile regulator of inflammation and autoimmune pathology. Autoimmun Rev 2015;14(3):223–30.
[7] McMurray RW. Estrogen, prolactin, and autoimmunity: actions and interactions. Int Immunopharm 2001;1(6):995–1008.
[8] Watad A, Azrielant S, Bragazzi NL, Sharif K, David P, Katz I, et al. Seasonality and autoimmune diseases: the contribution of the four seasons to the mosaic of autoimmunity. J Autoimmun 2017;82:13–30.
[9] Savino W. Prolactin: an immunomodulator in health and disease. Front Horm Res 2017;48:69–75.
[10] Chikanza IC. Prolactin and neuroimmunomodulation: in vitro and in vivo observations. Ann NY Acad Sci 1999;876:119–30.
[11] Freeman ME, Kanyicska B, Lerant A, Nagy G. Prolactin: structure, function, and regulation of secretion. Physiol Rev 2000;80(4):1523–631.
[12] Watad A, Versini M, Jeandel PY, Amital H, Shoenfeld Y. Treating prolactinoma can prevent autoimmune diseases. Cell Immunol 2015;294(2):84–6.
[13] Bole-Feysot C, Goffin V, Edery M, Binart N, Kelly PA. Prolactin (PRL) and its receptor: actions, signal transduction pathways and phenotypes observed in PRL receptor knockout mice. Endocr Rev 1998;19(3):225–68.

[14] Somers W, Ultsch M, De Vos AM, Kossiakoff AA. The X-ray structure of a growth hormone-prolactin receptor complex. Nature 1994;372(6505):478–81.

[15] Dimitrov S, Lange T, Fehm HL, Born J. A regulatory role of prolactin, growth hormone, and corticosteroids for human T-cell production of cytokines. Brain Behav Immun 2004;18(4):368–74.

[16] Carreno PC, Jimenez E, Sacedon R, Vicente A, Zapata AG. Prolactin stimulates maturation and function of rat thymic dendritic cells. J Neuroimmunol 2004;153(1–2):83–90.

[17] Saha S, Gonzalez J, Rosenfeld G, Keiser H, Peeva E. Prolactin alters the mechanisms of B cell tolerance induction. Arthritis Rheum 2009;60(6):1743–52.

[18] Athreya BH, Pletcher J, Zulian F, Weiner DB, Williams WV. Subset-specific effects of sex hormones and pituitary gonadotropins on human lymphocyte proliferation in vitro. Clin Immunol Immunopathol 1993;66(3):201–11.

[19] Kochendoerfer SK, Krishnan N, Buckley DJ, Buckley AR. Prolactin regulation of Bcl-2 family members: increased expression of bcl-xL but not mcl-1 or bad in Nb2-T cells. J Endocrinol 2003;178(2):265–73.

[20] Brand JM, Frohn C, Cziupka K, Brockmann C, Kirchner H, Luhm J. Prolactin triggers pro-inflammatory immune responses in peripheral immune cells. Eur Cytokine Netw 2004;15(2):99–104.

[21] Peeva E, Zouali M. Spotlight on the role of hormonal factors in the emergence of autoreactive B-lymphocytes. Immunol Lett 2005;101(2):123–43.

[22] Lahat N, Miller A, Shtiller R, Touby E. Differential effects of prolactin upon activation and differentiation of human B lymphocytes. J Neuroimmunol 1993;47(1):35–40.

[23] Krause I, Blumenfeld Z, Malchinsky M, Cohen S, Blank M, Eldor A, et al. Anti-endothelial cell antibodies in the sera of hyperprolactinemic women. Lupus 1998;7(6):377–82.

[24] Leanos-Miranda A, Pascoe-Lira D, Chavez-Rueda KA, Blanco-Favela F. Antiprolactin autoantibodies in systemic lupus erythematosus: frequency and correlation with prolactinemia and disease activity. J Rheumatol 2001;28(7):1546–53.

[25] Allen SH, Sharp GC, Wang G, Conley C, Takeda Y, Conroy SE, et al. Prolactin levels and antinuclear antibody profiles in women tested for connective tissue disease. Lupus 1996;5(1):30–7.

[26] Leanos A, Pascoe D, Fraga A, Blanco-Favela F. Anti-prolactin autoantibodies in systemic lupus erythematosus patients with associated hyperprolactinemia. Lupus 1998;7(6):398–403.

[27] Gutierrez MA, Molina JF, Jara LJ, Garcia C, Gutierrez-Urena S, Cuellar ML, et al. Prolactin-induced immunoglobulin and autoantibody production by peripheral blood mononuclear cells from systemic lupus erythematosus and normal individuals. Int Arch Allergy Immunol 1996;109(3):229–35.

[28] Shoenfeld Y, Blank M. Autoantibodies associated with reproductive failure. Lupus 2004;13(9):643–8.

[29] Peeva E, Michael D, Cleary J, Rice J, Chen X, Diamond B. Prolactin modulates the naive B cell repertoire. J Clin Investig 2003;111(2):275–83.

[30] Tomio A, Schust DJ, Kawana K, Yasugi T, Kawana Y, Mahalingaiah S, et al. Prolactin can modulate CD4+ T-cell response through receptor-mediated alterations in the expression of T-bet. Immunol Cell Biol 2008;86(7):616–21.

[31] Mellai M, Giordano M, D'Alfonso S, Marchini M, Scorza R, Danieli MG, et al. Prolactin and prolactin receptor gene polymorphisms in multiple sclerosis and systemic lupus erythematosus. Hum Immunol 2003;64(2):274–84.

[32] Adamson AD, Friedrichsen S, Semprini S, Harper CV, Mullins JJ, White MR, et al. Human prolactin gene promoter regulation by estrogen: convergence with tumor necrosis factor-alpha signaling. Endocrinology 2008;149(2):687–94.

[33] Brennan P, Hajeer A, Ong KR, Worthington J, John S, Thomson W, et al. Allelic markers close to prolactin are associated with HLA-DRB1 susceptibility alleles among women with rheumatoid arthritis and systemic lupus erythematosus. Arthritis Rheum 1997;40(8):1383–6.

[34] Lee YH, Bae SC, Song GG. Meta-analysis of associations between functional prolactin -1149 G/T polymorphism and susceptibility to rheumatoid arthritis and systemic lupus erythematosus. Clin Rheumatol 2015;34(4):683–90.

[35] Treadwell EL, Wiley K, Word B, Melchior W, Tolleson WH, Gopee N, et al. Prolactin and dehydroepiandrosterone levels in women with systemic lupus erythematosus: the role of the extrapituitary prolactin promoter polymorphism at -1149G/T. J Immunol Res 2015;2015:435658.

[36] Shoenfeld Y, Isenberg DA. The mosaic of autoimmunity. Immunol Today 1989;10(4):123–6.

[37] Amital H, Gershwin ME, Shoenfeld Y. Reshaping the mosaic of autoimmunity. Semin Arthritis Rheum 2006;35(6):341–3.

[38] Anaya JM, Shoenfeld Y. Multiple autoimmune disease in a patient with hyperprolactinemia. Isr Med Assoc J 2005;7(11):740–1.

[39] Orbach H, Zandman-Goddard G, Amital H, Barak V, Szekanecz Z, Szucs G, et al. Novel biomarkers in autoimmune diseases: prolactin, ferritin, vitamin D, and TPA levels in autoimmune diseases. Ann NY Acad Sci 2007;1109:385–400.

[40] De Bellis A, Bizzarro A, Pivonello R, Lombardi G, Bellastella A. Prolactin and autoimmunity. Pituitary 2005;8(1):25–30.

[41] Szyper-Kravitz M, Zandman-Goddard G, Lahita RG, Shoenfeld Y. The neuroendocrine-immune interactions in systemic lupus erythematosus: a basis for understanding disease pathogenesis and complexity. Rheum Dis Clin N Am 2005;31(1):161–75.

[42] Mok MY, Shoenfeld Y. Recent advances and current state of immunotherapy in systemic lupus erythematosus. Expet Opin Biol Ther 2016;16(7):927–39.

[43] Peeva E. Reproductive immunology: a focus on the role of female sex hormones and other gender-related factors. Clin Rev Allergy Immunol 2011;40(1):1–7.

[44] Orbach H, Shoenfeld Y. Hyperprolactinemia and autoimmune diseases. Autoimmun Rev 2007;6(8):537–42.

[45] Jara LJ, Gomez-Sanchez C, Silveira LH, Martinez-Osuna P, Vasey FB, Espinoza LR. Hyperprolactinemia in systemic lupus erythematosus: association with disease activity. Am J Med Sci 1992;303(4):222–6.

[46] Buskila D, Lorber M, Neumann L, Flusser D, Shoenfeld Y. No correlation between prolactin levels and clinical activity in patients with systemic lupus erythematosus. J Rheumatol 1996;23(4):629–32.

[47] Karimifar M, Tahmasebi A, Bonakdar ZS, Purajam S. Correlation of serum prolactin levels and disease activity in systematic lupus erythematosus. Rheumatol Int 2013;33(2):511–6.

[48] Legorreta-Haquet MV, Flores-Fernandez R, Blanco-Favela F, Fuentes-Panana EM, Chavez-Sanchez L, Hernandez-Gonzalez R, et al. Prolactin levels correlate with abnormal B cell maturation in MRL and MRL/lpr mouse models of systemic lupus erythematosus-like disease. Clin Dev Immunol 2013;2013:287469.

[49] McMurray R, Keisler D, Kanuckel K, Izui S, Walker SE. Prolactin influences autoimmune disease activity in the female B/W mouse. J Immunol (Baltimore Md 1950) 1991;147(11):3780–7.

[50] McMurray RW. Prolactin in murine systemic lupus erythematosus. Lupus 2001;10(10):742–7.

[51] Jacobi AM, Rohde W, Ventz M, Riemekasten G, Burmester GR, Hiepe F. Enhanced serum prolactin (PRL) in patients with systemic lupus erythematosus: PRL levels are related to the disease activity. Lupus 2001;10(8):554–61.

[52] Orbach H, Zandman-Goddard G, Boaz M, Agmon-Levin N, Amital H, Szekanecz Z, et al. Prolactin and autoimmunity: hyperprolactinemia correlates with serositis and anemia in SLE patients. Clin Rev Allergy Immunol 2012;42(2):189–98.

[53] Vera-Lastra O, Mendez C, Jara LJ, Cisneros M, Medina G, Ariza R, et al. Correlation of prolactin serum concentrations with clinical activity and remission in patients with systemic lupus erythematosus. Effect of conventional treatment. J Rheumatol 2003;30(10):2140–6.

[54] Gutierrez MA, Molina JF, Jara LJ, Cuellar ML, Garcia C, Gutierrez-Urena S, et al. Prolactin and systemic lupus erythematosus: prolactin secretion by SLE lymphocytes and proliferative (autocrine) activity. Lupus 1995;4(5):348–52.

[55] Ferreira C, Paes M, Gouveia A, Ferreira E, Padua F, Fiuza T. Plasma homovanillic acid and prolactin in systemic lupus erythematosus. Lupus 1998;7(6):392–7.

[56] Pacilio M, Migliaresi S, Meli R, Ambrosone L, Bigliardo B, Di Carlo R. Elevated bioactive prolactin levels in systemic lupus erythematosus–association with disease activity. J Rheumatol 2001;28(10):2216–21.

[57] Jeganathan V, Peeva E, Diamond B. Hormonal milieu at time of B cell activation controls duration of autoantibody response. J Autoimmun 2014;53:46–54.

[58] DeGiorgio LA, Konstantinov KN, Lee SC, Hardin JA, Volpe BT, Diamond B. A subset of lupus anti-DNA antibodies cross-reacts with the NR2 glutamate receptor in systemic lupus erythematosus. Nat Med 2001;7(11):1189–93.

[59] Walker SE. Treatment of systemic lupus erythematosus with bromocriptine. Lupus 2001;10(3):197–202.

[60] Blank M, Krause I, Buskila D, Teitelbaum D, Kopolovic J, Afek A, et al. Bromocriptine immunomodulation of experimental SLE and primary antiphospholipid syndrome via induction of nonspecific T suppressor cells. Cell Immunol 1995;162(1):114–22.

[61] Tincani A, Andreoli L, Shoenfeld Y. Anti-phospholipid antibodies. Rheumatol (Oxf) 2014;53(2):201–2.

[62] Meroni PL, Shoenfeld Y. Predictive, protective, orphan autoantibodies: the example of anti-phospholipid antibodies. Autoimmun Rev 2008;7(8):585–7.

[63] Praprotnik S, Agmon-Levin N, Porat-Katz BS, Blank M, Meroni PL, Cervera R, et al. Prolactin's role in the pathogenesis of the antiphospholipid syndrome. Lupus 2010;19(13):1515–9.

[64] Mon SY, Alkabbani A, Hamrahian A, Thorton JN, Kennedy L, Weil R, et al. Risk of thromboembolic events in patients with prolactinomas compared with patients with nonfunctional pituitary adenomas. Pituitary 2013;16(4):523–7.

[65] Yilmaz O, Calan M, Kume T, Temur M, Yesil P, Senses MY. The effect of prolactin levels on MPV in women with PCOS. Clin Endocrinol 2015;82(5):747–52.

[66] Sherer Y, Blank M, Shoenfeld Y. Immunomodulation of experimental antiphospholipid syndrome. Scand J Rheumatol Suppl 1998;107:48–52.

[67] Ziporen L, Shoenfeld Y. Anti-phospholipid syndrome: from patient's bedside to experimental animal models and back to the patient's bedside. Hematol Cell Ther 1998;40(5):175–82.

[68] Shor DB, Shoenfeld Y. Autoimmunity: will worms cure rheumatoid arthritis? Nat Rev Rheumatol 2013;9(3):138–40.

[69] Lee YC, Raychaudhuri S, Cui J, De Vivo I, Ding B, Alfredsson L, et al. The PRL -1149 G/T polymorphism and rheumatoid arthritis susceptibility. Arthritis Rheum 2009;60(5):1250–4.

[70] Reyes-Castillo Z, Pereira-Suarez AL, Palafox-Sanchez CA, Rangel-Villalobos H, Estrada-Chavez C, Oregon-Romero E, et al. The extrapituitary prolactin promoter polymorphism is associated with rheumatoid arthritis and anti-CCP antibodies in Mexican population. Gene 2013;525(1):130–5.

[71] Ram S, Blumberg D, Newton P, Anderson NR, Gama R. Raised serum prolactin in rheumatoid arthritis: genuine or laboratory artefact? Rheumatol (Oxf) 2004;43(10):1272–4.

[72] Seriolo B, Ferretti V, Sulli A, Fasciolo D, Cutolo M. Serum prolactin concentrations in male patients with rheumatoid arthritis. Ann NY Acad Sci 2002;966:258–62.

[73] Olsen NJ, Kovacs WJ. Hormones, pregnancy, and rheumatoid arthritis. J Gend Specif Med 2002;5(4):28–37.

[74] Harbuz MS, Korendowych E, Jessop DS, Crown AL, Li pdfan SL, Kirwan JR. Hypothalamo-pituitary-adrenal axis dysregulation in patients with rheumatoid arthritis after the dexamethasone/corticotrophin releasing factor test. J Endocrinol 2003;178(1):55–60.

[75] Jorgensen C, Bressot N, Bologna C, Sany J. Dysregulation of the hypothalamo-pituitary axis in rheumatoid arthritis. J Rheumatol 1995;22(10):1829–33.

[76] Zoli A, Lizzio MM, Ferlisi EM, Massafra V, Mirone L, Barini A, et al. ACTH, cortisol and prolactin in active rheumatoid arthritis. Clin Rheumatol 2002;21(4):289–93.

[77] Fojtikova M, Tomasova Studynkova J, Filkova M, Lacinova Z, Gatterova J, Pavelka K, et al. Elevated prolactin levels in patients with rheumatoid arthritis: association with disease activity and structural damage. Clin Exp Rheumatol 2010;28(6):849–54.

[78] Peri Y, Agmon-Levin N, Theodor E, Shoenfeld Y. Sjogren's syndrome, the old and the new. Best Pract Res Clin Rheumatol 2012;26(1):105–17.

[79] Colafrancesco S, Perricone C, Priori R, Valesini G, Shoenfeld Y. Sjogren's syndrome: another facet of the autoimmune/inflammatory syndrome induced by adjuvants (ASIA). J Autoimmun 2014;51:10–6.

[80] Tishler M, Aharon A, Ehrenfeld M, Avni I, Bendet E, Bombardieri S, et al. Sjogren's syndrome in Israel: primary versus secondary disease. Clin Rheumatol 1994;13(3):438–41.

[81] Haga HJ, Rygh T. The prevalence of hyperprolactinemia in patients with primary Sjogren's syndrome. J Rheumatol 1999;26(6):1291–5.

[82] Jara LJ, Vera-Lastra O, Miranda JM, Alcala M, Alvarez-Nemegyei J. Prolactin in human systemic lupus erythematosus. Lupus 2001;10(10):748–56.

[83] Gutierrez MA, Anaya JM, Scopelitis E, Citera G, Silveira L, Espinoza LR. Hyperprolactinaemia in primary Sjogren's syndrome. Ann Rheum Dis 1994;53(6):425.

[84] El Miedany YM, Ahmed I, Moustafa H, El Baddini M. Hyperprolactinemia in Sjogren's syndrome: a patient subset or a disease manifestation? Joint Bone Spine revue du rhumatisme 2004;71(3):203–8.

[85] Proenca H, Ferreira C, Miranda M, Castanheira-Dinis A, Monteiro-Grillo M. Serum prolactin levels and Behcet disease. Eur J Ophthalmol 2007;17(3):404–7.

[86] Atasoy M, Karatay S, Yildirim K, Kadi M, Erdem T, Senel K. The relationship between serum prolactin levels and disease activity in patients with Behcet's disease. Cell Biochem Func 2006;24(4):353–6.

[87] Keser G, Oksel F, Ozgen G, Aksu K, Doganavsargil E. Serum prolactin levels in Behcet's Syndrome. Clin Rheumatol 1999;18(4):351–2.

[88] Houman H, Ben Ghorbel I, Lamloum M, Feki M, Khanfir M, Mebazaa A, et al. Prolactin levels in Behcet's disease: no correlation with disease manifestations and activity. Ann Med Interne 2001;152(3):209–11.

[89] de Vlam K, Gottlieb AB, Mease PJ. Current concepts in psoriatic arthritis: pathogenesis and management. Acta Derm Venereol 2014;94(6):627–34.

[90] Tang MW, Reedquist KA, Garcia S, Fernandez BM, Codullo V, Vieira-Sousa E, et al. The prolactin receptor is expressed in rheumatoid arthritis and psoriatic arthritis synovial tissue and contributes to macrophage activation. Rheumatol (Oxf) 2016;55(12):2248–59.

[91] Tang MW, Reedquist KA, Garcia S, Gerlag DM, Tak PP. 1.57 Prolactin is locally produced in the synovium of patients with inflammatory arthritic diseases and promotes macrophage activation. Ann Rheum Dis 2014;73(Suppl. 1):A24.

[92] Buskila D, Sukenik S, Holcberg G, Horowitz J. Improvement of psoriatic arthritis in a patient treated with bromocriptine for hyperprolactinemia. J Rheumatol 1991;18(4):611–2.

[93] Eulry F, Bauduceau B, Mayaudon H, Lechevalier D, Ducorps M, Magnin J. Therapeutic efficacy of bromocriptine in psoriatic arthritis (two case-reports). Revue du rhumatisme (English ed) 1995;62(9):607–8.

[94] Eulry F, Mayaudon H, Lechevalier D, Bauduceau B, Ariche L, Ouakil H, et al. Treatment of rheumatoid psoriasis with bromocriptine. Presse Med 1995;24(35):1642–4.

[95] Kokot I, Pawlik-Sobecka L, Placzkowska S, Piwowar A. [Prolactin as an immunomodulatory factor in psoriatic arthritis]. Postępy Higieny Medycyny Doświadczalnej 2013;67:1265–72.

[96] Chighizola C, Shoenfeld Y, Meroni PL. Systemic sclerosis. Introduction. Autoimmun Rev 2011;10(5):239–40.

[97] Renaudineau Y, Revelen R, Levy Y, Salojin K, Gilburg B, Shoenfeld Y, et al. Anti-endothelial cell antibodies in systemic sclerosis. Clin Diagn Lab Immunol 1999;6(2):156–60.

[98] Steen VD. Pregnancy in women with systemic sclerosis. Obstet Gynecol 1999;94(1):15–20.

[99] Fojtikova M, Cejkova P, Becvar R, Vencovsky J, Tomasova Studynkova J, Cerna M. Polymorphism of the extrapituitary prolactin promoter and systemic sclerosis. Rheumatol Int 2010;30(12):1691–3.

[100] Hilty C, Bruhlmann P, Sprott H, Gay RE, Michel BA, Gay S, et al. Altered diurnal rhythm of prolactin in systemic sclerosis. J Rheumatol 2000;27(9):2160–5.

[101] Jara LJ, Medina G, Saavedra MA, Vera-Lastra O, Navarro C. Prolactin and autoimmunity. Clin Rev Allergy Immunol 2011;40(1):50–9.

[102] Shahin AA, Abdoh S, Abdelrazik M. Prolactin and thyroid hormones in patients with systemic sclerosis: correlations with disease manifestations and activity. Zeitschrift fur Rheumatologie 2002;61(6):703–9.

[103] Czuwara-Ladykowska J, Sicinska J, Olszewska M, Uhrynowska-Tyszkiewicz I, Rudnicka L. Prolactin synthesis by lymphocytes from patients with systemic sclerosis. Biomed Pharmacother 2006;60(4):152–5.

[104] La Montagna G, Baruffo A, Pasquali D, Bellastella A, Tirri G, Sinisi AA. Assessment of pituitary gonadotropin release to gonadotropin releasing hormone/thyroid-stimulating hormone stimulation in women with systemic sclerosis. Rheumatology (Oxf) 2001;40(3):310–4.

[105] Vera-Lastra O, Jara LJ, Medina G, Rojas JL, Velaquez F, Ariza R, et al. Functional hyperprolactinemia and hypophyseal microadenoma in systemic sclerosis. J Rheumatol 2006;33(6):1108–12.

[106] Belbasis L, Bellou V, Evangelou E, Ioannidis JP, Tzoulaki I. Environmental risk factors and multiple sclerosis: an umbrella review of systematic reviews and meta-analyses. Lancet Neurol 2015;14(3):263–73.

[107] Steinman L. Immunology of relapse and remission in multiple sclerosis. Annu Rev Immunol 2014;32:257–81.

[108] Nagy E, Berczi I, Wren GE, Asa SL, Kovacs K. Immunomodulation by bromocriptine. Immunopharmacology 1983;6(3):231–43.

[109] Riskind PN, Massacesi L, Doolittle TH, Hauser SL. The role of prolactin in autoimmune demyelination: suppression of experimental allergic encephalomyelitis by bromocriptine. Ann Neurol 1991;29(5):542–7.

[110] Canonico PL, Sortino MA, Favit A, Aleppo G, Scapagnini U. Dihydroergocryptine protects from acute experimental allergic encephalomyelitis in the rat. Funct Neurol 1993;8(3):183–8.

[111] Dijkstra CD, van der Voort ER, De Groot CJ, Huitinga I, Uitdehaag BM, Polman CH, et al. Therapeutic effect of the D2-dopamine agonist bromocriptine on acute and relapsing experimental allergic encephalomyelitis. Psychoneuroendocrinology 1994;19(2):135–42.

[112] Shelly S, Boaz M, Orbach H. Prolactin and autoimmunity. Autoimmun Rev 2012;11(6–7):A465–70.

[113] Azar ST, Yamout B. Prolactin secretion is increased in patients with multiple sclerosis. Endocr Res 1999;25(2):207–14.

[114] Correale J, Farez MF, Ysrraelit MC. Role of prolactin in B cell regulation in multiple sclerosis. J Neuroimmunol 2014;269(1–2):76–86.

[115] Safarinejad MR. Evaluation of endocrine profile, hypothalamic-pituitary-testis axis and semen quality in multiple sclerosis. J Neuroendocrinol 2008;20(12):1368–75.

[116] Da Costa R, Szyper-Kravitz M, Szekanecz Z, Csepany T, Danko K, Shapira Y, et al. Ferritin and prolactin levels in multiple sclerosis. Isr Med Assoc J 2011;13(2):91–5.

[117] Nociti V, Frisullo G, Tartaglione T, Patanella AK, Iorio R, Tonali PA, et al. Multiple sclerosis attacks triggered by hyperprolactinemia. J Neurooncol 2010;98(3):407–9.

[118] Bissay V, De Klippel N, Herroelen L, Schmedding E, Buisseret T, Ebinger G, et al. Bromocriptine therapy in multiple sclerosis: an open label pilot study. Clin Neuropharmacol 1994;17(5):473–6.

[119] Yi JS, Guptill JT, Stathopoulos P, Nowak RJ, O'Connor KC. B cells in the pathophysiology of myasthenia gravis. Muscle Nerve 2018;57:172–84.

[120] Worwood M, Raha Chowdhury R, Robson KJ, Pointon J, Shearman JD, Darke C. The HLA A1-B8 haplotype extends 6 Mb beyond HLA-A: associations between HLA-A, B, F and 15 microsatellite markers. Tissue Antigens 1997;50(5):521–6.

[121] Garchon HJ. Genetics of autoimmune myasthenia gravis, a model for antibody-mediated autoimmunity in man. J Autoimmun 2003;21(2):105–10.

[122] Harris SM, Leong HM, Chowdhury R, Ellis C, Brennan J, Scobie IN. Concomitant myasthenia gravis and macroprolactinoma: the immunomodulatory role of prolactin and its potential therapeutic use. Endocrine 2014;45(1):9–14.

[123] Shapiro MS, Weiss E, Kott E, Taragan R, Shenkman L. Gonadotropin, prolactin and TSH secretion in patients with myasthenia gravis. J Endocrinol Investig 1984;7(6):579–83.

[124] Lysenko GI, Shevniuk MM, Shatrova KM, Pshenichnaia VA. Hypophyseal-adreno-gonadal system function in myasthenia patients with tumorous and nontumorous pathology of the thymus. Likars'ka sprava 1998;6:79–82.

[125] Parra-Medina R, Molano-Gonzalez N, Rojas-Villarraga A, Agmon-Levin N, Arango MT, Shoenfeld Y, et al. Prevalence of celiac disease in Latin america: a systematic review and meta-regression. PLoS One 2015;10(5):e0124040.

[126] Reifen R, Buskila D, Maislos M, Press J, Lerner A. Serum prolactin in coeliac disease: a marker for disease activity. Arch Dis Child 1997;77(2):155–7.

[127] Kapur G, Patwari AK, Narayan S, Anand VK. Serum prolactin in celiac disease. J Trop Pediatr 2004;50(1):37–40.

[128] Delvecchio M, Faienza MF, Lonero A, Rutigliano V, Francavilla R, Cavallo L. Prolactin may be increased in newly diagnosed celiac children and adolescents and decreases after 6 months of gluten-free diet. Horm Res Paediatr 2014;81(5):309–13.

[129] Dong YH, Fu DG. Autoimmune thyroid disease: mechanism, genetics and current knowledge. Eur Rev Med Pharmacol Sci 2014;18(23):3611–8.

[130] Yamamoto M, Iguchi G, Takeno R, Okimura Y, Sano T, Takahashi M, et al. Adult combined GH, prolactin, and TSH deficiency associated with circulating PIT-1 antibody in humans. J Clin Investig 2011;121(1):113–9.

[131] Madala J, Bashamalla R, Kumar MP. Current concepts of pemphigus with a deep insight into its molecular aspects. J Oral Maxillofac Pathol 2017;21(2):260–3.

[132] Sagi L, Baum S, Barzilai O, Ram M, Bizzaro N, SanMarco M, et al. Novel antiphospholipid antibodies in autoimmune bullous diseases. Hum Antibodies 2014;23(1–2):27–30.

[133] Fine JD. Prevalence of autoantibodies to bullous pemphigoid antigens within the normal population. Arch Dermatol 2010;146(1):74–5.

[134] Mihai S, Sitaru C. Immunopathology and molecular diagnosis of autoimmune bullous diseases. J Cell Mol Med 2007;11(3):462–81.

[135] Khandpur S, Reddy BS. An unusual association of pemphigus vulgaris with hyperprolactinemia. Int J Dermatol 2002;41(10):696–9.

[136] Yousefi M, Mozafari N, Hosseini MS, Gholamin S, Razavi SM, Namazi MR, et al. Evaluating serum prolactin and serum dehydroepiandrosterone sulfate levels in patients with pemphigus. Int J Dermatol 2016;55(6):e332–7.

[137] Botezatu D, Tovaru M, Georgescu SR, Leahu OD, Giurcaneanu C, Curici A. Interplay between prolactin and pathogenesis of psoriasis vulgaris. Maedica 2016;11(3):232–40.

[138] Rathika S, Rajappa M, Chandrashekar L, Munisamy M, Thappa DM. Effect of treatment on prolactin levels in patients with psoriasis vulgaris. Clin Chim Acta 2014;429:212–4.

[139] Kanda N, Watanabe S. Prolactin enhances interferon-gamma-induced production of CXC ligand 9 (CXCL9), CXCL10, and CXCL11 in human keratinocytes. Endocrinology 2007;148(5):2317–25.

[140] Kanda N, Shibata S, Tada Y, Nashiro K, Tamaki K, Watanabe S. Prolactin enhances basal and IL-17-induced CCL20 production by human keratinocytes. Eur J Immunol 2009;39(4):996–1006.

[141] Weber G, Frey H. Treatment of psoriatic arthritis with bromocriptine. J Am Acad Dermatol 1987;16(2 Pt 1):388–9.

[142] Guilhou JJ, Guilhou E. Bromocriptine treatment of psoriasis. Arch Dermatol Res 1982;273(1–2):159–60.

[143] Papotto PH, Marengo EB, Sardinha LR, Goldberg AC, Rizzo LV. Immunotherapeutic strategies in autoimmune uveitis. Autoimmun Rev 2014;13(9):909–16.

[144] Proenca H, Ferreira C, Miranda M, Castanheira-Dinis A, Monteiro-Grillo M. Serum prolactin levels in HLA-B27-associated uveitis. Eur J Ophthalmol 2008;18(6):929–33.

[145] Pleyer U, Gupta D, Weidle EG, Lisch W, Zierhut M, Thiel HJ. Elevated prolactin levels in human aqueous humor of patients with anterior uveitis. Graefe's Arch Clin Exp Ophthalmol=Albrecht von Graefes Archiv fur klinische und experimentelle Ophthalmologie 1991;229(5):447–51.

[146] Palestine AG, Nussenblatt RB, Gelato M. Therapy for human autoimmune uveitis with low-dose cyclosporine plus bromocriptine. Transplant Proc 1988;20(3 Suppl. 4):131–5.

[147] Zierhut M, Thiel HJ, Pleyer U, Waetjen R, Weidle EG. [Bromocriptine in therapy of chronic recurrent anterior uveitis]. Fortschritte Ophthalmol Z Dtsch Ophthalmol Ges 1991;88(2):161–4.

[148] Arany Z. Understanding peripartum cardiomyopathy. Annu Rev Med 2018;69(1):165–76.

[149] Hilfiker-Kleiner D, Sliwa K. Pathophysiology and epidemiology of peripartum cardiomyopathy. Nat Rev Cardiol 2014;11(6):364–70.

[150] Haghikia A, Podewski E, Libhaber E, Labidi S, Fischer D, Roentgen P, et al. Phenotyping and outcome on contemporary management in a German cohort of patients with peripartum cardiomyopathy. Basic Research in Cardiology 2013;108(4):366.

[151] Hilfiker-Kleiner D, Kaminski K, Podewski E, Bonda T, Schaefer A, Sliwa K, et al. A cathepsin D-cleaved 16 kDa form of prolactin mediates post-partum cardiomyopathy. Cell 2007;128(3):589–600.

[152] Karaye KM, Henein MY. Peripartum cardiomyopathy: a review article. Int J Cardiol 2013;164(1):33–8.

[153] Haghikia A, Kaya Z, Schwab J, Westenfeld R, Ehlermann P, Bachelier K, et al. Evidence of autoantibodies against cardiac troponin I and sarcomeric myosin in peripartum cardiomyopathy. Basic Res Cardiol 2015;110(6):60.

[154] Ansari AA, Fett JD, Carraway RE, Mayne AE, Onlamoon N, Sundstrom JB. Autoimmune mechanisms as the basis for human peripartum cardiomyopathy. Clin Rev Allergy Immunol 2002;23(3):301–24.

[155] Sundstrom JB, Fett JD, Carraway RD, Ansari AA. Is peripartum cardiomyopathy an organ-specific autoimmune disease? Autoimmun Rev 2002;1(1–2):73–7.

[156] Hilfiker-Kleiner D, Haghikia A, Berliner D, Vogel-Claussen J, Schwab J, Franke A, et al. Bromocriptine for the treatment of peripartum cardiomyopathy: a multicentre randomized study. Eur Heart J 2017;38(35):2671–9.

[157] Arrigo M, Blet A, Mebazaa A. Bromocriptine for the treatment of peripartum cardiomyopathy: welcome on BOARD. Eur Heart J 2017;38(35):2680–2.

[158] Horn P, Saeed D, Akhyari P, Hilfiker-Kleiner D, Kelm M, Westenfeld R. Complete recovery of fulminant peripartum cardiomyopathy on mechanical circulatory support combined with high-dose bromocriptine therapy. ESC Heart Fail Nov 2017;4(4):641–4.

[159] Melo MA, Carvalho JS, Feitosa FE, Araujo Junior E, Peixoto AB, Costa Carvalho FH, et al. Peripartum cardiomyopathy treatment with dopamine agonist and subsequent pregnancy with a satisfactory outcome. Rev Bras Ginecol Obstet 2016;38(6):308–13.

[160] Rybakowski JK, Dmitrzak-Weglarz M, Kapelski P, Hauser J. Functional -1149 g/t polymorphism of the prolactin gene in schizophrenia. Neuropsychobiology 2012;65(1):41–4.

[161] Riecher-Rossler A, Rybakowski JK, Pflueger MO, Beyrau R, Kahn RS, Malik P, et al. Hyperprolactinemia in antipsychotic-naive patients with first-episode psychosis. Psychol Med 2013;43(12):2571–82.

[162] Bloemen OJ, de Koning MB, Gleich T, Meijer J, de Haan L, Linszen DH, et al. Striatal dopamine D2/3 receptor binding following dopamine depletion in subjects at Ultra High Risk for psychosis. Eur Neuropsychopharmacol 2013;23(2):126–32.

[163] Montalvo I, Gutierrez-Zotes A, Creus M, Monseny R, Ortega L, Franch J, et al. Increased prolactin levels are associated with impaired processing speed in subjects with early psychosis. PLoS One 2014;9(2):e89428.

[164] Gragnoli C, Reeves GM, Reazer J, Postolache TT. Dopamine–prolactin pathway potentially contributes to the schizophrenia and type 2 diabetes comorbidity. Transl Psychiatry 2016;6(4):e785.

[165] McMurray RW. Bromocriptine in rheumatic and autoimmune diseases. Semin Arthritis Rheum 2001;31(1):21–32.

[166] Buskila D, Shoenfeld Y. Prolactin, bromocriptine and autoimmune diseases. Isr J Med Sci 1996;32(1):23–7.

Chapter 41

Cancer and Autoimmune Diseases

Eitan Giat[1], Michael Ehrenfeld[1], Yehuda Shoenfeld[2,3]

[1]Zabludowicz Center for Autoimmune Diseases, Sheba Medical Center, Tel-Hashomer, Israel; [2]Zabludowicz Center for Autoimmune Diseases, Sheba Medical Center, affiliated to Sackler Faculty of Medicine, Tel Aviv University, Tel Aviv, Israel; [3]Laboratory of the Mosaics of Autoimmunity, Saint-Petersburg University, Saint-Petersburg, Russian Federation

INTRODUCTION

The association between cancer and autoimmune disorders (AID) is bidirectional. On one hand, an increased risk of malignancies, both hematological and nonhematological, has been observed in different AID. On the other hand, some malignancies may increase the risk of developing an AID. Furthermore, some cancers may present with clinical features resembling an AID. This review discusses the association of malignancies with common AID such as rheumatoid arthritis (RA), systemic lupus erythematosus (SLE), primary Sjogren's syndrome (pSS), inflammatory myopathies, systemic sclerosis (Sc), vasculitis, and other AID. This topic has been reviewed previously [1], and this chapter is an update of this topic reviewing literature published in the past years.

RHEUMATOID ARTHRITIS

Early studies have suggested an increased prevalence of malignancies among RA patients. The pathogenesis of RA involves a dysregulation of different aspects of the innate immune system including cytokines and cells that have been implicated in tumor formation [2], suggesting that the dysregulated immune system may be prooncogenic. Over the years, RA was associated with an increased risk of both hematological and solid malignancies [1]. An increased risk of cancer was also implicated in the treatment of DMARDs and biologic therapy.

Large trials assessing the association of RA and its treatment with cancer among different populations have been published in the past years (Table 41.1). Recently, a retrospective Korean cohort study [3], following 2104 RA patients over a mean follow-up duration of 7.4 years and 17,436 person-years, showed that RA patients have an increased risk of non-Hodgkin's lymphoma (NHL) (standardized incidence ratio [SIR] = 3.387, 95% CI = 1.462–6.673), but a lower risk for gastric cancer (SIR = 0.663, 95% CI = 0.327–0.998). Similarly, a larger nationwide Japanese cohort database [4], between 2003 and 2012, composed of 66,953 patient-years yielded an overall incidence of malignancies in patients with RA, which was slightly lower than in the general population (SIR 0.89, 95% CI 0.82–0.97). A reduced risk was noted in malignancies of the rectum and the kidney in males, in stomach and rectal cancer in females, and in liver malignancies among both males and females. Nevertheless, the risk of lymphoma was significantly higher (SIR 3.43, 95% CI 2.59–4.28) among RA patients of both sexes, but the incidence of leukemia was markedly reduced in RA females [5].

Similar results were observed in a nationwide dynamic cohort study in Taiwan [6] following 30,504 patients with no history of cancer who were newly diagnosed with RA between 1996 and 2008 and followed up to 2010 (225,432 person-years of follow-up). The overall risk for malignancy was reduced (SIR = 0.93, 95% CI 0.88–0.97); among site-specific solid cancers, only colorectal cancer was significantly reduced (SIR = 0.71, 95% CI 0.61–0.82), while an increased risk was shown for Hodgkin's lymphoma (SIR 3.31, 95% CI 1.24–8.81) and NHL (SIR 3.18, 95% CI 2.64–3.83). Further analysis of this cohort revealed increased risk for both lymphoid and myeloid malignancies in male and for lymphoid malignancies female RA patients.

Surprisingly, another recently published study from a cohort of 3499 Danish RA patients [7] found that neither recent onset nor long-standing RA was associated with the incidence of solid tumors or lymphoproliferative malignancies after adjusting for confounders, but the follow-up period in this cohort was only 4 years.

In a similar accord, a nationwide population-based prospective cohort study from Sweden found that RA patients who have not been treated with biological drugs do not exhibit an increased risk of melanoma compared with the general population. Yet another study from Sweden [8], following 125,117 RA patients from 1964 to 2010 (1,212,967 person-years, mean follow-up 9.7 years), found a twofold increase in NHL. Analysis from the Swedish register also found [9] higher rates of cytology screening, CIN I–II, and CIN III among biologic-naive RA patients compared with the general population

TABLE 41.1 Large Trials Assessing the Association of Rheumatoid Arthritis (RA) and Its Treatment With Cancer

Study	Location	Details	Results
Chang et al. [3]	Korea	Mean follow-up duration of 7.4 years and 17,436 person-years	An increased risk of non-Hodgkin's lymphoma (SIR=3.387, 95% CI=1.462–6.673), but a lower risk for gastric cancer (SIR=0.663, 95% CI=0.327–0.998)
Hashimoto et al. [4]	Japan	66,953 patient-years, between 2003 and 2012	Lower overall incidence of malignancies (SIR 0.89, 95% CI 0.82–0.97), lower incidence of rectum and the kidney cancer in males, leukemia, stomach, and rectal cancer in females, and liver cancer in both males and females Lymphoma risk was higher (SIR 3.43, 95% CI 2.59–4.28)
Huang et al. [6]	Taiwan	30,504 newly diagnosed RA patients (between 1996 and 2008), followed up to 2010,225,432 person-years of follow-up	Reduced overall risk (SIR=0.93, 95% CI 0.88–0.97)
Lin et al. [5]	Taiwan	Nationwide retrospective cohort study, 17,472 patients, 87,360 controls from the Taiwan National Health Insurance Database covering 1997–2008	Higher incidences of both lymphoid and myeloid malignancies in male RA patients (SIR 3.36, 95% CI=2.03–5.57, and SIR: 3.69, 95% CI=2.46–5.53)
			A significantly increased overall incidence risk in lymphoid malignancies (SIR 3.00, 95% CI=2.22–4.05) but not significantly increased in myeloid malignancies (SIR 1.54, 95% CI=0.95–2.50) in female RA
Andersen et al. [7]	Denmark	921 patients with recent onset RA and 2578 with long disease duration from the Copenhagen Primary Care Differential Count (CopDiff) Database nationwide population-based prospective cohort study following RA patients treated (n=10,878) or not (n=42,198) with TN general population comparators in Swedish registers through 2001–2010	Neither recent onset nor long-standing RA was associated with incident lymphoproliferative malignancies or solid cancers
Raaschou et al. [28]	Sweden		RA patients not treated with biological drugs were not at increased risk of melanoma compared with the general population (hazard ratio 1.2, 95% CI 0.9–1.5)
			RA patients treated with TNF inhibitors had an increased risk of melanoma compared with RA patients not treated with biological drugs (hazard ratio 1.5, 1.0–2.2; 20 additional cases per 100,000 person-years) and a nonsignificant increased risk for a second primary melanoma was increased (hazard ratio 3.2, 0.8–13.1; n=3 v 10)
Fallah et al. [8]	Sweden	Average of 9.4-year follow-up of 878,161 Swedish patients with AID diagnosed in 1964–2010 with 33 different AID	Significantly increased risk for non-Hodgkin lymphoma
Fallah et al. [96]	Sweden	Average of 9.4-year follow-up of 878,161 Swedish patients diagnosed in 1964–2010 with 33 different AID	Significantly increased risk 3.2 (2.6–3.9) for Hodgkin lymphoma

TABLE 41.1 Large Trials Assessing the Association of Rheumatoid Arthritis (RA) and Its Treatment With Cancer—cont'd

Study	Location	Details	Results
Raaschou et al. [110]	Sweden	Cohort study (ARTIS) based on nation-wide prospectively recorded data from Sweden assessing risk of squamous cell and basal cell skin cancer	Basal cell cancer: Biologic-naïve patients: HR = 1.22 (1.07–1.41) treatment with TNF inhibitors did not increase this risk
			Squamous cell cancer: Biologic-naïve patients: HR = 1.88 (1.74–2.03)
			TNF inhibitors treated patients: 1.30 (1.10–1.55; 191 v 847 events) compared with biologic-naive patients;
			Among people with a history of squamous cell or basal cell cancer, TNF inhibitors did not further increase risks
Mercer et al. [11]	Britain	3771 biologic-naïve RA subjects recruited to the British register BSRBR from 2002 to 2009 (13,315 person-years of follow-up)	Increased overall risk of cancer (SIR = 1.28, 95% CI 1.10–1.48). An increased risk was noted in lung cancer (SIR 2.39, 95% CI 1.75, 3.19), Hodgkin lymphoma (SIR 12.82, 95% CI 4.16, 29.92), and non-Hodgkin lymphoma (SIR 3.12, 95% CI 1.79, 5.07), while the risk of prostate cancer (SIR 0.35, 95% CI 0.11, 0.82) and gynecological cancers (SIR 0.35, 95% CI 0.10, 0.90) was reduced. Current or previous smoking increased the risk twofold. The addition of TNF inhibitors to DMARDs does not alter the risk of cancer in RA patients selected for TNF inhibitors in the United Kingdom
Mercer et al. [27]	Britain	Rates of solid cancers in 11,767 patients from the BSRBR without prior cancer who received TNFi were compared with those in 3249 patients without prior cancer treated with sDMARDs	
Mercer et al. [29]	11 Biologic registers from 9 European countries	130,315 RA patients, contributing 579,983 person-years	287 developed a first melanoma. Pooled SIRs for biologic-naïve, TNFi, and rituximab-exposed patients were 1.1 (95% CI 0.9 to 1.4), 1.2 (0.99–1.6), and 1.3 (0.6–2.6), respectively.
			Incidence rates in tocilizumab and abatacept-exposed patients were also not significantly increased. Incidence rate ratios versus biologic-naïve patients were: TNFi 1.1 (95% CI 0.8 to 1.6); rituximab 1.2 (0.5–2.9).
Buchbinder et al. [111]	Australian database	Comparing cancer incidence between TNFi-treated RA patients (2145 patients, 5752 person-years) and biologic-naïve group (803 patients, 1682 patient-years)	No overall increased risk of malignancy in TNFi-treated RA patients compared with the general population or with biologic-naïve RA patients. The risk of melanoma was increased for both biologic-naïve and TNFi-treated patients when compared with the general population (SIR 2.72 (95% CI 1.13 to 6.53) and SIR 2.03 (95% CI 1.09 to 3.78), respectively). The relative risk of melanoma was not increased in the TNFi-exposed group compared with biologic-naïve patients (RR 0.54, 95% CI 0.12, 2.40).

AID, autoimmune disorders; *SIR,* standardized incidence ratio.

cohort, albeit no difference in invasive cervical cancer rates. Similar results were found in a smaller Canadian prospective study [10]. Conversely, an increased risk of cancer was observed among biologic-naïve RA subjects receiving nonbiologic DMARD therapy recruited to the British Society for Rheumatology Biologics Register (BSRBR) from 2002 to 2009 [11]. This cohort comprising 3771 RA patients (13,315 person-years of follow-up) revealed an overall increased risk of cancer (SIR = 1.28, 95% CI 1.10–1.48). An increased risk was noted in lung cancer (SIR 2.39, 95% CI 1.75, 3.19), Hodgkin lymphoma (SIR 12.82, 95% CI 4.16, 29.92), and non-Hodgkin lymphoma (SIR 3.12, 95% CI 1.79, 5.07), whereas the risk of prostate cancer (SIR 0.35, 95% CI 0.11, 0.82) and gynecological cancers (SIR 0.35, 95% CI 0.10, 0.90) was reduced. Current or previous smoking habit increased the risk twofold.

The discrepancy between these results could be explained by an intercountry variance in environment, genetic risk factors, the prevalence of comorbidities, patient compliance, and prevention [12]. For example, a metaanalysis performed by Tian et al. [13] found no increased breast cancer risk in RA patients However, the subgroup analysis showed that while the risk was reduced in Caucasians (SIR = 0.82, 95% CI = 0.73–0.93), non-Caucasians exhibited an increased risk (SIR = 1.21, 95% CI = 1.19–1.23). In the same metaanalysis, hospital-based case subjects also showed a reduced risk, suggesting that these subjects also showed a reduced risk severity of the disease and its course may modify the risk of cancer.

Smitten et al. [14] have conducted a metaanalysis in 2008 reviewing incidence of malignancies in RA patient. This was recently updated by Simon et al. [15], supporting their previous data showing increased risk for lymphomas, and to a lower degree, lung cancer, but not for other malignancies. This observational metaanalysis reviewed published studies between January 1, 2008 and November 30, 2014 and found a modest increased risk in overall malignancy. An increased risk was found for lymphoma and lung cancer compared with the general population, while colorectal and breast cancers showed a decrease in risk. Cervical cancer, prostate cancer, and melanoma appeared to show no consistent trend in risk in this metaanalysis.

Similarly, Askling et al. compared different registries across the world, finding high consistency in overall cancer rates, excluding nonmelanoma skin cancer (NMSC), across five large registries from the United States, United Kingdom, Japan, Sweden, and others, following age/sex standardization. SIR of overall malignancy excluding NMSC varied from 0.56 to 0.87 per 100 person-years.

Cancer Outcomes

Besides the risk for cancer, RA also has an impact on cancer survival in RA patients with cancer. Mortality was increased by 40% and 50%, respectively, in elderly patients with RA who developed breast or prostate cancer in a population-based study [16], but this association was not seen for cancers for shorter survival (colorectal or lung). Others have found higher mortality also in patients with lung cancer [17]. Similarly, analysis of the Swedish register data [18] suggests that the increase in mortality among RA patients diagnosed with cancer seems to result from an RA effect and is independent of the cancer.

Therapy of Rheumatoid Arthritis and Cancer

Disease-Modifying Antirheumatic Drugs

Recent studies show that the RA treatment may also increase cancer risk. Among synthetic disease-modifying antirheumatic drugs (sDMARDs), methotrexate (MTX) is an important part of RA treatment. A recent systematic Cochrane review [19] failed to show any increase in cancer risk, but this review was limited to a small number of patients and a short follow-up period. On the other hand, MTX has been shown to increase the risk for nonmelanoma skin cancer by 60% [20] in a large Medicare based study.

Anti-TNF Therapy in Rheumatoid Arthritis and Cancer

The introduction of biologics in RA, especially anti-TNF therapy, has raised the possibility of an increased risk of cancer. TNF has been found to have both proliferation and antiproliferative effects. Most RCT metaanalyses of anti-TNF and other biological agents in RA [13,21–24] do not show significant differences in the incidence of cancer and lymphoma between biologics and control treatments, but a nonsignificant increase in some cancers warrants further research [25].

Observational data from large registries have provided similar results. A nationwide cohort study between 1997 and 2011 in Taiwan showed a significant risk adjusted reduction for solid tumors among RA patients taking anti-TNF therapy (adjusted HR 0.63, 95% CI 0.49–0.80, $P < .001$), albeit a nonstatistically significant increased risk for hematologic malignancies [26]. Similarly, the BSRBR national prospective cohort reported no difference in risk of solid cancers among RA patients treated with any of the anti-TNF compared to sDMARD-treated patients [27]. Similarly, US-based cohorts, such as the Safety Assessment of Biological Therapeutics study (Haynes 2013), also showed no increased risk for solid tumors.

On the other hand, the Swedish ARTIS nationwide prospective cohort study [28] found that anti-TNF therapy was associated with an increased risk for new onset of melanoma (hazard ratio 1.5, 1.0–2.2; 20 additional cases per 100,000 person-years). It is true that this risk was not confirmed when combining 11 different registries from different European countries [29], but this does not rule out a population or geographical dependent risk. Similarly, a study from the Netherlands [30] following 365 RA patients treated with anti-TNF therapy found a slightly higher risk in both solid and hematological cancers, although this study compared the cancer risk rates with risk rates among the general population and not to risk rates among biologic-naïve RA patients, therefore making it impossible to draw any conclusions about the contributory effect of anti-TNF therapy.

Among RA patients with prior malignancy, treatment with anti-TNF therapy does not seem to increase recurrence rates, despite current guidelines, which require at least 5 years of remission. Analysis of the BSRBR data found lower rates of a new malignancy among patients treated with anti-TNF and rituximab compared with sDMARDs [31], although this study included only 425 patients.

Despite evidence from registries, accumulating data from randomized controlled studies suggest that the association of anti-TNFs with cancer may have been overestimated [32]. It is also important to point that the identification of any increased risk of malignancy among anti-TNF–treated RA patients does not necessarily apply to patients treated with anti-TNFs for other indications such as ankylosing spondylitis (AS), psoriatic arthritis (PsA), or inflammatory bowel disease (IBD).

Other Biologics

Experience from biologics other than anti-TNF is lacking, although some of the registries included different biologics. In general, data from clinical trials do not show an increased incidence of malignancies. Rituximab, tocilizumab, and tofacitinib do not increase the incidence of cancer in clinical trials [33–35]. Abatacept, a CTLA4 fusion protein, suppresses T cell activation, which is an important component in the immune response to cancer. The T cells through CTLA4 inhibitor is the therapeutic target of Ipilimumab, an anticancer agent. This raises the possibility of abatacept hampering the immune response to potential malignancies in RA. Nevertheless, the incidence rates of total malignancy (excluding NMSC), breast, colorectal, lung cancers, and lymphoma in abatacept-treated patients in clinical trials were consistent with those in a comparable RA population [36].

Put together, it seems that, in general, biologic therapy does not significantly increase the risk of malignancy in RA patients, although there may be regional variations resulting from different ethnic or environmental backgrounds.

PSORIATIC ARTHRITIS, ANKYLOSING SPONDYLITIS, AND OTHER SERONEGATIVE SPONDYLOARTHROPATHIES

Studies concerning PsA and AS cancer risk are scarce and provide conflicting results. Similar to RA, an increased prevalence of cervical cancer was reported among PsA patients in a Canadian cohort [10]. Analysis of data from the USA-based CORONA registry (2970 patients with PsA, 7133 patient-years of follow-up, and 19,260 patients with RA 53,864 patient-years of follow-up) cohort compared and found no difference between PsA and RA risks for malignancy [37]. In contrary, a recent analysis of the data from the Swedish National Patient registry of 8708 AS patients and 19,283 PsA patients [38] assessed the risk for lymphoma among PsA and AS patients compared with RA patients. Compared with the general population, the hazard ratio for lymphoma was 0.9 (95% CI 0.5–1.6) for AS patients, 1.2 (95% CI 0.9–1.7) for PsA patients, and 1.7 (95% CI 1.0–3.1) for PsA patients treated with MTX and/or sulfasalazine, leading the authors to conclude that in contrast to RA, the average risks of lymphoma in AS or PsA are not elevated. A recent metaanalysis suggests an increased risk for cancer in AS patients, which is increased among Asian AS patients [39]. Nevertheless, treatment with anti-TNF does not increase the risk among PsA or SpA in RCTs [32] or in registries and other cohorts [40,41].

ADULT-ONSET STILL'S DISEASE

Adult-onset Still's disease (AOSD) is a rare AID characterized by spiking fevers, rash, and arthritis, accompanied with leukocytosis and hyperferritinemia. A recent review of the literature [42] identified approximately 50 published cases of AOSD preceding a diagnosis of a malignancy, but it is unclear whether this observation is coincidental, results from a paraneoplastic AOSD-like syndrome, or reflects an inherent risk for malignancy in AOSD.

PRIMARY SJOGREN SYNDROME

Early studies in pSS have showed an increased incidence of different malignancies among pSS patients, including solid tumors and, most notably, NHL, where the risk may well exceed a tenfold increase in some reports. The NHL is typically B cell lymphoma, especially mucosa-associated lymphoid tissue lymphoma. Accordingly, different risk factors have been suggested to identify patients in high risk for developing cancer [1].

Extracting data from pSS studies is difficult because of different follow-up periods, heterogeneity in diagnostic criteria, and a relatively smaller number of studies from non-European countries. A recent metaanalysis [43] reviewing 14 studies involving >14,523 patients with pSS revealed significantly increased risks of overall cancer (RR 1.53; 95% CI 1.17–1.88), NHL (RR 13.76; 95% CI 8.53–18.99), and thyroid cancer (RR 2.58; 95% CI 1.14–4.03). Because of the small numbers and heterogeneity, subgroup analysis did not show significant results in other organ-specific cancers. In general, hospital-based cohorts revealed higher SIR compared with primary-based cohorts, suggesting a role for severe disease. An important drawback in this metaanalysis originates from the data originating from the Taiwanese cohort study-based National Health Insurance claims data of 7852 patients with pSS from 2000 to 2008. This non-European population-based study contributed more than half the patients but provided considerably different results from the other studies. The overall SIR for cancer was 1.04 (95% CI 0.91–1.18), though it was higher for patients aged 25–44 years 2.19 (95% CI 1.43–3.21). Only female patients with pSS had a higher risk of NHL (SIR 7.1, 95% CI 4.3–10.3), multiple myeloma (SIR 6.1, 95% CI 2.0–14.2), and thyroid gland cancer (SIR 2.6, 95% CI 1.4–4.3) and a lower risk of colon cancer (SIR 0.22, 95% CI 0.05–0.65). This cohort had multiple advantages, being large and nationwide, and being the only large study addressing male pSS patients, which were not found to be at any higher risk of developing cancer in particular sites. Nevertheless, the Taiwanese study had a short mean follow-up time, which could have resulted in an underestimation of the cancer risk. The authors excluded all patients who were diagnosed with cancer before pSS to avoid secondary Sjogren's syndrome, but this might have also excluded true pSS patients who were misdiagnosed prior to their cancer. True enough, the Taiwanese cohort revealed an increase of dental and ophthalmologic visits prior to the diagnosis, reflecting a considerable delay in diagnosis. Finally, the reporting structure of this study may have resulted in an overdiagnosis of pSS in primary care settings for insurance claims. In contrast, European studies were relatively nonheterogenic, consisted of longer follow-ups, and constantly showed a significant risk of different solid tumors. For instance, a recent retrospective study of long-term outcomes in 152 patients with pSS [44] showed that malignancy affected 28.3% of pSS patients compared with 2.9% in the Taiwanese cohort. Similarly, this study showed that 10.5% of pSS patients developed NHL compared with <0.5% in the Taiwanese cohort. Vasculitis and the presence of glandular complications (parotid swelling, lymphadenopathy) were the strongest risk factors for developing NHL. Of note, the small percentage of male patients in pSS in all cohorts prevents drawing any conclusions for this population, warranting further research. For example, Taiwanese male pSS patients had an observed rate three times higher than expected rate of NHL, but because of a small number, this rate did not reach statistical significance.

Predictors of Lymphoma in Primary Sjogren Syndrome

Different markers and symptoms have been described as prognostic factors in predicting lymphoma risk. A recent study has assessed the prognostic value of routinely performed minor salivary gland biopsy assessments in pSS patients. A lymphocytic focus score equal or higher than 3 was found to have a positive predictive value of 16% and a negative predictive value of 98% to develop NHL, suggesting that routine histopathological minor salivary gland assessment may have a role in assessing cancer risk. Another study [45] based on the ASSESS cohort has shown BAFF and beta2-microglobulin to be higher in pSS patients with lymphoma (1173.3(873.1–3665.5) versus 898.9 (715.9–1187.2) pg/mL, $P = .01$ and 2.6 (2.2–2.9) versus 2.1 (1.8–2.6) mg/L, $P = .04$, respectively). Another study [46] has shown the development of purpura, peripheral neuropathy, and glomerulonephritis concurring with lymphoma, but not later on, suggesting these may be paraneoplastic manifestations of the NHL. A recent study [47] analyzing 77 pSS patients who developed NHL found that the EULAR Sjögren's syndrome disease activity index is an important independent poor prognostic factor. Subsequently, a recent review article by the same group [48] analyzed risk factors for the development of lymphoma. Clinical symptoms such as parotid gland enlargement, purpura, lymphadenopathy, glomerulonephritis, peripheral neuropathy, or splenomegaly were associated with an increased risk and other histologic and laboratory factors (neutropenia, CD-4 T cell lymphopenia, lymphocytic focal score, germinal centers, serum BAFF levels, and more). Recently, a metaanalysis [49] identified lymphadenopathy, parotid enlargement, palpable purpura, low C4 serum levels, and cryoglobulins to be the most consistent non-Hodgkin's lymphoma/lymphoproliferative disease predictors. Still, these findings await further studies to determine whether they have any screening value.

Taken together, current evidence strongly suggests that pSS, especially a severe disease, procures an increased risk of cancer, especially NHL. The risk is pronounced in European patients and in females, and further research is warranted for Asian and male patients.

SYSTEMIC LUPUS ERYTHEMATOSUS AND CANCER

SLE has been associated with different types of cancer, including hematological malignancies and other organ-specific tumors [1]. Extensive studies have been undertaken to identify types of lupus and other comorbidities that are common among SLE patients who develop cancer.

Overall Risk

A recent systematic review of publications [50] assessing the risk of malignancies after SLE through February 2015 was recently published. This study reviewed 18 studies from different countries from Asia, Europe, and America. SLE patients had an increased risk of developing cancer, particularly among Asians and females. Age and SLE duration were found to be inversely associated with the risk of overall malignancies, reflecting the increasing risk with age among the non-SLE population. An increased incidence ratio (IR) of malignancies was observed in NHL, vagina/vulva, hematology, head/neck, leukemia, thyroid, liver/gallbladder, kidney, anal, cervix, esophagus, lung, and pancreas. A decreased IR of malignancies was observed in ovary and colon/rectum. This review supports the results of an earlier metaanalysis that showed an increased risk of cancer, particularly lung, bladder, and liver, albeit a decreased risk for prostate cancer [51].

A recent retrospective cohort study using the UK Clinical Practice Research Datalink (CPRD) estimating the co-morbidity associated with SLE in the United Kingdom during 1999–2012 [52] compared 7732 prevalent cases of SLE with 28,079 matched controls. This study found SLE patients to have an incidence rate ratios for cancer of 1.28 (95% CI: 1.17, 1.40), being slightly higher in males.

Breast Cancer

Contrary to earlier data suggesting SLE may be protective against breast cancer, a Medicare claims data-based cohort [53] found a 2.23 (95% CI 1.94–2.55) age-adjusted risk per 100 women for breast cancer in women with SLE compared with 2.14 (95% CI 1.96–2.34) in controls, suggesting that there is no decreased risk for breast cancer among SLE women.

A small study from Brazil [54] followed 395 SLE patients for 10 years in an outpatient clinic and found that breast and uterine cervix tumors were more common in SLE compared with the general population. In contrary, a large international cohort study [55] and review [56] shows decreased rates of breast and prostate cancer, but a recent multicenter international study conducted by the same group [57] could not identify any associated SLE-related factor that might explain this relationship.

Thyroid Cancer

A recent metaanalysis reviewed the association of SLE and thyroid cancer. The pooled SIR was 2.22 (95% CI 2.11–2.34), but because of lack of data, this review did not adjust for confounding factors, such as age, environmental triggers, etc., or was not able to determine the relationship of thyroid carcinoma to autoimmune thyroiditis [58].

Subpopulations

The risk in different lupus subpopulations has been also studied. It seems that cancer risk is increased in pediatric SLE as well [59]. A nationwide population-based study from Taiwan [60] reviewed 904 SLE pediatric patients followed for 6 years in Taiwan's registry and found that children with SLE were more susceptible to malignancy, compared with the non-SLE pediatric population.

Only limited data exist for small lupus subsets. Case reports of squamous cell carcinoma have been reported in discoid lupus [61]. A recent small study [62] (Singh ACR abstr 2628) including 66 cutaneous SLE (SCLE) suggests that the risk of cancer may not be increased in SCLE. These findings await confirmation from larger cohorts.

Finally, despite the clear increased risk for cancer, a recent review [63] found no original study addressing the necessity of specific cancer screening strategies for lupus patients. The authors recommend adhering to the usual screening guidelines as in the general population. This may be because of the fact that despite the increased risk for cancer, cancer remains to be a rare event in lupus patients. Alternatively, despite the clear increase in both hematological and solid malignancies, the extent of this increased risk is yet to be determined in larger studies before determining cost-effective preventive measures.

CANCER AND SYSTEMIC SCLEROSIS

Early studies have suggested an increased risk for cancer among Sc patients, particularly breast and lung cancer [1]. A recent cohort analysis of 1044 patients [64] from the John Hopkins Scleroderma Center database identified significant risk factors for the development of cancer, including age in years at onset of Sc (OR 1.04) and white race (OR 2.71). Previous work by this group has shown that cancer risk is associated with the presence of anti-RNA polymerase III subunit, but not other antibodies such as anti-Scl70 [65], contradicting previous data from an Italian cohort that found a relationship between Scl-70 and lung cancer [66]. While this finding can be explained by the higher prevalence of lung disease associated with anti-Scl-70, the Italian group also found a twofold increase in breast cancer risk, which was not associated to a specific antibody [67]. Further research by John Hopkins group revealed that tumors from patients who were diagnosed with cancer more or less concurrently with the diagnosis of Sc were found to harbor mutations in the polymerase III polypeptide A (POLR3A) gene, suggesting a role and a novel mechanism for cancer in the pathogenesis of Sc.

Anti-RNA polymerase III may not be the only antibodies associated with cancer. A recent report [68] found a prevalence of 20% of cancer in a cohort of 70 systemic sclerosis patients with anti-PM/Scl-100 antibodies. The cancer onset in these patients was within 36 months of the diagnosis of Sc. Furthermore, this group described the resolution of Sc symptoms following the disappearance of paraneoplastic anti-PM/Scl-100 antibodies after a curative resection of a pancreatic tumor, suggesting a similar mechanism as in POLR3A antibodies.

CANCER ASSOCIATED WITH POLYMYOSITIS AND DERMATOMYOSITIS

The association of polymyositis (PM)/dermatomyositis (DM) with cancer was recognized in the beginning of the 20th century [69], though metaanalyses addressing the magnitude of this risk are few. The strong association of cancer with the anti-p155/140 antibody targeting transcriptional intermediary factor 1-γ (TIF1-γ) [70] suggests a probable role for cancer in the pathogenesis of myositis among these patients, similar to the mechanism found in systemic sclerosis. True enough, a TIF1γ-overexpressing, highly progressive endometrial carcinoma was reported in a patient with DM positive for malignancy-associated anti-p155/140 autoantibody [71]. A recent systematic review [72] including 20 original studies from different countries assessed the risk of DM or PM for different malignancies, providing interesting results. The SIR for malignancy in PM was 1.62 (95% CI 1.19–2.04), 5.50 (4.31–6.70) for DM, and 4.07 (3.02–5.12) for PM/DM combined. Increased risks were more significant in patients within the first year of myositis diagnosis and in male patients. A significant association was also found between PM or DM and most site-specific malignancies with the exception of stomach and prostate cancers. This metaanalysis did not include a recently published study from southern China [73], which followed 246 DM patients from 2003 to 2012. Sixty patients (24.4%) had cancer, mostly (65%) within 1 year of diagnosis, and all cancer cases occurred within 3 years of diagnosis. Nasopharyngeal carcinoma and ovarian carcinoma were most common, accounting for 35% (21/60) and 15% (9/60) of malignancies, respectively, followed by lung and colon cancer. Another recent metaanalysis [74] supports these results, demonstrating the cancer risk in DM to be 17.29 in the first year, 2.7 between 1 and 5 years, and 1.37 after 5 years.

The types of cancers seem to vary geographically. For instance, nasopharyngeal cancer seems to be common among Chinese and Korean populations, but other cancers predominate among other populations [72]. Surprisingly, a small cohort [75] from Jordan, including 94 PM/DM patients, found a relatively low prevalence (4 patients) of malignancy among patients with PM/DM. Interestingly, however, in this cohort, two of these patients (50%) had nasopharyngeal cancer. These studies suggest that environmental and geographical factors may play a role in the development of PM/DM in different types of cancer.

CANCER AND ANCA-ASSOCIATED VASCULITIS

Few data are available assessing the association between cancer and granulomatosis with polyangiitis (GPA), eosinophilic granulomatosis with polyangiitis, and microscopic polyangiitis. A recent metaanalysis [76] reviewing 2578 ANCA-associated vasculitis patients found increased risk for nonmelanoma skin cancer (SIR 5.18), leukemia (SIR 4.89), and bladder cancer (3.84), lymphoma (SIR 3.79), liver (SIR 3.5), and lung (SIR 1.67). The vast majority of these patients had GPA and received cyclophosphamide, and the increased risk probably reflects the oncogenic side effects of the drug rather than an association to the disease. This is further emphasized by a recent Dutch cohort [77] that did not find an increase in patients who did not receive cyclophosphamide more than a year.

CANCER AND OTHER AUTOIMMUNE DISEASES

The association of cancer with polymyalgia rheumatica (PMR) and giant cell arteritis (GCA) is not clear. In the first 6 months after diagnosis of PMR patients were significantly more likely to receive a cancer diagnosis (adjusted risk 1.69 [1.18–2.42]) according to an analysis of the UK General Practice Research Database [78]. Similarly, patients hospitalized for PMR and GCA were found to have a marginally increased risk of cancer [79]. On the other hand, population-based case–control studies suggest no risk [80], or even a reduced risk [81] for malignancies in GCA, and a recent similar study found no risk for cancer in PMR [82].

Autoimmune pancreatitis does not seem to confer any risk for cancer [83]. Nodules in autoimmune thyroiditis have been connected to cancer in surgical series, but this may reflect a selection bias [84].

An increased risk for malignancies among patients with IGG4-related disease (IG4RD) has been suggested by some [85], but this has been recently disputed by a cohort study of 113 patients [86]. Yet this study excluded malignancies that were diagnosed at the time of the IgG4RD onset. Similarly, cancer was infrequent among 55 patients from a Spanish register [87]. On the contrary, a recent cohort-based study [88] found a twofold increased risk for cancer among IG4RD patients, and this increase was higher within the first year of diagnosis (3.53, 95% CI 1.23–5.83), suggesting a direct link between cancer and this disorder. One must take into account that some IGG4RD may be erroneously considered as metastases, which may lead to underreporting of this disorder.

Behcet's disease (BD), a common vasculitis in endemic areas, may increase cancer risk. The Taiwanese Health Insurance Research Database (including 1314 BD patients) found that female BD patients have a higher risk of overall cancer (SIR = 1.8). A high risk was noted for NHL (SIR 8.3), hematological malignancy (SIR 4.2), and breast cancer (SIR 2.2). This increase was highest within the first year, as 75% of the hematological malignancies were found within the first year [89].

The risk of cancer in sarcoidosis has been assessed in a cohort of Olmsted County, Minnesota [90]. Overall, the risk of malignancy was similar among sarcoidosis patients compared with nonsarcoidosis controls. However, the risk of incident hematologic malignancy was significantly higher among patients with sarcoidosis with extrathoracic involvement compared with patients without extrathoracic disease.

AUTOIMMUNE DISORDERS IN MALIGNANCIES

It seems that AID patients are prone to develop certain types of cancer. For example, in a single center in New York, one-fifth of all chronic myelomonocytic leukemia patients had at least one AID, while patients with myelodysplastic syndrome (MDS) had AID rates similar to the general population [91]. The authors suggested that MDS may have evolved through an immune mediated process. Similarly, in another study group of 1408 MDS patients, 28% had an autoimmune disease [92]. On the other hand, others [93] described eight cases of MDS presenting with autoimmune symptoms, including seronegative RA, which responded to MTX, pyoderma gangrenosum, cutaneous vasculitis, SLE, IBD, and hemophagocytic lymphohistiocytosis. In another cohort [94], 4.4% of MDS patients presented with AID around MDS diagnosis, suggesting AID as a paraneoplastic manifestation of MDS.

According to one center's experience, half of marginal zone lymphoma patients had an AID, with significantly increased rates for immune thrombocytopenia, autoimmune hemolytic anemia, Hashimoto thyroiditis, and RA [95]. Similarly, a study from the Swedish Cancer Registry [96] found that the overall incidence of non-Hodgkin lymphoma was increased after AID (SIR 1.6), especially in autoimmune hemolytic anemia (SIR = 27.2), immune thrombocytopenic purpura (SIR = 7.5), pSS (SIR = 4.9), SLE (SIR = 4.4), PM/DM (SIR = 4.1), primary biliary cirrhosis (SIR = 3.9), and polyarteritis nodosa, discoid lupus erythematosus, sarcoidosis, myasthenia gravis, Crohn's, Sc, RA, BD, rheumatic fever, ulcerative colitis, PMR, Hashimoto, and psoriasis. The SIR was higher in younger age groups and was increased for all histology subtypes, suggesting that autoimmunity in general increases the risk for developing cancer.

The risk for solid tumors may also be related to local autoimmunity. A Swedish national-based dataset study [97] found an increased risk for primary liver and gallbladder cancer among AID, including primary biliary cirrhosis, IBD, and Celiac disease, suggesting a role for a local autoimmune process.

Can cancer trigger autoimmunity? The development of systemic sclerosis in cancer patients harboring the relatively rare POLR3A cancer mutation suggests that cancer may directly induce AID [98]. Malignancies may induce AID such as myositis, which has a clear association with cancer, and other miscellaneous AID such as autoimmune hemolytic anemia [99], hepatitis [100], and neurological syndromes [101]. Similarly, specific autoantibodies (i.e., antitopoisomerase, anti-PM-Scl, anti-TIF, etc.) in Sc or PM/DM patients are related to an increased risk for cancer. The role of cancer as an inducer of AID is also implied by paraneoplastic autoimmune syndromes such as paraneoplastic pemphigus, Eaton-Lambert syndrome, paraneoplastic polyarthritis, periostitis related to hypertrophic osteoarthropathy, and palmar fasciitis (reviewed by Manger and Schett [102]). Similarly, childhood cancer survivors are at increased risk for AID [103], though this may be related to cancer therapy. Autoantibodies targeting tumors have been suggested as biomarkers for the early detection of esophageal [104], gastric [105], colorectal [106] ovarian [107], and breast [108] cancers. Finally, alarmins, such as HMGN1, have been proposed as antitumor mediators that might contribute to autoimmunity [109].

SUMMARY

In summary, AID have a clear association with cancer, though the strength of this association varies between different AID, different types of malignancies, and different populations. Therapy of AID may also contribute to this association. This variance may pose a challenge when inferring conclusions from metaanalyses and reviews and should encourage policymakers to create local cohorts and registries. Recent evidence has contributed to our understanding of the mechanisms involved in this association, suggesting that while on one hand AID may procure an increased risk for cancer, on the other hand cancer may also cause autoimmunity in different mechanisms. Hopefully, the elucidation of these mechanisms in the future might allow us to exploit these mechanisms to detect and treat both cancer and AID.

REFERENCES

[1] Ehrenfeld M. Cancer and autoimmunity. In: Anaya JM, Cervera R, Levy RA, Rojas- Villarraga A, Shoenfeld Y, editors. Autoimmunity: from bench to bedside. El Rosario University Press, Center for Autoimmune Diseases Research, CREA Texts Collection, School of Medicine and Health Sciences, El Rosario University; 2013. p. 683–9.

[2] Dranoff G. Cytokines in cancer pathogenesis and cancer therapy. Nat Rev Cancer 2004;4:11–22.

[3] Chang SH, Park JK, Lee YJ, Yang JA, Lee EY, Song YW, et al. Comparison of cancer incidence among patients with rheumatic disease: a retrospective cohort study. Arthritis Res Ther 2014;16:428.

[4] Hashimoto A, Chiba N, Tsuno H, Komiya A, Furukawa H, Matsui T, et al. Incidence of malignancy and the risk of lymphoma in Japanese patients with rheumatoid arthritis compared to the general population. J Rheumatol 2015;42:564–71.

[5] Lin YC, Chou HW, Tsai WC, Yen JH, Chang SJ, Lin YC. The age-risk relationship of hematologic malignancies in patients with rheumatoid arthritis: a nationwide retrospective cohort study. Clin Rheumatol 2015;34:1195–202.

[6] Huang WK, Chiou MJ, Kuo CF, Lin YC, Yu KH, See LC. No overall increased risk of cancer in patients with rheumatoid arthritis: a nationwide dynamic cohort study in Taiwan. Rheumatol Int 2014;34:1379–86.

[7] Andersen CL, Lindegaard H, Vestergaard H, Siersma VD, Hasselbalch HC, de Fine Olivarius N, et al. Risk of lymphoma and solid cancer among patients with rheumatoid arthritis in a primary care setting. PLoS One 2014;9:e99388.

[8] Fallah M, Liu X, Ji J, Forsti A, Sundquist K, Hemminki K. Autoimmune diseases associated with non-Hodgkin lymphoma: a nationwide cohort study. Ann Oncol 2014;25:2025–30.

[9] Wadström H, Frisell T, Askling J. FRI0061 cervical dysplasia and cervical cancer in women with rheumatoid arthritis. Ann Rheum Dis 2015;74:441.

[10] Khraishi M, Aslanov R, Khraishi S. 2014 ACR/ARHP annual meeting abstract supplement. Arthritis Rheumatol 2014;66:S1–1402.

[11] Mercer LK, Davies R, Galloway JB, Low A, Lunt M, Dixon WG, et al. Risk of cancer in patients receiving non-biologic disease-modifying therapy for rheumatoid arthritis compared with the UK general population. Rheumatology 2013;52:91–8.

[12] Dougados M, Soubrier M, Antunez A, Balint P, Balsa A, Buch MH, et al. Prevalence of comorbidities in rheumatoid arthritis and evaluation of their monitoring: results of an international, cross-sectional study (COMORA). Ann Rheum Dis 2014;73:62–8.

[13] Tian G, Liang JN, Wang ZY, Zhou D. Breast cancer risk in rheumatoid arthritis: an update meta-analysis. Biomed Res Int 2014;2014:453012.

[14] Smitten AL, Simon TA, Hochberg MC, Suissa S. A meta-analysis of the incidence of malignancy in adult patients with rheumatoid arthritis. Arthritis Res Ther 2008;10:R45.

[15] Simon TA, Thompson A, Gandhi KK, Hochberg MC, Suissa S. Incidence of malignancy in adult patients with rheumatoid arthritis: a meta-analysis. Arthritis Res Ther 2015;17:212.

[16] Nayak P, Luo R, Elting L, Zhao H, Suarez-Almazor ME. Impact of rheumatoid arthritis on the mortality of elderly patients who develop cancer: a population-based study. Arthritis Care Res 2017;69(1):75–83.

[17] Park JK, Yang JA, Ahn EY, Chang SH, Song YW, Curtis JR, et al. Survival rates of cancer patients with and without rheumatic disease: a retrospective cohort analysis. BMC Canc 2016;16:381.

[18] Simard JF, Ekberg S, Johansson AL, Askling J. What is the impact of chronic systemic inflammation such as rheumatoid arthritis on mortality following cancer? Ann Rheum Dis 2016;75:862–6.

[19] Lopez-Olivo MA, Siddhanamatha HR, Shea B, Tugwell P, Wells GA, Suarez-Almazor ME. Methotrexate for treating rheumatoid arthritis. Cochrane Database Syst Rev 2014:CD000957.

[20] Scott FI, Mamtani R, Brensinger CM, Haynes K, Chiesa-Fuxench ZC, Zhang J, et al. Risk of nonmelanoma skin cancer associated with the use of immunosuppressant and biologic agents in patients with a history of autoimmune disease and nonmelanoma skin cancer. JAMA Dermatol 2016;152:164–72.

[21] Lopez-Olivo MA, Tayar JH, Martinez-Lopez JA, Pollono EN, Cueto JP, Gonzales-Crespo MR, et al. Risk of malignancies in patients with rheumatoid arthritis treated with biologic therapy: a meta-analysis. JAMA 2012;308:898–908.

[22] Bongartz T, Warren FC, Mines D, Matteson EL, Abrams KR, Sutton AJ. Etanercept therapy in rheumatoid arthritis and the risk of malignancies: a systematic review and individual patient data meta-analysis of randomised controlled trials. Ann Rheum Dis 2009;68:1177–83.

[23] Leombruno JP, Einarson TR, Keystone EC. The safety of anti-tumour necrosis factor treatments in rheumatoid arthritis: meta and exposure-adjusted pooled analyses of serious adverse events. Ann Rheum Dis 2009;68:1136–45.

[24] Ramiro S, Gaujoux-Viala C, Nam JL, Smolen JS, Buch M, Gossec L, et al. Safety of synthetic and biological DMARDs: a systematic literature review informing the 2013 update of the EULAR recommendations for management of rheumatoid arthritis. Ann Rheum Dis 2014;73:529–35.

[25] Liu Y, Fan W, Chen H, Yu MX. Risk of breast cancer and total malignancies in rheumatoid arthritis patients undergoing TNF-alpha antagonist therapy: a meta-analysis of randomized control trials. Asian Pac J Cancer Prev 2014;15:3403–10.

[26] Wu CY, Chen DY, Shen JL, Ho HJ, Chen CC, Kuo KN, et al. The risk of cancer in patients with rheumatoid arthritis taking tumor necrosis factor antagonists: a nation-wide cohort study. Arthritis Res Ther 2014;16:449.

[27] Mercer LK, Lunt M, Low AL, Dixon WG, Watson KD, Symmons DP, et al. Risk of solid cancer in patients exposed to anti-tumour necrosis factor therapy: results from the British Society for Rheumatology Biologics Register for Rheumatoid Arthritis. Ann Rheum Dis 2015;74:1087–93.

[28] Raaschou P, Simard JF, Holmqvist M, Askling J, A.S. Group. Rheumatoid arthritis, anti-tumour necrosis factor therapy, and risk of malignant melanoma: nationwide population based prospective cohort study from Sweden. BMJ 2013;346:f1939.

[29] Mercer LK, Askling J, Raaschou P, Dixon WG, Dreyer L, Hetland ML, et al. Risk of invasive melanoma in patients with rheumatoid arthritis treated with biologics: results from a collaborative project of 11 European biologic registers. Ann Rheum Dis 2017;76(2):386–91.

[30] Berghen N, Teuwen LA, Westhovens R, Verschueren P. Malignancies and anti-TNF therapy in rheumatoid arthritis: a single-center observational cohort study. Clin Rheumatol 2015;34:1687–95.

[31] Silva-Fernandez L, Lunt M, Kearsley-Fleet L, Watson KD, Dixon WG, Symmons DP, et al. The incidence of cancer in patients with rheumatoid arthritis and a prior malignancy who receive TNF inhibitors or rituximab: results from the British Society for Rheumatology biologics register-rheumatoid arthritis. Rheumatology 2016;55(11):2033–9. Epub 2016 Aug 22.

[32] Bonovas S, Minozzi S, Lytras T, Gonzalez-Lorenzo M, Pecoraro V, Colombo S, et al. Risk of malignancies using anti-TNF agents in rheumatoid arthritis, psoriatic arthritis, and ankylosing spondylitis: a systematic review and meta-analysis. Expert Opin Drug Saf 2016;15:35–54.

[33] van Vollenhoven RF, Fleischmann RM, Furst DE, Lacey S, Lehane PB. Longterm safety of rituximab: final report of the rheumatoid arthritis global clinical trial program over 11 years. J Rheumatol 2015;42:1761–6.

[34] Rubbert-Roth A, Sebba A, Brockwell L, Kelman A, Porter-Brown B, Pulley J, et al. Malignancy rates in patients with rheumatoid arthritis treated with tocilizumab. RMD Open 2016;2:e000213.

[35] Curtis JR, Lee EB, Kaplan IV, Kwok K, Geier J, Benda B, et al. Tofacitinib, an oral Janus kinase inhibitor: analysis of malignancies across the rheumatoid arthritis clinical development programme. Ann Rheum Dis 2016;75:831–41.

[36] Simon TA, Smitten AL, Franklin J, Askling J, Lacaille D, Wolfe F, et al. Malignancies in the rheumatoid arthritis abatacept clinical development programme: an epidemiological assessment. Ann Rheum Dis 2009;68:1819–26.

[37] Gross RL, Schwartzman-Morris JS, Krathen M, Reed G, Chang H, Saunders KC, A, et al. Comparison of the malignancy incidence among patients with psoriatic arthritis and patients with rheumatoid arthritis in a large US cohort. Arthritis Rheumatol 2014;66:1472–81.

[38] Hellgren K, Smedby KE, Backlin C, Sundstrom C, Feltelius N, Eriksson JK, et al. Anky-losing spondylitis, psoriatic arthritis, and risk of malignant lymphoma: a cohort study based on nationwide prospectively recorded data from Sweden. Arthritis Rheumatol 2014;66:1282–90.

[39] Deng C, Li W, Fei Y, Li Y, Zhang F. Risk of malignancy in ankylosing spondylitis: a systematic review and meta-analysis. Sci Rep 2016;6:32063.

[40] Hellgren K, Dreyer L, Arkema EV, Glintborg B, Jacobsson LT, Kristensen LE, et al. Cancer risk in patients with spondyloarthritis treated with TNF inhibitors: a collaborative study from the ARTIS and DANBIO registers. Ann Rheum Dis 2017;76(1):105–11.

[41] Costa L, Caso F, Del Puente A, Di Minno MN, Peluso R, Scarpa R. Incidence of malignancies in a cohort of psoriatic arthritis patients taking traditional disease modifying Antirheumatic drug and tumor necrosis factor inhibitor therapy: an observational study. J Rheumatol 2016;43(12):2149–54. Epub 2016 Sep. 15.

[42] Hofheinz K, Schett G, Manger B. Adult onset Still's disease associated with malignancy-cause or coincidence? Semin Arthritis Rheum 2016;45:621–6.

[43] Liang Y, Yang Z, Qin B, Zhong R. Primary Sjogren's syndrome and malignancy risk: a systematic review and meta-analysis. Ann Rheum Dis 2014;73:1151–6.

[44] Abrol E, Gonzalez-Pulido C, Praena-Fernandez JM, Isenberg DA. A retrospective study of long-term outcomes in 152 patients with primary Sjogren's syndrome: 25-year experience. Clin Med 2014;14:157–64.

[45] Gottenberg JE, Seror R, Miceli-Richard C, Benessiano J, Devauchelle-Pensec V, Dieude P, et al. Serum levels of beta2-microglobulin and free light chains of immunoglobulins are associated with systemic disease activity in primary Sjogren's syndrome. Data at enrollment in the prospective ASSESS cohort. PLoS One 2013;8:e59868.

[46] Risselada AP, Kruize AA, Bijlsma JW. Clinical features distinguishing lymphoma development in primary Sjogren's syndrome — a retrospective cohort study. Semin Arthritis Rheum 2013;43:171–7.

[47] Papageorgiou A, Ziogas DC, Mavragani CP, Zintzaras E, Tzioufas AG, Moutsopoulos HM, et al. Predicting the outcome of Sjogren's syndrome-associated non-hodgkin's lymphoma patients. PLoS One 2015;10:e0116189.

[48] Papageorgiou A, Voulgarelis M, Tzioufas AG. Clinical picture, outcome and predictive factors of lymphoma in Sjgren syndrome. Autoimmun Rev 2015;14:641–9.

[49] Nishishinya MB, Pereda CA, Munoz-Fernandez S, Pego-Reigosa JM, Rua-Figueroa I, Andreu JL, et al. Identification of lymphoma predictors in patients with primary Sjogren's syndrome: a systematic literature review and meta-analysis. Rheumatol Int 2015;35:17–26.

[50] Mao S, Shen H, Zhang J. Systemic lupus erythematosus and malignancies risk. J Cancer Res Clin Oncol 2016;142:253–62.

[51] Ni J, Qiu LJ, Hu LF, Cen H, Zhang M, Wen PF, et al. Lung, liver, prostate, bladder malignancies risk in systemic lupus erythematosus: evidence from a meta-analysis. Lupus 2014;23:284–92.

[52] Rees F, Doherty M, Grainge M, Lanyon P, Davenport G, Zhang W. Burden of comorbidity in systemic lupus erythematosus in the UK, 1999–2012. Arthritis Care Res 2016;68:819–27.

[53] Khaliq W, Qayyum R, Clough J, Vaidya D, Wolff AC, Becker DM. Comparison of breast cancer risk in women with and without systemic lupus erythematosus in a Medicare population. Breast Cancer Res Treat 2015;151:465–74.

[54] Skare TL, da Rocha BV. Breast and cervical cancer in patients with systemic lupus erythematosus. Rev Bras Ginecol Obstet 2014;36:367–71.

[55] Bernatsky S, Ramsey-Goldman R, Labrecque J, Joseph L, Boivin JF, Petri M, et al. Cancer risk in systemic lupus: an updated international multi-centre cohort study. J Autoimmun 2013;42:130–5.

[56] Goobie GC, Bernatsky S, Ramsey-Goldman R, Clarke AE. Malignancies in systemic lupus erythematosus: a 2015 update. Curr Opin Rheumatol 2015;27:454–60.

[57] Bernatsky S, Ramsey-Goldman R, Petri M, Urowitz MB, Gladman DD, Fortin PF, et al. Breast cancer in systemic lupus. Lupus 2017;26(3):311–5.

[58] Zhang M, Li XM, Wang GS, Qian L, Tao JH, Ma Y, et al. Thyroid cancer in systemic lupus erythematosus: a meta analysis. Int J Clin Exp Pathol 2014;7:6270–3.

[59] Bernatsky S, Clarke AE, Labrecque J, von Scheven E, Schanberg LE, Silverman ED, et al. Cancer risk in childhood-onset systemic lupus. Arthritis Res Ther 2013;15:R198.

[60] Chan PC, Yu CH, Yeh KW, Horng JT, Huang JL. Comorbidities of pediatric systemic lupus erythematosus: a 6-year nationwide population-based study. J Microbiol Immunol Infect = Wei mian yu gan ran za zhi 2016;49:257–63.

[61] Flower C, Gaskin D, Bhamjee S, Bynoe Z. High-risk variants of cutaneous squamous cell carcinoma in patients with discoid lupus erythematosus: a case series. Lupus 2013;22:736–9.

[62] Singh AG, Crowson CS, Singh S, Davis MD, Maradit-Kremers H, Matteson EL, et al. Cancer risk in cutaneous lupus erythematosus: a population-based cohort study. Rheumatology 2016;55(11):2009–13. Epub 2016 Aug 12.

[63] Tessier-Cloutier B, Clarke AE, Pineau CA, Keeling S, Bissonauth A, Ramsey-Goldman R, et al. What investigations are needed to optimally monitor for malignancies in SLE? Lupus 2015;24:781–7.

[64] Shah AA, Hummers LK, Casciola-Rosen L, Visvanathan K, Rosen A, Wigley FM. Examination of autoantibody status and clinical features associated with cancer risk and cancer-associated scleroderma. Arthritis Rheumatol 2015;67:1053–61.

[65] Shah AA, Rosen A, Hummers L, Wigley F, Casciola-Rosen L. Close temporal relationship between onset of cancer and scleroderma in patients with RNA polymerase I/III antibodies. Arthritis Rheum 2010;62:2787–95.

[66] Colaci M, Giuggioli D, Sebastiani M, Manfredi A, Vacchi C, Spagnolo P, et al. Lung cancer in scleroderma: results from an Italian rheumatologic center and review of the literature. Autoimmun Rev 2013;12:374–9.

[67] Colaci M, Giuggioli D, Vacchi C, Lumetti F, Iachetta F, Marcheselli L, et al. Breast can-cer in systemic sclerosis: results of a cross-linkage of an Italian rheumatologic center and a population-based cancer registry and review of the literature. Autoimmun Rev 2014;13:132–7.

[68] Bruni C. Resolution of paraneoplastic PM/Scl-positive systemic sclerosis after curative resection of a pancreatic tumour. Rheumatology 2017;56(2):317–8.

[69] Ungprasert P, Bethina NK, Jones CH. Malignancy and idiopathic inflammatory myopathies. N Am J Med Sci 2013;5:569–72.

[70] Trallero-Araguas E, Rodrigo-Pendas JA, Selva-O'Callaghan A, Martinez-Gomez X, Bosch X, Labrador-Horrillo M, et al. Usefulness of anti-p155 autoantibody for diagnosing cancer-associated dermatomyositis: a systematic review and meta-analysis. Arthritis Rheum 2012;64:523–32.

[71] Kasuya A, Hamaguchi Y, Fujimoto M, Tokura Y. TIF1gamma-overexpressing, highly progressive endometrial carcinoma in a patient with derma-tomyositis positive for malignancy-associated anti-p155/140 autoantibody. Acta Derm Venereol 2013;93:715–6.

[72] Yang Z, Lin F, Qin B, Liang Y, Zhong R. Polymyositis/dermatomyositis and malignancy risk: a metaanalysis study. J Rheumatol 2015;42:282–91.

[73] Chen D, Yuan S, Wu X, Li H, Qiu Q, Zhan Z, et al. Incidence and predictive factors for malignancies with dermatomyositis: a cohort from southern China. Clin Exp Rheumatol 2014;32:615–21.

[74] Qiang JK, Kim WB, Baibergenova A, Alhusayen R. Risk of malignancy in dermatomyositis and polymyositis: a systematic review and meta-analysis. J Cutan Med Surg 2017;21(2):131–6.

[75] Mustafa KN, Al-Heresh AM, Khataybeh OY, Alawneh KM, Khader YS. Low prevalence of malignancy in patients with idiopathic inflammatory myopathies in Jordan. Clin Exp Rheumatol 2015;33:731–3.

[76] Shang W, Ning Y, Xu X, Li M, Guo S, Han M, et al. Incidence of cancer in ANCA-associated Vasculitis: a meta-analysis of observational studies. PLoS One 2015;10:e0126016.

[77] Rahmattulla C, Berden AE, Wakker SC, Reinders ME, Hagen EC, Wolterbeek R, et al. Incidence of malignancies in patients with Antineutrophil cytoplasmic antibody-associated vasculitis diagnosed between 1991 and 2013. Arthritis Rheumatol 2015;67:3270–8.

[78] Muller S, Hider SL, Belcher J, Helliwell T, Mallen CD. Is cancer associated with polymyalgia rheumatica? A cohort study in the general practice research database. Ann Rheum Dis 2014;73:1769–73.

[79] Ji J, Liu X, Sundquist K, Sundquist J, Hemminki K. Cancer risk in patients hospitalized with polymyalgia rheumatica and giant cell arteritis: a follow-up study in Sweden. Rheumatology 2010;49:1158–63.

[80] Kermani TA, Schafer VS, Crowson CS, Hunder GG, Gabriel SE, Ytterberg SR, et al. Malignancy risk in patients with giant cell arteritis: a population-based cohort study. Arthritis Care Res 2010;62:149–54.

[81] Kermani TA, Schafer VS, Crowson CS, Hunder GG, Ytterberg SR, Matteson EL, et al. Cancer preceding giant cell arteritis: a case-control study. Arthritis Rheum 2010;62:1763–9.

[82] Pfeifer EC, Crowson CS, Major BT, Matteson EL. Polymyalgia rheumatica and its association with cancer. Rheumatology 2015;(Suppl. 6).

[83] Hart PA, Law RJ, Dierkhising RA, Smyrk TC, Takahashi N, Chari ST. Risk of cancer in autoimmune pancreatitis: a case-control study and review of the literature. Pancreas 2014;43:417–21.

[84] Castagna MG, Belardini V, Memmo S, Maino F, Di Santo A, Toti P, et al. Nodules in autoimmune thyroiditis are associated with increased risk of thyroid cancer in surgical series but not in cytological series: evidence for selection bias. J Clin Endocrinol Metab 2014;99:3193–8.

[85] Yamamoto M, Takahashi H, Tabeya T, Suzuki C, Naishiro Y, Ishigami K, et al. Risk of malignancies in IgG4-related disease. Mod Rheumatol 2012;22:414–8.

[86] Hirano K, Tada M, Sasahira N, Isayama H, Mizuno S, Takagi K, et al. Incidence of malignancies in patients with IgG4-related disease. Intern Med 2014;53:171–6.

[87] Fernandez-Codina A, Martinez-Valle F, Pinilla B, Lopez C, DeTorres I, Solans-Laque R, et al. IgG4-related disease: results from a multicenter Spanish registry. Medicine 2015;94:e1275.

[88] Asano J, Watanabe T, Oguchi T, Kanai K, Maruyama M, Ito T, et al. Association between immunoglobulin G4-related disease and malignancy within 12 years after diagnosis: an analysis after longterm followup. J Rheumatol 2015;42:2135–42.

[89] Wang LH, Wang WM, Hsu SM, Lin SH, Shieh CC. Risk of overall and site-specific cancers in Behcet disease: a Nationwide population-based study in Taiwan. J Rheumatol 2015;42:879–84.

[90] Ungprasert P, Crowson CS, Matteson EL. Risk of malignancy among patients with sarcoidosis: a population-based cohort study. Arthritis Care Res 2017;69(1):46–50.

[91] Peker D, Padron E, Bennett JM, Zhang X, Horna P, Epling-Burnette PK, et al. A close association of autoimmune-mediated processes and autoimmune disorders with chronic myelomonocytic leukemia: observation from a single institution. Acta Haematol 2015;133:249–56.

[92] Komrokji RS, Kulasekararaj A, Al Ali NH, Kordasti S, Bart-Smith E, Craig BM, et al. Autoimmune diseases and myelodysplastic syndromes. Am J Hematol 2016;91:E280.

[93] Frietsch JJ, Dornaus S, Neumann T, Scholl S, Schmidt V, Kunert C, et al. Paraneoplastic inflammation in myelodysplastic syndrome or bone marrow failure: case series with focus on 5-azacytidine and literature review. Eur J Haematol 2014;93:247–59.

[94] Williamson BT, Foltz L, Leitch HA. Autoimmune syndromes presenting as a paraneoplastic manifestation of myelodysplastic syndromes: clinical features, course, treatment and outcome. Hematol Rep 2016;8:6480.

[95] Dasanu CA, Bockorny B, Grabska J, Codreanu I. Prevalence and pattern of autoimmune conditions in patients with marginal zone lymphoma: a single institution experience. Conn Med 2015;79:197–200.

[96] Fallah M, Liu X, Ji J, Forsti A, Sundquist K, Hemminki K. Hodgkin lymphoma after autoimmune diseases by age at diagnosis and histological subtype. Ann Oncol 2014;25:1397–404.

[97] Castro FA, Liu X, Forsti A, Ji J, Sundquist J, Sundquist K, et al. Increased risk of hepatobiliary cancers after hospitalization for autoimmune disease. Clin Gastroenterol Hepatol 2014;12:1038–45. [e7].

[98] Joseph CG, Darrah E, Shah AA, Skora AD, Casciola-Rosen LA, Wigley FM, et al. Association of the autoimmune disease scleroderma with an immunologic response to cancer. Science 2014;343:152–7.

[99] Rhodes EC, Parikh SP, Bhattacharyya N. Severe autoimmune hemolytic anemia with renal neoplasm. Pediatr Surg Int 2014;30:243–4.

[100] Mendogni P, Rosso L, Tosi D, Palleschi A, Righi I, Minonzio F, et al. Autoimmune hepatitis: an uncommon presentation of thymoma. Tumori 2016;11(Suppl. 2):102.

[101] Pittock SJ, Palace J. Paraneoplastic and idiopathic autoimmune neurologic disorders: approach to diagnosis and treatment. Handb Clin Neurol 2016;133:165–83.

[102] Manger B, Schett G. Paraneoplastic syndromes in rheumatology. Nat Rev Rheumatol 2014;10:662–70.

[103] Holmqvist AS, Olsen JH, Mellemkjaer L, Garwicz S, Hjorth L, Moell C, et al. Autoimmune diseases in adult life after childhood cancer in Scandinavia (ALiCCS). Ann Rheum Dis 2016;75:1622–9.

[104] Zhang H, Xia J, Wang K, Zhang J. Serum autoantibodies in the early detection of esophageal cancer: a systematic review. Tumour Biol 2015;36:95–109.

[105] Werner S, Chen H, Tao S, Brenner H. Systematic review: serum autoantibodies in the early detection of gastric cancer. Int J Cancer 2015;136:2243–52.

[106] Chen H, Werner S, Tao S, Zornig I, Brenner H. Blood autoantibodies against tumor-associated antigens as biomarkers in early detection of colorectal cancer. Cancer Lett 2014;346:178–87.

[107] Shi JX, Qin JJ, Ye H, Wang P, Wang KJ, Zhang JY. Tumor associated antigens or anti-TAA autoantibodies as biomarkers in the diagnosis of ovarian cancer: a systematic review with meta-analysis. Expert Rev Mol Diagn 2015;15:829–52.

[108] Xia J, Shi J, Wang P, Song C, Wang K, Zhang J, et al. Tumour-associated autoantibodies as diagnostic biomarkers for breast cancer: a systematic review and meta-analysis. Scand J Immunol 2016;83:393–408.

[109] Wei F, Yang D, Tewary P, Li Y, Li S, Chen X, et al. The Alarmin HMGN1 contributes to antitumor immunity and is a potent immunoadjuvant. Cancer Res 2014;74:5989–98.

[110] Raaschou P, Simard JF, Asker Hagelberg C, Askling J, A.S. Group. Rheumatoid arthritis, anti-tumour necrosis factor treatment, and risk of squamous cell and basal cell skin cancer: cohort study based on nationwide prospectively recorded data from Sweden. BMJ 2016;352:i262.

[111] Buchbinder R, Van Doornum S, Staples M, Lassere M, March L. Malignancy risk in Australian rheumatoid arthritis patients treated with anti-tumour necrosis factor therapy: analysis of the Australian Rheumatology Association Database (ARAD) prospective cohort study. BMC Musculoskelet Disord 2015;16:309.

Chapter 42

Autoimmune Syndromes in Cancer

Dr Lior Seluk[1], Dr Shaye Kivity[1,2,3]

[1]*Department of Medicine A, Ramat-Gan, Israel;* [2]*Sackler School of Medicine, Ramat Aviv, Israel;* [3]*The Zabludowicz Center for Autoimmune Diseases, Ramat-Gan, Israel*

MUSCULOSKELETAL-ASSOCIATED PARANEOPLASTIC SYNDROMES

Paraneoplastic Arthritis

Arthritis can precede and lead to the detection of cancer. A large cohort (n=65) of patients with paraneoplastic arthritis demonstrated a male predominance and initial presentation mainly with acute asymmetric arthritis [1,2].

Remitting Seronegative Symmetrical Synovitis with Pitting Edema (RS3PE)

This syndrome is characterized by distal swelling of the hands and feet and occurs mainly in the elderly. RS3PE patients respond very well to corticosteroids and have an excellent prognosis. Several small studies have demonstrated up to 30% of associated malignancy, especially those with a poor response to corticosteroids [2].

Dermatomyositis Associated With Malignancy

Dermatomyositis is associated with an underlying neoplastic disease in about 20% of all cases [2,3]. However, when clinical features overlap with other collagen vascular diseases (e.g., interstitial lung involvement, Raynaud's phenomenon) and the presence of various autoantibodies (AAbs) suggestive for connective tissue disease (antisynthetase, anti-Ro52, or systemic sclerosis–associated antibodies), tumor risk is not increased [2]. Up to 83% of dermatomyositis patients with malignancy have anti–NXP-2 and anti–TIF-1γ (anti-p155) antibodies [4].

Hypertrophic (Pulmonary) Osteoarthropathy

Hypertrophic osteoarthropathy (HOA) is characterized by clubbing of the distal phalanges of the fingers and/or toes with periostitis causing bone and joint pain and often synovitis. HOA can occur in relation to malignancies, mainly intrathoracic ones (1% of primary lung cancer) but not solely. It is suspected that platelet-derived growth factor or vascular endothelial growth factor produced by the tumor cells contributes to the pathogenesis of HOA [2].

HEMATOLOGICAL PARANEOPLASTIC SYNDROMES

Autoimmune Hemolytic Anemia

This syndrome is among the most prevalent paraneoplastic phenomena known. It is characterized by accelerated destruction of erythrocytes by circulating AAbs [5]. In a series of 175 patients with autoimmune hemolytic anemia (AIHA), up to 14% can be associated with malignancy in the background. Paraneoplastic-AIHA is mainly linked to hematological malignancies such as lymphomas and leukemia [6]; however, association with solid tumors such as bladder and ovarian cancer were described [7–9]. Most patients with paraneoplastic AIHA due to solid tumors suffer from advanced metastatic disease, yet respond to surgical resection [7,10]. In paraneoplastic AIHA, the AAbs are mainly of the "warm" type; however, "cold" AAbs have also been reported as well as mixed type [7,8].

Mosaic of Autoimmunity. https://doi.org/10.1016/B978-0-12-814307-0.00042-6

Autoimmune Thrombocytopenia

The main cause of thrombocytopenia in cancer patients is bone marrow aplasia due to cytotoxic chemotherapy or radiation. Less common causes are bone marrow infiltration by the tumor, drug-induced immune thrombocytopenia, or disseminated intravascular coagulation. A rare syndrome similar to idiopathic thrombocytopenic purpura (ITP) has been reported in patients with malignancies as well. It is the clinical course of 1%–5% of patients with chronic lymphocytic leukemia [6]. It is rare cause of thrombocytopenia in solid tumors: in a review of 68 cases of paraneoplastic thrombocytopenia, the most common tumor was lung (15 of 68 patients) and breast cancer (15 of 68 patients), followed by renal cell, ovarian and gastrointestinal cancers, and very rare in prostate cancer [11]. The syndrome occurred either before (with a median of 5 years), concurrent with, or after the diagnosis of the cancer. Patients respond to corticosteroids and splenectomy, as in treatment for primary ITP. In several cases the presence of antiplatelet AAbs has been detected.

Autoimmune Neutropenia

This is an extremely rare condition reported in patients with hematological malignancies [6]. A single case of paraneoplastic neutropenia and malignant melanoma was reported [12]. Before diagnosis is made, other secondary causes should be excluded such as systemic lupus erythematosus, rheumatoid arthritis, Sjogren syndrome, celiac disease, hyperthyroidism (Graves disease), Crohn disease, and other (auto) immune diseases as well as prior rituximab treatment [6].

VASCULITIS ASSOCIATED WITH MALIGNANCY

Vasculitis may be rarely associated with malignancy. The most prevalent histopathology type is cutaneous leukocytoclastic vasculitis. Hematologic malignancies are identified as a cause in more than half of the cases, with myelodysplasia and non-Hodgkin lymphoma being the most frequent diagnoses. Among solid tumors, lung, breast, and urogenital cancers are the most common causes of paraneoplastic vasculitis [2]. Instances of vasculitis have been reported to occur both before and after onset of malignancy. Greer et al. reported 13 patients with malignancy-related vasculitis, which were poorly responsive to therapy, and chemotherapy directed at the underlying malignancy was also generally ineffective [13].

NEUROLOGICAL PARANEOPLASTIC SYNDROMES

The paraneoplastic neurological syndromes (PNSs) are a heterogeneous group that may affect any part of the central and peripheral nervous system, the neuromuscular junction, or the muscles. These syndromes are rare and vary with the neurologic syndrome and tumor type. The main presentations are encephalomyelitis (pathological involvement of all parts of the central nervous system and peripheral nervous system), limbic encephalitis (pathological involvement in the amygdale and hippocampus), subacute cerebellar degeneration (pathological involvement in Purkinje cells), opsoclonus-myoclonus, subacute sensory neuronopathy (pathological involvement in the dorsal root ganglia), and Lambert–Eaton myasthenic syndrome [14,15]. There has been an attempt to divide the PNS into two groups, according to the location of the antigen that the antibodies target [16–18]. In the first group, antibodies are directed against intracellular neuronal proteins and can be detected in the serum and CSF. These antibodies have a strong association with underlying tumor (Table 42.1) and are

TABLE 42.1 "Well-Characterized" Paraneoplastic Antibodies, Associated Tumors, and Neurological Presentations

Antibody	Neurological Presentation	Tumor
Anti-HU (ANNA1)	Encephalomyelitis, sensory neuronopathy, chronic gastrointestinal pseudo-obstruction, paraneoplastic cerebellar degeneration (PCD), limbic encephalitis	Small cell lung cancer (SCLC)
Anti-Yo (PCA1)	Cerebellar degeneration	Ovary, breast
Anti-RI (ANNA2)	Brainstem encephalitis	SCLC, breast
Anti-amphiphysin	Stiff person syndrome	SCLC, breast
Anti-MA2 (Ta)	With limbic/diencephalic encephalitis, brainstem encephalitis/PCD	Testis, lung
Anti-CV2 (CRMP5)	encephalomyelitis, chorea, sensory neuronopathy, sensorimotor neuropathy, chronic gastrointestinal pseudo-obstruction, paraneoplastic cerebellar degeneration, limbic encephalitis	SCLC, thymoma

TABLE 42.2 Autoimmune Encephalitis Antibodies, Associated Tumors, and Neurological Presentations

Antibody	Neurological Presentation	Tumor
Anti-VKGC (Anti LGI-1; Anti-CASPR2)	Limbic encephalitis, Morvan's syndrome Creutzfeldt–Jakob disease-like syndrome	SCLC, Thymoma
NMDA receptor	Encephalitis with initial psychiatric features followed by catatonia, dystonia, aphasia, and hypoventilation	Ovarian teratoma
AMPA receptor	Limbic encephalitis Atypical psychosis	SCLC, breast, thymoma
GABA B receptor	Limbic encephalitis	SCLC
VGCC	Lambert–Eaton myasthenic syndrome (LEMS), paraneoplastic cerebellar degeneration (PCD)	SCLC

termed "well characterized" paraneoplastic or onconeuronal antibodies. The pathogenic mechanism is believed to be mediated by cytotoxic T-cells, and the antibodies are thought to be markers in most cases.

The second group (Table 42.2) of antibodies is directed against neuronal cell surface or synaptic proteins, including receptors and is detected in the serum and CSF as well [19,20]. Antibodies in this group are mainly associated with autoimmune encephalitis; however, overlap syndromes affecting CNS/peripheral nervous system also occur. The autoimmune encephalitis PNS may affect children [21,22] and are less associated with cancer than the "well characterized" PNS [20]. Studies suggest these antibodies have a direct pathogenic effect on the target antigens and a correlation between antibody titers and neurological outcome has been documented.

PNS may occur years before or after a detectable cancer and may occur with or without detectable antibodies. Serum antibodies may occur without neurological symptoms or NPS. Thus, diagnosis is mostly done by clinical suspicion and exclusion of secondary causes such as metastases, stroke, metabolic and nutritional deficits, infections, coagulopathy, and chemo/biological/radiotherapy side effects. Treatment is targeted both to remove the antigen source by treating the cancer, and suppression of the immune-mediated response (by plasma exchange, intravenous immunoglobulins, glucocorticoids, cyclophosphamide, and rituximab) [23,24].

AUTOANTIBODIES IN MALIGNANT DISEASES

AAbs are investigated for use as biomarkers of cancer screening, prognostic markers for disease staging, monitoring the efficacy of therapeutic response, and the identification of potential targets for personalized immunotherapy [25–28]. In some cases, an increase in serum levels of AAbs has been shown to precede the development of disease symptoms by several months to years and correlate with cancer incidence [25,28–30]. These AAbs are presented in early stages of carcinogenesis due to cancer immunosurveillance, the process by which the immune system recognizes and destroys invading pathogens as well as host cells that have become cancerous. These antigens are denoted collectively as tumor associated antigens (TAAs). The persistence and stability of antibodies against TAAs in the serum of cancer patients is an advantage over other potential markers, including the TAAs themselves, which are released by tumors but rapidly degraded [26]. Yet the general estimate even for the best TAAs is that they may evoke humoral response in only 5%–10% of cancer patients. One example of the potential of serologic AAbs to diagnose early-stage cancer is the discovery of the extracellular protein kinase A autoantibody as a universal cancer biomarker. This antibody was found to be elevated in a wide range of cancers of various stages [25]. Another example is the most investigated AAb anti-p53; these antibodies have been detected in the sera of workers exposed to vinyl chloride who developed angiosarcoma of the liver and in the sera of heavy smokers and uranium workers who developed lung cancer [27]. It has been reported that in patients with esophageal carcinoma, in which up to 60% of patients were detected with anti-p53, its levels had a potential of evaluating the response to the treatment and prognosis. However, the detection frequency at the time of diagnosis of other cancers has been reported in as little as 7%. To date, no single AAb biomarker has been used as a cancer biomarker due to the low sensitivity and specificity of single markers.

Antinuclear Antibodies

In several studies an increased titer of IgG and IgM antinuclear antibody (ANA) has been reported with a speckled pattern observed occasionally. In vitro, the AAbs react with both normal and malignant tissues [31]. In one series ANA was found in 19% of 342 patients with various cancers (vs. 1% in controls). The cancer most reported to correlate with positive ANA is breast cancer [32–34], in which positive ANA is also associated with a worse prognosis. There are also reports of positive ANA in patients with lung, gastrointestinal, uterus, hepatocellular carcinomas, and malignant melanomas and leukemia [35–37]. In contrast, several authors have not found increased levels of ANA in patients with lung carcinoma and chronic lymphatic leukemia. These discrepancies may be due to different techniques employed. It is noteworthy that anti-dsDNA and anti-Sm antibodies have been rarely associated with malignancy, whereas anti-ssDNA and antihistone antibodies have been described in patients with leukemias and other solid tumors [38,39].

Rheumatoid Factor

The association of rheumatoid factor (RF) and cancer has been reported to vary from 11% to 85%, perhaps due to different malignancies as well as different measuring techniques or positivity thresholds [36,40]. Higher RF frequency was also shown in association with a larger tumor burden. In a cohort of 295,837 participants RF was associated with a greater risk of cancer mortality; however, this association was not considerably different after hsCRP levels had also been adjusted for [41].

Antismooth Muscle Antibody

IgG and IgM antismooth muscle antibodies (ASMAs) were detected in the sera of patients with melanoma, breast, ovarian, lung, and cervical carcinoma. However, the association of ASMA with malignancy is controversial and most major studies are from the 1970s [33,34,42,43]. The presence of ASMA may be due to exposure of an actomyosin-like antigen on the membrane of the tumor cells [44].

REFERENCES

[1] Kisacik B, Onat AM, Kasifoglu T, Pehlivan Y, Pamuk ON, Dalkilic E, et al. Diagnostic dilemma of paraneoplastic arthritis: case series. Int J Rheum Dis July 2014;17(6):640–5.

[2] Manger B, Schett G. Rheumatic paraneoplastic syndromes - a clinical link between malignancy and autoimmunity. Clin Immunol January 2018;186:67–70.

[3] Zerdes I, Tolla M, Nikolaou M, Tsoukalas N, Velentza L, Hajiioannou J, et al. How can we effectively address the paraneoplastic dermatomyositis: diagnosis, risk factors and treatment options. J BUON July–August 2017;22(4):1073–80.

[4] Fiorentino DF, Chung LS, Christopher-Stine L, Zaba L, Li S, Mammen AL, et al. Most patients with cancer-associated dermatomyositis have antibodies to nuclear matrix protein NXP-2 or transcription intermediary factor 1gamma. Arthritis Rheum November 2013;65(11):2954–62.

[5] Hamblin TJ, Oscier DG, Young BJ. Autoimmunity in chronic lymphocytic leukaemia. J Clin Pathol July 1986;39(7):713–6.

[6] Visco C, Barcellini W, Maura F, Neri A, Cortelezzi A, Rodeghiero F. Autoimmune cytopenias in chronic lymphocytic leukemia. Am J Hematol November 2014;89(11):1055–62.

[7] Isotani S, Horiuchi A, Koja M, Noguchi T, Sugiura S, Shimoyama H, et al. Autoimmune hemolytic anemia associated with renal urothelial cancer: a case report and literature review. BMC Urol July 28, 2015;15:75.

[8] Loh KP, Kansagra A, Asik A, Ali S, Dahiya S. Paraneoplastic autoimmune hemolytic anemia in ovarian cancer: a marker of disease activity. Rare Tumors February 11, 2015;7(1):5598.

[9] Nenova IS, Valcheva MY, Beleva EA, Tumbeva DY, Yaneva MP, Rancheva EL, et al. Autoimmune phenomena in patients with solid tumors. Folia Med (Plovdiv) September 1, 2016;58(3):195–9.

[10] Barry KG, Crosby WH. Auto-immune hemolytic anemia arrested by removal of an ovarian teratoma: review of the literature and report of a case. Ann Intern Med November 1957;47(5):1002–7.

[11] Krauth MT, Puthenparambil J, Lechner K. Paraneoplastic autoimmune thrombocytopenia in solid tumors. Crit Rev Oncol Hematol January 2012;81(1):75–81.

[12] White JD, MacPherson IR, Evans TR. Auto-immune neutropenia occurring in association with malignant melanoma. Oncol Rep January–February 2003;10(1):249–51.

[13] Greer JM, Longley S, Edwards NL, Elfenbein GJ, Panush RS. Vasculitis associated with malignancy. Experience with 13 patients and literature review. Medicine (Baltim) July 1988;67(4):220–30.

[14] Darnell RB, Posner JB. Paraneoplastic syndromes involving the nervous system. N Engl J Med October 16, 2003;349(16):1543–54.

[15] Gozzard P, Woodhall M, Chapman C, Nibber A, Waters P, Vincent A, et al. Paraneoplastic neurologic disorders in small cell lung carcinoma: a prospective study. Neurology July 21, 2015;85(3):235–9.

[16] Kannoth S. Paraneoplastic neurologic syndrome: a practical approach. Ann Indian Acad Neurol January 2012;15(1):6–12.

[17] Graus F, Saiz A, Dalmau J. Antibodies and neuronal autoimmune disorders of the CNS. J Neurol April 2010;257(4):509–17.

[18] Graus F, Delattre JY, Antoine JC, Dalmau J, Giometto B, Grisold W, et al. Recommended diagnostic criteria for paraneoplastic neurological syndromes. J Neurol Neurosurg Psychiatry August 2004;75(8):1135–40.

[19] Leypoldt F, Armangue T, Dalmau J. Autoimmune encephalopathies. Ann NY Acad Sci March 2015;1338:94–114.

[20] Moscato EH, Jain A, Peng X, Hughes EG, Dalmau J, Balice-Gordon RJ. Mechanisms underlying autoimmune synaptic encephalitis leading to disorders of memory, behavior and cognition: insights from molecular, cellular and synaptic studies. Eur J Neurosci July 2010;32(2):298–309.

[21] Armangue T, Petit-Pedrol M, Dalmau J. Autoimmune encephalitis in children. J Child Neurol November 2012;27(11):1460–9.

[22] Florance NR, Davis RL, Lam C, Szperka C, Zhou L, Ahmad S, et al. Anti-N-methyl-D-aspartate receptor (NMDAR) encephalitis in children and adolescents. Ann Neurol July 2009;66(1):11–8.

[23] Titulaer MJ, McCracken L, Gabilondo I, Armangue T, Glaser C, Iizuka T, et al. Treatment and prognostic factors for long-term outcome in patients with anti-NMDA receptor encephalitis: an observational cohort study. Lancet Neurol February 2013;12(2):157–65.

[24] Lancaster E, Martinez-Hernandez E, Dalmau J. Encephalitis and antibodies to synaptic and neuronal cell surface proteins. Neurology July 12, 2011;77(2):179–89.

[25] Zaenker P, Ziman MR. Serologic autoantibodies as diagnostic cancer biomarkers--a review. Cancer Epidemiol Biomark Prev December 2013;22(12):2161–81.

[26] Zhu Q, Liu M, Dai L, Ying X, Ye H, Zhou Y, et al. Using immunoproteomics to identify tumor-associated antigens (TAAs) as biomarkers in cancer immunodiagnosis. Autoimmun Rev October 2013;12(12):1123–8.

[27] Dudas SP, Chatterjee M, Tainsky MA. Usage of cancer associated autoantibodies in the detection of disease. Cancer Biomark 2010;6(5–6):257–70.

[28] Jett JR, Peek LJ, Fredericks L, Jewell W, Pingleton WW, Robertson JF. Audit of the autoantibody test, EarlyCDT(R)-lung, in 1600 patients: an evaluation of its performance in routine clinical practice. Lung Cancer January 2014;83(1):51–5.

[29] Fortner RT, Damms-Machado A, Kaaks R. Systematic review: tumor-associated antigen autoantibodies and ovarian cancer early detection. Gynecol Oncol November 2017;147(2):465–80.

[30] Qiu J, Choi G, Li L, Wang H, Pitteri SJ, Pereira-Faca SR, et al. Occurrence of autoantibodies to annexin I, 14-3-3 theta and LAMR1 in prediagnostic lung cancer sera. J Clin Oncol November 1, 2008;26(31):5060–6.

[31] Burnham TK. Antinuclear antibodies in patients with malignancies. Lancet August 26, 1972;2(7774):436.

[32] Turnbull AR, Turner DT, Fraser JD, Lloyd RS, Lang CJ, Wright R. Autoantibodies in early breast cancer: a stage-related phenomenon? Br J Cancer September 1978;38(3):461–3.

[33] Mittra I, Perrin J, Kumaoka S. Thyroid and other autoantibodies in British and Japanese women: an epidemiological study of breast cancer. Br Med J January 31, 1976;1(6004):257–9.

[34] Wasserman J, Glas U, Blomgren H. Autoantibodies in patients with carcinoma of the breast. Correlation with prognosis. Clin Exp Immunol March 1975;19(3):417–22.

[35] Kiyosawa K, Daemer RJ, He LF, Bonino F, Prozesky OW, Purcell RH. The spectrum of complement-fixing antinuclear antibodies in patients with hepatocellular carcinoma. Hepatology July–August 1985;5(4):548–55.

[36] Schattner A, Shani A, Talpaz M, Bentwich Z. Rheumatoid factors in the sera of patient with gastrointestinal carcinoma. Cancer December 1, 1983;52(11):2156–61.

[37] Thomas PJ, Kaur JS, Aitcheson CT, Robinson WA, Tan EM. Antinuclear, antinucleolar, and anticytoplasmic antibodies in patients with malignant melanoma. Cancer Res March 1983;43(3):1372–80.

[38] Izui S, Lambert PH, Carpentier N, Miescher PA. The occurrence of antibodies against single-stranded DNA in the sera of patients with acute and chronic leukaemia. Clin Exp Immunol June 1976;24(3):379–84.

[39] Kostiala AA, Gripenberg M, Elonen E, Gripenberg G, Kostiala I. Follow-up of antibodies against single-stranded DNA in patients with haematological malignancies. Clin Exp Immunol July 1985;61(1):15–23.

[40] Giuliano AE, Irie R, Morton DL. Rheumatoid factor in melanoma patients: alterations of humoral tumor immunity in vitro. Cancer May 1979;43(5):1624–9.

[41] Ahn JK, Hwang J, Chang Y, Ryu S. Rheumatoid factor positivity increases all-cause and cancer mortality: a cohort study. Rheumatol Int July 2017;37(7):1135–43.

[42] McCarty GA, Rice JR, Fetter BF, Pisetsky DS. Lymphocytic lymphoma and systemic lupus erythematosus: their coexistence with antibody to the Sm antigen. Arch Pathol Lab Med April 1982;106(4):196–9.

[43] Hodson ME, Turner-Warwick M. Autoantibodies in patients with bronchial carcinoma. Thorax August 1975;30(4):367–70.

[44] Whitehouse JM, Holborow EJ. Smooth muscle antibody in malignant disease. Br Med J November 27, 1971;4(5786):511–3.

Classical Autoimmune Diseases

Chapter 43

Current Insights Into Systemic Lupus Erythematosus: From Pathogenesis to Biomarkers and Therapeutical Strategies

Fulvia Ceccarelli, Carlo Perricone, Guido Valesini, Fabrizio Conti

Rheumatology, Department of Internal Medicine, Sapienza University of Rome, Rome, Italy

INTRODUCTION

Systemic lupus erythematosus (SLE) is a systemic autoimmune disease, with an incidence approximately of 5–20 per 100,000 in the US population, with higher prevalence for people of African, Hispanic, or Asian ancestry, and a female/male ratio of 9:1 [1–3]. The disease is characterized by a wide heterogeneity in terms of production of autoantibodies, phenotypes, degrees of severity, and outcome. This variability parallels with complex pathogenesis, involving different mechanisms and pathways, not yet fully understood and leading to continuing researches. In the present chapter, we aimed at describing the current insights into SLE, moving from pathogenesis and biomarkers; moreover, we will be analyzing the more recent therapeutic strategies proposed for these patients.

Pathogenesis

The SLE pathogenesis moves from intricate disorders in the immune system, leading to production of autoantibodies and to enhancement of type I interferon (IFN) pathway and B-cell activating factor/B lymphocyte stimulator (BLyS) system [4]. These disorders originate from a multifactorial etiology, in which genetic factors interplay with environmental factors, determining disease susceptibility and features (Fig. 43.1).

The application of genome-wide association studies substantially increased the knowledge about SLE-associated genetic factors. In the last decades, more than 100 loci resulted strongly associated with disease susceptibility and/or phenotypes; frequently these variants were shared with other immune-mediated diseases, such as rheumatoid arthritis or Sjögren syndrome [5,6]. Briefly, the genetic variants involved in SLE development codify for protein implicated in innate and adaptive immune response (in particular, Toll-like receptors [TLRs] or IFN pathway), immune cells signaling or migration, mechanisms of apoptosis and autophagy, DNA repair, and lysosome function [5,7]. The identification of genetic factors is very important to better understand pathogenic mechanisms and to recognize new therapeutic approaches for SLE patients.

Environmental Factors

The complex interaction between environmental, genetic, and epigenetic factors contributing to SLE development leads to the *exposome* hypothesis [8]. The outcomes of research focusing on environmental exposure include the identification of causal risk factors potentially modifiable to reduce the burden of disease and to improve the knowledge of disease pathogenesis.

An epidemiological approach demonstrated a strong association between disease development and specific environmental factors. In particular, the exposure to UV light, infections, and estrogens are widely recognized as potential risk factors for SLE susceptibility [9]. In front of a strong epidemiological association, several questions remain unresolved about the pathogenic mechanisms linking the exposition to disease development. Several evidences underline that UV radiation exposure could induce SLE or exacerbate preexisting disease; however, the punctual mechanism leading UV to SLE pathogenesis is not yet fully understood. Data from experimental studies suggested the induction of reactive oxygen species after UV exposure, leading to the production of new autoantigens, deriving from DNA damage [10].

Mosaic of Autoimmunity. https://doi.org/10.1016/B978-0-12-814307-0.00043-8

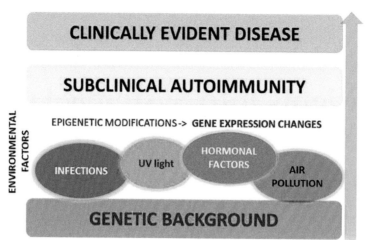

FIGURE 43.1 Pathogenic model for systemic lupus erythematosus.

Moreover, an impairment of immune response mechanisms, involving IFN system activation through TLRs, could explain the relationship between SLE development and infections. In particular, RNA- and DNA-containing antigens could activate an inflammatory cascade through the activation of TLR7 and 9, expressed at level of plasmacytoid dendritic cells. This mechanism could increase an IFN type I response that seems to be one of the most important pathway responsible for SLE development [11].

An epidemiological association between exogenous hormone use and increased SLE risk has been widely observed [12,13]. Moving on experimental data, hormones, such as estrogens, could influence the functions of immune system by specific receptors (ERα and ERβ) expressed on immune cells surface. These receptors play pro- and antiinflammatory functions, respectively; thus, the presence of one ER subtype could promote or reduce inflammatory process [14]. Our group identified the presence of autoantibodies directed against ERα in 45% of SLE patients, significantly associated with disease activity and presence of arthritis. Moreover, these antibodies resulted able to induce cell activation and apoptotic cell death in resting lymphocytes and proliferation of anti–CD3-stimulated T lymphocytes [15]. In the study conducted by Maselli and colleagues in 2016, a significantly lower intracellular expression of ERβ was identified in T cells of SLE patients with high disease activity in comparison with patients in low activity and healthy donors. Furthermore, ER-dependent signaling pathways were activated in T cells from active SLE patients, but not in those with low disease activity, when both membrane and intracellular ERs were stimulated by co-treatment with E2 and anti-ERα. Taken together, these results suggest that estrogens could modulate immune response and participate to disease pathogenesis [16].

In the last years, other possible environmental factors have been recognized, with specific attention to air pollution. Cigarette smoke includes several different components, such as nicotine, carbon monoxide, and polycyclic aromatic hydrocarbons. The exposure to these components could damage endogenous proteins and DNA, causing genetic mutations and gene activation. These modifications could be involved in SLE development, through the activation of immune response and the production of proinflammatory cytokines and autoantibodies [17]. Of note, current smokers condition resulted significantly associated with the presence of anti-dsDNA, suggesting the involvement of this environmental factor in the production of these antibodies and in pathogenesis of anti-dsDNA–related phenotypes [18]. Large population-based analysis suggested the possible role of silica exposure in increasing SLE risk [18]. By acting as immune adjuvant, crystalline silica could induce apoptotic phenomena with intracellular antigens release, increased production of proinflammatory cytokines, enhanced T cell response, reduction of number, and function of regulatory T cells [19].

More recently, it has been hypothesized that environmental stimuli could induce epigenetic modifications and changes in gene expression [20,21]. The role of epigenetic alterations in SLE pathogenesis became increasingly clear because of the evidence of their part in contributing to alteration in gene regulation and expression of co-receptors, cytokines, and intracellular signals [22]. In particular, impaired DNA methylation, hydroxyl methylation, and histone modifications could modify the accessibility to chromatin and the gene expression in SLE immune cells. This could contribute to uncontrolled expression of inflammatory mediators resulting in systemic inflammation and tissue damage [23].

Systemic Lupus Erythematosus, Microbiota, and Diet

Recent findings suggested an interaction between host microbiota and immune system, allowing the maintenance of tissue homeostasis in healthy individuals [23]. Modifications in the composition of host gut microbiota have been observed in several autoimmune diseases [24]. These modifications, probably influenced by nutritional factors, could induce immune-modulating effects, with increase of Th17 subset and reduction of T regulatory cells [25]. The interplay between micro-organisms and host develops through different mechanisms, including molecular mimicry, microbial translocation, or autoantigen overproduction due to proteolytic enzymes and host protein modification [26].

To date, few data are available concerning microbiota modifications in SLE. In 2014, Zhang and colleagues analyzed the gut microbiota in a classical SLE mouse model MRL/Mp-Faslpr (MRL/lpr): a marked depletion on *Lactobacilli* and an increase on *Lachnospiraceae* were observed. Moreover, an increased bacterial diversity was described in comparison with age-matched healthy controls. In this model, the treatment for lupus manifestations was able to restore the normal microbiota composition [27]. Hevia and coworkers performed a cross-sectional study aiming at evaluating the presence of SLE-associated gut dysbiosis in patients without active disease. The study included the analysis of fecal microbial profiles of 20 SLE patients in remission and 20 age- and sex-matched healthy control subjects. A lower *Firmicutes/Bacteroidetes* ratio was observed in SLE subjects, suggesting the presence of microbiota modifications regardless disease activity [28].

Current knowledge suggests a diet implication in SLE susceptibility and features by inducing changes in the composition and function of gut microbiota. These changes could lead to modulation of immunological pathways and induction of epigenetic changes [24,29].

In 2015, Cuervo and colleagues analyzed the role of fibers and polyphenol intake by performing a case-control study on 20 SLE women and 20 age-matched controls. Food intake was recorded by a food frequency questionnaire: in particular, the authors calculated the fibers intake by using Marlett tables and the polyphenol consumption by Phenol-Explorer. The results of this study suggested that the intake of these dietary compounds was able to modify the intestinal microbiota. In particular, in the SLE group, the authors identified positive associations between flavone intake and *Blautia*, *Flavanones*, and *Lactobacillus*, as well as between dihydrochalcones and *Bifidobacterium* [30].

More recently, the possible role of salt was explored moving from the results of two independent studies, reporting the modulation in T cells immune response in murine models following an increased salt intake [31,32]. Scrivo and colleagues analyzed 15 SLE patients who underwent a dietary regimen starting with a restricted daily sodium intake followed by a normal sodium daily ingestion. A progressive reduction in the percentage of Th17 cells and an increase in the percentage of T regulatory cells were found following the low-sodium dietary regimen, suggesting a possible role of salt in modulating immune response [33]. The role of other diet compounds has been investigated, among these, coffee, chocolate, and omega-3 fatty acids. These seem to be able to induce an increased proinflammatory production and a reduction in Th17 subset number and/or function [25].

Other compounds seem to play a protective role. Data from a metaanalysis demonstrated an inverse association between moderate alcohol intake and SLE risk (OR 0.72) [34]. This could be related to the ability of ethanol in decreasing cellular responses and suppressing proinflammatory cytokines production, demonstrated by in vivo and in vitro studies [35].

More evidence is available concerning the role of vitamin D in the pathogenesis of autoimmune diseases, including SLE. It acts on immune system homeostasis through a diffusely expressed nuclear receptor (vitamin D receptor [VDR]): polymorphisms of the VDR gene have been associated with SLE susceptibility [36,37]. Next to epidemiological association between SLE disease activity and low vitamin D levels, some data suggested a pathogenic link. In particular, vitamin D seems to be able to inhibit neutrophil extracellular trap formation in cultured cells from SLE patients, preventing endothelial damage and the progression of disease [38,39]. Moreover, a recent study described an increase of T regulatory cells number after vitamin D supplementation [40].

Biomarkers

A biomarker was defined as a characteristic that is objectively measured and evaluated and could be used as an indicator of normal or pathogenic biological process [41]. It is possible to distinguish different types of biomarkers: in particular, diagnostic biomarkers (able to confirm a disease or a specific disease subtype), prognostic biomarkers (to identify a specific disease manifestation or individuals at risk for disease development), predictive biomarkers (to predict a specific outcome moving from the baseline measure), and pharmacodynamics biomarkers (to determine optimal therapeutic doses) [42].

SLE is a complex and heterogeneous disease in which different clinical manifestations and therapeutic responses may be determined by distinct pathogenic mechanisms: this complexity leads to the difficulty in the identification of useful biomarkers, able to diagnose disease, to discriminate different phenotypes and severity degrees, and to predict response to treatment. The ideal SLE biomarker should be specific not only for the disease but also for the different disease phenotypes; moreover, it should be characterized by a good correlation with disease activity and able to capture disease flare, to stratify disease severity and/or prognosis. Finally, a good biomarker should be sensitive to change [42].

Despite a large number of studies aiming at identifying new SLE biomarker, to date anti-dsDNA antibodies remain the most important biomarker in terms of sensitivity and specificity (70% and 95%, respectively). A review published by Arriens and colleagues in 2016, by using the Implicit Relationship Identification by in-Silico Construction of an Entity-Based Network from Text approach, demonstrated for anti-dsDNA the higher strength of association, in terms of degree of mutual information, in comparison with other biomarkers, including complement levels, BLys, and INF-α level [43].

Anti-dsDNAs play a pathogenic role, in particular a nephritogenic role, as demonstrated by their ability in causing SLE manifestations by immune complex formation or cross-reactive binding. Finally, anti-dsDNAs are capable to induce proinflammatory cytokines production, leading to INF pathway stimulation [44].

Nevertheless, some aspects must be considered. Although anti-dsDNA antibodies are traditionally linked to SLE in terms of diagnostic and classification factors, a pathogenic link between these antibodies and specific disease manifestation has been demonstrated only for nephritis and in certain forms of neuropsychiatric features. Moreover, in absence of a gold standard, different methodological approaches are available to determine the presence of anti-dsDNA (such as *Crithidia luciliae* immunofluorescence test, FARR, ELISA) with different levels of sensitivity and specificity. Finally, it should be considered the possible production of antibodies DNA binding in other than SLE pathological conditions [45]. In particular, 7.6% of healthy elderly Italian individuals had positive anti-dsDNA results [46]; moreover, the study conducted by Attar and colleagues in 2010 reported that 58.8% of patients with a positive anti-dsDNA had SLE, yet 41.5% presented with other rheumatological diseases, malignancies, infections, hepatitis, or endocrine disorders [47].

The presence of anti-dsDNA seems to identify patients with different disease subsets. The comparison between patients with and without these antibodies demonstrated a significantly higher prevalence of serositis in anti-dsDNA negative subjects [48]. Furthermore, SLE patients showed positivity for several other antibodies that could be associated with different disease features. This happens when considering SSA antibodies, associated with subacute cutaneous lupus, neonatal lupus, and interstitial lung disease. However, on the other side of the coin, it should be considered that different antibodies could be associated with the same clinical manifestation, as demonstrated for kidney involvement, associated with positivity for anti-dsDNA, anti-C1q, and antinucleosome [49].

Some attempts have been made to identify specific biomarkers able to identify specific disease subtype or manifestations. In particular, some data are available for joint involvement, one of the most frequent disease feature, potentially involving up to 90% of SLE patients [50]. To identify patients at risk to develop more aggressive phenotype has been investigated the role of antibodies associated with erosive damage in other inflammatory arthropathy, such as rheumatoid arthritis. The presence of antibodies directed against citrullinated peptides resulted associated with bone damage also in SLE patients [50]. More recently, the role of anti–carbamylated protein antibodies (anti-CarP) has been tested: these antibodies resulted associated with SLE-related joint involvement and with the presence of erosive arthritis [51,52].

As above-reported, biomarkers could be applied to identify patients at risk to develop a specific disease. Data from the literature suggest that first-degree relatives (FDR) of SLE patients showed higher risk to develop an autoimmune disease. In particular, the risk of SLE increased with increasing number of FDR with an autoimmune disease (one FDR affected, OR 4.1, 95% CI 1.7–10.1; two or more FDR affected, OR 11.3, 95% CI 1.3–92.1; $P < .01$) [53]. Moreover, family history of SLE is associated with a clearly elevated risk of SLE and, to a much lesser degree, of rheumatoid arthritis and other autoimmune diseases [54]. Moreover, healthy individuals positive for antinuclear antibodies (especially high titer) showed an increased risk to develop SLE: this is in agreement with the presence of autoantibodies many years before the diagnosis of SLE, with a progressive accumulation before the onset of SLE, while patients are still asymptomatic [55]. In these asymptomatic subjects, IgM isotype is more prevalent than IgG; environmental factors, such as gonadal steroid hormones, probably contributing to antibody class switch mechanisms, and increasing IgG levels. Due to higher pathogenic action of these antibodies, autoimmune clinical manifestations become apparent [56]. In the last years, some studies have evaluated the role of other than antibodies molecules in identifying at risk subjects. The study conducted by Munroe and colleagues suggests the possible role of BLys and stem cell factor: their levels at baseline were significantly higher in patients developing SLE during the follow-up [57].

In the light of many unanswered questions about biomarkers in SLE, in the last years some attempts have been made to evaluate the possible role of genomics, transcriptomics, proteomics, and metabolomics: probably the studies conducted on this field will represent the future of biomarkers [58].

New Therapeutic Strategies

Moving from the increased knowledge about SLE pathogenesis, biological drugs have been introduced in the disease treatment, representing the most important innovation occurring in the last years. Biological drugs act by interacting with different molecules and consequently by modulating different pathways and interfering with chronic inflammation. Considering the key role exerted by B cells, several drugs work by interacting with B cell–related molecules (Fig. 43.2).

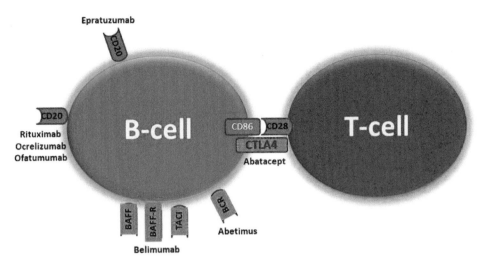

FIGURE 43.2   B cell depletion in treatment of systemic lupus erythematosus.

Belimumab is the first drug approved and registered for SLE patients. By blocking BLys, it alters B cell maturation and function, leading to reduction in antibodies production. After 5 years from the registration, data from the real life confirmed the good results obtained from BLISS-52 or BLISS-76 randomized controlled trials [59,60].

In a real-life setting, the study conducted by Iaccarino and colleagues on 188 SLE patients demonstrated the achievement of SLE Responder Index −4 on 77.0% of patients at 12 months and 68.7% at 24 months of follow-up. Moreover, basal SLEDAI-2K ≥ 10 and polyarthritis were the independent predictors for response at the same time points [61]. Belimumab results not only in controlling disease activity but also chronic damage progression: Bruce and colleagues observed that 85.1% of patients treated by this drug had no change from baseline in SLICC Damage Index (SDI) score after 5 years of follow-up [62]. However, the effectiveness of belimumab in renal and neuropsychiatric manifestations is unknown because of the exclusion of these subsets from the randomized controlled trials; moreover, in real life, belimumab was prevalently used for musculoskeletal and skin manifestations [59–61].

Besides belimumab, the B cell inhibition represents one of the most important targets for SLE treatment. As known, Rituximab, a monoclonal antibody directed against CD20 acting on mature B cells, is not registered for SLE treatment. Nonetheless, several observational studies demonstrated its effectiveness in refractory SLE patients: of note, this drug was used in patients with renal and neuropsychiatric manifestations resistant to conventional therapies with encouraging results [63]. However, because of the off-label use, data from the International Registry for Biologics in SLE reported the estimated off-label use of Rituximab resulted limited to 0.5%–1.5% of SLE patients [64]. The lack of Rituximab registration for SLE patients derives from the failure of randomized controlled trials LUNAR and EXPLORER, enrolling patients with nephritis and nonrenal SLE, respectively [65,66]. The failure could be related to several reasons, including disease activity indices and outcomes employed, placebo effect, and patients enrolled. Despite these negative results, the recommendations published by the European League Against Rheumatism (EULAR) suggest the use of rituximab as last resort therapy in lupus nephritis patients [67]. Other anti-CD20 treatments have been evaluated by randomized controlled trials, with contrasting results: in particular, two studies (BELONG, BEGIN) assessed the efficacy and safety of ocrelizumab, a fully humanized anti-CD20 antibody; these studies are early terminated because of significant increases in severe infections in the ocrelizumab group [67]. An attempt to target CD22 has been made by using epratuzumab, a humanized anti-CD22 antibody: the promising results obtained in the EMBLEM phase II trials were not confirmed in the phase III EMBODY trials, leading to stop further development of this promising drug [68].

More recently, other therapeutic targets have been tested: among these, sifalimumab and rontalizumab, acting as IFN-alpha blockers. The efficacy of rontalizumab, a monoclonal antibody targeted IFN-alpha, has been investigated in a large phase II trial including 238 patients with active SLE, demonstrating a significant improvement in BILAG and SRI [69].

In the era of oral treatment, the use of drugs acting on kinases has been proposed also for SLE patients. In particular, a growing interest has been addressed on Btk, an intracellular kinase activated after B Cell Receptor (BCR) activation and leading to the recruitment of NfkB to the nucleus of B cells. The small molecule inhibitor MSC2364447C (M2951) has been evaluated in a phase Ib trial (NCT02537028) in mild to moderate SLE patients to asses drug efficacy [70]. Waiting for further studies, Btk inhibition could potentially represent an interesting therapeutical approach, thanks to the role exerted by this kinase in antibody production [70]. Moreover, the inhibition of proteasome has been suggested to treat SLE patients.

After encouraging results deriving from mouse model, 12 refractory SLE patients were treated with bortezomib, a proteasome inhibitor: this treatment determines the reduction of autoantibody levels and plasma cell numbers. Moreover, a significant improvement in disease activity was observed in almost all of the involved organ/systems. However, the drug was associated with neurological side effects (in particular neuropathy) that could potentially limit their usefulness, especially in long-term treatment [71].

CONCLUSIONS

In the last years, several advances have been observed regarding the understanding of SLE pathogenesis, focusing on role exerted by environmental factors in determining disease development in genetically susceptible individuals. These advances lead to the identification of new biomarkers and therapeutical approaches.

REFERENCES

[1] Lim SS, Bayakly AR, Helmick CG, et al. The incidence and prevalence of systemic lupus erythematosus, 2002-2004: the Georgia Lupus Registry. Arthritis Rheumatol 2014;66:357e68.

[2] Somers EC, Marder W, Cagnoli P, et al. Population-based incidence and prevalence of systemic lupus erythematosus: the Michigan Lupus Epidemiology and Surveillance program. Arthritis Rheumatol 2014;66:369e78.

[3] Mccarty DJ, Manzi S, Medsger TA, et al. Incidence of systemic lupus erythematosus race and gender differences. Arthritis Rheumatol 1995;38(9):1260e70.

[4] Wahren-Herlenius M, Dorner T. Immunopathogenic mechanisms of systemic autoimmune disease. Lancet 2013;382(9894):819e31.

[5] Deng Y, Tsao BP. Updates in lupus genetics. Curr Rheumatol Rep October 5, 2017;19(11):68.

[6] Ceccarelli F, Perricone C, Borgiani P, Ciccacci C, Rufini S, Cipriano E, et al. Genetic factors in systemic lupus erythematosus: contribution to disease phenotype. J Immunol Res. 2015;2015:745647.

[7] Valesini G, Gerardi MC, Iannuccelli C, Pacucci VA, Pendolino M, Shoenfeld Y. Citrullination and autoimmunity. Autoimmun Rev June 2015;14(6):490–7.

[8] Wild CP. Complementing the genome with an "Exposome": the outstanding challenge of environmental exposure measurement in molecular epidemiology. Cancer Epidemiol Prev Biomark August 1, 2005;14(8):1847e50.

[9] Miller FW, Alfredsson L, Costenbader KH, et al. Epidemiology of environmental exposures and human autoimmune diseases: findings from a national Institute of environmental health sciences expert panel workshop. J Autoimmun 2012;39(4):259e71.

[10] Rünger TM, Epe B, Moller K. Processing of directly and indirectly ultraviolet-induced DNA damage in human cells. Recent Results Cancer Res 1995;139:31e42.

[11] Vollmer J, Tluk S, Schmitz C, et al. Immune stimulation mediated by autoantigen binding sites within small nuclear RNAs involves toll-like receptors 7 and 8. J Exp Med 2005;202:1575e85.

[12] Costenbader KH, Feskanich D, Stampfer MJ, et al. Reproductive and menopausal factors and risk of systemic lupus erythematosus in women. Arthritis Rheum 2007;56:1251e62.

[13] Lateef A, Petri M. Hormone replacement and contraceptive therapy in autoimmune diseases. J Autoimmun 2012;38:J170e6.

[14] Cutolo M, Sulli A, Straub RH. Estrogen metabolism and autoimmunity. Autoimmun Rev 2012;11:A460–4.

[15] Colasanti T, Maselli A, Conti F, Sanchez M, Alessandri C, Barbati C, et al. Autoantibodies to estrogen receptor α interfere with T lymphocyte homeostasis and are associated with disease activity in systemic lupus erythematosus. Arthritis Rheum 2012;64:778–87.

[16] Maselli A, Capoccia S, Pugliese P, Raggi C, Cirulli F, Fabi A, et al. Autoantibodies specific to estrogen receptor alpha act as estrogen agonists and their levels correlate with breast cancer cell proliferation. OncoImmunology 2015;5:e1074375.

[17] Perricone C, Versini M, Ben-Ami D, Gertel S, Watad A, Segel MJ, et al. Smoke and autoimmunity: the fire behind the disease. Autoimmun Rev 2016;15:354–74.

[18] Blanc PD, Jarvholm B, Toren K. Prospective risk of rheumatologic disease associated with occupational exposure in a cohort of male construction workers. Am J Med 2015;128(10):1094e101.

[19] Pollard KM. Silica, silicosis, and autoimmunity. Front Immunol 2016;7:1e7.

[20] Somers EC, Richardson BC. Environmental exposures, epigenetic changes and the risk of lupus. Lupus 2014;23(6):568e76.

[21] Oaks Z, Perl A. Metabolic control of the epigenome in systemic Lupus erythematosus. Autoimmunity 2014;47(4):256e64.

[22] Hedrich CM. Mechanistic aspects of epigenetic dysregulation in SLE. Clin Immunol 2018. S1521–6616(18)30007-X.

[23] Kamada N, Seo SU, Chen GY, Nunez G. Role of the gut microbiota in immunity and inflammatory disease. Nat Rev Immunol 2013;13(5):321–35.

[24] Vieira SM, Pagovich OE, Kriegel MA. Diet, microbiota and autoimmune diseases. Lupus 2014;23(6):518–26.

[25] Dahan S, Segal Y, Shoenfeld Y. Dietary factors in rheumatic autoimmune diseases: a recipe for therapy? Nat Rev Rheumatol 2017;13:348–58.

[26] Chen X, Liu S, Tan Q, Shoenfeld Y, Zeng Y. Microbiome, autoimmunity, allergy, and helminth infection: the importance of the pregnancy period. Am J Reprod Immunol 2017;78.

[27] Zhang H, Liao X, Sparks JB, Luo XM. Dynamics of gut microbiota in autoimmune lupus. Appl Environ Microbiol 2014;80(24):7551–60.

[28] Hevia A, Milani C, Lopez P, Cuervo A, Arboleya S, Duranti S, et al. Intestinal dysbiosis associated with systemic lupus erythematosus. mBio 2014;5(5). e1548–1514.

[29] Somers EC, Richardson BC. Environmental exposures, epigenetic changes and the risk of lupus. Lupus 2014;23(6):568–76.

[30] Cuervo A, Hevia A, Lopez P, Suarez A, Sanchez B, Margolles A, et al. Association of polyphenols from oranges and apples with specific intestinal microorganisms in systemic lupus erythematosus patients. Nutrients 2015;7(2):1301–17.

[31] Kleinewietfeld M, Manzel A, Titze J, Kvakan H, Yosef N, Linker RA, et al. Sodium chloride drives autoimmune disease by the induction of pathogenic TH17 cells. Nature April 25, 2013;496(7446):518–22.

[32] Wu C, Yosef N, Thalhamer T, Zhu C, Xiao S, Kishi Y, et al. Induction of pathogenic TH17 cells by inducible salt-sensing kinase SGK1. Nature April 25, 2013;496(7446):513–7.

[33] Scrivo R, Massaro L, Barbati C, Vomero M, Ceccarelli F, Spinelli FR, Riccieri V, Spagnoli A, Alessandri C, Desideri G, Conti F, Valesini G. The role of dietary sodium intake on the modulation of T helper 17 cells and regulatory T cells in patients with rheumatoid arthritis and systemic lupus erythematosus. PLoS One 2017;12:e0184449.

[34] Wang J, Pan HF, Ye DQ, et al. Moderate alcohol drinking might be protective for systemic lupus erythematosus: a systematic review and meta-analysis. Clin Rheum 2008;27(12):1557e63.

[35] Waldschmidt TJ, Cook RT, Kovacs EJ. Alcohol and inflammation and immune responses: summary of the 2006 alcohol and immunology research interest group (AIRIG) meeting. Alcohol 2008;42(2):137e42.

[36] Perricone C, Agmon-Levin N, Colafrancesco S, Shoenfeld Y. Vitamins and systemic lupus erythematosus: to D or not to D. Expert Rev Clin Immunol 2013;9:397–9.

[37] Carvalho C, Marinho A, Leal B, Bettencourt A, Boleixa D, Almeida I, et al. Association between vitamin D receptor (VDR) gene polymorphisms and systemic lupus erythematosus in Portuguese patients. Lupus 2015;24(8):846–53.

[38] Handono K, Sidarta YO, Pradana BA, Nugroho RA, Hartono IA, Kalim H, et al. Vitamin D prevents endothelial damage induced by increased neutrophil extracellular traps formation in patients with systemic lupus erythematosus. Acta Med Indones 2014;46(3):189–98.

[39] Smith CK, Kaplan MJ. The role of neutrophils in the pathogenesis of systemic lupus erythematosus. Curr Opin Rheumatol 2015;27(5):448–53.

[40] Andreoli L, Dall'Ara F, Piantoni S, Zanola A, Piva N, Cutolo M, et al. A 24-month prospective study on the efficacy and safety of two different monthly regimens of vitamin D supplementation in pre-menopausal women with systemic lupus erythematosus. Lupus 2015;24(4–5):499–506.

[41] Biomarkers Definitions Working Group. Biomarkers and surrogate endpoints: preferred definitions and conceptual framework. Clin Pharmacol Ther 2001;69:89–95.

[42] Mok CC. Towards new avenues in the management of lupus glomerulonephritis. Nat Rev Rheumatol 2016;12:221–34.

[43] Arriens C, Wren JD, Munroe ME, Mohan C. Systemic lupus erythematosus biomarkers: the challenging quest. Rheumatology (Oxf) April 1, 2017;56(Suppl. 1):i32–45.

[44] Pisetsky DS. Anti-DNA antibodies–quintessential biomarkers of SLE. Nat Rev Rheumatol 2016;12:102–10.

[45] Rekvig OP. The anti-DNA antibody: origin and impact, dogmas and controversies. Nat Rev Rheumatol 2015;11:530–40.

[46] Ruffatti A, Calligaro A, Del Ross T, Bertoli MT, Doria A, Rossi L, et al. Anti-double-stranded DNA antibodies in the healthy elderly: prevalence and characteristics. J Clin Immunol 1990;10:300–3.

[47] Attar SM, Koshak EA. Medical conditions associated with a positive anti-double-stranded deoxyribonucleic acid. Saudi Med J 2010;31:781–7.

[48] Conti F, Ceccarelli F, Perricone C, Massaro L, Marocchi E, Miranda F, et al. Systemic lupus erythematosus with and without anti-dsDNA antibodies: analysis from a large monocentric cohort. Mediators Inflamm 2015;2015:328078.

[49] Kaul A, Gordon C, Crow MK, Touma Z, Urowitz MB, van Vollenhoven R, et al. Systemic lupus erythematosus. Nat Rev Dis Primers 2016;2:16039.

[50] Ceccarelli F, Perricone C, Cipriano E, Massaro L, Natalucci F, Capalbo G, et al. Joint involvement in systemic lupus erythematosus: from pathogenesis to clinical assessment. Semin Arthritis Rheum 2017;47:53–64.

[51] Massaro L, Ceccarelli F, Colasanti T, Pendolino M, Perricone C, Cipriano E, et al. Anti-carbamylated protein antibodies in systemic lupus erythematosus patients with articular involvement. Lupus 2018;27:105–11.

[52] Ceccarelli F, Perricone C, Colasanti T, Massaro L, Cipriano E, Pendolino M, et al. Anti-carbamylated protein antibodies as a new biomarker of erosive joint damage in systemic lupus erythematosus. Arthritis Res Ther 2018;20:126.

[53] Priori R, Medda E, Conti F, Cassara EA, Danieli MG, Gerli R, et al. Familial autoimmunity as a risk factor for systemic lupus erythematosus and vice versa: a case-control study. Lupus 2003;12(10):735–40.

[54] Ulff-Møller CJ, Simonsen J, Kyvik KO, Jacobsen S, Frisch M. Family history of systemic lupus erythematosus and risk of autoimmune disease: nationwide Cohort Study in Denmark 1977-2013. Rheumatology 2017;56:957–64.

[55] Arbuckle MR, McClain MT, Rubertone MV, Scofield RH, Dennis GJ, James JA, et al. Development of autoantibodies before the clinical onset of systemic lupus erythematosus. N Engl J Med 2003;349:1526–33.

[56] Olsen NJ, Karp DR. Autoantibodies and SLE: the threshold for disease. Nat Rev Rheumatol 2014;10:181–6.

[57] Munroe ME, Lu R, Zhao YD, Fife DA, Robertson JM, Guthridge JM, et al. Altered type II interferon precedes autoantibody accrual and elevated type I interferon activity prior to systemic lupus erythematosus classification. Ann Rheum Dis 2016;75:2014–202.

[58] Arriens C, Mohan C. Systemic lupus erythematosus diagnostics in the 'omics' era. Int J Clin Rheumtol 2013;8:671–87.

[59] Navarra SV, Guzmán RM, Gallacher AE, Hall S, Levy RA, Jimenez RE, et al. Efficacy and safety of belimumab in patients with active systemic lupus erythematosus: a randomised, placebo-controlled, phase 3 trial. Lancet 2011;377:721–31.

[60] Furie R, Petri M, Zamani O, Cervera R, Wallace DJ, Tegzová D, et al. A phase III, randomized, placebo-controlled study of belimumab, a monoclonal antibody that inhibits B lymphocyte stimulator, in patients with systemic lupus erythematosus. Arthritis Rheum 2011;63:3918–30.

[61] Iaccarino L, Andreoli L, Bocci EB, Bortoluzzi A, Ceccarelli F, et al. Clinical predictors of response and discontinuation of belimumab in patients with systemic lupus erythematosus in real life setting. Results of a large, multicentric, nationwide study. J Autoimmun 2018;86:1–8.

[62] Bruce IN, Urowitz M, van Vollenhoven R, Aranow C, Fettiplace J, Oldham M, et al. Long-term organ damage accrual and safety in patients with SLE treated with belimumab plus standard of care. Lupus June 2016;25(7):699–709.

[63] Duxbury B, Combescure C, Chizzolini C. Rituximab in systemic lupus erythematosus: an updated systematic review and meta-analysis. Lupus December 2013;22(14):1489–503.

[64] Rydén-Aulin M, Boumpas D, Bultink I, Callejas Rubio JL, Caminal-Montero L, Castro A, et al. Off-label use of rituximab for systemic lupus erythematosus in Europe. Lupus Sci Med 2016;3:e000163.

[65] Rovin BH, Furie R, Latinis K, Looney RJ, Fervenza FC, Sanchez-Guerrero J, et al. LUNAR Investigator Group. Efficacy and safety of rituximab in patients with active proliferative lupus nephritis: the Lupus Nephritis Assessment with Rituximab study. Arthritis Rheum 2012;64:1215–26.

[66] Merrill JT, Neuwelt CM, Wallace DJ, Shanahan JC, Latinis KM, Oates JC, et al. Efficacy and safety of rituximab in moderately-to-severely active systemic lupus erythematosus: the randomized, double-blind, phase II/III systemic lupus erythematosus evaluation of rituximab trial. Arthritis Rheum 2010;62:222–33.

[67] Kamal A, Khamashta M. The efficacy of novel B cell biologics as the future of SLE treatment: a review. Autoimmun Rev 2014;13:1094–101.

[68] Clowse ME, Wallace DJ, Furie RA, Petri MA, Pike MC, Leszczyński P, et al. Efficacy and safety of epratuzumab in moderately to severely active systemic lupus erythematosus: results from two phase III randomized, double-blind, placebo-controlled trials. Arthritis Rheumatol 2017;69:362–75.

[69] Kalunian KC, Merrill JT, Maciuca R, McBride JM, Townsend MJ, Wei X, et al. A Phase II study of the efficacy and safety of rontalizumab (rhuMAb interferon-α) in patients with systemic lupus erythematosus (ROSE). Ann Rheum Dis 2016;75:196–202.

[70] Paz Z, Tsokos GC. New therapeutics in systemic lupus erythematosus. Curr Opin Rheumatol May 2013;25(3):297–303.

[71] Alexander T, Sarfert R, Klotsche J, Kühl AA, Rubbert-Roth A, Lorenz HM, et al. The proteasome inhibitior bortezomib depletes plasma cells and ameliorates clinical manifestations of refractory systemic lupus erythematosus. Ann Rheum Dis 2015;74:1474–8.

Chapter 44

Antiphospholipid Syndrome

Vinicius Domingues[1], Gustavo Guimarães Moreira Balbi[2,3], Guilherme Ramires de Jesús[4], Flavio Signorelli[2,5], Roger Abramino Levy[2,6]

[1]Florida State University, College of Medicine Daytona Beach, FL, United States; [2]Department of Rheumatology, Hospital Universitário Pedro Ernesto, Universidade do Estado do Rio de Janeiro, Rio de Janeiro, Brazil; [3]Department of Rheumatology, Hospital Universitário, Universidade Federal de Juiz de Fora, Juiz de Fora, Brazil; [4]Department of Obstetrics, Hospital Universitário Pedro Ernesto, Universidade do Estado do Rio de Janeiro, Rio de Janeiro, Brazil; [5]Department of Internal Medicine, Hospital Universitário Clementino Fraga Filho, Universidade Federal do Rio de Janeiro, Rio de Janeiro, Brazil; [6]Global Medical Expert, GSK, Upper Providence, PA, United States

INTRODUCTION

Antiphospholipid syndrome (APS) is an acquired, immune-mediated thrombophilia. It is characterized by the occurrence of thrombosis in any vascular bed and gestational morbidity, associated with the identification of circulating antiphospholipid antibodies (aPL), namely lupus anticoagulant (LA), anticardiolipin (aCL) IgG and IgM, and anti-β2-glycoprotein I (aβ2GPI) IgG and IgM [1].

The aim of this chapter is to review the most relevant aspects of APS and provide evidence-based information for a better understanding and treatment of this complex disease.

PATHOGENESIS

The etiopathogenesis of APS is not fully understood. Several different mechanisms of disease have been proposed, including triggering factors, molecular mimicry, direct participation of aPL, activation of endothelial cells, increased oxidative stress, impaired function of endothelial nitric oxide synthase, increased expression of Toll-like receptors (TLR) 4, antibody-mediated activation of complement C3 and C5, disruption of the annexin A5 shield, and many others [2]. Nonetheless, no single factor was identified as capable of causing APS and probably many of these are implied. In fact, neither the positivity of aPL alone was capable of inducing clot formation in animal models [3,4]. The presence of a "second hit" is required for the development of thrombosis, such as cigarette smoking, infections, and malignancies [5–7]. These two latter may also be involved in mechanisms of molecular mimicry in the pathogenesis of APS [8–12].

β2-glycoprotein I (β2GPI) is a cationic glycoprotein that binds to negatively charged phospholipids through its fifth domain. It has an important role as a natural circulating anticoagulant and is capable of interfering in the protein C/S system. LA because of the presence of aβ2GPI antibodies is more strongly associated with thrombosis than does LA due to antiprothrombin antibodies, and the domain I of the aβ2GPI confers the highest risk [2]. This indicates that β2GPI is probably the most relevant targeted antigen in the pathogenesis of APS. These autoantibodies bind directly to β2GPI and induce an NF-kB–dependent endothelial cells activation, with increased adhesion molecules expression (elevated levels of E-selectin, VCAM-1, and ICAM-1), cytokine secretion (elevated levels of IL-6), and arachidonic acid metabolism (elevated levels of 6-keto-PGF1-alpha, a metabolic of arachidonic acid) [13–15]. Consequently, it creates a prothrombotic state; it can also interact with von Willebrand factor receptor and cross-activate platelets, releasing thromboxane A2, which subsequently increases platelet adhesiveness [2].

Because both adaptive and innate immunity are involved in the pathogenesis of APS, it is probable that a predisposing genetic background exists. Several genetic HLA class II polymorphisms were associated with aPL production and the development of APS, such as HLA-DRB1*04, DRB1*07 (0701), DRB1*1302, DQB1*0301 (DQ7), DQB1*0302, and DQB1*0303. HLA-BDPB1 alleles, HLA-DM polymorphisms, and valine/leucine247 polymorphisms of β2GPI may also be involved [7,16,17]. In a recently published genome-wide association study, Sugiura-Ogasawara et al. found that the presence of TSHR and C1D genes were associated with obstetric APS (ObAPS) [18].

TABLE 44.1 APS Classification Criteria

Clinical Criteria	Laboratory Criteria
• Vascular thrombosis One or more clinical episodes of arterial, venous, or small vessel thrombosis, in any tissue or organ, supported by unequivocal findings of appropriate imaging studies or histopathology. For histopathological support, it should be present without substantial evidence of inflammation in the vessel wall.	Lupus anticoagulant present in plasma: • Two or more occasions • At least 12 weeks apart • Detected according to the guidelines of the International Society on Thrombosis and Hemostasis.
• Gestacional morbidity One or more unexplained deaths of a morphologically healthy fetus at or beyond the 10th week of gestation, with healthy fetal morphology documented by ultrasound or by direct examination of the fetus. One or more premature births of a morphologically healthy newborn baby before the 34th week of gestation due to eclampsia, severe preeclampsia, or placental failure. Three or more unexplained consecutive spontaneous abortions before the 10th week of gestation, with maternal anatomical or hormonal abnormalities and paternal and maternal chromosomal causes excluded.	Anticardiolipin antibody in serum or plasma: • IgG or IgM isotype, or both • Medium or high titers (i.e., >40 GPL or MPL, or greater than the 99th percentile) • Two or more occasions • At least 12 weeks apart • Measured by a standardized ELISA. Anti-β2-glycoprotein 1 antibody in serum or plasma: • IgG or IgM isotype, or both • Titers greater than the 99th percentile • Two or more occasions • At least 12 weeks apart • Measured by a standardized ELISA, according to recommended procedures.

For the diagnosis of APS, at least one clinical and one laboratory criteria are required.
Adapted from Miyakis S, Lockshin MD, Atsumi T, Derksen RHWM, de Groot PG, Koike T. International consensus statement on an update of the classification criteria for definite antiphospholipid syndrome. J Thromb Haemost 2006;4:295–306. (August 2005).

CLINICAL MANIFESTATIONS

There is a wide array of clinical manifestations of APS and the hallmark of the syndrome is thrombosis [19]. However, in contrast with thromboses associated with congenital thrombophilias, those associated with APS might occur in any vascular bed [20]. Deep vein thrombosis is the most common venous thrombosis followed by pulmonary emboli [20]. In the arterial bed, the central nervous system (CNS) is the most affected with stroke and transient ischemic attacks; however, myocardial infarction is seen but less frequently [20]. Small vessel thrombosis can occur in the form of thrombotic microangiopathy (TMA). The current classification criteria for APS are outlined at Table 44.1 [1].

Recently, there has been a lot of attention on the noncriteria manifestations of APS, which resembles more of an inflammatory pathology than a thrombotic one per se [21]. CNS manifestations such as myelopathy, migraine, and epilepsy, which are refractory to standard treatment, have also been associated with aPL [22]. Mild cognitive impairment has been recorded in more than 40% of the patients with APS with a strong association with white matter lesions and multiple sclerosis–like CNS lesions and compatible clinical presentation [23–26].

aPL has been very closely associated with cardiac valvular disease with mitral most frequently affected followed by aortic valve [27]. Regurgitation is more common than stenosis and many patients remain asymptomatic for years until it is found by imaging a verrucous pattern lesion in the valve leaflets [27]. A recent metaanalysis also showed that the presence of aPL is strongly associated with pulmonary hypertension in systemic lupus erythematosus (SLE) patients [28].

Renal involvement in APS was first described in 1992 [29]. TMA is the most characteristic finding in APS nephropathy (APSN); however, fibrous intimal hyperplasia, focal cortical atrophy, and arterial occlusions have also been described [29]. Hypertension with proteinuria (often subnephrotic) and renal insufficiency are typical presentations of APSN [30]. Renal artery stenosis can also present as refractory hypertension [31]. Hematologic manifestations include thrombocytopenia that can be moderate to severe with bleeding and clotting and hemolytic anemia [21].

Livedo reticularis, a mottled reticulated vascular pattern that appears as a lace-like purplish discoloration of the skin, is present in about 25% of patients with APS and is associated with greater risk for arterial thrombosis [32]. Skin ulcers are frequently seen around and predominantly in lower extremities. Those ulcers are typically refractory to wound care and may take years to heal adequately [32]. Avascular necrosis, adrenal insufficiency, and diffuse alveolar hemorrhage are reported but seen less frequently [21].

The most severe and fortunately infrequent form of APS is catastrophic APS (CAPS). This form is characterized by widespread small vessel thrombosis with multiorgan failure and carries a mortality of up to 50% [7].

OBSTETRIC MANIFESTATIONS

Besides vascular thrombosis, APS can also present with obstetric morbidity, which some authors call "ObAPS." Recurrent miscarriages, fetal loss, placental insufficiency, or preeclampsia has been related to aPL and is part of International Consensus Statement on classification criteria for APS [1]. Those obstetric complications can occur in patients with previous vascular thrombotic events, precede thrombotic events, or be the only type of manifestation of the disease.

The first obstetric criteria described in International Consensus is "One or more unexplained deaths of a morphologically normal fetus at or beyond the 10th week of gestation, with normal fetal morphology documented by ultrasound or by direct examination of the fetus" and is considered the most specific criterion for ObAPS [1]. Two recently published multicenter studies support this association, with the first one reporting that elevated levels of aCL and anti-β2-glycoprotein-I antibodies were associated with a three- to fivefold increased odds of stillbirth [33], while the other one described LA as the primary predictor of adverse pregnancy outcome after 12 weeks, including fetal death [34].

Another criterion related to pregnancy loss is associated with early miscarriage: *Three or more unexplained consecutive spontaneous abortions before the 10th week of gestation, with maternal anatomic or hormonal abnormalities and/or paternal and maternal chromosomal causes excluded.* Recurrent early abortion has been classified by some authors and also by International Consensus [1] as the most sensitive obstetric criterion, although not very specific. In the same way that occurs with fetal death, it is important to exclude other causes that may be related to the miscarriage. Recent studies [34] reported that abnormal embryonic karyotype is the most frequent cause of recurrent miscarriage, in a similar frequency that occurs in single spontaneous abortions, but this investigation is not frequent in clinical practice considering the high cost of the procedure.

This inability to adequately exclude other causes of recurrent abortion, combined with different inclusion criteria, may explain the conflicting results in observational studies and clinical trials performed in this group of patients [35]. Additionally, well-designed studies following strictly the International Consensus are lacking, and some authors are questioning the association between recurrent early miscarriage and aPL [36].

Patients with APS develop preeclampsia more frequently than general population, which occurs in 5%–10% of pregnancies. The real frequency of aPL in patients with preeclampsia is still unknown, but most of the studies reported a significant association with early-onset and severe cases [37]. Considering that both preeclampsia and placental insufficiency can have the same underlying mechanism, i.e., abnormal trophoblastic invasion, it is not surprising that both complications can affect the same pregnancy. Some authors have described between 15 and up to almost 40% [38,39] of small for gestational age neonates (below the 10th percentile) in pregnant patients with APS.

The exclusion of other justifiable causes of placental insufficiency should be pursued to confirm its relationship to aPL, but sometimes it may be impossible in the clinical or even in the research settings as more than one confounding factor can be present. This prevents an adequate estimate of aPL frequency among patients with placental failure.

To improve the specificity, the International Consensus recommends including only cases that required delivery before 34 weeks of pregnancy, usually more severe than those that develop close to term. However, the criteria's authors report that this criterion may be relatively insensitive or nonspecific. It is also important to notice that delivery usually occurs by medical intervention because of those obstetric complications because spontaneous preterm delivery is not usual in patients with ObAPS [35].

Other pregnancy morbidities not present in International Consensus have been associated to aPL, but there is lack of consensus in this topic. HELLP syndrome, an acronym for *h*emolysis, *e*levated *l*iver enzymes, and *l*ow *p*latelet count, usually occurs as a severe form of preeclampsia. The substantial increase in the incidence of preeclampsia in patients with APS may result in an increased frequency of cases of HELLP syndrome, but sometimes differential diagnosis between APS and HELLP syndrome can be difficult, as overlapping clinical findings can develop [40]. Placental abruption is also related to hypertensive disorders of pregnancy, which is clearly a confounding factor to associate this disease with aPL. To date, there is no described underlying mechanism that can justify an increased incidence of placental abruption related to aPL.

Infertility is a common gynecologic condition and has been tentatively linked to aPL for decades. In vitro studies have proposed some pathophysiological mechanisms [41], but clinical studies in this topic failed to prove such an effect. Although some authors identified more aPL in patients than controls, the results are arguable considering heterogeneity of clinical and methodological aspects, such as definition of positivity different from International Consensus or small number of participants. In addition, several studies included noncriteria aPL tests, which have controversial clinical significance [42]. A recent review of the subject reported a lack of association between aPL and assisted reproductive therapy (ART) outcome and no benefit on ART outcome when treating aPL-positive women [41], conclusions that are supported by the American Society of Reproductive Medicine [43].

DIAGNOSIS AND CLASSIFICATION

There are three criteria antibodies in APS classification: LA, aCL, and aβ2GPI. LA should be detected according to the guidelines of the International Society on Thrombosis and Hemostasis. aCL of IgG and/or IgM isotype in serum or plasma should be present in medium or high titer (>40 GPL or MPL [IgG and IgM phospholipid units], or >the 99th percentile), measured by a standardized ELISA. Finally, aβ2GPI of IgG and/or IgM isotype should be present in serum or plasma (in titer >the 99th percentile), measured by a standardized ELISA. They should be detected in plasma on two or more occasions at least 12 weeks apart. Additionally, classification of APS should be avoided if the positive aPL test and the clinical manifestation are separated for more than 5 years [1]. Accordingly to the presence of one or more laboratory criteria, APS patients can be further classified into one of the following categories: I—more than one laboratory criteria present (any combination); IIa—LA present alone; IIb—aCL antibody present alone; IIc—aβ2GPI present alone [1].

LABORATORY PITFALLS

LA detection is technically laborious, envisaging screening, mixing, and confirming tests [44]. A weak LA should be considered a positive test [42], but there is still some concern about the clinical relevance of this result [45]. Another critical point is the equivocal laboratory results in patients under anticoagulation. LA can be falsely positive in patients treated with heparin, vitamin K antagonists (VKA), and direct oral anticoagulants (DOACs) [46]. When international normalized ratio (INR) is >3.5, the LA testing is unworkable [1]. Likewise, pregnancy and oral contraceptive pills can lead to aCL and aβ2GPI transiently positive [46].

Interpretation and confirmation of aPL is another challenge. When both aCL and aβ2GPI ELISAs are positive in the same patient, they should be both positive for the same isotype (IgG or IgM). Triple positivity (LA+; aCL+; and aβ2GPI+, same isotype) is the most reliable profile and always confirmed after 12 weeks. On the other hand, single positivity is confirmed after 12 weeks in less than 50% [45].

Noncriteria Antiphospholipid Antibody Tests

Current APS classification criteria identify a homogeneous group of APS patients but exclude patients with clinical manifestations highly suggestive of APS. Therefore, "noncriteria" aPL that target other plasma proteins or phospholipid-bound proteins complexes may help to classify additional APS patients recognized as "seronegative" [47]. Using 11 noncriteria markers, including aCL IgA e aβ2GPTN I IgA; aβ2GPI DI; antibodies to phosphatidylserine (aPS) IgM, IgG and IgA; antibodies to the phosphatidylserine–prothrombin complex (aPS/PT) IgG and IgM; antiphosphatidylethanolamine (aPE) IgG and IgM; aCL/vimentin antibodies IgG, a recent study could reclassify combining the results, 25 out of 68 seronegative patients into seropositive (36.8%). Conversely, seropositive patients were positive for at least one non–antibody criteria in 83.2% of cases [47]. We will discuss below the most relevant noncriteria aPL.

IgA Isotypes (aCL IgA e aβ2GPTN I IgA)

The heterogeneity in different study designs and the use of various nonstandardized assays is troublesome to make a recommendation. Besides, positive IgA aPL are usually associated with other isotypes in the presence of the major manifestations of APS, making it difficult to understand the role of IgA alone [48]. IgA aPL is the dominant isotype in Afro-Caribbeans and in Afro-Americans. However, they are probably not associated with clinical manifestations in these ethnic groups, besides being usually transient and present at low or moderate titers [49].

The SLICC classification criteria for SLE included as a new aPL criterion both IgA aCL and IgA aβ2GPI [48]. It seems that IgA aβ2GPI is highly prevalent in SLE patients and associated particularly with arterial thrombosis, making them a relevant test in this group of patients [42]. IgA aPL antibodies are also linked to skin ulcers, Raynaud's phenomenon, livedo, or cutaneous vasculitis. Furthermore, in pretransplant patients, IgA aβ2GPI was correlated with lower graft and patient survival at 6 months and may be an early transplant failure biomarker [49].

In summary, testing for IgA aPL could contribute to the assessment of risk for thrombosis and/or pregnancy morbidity, especially in SLE patients, when there is a strong suspicion of APS but other aPL tests are negative [42].

Antibodies Against Specific Domains of aβ2GPI

β2GPI is a glycoprotein with five domains (DI–DV) and the most relevant epitope is located in DI in patients with autoimmune diseases. Domain I is responsible for binding with the aPL, and DV in turn is responsible for binding the complex β2GPI-aPL with the phospholipid on the cell surface. aβ2GPI DI antibodies carry at high specificity and low sensitivity, putting their clinical utility doubtful. A large cohort of patients demonstrated that IgG targeting DI represents the prevalent aβ2GPI antibody subpopulation among patients with APS and with autoimmune conditions without any clinical feature suggestive of APS. On the other hand, anti-DIV/V antibodies were in asymptomatic aPL carriers or those without any underlying autoimmune disease. It means that the ratio between antibodies to DI and DIV/V may be a predictor for systemic autoimmunity [49].

Antibodies to the Phosphatidylserine–Prothrombin Complex

Antiprothrombin antibodies are a heterogeneous population including antibodies against prothrombin alone (aPT-A) and antibodies to the phosphatidylserine–prothrombin complex (aPS/PT) detected by ELISA [1].

There is a strong association between aPS/PT and the LA. In fact, up to 86.7% of patients with aPS/PT are also LA positive [47], suggesting that aPS/PT can serve as a confirmatory assay for LA [1] or to replace it when clotting test cannot be performed because of technical limitations [50]. Still, aPS/PT has been shown to be useful in establishing the thrombotic risk, irrespective of the site and type of thrombosis, in patients with previous thrombotic events and/or systemic autoimmune diseases [49]. Measurement of the three criteria aPL, in conjunction with IgG aPS/PT, might contribute to a better and more complete identification of patients at risk of thrombotic complications [50]. The aPS/PT inclusion as a laboratory criterion for the APS should be strongly considered [49].

Antibodies as Prognostic Biomarkers

The aPL most strongly related to thrombosis is LA. In addition, multiple positive aPL or high-titer aPL correlate to thrombotic events [51]. Ruiz-Irastorza et al. defined three high-risk serological features in patients with APS: LA positivity, triple positivity, and isolated persistently positive aCL at medium–high titers (the last only studied in patients with SLE) [51].

The need of thrombotic risk stratification in APS patients has led to the emergence of two important scores: the Antiphospholipid Score (aPL-S) and the Global Antiphospholipid Syndrome Score (GAPSS). Both have shown a degree of accuracy in identifying high-risk APS patients, especially those at a high risk of thrombosis [52]. GAPSS includes the testing for aPS/PT, an assay that is not commercially available and consequently not routinely performed. Therefore, an adjusted score was created, excluding the aPS/PT, the aGAPSS; it is calculated by adding the points corresponding to the risk factors, based on a linear transformation derived from the β-regression coefficient as follows: 3 for hyperlipidemia, 1 for arterial hypertension, 5 for aCL IgG/IgM, 4 for aβ2GPI IgG/IgM, and 4 for LA [53]. Radin et al. demonstrated that higher aGAPSS values were observed in patients with acute myocardial infarction and this finding could aid to the risk stratification of APS patients younger than 50 years old for the likelihood of developing coronary thrombotic events [53].

In the field of pregnancy morbidity, the PROMISSE study (Predictors of Pregnancy Outcome: Biomarkers in APL Syndrome and SLE) independently confirmed in a group of aPL-positive patients that LA is the only aPL predictor of poor pregnancy outcomes after the first trimester of pregnancy [54].

TREATMENT

Thrombotic Antiphospholipid Syndrome

The current recommendation for thrombotic APS is lifelong treatment oral anticoagulation with VKA. There is much controversy related to the INR range to target, especially in those with recurrent venous events in spite of treatment and those with arterial thrombosis, low-intensity anticoagulation (INR 2–3) against high-intensity anticoagulation (INR 3–4). Against the high intensity, there are difficulties in keeping a stable INR over 3 and there is also a possibility for interference by aPL on the thromboplastins used for INR measurement. Additionally, bleeding is a major concern, although studies are not concordant in reporting an increased risk of bleeding when high-intensity regimen is compared with the low-intensity group [55]. Moreover, INR equal or over 3.0 dramatically reduced recurrent thrombosis [56]. In summary, for practical issues, venous thrombosis is treated with anticoagulation targeting INR 2–3. When there are arterial thromboses or venous recurrent thrombosis with a target INR between 2 and 3, we recommend that the treatment should aim an INR of 3–4 or LDA (low-dose aspirin) plus VKA. These recommendations are based on two randomized controlled trials (RCTs) of limited quality and a systematic review (observational studies) for venous thrombosis and on observational studies and one RCT of low quality for arterial thrombosis. There are no studies available regarding triple aPL positivity and anticoagulation should follow according to the type of thrombosis (venous or arterial) as mentioned or may be based on clinical judgment [57].

The cessation of anticoagulation in APS patients who became aPL negative has been questioned. Khamashta et al. showed that the rate of thrombosis recurrence was highest (1.30 per patient year) during the first 6 months after the cessation of warfarin therapy [56]. A retrospective study was conducted in 44 APS patients who interrupted oral anticoagulation for various reasons, including prolonged disappearance of aPL. Results demonstrated that 11 (25%) patients developed a recurrent thrombotic event after oral anticoagulation cessation. Three had CAPS and one died because of lower limb ischemia [58]. Another study showed that 11 out of 24 (45.8%) patients still developed recurrent thrombosis despite oral anticoagulation with a follow-up of 60 months since aPL disappearance [59]. The current recommendation is lifelong oral anticoagulation unless contraindicated.

Regarding the DOACs, only one trial is completed. RAPS (Rivaroxaban in APS) was a prospective, randomized, controlled, noninferiority, phase 2/3 clinical trial of rivaroxaban versus warfarin in APS patients (primary APS or with SLE) with venous thrombosis. The primary outcome was not clinical focused in the percentage change in endogenous thrombin potential assessed using thrombin generation testing. Rivaroxaban failed to reach the noninferiority threshold [60]. To date, there are four other DOACs trials ongoing, being three with rivaroxaban and one with apixaban. TRAPS (Trial on Rivaroxaban in Antiphospholipid Syndrome) was designed to evaluate the efficacy and safety of rivaroxaban in high-risk APS patients with triple-positive thrombotic APS patients regardless of the presence of arterial events [61]. ASTRO-APS (Apixaban for the Secondary Prevention of Thrombosis Among Patients With Antiphospholipid Syndrome) is a pilot phase 3 trial, which will analyze secondary prevention of thrombosis as a secondary outcome in patients with venous thrombosis [62].

Hydroxychloroquine (HCQ) has been controversial but a promising adjuvant therapy in APS. A prospective nonrandomized trial compared oral anticoagulation plus HCQ (400 mg daily) versus oral anticoagulation alone in primary APS patients. All patients were off antiplatelet aggregation therapy. Six patients (30%) in the monotherapy group (N=20) had venous events despite therapeutic range INR in contrast to none in the HCQ group (N=20) during the 6 month and 36 month follow-up, respectively. HCQ should be prescribed in all aPL-positive SLE patients. There are no strong data to recommend HCQ in persistently aPL-positive patients without other autoimmune diseases [63].

Gestational Antiphospholipid Syndrome

Current treatment for recurrent abortions or fetal loss in patients with APS is based on RCTs developed in the late 90s and in the early years of this century. The results are conflicting and this can be attributed to different inclusion criteria, especially concerning aPL profile [64]: LDA alone was found to be inferior to LDA plus heparin in two studies [65,66], whereas other studies reported similar results when those treatment groups were compared [67,68]. Due to this discrepancy, there is no consensus on a treatment recommendation for recurrent abortion before 10 weeks of pregnancy, when LDA alone or LDA plus heparin can be used for recurrent miscarriage related to APS, with the latter usually being preferred by specialists.

In the same fashion, most of authors recommend LDA plus prophylactic dose heparin in patients with fetal loss (after 10 weeks of pregnancy) throughout pregnancy until 6 weeks postpartum [69], although trials with this specific group of patients are lacking. There is, however, a significant increase in live birth rates from as low as 4% [70] before the diagnosis and treatment of ObAPS to up to 85% after treatment [38,70].

If pregnancy failure occurs despite recommended medications, there is no study to support the use of any different drug and suggested treatments rely on expert's opinion. Prednisone, intravenous immunoglobulin (IVIG), HCQ, and anti-TNF drugs have been proposed to be used in patients with APS and pregnancy losses, but there are no evidences to support the use of any of them [71]. Actually, few drugs, such as prednisone, have been associated with more adverse pregnancy results [72] and should be used with caution.

Considering patients with definite APS, there are no RCTs that included patients with exclusively severe preeclampsia or eclampsia and premature birth before the 34th week, as stated by the classification criteria [64]. Therefore, recommended treatment for this group of patients (LDA plus heparin) is the same as for the patients with pregnancy loss; however, the real efficacy is unknown. The main question is if the treatment can prevent the development of preeclampsia and intrauterine growth restriction in aPL-positive patients, as some authors have reported a high incidence of these complications despite appropriate treatment for APS [37].

High prevalence of preeclampsia in APS patients despite treatment may represent a different pathway of non-aPL–related hypertensive disorder of pregnancy. For example, LDA, used in all recommended protocols for APS, reduced the occurrence of preeclampsia in 53% of non-APS high-risk patients when started before 16 weeks of pregnancy, with a reduction of almost 80% of the severe cases [73]. Although studies in APS patients are still lacking, we do not seem to be closer to those numbers with the current treatment.

In addition to preeclampsia, IUGR is commonly found in pregnant women with APS before and after treatment. A publication evaluating the efficacy of prophylaxis using LDA and unfractionated heparin (UFH) in the prevention of IUGR in patients with APS provided negative results. Of the study group, 32.3% had low birth weight newborns (below 10th percentile) compared with 2.5% of the control group. The mean birth weight of the newborn babies of the study group was also smaller than controls (2798 vs. 3124 g, respectively) [74].

Patients with previous thrombosis using long-term anticoagulants should change warfarin to full-dose heparin (preferably low molecular weight heparin) and LDA during pregnancy, which can be switched back after delivery. Warfarin during pregnancy has been associated with congenital malformations (warfarin embryopathy) and fetal bleeding, so it should be avoided [37].

Noncriteria Manifestations

Different noncriteria manifestations have been described in APS. Their treatments are mainly based on case series and open-label studies, and some of them are extrapolated from SLE patients' data [57].

Steroids, IVIG (in cases refractory to steroids), azathioprine, and rituximab are the most common medications used for the treatment of APS-related thrombocytopenia and autoimmune hemolytic anemia. In patients with aPL-related thrombocytopenia, primary thromboprophylaxis with LDA and/or HCQ should be considered [57].

When there are neurological manifestations, such as chorea, myelitis, and multiple sclerosis–like disease, steroids and immunosuppressive agents (i.e., cyclophosphamide), in addition to anticoagulation therapy, may be considered, especially in cases associated with SLE [57].

The treatment of aPL-associated nephropathy includes antiplatelet and/or anticoagulation therapy, with variable results. Angiotensin-converting enzyme inhibitors or angiotensin receptor blockers should be prescribed for controlling hypertension and proteinuria [57].

Patients with symptomatic heart disease must undergo anticoagulation therapy, as they are at high risk of thromboembolic events. Asymptomatic disease is treated with LDA. Infective endocarditis prophylaxis is not currently recommended [57].

Catastrophic Antiphospholipid Syndrome

Treatment of CAPS is directed to the two most important mechanisms of disease: controlling the thrombotic events and suppressing the inflammation/cytokine cascade [7].

According to the 14th International Congress on Antiphospholipid Antibodies Task Force Report on CAPS, glucocorticoids (GC) and anticoagulation are the "backbone of therapy" for CAPS. In addition to the combination of GC plus anticoagulation, IVIG and/or plasma exchange (PE) should always be considered, especially in life-threatening disease because it was associated with reduction in mortality, when compared with strategies that not included IVIG and/or PE ($P = .04$) [7]. In the last CAPS Registry analysis, triple therapy was associated with a mortality rate of 27.9% (vs. 40.6% with other combination and 75% with no treatment) [75].

Anticoagulation remains the most important therapeutic intervention in CAPS. Although no difference between unfractionated heparin and low molecular weight heparin has been reported, intravenous unfractionated heparin is the therapy of choice because of its reversibility [76]. There is no data supporting the use of DOACs, fibrinolytics, or antiplatelet therapy in CAPS [76,77].

GC are usually prescribed in pulse therapy (p.e. methylprednisolone 500–1000 mg, 1–3 days) or at doses of 1–2 mg/kg per day of prednisone or equivalent [75]. IVIG is used in a dose of 2 g/kg, given in 5 days (i.e., 0.4 g/kg per day for 5 days). PE is used to remove aPL, proinflammatory cytokines (such as TNF-alpha), and complement components. In the majority of cases reported, the replacement fluid used was fresh frozen plasma, which contains natural anticoagulants (p.e. antithrombin III) and procoagulant factors. It is unclear if the use of albumin as replacement fluid results in different outcomes [78].

Immunosuppressive drugs (IS) are reserved for patients with SLE or other autoimmune diseases. Cyclophosphamide is the most common IS prescribed (65 patients), followed by azathioprine (4 patients), cyclosporine (2 patients), and mycophenolate mofetil (1 patient). Nonetheless, no evidence-based data support the choice of one over another. The use of IS in CAPS because of primary APS is not established [7]. Rituximab and eculizumab have been used with success in refractory CAPS cases [7,76,79–81].

Novel and Upcoming Treatments

Different new treatments are being developed for APS, as the current ones do not meet all the patients' needs. HCQ, statins, rituximab, belimumab, eculizumab, antiplatelets glycoprotein receptor inhibitors, protease-activated receptor (PAR) antagonists, peptide therapies, coenzyme Q10, TLR-4 inhibitors, tissue factor inhibitors, mTOR inhibitors, intracellular signaling blockade, and others are under investigation. The various aspects of these medications will be discussed elsewhere [82].

REFERENCES

[1] Miyakis S, Lockshin MD, Atsumi T, Derksen RHWM, de Groot PG, Koike T. International consensus statement on an update of the classification criteria for definite antiphospholipid syndrome. J Thromb Haemost 2006;4:295–306 (August 2005).

[2] Giannakopoulos B, Krilis SA. The pathogenesis of antiphospholipid syndrome. N Engl J Med 2013;368:1033–44.

[3] Fischetti F, Durigutto P, Pellis V, Debeus A, Macor P, Bulla R, et al. Thrombus formation induced by antibodies to ß2-glycoprotein I is complement dependent and requires a priming factor. Blood 2005;106:2340–7.

[4] Arad A, Proulle V, Furie RA, Furie BC, Furie B. ß2-glycoprotein-1 autoantibodies from patients with antiphospholipid syndrome are sufficient to potentiate arterial thrombus formation in a mouse model. Blood 2011;117:3453–60.

[5] Bordin G, Boldorini R, Meroni P. The two hit hypothesis in the antiphospholipid syndrome: acute ischaemic heart involvement after valvular replacement despite anticoagulation in a patient with secondary APS. Lupus 2003;12:851–3.

[6] Meroni PL, Riboldi P. Pathogenic mechanisms mediating antiphospholipid syndrome. Curr Opin Rheumatol 2001;13:377–82.

[7] Cervera R, Rodríguez-Pintó I, Colafrancesco S, Conti F, Valesini G, Rosário C, et al. 14th international congress on antiphospholipid antibodies task force report on catastrophic antiphospholipid syndrome. Autoimmun Rev 2014;13:699–707.

[8] Shoenfeld Y, Blank M, Cervera R, Font J, Raschi E, Meroni P-L. Infectious origin of the antiphospholipid syndrome. Ann Rheum Dis 2006;65:2–6.

[9] Santiago M, Cossermelli W, Tuma M, Pinto M, Oliveira R. Anticardiolipin antibodies in patients with infectious disease. Clin Rheumatol 1998;8:23–8.

[10] Zuckerman E, Toubi E, Golan TD, Sabo E, Shmuel Z. Increased thromboembolic incidence in anti-cardiolipin-positive patients with malignancy. Br J Cancer 1995;72:447–51.

[11] De ME, Brandão BC, Capella FC, Garcia JAP, Gregory SC. Catastrophic antiphospholipid syndrome in cancer patients: an interaction of clotting, autoimmunity and tumor growth? Isr Med Assoc J 2014;16:544–7.

[12] Lazzaroni MG, Taglietti M, Tincani A. Malignancies: a possible "first hit" in the development of catastrophic antiphospholipid syndrome? Isr Med Assoc J 2014;16:2–3.

[13] Meroni PL, Raschi E, Camera M, Testoni C, Nicoletti F, Tincani A, et al. Endothelial activation by aPL: a potential pathogenetic mechanism for the clinical manifestations of the syndrome. J Autoimmun 2000;15:237–40.

[14] Del Papa N, Guidali L, Sala A, Buccellati C, Khamashta M, Ichikawa K, et al. Endothelial cells as target for antiphospholipid antibodies. Human polyclonal and monoclonal anti-ß2-glycoprotein I antibodies react in vitro with endothelial cells through adherent ß2-glycoprotein I and induce endothelial activation. Arthritis Rheum 1997;40:551–61.

[15] Dunoyer-geindre S, De Moerloose P, Rochemonteix BG, Reber G, Kruithof EKO. NF-κB is an essential intermediate in the activation of endothelial cells by anti- β 2glycoprotein I antibodies NF-κB is an essential intermediate in the activation of endothelial cells by anti-ß2 -glycoprotein I antibodies. Thromb Haemost 2002;88:851–7.

[16] Asherson R, Doherty D, Vergani D, Khamashta M, Hughes G. Major histocompatibility complex associations with primary antiphospholipid syndrome. Arthritis Rheum 1992;35:3–4.

[17] Caliz R, Atsumi T, Kondeatis E, Amengual O, Khamashta MA, Vaughan RW, et al. HLA class II gene polymorphisms in antiphospholipid syndrome: haplotype analysis in 83 Caucasoid patients. Rheumatology 2001;40:31–6.

[18] Sugiura ogasawara M, Omac Y, Kawashima M, Toyo-oka L, Khoi S, Sawai H, et al. The first genome-wide association study identifying new susceptibility loci for obstetric antiphospholipid syndrome. J Hum Genet 2017. [Internet]. Nature Publishing Group; ahead of p. 1–8. Available from: https://doi.org/10.1038/jhg.2017.46.

[19] Hughes G. The antiphospholipid syndrome: ten years on. Lancet 1993;342:341–4.

[20] Cervera R, Piette J, Font J, Kamashta M, Shoenfeld Y, Campos M, et al. Antiphospholipid Syndrome: clinical and immunologic manifestations and patterns of disease expression in a cohort of 1000 patients. Arthritis Rheum 2002;46:1019–27.

[21] Abreu MM, Danowski A, Wahl D, Amigo M, Tektonidou M, Pacheco M, et al. The relevance of "non-criteria": clinical manifestations of antiphospholipid syndrome: 14th international congress on antiphospholipid antibodies technical task force report on antiphospholipid syndrome clinical features. Autoimmun Rev 2015;5:401–14.

[22] Sanna G, Bertolaccini M, Cuadrado M, Kamashta M, Hughes G. Central nervous system involvement in the antiphospholipid syndrome. Rheumatology 2003;42:200–13.

[23] Menon S, Jameson-Shortall E, Newman S, Hall-Crags M, Chinn R, Isenberg D. A longitudinal study of anticardiolipin antibody levels and cognitive functioning in systemic lupus erythemathosus. Arthritis Rheum 1999;4:735–41.

[24] Hanly J, Hong C, Smith S, Fisk J. A prospective analysis of cognitive function and anticardiolipin in systemic lupus erythemathosus. Arthritis Rheum 1999;42:728–34.

[25] Tektonidou M, Varsou N, Katoulas G, Antoniou A, Moutsopoulos H. Cognitive deficits on patients with antiphospholipid syndrome: association with clinical, laboratory, and brain magnetic resonance imaging findings. Arch Intern Med 2006;166:2278–84.

[26] Cuadrado M, Kamashta M, Ballesteros A, Godfrey T, Simon M, Hughes G. Can neurologic manifestations of Hughes (antiphospholipid) syndrome be distinguished from multiple sclerosis? Analysis of 27 patients and review of literature. Medicine 2000;79:57–68.

[27] Lockshin M, Tenedios F, Petri M, McCarty G, Forastiero R, Krilis S, et al. Cardiac disease in the antiphospholipid syndrome: recommendations for treatment. Committee consensus report. Lupus 2003;12:518–23.

[28] Zuily S, Domingues V, Suty-Selton C, Eschwège V, Bertoletti L, Chaouat A, et al. Antiphospholipid antibodies can identify lupus patients at risk for pulmonary hypertension: a systematic review and meta-analysis. Autoimmun Rev 2017;16:576–86.

[29] Amigo M, Garcia-Torres R, Robles M, Bochicchio T, Reyes P. Renal involvement in primary antiphospholipid syndrome. J Rheumatol 1992;9:181–5.

[30] Tektonidou M, Sotisou F, Nakapoulou L, Vlachoyiannopoulos P, Moutsopoulos H. Antiphospholipid syndrome nephropathy in patients with systemic lupus erythematosus and antiphospholipid antibodies: prevalence, clinical associations and long-term outcome. Arthritis Rheum 2004;50:2569–79.

[31] Paul S, Sangle S, Bennett A, El-Hachmi M, Hangartner R, Hughes G, et al. Vasculitis, antiphospholipid antibodies, and renal artery stenosis. Ann Rheum Dis 2005;62:1800–2.

[32] Francès C, Niang S, Laffitte E, Pelletier F, Costedoat N, Piette J. Dermatologic manifestations of the antiphospholipid syndrome: two hundred consecutive cases. Arthritis Rheum 2005;52:1785–93.

[33] Lockshin M, Kim M, Laskin C, Guerra M, Branch D, Merrill J, et al. Prediction of adverse pregnancy outcome by the presence of lupus anticoagulant, but not anticardiolipin antibody, in patients with antiphospholipid antibodies. Arthritis Rheum 2012;64:2311–8.

[34] Sugiura-Ogasawara M, Ozaki Y, Katano K, Suzumori N, Kitaori T, Mizutani E. Abnormal embryonic karyotype is the most frequent cause of recurrent miscarriage. Hum Reprod 2012;27:2297–303.

[35] de Jesus GR, Agmon-levin N, Andrade CA, Andreoli L, Chighizola CB, Porter TF, et al. 14th international congress on antiphospholipid antibodies task force report on obstetric antiphospholipid syndrome. Autoimmun Rev 2014;13:795–813.

[36] Wong L, Porter T, de Jesús G. Recurrent early pregnancy loss and antiphospholipid antibodies: where do we stand? Lupus 2014;23:1226–8.

[37] De Jesús GR, Rodrigues G, De Jesús NR, Levy RA. Pregnancy morbidity in antiphospholipid syndrome: what is the impact of treatment? Curr Rheumatol Rep 2014;16:403–11.

[38] Serrano F, Nogueira I, Borges A, Branco J. Primary antiphospholipid syndrome: pregnancy outcome in a Portuguese population. Acta Reumatol Port 2009;34:492–7.

[39] Bramham K, Hunt B, Germain S, Calatayud I, Khamashta M, Bewley S, et al. Pregnancy outcome in different clinical phenotypes of antiphospholipid syndrome. Lupus 2010;19:58–64.

[40] Pourrat O, Coudroy R, Pierre F. Differentiation between severe HELLP syndrome and thrombotic microangiopathy, thrombotic thrombocytopenic purpura and other imitators. Eur J Obstet Gynecol Reprod Biol 2015;189:68–72.

[41] Chighizola C, de Jesús G, Branch D. The hidden world of anti-phospholipid antibodies and female infertility: a literature appraisal. Autoimmun Rev 2016;15:493–500.

[42] Bertolaccini ML, Amengual O, Andreoli L, Atsumi T, Chighizola CB, Forastiero R, et al. 14th international congress on antiphospholipid antibodies task force. Report on antiphospholipid syndrome laboratory diagnostics and trends. Autoimmun Rev 2014;13:917–30.

[43] Practice Committee of American Society for Reproductive Medicine. Anti-phospholipid antibodies do not affect IVF success. Fertil Steril 2008;90:S172–3.

[44] Chighizola C, Raschi E, Banzato A, Borghi M, Pengo V, Meroni P. The challenges of lupus anticoagulants. Expert Rev Hematol 2016;9:389–400.

[45] Pengo V, Bison E, Zoppellaro G, Jose S, Denas G, Hoxha A, et al. APS - diagnostics and challenges for the future. Laboratory testing for antiphospholipid syndrome. Autoimmun Rev 2016;15:1031–3.

[46] Pruthi RK. Optimal utilization of thrombophilia testing. Int J Lab Hematol 2017;39:104–10.

[47] Zohoury N, Bertolaccini M, Rodriguez-Garcia J, Shums Z, Ateka-Barrutia O, Sorice M, et al. Closing the serological gap in the antiphospholipid syndrome: the value of "non-criteria" antiphospholipid antibodies. J Rheumatol 2017. https://doi.org/10.3899/jrheum.170044. Ahead of print.

[48] Andreoli L, Fredi M, Nalli C, Piantoni S, Reggia R, Dall'Ara F, et al. Clinical significance of IgA anti-cardiolipin and IgA anti-β2glycoprotein I antibodies. Curr Rheumatol Rep 2013;15:343.

[49] Bertolaccini ML, Sanna G. The clinical relevance of noncriteria antiphospholipid antibodies. Semin Thromb Hemost 2018;44(5):453–57.

[50] Amengual O, Forastiero R, Sugiura-Ogasawara M, Otomo K, Oku K, Favas C, et al. Evaluation of phosphatidylserine-dependent antiprothrombin antibody testing for the diagnosis of antiphospholipid syndrome: results of an international multicentre study. Lupus 2017;26:266–76.

[51] Ruiz-Irastorza G, Cuadrado M, Ruiz-Arruza I, Brey R, Crowther M, Derksen R, et al. Evidence-based recommendations for the prevention and long-term management of thrombosis in antiphospholipid antibody-positive patients: report of a task force at the 13th international congress on antiphospholipid antibodies. Lupus 2011;20:206–18.

[52] Oku K, Amengual O, Yasuda S, Atsumi T. How to identify high-risk APS patients: clinical utility and predictive values of validated scores. Curr Rheumatol Rep 2017;19:51.

[53] Radin M, Schreiber K, Costanzo P, Cecchi I, Roccatello D, Baldovino S, et al. The adjusted Global AntiphosPholipid Syndrome Score (aGAPSS) for risk stratification in young APS patients with acute myocardial infarction. Int J Cardiol 2017;240:72–7. [Internet]. Elsevier B.V. Available from: https://doi.org/10.1016/j.ijcard.2017.02.155.

[54] Yelnik C, Laskin C, Porter T, Branch D, Buyon J, Guerra M, et al. Lupus anticoagulant is the main predictor of adverse pregnancy outcomes in aPL-positive patients: validation of PROMISSE study results. Lupus Sci Med 2016;3:e000131.

[55] Pengo V, Ruiz-Irastorza G, Denas G, Andreoli L, Khamashta M, Tincani A. High intensity anticoagulation in the prevention of the recurrence of arterial thrombosis in antiphospholipid syndrome: "PROS" and "CONS". Autoimmun Rev 2012;11:577–80.

[56] Khamashta M, Cuadrado M, Mujic F, Taub N, Hunt B, Hughes G. The management of thrombosis in the antiphospholipid-antibody syndrome. N Engl J Med 1995;332:993–7.

[57] Espinosa G, Cervera R. Current treatment of antiphospholipid syndrome: lights and shadows. Nat Rev Rheumatol 2015;11:586–96.

[58] Camarmond C, Jego P, Veyssier-Belot C, Marie I, Mekinian A, Elmaleh-Sachs A, et al. Cessation of oral anticoagulants in antiphospholipid syndrome. Lupus 2017;26:1291–6.

[59] Medina G, Briones-Garcia E, Cruz-Domingues M, Flórez-Durante O, Jara L. Antiphospholipid antibodies disappearance in primary antiphospholipid syndrome: thrombosis recurrence. Autoimmun Rev 2017;16:352–4.

[60] Cohen H, Hunt BJ, Efthymiou M, Arachchillage DRJ, Mackie IJ, Clawson S, et al. Rivaroxaban versus warfarin to treat patients with thrombotic antiphospholipid syndrome, with or without systemic lupus erythematosus (RAPS): a randomised, controlled, open-label, phase 2/3, non-inferiority trial. Lancet Haematol 2016;3:e426–36. [Internet]. The Author(s). Published by Elsevier Ltd. This is an Open Access article under the CC BY license, Available from: https://doi.org/10.1016/S2352-3026(16)30079-5.

[61] Pengo V, Banzato A, Bison E, Zoppellaro G, Jose SP, Denas G. Efficacy and safety of rivaroxaban vs warfarin in high-risk patients with antiphospholipid syndrome: rationale and design of the Trial on Rivaroxaban in AntiPhospholipid Syndrome (TRAPS) trial. Lupus 2016;25:301–6.

[62] Woller SC, Stevens SM, Kaplan DA, Branch DW, Aston VT, Wilson EL, et al. Apixaban for the secondary prevention of thrombosis among patients with antiphospholipid syndrome: study rationale and design (ASTRO-APS). Clin Appl Thromb Hemost 2016;22:239–47.

[63] Erkan D, Aguiar CL, Andrade D, Cohen H, Cuadrado MJ, Danowski A, et al. 14th international congress on antiphospholipid antibodies task force report on antiphospholipid syndrome treatment trends. Autoimmun Rev 2014;13:685–96.

[64] Andreoli L, Chighizola C, Banzato A, Pons-Estel G, de Jesus G, Erkan D. Estimated frequency of antiphospholipid antibodies in patients with pregnancy morbidity, stroke, myocardial infarction, and deep vein thrombosis: a critical review of the literature. Arthritis Rheum 2013;65:1869–73.

[65] Rai R, Cohen H, Dave M, Regan L. Randomised controlled trial of aspirin and aspirin plus heparin in pregnant women with recurrent miscarriage associated with phospholipid antibodies (or antiphospholipid antibodies). BMJ 1997;314:253–7.

[66] Kutteh W, Ermel L. A clinical trial for the treatment of antiphospholipid antibody-associated recurrent pregnancy loss with lower dose heparin and aspirin. Am J Reprod Immunol 1996;35:402–7.

[67] Farquharson R, Quenby S, Greaves M. Antiphospholipid syndrome in pregnancy: a randomized, controlled trial of treatment. Obstet Gynecol 2002;100:408–13.

[68] Laskin C, Spitzer K, Clark C, Crowther M, Ginsberg J, Hawker G, et al. Low molecular weight heparin and aspirin for recurrent pregnancy loss: results from the randomized, controlled HepASA Trial. J Rheumatol 2009;36:279–87.

[69] de Jesús G, dos Santos F, Oliveira C, Mendes-Silva W, de Jesús N, Levy R. Management of obstetric antiphospholipid syndrome. Curr Rheumatol Rep 2012;14:79–86.

[70] Dadhwal V, Sharma A, Deka D, Gupta B, Mittal S. The obstetric outcome following treatment in a cohort of patients with antiphospholipid antibody syndrome in a tertiary care center. J Postgrad Med 2011;57:16–9.

[71] Alijotas-Reig J. Treatment of refractory obstetric antiphospholipid syndrome: the state of the art and new trends in the therapeutic management. Lupus 2013;22:6–17.

[72] Laskin C, Bombardier C, Hannah M, Mandel F, Ritchie J, Farewell V, et al. Prednisone and aspirin in women with autoantibodies and unexplained recurrent fetal loss. N Engl J Med 1997;337:148–54.

[73] Roberge S, Giguère Y, Villa P, Nicolaides K, Vainio M, Forest J, et al. Early administration of low-dose aspirin for the prevention of severe and mild preeclampsia: a systematic review and meta-analysis. Am J Perinatol 2012;29:551–6.

[74] Spegiorin L, Galão E, De Godoy J, Bagarelli L, Oliani A. Antiphospholipid antibodies and growth retardation in intrauterine development. Prague Med Rep 2007;108:185–90.

[75] Rodriguez-Pintó I, Espinosa G, Erkan D, Shoenfeld Y, Cervera R. The effect of "triple therapy" with anticoagulation plus corticosteroids plus plasma exchange and/or intravenous immunoglobulins on the mortality of catastrophic antiphospholipid syndrome (CAPS) patients. Ann Rheum Dis 2017;76(Suppl. 2):OP0231.

[76] Kazzaz NM, Mccune WJ, Knight JS. Treatment of catastrophic antiphospholipid syndrome. Curr Opin Rheumatol 2016;28:218–27.

[77] Signorelli F, Nogueira F, Domingues V, Mariz HA, Levy RA. Thrombotic events in patients with antiphospholipid syndrome treated with rivaroxaban: a series of eight cases. Clin Rheumatol 2016;35:801–5.

[78] Bucciarelli S, Erkan D, Espinosa G, Cervera R. Catastrophic antiphospholipid syndrome: treatment, prognosis, and the risk of relapse. Clin Rev Allergy Immunol 2009;36:80–4.

[79] Erkan D, Vega J, Ramo G, Kozora E, Lockshin MD. A pilot open-label phase II trial of rituximab for non-criteria manifestations of antiphospholipid syndrome. Arthritis Rheum 2013;65:464–71.

[80] Berman H, Rodríguez-pintó I, Cervera R, Morel N, Costedoat-chalumeau N, Erkan D, et al. Rituximab use in the catastrophic antiphospholipid syndrome: descriptive analysis of the CAPS registry patients receiving rituximab. Autoimmun Rev 2013;12:1085–90.

[81] Elazary AS, Klahr PP, Hershko AY, Dranitzki Z, Rubinow A, Naparstek Y. Rituximab induces resolution of recurrent diffuse alveolar hemorrhage in a patient with primary antiphospholipid antibody syndrome. Lupus 2015;21:438–40.

[82] Andrade D, Tektonidou M. Emerging therapies in antiphospholipid syndrome. Curr Rheumatol Rep 2016;18:22.

Chapter 45

Catastrophic Antiphospholipid Syndrome

Ricard Cervera, Ignasi Rodríguez-Pintó, Gerard Espinosa

Department of Autoimmune Diseases, Hospital Clínic, Barcelona, Spain

INTRODUCTION

The descriptive adjective "catastrophic" was added to the term antiphospholipid syndrome (APS) to highlight an accelerated form of this syndrome resulting in multiorgan failure [1,2]. Patients with catastrophic APS have in common (1) clinical evidence of multiple organ involvement developing over a very short period; (2) histopathological evidence of multiple small-vessel occlusions; and (3) laboratory confirmation of the presence of antiphospholipid antibodies (aPL), usually in high titer [3–5].

Although less than 1% of patients with the APS develop this complication [6], its potentially lethal outcome emphasizes its importance in clinical medicine today. The majority of patients with catastrophic APS end up in intensive care units (ICU) with multiorgan failure. The reason why some patients develop recurrent thromboses, mainly of large vessels (simple or classic APS), while others develop rapidly recurrent vascular occlusions, predominantly affecting small vessels (catastrophic APS), is still unclear [7–10].

Because of the rarity of this syndrome, an international registry of patients with catastrophic APS ("CAPS Registry") was created in 2000 [11]. Currently, it documents the clinical, laboratory, and therapeutic data of more than 500 patients with catastrophic APS. The periodical analysis of these data has allowed not only the description of the clinical and laboratory characteristics of this syndrome but also the elaboration of classification criteria, diagnostic algorithms, and therapeutic guidelines [7–10].

CLASSIFICATION AND DIAGNOSIS

The heterogeneity of the different clinical presentations in catastrophic APS led to the development of consensus criteria for the definition and classification of these patients [7] that were later validated [8].

However, when patients present with multiple organ thromboses in a "real-world" setting, especially in ICU, multiple factors can impede the timely diagnosis of catastrophic APS and, at times, the differential diagnosis cannot be narrowed to a single disease. It has been suggested that a *continuum* of conditions, all demonstrating aPL, might exist comprising some patients with thrombotic thrombocytopenic purpura; hemolysis, elevated liver enzymes, low platelets syndrome; or catastrophic APS, and the term "microangiopathic" APS has been proposed to embrace this group of patients [12–16]. To address this problem, diagnostic algorithms have been delineated to help clinicians facing patients with multiorgan thromboses in whom the catastrophic APS is suspected [9,10].

CLINICAL AND LABORATORY FEATURES

Five hundred patients accounting for 522 episodes of catastrophic APS were included in the most recent analysis of the "CAPS Registry" [17]. 483 patients had only one episode, while 17 patients had several recurrent episodes: 12 (3.3%) patients developed two episodes and 5 (1%) patients developed three episodes. Most cases are described in young women. The main demographic results can be seen in Table 45.1.

Precipitating Factors

Typically, this overwhelming situation is triggered by precipitating factors. Precipitating factors were identified in 65% of the episodes. The most frequent factors were infections (49% of episodes) mainly in the respiratory tract (33%), followed by the urinary tract (19%) and the skin (13%).

Mosaic of Autoimmunity. https://doi.org/10.1016/B978-0-12-814307-0.00045-1

TABLE 45.1 Demographic Characteristics and Precipitating Factors of Patients With Catastrophic Antiphospholipid Syndrome (APS) [17]

	%
Mean age at diagnosis (years)	38 (17)[a]
Sex (female)	343 (69%)[a]
CAPS as first manifestation of APS	50[a]
Diagnosis	
Primary APS	60[a]
Associated SLE	30[a]
SLE-like	4[a]
Others	6[a]
Precipitating factors (N = 481)[b]	65
Infections	49
Surgery	17
Malignancy	16
Contraceptives	10
Pregnancy related	8
Drugs	5
SLE flare	3
Trauma	2
Others	13

CAPS, catastrophic antiphospholipid syndrome; *SLE*, systemic lupus erythematosus.
Results presented as percentages from the total number of episodes expect when otherwise stated.
[a]*Frequency calculated excluding recurrent episodes.*
[b]*In 13% of episodes, more than one precipitating factor was identified.*

Clinical Features

The clinical picture of catastrophic APS was characterized by renal involvement (73%), with variable degree of renal failure, and lung involvement (60%) in the form of acute respiratory distress syndrome or pulmonary embolism (26%). Up to 56% of patients showed central nervous system manifestations because of stroke or encephalopathy. Catastrophic APS affected the heart in half of episodes, mainly because of myocardial infarction or valvulopathy. Libman-Sacks endocarditis was reported in 13% of catastrophic APS episodes with heart involvement. Skin complications in form of *livedo reticularis* were frequently observed while other skin manifestations were less often (Table 45.2).

Laboratory Features

Laboratory features of hemolytic anemia were also often shown (37%), sometimes associated with schistocytes (22%). Thrombotic microangiopathy was less often reported (19%). Additionally, some patients developed disseminated intravascular coagulation [18–20].

MANAGEMENT APPROACH

The optimal management of catastrophic APS has been a challenge since its description. Today, catastrophic APS mortality continues to be extremely high despite therapy [21–23]. Due to this high mortality rate, early diagnosis and aggressive treatment are essential clues in its successful management. The analysis of patients with this condition included in the "CAPS Registry" has allowed the evaluation of several therapeutic combinations and to propose the current therapeutic approach [24].

TABLE 45.2 Clinical Manifestations and Laboratory Features[a] of Patients With Catastrophic Antiphospholipid Syndrome (APS) [17]

Clinical Manifestation	%
Organ Involved	
Kidney (N=518)	**73**
Renal failure	77
Proteinuria	29
Arterial hypertension	24
Hematuria	16
Lung (N=517)	**60**
Acute respiratory distress syndrome	36
Pulmonary embolism	26
Alveolar hemorrhage	12
Pulmonary edema	8
Brain (N=515)	**56**
Stoke	40
Encephalopathy	39
Seizures	15
Headache	8
Heart (N=515)	**50**
Heart failure	44
Myocardial infarction	30
Valvulopathy	28
Libman-Sacks endocarditis	13
Skin (N=517)	**17**
Livedo reticularis	43
Cutaneous necrosis	26
Cutaneous ulcers	24
Purpura	14
Liver (N=515)	**39**
Elevated liver enzymes	63
Hepatomegaly	10
Liver failure	9
Jaundice	7
Peripheral Vessel (N=515)	**37**
Peripheral venous thrombosis	69
Peripheral arterial thrombosis	46
Gastrointestinal Involvement	**24**
Gastrointestinal bleeding	18
Ileus	4

Continued

TABLE 45.2 Clinical Manifestations and Laboratory Features[a] of Patients With Catastrophic Antiphospholipid Syndrome (APS) [17]—cont'd

Clinical Manifestation	%
Spleen (N=513)	**18**
Adrenal Glands (N=510)	**10**
Laboratory Features	
Thrombocytopenia	67
Schistocytes	22
Thrombotic microangiopathy[b]	14
Disseminated intravascular coagulation[c]	11
Lupus anticoagulant	83
aCL IgG	81
aCL IgM	49
aβ2GPI IgG	78
aβ2GPI IgM	40
Antinuclear antibodies	57
Anti-DNA antibodies	32
Anti-ENA	10

[a]Results presented as percentages from the total number of episodes
[b]Thrombotic microangiopathy defined as those patients with low platelet count, hemolysis features, and schistocytes.
[c]Disseminated intravascular coagulation defined as those patients with low platelet count, d-dimer increase, and low prothrombin time.

These guidelines state that specific therapy together with precipitating factor treatment and supportive treatment should be administered to patients with clinical suspicion of catastrophic APS. Current knowledge supports the treatment with the combination of high doses of glucocorticoids (GC) and anticoagulation (AC) with heparin as first-line treatment. Additionally, adding plasma exchange (PE) and/or intravenous immunoglobulins (IVIG) should be considered in cases with associated life-threatening situation. Intravenous cyclophosphamide is recommended in patients in whom catastrophic APS is associated to SLE [25].

Furthermore, rituximab, as an add-on therapy in the first-line treatment of catastrophic APS patients refractory to conventional treatment or recurrent cases, has shown a benefit [26]. More recently, some authors have reported success in the treatment of catastrophic APS with eculizumab [27,28].

Supportive General Measures

According to the patient medical condition, appropriate supportive care should be established and, often, it includes ICU admission. External ventilation support and hemodialysis might be necessary, but mostly only tight control is necessary. Classical thrombotic risk factors should be controlled or avoided when possible. It might include the use of external pneumatic compression devices when immobility is a concern. Any surgery should be postponed when its aim is not to remove necrotic tissue to control the cytokine storm. Additionally, catastrophic APS patients may benefit from glycemic control, stress ulcer prophylaxis, and blood pressure control [29].

Trigger-Guided Therapy

When an infection is suspected, any effort should be undertaken to recover responsible microorganism. At the same time, removing necrotic tissue or limb amputation is advised with the aim of controlling systemic inflammatory response [30].

The perioperative management of patients with APS or aPL carriers should be very cautious with the purpose of decreasing thrombotic recurrence risk or the development of a catastrophic episode. Thus, careful bridging between oral anticoagulant to heparin is required. Probably, a multidisciplinary approach with a hemostasis specialist to each case might be necessary. Additionally, puerperium should be adequately covered for a minimum of 6 weeks with parenteral anticoagulants.

Anticoagulation

AC with heparin is the mainstay catastrophic APS treatment. The main reason for its use is the inhibition of ongoing clotting and its ability to break up existing clots that may contribute to the ongoing thrombosis [31]. Moreover, although its pharmacodynamic mechanisms are not completely understood, antiinflammatory activity of heparin seems to account for its extraordinary usefulness in catastrophic APS [32] and, additionally, heparin seems to inhibit aPL binding to their target on the cell surface [33]. Most catastrophic APS patients are initially treated with unfractionated heparin because nonfractionated heparin enables throwing back its effect in case of requirement. This is often a need during ICU period either because electively to perform invasive procedures or of bleeding. Later, nonfractionated heparin can be switched to low molecular weight heparin and finally to oral AC. However, physicians should not rush to change heparin to other AC because a long time under heparin treatment favors clot fibrinolysis. A 7–10 days course under heparin treatment is recommended. However, heparin should not be withdrawn before achieving a correct international normalized ratio between 2 and 3 with oral AC treatment.

Steroids

GC are the most commonly used antiinflammatory drugs in the treatment of autoimmune diseases. GC bind to a cytoplasmic receptor that, subsequently, binds to the chromosomic material and modulates gene expression. In this sense, GC are used to overcome the excessive inflammatory response triggered by multiple blood flow occlusions and resultant ischemic necrotic tissue.

Although no direct evidence supports GC use in patients with severe infections or in catastrophic APS, unless patients develop adrenal insufficiency, strong rational arguments drive investigators to think that this lack of evidence is attributable to underpowered studies. Thus, GC are recommended in patients with catastrophic APS, although the best initial dose, the route of administration, and the tapering strategies are still an investigation field. Data from the "CAPS Registry" showed that GC are given as intravenous pulses of 500–1000 mg/d for 1–3 d in one-third of episodes and as oral or intravenous dosages of 1–2 mg/kg/d in another third. Nevertheless, most physicians continue GC treatment until patient is discharged in a daily oral dose and then taper the dose until it is being administered in low doses.

Plasma Exchange

PE is a technique designed to remove large molecular weight molecules from plasma. It consists in removing large quantities of plasma (usually 2–5 L) and replacement by either fresh frozen or stored plasma. Its use in catastrophic APS relies on the rational that PE removes aPL and cytokines from the patient while volume replacement with fresh frozen plasma would restore natural anticoagulants such as antithrombin-III. Its use comes by analogy to the management of classical microangiopathic conditions where this treatment has shown its beneficial effects in randomized controlled trials [34]. Therefore, PE is specially suitable in those patients with catastrophic APS who present serological features of microangiopathy (schistocytes) [35].

The use of therapeutic PE in catastrophic APS is recommended with a grade of evidence of 2C by the American Society for Apheresis (ASA) [36]. It is indicated when a patient with catastrophic APS evolves to a life-threatening situation as an add-on therapy to effective AC with intravenous heparin and high-dose steroids.

There is no consensus on the replacement fluid of choice for therapeutic PE in catastrophic APS, and fresh frozen plasma, human albumin, and solvent/detergent plasma have been used. Following ASA recommendations, a combination of plasma and albumin would provide the necessary benefit of therapeutic PE and minimize potentially serious and undesirable side effects from excessive exposure to plasma.

There is no recommendation about the duration of this procedure. It is generally continued for a minimum of 3–5 days; however, clinical response is the main parameter that should dictate discontinuation of the therapy.

Intravenous Immunoglobulins

IVIG are used in a wide variety of autoimmune and inflammatory conditions, although the mechanisms of action by which IVIG exert its immunomodulatory and antiinflammatory effects remain unclear. Probably, high intravenous antibodies concentration leads to Fc receptor overload, thus inhibiting pathologic autoantibody to develop their detrimental effects and increasing their clearance. At the same time, it might increase Tregs downregulating cytokine storm [37]. Only recently, the beneficial effects of IVIG in primary APS have been proved by decreasing aPL titers and, therefore, reducing the thrombotic risk of these patients [38,39]. Thus, rationally IVIG may be effective to achieve a prompt reduction of aPL titters and downregulate proinflammatory levels in patients with catastrophic APS.

There is no established recommendation on the dose that might be beneficial in patients with catastrophic APS. Although by analogy to other autoimmune diseases, they have been used following two different schemes: 400 mg/kg daily for 5 d and a total dose of 2 g/kg of body weight infused over a period of 2–5 d. However, when PE is performed, IVIG are administered after PE session and, additionally, often an extra IVIG dose is administered after PE to replace IVIG removed by it.

IVIG are usually well-tolerated, but there are some reports of thromboembolic events and acute renal failure after IVIG, especially in those cases of catastrophic APS to whom AC has to be stopped because of bleeding. Thus, IVIG should be administered slowly, especially in elderly patients with high blood pressure, diabetes, or hypercholesterolemia. Anyhow, an eye should be kept for early detection of any complication.

Rituximab

The evidence for the use of rituximab in patients with catastrophic APS comes from the recent review performed recently by our group [26]. In this review, we identified 20 out of 441 (4.6%) patients included in the "CAPS Registry" as of May 2013 who were treated with rituximab.

Considering the outcome, 16 (80%) patients recovered from the acute catastrophic APS episode and 4 (20%) died at the time of the event. Two of the patients who died had received rituximab as a first-line therapy. Regarding the effect of rituximab in aPL profile, these data were available in only 8 patients. Overall, half of patients remained with persistent aPL in the follow-up with positive lupus anticoagulant (LA) at 11 weeks and LA plus anticardiolipin antibodies at 2, 3, and 5 months of follow-up, respectively. In the remaining 4 patients (50%), aPL became negative.

Eculizumab

Eculizumab is a monoclonal antibody that binds with high affinity to complement protein C5, inhibiting its cleavage and, thus, preventing C5a formation and its chemoattractant function so as the membrane attack complex assembly. It is approved by the US Food and Drug Administration for the treatment of paroxysmal nocturnal hemoglobinuria and for atypical hemolytic uremic syndrome. Recently, some authors reported success with eculizumab use in patients with refractory episodes of catastrophic APS [27,28,40,41]. Dosage has been taken over from the experience on other thrombotic microangiopathies. Weekly doses of 900–1200 mg of eculizumab have been used in the acute phase decreasing its frequency after effervescence to 900 mg administered every 2 wks. However, there is no known clue to decide the duration of the treatment and, then, often, not only effectivity has to be taken into consideration but also its efficiency.

Eculizumab seems to be an attractive promising treatment for patients with catastrophic APS or at least to prevent its recurrence in high-risk situations, although a larger experience is needed to define eculizumab place in catastrophic APS treatment. However, its high cost throws back many initiatives to use it. Probably, expected future economic cost drop will increase its use in catastrophic APS providing the required experience.

CONCLUSIONS

Catastrophic APS is a rare disorder. Its rarity, the lack of knowledge or orientation among the treating physicians (mostly, ICU physicians), and the absence of animal model make it difficult to develop an evidence-based model of its pathogenesis. Our knowledge mainly comes from the data analyzed from the "CAPS Registry." Hopefully, with a more widespread recognition of this condition, more patients will be identified and investigated, elaborating our knowledge on molecular pathways leading to catastrophic APS.

Unfortunately, despite currently used approach, catastrophic APS mortality remains unacceptable high and optimizing current available therapy is a need. Regardless some promising results with new therapies (i.e., eculizumab), more experience is still required.

REFERENCES

[1] Asherson RA. The catastrophic antiphospholipid syndrome. J Rheumatol 1992;19:508–12.

[2] Piette J-C, Cervera R, Levy RA, Nasonov EL, Triplett DA, Shoenfeld Y. The catastrophic antiphospholipid syndrome–Asherson's syndrome. Ann Méd Interne 2003;154:195–6.

[3] Asherson RA, Cervera R, Piette JC, Font J, Lie JT, Burcoglu A, et al. Catastrophic antiphospholipid syndrome. clinical and laboratory features of 50 patients. Medicine 1998;77:195–207.

[4] Asherson RA, Cervera R, Piette JC, Shoenfeld Y, Espinosa G, Petri MA, et al. Catastrophic antiphospholipid syndrome: clues to the pathogenesis from a series of 80 patients. Medicine 2001;80:355–77.

[5] Bucciarelli S, Cervera R, Espinosa G, Gómez-Puerta JA, Ramos-Casals M, Font J, et al. Mortality in the catastrophic antiphospholipid syndrome: causes of death and prognostic factors. Autoimmun Rev 2006;6:72–5.

[6] Cervera R, Piette J-C, Font J, Khamashta MA, Shoenfeld Y, Camps MT, et al. Antiphospholipid syndrome: clinical and immunologic manifestations and patterns of disease expression in a cohort of 1,000 patients. Arthritis Rheum 2002;46:1019–27.

[7] Asherson R, Cervera R, de Groot PG, Boffa MC, Piette JC, Khamashta MA, et al. Catastrophic antiphospholipid syndrome: international consensus statement on classification criteria and treatment guidelines. Lupus 2003;12:530–4.

[8] Cervera R, Font J, Gómez-Puerta JA, Espinosa G, Cucho M, Bucciarelli S, et al. Validation of the preliminary criteria for the classification of catastrophic antiphospholipid syndrome. Ann Rheum Dis 2005;64:1205–9.

[9] Cervera R, Tektonidou MG, Espinosa G, Cabral AR, González EB, Erkan D, et al. Task force on catastrophic antiphospholipid syndrome (APS) and non-criteria aps manifestations (i): catastrophic APS, APS nephropathy and heart valve lesions. Lupus 2011;20:165–73.

[10] Erkan D, Espinosa G, Cervera R. Catastrophic antiphospholipid syndrome: updated diagnostic algorithms. Autoimmun Rev 2010;10:74–9.

[11] Cervera R, Tincani A. European Working Party on systemic lupus erythematosus and European Forum on antiphospholipid antibodies: two networks promoting European research on autoimmunity. Lupus 2009;18:863–8.

[12] Asherson RA, Pierangeli SS, Cervera R. Is there a microangiopathic antiphospholipid syndrome? Ann Rheum Dis 2007;66:429–32.

[13] Asherson RA, Pierangeli S, Cervera R. Microangiopathic antiphospholipid-associated syndromes revisited new concepts relating to antiphospholipid antibodies and syndromes. J Rheumatol 2007;34:1793–5.

[14] Asherson RA, Cervera R. Microvascular and microangiopathic antiphospholipid-associated syndromes ("MAPS"): semantic or antisemantic? Autoimmun Rev 2008;7:164–7.

[15] Asherson RA, Cervera R, Font J. Multiorgan thrombotic disorders in systemic lupus erythematosus: a common link? Lupus 1992;1:199–203.

[16] Cervera R, Bucciarelli S, Plasín MA, Gómez-Puerta JA, Plaza J, Pons-Estel G, et al. Catastrophic antiphospholipid syndrome (CAPS): descriptive analysis of a series of 280 patients from the "caps registry". J Autoimmun 2009;32:240–5.

[17] Rodríguez-Pintó I, Moitinho M, Santacreu I, Shoenfeld Y, Erkan D, Espinosa G, et al. Catastrophic antiphospholipid syndrome (CAPS): descriptive analysis of 500 patients from the International CAPS Registry. Autoimmun Rev 2016;15:1120–4.

[18] Bucciarelli S, Espinosa G, Cervera R, Erkan D, Gómez-Puerta JA, Ramos-Casals M, et al. Mortality in the catastrophic antiphospholipid syndrome: causes of death and prognostic factors in a series of 250 patients. Arthritis Rheum 2006;54:2568–76.

[19] Asherson RA, Espinosa G, Cervera R, Gómez-Puerta JA, Musuruana J, Bucciarelli S, et al. Disseminated intravascular coagulation in catastrophic antiphospholipid syndrome: clinical and haematological characteristics of 23 patients. Ann Rheum Dis 2005;64:943–6.

[20] Espinosa G, Bucciarelli S, Cervera R, Lozano M, Reverter JC, de la Red G, et al. Thrombotic microangiopathic haemolytic anaemia and antiphospholipid antibodies. Ann Rheum Dis 2004;63:730–6.

[21] Rodríguez-Pintó I, Espinosa G, Cervera R. Catastrophic antiphospholipid syndrome – 20 years later. Curr Rheumatol Rev 2013;9:73–80.

[22] Rodríguez-Pintó I, Espinosa G, Cervera R. Catastrophic APS in the context of other thrombotic microangiopathies. Curr Rheumatol Rep 2015;17:1–10.

[23] Cervera R, Rodríguez-Pintó I, Colafrancesco S, Conti F, Valesini G, Rosário C, et al. 14th International Congress on antiphospholipid antibodies task force report on catastrophic antiphospholipid syndrome. Autoimmun Rev 2014;13:699–707.

[24] Rodríguez-Pintó I, Espinosa G, Cervera R. Catastrophic antiphospholipid syndrome: the current management approach. Best Pract Res Clin Rheumatol 2016;30:239–49.

[25] Bayraktar UD, Erkan D, Bucciarelli S, Espinosa G, Asherson R. The clinical spectrum of catastrophic antiphospholipid syndrome in the absence and presence of lupus. J Rheumatol 2007;34:346–52.

[26] Berman H, Rodríguez-Pintó I, Cervera R, Morel N, Costedoat-Chalumeau N, Erkan D, et al. Rituximab use in the catastrophic antiphospholipid syndrome: descriptive analysis of the CAPS registry patients receiving rituximab. Autoimmun Rev 2013;12:1085–90.

[27] Kronbichler A, Frank R, Kirschfink M, Szilágyi Á, Csuka D, Prohászka Z, et al. Efficacy of eculizumab in a patient with immunoadsorption-dependent catastrophic antiphospholipid syndrome. Medicine (Baltim) 2014;93:e143.

[28] Shapira I, Andrade D, Allen SL, Salmon JE. Induction of sustained remission in recurrent catastrophic antiphospholipid syndrome via inhibition of terminal complement with eculizumab. Arthritis Rheum 2012;64:2719–23.

[29] Rodríguez-Pintó I, Soriano A, Espinosa G, Shoenfeld Y, Cervera R. Catastrophic antiphospholipid syndrome: an orchestra with several musicians. IMAJ 2014;16:585–6.

[30] Amital H, Levy Y, Davidson C, Lundberg I, Harju A, Kosach Y, et al. Catastrophic antiphospholipid syndrome: remission following leg amputation in 2 cases. Semin Arthritis Rheum 2001;31:127–32.

[31] Ortel TL, Kitchens CS, Erkan D, Brandão LR, Hahn S, James AH, et al. Clinical causes and treatment of the thrombotic storm. Expert Rev Hematol 2012;5:653–9.

[32] Levi M, van der Poll T. Inflammation and coagulation. Crit Care Med 2010;38:S26–34.

[33] Franklin RD, Kutteh WH. Effects of unfractionated and low molecular weight heparin on antiphospholipid antibody binding in vitro. Obstet Gynecol 2003;101:455–62.

[34] Rock GA, Shumak KH, Buskard NA, Blanchette VS, Kelton JG, Nair RC, et al. Comparison of plasma exchange with plasma infusion in the treatment of thrombotic thrombocytopenic purpura. Canadian Apheresis Study Group. N Engl J Med 1991;325:393–7.

[35] Espinosa G, Cervera R. Current treatment of antiphospholipid syndrome: lights and shadows. Nat Rev Rheumatol 2015;11:586–96.

[36] Schwartz J, Winters JL, Padmanabhan A, Balogun RA, Delaney M, Linenberger ML, et al. Guidelines on the use of therapeutic apheresis in clinical practice-evidence-based approach from the Writing Committee of the American Society for Apheresis: the sixth special issue. J Clin Apher 2013;28:145–284.

[37] Gelfand E. Intravenous immune globulin in autoimmune and inflammatory diseases. N Engl J Med 2012;367:2015–25.

[38] Sciascia S, Giachino O, Roccatello D. Prevention of thrombosis relapse in antiphospholipid syndrome patients refractory to conventional therapy using intravenous immunoglobulin. Clin Exp Rheumatol 2012;30:409–13.

[39] Tenti S, Guidelli GM, Bellisai F, Galeazzi M, Fioravanti A. Long-term treatment of antiphospholipid syndrome with intravenous immunoglobulin in addition to conventional therapy. Clin Exp Rheumatol 2013;31:877–82.

[40] Lonze BE, Singer AL, Montgomery R. Eculizumab and renal transplantation in a patient with CAPS. N Engl J Med 2010;362:1744–5.

[41] Lonze BE, Zachary AA, Magro CM, Desai NM, Orandi BJ, Dagher NN, et al. Eculizumab prevents recurrent antiphospholipid antibody syndrome and enables successful renal transplantation. Am J Transplant 2014;14:459–65.

Chapter 46

Rheumatoid Arthritis

Stefano Alivernini, Barbara Tolusso, Luca Petricca, Gianfranco Ferraccioli, Elisa Gremese
Institute of Rheumatology, Fondazione Policlinico Universitario A. Gemelli - IRCCS – Catholic University of the Sacred Heart, Rome, Italy

INTRODUCTION

Rheumatoid arthritis (RA) is a chronic autoimmune disease that affects nearly 0.5%–1% of the world's population. It is characterized by synovial tissue inflammation with symmetric polyarticular distribution. This inflammation leads to pain and stiffness and can result in progressive joint damage, deformities, and loss of function (Fig. 46.1). RA is associated to organ damage having extra-articular manifestations whose development contributes to severe disability. Over the past 2 decades, the knowledge about biological mechanisms in RA pathogenesis has significantly increased promoting the development of specific drugs which effectively may target them.

EPIDEMIOLOGY

RA is the third most common type of arthritis behind osteoarthritis (prevalence 26.9 million) and gout (prevalence 6.1 million). RA affects approximately 1.3 million in the United States [1] and is one of the most common autoimmune diseases, with rates higher than a number of other conditions, including psoriasis, Crohn's disease, type I (insulin-dependent) diabetes, lupus and multiple sclerosis [1]. RA is a chronic disease that affects about 1% of the world population. The prevalence and incidence (new cases per year) of RA appears to have declined since the early 1960s [2]. One study conducted in Rochester, Minnesota, found that the incidence of RA had declined for both men and women over a 40-year period [3].

Even with these declines, RA occurs at twice the rate in women compared with men, with a prevalence of 1.06% in women (as a percentage of the total population) compared with 0.61% in men [1]. The incidence (new cases per year) of RA increases with increasing age in most populations until about the eighth decade of life, when it declines. Results from the same Rochester, Minnesota, study mentioned above found that the average yearly incidence among different age groups increased until about ages 74–84 and decreased thereafter. The incidence peaked earlier for women than men at about ages 55–64 years for women compared with 75–84 years for men [3].

PATHOGENESIS

The last decades of research have dramatically increased our knowledge about RA pathogenesis and disease course. This has led to the development of potent new biologic and small molecules therapies. As shown in Fig. 46.2, it is possible to identify a preclinical phase of the disease before any clinical symptoms manifestation, during which the loss of immunological tolerance is promoted by different trigger factors. Among them, the complex interplay between the innate and adaptive immune system has a critical role in the onset and perpetuation of synovial tissue inflammation in RA [4]. The presence of autoantibodies in the sera of asymptomatic individuals up to 10 years before the onset of clinical disease clearly supports the notion that the clinical manifestation of the pathology represents an already advanced step in the disease course. In this context, the genetic background characterized by markers able to predict the onset or severity of RA suggests that these biological processes might be operative over the lifetime of an individual [5]. Twin studies, aiming to dissect the role of the genotype in RA development, showed a concordance rate of 15%–30% among monozygotic twins and nearly 5% among dizygotic twins [6]. The association with the human leukocyte antigen (HLA)-DRB1 locus was demonstrated in multiple populations, mainly in RA patients seropositive for rheumatoid factor (RF) or anticitrullinated peptide antibodies (ACPA) [7], called the "shared epitope." To date other risk alleles have been identified in ACPA-positive RA patients, functionally linked with the immune regulation including T cell stimulation, activation and functional differentiation (i.e., PTPN22 and CTLA4) [8–10]. Studies of gene–environment interaction showed that smoking and other forms of bronchial stress are

Mosaic of Autoimmunity. https://doi.org/10.1016/B978-0-12-814307-0.00046-3

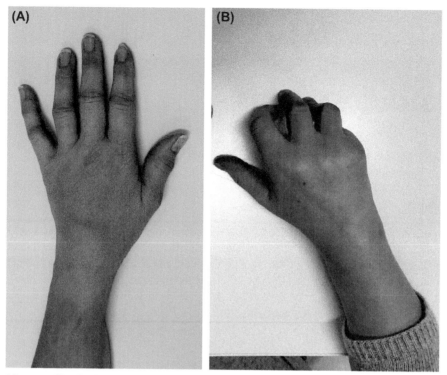

FIGURE 46.1 **Clinical features of hands of RA patients based on disease duration.** (A) Swollen II–III MCP, II–III PIP joints, and wrist in patient with ACPA/RF+ RA after 3 months from disease onset. (B) Joint deformities of the hand of patient with ACPA/RF+ long-standing RA. Property of the Biopsy Unit of the Institute of Rheumatology – Fondazione Policlinico Universitario A. Gemelli - IRCCS – Catholic University of the Sacred Heart, Rome – Italy. *ACPA*, anticitrullinated peptide antibodies; *MCP*, metacarpophalangeal; *PIP*, proximal interphalangeal; *RA*, rheumatoid arthritis; *RF*, rheumatoid factor.

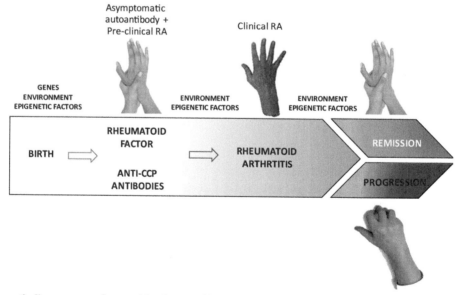

FIGURE 46.2 **Schematic disease course of seropositive rheumatoid arthritis (RA).** Seropositive RA is a chronic inflammatory disease characterized by the presence of autoantibodies (as anticitrullinated peptide antibodies and rheumatoid factor). Both genetic and environmental factors have an important role in RA pathogenesis because in genetically susceptible individual, environmental challenges (such as microorganisms in the mucosal sites) could lead to local inflammatory changes and immune activation resulting in the loss of immunological tolerance and the generation of autoantibodies. This aberrant mechanism is under epigenetic control because of DNA and histone modifications, as well as microRNA network effect. This process can occur several years before the onset of joint disease during which the titer of autoantibodies gradually increases undergoing to epitope spreading able to result in bone loss and pain before the clinical onset of the disease. Therefore, based on the current theories, in the presence of autoantibodies and antibodies-induced bone damage, minor joint challenges, which normally resolve without consequences, will instead lead to chronic inflammation. Once the disease is clinically evident, multiple immunological, genetic, and epigenetic factors play a crucial role in the determinism of disease prognosis toward clinical remission of disease progression with bone damage.

linked to increased risk of RA development in HLA-DR4 carriers [11]. Moreover, smoking and HLA-DRB1 alleles synergistically increase one's risk of having ACPA [12].

Among the environmental factors, a high body mass index has been studied as having a potential role [13,14]. The prevalence of obesity has risen dramatically, mostly in the Western countries, having a role also in the growing incidence of RA observed in the last years [14,15], even if there were no conclusive data possibly because of the influence of other confounders as lifestyle factors.

The association between an excess of white adipose tissue (WAT) and RA onset and progression may be explained by the fact that WAT is an active endocrine organ, playing a role not only on metabolism but also on immune and inflammatory processes by releasing several adipokines and proinflammatory mediators [16–18]. Recently, Qin et al. reviewed the published data, concluding that being overweight or obese is associated with a significantly increased risk (1.15 and 1.31, respectively) of RA development [15]. This association was even stronger among women diagnosed at younger ages, i.e., <55 years. Interestingly, also the "exposure time" to obesity seems to influence the RA risk in woman aged 55 or younger, with a 37% increased risk of RA with a history of 10 years of being obese [14,19]. Finally, data from three different cohorts of patients seem to indicate that obesity is associated with a likelihood of developing a seronegative RA, with a relative risk between 1.6 and 3.5 [20–22]. Obesity itself seems to influence disease phenotype also in terms of activity and severity, even if few data are available at the earliest stage of the disease. Controversial data provided by randomized controlled trials and observational studies were found on the association between obesity and inflammatory parameters or disease activity in early RA at the time of diagnosis, despite obese patients characterized by more severe disease in terms of Health Assessment Questionnaire, pain, and global health assessment [17,23,24]. The association between obesity and worst disease activity and disability has been also observed in cohorts of patients with established RA [25,26].

As previously stated, a critical observation about the genetic influence on RA susceptibility is that the concordance rate among monozygotic twins is only nearly 15% [27]. Therefore, other factors as epigenetic changes may have a major contribution. Epigenetic mechanisms are potentially heritable and regulate gene expression without DNA sequence changes. They include covalent modification of DNA (methylation of cytosine at position C5 in CpG pairs mainly in regulatory regions), histones modifications (methylation and acetylation) able to remodel chromatin leading to activation, or silencing of gene transcription [28]. Other epigenetic mechanisms are microRNA (miRNA), which are posttranscriptional regulators of gene expression by binding to complementary target mRNA leading to their degradation [29]. Among them, increasing evidences have been produced demonstrating the crucial role of some miRNA species as miR-155 whose expression is aberrantly regulated in inflammatory cells of the innate [30] and the adaptive [31] immune system in RA patients mirroring the disease activity [32]. In particular, miR-155 knockout mice are resistant to collagen-induced arthritis, bone damage, and autoantibody production by B cells [30]. This is because of the repressive action by miR-155 on antiinflammatory molecular as phosphatidylinositol-3,4,5-trisphosphate 5-phosphatase 1 (SHIP-1) in macrophages [30] and PU.1 in B lymphocytes, which is a crucial transcription factor for B cell maturation and antibody production [31], whose expression was confirmed to be significantly repressed in RA patients.

RA is characterized by inflammation of the synovial tissue that displays as synovial lining layer hyperplasia, sublining infiltration with mononuclear cells, increased vascularity, and fibrin deposition. These features can be very heterogeneous among RA patients from pauci-immune or diffuse infiltrate till the formation of lymphoid structures within the synovium (follicular synovitis) [31] (Fig. 46.3). Synovial tissue inflammation (synovitis) occurs when leukocytes infiltrate the synovial compartment because of an increase of their migration within the tissue. Inflammatory cells migration is enabled by endothelial cells activation in synovial vessels which are increased in number and show an overexpression of adhesion molecules (as integrins and selectins) and lead the release of cytokines and chemokines [33].

Innate Immune System

Several inflammatory cells of the innate immune system are found in the synovial membrane of RA patients, including macrophages, mast cells, and natural killer cells. Among them, macrophages play a central role in promoting synovial tissue inflammation through the release of inflammatory cytokines (tumor necrosis factor alpha [TNF-α] and interleukin [IL] 1, IL-6, IL-12, IL-15, IL-18, and IL-23), reactive oxygen products, and matrix-degrading enzymes [34]. Macrophages are activated by a wide range of signals as Toll-like receptors (TLR) and nucleotide-binding oligomerization domain–like receptors which enable the recognition of pathogen- and damage-associated molecular patterns including bacterial, viral, and endogenous ligands [35]. In particular, the synovial molecular microenvironment is responsible for macrophages reprogramming that can be divided into classical and alternative activation leading to M1 and M2 phenotypes, respectively [36]. Classically activated M1 macrophages play a crucial role in the initiation and development of inflammation by producing a large number of proinflammatory factors as IL-6 and TNF [37], as well as IL-12 and IL-23 [38]. M1 phenotype

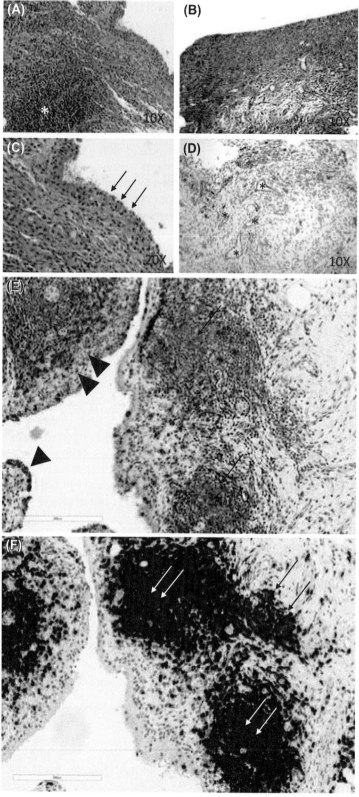

FIGURE 46.3 Histopathology of rheumatoid arthritis (RA) synovitis. (A) Lymphoid aggregate; (B) diffuse lymphocytes infiltrate; (C) hyperplasia of the lining layer (thin *black arrows*); (D) immunohistochemistry for CD31 (DAB) marking synovial vessels (*black asterisk*); (E) double immunohisto-chemistry for CD68 (RED) and CD21 (DAB) for macrophages (*black arrow heads*) and follicular dendritic cells (*thin black arrows*) in synovial tissue of RA patient; (F) double immunohistochemistry for CD3 (RED) and CD20 (DAB) for T lymphocytes (*thin black arrows*) and B lymphocytes (*thin white arrows*) cells in synovial tissue of RA patient. Property of the Biopsy Unit of the Institute of Rheumatology – Fondazione Policlinico Universitario A. Gemelli - IRCCS – Catholic University of the Sacred Heart, Rome – Italy.

macrophages actively promote the recruitment of Th1 and natural killer cells within the inflamed tissue and show high surface expression of TLR4, CD86, MHC-II, CCL2, and CCL5. Conversely M2 macrophages are usually induced by Th2 cytokines as IL-4 and IL-10 and show high surface expression of CD206 and CD163. Moreover, M2 macrophages have been divided into M2a, M2b, M2c, and M2d, based on the major promoting factor as IL-4, TLR/IL-1R, IL-10/TGF-β, and adenosine A2A receptor, respectively, with phenotype-specific cell functions [36,37].

Even neutrophils, which are abundantly found in the synovial fluid of RA patients, act as crucial cells in the promotion of synovial tissue inflammation synthesizing prostaglandins, proteases, and reactive oxygen species. Moreover, it has been demonstrated that neutrophils are sensitive to the release of IL-8 from macrophages, which enhances their tissue homing already in the preclinical phases of the disease [39] promoting the development of pain and subclinical bone damage [39].

Autoimmunity

RA is characterized by the positivity of various antibodies as autoantibodies against citrullinated antigens. Citrulline derives from arginine by posttranslational modification induced by peptidylarginine deiminases activity [40]. These antibodies were first identified in 1964 as antibodies against perinuclear granules in the superficial cells of the human buccal mucosa epithelium (antiperinuclear antibodies, APF) [41]. In 1979, antikeratin antibodies (AKA) were described and in 1995 it was shown that filaggrin is the common antigen targeted by both APF and AKA [42]. This led to the development of ELISA tests: CCP-1 using filaggrin-derived cyclic peptide [43] and currently CCP-2 which utilizes a mixture of cyclic citrullinated peptides and made commercially available in 2002 [44]. Several other assays were also developed (CCP-3, MCV) [45]. ACPA are present in nearly two-third of RA patients and are more specific than the RF for RA [46–49]. In many cases, the diagnosis of RA is made clinically and is often delayed by an initial period of nonspecific symptoms. However, it is generally accepted that there is a window of opportunity for an early aggressive management of RA and that the disease management delay may result in increase of joint damage and disability [50].

In this contest, Brink M et al. analyzed a wide cohort of individuals at risk of developing RA showing that the development of an immune response toward citrullinated peptides is initially restricted but expands with time to induce a more specific response, with autoantibodies levels increasing during the predating time period closer to the onset of clinical symptoms [51]. Moreover, Sokolove J and coworkers observed a time-dependent expansion of ACPA specificity with an increase of ACPA subtypes suggesting an accumulation of multiple autoantibody specificities reflecting the process of epitope spreading [52]. In addition, years before RA onset, antibodies positivity is associated with inflammatory cytokines deregulation [53,54] (including TNF-α, IL-6, IL-12p70, and IFN-γ), suggesting that the autoimmune processes leading to clinical manifestation of arthritis is tightly related to the proinflammatory status. Therefore, ACPA role in the preclinical phase of RA seems to be limited not only to their high specificity for RA but also by their well-established association with a severe erosive phenotype [55–58]. Moreover, a qualitative change in the ACPA response before disease onset was found as the Fc fragment glycosylation enhancing the inflammatory activity of IgG [59]. In particular, Rombouts et al. found a decrease of galactosylation and an increase of core fucosylation of serum ACPA-IgG1 before the onset of RA [60]. Despite autoantibodies positivity in this early period, ACPA do not cause apparent pathology because individuals at risk of RA development (ACPA and/or RF positive) do not show evidence of histologically proven synovitis in the preclinical phase, in terms of CD3+, CD22+, CD55+, CD68+, and CD138+ cells [61]. However, ACPA positivity fosters a wide range of systemic and local inflammatory processes [62] as enhancement of osteoclastogenesis, osteoclasts differentiation, and bone resorption, respectively [63]. In particular, a rapid radiographic progression was shown to be predicted by high ACPA titers in the ESPOIR cohort and a reduction of systemic bone mineral density in RA patients at disease onset mainly in ACPA/RF seropositive patients [64,65]. In this contest, Krishnamurty et al. found that ACPA, binding to osteoclast precursors, induce the expression and release of TNF-α together with an increase of IL-8 able to promote osteoclastogenesis in a dose-dependent manner [66]. These findings provide the biological basis for the detection of erosive damage in asymptomatic individuals at risk of developing RA before any clinical manifestation [67]. ACPA-positive individuals showed changes in periarticular bone as thinning and fenestration of the cortical bone as well as milder changes in the trabecular bone [67]. These findings challenged the concept that bone damage in RA is exclusively led by inflammation. Moreover, the observation that the first bone change in at-risk individuals is the cortical fenestration providing a direct anatomical connection between the bone marrow and the joint space is interesting because it is still unknown where ACPA-producing plasma cells are firstly located. In fact, despite it is known that citrullination of proteins may occur at anatomical sites far from the joint, as lung epithelium [63] and gingival mucosa [68], it is still unknown where and how the loss of immunological tolerance takes place and where the ACPA production by autoreactive plasma cells firstly occurs [69]. ACPA positivity is more specific than IgM-RF, IgG-RF, or IgA-RF positivity for RA and is more specific than IgM-RF for early RA, with similar sensitivity (sensitivity of 67% and specificity of 95%) [70], despite anti-CCP2 test has a low sensitivity to be used as a screening test. However, in daily practice, a positive test is highly specific for RA and anti-CCP2 appears to be highly predictive of the future development of RA in both normal individuals and patients with undifferentiated arthritis [71,72]. Therefore, these tests appear to provide the best predictive assay to foresee which patients with recent onset of clinical synovitis would develop RA (see the diagnosis section below).

Adaptive Immune System

The presence of autoantibodies clearly places the adaptive immune cells at the center of RA pathogenesis. The synovial tissue of RA patients contains abundant myeloid cells and plasmacytoid dendritic cells that express cytokines as IL-12, IL-15, and IL-23, HLA class II molecules and co-stimulatory molecules that are crucial for antigen presentation, loss of immunological tolerance, and T cell activation [73,74]. Moreover, there are increasing evidences about the presence of synovial T cell oligoclonality and B cell hypermutation already in the preclinical phases with increasing rate close to the disease onset suggesting the aberrant activation of the adaptive immune system as early phenomenon contributing to the disease [75–78].

Despite RA being conventionally considered a type 1 helper-mediated disease, there are increasing evidences about the role of type 17 helper T cells (the so-called Th17), which represent a T cell subset that produces IL-17A and IL-22 as well as TNF-α [79,80]. Macrophage and dendritic cell–derived inflammatory molecules (as IL-1β, IL-21, and IL-23) create an inflammatory milieu able to support Th17 differentiation and suppress the development of regulatory T cells (Treg). In particular, Treg cells have been detected in tissue of RA patients with impaired regulatory properties [81]. This imbalance between Th17 and Treg cells may reflect the local production of TNF-α [81,82]. Synovial B cells are localized mainly within the synovial aggregates with the formation of ectopic lymphoid follicles that have been shown to support the production of autoantibodies [76]. Moreover, it has been demonstrated that B cells undergo clonal expansion within the synovial tissue which harbors populations of expanded B cell clones mirrored in the draining lymphoid organs (lymph nodes) [78].

CLINICAL MANIFESTATIONS

RA is a chronic, systemic, inflammatory disorder that primarily involves synovial joints with symmetrical synovitis of diarthrodial joints that usually leads, if uncontrolled, to their destruction because of erosion of cartilage and bone. This process causes joint deformities, resulting in significant disability in patients who do not start or fully respond to pharmacological treatment. Thus an early diagnosis is of crucial importance. However, recognizing the clinical features of early RA can be challenging. Multiple studies have showed the value of early diagnosis in RA patients, which avoids the development of irreversible joint damage and functional disability [83]. In fact, the course of established, long-standing RA can range from mild disease to rapidly multisystem inflammation. The majority of patients show an insidious disease, whereas 20% of patients have an intermediate onset and 10% have a sudden acute onset [84]. Different patterns of activity have been described for RA, with some patients having a course referred as "palindromic rheumatism" that may last for several years before the chronic, persistent RA becomes clear. Palindromic rheumatism is characterized by acute, recurrent "palindromic" oligoarthritis without bone or cartilage destruction development and generally with a favorable long-term prognosis [85]. The issue of RA in the elderly (with onset at age 60 years or older) has been the subject of debate as to whether it is a distinct disease from classic, younger-onset RA. In the differential diagnosis, the so-called "RS3PE" (remitting seronegative symmetric synovitis with pitting edema) must be considered because it is characterized by an acute onset of symmetric polyarthritis involving peripheral joints and flexor digitorum tendons associated with pitting edema of hands and feet [86].

Adult-onset Still's disease can mimic RA when patients present with arthritis, but the typical patient comes to medical attention with major systemic signs and symptoms of high spiking fever, evanescent salmon pink–colored rash associated with the fever, leukocytosis and thrombocytosis, and with the minor criteria of sore throat, lymphadenopathy, splenomegaly, liver dysfunction, seronegativity for RF and ACPA, and elevated levels of ferritin and glycosylated ferritin [87,88].

One of the most common complaints of RA patients at disease onset is morning stiffness together with pain and swelling of peripheral joints. Joint *stiffness* is considered to be relevant if lasts more than 30 min and is markedly worse in the morning or after long periods of inactivity and requires a few hours of movement to loosen it up. The physical examination of the joints reveals tenderness of the joint sites, synovial thickening, and/or joint effusion. Generally, RA begins in one or a few joints and evolves in an additive pattern. More than half of RA patients show initial involvement in the upper extremities with multiple joints affected in one-third and hand-only involvement in about one-quarter of the cases. Articular symptoms are symmetric at disease onset in 70% of cases and become symmetric within 1 year after disease onset in 85% of cases [89]. The most commonly affected joints are the proximal interphalangeal (PIP) and metacarpophalangeal (MCP) joints of the hands and wrists, followed by the metatarsophalangeal (MTP) joints of the feet, ankles, and shoulders [90].

ARTICULAR MANIFESTATIONS

Upper Extremity

RA affecting the hands generally presents with pain and swelling of the MCP and PIP joints and patients may report decreased grip strength [91]. RA patients can also experience tendon ruptures because of tendons rubbing against bony prominences from eroded bone, resulting in loss of extension or flexion. The most frequent site for extensor tendon rupture is at the distal end of the ulna with loss of movement of the third, fourth, and/or fifth fingers, respectively. Late manifestations of RA of the hands are anatomic disruptions of the integrity of the joint surfaces causing the visible joint deformities that subsequently lead to loss of function and disability. Abnormal alignment results from the changing biomechanical forces affecting tendons and ligaments along eroded bone, thus resulting in subluxations at the MCP joints, the boutonniere and swan neck deformities, and the Z deformity of the thumb. The *boutonnière* deformity is a nonreducible flexion at the PIP joint with hyperextension at the distal interphalangeal (DIP) joint. This process occurs when the central extensor tendon is stretched, the PIP is pulled through the tendon, and the lateral bands are displaced. With time the tendon shortens and the DIP becomes hyperflexed. The *swan neck* deformity is the opposite of the *boutonnière*. It is hyperextension at the PIP joint and flexion of the DIP joint; this process takes place either when the extensor tendon is affected and a shortening of the central extensor tendon occurs or when the PIP joint capsule herniates from weakening because of synovitis [92] (Fig. 46.4).

The involvement of the wrist is a common early clinical manifestation of RA leading to the loss of wrist extension [93]. In the wrist, tenosynovitis can be present in the common sheath of the abductor pollicis longus and extensor pollicis brevis tendons, respectively (the so-called de Quervain's tenosynovitis). Moreover, ongoing inflammation can lead to nerve compression and erosions promoting carpal tunnel syndrome (median nerve entrapment) and ulnar nerve entrapment development, which can lead to motor loss and thenar muscle atrophy if long-standing.

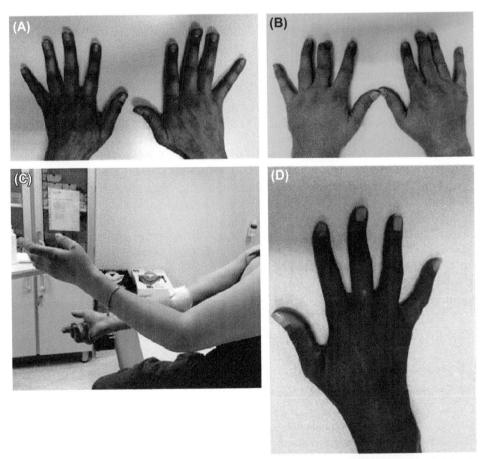

FIGURE 46.4 **Joint involvement in rheumatoid arthritis patients.** (A) Ulnar subluxation of the fingers; (B) swan neck deformities; (C) limitation in extension of the elbow; (D) Z deformity of the thumb and Boutonniere deformity. Property of the Biopsy Unit of the Institute of Rheumatology - IRCCS – Fondazione Policlinico Universitario A. Gemelli – Catholic University of the Sacred Heart, Rome – Italy.

In RA patients, chronic inflammation at the wrist leads to further deformities: a zigzag deformity is formed by the combination of the ulnar deviation of the phalanges at the metacarpal–phalangeal joints coupled with rotation of the navicular bone and radial deviation of the carpal bones at the distal radius and ulna articulations. RA patients also display an increased rate of collapse of the carpal height with an associated decrease in the ratio of carpal height to radial width [94]. In RA patients the involvement of the elbow may lead to loss of full extension (Fig. 46.4). RA patients can be often unaware of this as they compensate for overall arm function and movement with the wrists and shoulder, respectively [95].

Involvement of articular and periarticular tissues of the shoulder is extremely common and is one of the most disabling features in patients, especially because of its effect on sleep. Patients may present with shoulder pain and stiffness, decreased range of motion, and, less commonly, swollen, warm joints. The shoulder joint, rotator cuff muscles, and shoulder bursa can be affected with the initial symptoms, usually a result of a combination of synovitis, tendonitis, and/or bursitis. Bicipital tendonitis is common and, following the feared complication of tendon rupture, it is possible to observe the "popeye" sign, the contraction of the belly of the biceps muscle [96].

Lower Extremity

Initial involvement of the feet and ankles is quite common during the course of disease. It has been demonstrated that nearly 90% of RA patients will have such involvement [97]. RA patients often complain of pain on weight-bearing movement and walking with the forefoot as the most common painful area [98]. RA patients may experience an acute pain by a light squeeze across the MTP joints (squeeze test). Patients may complain of paresthesia if synovitis compresses the tarsal tunnel where the posterior tibial nerve runs. They may not be able to do a heel-rise if there is edema or swelling of the posterior tibialis tendon [98]. At the level of the small joints of the feet, it is possible to observe different joint deformities: *Hallux valgus* of the first MTP joint is an early manifestation in the rheumatoid foot [99]. *Hammer/mallet* or *claw toe* deformities that are due to a decreased stabilization in the MTPs because of a chronic inflammation of these joints with a subsequent weakening of the capsular and ligamentous structures. With the continued dorsiflexion during walking, the second to fifth MTP joints begin to sublux and eventually the extensor tendons shorten and the proximal phalanges can dislocate entirely [97].

At the ankle level, with persistent inflammation, the talonavicular bone collapses and causes the valgus flat foot deformity [100]. The insertion of the Achilles tendon can itself become inflamed and thickened, or it is possible to observe the sub-Achilles bursitis [99,101].

Early symptoms of knee involvement are due to synovial proliferation and effusion that lead to a limit flexion of the knee associated with patients' complaints of restriction of movement. It is possible to palpate synovial hypertrophy, and effusions can be observed by patellar tap or the bulge sign. Persistent knee inflammation may cause progressive cartilage damage, ligamentous laxity and quadriceps muscle atrophy, eventually leading to weakness, contractures, and difficulty in walking and progressive valgus or varus deformities may occur.

Increasing synovial fluid causes increased intraarticular pressure in the joint, leading to an outpouching of the synovial capsule forming the Baker's cysts. These cysts have been shown to be connected to the joint by a one-way valvular mechanism with a posterior accumulation of the fluid from the knee joint. One of the most serious complications is their rupture which clinically mimics acute thrombophlebitis with a painful and swollen thigh or calf [102]. Of course, even the hip may be site of inflammation in RA patients and its involvement seems to be a factor associated with more destructive peripheral joint disease [103]. At the physical examination, RA patients may display stiffness and limited range of motion of internal rotation, groin, or medial knee pain that is referred from the hip. With the progression of inflammation and erosive disease, the femoral head and acetabulum can erode into and protrude medially through the pelvis leading to the so-called "protrusio acetabuli." Moreover, RA patients may experience hip osteonecrosis or avascular necrosis particularly related to a previous history of corticosteroid exposure.

Spine and Axial Joints

From early studies the prevalence of cervical involvement was reported till 80%; however, recent studies conducted on early RA cohorts show that its prevalence is much lower, as suggested by earlier aggressive treatment contributing to this improvement [104]. Polyarticular severe involvement (especially of the hands), presence of rheumatoid nodules, high-titer autoantibody, high-dose steroid treatment, longer disease duration, presence of radiographic erosions in hands and feet, and the presence of extra-articular manifestations are risk factors for cervical spine abnormalities [105]. The most frequently involved cervical segments are the occipito-atlantal and atlanto-axial (C1–C2) joints causing cervical instability because of atlantoaxial subluxation. Synovial tissue thickening can cause spinal canal stenosis resulting in cord compression.

The earliest symptoms of cervical spine instability are pain in the neck, occiputs, and in the retro-orbital or temporal areas. Severe cervical instability will lead to cord compression with the development of myelopathy with weakness, heaviness sensation in the lower extremities, gait disturbances, hand clumsiness, bowel/bladder abnormalities, increased deep tendon reflexes, or Babinski sign. Moreover, the association with vertebral-basilar insufficiency can lead to additional symptoms such as tinnitus, vertigo, diplopia, or loss of proprioception [106]. The development of odontoid erosions or laxity of the transverse, alar, and apical ligaments of the first cervical vertebra may lead to the posterior slippage of the odontoid process [106,107]. In addition, when there is the development of bone and cartilage erosions, the skull can descend on the cervical spine and the odontoid can enter the foramen magnum causing basilar invagination, leading to brain stem or cord compression, vertebral artery insufficiency and sudden death [106].

Other Joints

Among other joint, the sternoclavicular involvement occurs in about one-third of RA patients, is usually asymmetric, and is characterized by swelling, crepitus, tenderness, hypertrophy, pain, or limitation of motion [108,109]. The temporomandibular joint involvement manifests clinically with pain, swelling, crepitus, and stiffness on mouth opening with limitation of motion and it is observed in patients with severe and long-standing disease [110]. Finally, the cricoarytenoid joint involvement is characterized by arthritis of the arytenoid cartilage, cricoid cartilage, subchondral bone, joint capsule and/or the surrounding ligaments which may be very difficult to notice at the beginning of the disease. The long-term complications are the joint space narrowing with joints ankylosis leading to upper airway obstruction. The most common clinical manifestations are the sensation of a foreign body or pharyngeal fullness in the throat, which is worse during swallowing or speaking [111,112].

EXTRA-ARTICULAR MANIFESTATIONS

RA is a systemic, inflammatory disease, so systemic symptoms may also be present in these patients. The extra-articular manifestations can occur in about 40% of patients, either at the disease onset or during the disease course [113]. Generally, extra-articular manifestations of RA are more frequently seen in patients with severe and active disease and are associated with increased mortality: in particular, RA patients are at an increased risk of developing cardiovascular disease (CVD), malignancy (non-Hodgkin's lymphoma), or severe infections [114,115].

Severe extra-articular manifestations share immunologic and inflammatory disease mechanisms, although local factors may also influence organ involvement. Predictors of developing severe extra-articular manifestations include clinical, serologic (autoantibody positivity), and genetic markers (double copies of HLA-DRB1*04 shared epitope alleles). Even environmental factors, such as smoking habit, are associated with early rheumatoid nodules onset and development of severe extra-articular manifestation, in addition to being a risk factor for the development of RA itself [116].

In general, in up to one-third of RA patients, the acute onset of arthritis is associated with constitutional symptoms such as prominent myalgia, fatigue, low-grade fever, weight loss and depression. Therefore, uncontrolled systemic inflammation in RA is associated with several long-term complications. For example, rheumatoid cachexia, with a loss of lean body mass, is often a feature of long-standing, severe systemic disease. Persistent elevation of inflammatory biomarker (erythrocyte sedimentation rate [ESR] and C-reactive protein [CRP]) levels and high disease activity are associated with tissue amyloidosis and organ damage [117].

Rheumatoid nodules are the most frequent extra-articular *skin manifestations* (with an incidence of around 20%) [118] and are characterized by painless subcutaneous lumps that develop most commonly on pressure areas, including the elbows, finger joints, ischial and sacral prominences, occipital scalp and Achilles tendon. Moreover, they can also occur in internal organ tissue, such as the myocardium, the meninges, and lung tissue [119]. At physical examination, these nodules may move easily when touched, or they may be fixed to deeper tissues. They occur mainly in autoantibody (ACPA or RF) positive RA patients and their presence may reflect the level of disease activity but can occur in cases of relatively quiescent joint disease. Moreover, RA patients with early diagnosis having rheumatoid nodules at the time of diagnosis are at an increased risk of developing more severe extra-articular manifestations [120]. The etiology of rheumatoid nodules is uncertain but it is believed to occur as a result of small vessel vasculitis: histologically there is a central focal fibrinoid necrosis with surrounding fibroblasts encapping areas of tissue characterized by granulomatous inflammation [121]. Other manifestations of RA small vessel vasculitis may present with involvement of small- and medium-sized vessels of the skin (causing nail fold infarcts, leg ulcers, purpura, and digital gangrene) together with a progressive sensory motor neuropathy. This may lead to mononeuritis multiplex being involved in the development of severe vasculitis. Vasculitis during RA may involve mesenteric (leading to intestinal infarction with acute abdominal pain, intestinal bleeding, and perforation), coronary and cerebral arteries and be associated with severe eye involvement [122]. RA patients with vasculitis are usually characterized by high serum titers of autoantibodies, cryoglobulins and low levels of complement because of its degradation [123]. Digital gangrene and sharply demarcated ulcerations appear mostly at the lower extremities or in sites of skin pressure. Lower extremities ulcers are clinical manifestation of severe, generally in patients with long-standing disease. As previously mentioned, the pathogenesis of leg ulcers is thought to be due to an underlying vasculitis that initiates the lesions, but ulcer expansion and its chronicity may be influenced by other features, including concomitant venous insufficiency, arterial insufficiency, tissue edema, trauma, superimposed infection, and long-term use of glucocorticoids [124]. Skin manifestations are frequently associated with episcleritis, pleural, and pericardial effusion. Episcleritis is a common *ocular involvement* of RA which causes an inflammation of the superficial layer to the sclera and it occurs in less than 1% of patients with RA and is generally a self-limiting condition. Scleritis represents a more aggressive process characterized by an intensely painful inflammation of the sclera. The most frequent ocular manifestation is keratoconjunctivitis sicca which is frequently associated with xerostomia (oral dryness) in a secondary Sjögren's syndrome with salivary gland swelling more rarely found.

RA patients may present with *hematological abnormalities* either at the time of diagnosis or during the course of the disease. In particular, it is possible to find anemia, neutropenia, thrombocytopenia, thrombocytosis, eosinophilia, and hematological malignancies [125]. Anemia is one of the most common extra-articular symptoms of RA and its cause is multifactorial: disease activity drug-induced, nutritional, gastrointestinal bleeding, bone marrow suppression may be due to immunosuppressive therapy and ineffective erythropoiesis [126]. Anemia of chronic disease observed in RA patients usually correlates with disease activity (particular the degree of articular inflammation) and is normochromic/normocytic. Active RA is associated with lymphadenopathy and also with an increased risk of non-Hodgkin lymphoma compared with the general population whose most frequent subtype is large-cell, B cell lymphoma [127]. Chronic neutropenia with splenomegaly in the absence of lymphoma-associated disease occurs in patients with Felty's syndrome (with an incidence of less than 1% of RA patients). As other systemic extra-articular manifestations, Felty's syndrome usually develops in RA patients with long-standing, seropositive, nodular, deforming RA [128]. *Pulmonary involvement* in RA is one of the most frequent extra-articular manifestations, although not always clinically recognized at the first clinical examination. It includes rheumatoid pleuritis, RA-associated interstitial pneumonitis, cryptogenic organizing pneumonia, obliterative bronchiolitis, and intrapulmonary rheumatoid nodules. Pleural disease is common but usually asymptomatic and it is detected only at routine chest X-ray assessment or at autopsy (interestingly autoptic studies reported pleural involvement in nearly 50% of cases, 10% of whom were clinically previously detected) [129]. Pleural effusions are usually exudates with mixed cell counts and high protein concentration with the presence of multinucleated giant cells which are highly specific for RA. The lung involvement in RA patients is frequently associated with exudative pericarditis and with interstitial lung disease. Parenchymal pulmonary nodules generally are asymptomatic and found in autoantibody-positive patients with concomitant rheumatoid nodules elsewhere. During the disease course they can cavitate and cause pleural effusions. Pathological examination of the nodules reveals a central necrotic zone surrounded by a cellular area of proliferating fibroblasts [130]. Interstitial lung disease during RA has an undefined prevalence and natural history because of the heterogeneity in study cohorts and in the diagnostic methods used for its detection and evaluation. The clinical presentation and evolution of RA-associated interstitial lung disease seems to be similar to that of idiopathic pulmonary fibrosis, but with a better response to immunosuppression [131]. The most common radiographic finding is bilateral basilar interstitial abnormalities, which are often asymmetric. Initially, these may appear as patchy alveolar infiltrates until a reticulonodular pattern is seen in patients with progressive disease [132] (Fig. 46.5). High-resolution computed tomography and open lung biopsy are considered the gold standard methods for the diagnosis of interstitial lung disease. The bronchoalveolar lavage can be variable and it can range from lymphocytic alveolitis to neutrophilic inflammation, while histologic findings may show an inflammatory infiltrate with lymphocytes, plasma cells, and histiocytes with varying degrees of fibrosis, and may be classified as usual interstitial pneumonia (UIP) or nonspecific interstitial pneumonia (NSIP) [133]. RA-associated UIP must be distinguished from methotrexate (MTX)–induced lung toxicity, which usually has a subacute onset with rapidly progressive respiratory symptoms, less radiographic evidence of fibrosis and a histologic pattern dominated by eosinophilia and type II pneumocyte hyperplasia [134]. The possibility of a superimposed respiratory tract infection must be considered in the setting of rapid progression of pulmonary symptoms in patients with suspected RA-associated or treatment-related lung involvement.

Pericarditis is one of the most common *cardiac manifestations* in RA, and although symptomatic pericarditis is relatively uncommon, autoptic studies revealed the presence of pericardial inflammation in nearly 50% of RA patients. It usually occurs in autoantibody-positive RA patients with nodules, and analysis of pericardial fluid reveals changes similar to those found in RA-related pleural effusions [135]. Myocarditis (even with the presence of rheumatoid nodules within the myocardium) has been observed in autoptic studies, and myocardial fibrosis can lead to conduction abnormalities. In addition, myocarditis and endocarditis have been observed in autoptic studies with the formation of rheumatoid nodules in the aortic or mitral valves edges that can lead to valvular dysfunction. Arterial stiffness is an important factor in cardiovascular

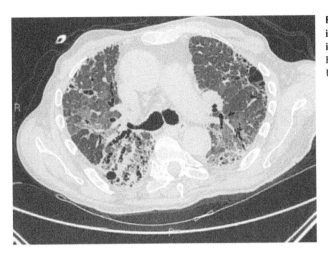

FIGURE 46.5 **CT scan of the lungs of anticitrullinated peptide antibodies/rheumatoid factor–positive rheumatoid arthritis patient with lung involvement.** Property of the Biopsy Unit of the Institute of Rheumatology – Fondazione Policlinico Universitario A. Gemelli - IRCCS – Catholic University of the Sacred Heart, Rome – Italy.

comorbidity in patients with RA and it has been observed that the decreased arterial distensibility correlates with disease severity [136]. RA patients are also more prone to heart conditions such as the thickening of the artery walls (atherosclerosis) and heart attacks [137]. The risk for myocardial infarction in female RA patients is twice that of women without RA, and in long-standing disease of at least 10 years, the risk is three times higher. Among the different factors associated with CVD development in RA patients, the seropositivity for ACPA arose to be associated with the development of ischemic heart disease in RA [138,139]. Interestingly, ACPA positivity is associated with subclinical atherosclerosis in RA patients measured as the carotid intima-media thickness [140], suggesting the pathological role of ACPA antibodies in the disruption of atherosclerotic plaques causing the release of peroxides and peroxynitrites products by neutrophils secondary to the increase of mitochondria depolarization [141].

Kidney involvement in RA (developing as glomerulonephritis and interstitial renal disease) is a rare extra-articular manifestation and may represent the expression of an underlying vasculitis. However, kidney function abnormalities are frequently iatrogenic in RA patients. The most common histological finding is represented by mesangial glomerulonephritis associated with variable levels of interstitial inflammation. Amyloidosis is the most common finding among RA patients with nephritic/nephrotic syndrome [142].

CLINICAL ASSESSMENT

Disease activity is a central aspect in the evaluation of RA patients because it evaluates, at the time of the clinical assessment, signs and symptoms of the disease (i.e., inflammatory pain, swelling, and stiffness). Based on that, the reduction of disease activity is the major target of therapeutic interventions (see below). The overall assessment of the disease activity consists of a complete set of parameters that include counts of swollen and tender joints, patient assessment of pain, patient and evaluator global assessment of disease activity, and measure of the acute-phase response.

Joint Counts

Joint involvement is typically evaluated for soft tissue swelling and effusion (swollen joint count, SJC) and tenderness on pressure or motion (tender joint count, TJC). Several joint indices and counts have been developed over the past 50 years [143] differing mainly for the number of the assessed joints. The comprehensive 66/68-joint count, as suggested by the American Rheumatism Association (ARA; now American College of Rheumatology, ACR) in 1965 [144], is time-consuming, with limited usage in clinical practice. Another index, the Ritchie Articular Index, assesses graded tenderness in 26 joint areas [145,146].

Simplifications of the extensive ACR joint count have been developed over time, reducing the number of assessed joints to 28 [147]. Despite their validity and reliability compared with comprehensive joint counts [148,149], the 28 joints count excludes the assessment of the foot and ankle joints because swelling and tenderness in these joints are frequently present in disorders other than RA [147]. In fact, the 28-joint count became widely accepted and generally used in almost all clinical trials for RA. *VAS pain:* Pain is clearly the predominant symptom in RA patients and its assessment is important in the understanding of the disease impact on patients' life. Most commonly pain is measured on 100-mm horizontal visual analog scales (VASs) on which patients are asked to estimate their feeling based on the previous week because of the fluctuating nature of pain [150].

General Health/Global Health

General health/global health (GH) is a patient self-report "global measure" and it is part of the ACR core data set and a component of multiple composite indices used for RA activity assessment and treatment response. Patients are asked to estimate their health condition from 0 "very well" to 10 "very poor."

Patient Global Assessment

Similarly to pain, the global level of disease activity can be directly rated by the patient ("patient global assessment," PGA). In contrast to pain, it is often valuable to use the rating of a physician and/or an evaluator on the global assessment of disease activity (MD global, EGA). Typically, both are presented together and are measured by using 100-mm VASs.

Composite Indices

RA is a prototype of a multifaceted disease in which the evaluation of any of the available measures does not allow the clinician to reliably identify a patient's disease activity or the response to therapy. Pooled indices combine a number of disease activity measures and have been developed to overcome the previously cited limitations [151–153]. Pooled indices were developed to be used for standardized clinical assessment in clinical trials; however, they have been shown to be very useful in following patients in clinical practice in outpatient settings [154].

The disease activity score (DAS) was developed in 1990 [155]. It is derived by a complex formula which takes into account the Ritchie articular index, SJC over 44 joints, ESR, and GH (not equal to PGA). As the complex Ritchie index for tenderness and the 44 SJC are rarely used in clinical practice and trials, the joint assessment was simplified in 1993 to include the 28-joint counts for both tenderness and swelling (TJC28, SJC28). This index, the DAS28 [148], is calculated with a complex formula using the following parameters: TJC28 (TJC based on 28 joints), SJC28 (SJC based on 28 joints), ESR, and GH.

Currently, there are several modifications of the DAS and the DAS28 available: one modification is the use of CRP instead of ESR (DAS-CRP and DAS28-CRP); another modification is the exclusion of GH. To overcome the major practical limitations of the DAS-based indices, simpler indices have been recently developed. The simplified disease activity index (SDAI) [156] was the first index to include a sum of variables that were untransformed and unweighted. It is characterized by a simple formula (SDAI = SJC28 + TJC28 + PGA [cm] + EGA [cm] + CRP mg/dL) and it has been widely validated using clinical trial data, as well as in daily outpatient settings. The SDAI, DAS, and DAS28 all require laboratory measures (CRP or ESR), which might constitute a limitation in clinical practice because it frequently prevents the immediate assessment because of waiting time for lab results (if available at all). To overcome this issue, the CDAI (clinical disease activity index), which is a simplified index, based solely on clinical measures (CDAI = SJC28 + TJC28 + PGA [cm] + EGA [cm]), has been validated [157]. The CDAI allows making prompt assessment of disease activity, facilitating immediate treatment decisions [158]. The DAS, DAS28, SDAI, and CDAI not only allow us to determine the level of a patient's disease activity but also to categorize disease activity states as high, moderate, and low disease activity and remission. Although they are more similar in patients with severe disease activity, the remission criteria of the SDAI and CDAI are more stringent than those of the DAS28 [159,160] (Table 46.1). Recently an additional more stringent remission definition was created to be used in the assessment of RA patients: the Boolean remission. Based on this definition, an RA patient is classified as having reached the Boolean remission if, at any time, the following parameters are satisfied: TJC and SJC (over 28) ≤ 1 and CRP ≤ 1 mg/dL and PGA ≤ 1 (on a 0–10 scale).

TABLE 46.1 Disease Activity Evaluation With Pooled Indices (DAS, DAS28, SDAI, and CDAI) in Rheumatoid Arthritis Patients

	DAS	DAS28	SDAI	CDAI
Remission	<1.6	≤2.6	≤3.3	≤2.8
Low disease activity	≤2.4	> 2.6 and ≤3.2	≤ 11	≤ 10
Moderate disease activity	>2.4 and ≤3.7	>3.2 and ≤5.1	≤26	≤22
High disease activity	>3.7	>5.1	>26	>22

CDAI, clinical disease activity index; *DAS*, disease activity index; *SDAI*, simplified disease activity index.

DIAGNOSIS

In the last 60 years different classification criteria for RA have been proposed and used worldwide. In 1956 a subcommittee of the ARA developed a set of criteria for RA [161,162], which was subsequently revised in 1958. Disease characteristics (including joint involvement, symptoms duration, and autoimmunity) that showed high specificity (for definite/probable RA) or high sensitivity (for possible RA) were included in this criteria set [162]. Therefore, the 1958 Criteria set was widely used for almost 30 years. However, because of the increasing knowledge in RA pathogenesis and the incoming need to distinguish other forms of seronegative arthritides as spondyloarthritis, calcium pyrophosphate deposition disease, Lyme arthritis, and polymyalgia rheumatic from seronegative RA, the ACR proposed the development of new classification criteria in 1987 [163]. However, it was generally accepted that the 1987 criteria were more specific but less sensitive than the 1958 criteria. Moreover, one consistent criticism of the 1987 criteria was its poor performance mainly related to the low sensitivity in patients with early inflammatory arthritis.

Based on this, and mainly because it was widely recognized that early therapeutic intervention significantly improves the clinical outcomes and reduces joint damage and disability in RA patients [164–166], a new set of classification criteria for RA was developed by a collaborative initiative between ACR and the European League Against Rheumatism (EULAR) in 2010 [167]. As shown in Table 46.2, the 2010 classification criteria can be applied to any patient or otherwise healthy

TABLE 46.2 2010 ACR/EULAR Classification Criteria for Rheumatoid Arthritis

	Score
Target population (who should be tested?): patients who	
1. Have at least 1 joint with definite clinical synovitis (swelling) 2. With the synovitis not better explained by another disease	
Classification criteria for RA (score-based algorithm: add score of categories A–D; a score of ≥6/10 is needed for classification of a patient as having definite RA)	
A. Joint involvement	
1 Large joint	0
2–10 Large joints	1
1–3 Small joints (with or without involvement of large joints)	2
4–10 Small joints (with or without involvement of large joints)	3
>10 Joints (at least 1 small joint)	5
B. Serology (at least 1 test result is needed for classification)	
Negative RF and negative ACPA	0
Low-positive RF or low-positive ACPA	2
High-positive RF or high-positive ACPA	3
C. Acute-phase reactants (at least 1 test result is needed for classification)	
Normal CRP and normal ESR	0
Abnormal CRP or abnormal ESR	1
D. Duration of symptoms	
<6 weeks	0
≥6 weeks	1

Large joints refer to shoulders, elbows, hips, knees, and ankles, whereas small joints refer to the metacarpophalangeal joints, proximal interphalangeal joints, second through fifth metatarsophalangeal joints, thumb interphalangeal joints, and wrists. Negative refers to IU values that are less than or equal to the upper limit of normal (ULN) for the laboratory and assay; low-positive refers to IU values that are higher than the ULN but three times the ULN for the laboratory and assay; high-positive refers to IU values that are three times the ULN for the laboratory and assay. Normal/abnormal is determined by local laboratory standards. Duration of symptoms refers to patient self-report of the duration of signs or symptoms of synovitis (e.g., pain, swelling, tenderness) of joints that are clinically involved at the time of assessment, regardless of treatment status. *ACPA*, anticitrullinated protein antibody; *CRP*, C-reactive protein; *ESR*, erythrocyte sedimentation rate; *RA*, rheumatoid arthritis; *RF*, rheumatoid factor.

individual, as long as two mandatory requirements are met: first, there must be evidence of currently active clinical synovitis (i.e., swelling) in at least 1 joint as determined by an expert assessor. Second, the criteria may be applied only to those patients in whom the observed synovitis is not better explained by another diagnosis. Additional criteria (autoimmunity, acute-phase reactants, joint involvement, and symptoms duration) are then applied to eligible patients providing a score of 0–10, with a score ≥6 being indicative of the presence of definite RA [167].

In clinical practice, to maximize sensitivity, most rheumatologists recommend measuring ACPA together with RF because ACPA have moderate sensitivity, especially for early RA [168]. The simultaneous evaluation of ACPA and RF provides a trade-off between overall sensitivity and specificity. If the clinician wants to maximize sensitivity, then testing for both analytes is recommended, although this may lead to treat patients who are ACPA negative but RF positive and then risking to treat individuals with false-positive results who do not have RA [169]. On the contrary, ACPA alone seems to be a reasonable strategy when the probability of RA is relatively low, such as in patients who have monoarticular involvement only in primary care. However, in rheumatology outpatient setting, in which the probability of RA development is relatively high, measuring ACPA and/or IgM-RF seems to be a reasonable strategy that avoids missing potentially treatable patients [170]. Moreover, it is interesting to note that a relatively extensive isotype usage in the ACPA response was detected in patients with recent onset arthritis and that the presence of IgM ACPA in follow-up samples obtained from RA patients suggests an ongoing activation of new clones of ACPA-producing B cells, reflecting a continuous (re)activation of the RA-specific ACPA response during the course of ACPA-positive RA [171–174]. Therefore, in the diagnostic setting, testing for anti–CCP-2 antibodies represents the gold standard of testing for ACPA with the highest sensitivity and specificity balance in the contest of all the known RA-related autoantibodies.

TREATMENT

Over the past several decades the treatment of RA has been revolutionized by the development of powerful biologic disease-modifying antirheumatic drugs (DMARDs) and by better understanding of how to effectively use conventional DMARDs. A drug can be classified as a DMARD if it (1) has an effect on clinical signs and symptoms, (2) causes a reduction of acute-phase reactants, (3) induces an improvement in the patient's functional status, and (4) reduces the rate of radiographic progression measured by standardized radiological scores. Several lines of evidences have been produced showing that a "treatment window" exists in early RA, during which optimal treatment provides a better long-term outcome. A delay in the administration of DMARD therapy reduces the likelihood of RA patients achieving disease remission and is associated with more rapid radiological progression and worse functional outcomes [175]. Different strategies are available for the treatment of RA: combination therapy can involve a step-up approach, a parallel approach, or a step-down approach (Fig. 46.6). Because early intervention represents one of the most important factors associated with good clinical response in RA patients, the EULAR and ACR developed recommendations for standardization of RA management (see below).

FIGURE 46.6 Therapeutic strategies in the treatment of rheumatoid arthritis patients. In the step-up regimen, treatment begins using one DMARD, and other DMARDs are sequentially added if the patients do not reach an optimal response. In the parallel approach, multiple DMARDs are simultaneously used from the beginning of the therapeutic regimen. In the step-down approach, multiple DMARDs are initially simultaneously used but are subsequently sequentially withdrawn according to the reached clinical response.

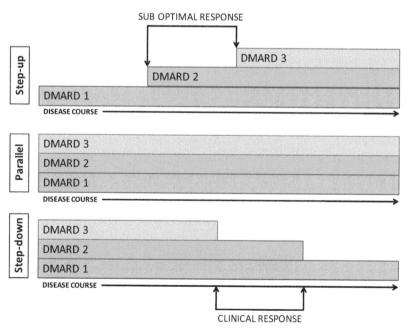

Conventional DMARDs

To date, different conventional DMARDs are available for the treatment of RA such as MTX, sulfasalazine, and leflunomide.

Methotrexate

MTX is widely considered the cornerstone and the drug of first choice in the treatment of RA and may be used as monotherapy as well as in combination with other agents. MTX has demonstrated to be efficacious in the management of RA in multiple studies including both in radiographic and clinical outcomes. It is the first DMARD prescribed following the diagnosis of RA because significant percentage of patients responds favorably to it. MTX inhibits dihydrofolate reductase, an important enzyme for the synthesis of DNA mainly in actively dividing cells. MTX can be given orally or parentally in a once-a-week regimen with a better long-term efficacy and tolerability profile compared with other DMARDs. MTX should be started early in the disease course and rapidly increased to maximal tolerated dose during the first 3–6 months to exert its effects. Furthermore, folate supplementation is recommended with MTX therapy and reduces the frequency and severity of side effects without affecting efficacy.

MTX has a favorable long-term safety profile, and withdrawal of treatment for toxicity is less common than for other DMARDs. Almost 20% of RA patients develop transient elevation of hepatic transaminases but it rarely necessitates treatment discontinuation. Myelosuppression and oral ulcerations may occur, generally responding to folate supplementation. Pulmonary toxicity from MTX may include a hypersensitivity pneumonitis, interstitial fibrosis, pleuritis, pleural effusions, and pulmonary nodules. Hypersensitivity pneumonitis is a rare but life-threatening complication, occurring in less than 0.5% of RA patients. Moreover, being teratogenic, MTX should be discontinued in women who are considering conception. Despite this, the most common reason for discontinuation has been shown to be lack of efficacy rather than toxicity, and retention rates for MTX are higher than those of other DMARDs. Even when biologic agents are used in the management of RA, MTX is generally continued, as it slightly increases circulating levels of infliximab and adalimumab, as well as reduces immunogenicity of the biologic agents [176].

Sulfasalazine

Sulfasalazine is a conventional DMARD that after oral administration undergoes reduction by colonic bacteria into sulfapyridine and 5-aminosalicylic acid. Both derivatives act by inhibiting T cell proliferation, reducing IL-2 production, and enhancing T cell apoptosis. Moreover, sulfasalazine reduces the production of IL-1, IL-6, and TNF-α by monocytes and macrophages. Multiple features make it an acceptable drug to both patient and physician such as being effective in different age groups and in both RF-positive and negative RA patients. Sustained improvement data have been shown over 5–10 years for both clinical and laboratory variables of disease activity. It has been shown to be superior to hydroxychloroquine but equivalent to gold and leflunomide. Several studies analyzed the efficacy of sulfasalazine monotherapy and others its efficacy in combination with other DMARDs using parallel, step-down, or step-up strategies in RA. Studies comparing dual treatment (sulfasalazine and MTX or hydroxychloroquine) to triple therapy (sulfasalazine, MTX, and hydroxychloroquine) showed a significant superiority of the latter [177]. The ability of sulfasalazine in reducing bone damage in RA patients was confirmed as well.

It's thought that nearly 30% of RA patients discontinue sulfasalazine treatment because of side effect. Most of them occur within the first few months of treatment, although not all of them are serious requiring withdrawal. Gastrointestinal manifestations are common with nausea, loss of appetite, and more rarely diarrhea. Even mucocutaneous reactions can occur such as maculopapular rashes, urticaria, and photosensitivity. Moreover, up to 3% of patients can develop leukopenia because of either lymphopenia or neutropenia. Occasionally treated patients may develop minor rises in transaminases level whereas rare is an eosinophilic pneumonia. Although sulfasalazine can be safely continued by women who wish to conceive, a reversible decline in sperm number and morphology can lead in infertility in men even if no association with teratogenicity has been described.

Leflunomide

Leflunomide is an antimetabolite with antiproliferative effects on T lymphocytes through the inhibition of pyrimidine synthesis. Leflunomide effectively blocks the proliferation of human lymphocytes, which are highly dependent on this pathway for nucleotide synthesis [178] leading to the arrest in the G1/S phase of the cell cycle, interrupting the T lymphocytes clonal expansion. Moreover, leflunomide has been shown to inhibit the activation of NF-kB being able to block TNF-mediated NF-kB activation in a dose- and time-dependent manner [179] with an inhibitory effect not limited to cell type, as NF-kB activation was inhibited in myeloid and epithelial cells as well as in T lymphocytes. Leflunomide also inhibits the expression of cell adhesion molecules, which facilitate cellular interactions and diapedesis within the inflamed synovial tissue. Studies on synovial tissues in RA patients receiving leflunomide showed a reduction in synovial macrophages as well as intracellular adhesion molecule-1 and vascular cell adhesion molecule-1 expression with a decreased ratio of matrix metalloproteinase-1 to tissue inhibitor of metalloproteinases-1 [180]. Leflunomide was tested against placebo [181] and against MTX [182] showing that the onset of effect was estimated to occur at a mean of 8.6 weeks for RA patients treated with leflunomide compared with 9.5 weeks for those in MTX treatment. The improvement in tender and SJCs was similar in both groups and the radiographic analyses showed significantly less structural damage in both treatment groups compared with placebo [183]. The ease of administration, its efficacy, and mechanism of action make it a useful alternative to MTX in monotherapy and in combination therapy even with anti–TNF-α agents (see below).

BIOLOGICAL AGENTS

The introduction of biologic agents represented an important advance for the treatment of RA. These agents are efficacious options for patients who did not respond to or are intolerant of conventional DMARDs, allowing not only to improve signs and symptoms of the disease but also to prevent joint damage and future disease severity. They target specific immunological pathways that have been demonstrated being crucial in the pathogenesis of the disease. Biologics can be divided into different categories on the basis of their structure: soluble receptors, monoclonal antibodies, receptor antagonists, and synthetic biologics. Soluble receptors are fusion proteins that combine the ligand-binding regions of receptors normally found on the cells' surface with an immunoglobulin Fc region. Once a cytokine is bound to the soluble receptor, this link prevents it from binding the normal receptor on the cell. Monoclonal antibodies can bind to cytokines in the circulation or to proteins present on the cell surface and once bound, this linkage clears the cytokine from the circulation and prevents its linkage to the target receptor. Moreover, monoclonal antibodies directed against specific proteins on the cell surface can deplete those cells through apoptosis, complement-mediated cell lysis, or Fc receptor–mediated clearance. The receptor antagonist can mimic the function of native proteins and is able to occupy a cell surface receptor preventing the engagement and binding by its specific natural ligand. Finally, the synthetic biologic can mimic the structure of cellular derivatives (i.e., ATP) competing with them in the normal cellular function.

Tumor Necrosis Factor Alpha Inhibitors

TNF-α is a proinflammatory cytokine mainly produced by monocytes and macrophages involved in the normal inflammatory response. It has been found elevated in different rheumatic pathological conditions and in the joint and in the circulation of RA patients. Among its functions, TNF-α recruits inflammatory cells, increases vasodilation and bone damage, and stimulates the production of prostaglandins and collagenase [184]. Among them, infliximab, etanercept, adalimumab, certolizumab, and golimumab are currently available for the treatment of RA. *Infliximab* (Remicade) is a chimeric monoclonal antibody against TNF-α and is used to treat not only RA but also other autoimmune conditions as Crohn's disease, ulcerative colitis, psoriasis, psoriatic arthritis, and ankylosing spondylitis. Infliximab is an artificial antibody. It was originally developed in mice as a mouse antibody. To avoid immune reactions to mouse proteins, the mouse common domains have been replaced with similar human antibody domains. They are monoclonal antibodies and have identical structures and affinities to the target. Recently, infliximab biosimilars have been approved in the European Union (2013), Japan (2014), and United States (2016), respectively (Remsima and Inflectra). *Etanercept* (Enbrel) is a dimeric fusion protein consisting of the extracellular ligand-binding portion of the human 75 kDa (p75) tumor necrosis factor receptor (TNFR) linked to the Fc portion of human IgG1. The Fc component of etanercept contains the CH2 domain, the CH3 domain, and hinge region, but not the CH1 domain of IgG1. Etanercept is produced by recombinant DNA technology in a Chinese hamster ovary mammalian cell expression system and has indication for the treatment of RA, juvenile RA, psoriatic arthritis, plaque psoriasis, and ankylosing spondylitis [185]. Recently, etanercept biosimilar has been approved (Benepali). Etanercept recommended dose for RA is 50 mg weekly. *Adalimumab* (Humira) is a fully human monoclonal antibody against TNF. It binds specifically to TNF-α and blocks its interaction with the p55 and p75 cell surface TNFRs. Adalimumab also lyzes surface TNF expressing cells in vitro in the presence of complement. However, it does not bind or inactivate lymphotoxin (TNF-β). It had been approved by the FDA for the treatment of RA, psoriatic arthritis, ankylosing spondylitis, Crohn's disease, moderate to severe chronic psoriasis, and juvenile idiopathic arthritis. Adalimumab recommended dose for RA is 40 mg every other week. *Certolizumab pegol* (Cimzia) is a recombinant, humanized antibody Fab fragment conjugated to polyethylene glycol (PEG), specific for human TNF-α. The PEG portion is an inert molecule that increases the plasma half-life of the drug. Certolizumab is unable to activate complement or initiate antibody-dependent cellular cytotoxicity (ADCC) because it is structurally different from other anti–TNF-α [186–189]. It can be administered as combination therapy with MTX or as monotherapy. The recommended dose for patients with active RA is 400 mg initially and at weeks 2 and 4, followed by 200 mg every other week. *Golimumab* (Simponi) is a human immunoglobulin G1-kappa monoclonal antibody that is specific for TNF-α and binds to both the soluble and transmembrane forms of human TNF-α. It is a fully human monoclonal antibody with the amino acid sequences of the light and heavy chains identical to those of infliximab [190]. In RA patients the approved dosage of golimumab for the treatment of RA is 50 mg, given subcutaneously once a month [191].

Non-antiTNF agents (Rituximab, Abatacept, Tocilizumab): Both B and T cells are known to play an important role in the pathogenesis of RA. Different randomized control trials have shown that therapies targeting either B or T cells are efficacious in RA treatment. *Anti-CD20 depletion therapy*: B cells role in the pathogenesis of RA is shown by the presence of RF and ACPA in blood and synovial fluid of RA patients. These autoantibodies are already present in the earliest disease stages and may precede disease onset by several years. CD20 is a surface antigen on B cells except for stem cells, early pre-B cells, or plasma cells. *Rituximab* (Rituxan, Mabthera), a genetically engineered chimeric anti-CD20 monoclonal antibody, can deplete CD20 positive cells. Rituximab is able to induce depletion of B cells by different mechanisms. Fc domain of rituximab is recognized by phagocytes, as macrophages, through Fcγ receptor causing the ADCC. Rituximab bound to CD20 on B cells can also cause the activation of complement, which eventually leads to the formation of membrane attack complex and complement-dependent lysis of B cells. In 2001, there was the first report of efficacy of B cells depletion therapy in RA. The precise effect of rituximab was firstly unclear because all the patients, in the previous study, were concomitantly treated with high doses of steroids and cyclophosphamide [192]. To clarify this issue, the first multicentre, randomized, double-blind, placebo-controlled trial was conducted on active RA patients showing that the clinical efficacy was higher in the rituximab groups compared with controls [193]. Subsequently, in the Dose-Ranging Assessment International Clinical Evaluation of Rituximab in RA (DANCER) study, more than 450 seropositive RA patients randomly received placebo, 500 or 1000 mg of rituximab 2 weeks apart. The ACR20 clinical response was higher in the study groups compared with controls (28%, 55%, and 54% of patients in the placebo, 500 and 1000 mg rituximab groups, respectively) and 20% of the patients in the 1000 mg rituximab group reached the ACR70 response [194]. To date, rituximab is approved as a therapeutic choice for RA patients who failed a course of TNF-α blockade therapy (in Italy) (in other countries even approved to be used as a first-line biologic). *Co-stimulation blockade*: The proliferation and the full activation of an antigen-specific T cell need a signal mediated by the specific T cell receptor and at least one co-stimulatory signal by an antigen-presenting cell. Among co-stimulatory molecules, one of the most important involves the interactions between the CD28 and CTLA4 (CD152) molecules and their ligands CD80 (B7-1) and CD86 (B7-2) on the T cell and antigen-presenting cell membrane, respectively. *Abatacept* (Orencia) is a fusion protein made by combining the external domain of human CTLA4 to the heavy chain constant region of the human IgG1. This molecule is able to bind both CD80 and CD86 with high avidity preventing these molecules from linking CD28 on T cells. Different studies have demonstrated that abatacept is efficacious in RA naive/nonnaive to MTX as well as no responder to TNF-α blockade. In MTX-naïve patients with early RA and poor prognostic factors [195], the ACR50 was reached in 57.4% of the active than in 42.3% in the placebo group as well as a less radiographic progression after 1 year. Moreover, in RA patients who failed MTX treatment, abatacept has been shown to be efficacious in achieving the ACR20 response compared with placebo group maintaining this response after 2 or 5 years. Finally, RA patients who had an inadequate response to anti–TNF-α therapy showed an ACR20 response in 50.4% of patients in the abatacept group and only 19.5% of patients in the placebo one after 6 months. Additionally, 10% of patients in the abatacept group reached DAS-defined remission, whereas less than 1% of patients in the placebo were able to reach this endpoint [196]. *Anti–IL-6 receptor*: IL-6 is a pleiotropic proinflammatory cytokine produced by T cells, B cells, lymphocytes, and monocytes in areas affected by inflammation, with a role in T cell activation and immunoglobulin secretion. Its signal transduction is mediated by membrane-bound and soluble IL-6 receptors. *Tocilizumab* (Actemra) is a humanized antihuman IL-6 receptor IgG1 monoclonal antibody against the IL-6 receptor. The efficacy and safety of tocilizumab monotherapy compared with MTX was demonstrated in patients with active RA [197]. The SATORI [198] study confirmed its efficacy and safety in monotherapy in patients with active RA with an inadequate response to MTX. Moreover, the ability of tocilizumab monotherapy to inhibit the progression of structural joint damage was demonstrated in early RA patients showing a significant less progression in the tocilizumab group than the placebo one after 52 weeks of follow-up [199]. Because of the use of TNF-α inhibitor therapy in the therapeutic armamentarium, tocilizumab was tested even in [200] active RA patients refractory to TNF-α blockers. It was shown that the ACR20 response at week 24 was reached by 50% for tocilizumab at the dose of 8 mg/kg and 30.4% for tocilizumab at 4 mg/kg compared with 10.1% for placebo. Tocilizumab is generally well tolerated and the most commonly reported adverse events were upper respiratory tract infections, nasopharyngitis, headache, hypertension, and increased transaminases. The infusion-related events were reported in 7%–8% of patients in tocilizumab-DMARD combination and 5% on the placebo-DMARD combination with headache and skin reactions as the most commonly reported events within the first 24 h of infusion. 1% of patients experienced hypertension for both doses and a clinically significant hypersensitivity reaction was documented in 0.2% of patients. 2% of patients developed antitocilizumab antibodies. Neutropenia (neutrophils count <1000/mm^3) occurred in nearly 3% in the combination DMARD group and 0.1% in the placebo group. Even platelets decrease (platelets count <100,000/mm^3) was found in 1.3% (4 mg/kg) and 1.7% (8 mg/kg) of patients, whereas only in 0.5% of patients in the placebo group, with no bleeding events in any of the groups. Evaluating the incidence of malignancies during tocilizumab treatment, the exposure-adjusted incidence was 1.32 events per 100 patient-years for the tocilizumab groups and 1.37 events per 100 patient-years for the placebo-DMARD groups.

JAK Inhibitors

The Janus kinase (JAK) family of tyrosine kinases includes JAK1, JAK2, JAK3, and TYK2 and is required for signaling through type I and type II cytokine receptors. Once activated, JAKs phosphorylate the signal transducers and activators of transcription (STAT) that subsequently induce the expression of many genes. This pathway is involved in the pathogenesis of RA. Among them, JAK3 is predominantly expressed in cells of the immune system and plays a crucial role for signal transduction from receptors for different cytokines involved in lymphocyte activation, function, and proliferation. *Tofacitinib* (Xeljanz) is a pan-JAK inhibitor that primarily inhibits JAK1 and JAK3. It is the first oral targeted synthetic biological DMARD. In 2012, tofacitinib was approved by the FDA, in monotherapy or in association with other cDMARDs, for treatment of moderate to severe RA in patients with inadequate response or intolerance to MTX. Boyle et al. studied the effects of tofacitinib on synovial pathobiology in a randomized, double-blind, phase II study. They enrolled patients with RA in therapy with MTX but with an inadequate response to this drug. Patients were randomized to receive tofacitinib 10 mg twice a day or placebo for 28 days. A synovial biopsy was performed at day 7 and at day 28 and disease activity was evaluated by DAS28 and EULAR response. In the tofacitinib group, they observed, besides a good clinical response, a reduction in metalloproteinase and interferon-regulated gene expression in rheumatoid synovium. Moreover, they found that reduction in synovial phosphorylation of STAT1 and STAT3 correlated with clinical improvement [201]. Of interest tofacitinib was able to improve patients reported outcomes compared with placebo [202,203]. The recommended dose of tofacitinib for the treatment of RA is 5 mg twice a day. In addition to tofacitinib, other JAK inhibitor molecules have also been studied in RCTs. These molecules show different degrees of specificity toward the four JAKs. Among these new drugs, *Baricitinib* (Olumiant), which is an oral, selective, and reversible inhibitor of JAK1 and JAK2, was approved for the treatment of RA. Baricitinib has been successfully tested in different population of RA patients. In particular, baricitinib was found to be effective in naive and MTX no responder RA patients [204–206]. Moreover, in RA patients, insufficient responder to MTX baricitinib was found to be superior to standard of care as adalimumab [207]. The recommended dose of baricitinib for the treatment of RA is 4 mg daily.

PRACTICE AND PROCEDURE

There is an agreement among rheumatologists that in RA patients the first treatment approach should include synthetic DMARDs because a significant proportion of patients can reach a state of very low disease activity or remission (Fig. 46.7) [208]. Moreover, because any delay in the start of DMARD treatment in RA patients may lead to a worse outcome in comparison with an early start of treatment, a DMARD should be started as soon as a diagnosis of RA has been made. Disease clinical remission is the primary therapeutic aim, especially in early RA, although low disease activity may be an appropriate alternative, especially in patients with long-standing RA. A well-structured follow-up is crucial because it has been shown that reaching a low disease activity or remission by adjusting treatment every 1–3 months in conjunction with strict monitoring is associated with a better clinical, radiographic, and functional outcome. As a general approach, the treatment target should be almost reached, within 3 months and definitely by a maximum of 6 months. This choice comes from the use of a 1–3 months' period for switching treatments in several strategy trials and on data showing that disease activity status at 3–6 months after treatment initiation predicts outcome at later time points [209]. This therapeutic strategy is called "treat to target" strategy.

MTX is considered to be the first choice DMARD in the treatment of RA, both on the basis of its efficacy as monotherapy and on its ability to increase the efficacy of biological DMARDs when used in combination, as well as its beneficial long-term safety profile. To date there is no clear evidence that leflunomide or sulfasalazine is less efficacious compared with MTX. However, because of the more extensive data about MTX efficacy and safety profile, other DMARDs should be used instead of MTX at first, mainly if there are contraindications to (or intolerance of) MTX.

The presence of prognostic markers is an important step in the decision-making phase. Independent factors that can predict a bad outcome are RF and/or ACPA antibodies at high levels, a high disease activity, and early occurrence of erosions.

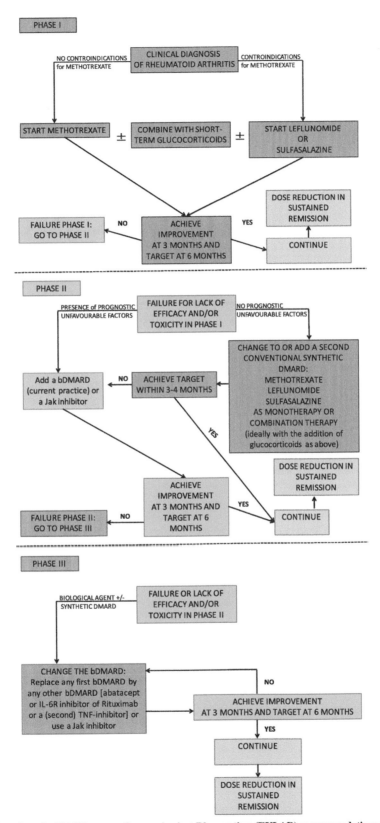

FIGURE 46.7 **Algorithm based on the 2016 European League Against Rheumatism (EULAR) recommendations on rheumatoid arthritis (RA) management.** *ACR*, American College of Rheumatology; *bDMARD*, biological DMARD; *csDMARDs*, conventional synthetic DMARDs; *DMARDs*, disease-modifying antirheumatic drugs; *IL*, interleukin; *TNF*, tumor necrosis factor; *tsDMARDs*, targeted synthetic DMARDs.

According to this, RA patients who failed to reach the treatment target on an initial strategy with synthetic DMARDs, negative for the cited poor prognostic markers should be switched to another synthetic DMARDs strategy for 3–6 months. On the contrary, patients for whom an initial DMARD failed and who have poor prognostic markers should have the opportunity to receive a biological DMARD, in addition to their synthetic DMARDs.

To date, TNF inhibitors (adalimumab, certolizumab pegol, etanercept, golimumab, infliximab, and the EMA/FDA-approved biosimilars), abatacept, IL-6 inhibitors, or rituximab, if approved for such indication, can be started after MTX insufficient response. In RA patients who cannot use conventional DMARDs as comedication, IL-6R inhibitor and synthetic bDMARDs have some advantages. According to the 2016 updated recommendation for the management of RA, the current practice would be to start with a bDMARD (in combination with MTX or another conventional DMARD) because of the long-term experience compared with synthetic DMARDs (JAK inhibitors) (Fig. 46.5).

As stated in the 2016 ACR/EULAR recommendation for the management of RA, stable disease remission represents the main goal in the treatment of RA patients. The updated version of the recommendations now includes the possibility to taper the pharmacological treatment in RA patients reaching the good clinical outcome [208,209]. It's well accepted that despite clinical remission, RA patients may have sign of subclinical synovitis in more that 50% of case and bone damage progression in one-third of patients [210,211]. Moreover, RA patients in stable clinical remission may display signs of synovial inflammation through the ultrasonographic assessment, as Power Doppler signal, whose presence was associated with less success in maintaining disease control after treatment tapering or discontinuation [212–214].

REFERENCES

[1] Gibofsky A. Overview of epidemiology, pathophysiology, and diagnosis of rheumatoid arthritis. Am J Manag Care 2012;18:S295–302.

[2] Helmick CG, Felson DT, Lawrence RC, et al. Estimates of the prevalence of arthritis and other rheumatic conditions in the United States. Part I. Arthritis Rheum 2008;58:15–25.

[3] Doran MF, Pond GR, Crowson CS, et al. Trends in incidence and mortality in rheumatoid arthritis in Rochester, Minnesota, over a forty-year period. Arthritis Rheum 2002;46:625–31. 3.

[4] McInnes IB, Schett G. Pathogenetic insights from the treatment of rheumatoid arthritis. Lancet 2017;10(389):2328–37.

[5] Raychaudhuri S. Recent advances in the genetics of rheumatoid arthritis. Curr Opin Rheumatol 2010;22:109–18.

[6] MacGregor AJ, Snieder H, Rigby AS, et al. Characterizing the quantitative genetic contribution to rheumatoid arthritis using data from twins. Arthritis Rheum 2000;43:30–7.

[7] Gregersen PK, Silver J, Winchester RJ. The shared epitope hypothesis: an approach to understanding the molecular genetics of susceptibility to rheumatoid arthritis. Arthritis Rheum 1987;30:1205–13.

[8] Begovich AB, Carlton VE, Honigberg LA, et al. A missense single-nucleotide polymorphism in a gene encoding a protein tyrosine phosphatase (PTPN22) is associated with rheumatoid arthritis. Am J Hum Genet 2004;75:330–7.

[9] Kurreeman FA, Padyukov L, Marques RB, et al. A candidate gene approach identifies the TRAF1/C5 region as a risk factor for rheumatoid arthritis. PLoS Med 2007;4(9):e278. [Erratum, PLoS Med 2007;4(12):e358.].

[10] Plenge RM, Cotsapas C, Davies L, et al. Two independent alleles at 6q23 associated with risk of rheumatoid arthritis. Nat Genet 2007;39:1477–82.

[11] Symmons DP, Bankhead CR, Harrison BJ, et al. Blood transfusion, smoking, and obesity as risk factors for the development of rheumatoid arthritis: results from a primary care-based incident case-control study in Norfolk, England. Arthritis Rheum 1997;40:1955–61.

[12] Klareskog L, Stolt P, Lundberg K, et al. A new model for an etiology of rheumatoid arthritis: smoking may trigger HLA-DR (shared epitope)-restricted immune reactions to autoantigens modified by citrullination. Arthritis Rheum 2006;54:38–46.

[13] Gremese E, Tolusso B, Gigante MR, et al. Obesity as a risk and severity factor in rheumatic diseases (autoimmune chronic inflammatory diseases). Front Immunol 2014;11(5):576.

[14] Tolusso B, Alivernini S, Gigante MR, et al. Biomolecular features of inflammation in obese rheumatoid arthritis patients: management considerations. Expert Rev Clin Immunol 2016;12:751–62.

[15] Crowson CS, Matteson EL, Davis 3rd JM, et al. Contribution of obesity to the rise in incidence of rheumatoid arthritis. Arthritis Care Res 2013;65:71–7.

[16] Qin B, Yang M, Fu H, et al. Body mass index and the risk of rheumatoid arthritis: a systematic review and dose-response meta-analysis. Arthritis Res Ther 2015;17:86–98.

[17] Kaufmann J, Kielstein V, Killan S, et al. Relation between body mass index and radiological progression in patients with rheumatoid arthritis. J Rheumatol 2003;30:2350–5.

[18] Ajeganova S, Andersson ML. Hafstrom I for the Barfot Study Group. Association of obesity with worse disease severity in Rheumatoid Arthritis as well as with comorbidities: a long-term followup from disease onset. Arthritis Care Res 2013;65:78–87.

[19] Wolfe F, Michaud K. Effect of body mass index on mortality and clinical status in rheumatoid arthritis. Arthritis Care Res 2012;64:1471–9.

[20] Lu B, Hiraki LT, Sparks JA, et al. Being overweight or obese and risk of developing rheumatoid arthritis among women: a prospective cohort study. Ann Rheum Dis 2014;73:1914–22.

[21] Pedersen M, Jacobsen S, Klarlund M, et al. Environmental risk factors differ between rheumatoid arthritis with and without auto-antibodies against cyclic citrullinated peptides. Arthritis Res Ther 2006;8:R133.

[22] Wesley A, Bengtsson C, Elkan AC, et al. Association between body mass index and anti- citrullinated protein antibody-positive and anti-citrullinated protein antibody-negative rheumatoid arthritis: results from a population-based case-control study. Arthritis Care Res 2013;65:107–12.

[23] Lahiri M, Luben RN, Morgan C, et al. Using lifestyle factors to identify individuals at higher risk of inflammatory polyarthritis (results from the European prospective investigation of cancer- Norfolk and the Norfolk arthritis register–the EPIC-2-NOAR study). Ann Rheum Dis 2014;73:219–26.

[24] Heimans L, van den Broek M, le Cessie S, et al. Association of high body mass index with decreased treatment response to combination therapy in recent-onset rheumatoid arthritis patients. Arthritis Care Res 2013;65:1235–42.

[25] Gremese E, Fedele AL, Gigante MR, et al. The body mass index: a determinant of remission in early rheumatoid arthritis. Ann Rheum Dis 2013;72:A113.

[26] Jawaheer D, Olsen J, Lahiff M, et al. Gender, body mass index and rheumatoid arthritis disease activity: results from the QUEST-RA study. Clin Exp Rheumatol 2010;28:454–61.

[27] Stavropoulos-Kalinoglou A, Metsios GS, Panoulas VF, et al. Underweight and obese states both associate with worse disease activity and physical function in patients with established rheumatoid arthritis. Clin Rheumatol 2009;28:439–44.

[28] van der Woude D, Houwing-Duistermaat JJ, Toes RE, et al. Quantitative heritability of anti-citrullinated protein antibody-positive and anti-citrullinated protein antibody-negative rheumatoid arthritis. Arthritis Rheum 2009;60:916–23.

[29] Richardson B. Primer: epigenetics of autoimmunity. Nat Clin Pract Rheumatol 2007;3:521–7.

[30] Filipowicz W, Bhattacharyya SN, Sonenberg N. Mechanisms of post-transcriptional regulation by microRNAs: are the answers in sight? Nat Rev Genet 2008;9:102–14.

[31] Kurowska-Stolarska M, Alivernini S, Ballantine LE, et al. MicroRNA-155 as a proinflammatory regulator in clinical and experimental arthritis. Proc Natl Acad Sci USA 2011;5(108):11193–8.

[32] Alivernini S, Kurowska-Stolarska M, Tolusso B, et al. MicroRNA-155 influences B-cell function through PU.1 in rheumatoid arthritis. Nat Commun 2016;27(7):1297.

[33] Elmesmari A, Fraser AR, Wood C, et al. MicroRNA-155 regulates monocyte chemokine and chemokine receptor expression in Rheumatoid Arthritis. Rheumatology (Oxford) 2016;55:2056–65.

[34] McInnes IB, Schett G, The pathogenesis of rheumatoid arthritis. N Engl J Med 2011;55:2205–19.

[35] Haringman JJ, Gerlag DM, Zwinderman AH, et al. Synovial tissue macro-phages: a sensitive biomarker for response to treatment in patients with rheumatoid arthritis. Ann Rheum Dis 2005;64:834–8.

[36] Seibl R, Birchler T, Loeliger S, et al. Expression and regulation of Toll-like receptor 2 in rheumatoid arthritis synovium. Am J Pathol 2003;162:1221–7.

[37] Murray PJ, et al. Macrophage activation and polarization: nomenclature and experimental guidelines. Immunity 2014;41:14–20.

[38] Lawrence T, Natoli G. Transcriptional regulation of macrophage polarization: enabling diversity with identity. Nat Rev Immunol 2011;11:750–61.

[39] Verreck FA, de Boer T, Langenberg DM, et al. Human IL-23-producing type 1macrophages promote but IL-10-producing type2 macrophages subvert immunity to (myco) bacteria. Proc Natl Acad Sci USA 2004;13:4560–5.

[40] Catrina AI, Svensson CI, Malmström V, et al. Mechanisms leading from systemic autoimmunity to joint-specific disease in rheumatoid arthritis. Nat Rev Rheumatol 2017;13:79–86.

[41] Alivernini S, Fedele AL, Cuoghi I, et al. Citrullination: the loss of tolerance and development of autoimmunity in rheumatoid arthritis. Reumatismo 2008;60:85–94.

[42] Nienhuis RL, Mandema E. A new serum factor in patients with rheumatoid arthritis: the antiperinuclear factor. Ann Rheum Dis 1964;23:302–5.

[43] Sebbag M, et al. The antiperinuclear factor and the so-called antikeratin antibodies are the same rheumatoid arthritis-specific autoantibodies. J Clin Investig 1995;95:2672–9.

[44] Schellekens GA, et al. The diagnostic properties of rheumatoid arthritis antibodies recognizing a cyclic citrullinated peptide. Arthritis Rheum 2000;43:155–63.

[45] Wiik AS, van Venrooij WJ, Pruijn GJ. All you wanted to know about anti-CCP but were afraid to ask. Autoimmun Rev 2010;10:90–3.

[46] Schellekens GA, Visser H, de Jong BA, et al. The diagnostic properties of rheumatoid arthritis antibodies recognizing a cyclic citrullinated peptide. Arthritis Rheum 2000;43:155–63.

[47] Nielen MM, van der Horst AR, van Schaardenburg D, et al. Antibodies to citrullinated human fibrinogen (ACF) have diagnostic and prognostic value in early arthritis. Ann Rheum Dis 2005;64:1199–204.

[48] Rantapaa-Dahlqvist S, de Jong BA, Berglin E, et al. Antibodies against cyclic citrullinated peptide and IgA rheumatoid factor predict the development of rheumatoid arthritis. Arthritis Rheum 2003;48:2741–9.

[49] Majka DS, Deane KD, Parrish LA, et al. Duration of preclinical rheumatoid arthritis-related autoantibody positivity increases in subjects with older age at time of disease diagnosis. Ann Rheum Dis 2008;67:801–7.

[50] O'Dell JR. Treating rheumatoid arthritis early: a window of opportunity? Arthritis Rheum 2002;46:283–5.

[51] Brink M, Hansson M, Mathsson L, et al. Multiplex analyses of antibodies against citrullinated peptides in individuals prior to development of rheumatoid arthritis. Arthritis Rheum 2013;65:899–910.

[52] Sokolove J, Bromberg R, Deane KD, et al. Autoantibody epitope spreading in the pre-clinical phase predicts progression to rheumatoid arthritis. PLoS One 2012;7:e35296.

[53] Deane KD, O'Donnell CI, Hueber W, et al. The number of elevated cytokines/chemokines in pre-clinical seropositive rheumatoid arthritis predicts time to diagnosis in an age-dependent manner. Arthritis Rheum 2010;62:3161–728.

[54] Kokkonen H, Soderstrom I, Rocklov J, et al. Up-regulation of cytokines and chemokines predates the onset of rheumatoid arthritis. Arthritis Rheum 2010;62:383–91.

[55] Clavel C, Nogueira L, Laurent L, et al. Induction of macrophage secretion of tumor necrosis factor alpha through Fcgamma receptor IIa engagement by rheumatoid arthritis-specific autoantibodies to citrullinated proteins complexed with fibrinogen. Arthritis Rheum 2008;58:678–88.

[56] Sokolove J, Zhao X, Chandra PE, et al. Immune complexes containing citrullinated fibrinogen costimulate macrophages via Toll-like receptor 4 and Fcgamma receptor. Arthritis Rheum 2011;63:53–62.

[57] Trouw LA, Haisma EM, Levarht EW, et al. Anti-cyclic citrullinated peptide antibodies from rheumatoid arthritis patients activate complement via both the classical and alternative pathways. Arthritis Rheum 2009;60:1923–31.

[58] Harre U, Georgess D, Bang H, et al. Induction of osteoclastogenesis and bone loss by human autoantibodies against citrullinated vimentin. J Clin Investig 2012;122:1791–802.

[59] Arnold JN, Wormald MR, Sim RB, et al. The impact of glycosylation on the biological function and structure of human immunoglobulins. Annu Rev Immunol 2007;25:21–50.

[60] Rombouts Y, Ewing E, van de Stadt LA, et al. Anti-citrullinated protein antibodies acquire a pro-inflammatory Fc glycosylation phenotype prior to the onset of rheumatoid arthritis. Ann Rheum Dis 2015;74:234–41.

[61] van de Sande MG, de Hair MJ, van der Leij C, et al. Different stages of rheumatoid arthritis: features of the synovium in the preclinical phase. Ann Rheum Dis 2011;70:772–7.

[62] England BR, Thiele GM, Mikuls TR. Anticitrullinated protein antibodies: origin and role in the pathogenesis of rheumatoid arthritis. Curr Opin Rheumatol 2017;29:57–64.

[63] Malmström V, Catrina AI, Klareskog L. The immunopathogenesis of Seropositive rheumatoid arthritis: from triggering to targeting. Nat Rev Immunol 2017;17:60–75.

[64] Bosello S, Fedele AL, Peluso G, et al. Very early rheumatoid arthritis is the major predictor of major outcomes: clinical ACR remission and radiographic non-progression. Ann Rheum Dis July 2011;70(7):1292–5.

[65] Llorente I, Merino L, Ortiz AM, et al. Anti-citrullinated protein antibodies are associated with decreased bone mineral density: baseline data from a register of early arthritis patients. Rheumatol Int 2017;37:799–806.

[66] Degboé Y, Constantin A, Nigon D, et al. Predictive value of autoantibodies from anti-CCP2, anti-MCV and anti-human citrullinated fibrinogen tests, in early rheumatoid arthritis patients with rapid radiographic progression at 1 year: results from the ESPOIR cohort. RMD Open 2015;1:e000180.

[67] Krishnamurthy A, Joshua V, Haj Hensvold A, et al. Identification of a novel chemokine-dependent molecular mechanism underlying rheumatoid arthritis-associated autoantibody-mediated bone loss. Ann Rheum Dis 2016;75:721–9.

[68] Kleyer A, Finzel S, Rech J, et al. Bone loss before the clinical onset of rheumatoid arthritis in subjects with anticitrullinated protein antibodies. Ann Rheum Dis 2014;73:854–60.

[69] Li S, Yu Y, Yue Y, et al. Autoantibodies from single circulating plasmablasts react with citrullinated antigens and porphyromonas gingivalis in rheumatoid arthritis. Arthritis Rheumatol 2016;68:614–26.

[70] Jimenez-Boj E, Redlich K, Türk B, et al. Interaction between synovial inflammatory tissue and bone marrow in rheumatoid arthritis. J Immunol 2005;175:2579–88.

[71] Nishimura K, Sugiyama D, Kogata Y, et al. Meta-analysis: diagnostic accuracy of anti-cyclic citrullinated peptide antibody and rheumatoid factor for rheumatoid arthritis. Ann Intern Med 2007;146:797–808.

[72] Riedemann JP, Muñoz S, Kavanaugh A. The use of second generation anti-CCP antibody (anti-CCP2) testing in rheumatoid arthritis—a systematic review. Clin Exp Rheumatol 2005;23:S69–76.

[73] Pietrapertosa D, Tolusso B, Gremese E, et al. Diagnostic performance of anti-citrullinated peptide antibodies for the diagnosis of rheumatoid arthritis: the relevance of likelihood ratios. Clin Chem Lab Med 2010;48:829–34.

[74] Lebre MC, Jongbloed SL, Tas SW, et al. Rheumatoid arthritis synovium contains two sub-sets of CD83-DC-LAMP-dendritic cells with distinct cytokine profiles. Am J Pathol 2008;172:940–50.

[75] Schröder AE, Greiner A, Seyfert C, et al. Differentiation of B cells in the nonlymphoid tissue of the synovial membrane of patients with rheumatoid arthritis. Proc Natl Acad Sci USA 1996;93:221–5.

[76] Cantaert T, Brouard S, Thurlings RM, et al. Alterations of the synovial T cell repertoire in anti-citrullinated protein anti-body-positive rheumatoid arthritis. Arthritis Rheum 2009;60:1944–56.

[77] Humby F, Bombardieri M, Manzo A, et al. Ectopic lymphoid structures support ongoing production of class-switched autoantibodies in rheumatoid synovium. PLoS Med 2009;6(1):e1.

[78] Tak PP, Doorenspleet ME, de Hair MJH, et al. Dominant B cell receptor clones in peripheral blood predict onset of arthritis in individuals at risk for rheumatoid arthritis. Ann Rheum Dis November 2017;76(11):1924–30.

[79] Doorenspleet ME, Klarenbeek PL, de Hair MJ, et al. Rheumatoid arthritis synovial tissue harbours dominant B-cell and plasma-cell clones associated with autoreactivity. Ann Rheum Dis April 2014;73(4):756–62.

[80] Chabaud M, Fossiez F, Taupin JL, et al. Enhancing effect of IL-17 on IL-1-induced IL-6 and leukemia inhibitory factor production by rheumatoid arthritis synoviocytes and its regulation by Th2 cytokines. J Immunol 1998;161:409–14. 34.

[81] Miossec P, Korn T, Kuchroo VK. Interleukin-17 and type 17 helper T cells. N Engl J Med 2009;361:888–98.

[82] Behrens F, Himsel A, Rehart S, et al. Imbalance in distribution of functional autologous regulatory T cells in rheumatoid arthritis. Ann Rheum Dis 2007;66:1151–6.

[83] Nadkarni S, Mauri C, Ehrenstein MR. Anti-TNF-alpha therapy induces a distinct regulatory T cell population in patients with rheumatoid arthritis via TGF-beta. J Exp Med 2007;204:33–9. [Erratum, J Exp Med 2007;204:205.].

[84] Goekoop-Ruiterman YP, de Vries-Bouwstra JK, Allaart CF, et al. Clinical and radiographic outcomes of four different treatment strategies in patients with early rheumatoid arthritis (the BeSt study): a randomized, controlled trial. Arthritis Rheum 2005;52(11):3381–90.

[85] Fleming A, Crown JM, Corbett M. Early rheumatoid disease. I. Onset. Ann Rheum Dis 1976;35(4):357–60.

[86] Guerne PA, Weisman MH. Palindromic rheumatism: part of or apart from the spectrum of rheumatoid arthritis. Am J Med 1992;93(4):451–60.

[87] McCarty DJ, O'Duff y JD, Pearson L, et al. Remitting seronegative symmetrical synovitis with pitting edema. RS3PE syndrome. JAMA 1985;254(19):2763–7.

[88] Yamaguchi M, Ohta A, Tsunematsu T, et al. Preliminary criteria for classification of adult Still's disease. J Rheumatol 1992;19(3):424–30.

[89] Fautrel B, Le Moël G, Saint-Marcoux B, et al. Diagnostic value of ferritin and glycosylated ferritin in adult onset Still's disease. J Rheumatol 2001;28(2):322–9.

[90] Lee DM, Weinblatt ME. Rheumatoid arthritis. Lancet 2001;358(9285):903–11.

[91] Fleming A, Benn RT, Corbett M, et al. Early rheumatoid disease. II. Patterns of joint involvement. Ann Rheum Dis 1976;35(4):361–4.

[92] Gray RG, Gottlieb NL. Hand flexor tenosynovitis in rheumatoid arthritis. Prevalence, distribution, and associated rheumatic features. Arthritis Rheum 1977;20(4):1003–8.

[93] Soeroso J. Review article: hand deformities in rheumatoid arthritis. Folia Med Indones 2006;42(4):262–9.

[94] Hastings DE, Evans JA. Rheumatoid wrist deformities and their relation to ulnar drift. J Bone Joint Surg Am 1975;57(7):930–4.

[95] Read GO, Solomon L, Biddulph S. Relationship between finger and wrist deformities in rheumatoid arthritis. Ann Rheum Dis 1983;42(6):619–25.

[96] Dorfman HD, Norman A, Smith RJ. Bone erosion in relation to subcutaneous rheumatoid nodules. Arthritis Rheum 1970;13(1):69–73.

[97] Roddy E, Lim V, Fairbairn KJ, et al. Ruptured "Baker's-type cyst" of the arm-a case study. Rheumatology (Oxford) 2003;42(5):704–5.

[98] Burra G, Katchis SD. Rheumatoid arthritis of the forefoot. Rheum Dis Clin North Am 1998;24(1):173–80.

[99] Trieb K. Management of the foot in rheumatoid arthritis. J Bone Joint Surg Br 2005;87(9):1171–7.

[100] Calabro JJ. A critical evaluation of the diagnostic features of the feet in rheumatoid arthritis. Arthritis Rheum 1962;5:19–29.

[101] Miyamoto N, Senda M, Hamada M, et al. Talo-navicular joint abnormalities and walking ability of patients with rheumatoid arthritis. Acta Med Okayama 2004;58(2):85–90.

[102] Rask MR. Achilles tendon rupture owing to rheumatoid disease. Case report with a nine-year follow-up. JAMA 1978;239(5):435–6.

[103] Jayson MI, Dixon AS. Valvular mechanisms in juxta-articular cysts. Ann Rheum Dis 1970;29(4):415–20.

[104] Lehtimaki MY, Kautiainen H, Hämäläinen MM, et al. Hip involvement in seropositive rheumatoid arthritis. Survivorship analysis with a 15-year follow-up. Scand J Rheumatol 1998;27(6):406409.

[105] van Eijk IC, Nielen MM, van Soesbergen RM, et al. Cervical spine involvement is rare in early arthritis. Ann Rheum Dis 2006;65(7):973–4.

[106] Zhu S, Xu W, Luo Y, et al. Cervical spine involvement risk factors in rheumatoid arthritis: a meta-analysis. Int J Rheum Dis May 2017;20(5):541–9.

[107] Rawlins BA, Girardi FP, Boachie-Adjei O. Rheumatoid arthritis of the cervical spine. Rheum Dis Clin North Am 1998;24(1):55–65.

[108] Aggarwal A, Kulshreshtha A, Chaturvedi V, et al. Cervical spine involvement in rheumatoid arthritis: prevalence and relationship with overall disease severity. J Assoc Physicians India July 1996;44(7):468–71.

[109] Khong TK, Rooney PJ. Manubriosternal joint subluxation in rheumatoid arthritis. J Rheumatol 1982;9(5):712–5.

[110] Yood RA, Goldenberg DL. Sternoclavicular joint arthritis. Arthritis Rheum 1980;23(2):232–9.

[111] Goupille P, Fouquet B, Goga D, et al. The temporomandibular joint in rheumatoid arthritis: correlations between clinical and tomographic features. J Dent 1993;21(3):141–6.

[112] Kolman J, Morris I. Cricoarytenoid arthritis: a cause of acute upper airway obstruction in rheumatoid arthritis. Can J Anaesth 2002;49(7):729–32.

[113] Chen JJ, Branstetter BFT, Myers EN. Cricoarytenoid rheumatoid arthritis: an important consideration in aggressive lesions of the larynx. Am J Neeuroradiol 2005;26(4):970–2.

[114] Cimmino MA, Salvarani C, Macchioni P, et al. Extra-articular manifestations in 587 Italian patients with rheumatoid arthritis. Rheumatol Int 2000;19(6):213–7.

[115] Turesson C, McClelland RL, Christianson TJ, et al. Severe extra-articular disease manifestations are associated with an increased risk of first ever cardiovascular events in patients with rheumatoid arthritis. Ann Rheum Dis 2007;66:70–5.

[116] Doran MF, Crowson CS, Pond GR, et al. Predictors of infection in rheumatoid arthritis. Arthritis Rheum 2002;46:2294–300.

[117] Turesson C, Schaid DJ, Weyand CM, et al. Association of smoking and HLA-C3 with vasculitis in patients with rheumatoid arthritis. Arthritis Rheum 2006;54:2776–83.

[118] Schneider F. AA amyloidosis in inflammatory rheumatic diseases. A report of clinical experiences. Z Rheumatol 1992;51:177–82.

[119] Cojocaru M, Cojocaru IM, Silosi I, et al. Extra-articular manifestations in rheumatoid arthritis. Maedica (Buchar) December 2010;5(4):286–91.

[120] Raven RW, Weber FP, Price LW. The necrobiotic nodules of rheumatoid arthritis. Ann Rheum Dis 1948;7:63–75.

[121] Turesson C, Jacobsson L, Bergström U, et al. Predictors of extra-articular manifestations in rheumatoid arthritis. Scand J Rheumatol 2000;29:358–64.

[122] Sokoloff L, McCluskey RT, Bunim JJ. Vascularity of the early subcutaneous nodule in rheumatoid arthritis. Arch Pathol 1953;55:475–95.

[123] Foster AC, Forstot SL, Wilson LA. Mortality rate in rheumatoid arthritis patients developing necrotizing scleritis or peripheral ulcerative keratitis: effects of systemic immunosuppression. Ophthalmology 1984;91:1253–63.

[124] Scott DG, Bacon PA, Allen C, et al. IgG rheumatoid factor, complement and immune complexes in rheumatoid synovitis and vasculitis: comparative and serial studies during cytotoxic therapy. Clin Exp Immunol 1981;43:54–63.

[125] Pun YL, Barraclough DR, Muirden KD. Leg ulcers in rheumatoid arthritis. Med J Aust 1990;153:585–7.

[126] Bowman SJ. Hematological manifestations of rheumatoid arthritis. Scand J Rheumatol 2002;31(5):251–9.

[127] Agrawal S, Misra R, Aggarwal A. Anemia in rheumatoid arthritis: high prevalence of iron-deficiency anemia in Indian patients. Rheumatol Int October 2006;26(12):1091–5.

[128] Baecklund E, Iliadou A, Askling J, et al. Association of chronic inflammation, not its treatment, with increased lymphoma risk in rheumatoid arthritis. Arthritis Rheum 2006;54:692–701.

[129] Saway PA, Prasthofer EF, Barton JC. Prevalence of granular lymphocyte proliferations in patients with rheumatoid arthritis and neutropenia. Am J Med 1989;86:303–7.

[130] Turesson C, O'Fallon WM, Crowson CS, et al. Occurrence of extra-articular disease manifestations is associated with excess mortality in a community based cohort of patients with rheumatoid arthritis. J Rheumatol 2002;29:62–7.

[131] Highton J, Hung N, Hessian P, et al. Pulmonary rheumatoid nodules demonstrating features usually associated with rheumatoid synovial membrane. Rheumatology (Oxford) 2007;34(13):997–1004.

[132] Scott DG, Bacon PA. Response to methotrexate in fibrosing alveolitis associated with connective tissue disease. Thorax 1980;35:725–31.

[133] Tanoue LT. Pulmonary manifestations of rheumatoid arthritis. Clin Chest Med 1998;19:667–85.

[134] Kim DS. Interstitial lung disease in rheumatoid arthritis: recent advances. Curr Opin Pulm Med 2006;12:346–53.

[135] Kremer JM, Alarcón GS, Weinblatt ME, et al. Clinical, laboratory, radiographic, and histopathologic features of methotrexate-associated lung injury in patients with rheumatoid arthritis: a multicenter study with literature review. Arthritis Rheum 1997;40:1829–37.

[136] Van Doornum S, McColl G, Wicks IP. Accelerated atherosclerosis: an extra-articular feature of rheumatoid arthritis? Arthritis Rheum 2002;46:862–73. 49.

[137] Liang KP, Kremers HM, Crowson CS. Autoantibodies and the risk of cardiovascular events. J Rheumatol 2009;36(11):2378–9.

[138] Solomon DH, Karlson EW, Rimm EB. Cardiovascular morbidity and mortality in women diagnosed with rheumatoid arthritis. Circulation 2003;107:1303–7.

[139] Sokolove J, Brennan MJ, Sharpe O, et al. Brief report: citrullination within the atherosclerotic plaque: a potential target for the anti-citrullinated protein antibody response in rheumatoid arthritis. Arthritis Rheum July 2013;65(7):1719–24.

[140] López-Longo FJ, Oliver-Miñarro D, de la Torre I, et al. Association between anti-cyclic citrullinated peptide antibodies and ischemic heart disease in patients with rheumatoid arthritis. Arthritis Rheum April 15, 2009;61(4):419–24.

[141] Barbarroja N, Pérez-Sanchez C, Ruiz-Limon P, et al. Anticyclic citrullinated protein antibodies are implicated in the development of cardiovascular disease in rheumatoid arthritis. Arterioscler Thromb Vasc Biol December 2014;34(12):2706–16.

[142] Vázquez-Del Mercado M, Nuñez-Atahualpa L, Figueroa-Sánchez M, et al. Serum levels of anticyclic citrullinated peptide antibodies, interleukin-6, tumor necrosis factor-α, and C-reactive protein are associated with increased carotid intima-media thickness: a cross-sectional analysis of a cohort of rheumatoid arthritis patients without cardiovascular risk factors. Biomed Res Int 2015;2015:342649.

[143] Ward MM. Clinical and laboratory measures. In: St Clair EW, Pisetsky DS, Haynes BF, editors. Rheumatoid arthritis. Philadelphia: Lippincott Williams & Wilkins; 2004. p. 51–63.

[144] Deandrade JR, Casagrande PA. A seven-day variability study of 499 patients with peripheral rheumatoid arthritis. Arthritis Rheum 1965;19:302–34.

[145] Ritchie DM, Boyle JA, McInnes IM, et al. Clinical studies with an articular index for the assessment of joint tenderness in patients with rheumatoid arthritis. Q J Med 1968;37:393–406.

[146] Hart LE, Tugwell P, Buchanan WW, et al. Grading of tenderness as a source of interrater error in the Ritchie articular index. J Rheumatol 1985;12:716–7.

[147] Fuchs HA, Brooks RH, Callahan LF, et al. A simplified twenty-eight joint quantitative articular index in rheumatoid arthritis. Arthritis Rheum 1989;32:531–7.

[148] Prevoo ML, van Riel PL, van't Hof MA, et al. Validity and reliability of joint indices: a longitudinal study in patients with recent onset rheumatoid arthritis. Br J Rheumatol 1993;32:589–94.

[149] Smolen JS, Breedveld FC, Eberl G, et al. Validity and reliability of the twenty-eight-joint count for the assessment of rheumatoid arthritis activity. Arthritis Rheum 1995;38:38–43.

[150] Carlsson AM. Assessment of chronic pain. I. Aspects of the reliability and validity of the visual analogue scale. Pain 1983;16:87–101. 25.

[151] Tugwell P, Bombardier C. A methodologic framework for developing and selecting endpoints in clinical trials. J Rheumatol 1982;9:758–62.

[152] Goldsmith CH, Smythe HA, Helewa A. Interpretation and power of a pooled index. J Rheumatol 1993;20:575–8.

[153] Schulz KF, Grimes DA. Multiplicity in randomised trials I: endpoints and treatments. Lancet 2005;365:1591–5.

[154] Grigor C, Capell H, Stirling A, et al. Effect of a treatment strategy of tight control for rheumatoid arthritis (the TICORA study): a single-blind randomised controlled trial. Lancet 2004;364:263–9.

[155] van der Heijde DM, van't Hof MA, van Riel PL, et al. Judging disease activity in clinical practice in rheumatoid arthritis: first step in the development of a disease activity score. Ann Rheum Dis 1990;49:916–20.

[156] Smolen JS, Breedveld FC, Schiff MH, et al. A simplified disease activity index for rheumatoid arthritis for use in clinical practice. Rheumatology (Oxford) 2003;42:244257.

[157] Aletaha D, Nell VP, Stamm T, et al. Acute phase reactants add little to composite disease activity indices for rheumatoid arthritis: validation of a clinical activity score. Arthritis Res Ther 2005;7:R796–806.

[158] Grigor C, Capell H, Stirling A, et al. Effect of a treatment strategy of tight control for rheumatoid arthritis (the TICORA study): a single-blind randomised controlled trial. Lancet 2004;364:263–9.

[159] Aletaha D, Ward MM, Machold KP, et al. Remission and active disease in rheumatoid arthritis: defining criteria for disease activity states. Arthritis Rheum 2005;52:2625–36.

[160] Mierau M, Schoels M, Gonda G, et al. Assessing remission in clinical practice. Rheumatology (Oxford) 2007;46:975–9.

[161] Bongartz T, Cantaert T, Atkins SR, etal. Citrullination in extra-articular manifestations of rheumatoid arthritis. Rheumatology (Oxford) 2007;46(1):70–5.

[162] Bennett GA, Cobb S, Jacox R, et al. Proposed diagnostic criteria for rheumatoid arthritis. Bull Rheum Dis 1956;7(4):121–4.

[163] Ropes MW, Bennett GA, Cobb S, et al. Proposed diagnostic criteria for rheumatoid arthritis. Ann Rheum Dis 1957;16(1):118–25.

[164] Arnett FC, Edworthy SM, Bloch DA, et al. The American Rheumatism Association 1987 revised criteria for the classification of rheumatoid arthritis. Arthritis Rheum 1988;31:315–24.

[165] Van der Heide A, Jacobs JW, Bijlsma JW, et al. The effectiveness of early treatment with "second-line" antirheumatic drugs: a randomized, controlled trial. Ann Intern Med 1996;124:699–707.

[166] Bukhari MA, Wiles NJ, Lunt M, et al. Influence of disease-modifying therapy on radiographic outcome in inflammatory polyarthritis at five years: results from a large observational inception study. Arthritis Rheumatol 2003;48:46–53.

[167] Van Dongen H, van Aken J, Lard LR, et al. Efficacy of methotrexate treatment in patients with probable rheumatoid arthritis: a double-blind, randomized, placebo-controlled trial. Arthritis Rheum 2007;56:1424–32.

[168] Aletaha D, Neogi T, Silman AJ, et al. 2010 rheumatoid arthritis classification criteria. An Merican College of rheumatology/European League against rheumatism collaborative initiative. Arthritis Rheumatol 2010;62(9):2569–81.

[169] Bas S, Genevay S, Meyer O, et al. Anti-cyclic citrullinated peptide antibodies, IgM and IgA rheumatoid factors in the diagnosis and prognosis of rheumatoid arthritis. Rheumatology 2003;42:677–80.

[170] Nishimura K, Sugiyama D, Kogata Y, et al. Meta-analysis: diagnostic accuracy of anti-cyclic citrullinated peptide antibody and rheumatoid factor for rheumatoid arthritis. Ann Intern Med 2007;146:797–808.

[171] Nell VP, Machold KP, Stamm TA, et al. Autoantibody profiling as early diagnostic and prognostic tool for rheumatoid arthritis. Ann Rheum Dis 2005;64:1731–6.

[172] Verpoort KN, Jol-van der Zijde CM, Papendrecht-van der Voort EA, et al. Isotype distribution of anti-cyclic citrullinated peptide antibodies in undifferentiated arthritis and rheumatoid arthritis reflects an ongoing immune response. Arthritis Rheumatol 2006;54:3799–808.

[173] Ärlestig L, Mullazehi M, Kokkonen H, et al. Antibodies against cyclic citrullinated peptides of IgG, IgA and IgM isotype and rheumatoid factor of IgM and IgA isotype are increased in unaffected members of multicase rheumatoid arthritis families from northern Sweden. Ann Rheum Dis 2012;71:825–9.

[174] Ramos-Remus C, Castillo-Ortiz JD, Aguilar-Lozano L, et al. Autoantibodies in prediction of the development of rheumatoid arthritis among healthy relatives of patients with the disease. Arthritis Rheumatol 2015;67:2837–44.

[175] Hensvold AH, Frisell T, Magnusson PK, et al. How well do ACPA discriminate and predict RA in the general population: a study based on 12 590 population-representative Swedish twins. Ann Rheum Dis 2017;76:119–25.

[176] Dale J, Alcorn N, Capell H, et al. Combination therapy for rheumatoid arthritis: methotrexate and sulfasalazine together or with other DMARDs. Nat Clin Pract Rheumatol 2007;3:450–8.

[177] Visser K, Katchamart W, Loza E, et al. Multinational evidence-based recommendations for the use of methotrexate in rheumatic disorders with a focus on rheumatoid arthritis: integrating systematic literature research and expert opinion of a broad international panel of rheumatologists in the 3E Initiative. Ann Rheum Dis 2009;68:1086–93.

[178] O'Dell JR, Leff R, Paulsen G, et al. Treatment of rheumatoid arthritis with methotrexate and hydroxychloroquine, methotrexate and sulfasalazine, or a combination of the three medications: results of a two-year, randomized, double-blind, placebo-controlled trial. Arthritis Rheum 2002;46:1164–70.

[179] Davis JP, Kain GA, Pitts WJ, et al. The immunosuppressive metabolite of leflunomide is a potent inhibitor of human dihydro-orotate dehydrogenase. Biochemestry 1996;35:1270–3.

[180] Manna SK, Aggarwal BB. Immunosuppressive leflunomide metabolite (A77 1726) blocks TNF-dependent nuclear factor-kB activation and gene expression. J Immunol 1999;162:2095–102.

[181] Kraan MC, Smeets TJ, Van Loon MJ, et al. Differential effects of leflunomide and methotrexate on cytokine production on Rheumatiod Arthritis. Ann Rheum Dis 2004;63:1056–61.

[182] Mladenovic V, Domljan Z, Rozman B, et al. Safety and effectiveness of leflunomide in the treatment of patients with active rheumatoid arthritis. Results of a randomized, placebo-controlled, phase II study. Arthritis Rheum 1995;38:1595–603.

[183] Strand V, Cohen S, Schiff M, et al. Treatment of active rheumatoid arthritis with leflunomide compared with placebo and methotrexate. Leflunomide Rheumatoid Arthritis Investigators Group. Arch Intern Med 1999;22(159):2542–50.

[184] Emery P, Breedveld FC, Lemmel EM, et al. A comparison of the efficacy and safety of leflunomide and methotrexate for the treatment of rheumatoid arthritis. Rheumatology (Oxford) 2000;39:655–65.

[185] Feldmann M, Maini RN. TNF defined as a therapeutic target for rheumatoid arthritis and other autoimmune diseases. Nat Med 2003;9:1245–50.

[186] Peppel K. A tumor necrosis factor (TNF) receptor-IgG heavy chain chimeric protein as a bivalent antagonist of TNF activity. J Exp Med 1991;174(6):1483–9.

[187] Keystone E, Heijde D, Mason Jr D, et al. Certolizumab pegol plus methotrexate is significantly more effective than placebo plus methotrexate in active rheumatoid arthritis: findings of a fifty-two-week, phase III, multicenter, randomized, double-blind, placebo-controlled, parallel-group study. Arthritis Rheumatol 2008;58:3319–29.

[188] Smolen J, Landewe RB, Mease P, et al. Efficacy and safety of certolizumab pegol plus methotrexate in active rheumatoid arthritis: the RAPID 2 study. A randomised controlled trial. Ann Rheum Dis 2009;68:797–804.

[189] Fleischmann R, Vencovsky J, van Vollenhoven RF, et al. Efficacy and safety of certolizumab pegol monotherapy every 4 weeks in patients with rheumatoid arthritis failing previous disease-modifying antirheumatic therapy: the FAST4WARD study. Ann Rheum Dis 2009;68:805–11.

[190] Emery P, Fleischmann RM, Moreland LW, et al. Golimumab, a human anti-tumor necrosis factor alpha monoclonal antibody, injected subcutaneously every four weeks in methotrexate-naive patients with active rheumatoid arthritis: twenty-four-week results of a phase III, multicenter, randomized, double-blind, placebo-controlled study of golimumab before methotrexate as first-line therapy for early-onset rheumatoid arthritis. Arthritis Rheum 2009;60:2272–83.

[191] Smolen JS, Kay J, Doyle MK, et al. Golimumab in patients with active rheumatoid arthritis after treatment with tumour necrosis factor alpha inhibitors (GO-AFTER study): a multi- centre, randomised, double-blind, placebo-controlled, phase III trial. Lancet 2009;374:210–21.

[192] Edwards JC, Cambridge G. Sustained improvement in rheumatoid arthritis following a protocol designed to deplete B lymphocytes. Rheumatology (Oxford) 2001;40:205–11.

[193] Edwards JC, Szczepanski L, Szechinski J, et al. Efficacy of B cell targeted therapy with rituximab in patients with rheumatoid arthritis. N Engl J Med 2004;350:2572–81.

[194] Emery P, Fleischmann R, Filipowicz-Sosnowska A, et al. The efficacy and safety of Rituximab in patients with active rheumatoid arthritis despite methotrexate treatment. Results of a Phase IIB randomized double blind controlled dose ranging trial. Arthritis Rheumatol 2006;54:1390–400.

[195] Westhovens R, Robles M, Ximenes AC, et al. Clinical efficacy and safety of abatacept in methotrexate-naive patients with early rheumatoid arthritis and poor prognostic factors. Ann Rheum Dis 2009;68:1870–7.

[196] Genovese MC, Becker JC, Schiff M, et al. Abatacept for rheumatoid arthritis refractory to tumor necrosis factor a inhibition. N Engl J Med 2005;353:1114–23.

[197] Jones G, Sebba A, Gu J, et al. Comparison of tocilizumab monotherapy versus methotrexate monotherapy in patients with moderate to severe rheumatoid arthritis: the AMBITION study. Ann Rheum Dis 2010;69:88–96.

[198] Nishimoto N, Miyasaka N, Yamamoto K, et al. Study of active controlled tocilizumab monotherapy for rheumatoid arthritis patients with an inadequate response to methotrexate (SATORI): significant reduction in disease activity and serum vascular endothelial growth factor by IL-6 receptor inhibition therapy. Mod Rheumatol 2009;19:12–9.

[199] Nishimoto N, Hashimoto J, Miyasaka N, et al. Study of active controlled monotherapy used for rheumatoid arthritis, an IL-6 inhibitor (SAMURAI): evidence of clinical and radiographic benefit from an x ray reader-blinded randomised controlled trial of tocilizumab. Ann Rheum Dis 2007;66:1162–7.

[200] Emery P, Keystone E, Tony HP, et al. IL-6 receptor inhibition with tocilizumab improves treatment outcomes in patients with rheumatoid arthritis refractory to anti-tumour necrosis factor biologicals: results from a 24-week multicentre randomised placebo-controlled trial. Ann Rheum Dis 2008;67:1516–23.

[201] Boyle DL, Soma K, Hodge J, et al. The JAK inhibitor Tofacitinib suppresses synovial JAK1-STAT signalling in rheumatoid arthritis. Ann Rheum Dis 2015;74:1311–6.

[202] Strand V, Kremer J, Wallenstein G, et al. Effects of tofacitinib monotherapy on patient-reported outcomes in a randomized phase 3 study of patients with active rheumatoid arthritis and inadequate responses to DMARDs. Arthritis Res Ther 2015;17:307.

[203] Strand V, Burmester GR, Zerbini CA, et al. Tofacitinib with methotrexate in third- line treatment of patients with active rheumatoid arthritis: patient-reported outcomes from a phase III trial. Arthritis Care Res (Hoboken) 2015;67:475–83.

[204] Smolen JS, Kremer JM, Gaich CL, et al. Patient-reported outcomes from a randomised phase III study of baricitinib in patients with rheumatoid arthritis and an inadequate response to biological agents (RA-BEACON). Ann Rheum Dis 2017;76(4):694–700.

[205] Dougados M, van der Heijde D, Chen YC, et al. Baricitinib in patients with inadequate response or intolerance to conventional synthetic DMARDs: results from the RA-BUILD study. Ann Rheum Dis 2017;76(1):88–95.

[206] Genovese MC, Kremer J, Zamani O, et al. Baricitinib in patients with refractory rheumatoid arthritis. N Engl J Med 2016;374(13):1243–52.

[207] Taylor PC, Keystone EC, van der Heijde D, et al. Baricitinib versus placebo or adalimumab in rheumatoid arthritis. N Engl J Med 2017;376(7):652–62.

[208] Smolen JS, Landewé R, Bijlsma J, et al. EULAR recommendations for the management of rheumatoid arthritis with synthetic and biological disease-modifying antirheumatic drugs: 2016 update. Ann Rheum Dis 2017;76(6):960–77.

[209] Aletaha D, Funovits J, Keystone EC, et al. Disease activity early in the course of treatment predicts response to therapy after one year in rheumatoid arthritis patients. Arthritis Rheum 2007;56:3226–35.

[210] Cohen G, Gossec L, Dougados M, et al. Radiological damage in patients with rheumatoid arthritis on sustained remission. Ann Rheum Dis 2007;66(3):358–63.

[211] Peluso G, Michelutti A, Bosello S, et al. Clinical and ultrasonographic remission determines different chances of relapse in early and long standing rheumatoid arthritis. Ann Rheum Dis 2011;70(1):172–5.

[212] Naredo E, Valor L, De la Torre I, et al. Predictive value of Doppler ultrasound-detected synovitis in relation to failed tapering of biologic therapy in patients with rheumatoid arthritis. Rheumatology (Oxford) 2015;54(8):1408–14.

[213] Alivernini S, Peluso G, Fedele AL, et al. Tapering and discontinuation of TNF-α blockers without disease relapse using ultrasonography as a tool to identify patients with rheumatoid arthritis in clinical and histological remission. Arthritis Res Ther 2016;3(18):39.

[214] Alivernini S, Tolusso B, Petricca L, et al. Synovial features of patients with rheumatoid arthritis and psoriatic arthritis in clinical and ultrasound remission differ under anti-TNF therapy: a clue to interpret different chances of relapse after clinical remission? Ann Rheum Dis 2017;76(7):1228–36.

Chapter 47

Psoriatic Arthritis

Francesco Caso, Luisa Costa, Rosario Peluso, Antonio Del Puente, Raffaele Scarpa
Rheumatology Unit, Department of Clinical Medicine and Surgery, School of Medicine and Surgery, University of Naples Federico II, Naples, Italy

INTRODUCTION

PsA represents an inflammatory arthropathy associated with psoriasis or its familiarity, belonging to the spondyloarthritis (SpAs) group [1,2].

Psoriatic skin lesions generally show as inflammatory hyperproliferative and erythematous cutaneous manifestations usually located on the extensor surfaces of the knees and elbows and other areas, more commonly represented by the scalp, intergluteal, and umbilical areas [3]. In addition, nails can be involved by inflammatory processes leading to psoriatic onychopathy [3]. Psoriasis occurs in 1%–3% of the population, and about 10%–40% of patients with psoriasis can develop PsA [3].

The average age at PsA onset is around the fourth decade, men and women can be affected equally [1]. Articular inflammatory processes can involve axial skeleton (spondylitis), peripheral joints (peripheral arthritis), insertion sites of tendons and ligaments into bone (enthesitis), and PIP and DIP joints, and soft tissue of digits (dactylitis). Any of these manifestations can occur alone or in any of the possible combinations [1–6].

PsA represents a significant health issue because of its high worldwide prevalence and implications both in terms of survival and social costs [2]. These are mainly correlated to alteration of functional status, disability, and negative impacts on patients' function and QOL and psychosocial aspects [7–12].

Diagnosis in early phases and immediate and effective therapy may be able to reduce disease severity, improving cutaneous, articular, QoL, and psychosocial outcomes [1,13].

ETIOPATHOGENESIS

Etiopathogenetic hypothesis of PsA includes a complex interaction of genetic, environmental, and immunological factors [14].

In the etiology of the disease, the familial aggregation of PsA supports a key role of genetic factors, most likely with a multifactorial inherited mechanism [14].

Environmental factors, particularly infections and trauma, have been called in cause as possible elements in triggering arthritis in genetically predisposed subjects [14].

The largest reported genetic association of psoriasis and PsA is represented by genetic loci localized within the major histocompatibility complex region [15–17].

The HLA allele, *B27*, has been reported as a PsA risk factor and key predictor of disease progression [18,19]. Frequency of *HLA-Cw*0602* is higher in psoriasis patients than among PsA ones [15–17,19]. In patients carrying *HLA-B*27* allele, PsA occurs more early and the temporal interval between psoriasis and arthritis is longer than in those without it. In patients with PsA carrying the *HLA-C*06* allele, the interval between the psoriasis and arthritis is longer than in those without it [20].

The pathogenic action of class I molecules belonging to the HLA complex remains unclarified. Among hypotheses, the pathogenetic role of HLA-B27 has been considered potentially linked to its possible ability of acting as a molecule presenting arthritogenic peptides to cytotoxic T cells [21–24].

Another mechanism provides a potential HLA-B27 misfolding with consequent endoplasmic reticulum accumulation, unfolded response, stress, and autophagy [21–24].

Furthermore, at level of cell surface, the binding of homodimers, constituted by β2-microglobulin-free HLA-B27 heavy chains, with immunoglobulin-like receptors on lymphocytes leads to inflammatory response [20–24].

Multiple and genome-wide association studies have investigated other genetic regions. Among numerous identified potential susceptible genes, the killer cell Ig-like receptors (KIR), KIR2DS2, expressed on natural killer cells, have been found to be significantly associated to PsA [24,25].

Mosaic of Autoimmunity. https://doi.org/10.1016/B978-0-12-814307-0.00047-5

Different studies have reported that different cytokines, especially TNF-α, interleukin (IL)-17, and IL-23, represent crucial proinflammatory molecules upregulated in peripheral blood, skin lesions, synovial membrane, and fluid of PsA patients [26–29].

TNF-α, expressed in the form of soluble cytokine (sTNF) and type II membrane-associated TNF (mTNF) protein, is a crucial molecule in pathogenesis of PsA [30–33].

TNF-α binds the TNF receptors, TNFR1 and TNFR2, present on various immune cell types. TNFR leads to activation of different kinases, phosphor-proteins and nuclear factor kappa B (NF-kB), proinflammatory genes transcription with consequent cytokines secretion, cytotoxic effects, and peripheral differentiation of T helper (Th) cell subsets [34].

In course of synovitis, overexpression of TNF-α by macrophages and other immune cells is able to promote unbalanced inflammatory response and articular damage [31–33]. Notably, the improved understanding of TNF-α mechanisms of action has represented the main factor in influencing the recent therapeutic approach to PsA patients by use of biological disease-modifying antirheumatic drugs (bDMARDs) [35,36].

Other proinflammatory molecules involved in the pathogenesis of the disease and representing therapeutic targets of new bDMARDs are represented by IL-12 and IL-23 produced by antigen-presenting cells. These cytokines are able to induce and activate Th1 and Th17 cells leading to the synthesis of type 1 cytokines [37].

In addition, Th-17 responses include dysregulation of the IL-17 axis cytokines. Among those, the proinflammatory cytokine, IL-17A, is crucial in the regulation of different innate and adaptive immune pathways [38–40]. It is produced by Th-17 cells and other innate immune cells as neutrophils, mast cells, CD8+, and T lymphocytes at sites of skin plaques and inflamed entheses, representing another pharmacologic target [38–40]. IL-17A, acting with other proinflammatory cytokines, including TNF-α, leads to upregulation of expression of different genes associated to inflammatory response in different cells, as well as keratinocytes and fibroblasts, leading to increased synthesis of proinflammatory molecules [38–41].

In the recent years, different studies have evidenced the important pathogenetic role of dysfunction of several regulating steps involving intracellular molecules [42–47]. They are represented by the signaling pathways involving transcription factors or enzymes, the JAK–signal transducer of activators of transcription (STAT) pathway [26,27], and PDE4 [42–47]. These represent also the target of several drugs known as tsDMARDs [35].

JAK/STAT molecules are activated by growth factors and interleukins and regulate intracellular inflammatory pathways and immune cell response by activation of proinflammatory genes [48].

PDE4 hydrolyzes cyclic adenosine monophosphate, leading to intracellular adenosine monophosphate increase [45–47] and consequent activation of protein kinase A, inhibition of antiinflammatory IL-10 and increased synthesis of proinflammatory molecules, including leukotriene B4, different chemokines (CXCL9, CXCL10, and CCL4), and the interleukins interferon-γ, TNF-α, IL-2, IL-8, IL-12, and IL-23 [45–47].

CLINICAL ASPECTS

Involvement of several domains represented by joints, entheses, digit, tendons, axial skeleton, skin, and nails leads to the wide heterogeneity of the disease [49–52]. Inflammatory involvement of sacroiliac joints and spine (axial pattern), asymmetrical oligoarthritis, DIP arthritis, symmetrical polyarthritis, dactylitis, enthesitis, and more rarely the mutilans form, in concomitance of psoriasis or its familial history, represent key clinical findings for addressing PsA diagnosis [49–52]. High specific (98.7%) and sensitive (91.4%) Classification Criteria for Psoriatic Arthritis (CASPAR) criteria are used to categorize research cohorts [53,54].

Laboratory evaluation shows usually negative serological test for rheumatoid factor (RF) and anticitrullinated peptide antibodies (ACPAs) [1]. Inflammatory markers, erythrocyte sedimentation rate (ESR), and C-reactive protein are found elevated in above half of PsA patients [1].

Diagnosis of PsA relies mainly on clinical aspects and imaging techniques can represent additional tools useful for addressing the diagnosis and are essential for monitoring joint involvement [55].

Plain radiography can detect erosive and bone proliferative changes in advanced phases and represents a key instrument for monitoring articular damage [55].

Main radiological findings can be represented by articular erosions, exuberant new bone formations, osteolysis, periostitis, enthesitis, nonmarginal syndesmophytes, and ankylosis [55].

In early and active phases of the disease, inflammatory aspects can be detected by use of MRI and ultrasonography, able to evidence active signs and staging articular and periarticular involvement (soft tissue and bone marrow) [56–61].

According to Moll and Wright classification, PsA can be divided into five subsets: axial PsA, symmetrical polyarthritis, asymmetrical oligoarthritis, DIP arthritis, and arthritis mutilans (Table 47.1) [14]. These subsets have been reported significantly different in terms of frequency and characteristics in several populations [62–65]. Additionally, PsA phenotypes

TABLE 47.1 Main Manifestations of the Five Psoriatic Arthritis (PsA) Subsets

	Main Articular Aspects	Possible Subset Overlap	Main X-Ray Findings
Axial involvement	Spondylitis; bilateral or more often unilateral sacroiliitis.	Peripheral arthritis.	Nonmarginal syndesmophytes distributed asymmetrically along the spine; bilateral or unilateral sacroiliitis.
Symmetrical polyarthritis	Symmetrical inflammatory involvement of ≥4 peripheral joints, resembling RA. Unlike RA, there is seronegativity for RF and ACPAs, involvement of DIP joints, concomitance of enthesopathies, dactylitis, spondylitis, and sacroiliitis.	Axial involvement; DIP arthritis.	Erosions are often associated with exuberant ankylosis, periostitis, and syndesmophytes.
Asymmetrical oligoarthritis	Oligoarthritis is characterized by asymmetrical involvement of less than four joints and dactylitis may represent a clinical expression. It can represent the onset phase of a symmetric polyarthritis.	Axial involvement; DIP arthritis.	Erosions are often associated with exuberant ankylosis, periostitis, and syndesmophytes.
DIP arthritis	Symmetrical or asymmetrical DIP arthritis can occur in more than 50% of patients with PsA. It can be associated with onychopathy and may occur more frequently in advanced phases.	DIP arthritis may occur as a single or combined manifestation of PsA both with axial involvement and with prevalent peripheral involvement (in course of symmetrical polyarthritis, asymmetrical oligoarthritis, and arthritis mutilans).	Presence of marginal erosions associated with adjacent bone proliferation; erosive modifications at first involve the margins of DIP joint and then centrally; lack of prominent juxtaarticular osteoporosis; resorption of the tufts of terminal phalanx both of hands and feet.
Arthritis mutilans	Digital shortening characterized by osteolysis of phalanx and metacarpals (opera glass).	It occurs in less than 1% of patients and generally as an isolated articular subset.	Osteolysis of phalangeal, metacarpal, and metatarsal bone (telescoping digits); periarticular and shaft periostitis; pencil-in-cup deformity.

ACPAs, anticitrullinated peptide antibodies; *DIP*, distal interphalangeal; *PsA*, psoriatic arthritis; *RA*, rheumatoid arthritis; *RF*, rheumatoid factor.

can change over time and peripheral arthritis, in particular polyarthritis and DIP arthritis may often occur in concomitance with axial involvement [62–65].

Furthermore, on the basis of the cutaneous manifestation, a PsA subset classified as "sine psoriasis" is recognized. It involves patients who have never suffered from psoriasis, but who present to the anamnesis psoriasis familiarity [66].

Axial Involvement

Axial involvement can show as spondylitis and bilateral or more often unilateral sacroiliitis. It can interest up to 70% of PsA, being associated or less with peripheral arthritis. Criteria match those used for ankylosing spondylitis (AS) [67–69].

PsA shows radiologic features which differentiate it from other SpAs, including AS [70–73].

Axial X-rays permit to identify peculiar nonmarginal syndesmophytes distributed asymmetrically along the spine. Syndesmophytes seem to emerge from spinal ligament and it is possible to detect an equal frequency of bulky marginal and paramarginal vertical syndesmophytes [70–73].

On the other hand, in AS, syndesmophytes are marginal, bridge the intervertebral discs, and are symmetric, progressing caudal to cranial [70–73].

Symmetrical Polyarthritis

Occurrence of symmetrical polyarthritis in PsA resembles that of rheumatoid arthritis (RA), and in the past, it has been recognized as rheumatoid-like form [64,74].

Findings characterizing psoriatic polyarthritis and useful in differentiating it from RA are mainly represented by RF and APCAs seronegativity, DIP involvement, concomitance of enthesopathies, dactylitis, spondylitis, and sacroiliitis [64,74].

In RA, progressive and bilateral involvement of small, medium, and large joints tends to be symmetric, differently from PsA. Furthermore, in RA, the involvement of DIP and of the spine is uncommon, except for cervical tract [75–78].

In addition, despite occasional detection in PsA of RF and APCAs, these are peculiar and specific markers of RA [79]. In PsA, APCAs seem to be correlated with severe polyarticular subset with a more and erosive disease course and more often in female patients [79].

Not at last, while in RA osteoporosis can represent a frequent finding both at a systemic level and at level of involved joints, and in PsA, mechanisms of bone loss are accompanied by bone formation with ankylosis, periostitis, and exuberant syndesmophytes [80,81].

Asymmetrical Oligoarthritis

Oligoarthritis is characterized by asymmetrical involvement of less than four joints and dactylitis may represent a typical clinical expression [74].

Oligoarthritis, as polyarthritis pattern, can occur isolated or less frequently in concomitance of axial involvement. Furthermore, it can represent the onset phases of a future symmetric polyarthritis [63,64,82,83].

Oligoarthritis, especially associated with inflammatory back pain, needs ruling out of other SpAs, such as enteroarthritis and reactive arthritis, mainly by the investigation on presence of inflammatory bowel diseases and recent gastrointestinal or urogenital infection by 1–6 weeks [84,85].

Distal Interphalangeal Arthritis

Symmetrical or asymmetrical DIP arthritis can be associated with onychopathy and may occur more frequently in advanced phases [52,86]. Erosive modifications at first involve the margins of DIP joint and then centrally [86].

DIP arthritis may occur as a single or combined manifestation of PsA [64,87].

In several cases, inflammatory DIP joints involvement occurring in PsA needs ruling out the erosive form of OA [88–91]. In uncertain cases, inflamed entheses with diffuse bone edema can address the PsA diagnosis and exclude OA, in which entheses are thickened and associated with osteophytes, cartilage loss and joint space narrowing [92].

Arthritis Mutilans

Arthritis mutilans represents a severe PsA phenotype in which osteolysis of phalanx and metacarpals represent the prominent findings (opera glass) [64,87]. It occurs in less than 1% of patients and generally as an isolated articular subset [64,87,93–95].

Psoriatic Arthritis Sine Psoriasis

PsA sine psoriasis is characterized by the presence of dactylitis and DIP arthritis and more rarely enthesitis, tenosynovitis, and axial involvement, in the absence of an overt skin and/or nail psoriasis and in presence of a familial history of psoriasis in first- and/or second-grade relatives [65,66]. HLA haplotypes showing *HLA-Cw*6* positivity can be useful for addressing the diagnosis [66].

LABORATORY AND INSTRUMENTAL FINDINGS

Markers of inflammation, such as ESR, show to be elevated up to 50% of the patients [96,97], and a peculiar finding is represented by the usual absence of RF, playing a significant role in cases where clinical aspects mime RA [98].

Although rarely, positivity of APCAs, a characteristic RA marker, can also be found in PsA and can correlate with a severe and erosive polyarthritis [99–103].

Main PsA indices measuring disease activity and remission are represented by minimal disease activity criteria, Composite Psoriatic Disease Activity Index, Psoriatic Arthritis Disease Activity Score, and Disease Activity Index for Psoriatic Arthritis [104].

In the routine practice, follow-up of axial involvement can be performed by the use of Bath Ankylosing Spondylitis Disease Activity Index and Bath Ankylosing Spondylitis Functional Index, whereas the count of swollen and tender joints, the tender entheseal count, and the Leeds Dactylitis Index represent PsA indices useful for monitoring of peripheral and entheseal involvement [104].

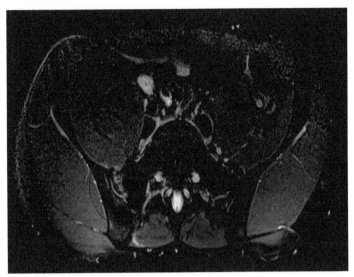

FIGURE 47.1 T2 weighted magnetic resonance imaging of the sacroiliac joints on coronal view shows a moderate increased signal intensity in joint space of the right sacroiliac joint and marrow edema, such as sacroiliitis (*red circle*).

With regard to skin, Psoriasis Area Severity Index (PASI) or body surface area and Nail Psoriasis Severity Index are used for the evaluation of the activity and extension of cutaneous involvement [104].

Plain film radiography has markedly contributed in describing PsA as a pathological entity different from RA [55,73]. Characteristic aspects are represented by the frequent asymmetric joint involvement, the involvement of DIP joints of fingers and toes; the presence of marginal erosions associated with adjacent bone proliferation; the lack of prominent juxtaarticular osteoporosis; the resorption of the tufts of terminal phalanx both of hands and feet; the osteolysis of phalangeal, metacarpal, and metatarsal bone (telescoping digits), in the case of arthritis mutilans; the periarticular and shaft periostitis; and pencil-in-cup deformity [55,73].

High-resolution ultrasonography, ultrasound combined with power Doppler, and MRI (Fig. 47.1) have been validated as sensitive techniques not only to detect the involvement of synovial membrane but also for the study of adjacent soft structures [55,73,105–109].

EXTRA-ARTICULAR MANIFESTATIONS

PsA has long been considered a disease with a low inflammatory profile, but recent studies have provided growing evidence of its multisystemic nature and association with extra-articular involvement in the form of colitis, uveitis, metabolic syndrome (MetS), and atherosclerosis [1,110].

Today, PsA, as well as psoriasis, is recognized under the most general term of psoriatic disease. It originated from a better understanding of pathogenetic mechanisms and systemic clinical manifestations of the disease [110].

Subclinical gut inflammation in patients with PsA has been reported as characterized by a specific histologic and immunologic signature represented by pronounced Paneth cell hyperplasia and Th17 and Th9 responses [111]. Th9 responses have been reported to be a specific PsA signature when compared with AS and Crohn's disease [111]. A possible link has also been hypothesized between intestinal and synovial inflammation through IL-9 overexpression and Th9 polarization that occur in synovitis and in the peripheral blood of patients with PsA. This could suggest a potential existence of a bowel joint migratory axis [111].

PsA can be characterized by ocular involvement [112]. Ophthalmic findings occur in 10% of patients with psoriasis [112,113] and in 31% of patients with PsA [114,115].

In PsA, recurrent acute anterior uveitis represents the most frequent manifestation of ocular involvement and it shows frequently bilateral [116].

In comparison with other spondyloarthropathies, PsA-associated uveitis has been reported more insidious in initial phases and chronic in duration [117]. Other ocular manifestations have been reported in course of PsA and among those conjunctivitis, followed by episcleritis, scleritis, keratitis, cystoid macular edema, glaucoma, and cataract [113–117].

In comparison with the general population, PsA patients show an increased risk of cardiovascular (CV) risk factors and CV events, in particular coronary heart disease (myocardial angina and infarction) and stroke [118–120].

PsA patients have been reported to have higher CV risk than those with psoriasis alone. Despite the significant contribution to CV morbidity and mortality of traditional risk factors, such as metabolic and lipid alterations, PsA per se should be considered as an independent CV risk factor [121].

An important role could be played by PsA inflammatory activity, metabolic components such as hypertension, dyslipidemia, and diabetes and the grade of systemic inflammation leading to accelerated atherosclerosis [122–129].

THERAPY

Inhibition of the structural radiological damage, clinical remission, and improvement of the patients' QOL represent the main aim of the treatment, as defined by international guidelines by the Group for Research and Assessment of Psoriasis and Psoriatic Arthritis (GRAPPA) and the European League Against Rheumatism (EULAR) [130–132].

The current treatment for nonsevere articular form consists initially of NSAIDs and intraarticular steroids injections, when these are appropriate [130–132]. csDMARDs, mainly methotrexate (MTX), sulfasalazine, and leflunomide, represent therapeutic options in refractory cases, but biologic agents (bDMARDs) are then recommended in resistant patients (Table 47.2) [130–134].

bDMARDs have been shown to be effective on all the clinical domains of the disease, including psoriasis, axial involvement enthesitis, dactylitis, joint pain, and swelling [130–132]. Inhibition of radiographic progression has been also reported under biological therapies [130–132].

The five anti-TNF-α agents available are infliximab, adalimumab, etanercept, golimumab, and certolizumab pegol (Table 47.2) [135–143].

In comparison with NSAIDs, glucocorticoids, and csDMARDs, a higher level of evidence has been reported on the efficacy of anti-TNF-α agents in treating both clinical aspects and in reducing radiographic progression [144,145].

The concomitant use of MTX has been reported well tolerated and able to prolong TNF inhibitor drug survival [146,147]. Combined therapy with MTX can be significantly useful to decrease prevalence of neutralizing antibodies to anti-TNF-α, and for this reason, MTX use should be strongly considered in patients with PsA under anti-TNF-α therapy [148–150].

With regard to anti-TNF safety profile, these agents have also been demonstrated to be reasonably safe in PsA [135,144,145].

A large metanalysis on anti-TNF-α has recently shown that the overall malignancy rates for PsA patients treated resulted similar to those expected from the general population and death rates are lower than, or equivalent to, those expected in the general population [151]. Randomized controlled trials (RCTs) safety data are confirmed by real-life studies and registries [152–155].

With regard to infectious risk, latent, acute, and chronic infections represent always a contraindication to use a biological therapy. In cases of Latent tuberculosis infection (LTBI), antitubercular prophylaxis can be considered in experienced and specialized rheumatologic units and in strong collaboration with related specialists [156–160]. In PsA patients, all related conditions need to be carefully evaluated to avoid microbial reactivation [161,162].

Several data have generally shown that switching to a second anti-TNF is safe and efficacious in patients with failure and inadequate response to the use of a previous TNF-α agent [163–165]. Fewer data are available about switching to a third anti-TNF-α [163–165].

Different mechanisms of blocking inflammatory pathways by therapy on mechanisms other than those TNF-α driven are important in patients refractory or developing loss of response to anti-TNF-α [166–168].

Among therapies able to inhibit precise cytokines other than TNF-α, ustekinumab (UST), a fully human monoclonal antibody blocking the common p40 chain shared by IL-12 and IL-23 (anti-IL-12p40), has been reported as an efficacious treatment for moderate-to-severe plaque psoriasis and active PsA (Table 47.2) [169,170].

Reports on two large phase III trials have shown that UST at dosage of 45 or 90 mg resulted more effective than placebo on cutaneous, articular, and radiological aspects as determined by significant improvement of PASI ≥75% response, American College of Rheumatology 20/50/70 rates, enthesitis and dactylitis scores, radiographic progression, and Health Assessment Questionnaire scores [171–174]. UST was generally safe and well tolerated, showing occasionally rare serious infections or CV events [171–174].

In addition to IL-12p40 and IL-23 blockage, targeting on IL-17 has been reported as a valid therapeutic option for PsA. IL-17A, acting with other proinflammatory cytokines, including TNF-α, leads to increased inflammatory response and its role in PsA seems to be significant [166,175,176].

Several direct and receptorial IL-17A inhibitors have shown promising results in several phase 2 clinical studies, and more recently in phase 3 RCTs on psoriasis and PsA [177–180].

TABLE 47.2 Structures and Administration Dosage of Disease-Modifying Antirheumatic Drugs Used in Psoriatic Arthritis (PsA) Therapy

DMARD		Drug Structure and Mechanism	Dose and Route Administration
csDMARDs			
MTX		Folate analog with inhibitory effects on proliferation and stimulation of apoptosis in immune and inflammatory cells	15–25 mg/wk; oral, or IM or SC
SSZ		Combined acetylsalicylic acid and sulfapyridine molecule with inhibitory effects on 5-lipoxygenase pathway	1–3 g/d; oral
LFN		Selective pyrimidine synthesis inhibitor	20 mg/d; oral
bDMARDs			
Anti-TNF-α agents	ADA	Fully human IgG1 anti-TNF-α monoclonal antibody	40 mg biweekly; SC
	CTZ-PEG	Human anti-TNF-α antibody Fab fragment linked to 40 kDa PEG	200 mg biweekly; SC
	ETN	Recombinant fusion protein consisting of the extracellular ligand-binding domain of the soluble 75 kD receptor (p75) for TNF-α and the Fc portion of human IgG1	50 mg weekly in a single administration or in two 25 mg administration; SC
	GOL	Fully human IgG1 kappa anti-TNF monoclonal antibody	50 mg, every 4 wks; SC
	IFX	Chimeric (human/murine) IgG1 anti-TNF-α monoclonal antibody	5 mg/kg at 2 and 6 wks after the first infusion and then every 8 wks; IV
Anti-IL12/23 agent	UST	Anti-IL-12/23 p40 fully human monoclonal antibody	45 mg/kg (for body weight of <100 kg) or 90 mg/kg (for body weight of ≥100 kg) at 0, 4, and 12 wk, then every 12 wks; SC
Anti-IL17 agent	SEC	Anti-IL-17A fully humanized IgG1k monoclonal antibody	150 mg weekly from 0 to 4 wk, then monthly; SC
tsDMARDs			
APR		Phosphodiesterase 4 inhibitor	30 mg twice per day; oral

ADA, adalimumab; *APR*, apremilast; *bDMARDs*, biologic disease-modifying antirheumatic drugs; *csDMARDs*, conventional synthetic disease-modifying antirheumatic drugs; *CTZ-PEG*, certolizumab pegol; *ETN*, etanercept; *GOL*, golimumab; *IFX*, infliximab; *IG*, immunoglobulin; *IL*, interleukin; *IM*, intramuscular; *IV*, intravenously; *LFN*, leflunomide; *MTX*, methotrexate; *PEbG*, polyethylene glycol; *PsA*, psoriatic arthritis; *SEC*, secukinumab; *SC*, subcutaneously; *SSZ*, sulfasalazine; *TNF*, tumor necrosis factor; *tsDMARDs*, targeted synthetic disease-modifying antirheumatic drugs; *UST*, ustekinumab.

The IL-17A inhibitor in PsA secukinumab (SEC) represents a fully human IgG1κ monoclonal antibody, which selectively neutralizes IL-17A. SEC has shown efficacy on skin manifestations and is significantly able to improve physical function in PsA patients (Table 47.2) [177–180].

The most frequently reported adverse events for agents targeting IL-17 are represented by upper respiratory tract infection, nasopharyngitis, and injection site erythema and neutropenia [177–180].

Among the emerging tsDMARDs, APR represents an oral molecule that inhibits the activity of PDE4, and data from clinical trials indicate its antiinflammatory effects (Table 47.2) [181–184]. Several trials both in psoriasis and PsA have shown APR as a safe and efficacious therapeutic option in the therapy of moderate-to-severe psoriasis and active PsA [181–184]. Furthermore, APR resulted well tolerated with an acceptable safety profile, while the most frequent adverse effects were represented by early onset of mild gastrointestinal complaints resolving with time, such as diarrhea, nausea, headache, upper respiratory tract infection, and nasopharyngitis [181–184].

With regard to APR position in the algorithm of the treatment of PsA, GRAPPA recommends its use for patients with peripheral PsA after failure of csDMARDs or if csDMARDs are contraindicated [130–132]. Furthermore, in the GRAPPA recommendations even if the effect on structural progression for APR is not established, it is taken into consideration before csDMARDs in definite cases with peripheral PsA, given its safety profile and ease of use [130–132].

On the other hand, because of lack of data on radiographic progression, moderate effect of APR on most disease outcomes, and the cost ratio benefit, the EULAR group recommends APR to patients who do not achieve targets with csDMARDs and for whom bDMARDs are contraindicated [130–132].

Among the emerging tsDMARDs, tofacitinib represents an oral JAK inhibitor [185]. A recent study has highlighted that tofacitinib regulates synovial inflammation in PsA, inhibiting activation of STAT molecules [186]. Several studies have shown that JAK inhibition by tofacitinib is able to suppress arthritic joint structural damage through decreased RANKL synthesis and inhibition of production of several proinflammatory cytokines [187–189]. In PsA, a coordinate increase of JAK1, STAT1, STAT3, and STAT5 phosphoproteins has been found in synovial fluid T cells [42].

Recent data have reported that the efficacy of tofacitinib was superior to that of placebo at month 3 in PsA patients who previously had an inadequate response to csDMARDs [190,191].

CONCLUSIONS

PsA represents a relevant health issue, being highly prevalent in worldwide population with severe implications both in terms of survival and of social costs [1]. Globally, psoriasis shows a high prevalence and arthritis can occur in about one-third of the affected patients [2–6]. PsA has been reported to be a disease that negatively impacts on patients' function and QOL; psychosocial expression of QOL and life satisfaction have been shown to be comparable to RA [11,12]. However, when diagnosed in early phases, PsA can show a less disabling arthropathy than early or established RA [13]. Anti-TNF-α therapies still represent the cornerstone for the treatment of moderate and severe PsA, making possible its adequate clinical control. These treatments have been shown to be effective on inhibition of radiographic progression and on all the clinical domains of the disease, including enthesitis, dactylitis, joint pain and swelling, axial involvement, and psoriasis [130–132]. Biologic therapies targeting molecules other than TNF-α and tsDMARDs have opened a large space in the therapeutic scenario of PsA, mainly both as first-line and in cases of primary nonresponse, loss of efficacy with time, intolerance, side effects, and contraindication to anti-TNF-α agents [192,193].

In the last years, progress in understanding pathogenetic mechanisms of PsA has contributed to better define the heterogeneous clinical expression of the disease. Furthermore, today it is also evident that in the pathogenesis of the disease, several cytokines and different inflammatory pathways likely contribute to induce and maintain PsA, and it is unlikely that blocking a single cytokine or a specific pathway or a defined cell line will resolve all cases of such a complex condition. The increasing development of agents targeting molecular pathways has never been more stimulating in PsA.

The clinical heterogeneity of the disease and the complexity of the pathogenetic aspects involving multiple cytokines, cell lines, and molecules need to be further investigated with a collaborative and translational effort for improving outcomes of patients affected by PsA.

KEY POINTS

- PsA represents an inflammatory arthropathy associated with psoriasis in which recently it has been recognized by its multisystemic nature and association with extra-articular involvement in the form of colitis, uveitis, metabolic syndrome, and atherosclerosis.
- In susceptible subjects through a complex interaction of a predisposing genetic background, an altered immune response, mainly mediated by proinflammatory cytokines, induces the inflammatory state.
- Articular inflammatory processes can involve axial skeleton (spondylitis), peripheral joints (peripheral arthritis), insertion sites of tendons and ligaments into bone (enthesitis), PIP and DIP joints, and soft tissue of digits (dactylitis). Any of these manifestations can occur alone or in any of the possible combinations.
- Inhibition of the structural radiological damage, clinical remission, and improvement of the patients' QOL represent the main aim of the treatment.
- The current treatment for nonsevere articular form consists initially of NSAIDs. csDMARDs represent therapeutic options in refractory cases, but biologic agents (bDMARDs), represented by TNF-α, IL-12/23R, and IL-17 inhibitors, are then recommended in resistant patients. Among the emerging tsDMARDs, APR, an inhibitor of PDE4, and tofacitinib, a Janus kinase inhibitor, have shown antiinflammatory effects.

REFERENCES

[1] Ritchlin CT, Colbert RA, Gladman DD. Psoriatic arthritis. N Engl J Med 2017;376:957–70.
[2] Gladman DD, Antoni C, Mease P, Clegg DO, Nash P. Psoriatic arthritis: epidemiology, clinical features, course, and outcome. Ann Rheum Dis 2005;64. ii14–i17.
[3] Boehncke WH, Schön MP. Psoriasis. Lancet 2015;386:983–94.

[4] Schaefer I, Rustenbach SJ, Zimmer L, Augustin M. Prevalence of skin diseases in a cohort of 48,665 employees in Germany. Dermatology 2008;217:169–72.

[5] Ferrándiz C, Bordas X, García-Patos V, Puig S, Pujol R, Smandía A. Prevalence of psoriasis in Spain (epiderma project: phase I). J Eur Acad Dermatol Venereol 2001;15:20–3.

[6] Rachakonda TD, Schupp CW, Armstrong AW. Psoriasis prevalence among adults in the United States. J Am Acad Dermatol 2014;70:512–6.

[7] Tsifetaki N, Migkos MP, Papagoras C, Voulgari PV, Athanasakis K, Drosos AA. Counting costs under severe financial constraints: a cost-of-illness analysis of spondyloarthropathies in a tertiary hospital in Greece. J Rheumatol 2015;42:963–7.

[8] Huscher D, Merkesdal S, Thiele K, Zeidler H, Schneider M, Zink A. German Collaborative Arthritis Centres. Cost of illness in rheumatoid arthritis, ankylosing spondylitis, psoriatic arthritis and systemic lupus erythematosus in Germany. Ann Rheum Dis 2006;65:1175–83.

[9] Zink A, Thiele K, Huscher D, Listing J, Sieper J, Krause A, et al. German Collaborative Arthritis Centres. Healthcare and burden of disease in psoriatic arthritis. A comparison with rheumatoid arthritis and ankylosing spondylitis. J Rheumatol 2006;33:86–90.

[10] Kawalec P, Malinowski KP. The indirect costs of psoriatic arthritis: systematic review and meta-analysis. Expert Rev Pharmacoecon Outcomes Res 2015;15:125–32.

[11] Borman P, Toy GG, Babaoğlu S, Bodur H, Ciliz D, Alli N. A comparative evaluation of quality of life and life satisfaction in patients with psoriatic and rheumatoid arthritis. Clin Rheumatol 2007;26:330–4.

[12] Sokoll KB, Helliwell PS. Comparison of disability and quality of life in rheumatoid and psoriatic arthritis. J Rheumatol 2001;28:1842–6.

[13] Picchianti-Diamanti A, Germano V, Ferlito C, Migliore A, D'Amelio R, Laganà B. Health-related quality of life and disability in patients with rheumatoid, early rheumatoid and early psoriatic arthritis treated with etanercept. Qual Life Res 2010;19:821–6.

[14] Moll JM, Wright V. Familial occurrence of psoriatic arthritis. Ann Rheum Dis 1973;32:181–201.

[15] Nograles KE, Brasington RD, Bowcock AM. New insights into the pathogenesis and genetics of psoriatic arthritis. Nat Clin Pract Rheumatol 2009;5:83–91.

[16] O'Rielly DD, Rahman P. Genetics of psoriatic arthritis. Best Pract Res Clin Rheumatol 2014;28:673–85.

[17] Rahman P, Elder JT. Genetics of psoriasis and psoriatic arthritis: a report from the GRAPPA 2010 annual meeting. J Rheumatol 2012;39:431–3.

[18] Gladman DD, Farewell VT. The role of HLA antigens as indicators of disease progression in psoriatic arthritis. Multivariate relative risk model. Arthritis Rheum 1995;38:845–50.

[19] Armstrong RD, Panayi GS, Welsh KI. Histocompatibility antigens in psoriasis, psoriatic arthropathy, and ankylosing spondylitis. Ann Rheum Dis 1983;42:142–6.

[20] Queiro R, Tejón P, Alonso S, Coto P. Age at disease onset: a key factor for understanding psoriatic disease. Rheumatology (Oxford) 2014;53:1178–85.

[21] Bowness P. HLA-B27. Annu Rev Immunol 2015;33:29–48.

[22] Colbert RA, Tran TM, Layh-Schmitt G. HLA-B27 misfolding and ankylosing spondylitis. Mol Immunol 2014;57:44–51.

[23] Queiro R, Morante I, Cabezas I, Acasuso B. HLA-B27 and psoriatic disease: a modern view of an old relationship. Rheumatology (Oxford) 2016;55:221–9.

[24] Reveille JD. Genetics of spondyloarthritis–beyond the MHC. Nat Rev Rheumatol 2012;8:296–304.

[25] Chandran V, Bull SB, Pellett FJ, Ayearst R, Pollock RA, Gladman DD. Killer-cell immunoglobulin-like receptor gene polymorphisms and susceptibility to psoriatic arthritis. Rheumatology 2014;53:233–9.

[26] Fiocco U, Martini V, Accordi B, Caso F, Costa L, Oliviero F, et al. Transcriptional network profile on synovial fluid T cells in psoriatic arthritis. Clin Rheumatol 2015;34:1571–80.

[27] Fiocco U, Accordi B, Martini V, Oliviero F, Facco M, Cabrelle A, et al. JAK/STAT/PKCδ molecular pathways in synovial fluid T lymphocytes reflect the in vivo T helper-17 expansion in psoriatic arthritis. Immunol Res 2014;58:61–9.

[28] van Kuijk AW, Reinders-Blankert P, Smeets TJ, Dijkmans BA, Tak PP. Detailed analysis of the cell infiltrate and the expression of mediators of synovial inflammation and joint destruction in the synovium of patients with psoriatic arthritis: implications for treatment. Ann Rheum Dis 2006;65:1551–7.

[29] Goodman WA, Levine AD, Massari JV, Sugiyama H, McCormick TS, Cooper KD. IL-6 signaling in psoriasis prevents immune suppression by regulatory T cells. J Immunol September 1, 2009;183(5):3170–6.

[30] Bazzoni F, Beutler B. The tumor necrosis factor ligand and receptor families. N Engl J Med 1996;334:1717–25.

[31] Tracey D, Klareskog L, Sasso EH, Salfeld JG, Tak PP. Tumor necrosis factor antagonist mechanisms of action: a comprehensive review. Pharmacol Ther 2008;117:244–79.

[32] Eissner G, Kolch W, Scheurich P. Ligands working as receptors: reverse signaling by members of the TNF superfamily enhance the plasticity of the immune system. Cytokine Growth Factor Rev 2004;15:353–66.

[33] Wong M, Ziring D, Korin Y, Desai S, Kim S, Lin J, et al. TNFalpha blockade in human diseases: mechanisms and future directions. Clin Immunol 2008;126:121–36.

[34] Pfeffer K. Biological functions of tumor necrosis factor cytokines and their receptors. Cytokine Growth Factor Rev 2003;14:185–91.

[35] Chimenti MS, Ballanti E, Perricone C, Cipriani P, Giacomelli R, Perricone R. Immunomodulation in psoriatic arthritis: focus on cellular and molecular pathways. Autoimmun Rev 2013;12:599–606.

[36] Coates LC, Ritchlin CT, Kavanaugh AF. GRAPPA treatment recommendations: an update from the GRAPPA 2013 Annual Meeting. J Rheumatol 2014;41:1237–9.

[37] Nestle FO, Turka LA, Nickoloff BJ. Characterization of dermal dendritic cells in psoriasis. Autostimulation of T lymphocytes and induction of Th1 type cytokines. J Clin Invest 1994;94:202–9.

[38] Kirkham BW, Kavanaugh A, Reich K. Interleukin-17A: a unique pathway in immune-mediated diseases: psoriasis, psoriatic arthritis and rheumatoid arthritis. Immunology 2014;141:133–42.

[39] Lynde CW, Poulin Y, Vender R, Bourcier M, Khalil S. Interleukin 17A: toward a new understanding of psoriasis pathogenesis. J Am Acad Dermatol 2014;71:141–50.

[40] Isailovic N, Daigo K, Mantovani A, Selmi C. Interleukin-17 and innate immunity in infections and chronic inflammation. J Autoimmun 2015;60:1–11.

[41] Reich K, Papp KA, Matheson RT, Tu JH, Bissonnette R, Bourcier M, et al. Evidence that a neutrophil-keratinocyte crosstalk is an early target of IL-17A inhibition in psoriasis. Exp Dermatol 2015;24:529–35.

[42] Fiocco U, Martini V, Accordi B, Caso F, Costa L, Oliviero F, et al. Ex vivo signaling protein mapping in T lymphocytes in the psoriatic arthritis joints. J Rheumatol Suppl 2015;93:48–52.

[43] Zippin JH, Chadwick PA, Levin LR, Buck J, Magro CM. Soluble adenylyl cyclase defines a nuclear cAMP microdomain in keratinocyte hyperproliferative skin diseases. J Invest Dermatol 2010;130:1279–87.

[44] Schafer PH, Truzzi F, Parton A, Wu L, Kosek J, Zhang LH, et al. Phosphodiesterase 4 in inflammatory diseases: effects of apremilast in psoriatic blood and in dermal myofibroblasts through the PDE4/CD271 complex. Cell Signal 2016;28:753–63.

[45] Perez-Aso M, Montesinos MC, Mediero A, Wilder T, Schafer PH, Cronstein B. Apremilast, a novel phosphodiesterase 4 (PDE4) inhibitor, regulates inflammation through multiple cAMP downstream effectors. Arthritis Res Ther 2015;17:249.

[46] McCann FE, Palfreeman AC, Andrews M, Perocheau DP, Inglis JJ, Schafer P, et al. Apremilast, a novel PDE4 inhibitor, inhibits spontaneous production of tumour necrosis factor-alpha from human rheumatoid synovial cells and ameliorates experimental arthritis. Arthritis Res Ther 2010;12. R107.

[47] Schafer PH, Parton A, Gandhi AK, Capone L, Adams M, Wu L, et al. Apremilast, a cAMP phosphodiesterase-4 inhibitor, demonstrates anti-inflammatory activity in vitro and in a model of psoriasis. Br J Pharmacol 2010;159:842–55.

[48] O'Shea JJ, Schwartz DM, Villarino AV, Gadina M, McInnes IB, Laurence A. The JAK-STAT pathway: impact on human disease and therapeutic intervention. Annu Rev Med 2015;66:311–28.

[49] Ogdie A, Weiss P. The epidemiology of psoriatic arthritis. Rheum Dis Clin N Am 2015;41:545–68.

[50] Caso F, Costa L, Atteno M, Del Puente A, Cantarini L, Lubrano E, Scarpa R. Simple clinical indicators for early psoriatic arthritis detection. Springerplus 2014;3:759.

[51] Marchesoni A, Atzeni F, Spadaro A, Lubrano E, Provenzano G, Cauli A, et al. Identification of the clinical features distinguishing psoriatic arthritis and fibromyalgia. J Rheumatol 2012;39:849–55.

[52] Gladman DD. Early psoriatic arthritis. Rheum Dis Clin N Am 2012;38:373–86.

[53] Taylor W, Gladman D, Helliwell P, Marchesoni A, Mease P, Mielants H. CASPAR Study Group. Classification criteria for psoriatic arthritis: development of new criteria from a large international study. Arthritis Rheum 2006;54:2665–73.

[54] Tillett W, Costa L, Jadon D, Wallis D, Cavill C, McHugh J, et al. The classification for Psoriatic ARthritis (CASPAR) criteria—a retrospective feasibility, sensitivity, and specificity study. J Rheumatol 2012;39:154–6.

[55] Sudoł-Szopińska I, Matuszewska G, Kwiatkowska B, Pracoń G. Diagnostic imaging of psoriatic arthritis. Part I: etiopathogenesis, classifications and radiographic features. J Ultrason 2016;16:65–77.

[56] Ficjan A, Husic R, Gretler J, Lackner A, Graninger WB, Gutierrez M, et al. Ultrasound composite scores for the assessment of inflammatory and structural pathologies in Psoriatic Arthritis (PsASon-Score). Arthritis Res Ther 2014;16:476.

[57] Fiocco U, Stramare R, Coran A, Grisan E, Scagliori E, Caso F, et al. Vascular perfusion kinetics by contrast-enhanced ultrasound are related to synovial microvascularity in the joints of psoriatic arthritis. Clin Rheumatol 2015;34:1903–12.

[58] Soscia E, Sirignano C, Catalano O, Atteno M, Costa L, Caso F, et al. New developments in magnetic resonance imaging of the nail unit. J Rheumatol Suppl 2012;89:49–53.

[59] Tan AL, Fukuba E, Halliday NA, Tanner SF, Emery P, McGonagle D. High-resolution MRI assessment of dactylitis in psoriatic arthritis shows flexor tendon pulley and sheath-related enthesitis. Ann Rheum Dis 2015;74:185–9.

[60] Gutierrez M, Filippucci E, De Angelis R, Filosa G, Kane D, Grassi W. A sonographic spectrum of psoriatic arthritis: "the five targets". Clin Rheumatol 2010;29:133–42.

[61] Fiocco U, Sfriso P, Oliviero F, Lunardi F, Calabrese F, Scagliori E, et al. Blockade of intra-articular TNF in peripheral spondyloarthritis: its relevance to clinical scores, quantitative imaging and synovial fluid and synovial tissue biomarkers. Joint Bone Spine 2013;80:165–70.

[62] Gladman DD. Clinical features and diagnostic considerations in psoriatic arthritis. Rheum Dis Clin N Am 2015;41:569–79.

[63] Jones SM, Armas JB, Cohen MG, Lovell CR, Evison G, McHugh NJ. Psoriatic arthritis: outcome of disease subsets and relationship of joint disease to nail and skin disease. Br J Rheumatol 1994;33:834–9.

[64] Scarpa R, Oriente P, Pucino A, Vignone L, Cosentini E, Minerva A, Biondi Oriente C. The clinical spectrum of psoriatic spondylitis. Br J Rheumatol 1988;27:133–7.

[65] Gladman DD, Shuckett R, Russell ML, Thorne JC, Schachter RK. Psoriatic arthritis (PSA)-an analysis of 220 patients. Q J Med 1987;62:127–41.

[66] Scarpa R, Cosentini E, Manguso F, Oriente A, Peluso R, Atteno M, et al. Clinical and genetic aspects of psoriatic arthritis "sine psoriasis". J Rheumatol 2003;30:2638–40.

[67] Gladman DD. Axial disease in psoriatic arthritis. Curr Rheumatol Rep 2007;9:455–60.

[68] Höhler T, Märker-Hermann E. Psoriatic arthritis: clinical aspects, genetics, and the role of T cells. Curr Opin Rheumatol 2001;13:273–9.

[69] Lubrano E, Parsons WJ, Marchesoni A, Olivieri I, D'Angelo S, Cauli A, et al. The definition and measurement of axial psoriatic arthritis. J Rheumatol Suppl 2015;93:40–2.

[70] Napolitano M, Caso F, Scarpa R, Megna M, Patrì A, Balato N, Costa L. Psoriatic arthritis and psoriasis: differential diagnosis. Clin Rheumatol 2016;35:1893–901.

[71] McEwen C, DiTata D, Lingg C, Porini A, Good A, Rankin T. Ankylosing spondylitis and spondylitis accompanying ulcerative colitis, regional enteritis, psoriasis and Reiter's disease. A comparative study. Arthritis Rheum 1971;14:291–318.

[72] Helliwell PS, Hickling P, Wright V. Do the radiological changes of classic ankylosing spondylitis differ from the changes found in the spondylitis associated with inflammatory bowel disease, psoriasis, and reactive arthritis? Ann Rheum Dis 1998;57:135–40.

[73] Poggenborg RP, Østergaard M, Terslev L. Imaging in psoriatic arthritis. Rheum Dis Clin N Am 2015;41:593–613.

[74] Kane D, Stafford L, Bresnihan B, FitzGerald O. A classification study of clinical subsets in an inception cohort of early psoriatic peripheral arthritis-'DIP or not DIP revisited'. Rheumatology (Oxford) 2003;42:1469–76.

[75] Jevtic V, Lingg G. Differential diagnosis of rheumatoid and psoriatic arthritis at an early stage in the small hand and foot joints using magnetic resonance imaging. Handchir Mikrochir Plast Chir 2012;44:163–70.

[76] Balakrishnan C, Madnani N. Diagnosis and management of psoriatic arthritis. Indian J Dermatol Venereol Leprol 2013;79:S18–24.

[77] Olivieri I, D'Angelo S, Palazzi C, Padula A. Advances in the management of psoriatic arthritis. Nat Rev Rheumatol 2014;10:531–42.

[78] Cervini C, Leardini G, Mathieu A, Punzi L, Scarpa R. Psoriatic arthritis: epidemiological and clinical aspects in a cohort of 1.306 Italian patients. Reumatismo 2005;57:283–90.

[79] Perez-Alamino R, Garcia-Valladares I, Cuchacovich R, Iglesias-Gamarra A, Espinoza LR. Are anti-CCP antibodies in psoriatic arthritis patients a biomarker of erosive disease? Rheumatol Int 2014;34:1211–6.

[80] Del Puente A, Esposito A, Parisi A, Atteno M, Montalbano S, Vitiello M, et al. Osteoporosis and psoriatic arthritis. J Rheumatol Suppl 2012;89:36–8.

[81] Del Puente A, Esposito A, Costa L, Benigno C, Del Puente A, Foglia F, et al. Fragility fractures in patients with psoriatic arthritis. J Rheumatol Suppl 2015;93:36–9.

[82] Helliwell PS, Hetthen J, Sokoll K, Green M, Marchesoni A, Lubrano E, et al. Joint symmetry in early and late rheumatoid and psoriatic arthritis: comparison with a mathematical model. Arthritis Rheum 2000;43:865–71.

[83] Khan M, Schentag C, Gladman DD. Clinical and radiological changes during psoriatic arthritis disease progression. J Rheumatol 2003;30:1022–6.

[84] van Tubergen A, Weber U. Diagnosis and classification in spondyloarthritis: identifying a chameleon. Nat Rev Rheumatol 2012;8:253–61.

[85] Colavite PM, Sartori A. Septic arthritis: immunopathogenesis, experimental models and therapy. J Venom Anim Toxins Incl Trop Dis 2014;20:19.

[86] Scarpa R, Oriente P, Pucino A, Torella M, Vignone L, Riccio A, Biondi Oriente C. Psoriatic arthritis in psoriatic patients. Br J Rheumatol 1984;23:246–50.

[87] Oriente P, Biondi-Oriente C, Scarpa R. Psoriatic arthritis. Clinical manifestations. Baillieres Clin Rheumatol 1994;8:277–94.

[88] Crain DC. Interphalangeal osteoarthritis. JAMA March 25, 1961;175:1049–53.

[89] Peter JB, Pearson CM, Marmor L. Erosive osteoarthritis of the hands. Arthritis Rheum 1966;9:365–88.

[90] Swezey RL, Alexander SJ. Erosive osteoarthritis and the main en lorgnette deformity (opera glass hand). Arch Intern Med 1971;128:269–72.

[91] Smukler NM, Edeiken J, Giuliano VJ. Ankylosis in osteoarthritis of the finger joints. Radiology 1971;100:525–30.

[92] McGonagle D, Hermann KG, Tan AL. Differentiation between osteoarthritis and psoriatic arthritis: implications for pathogenesis and treatment in the biologic therapy era. Rheumatology (Oxford) 2015;54:29–38.

[93] Haddad A, Johnson SR, Somaily M, Fazelzad R, Kron AT, Chau C, Chandran V. Psoriatic arthritis mutilans: clinical and radiographic criteria. A systematic review. J Rheumatol 2015;42:1432–8.

[94] Jadon DR, Shaddick G, Tillett W, Korendowych E, Robinson G, Waldron N, et al. Psoriatic arthritis mutilans: characteristics and natural radiographic history. J Rheumatol 2015;42:1169–76.

[95] Gudbjornsson B, Ejstrup L, Gran JT, Iversen L, Lindqvist U, Paimela L, et al. Psoriatic arthritis mutilans (PAM) in the Nordic countries: demographics and disease status. The Nordic PAM study. Scand J Rheumatol 2013;42:373–8.

[96] Prajzlerová K, Grobelná K, Pavelka K, Šenolt L, Filková M. An update on biomarkers in axial spondyloarthritis. Autoimmun Rev 2016;15:501–9.

[97] Chandran V, Gladman DD. Update on biomarkers in psoriatic arthritis. Curr Rheumatol Rep 2010;12:288–94.

[98] Moll JM, Wright V. Psoriatic arthritis. Semin Arthritis Rheum 1973;3:55–78.

[99] Pasquetti P, Morozzi G, Galeazzi M. Very low prevalence of anti-CCP antibodies in rheumatoid factor-negative psoriatic polyarthritis. Rheumatology (Oxford) 2009;48:315–6.

[100] Popescu C, Zofotă S, Bojincă V, Ionescu R. Anti-cyclic citrullinated peptide antibodies in psoriatic arthritis–cross-sectional study and literature review. J Med Life 2013;6:376–82.

[101] Schellekens GA, Visser H, de Jong BA, van den Hoogen FH, Hazes JM, Breedveld FC, van Venrooij WJ. The diagnostic properties of rheumatoid arthritis antibodies recognizing a cyclic citrullinated peptide. Arthritis Rheum 2000;43:155–63.

[102] Nijenhuis S, Zendman AJ, Vossenaar ER, Pruijn GJ, vanVenrooij WJ. Autoantibodies to citrullinated proteins in rheumatoid arthritis: clinical performance and biochemical aspects of an RA-specific marker. Clin Chim Acta 2004;350:17–34.

[103] Bogliolo L, Alpini C, Caporali R, Scirè CA, Moratti R, Montecucco C. Antibodies to cyclic citrullinated peptides in psoriatic arthritis. J Rheumatol 2005;32:511–5.

[104] Acosta Felquer ML, Ferreyra Garrott L, Marin J, Catay E, Scolnik M, Scaglioni V, et al. Remission criteria and activity indices in psoriatic arthritis. Clin Rheumatol 2014;33:1323–30.

[105] D'Angelo S, Palazzi C, Gilio M, Leccese P, Padula A, Olivieri I. Improvements in diagnostic tools for early detection of psoriatic arthritis. Expert Rev Clin Immunol 2016;12:1209–15.

[106] Michelsen B, Diamantopoulos AP, Hammer HB, Soldal DM, Kavanaugh A, Haugeberg G. Ultrasonographic evaluation in psoriatic arthritis is of major importance in evaluating disease activity. Ann Rheum Dis 2016;75:2108–13.

[107] Soscia E, Scarpa R, Cimmino MA, Atteno M, Peluso R, Sirignano C, et al. Magnetic resonance imaging of nail unit in psoriatic arthritis. J Rheumatol Suppl 2009;83:42–5.

[108] Healy PJ, Groves C, Chandramohan M, Helliwell PS. MRI changes in psoriatic dactylitis–extent of pathology, relationship to tenderness and correlation with clinical indices. Rheumatology (Oxford) 2008;47:92–5.

[109] Poggenborg RP, Eshed I, Østergaard M, Sørensen IJ, Møller JM, Madsen OR, Pedersen SJ. Enthesitis in patients with psoriatic arthritis, axial spondyloarthritis and healthy subjects assessed by 'head-to-toe' whole-body MRI and clinical examination. Ann Rheum Dis 2015;74:823–9.

[110] Scarpa R, Caso F, Costa L, Peluso R, Del Puente A, Olivieri I. Psoriatic disease 10 years later. J Rheumatol 2017;44:1298–301.

[111] Ciccia F, Guggino G, Ferrante A, Raimondo S, Bignone R, Rodolico V, et al. Interleukin-9 overexpression and Th9 polarization characterize the inflamed gut, the synovial tissue, and the peripheral blood of patients with psoriatic arthritis. Arthritis Rheumatol 2016;68:1922–31.

[112] Murray PI, Rauz S. The eye and inflammatory rheumatic diseases: the eye and rheumatoid arthritis, ankylosing spondylitis, psoriatic arthritis. Best Pract Res Clin Rheumatol 2016;30:802–25.

[113] Rehal B, Modjtahedi BS, Morse LS, Schwab IR, Maibach HI. Ocular psoriasis. J Am Acad Dermatol 2011;65:1202–12.

[114] Lambert JR, Wright V. Eye inflammation in psoriatic arthritis. Ann Rheum Dis 1976;35:354–6.

[115] Rosenbaum JT. Uveitis in spondyloarthritis including psoriatic arthritis, ankylosing spondylitis, and inflammatory bowel disease. Clin Rheumatol 2015;34:999–1002.

[116] Paiva ES, Macaluso DC, Edwards A, Rosenbaum JT. Characterisation of uveitis in patients with psoriatic arthritis. Ann Rheum Dis 2000;59:67–70.

[117] Abbouda A, Abicca I, Fabiani C, Scappatura N, Peña-García P, Scrivo R, Priori R, Paroli MP. Psoriasis and psoriatic arthritis-related uveitis: different ophthalmological manifestations and ocular inflammation features. Semin Ophthalmol 2016. https://doi.org/10.3109/08820538.2016.1170161.

[118] Atzeni F, Caso F, Masala IF, Sarzi-Puttini P. Cardiovascular involvement in psoriatic arthritis. Handbook of systemic autoimmune diseases. In: The heart in systemic autoimmune diseases, vol. 14. 2017. p. 409–26. Chapter 16.

[119] Eder L, Thavaneswaran A, Chandran V, Cook R, Gladman DD. Increased burden of inflammation over time is associated with the extent of atherosclerotic plaques in patients with psoriatic arthritis. Ann Rheum Dis 2015;74:1830–5.

[120] Han C, Robinson Jr DW, Hackett MV, Paramore LC, Fraeman KH, Bala MV. Cardiovascular disease and risk factors in patients with rheumatoid arthritis, psoriatic arthritis, and ankylosing spondylitis. J Rheumatol 2006;33:2167–72.

[121] Zhu TY, Li EK, Tam LS. Cardiovascular risk in patients with psoriatic arthritis. Int J Rheumatol 2012;2012:714321.

[122] Eder L, Wu Y, Chandran V, Cook R, Gladman DD. Incidence and predictors for cardiovascular events in patients with psoriatic arthritis. Ann Rheum Dis 2016;75:1680–6.

[123] Eder L, Jayakar J, Pollock R, Pellett F, Thavaneswaran A, Chandran V, et al. Serum adipokines in patients with psoriatic arthritis and psoriasis alone and their correlation with disease activity. Ann Rheum Dis 2013;72:1956–61.

[124] Costa L, Caso F, D'Elia L, Atteno M, Peluso R, Del Puente A, et al. Psoriatic arthritis is associated with increased arterial stiffness in the absence of known cardiovascular risk factors: a case control study. Clin Rheumatol 2012;31:711–5.

[125] Costa L, Caso F, Ramonda R, Del Puente A, Cantarini L, Darda MA, et al. Metabolic syndrome and its relationship with the achievement of minimal disease activity state in psoriatic arthritis patients: an observational study. Immunol Res 2015;61:147–53.

[126] Costa L, Caso F, Atteno M, Del Puente A, Darda MA, Caso P, et al. Impact of 24-month treatment with etanercept, adalimumab, or methotrexate on metabolic syndrome components in a cohort of 210 psoriatic arthritis patients. Clin Rheumatol 2014;33:833–9.

[127] Gentile M, Peluso R, Di Minno MND, Costa L, Caso F, de Simone B, et al. Association between small dense LDL and sub-clinical atherosclerosis in patients with psoriatic arthritis. Clin Rheumatol 2016;35:2023–9.

[128] Husted JA, Thavaneswaran A, Chandran V, Eder L, Rosen CF, Cook RJ, Gladman DD. Cardiovascular and other comorbidities in patients with psoriatic arthritis: a comparison with patients with psoriasis. Arthritis Care Res (Hoboken) 2011;63:1729–35.

[129] Sobchak C, Eder L. Cardiometabolic disorders in psoriatic disease. Curr Rheumatol Rep 2017;19:63.

[130] Coates LC, Kavanaugh A, Mease PJ, Soriano ER, Laura Acosta-Felquer M, Armstrong AW, et al. Group for research and assessment of psoriasis and psoriatic arthritis 2015 treatment recommendations for psoriatic arthritis. Arthritis Rheumatol 2016;68:1060–71.

[131] Gossec L, Smolen JS, Ramiro S, de Wit M, Cutolo M, Dougados M, et al. European League against Rheumatism (EULAR) recommendations for the management of psoriatic arthritis with pharmacological therapies: 2015 update. Ann Rheum Dis 2016;75:499–510.

[132] Gossec L, Coates LC, de Wit M, Kavanaugh A, Ramiro S, Mease PJ, Ritchlin CT, van der Heijde D, Smolen JS. Management of psoriatic arthritis in 2016: a comparison of EULAR and GRAPPA recommendations. Nat Rev Rheumatol 2016;12:743–50.

[133] Scarpa R, Costa L, Atteno M, Caso F, Lubrano E. Treatment options: NSAIDs and DMARDs. In: Advances in the management of Psoriatic Arthritis. 2013. p. 62–70. Chapter 5.

[134] Nash P, Clegg DO. Psoriatic arthritis therapy: NSAIDs and traditional DMARDs. Ann Rheum Dis 2005;64. ii74–i77.

[135] Lemos LL, de Oliveira Costa J, Almeida AM, Junior HO, Barbosa MM, Kakehasi AM, Acurcio FA. Treatment of psoriatic arthritis with anti-TNF agents: a systematic review and meta-analysis of efficacy, effectiveness and safety. Rheumatol Int 2014;34:1345–60.

[136] Caso F, Costa L, Del Puente A, Di Minno MN, Lupoli G, Scarpa R, Peluso R. Pharmacological treatment of spondyloarthritis: exploring the effectiveness of nonsteroidal anti-inflammatory drugs, traditional disease-modifying antirheumatic drugs and biological therapies. Ther Adv Chronic Dis 2015;6:328–38.

[137] Saad AA, Symmons DP, Noyce PR, Ashcroft DM. Risks and benefits of tumor necrosis factor-alpha inhibitors in the management of psoriatic arthritis: systematic review and metaanalysis of randomized controlled trials. J Rheumatol 2008;35:883–90. 157.

[138] Fransen J, Antoni C, Mease PJ, Uter W, Kavanaugh A, Kalden JR, Van Riel PL. Performance of response criteria for assessing peripheral arthritis in patients with psoriatic arthritis: analysis of data from randomised controlled trials of two tumour necrosis factor inhibitors. Ann Rheum Dis 2006;65:1373–8.

[139] Brodszky V, Pentek M, Gulacsi L. Efficacy of adalimumab, etanercept, and infliximab in psoriatic arthritis based on ACR50 response after 24 weeks of treatment. Scand J Rheumatol 2008;37:399–400.

[140] Braun-Moscovici Y, Markovits D, Rozin A, Toledano K, Nahir AM, Balbir-Gurman A. Anti-tumor necrosis factor therapy: 6 year experience of a single center in northern Israel and possible impact of health policy on results. Isr Med Assoc J 2008;10:277–81.

[141] Atteno M, Peluso R, Costa L, Padula S, Iervolino S, Caso F, et al. Comparison of effectiveness and safety of infliximab, etanercept, and adalimumab in psoriatic arthritis patients who experienced an inadequate response to previous disease-modifying antirheumatic drugs. Clin Rheumatol April 2010;29(4):399–403.

[142] Migliore A, Bizzi E, Broccoli S, Laganà B. Indirect comparison of etanercept, infliximab, and adalimumab for psoriatic arthritis: mixed treatment comparison using placebo as common comparator. Clin Rheumatol 2012;31:133–7.

[143] Saougou I, Markatseli TE, Papagoras C, Voulgari PV, Alamanos Y, Drosos AA. Sustained clinical response in psoriatic arthritis patients treated with anti-TNF agents: a 5-year open-label observational cohort study. Semin Arthritis Rheum 2011;40:398–406.

[144] Ramiro S, Smolen JS, Landewé R, van der Heijde D, Dougados M, Emery P, et al. Pharmacological treatment of psoriatic arthritis: a systematic literature review for the 2015 update of the EULAR recommendations for the management of psoriatic arthritis. Ann Rheum Dis 2016;75:490–8.

[145] Braun J. New targets in psoriatic arthritis. Rheumatology 2016;55. ii30-ii37.

[146] Behrens F, Cañete JD, Olivieri I, van Kuijk AW, McHugh N, Combe B. Tumour necrosis factor inhibitor monotherapy vs combination with MTX in the treatment of PsA: a systematic review of the literature. Rheumatology (Oxford) 2015;54:915–26.

[147] Costa L, Perricone C, Chimenti MS, Del Puente A, Caso P, Peluso R, Bottiglieri P, Scarpa R, Caso F. Switching between biological treatments in psoriatic arthritis: a review of the evidence. Drugs R D 2017. https://doi.org/10.1007/s40268-017-0215-7.

[148] De Simone C, Amerio P, Amoruso G, Bardazzi F, Campanati A, Conti A, et al. Immunogenicity of anti-TNFα therapy in psoriasis: a clinical issue? Expert Opin Biol Ther 2013;13:1673–82.

[149] Mok CC, van der Kleij D, Wolbink GJ. Drug levels, anti-drug antibodies, and clinical efficacy of the anti-TNFα biologics in rheumatic diseases. Clin Rheumatol 2013;32:1429–35.

[150] Zisapel M, Zisman D, Madar-Balakirski N, Arad U, Padova H, Matz H, et al. Prevalence of TNF-α blocker immunogenicity in psoriatic arthritis. J Rheumatol 2015;42:73–8.

[151] Burmester GR, Panaccione R, Gordon KB, McIlraith MJ, Lacerda AP. Adalimumab: long-term safety in 23 458 patients from global clinical trials in rheumatoid arthritis, juvenile idiopathic arthritis, ankylosing spondylitis, psoriatic arthritis, psoriasis and Crohn's disease. Ann Rheum Dis 2013;72:517–24.

[152] Costa L, Caso F, Del Puente A, Di Minno MN, Peluso R, Scarpa R. Incidence of malignancies in a cohort of psoriatic arthritis patients taking traditional disease modifying antirheumatic drug and tumor necrosis factor inhibitor therapy: an observational study. J Rheumatol 2016;43:2149–54.

[153] Saad AA, Ashcroft DM, Watson KD, Symmons DP, Noyce PR, Hyrich KL. BSRBR. Efficacy and safety of anti-TNF therapies in psoriatic arthritis: an observational study from the British Society for Rheumatology Biologics Register. Rheumatology (Oxford) 2010;49:697–705.

[154] Mariette X, Tubach F, Bagheri H, Bardet M, Berthelot JM, Gaudin P, et al. Lymphoma in patients treated with anti-TNF: results of the 3-year prospective French RATIO registry. Ann Rheum Dis 2010;69:400–8.

[155] Carmona L, Abasolo L, Descalzo MA, Pérez-Zafrilla B, Sellas A, de Abajo F, Gomez-Reino JJ. BIOBADASER Study Group; EMECAR Study Group. Cancer in patients with rheumatic diseases exposed to TNF antagonists. Semin Arthritis Rheum 2011;41:71–80.

[156] Adelzadeh L, Jourabchi N, Wu JJ. The risk of herpes zoster during biological therapy for psoriasis and other inflammatory conditions. J Eur Acad Dermatol Venereol 2014;28:846–52.

[157] Jung SM, Ju JH, Park MS, Kwok SK, Park KS, Kim HY, et al. Risk of tuberculosis in patients treated with anti-tumor necrosis factor therapy: a nationwide study in South Korea, a country with an intermediate tuberculosis burden. Int J Rheum Dis 2015;18:323–30.

[158] Kim YJ, Kim YG, Shim TS, Koo BS, Hong S, Lee CK, Yoo B. Safety of resuming tumour necrosis factor inhibitors in patients who developed tuberculosis as a complication of previous TNF inhibitors. Rheumatology (Oxford) 2014;53:1477–81.

[159] Atteno M, Costa L, Matarese A, Caso F, Del Puente A, Cantarini L, et al. The use of TNF-α blockers in psoriatic arthritis patients with latent tuberculosis infection. Clin Rheumatol 2014;33:543–7.

[160] Mongey AB, Doran JP, Kleinerova J, Fitzgerald O, McDonnell TJ. Late onset tuberculosis infection in patients receiving anti-TNFα therapy. QJM 2014;107:69–71.

[161] Caso F, Cantarini L, Morisco F, Del Puente A, Ramonda R, Fiocco U, et al. Current evidence in the field of the management with TNF-α inhibitors in psoriatic arthritis and concomitant hepatitis C virus infection. Expert Opin Biol Ther 2015;15:641–50.

[162] Costa L, Caso F, Atteno M, Giannitti C, Spadaro A, Ramonda R, et al. Long-term safety of anti-TNF-α in PsA patients with concomitant HCV infection: a retrospective observational multicenter study on 15 patients. Clin Rheumatol 2014;33:273–6.

[163] Rudwaleit M, Van den Bosch F, Kron M, Kary S, Kupper H. Effectiveness and safety of adalimumab in patients with ankylosing spondylitis or psoriatic arthritis and history of anti-tumor necrosis factor therapy. Arthritis Res Ther 2010;12. R117.

[164] Jani M, Macphie E, Rao C, Moore S, Mirjafari H, McLoughlin Y, et al. Effectiveness of switching between biologics in psoriatic arthritis- results of a large regional survey. Clin Med (Lond) 2014;14:95–6.

[165] Ohshima Y, Kinoshita Y, Akita Y, Tamada Y, Watanabe D. Psoriatic arthritis that responded dramatically when infliximab was switched to adalimumab. Ann Dermatol 2013;25:496–7.

[166] Caso F, Lubrano E, Del Puente A, Caso P, Peluso R, Foglia F, et al. Progress in understanding and utilizing TNF-α inhibition for the treatment of psoriatic arthritis. Expert Rev Clin Immunol 2016;12:315–31.

[167] Caso F, Del Puente A, Peluso R, Caso P, Girolimetto N, Del Puente A, et al. Emerging drugs for psoriatic arthritis. Expert Opin Emerg Drugs 2016;21:69–79.

[168] Costa L, Del Puente A, Peluso R, Tasso M, Caso P, Chimenti MS, et al. Small molecule therapy for managing moderate to severe psoriatic arthritis. Expert Opin Pharmacother 2017;18:1557–67.

[169] McKeage K. Ustekinumab: a review of its use in psoriatic arthritis. Drugs June 2014;74:1029–39.

[170] Almirall M, Rodriguez J, Mateo L, Carrascosa JM, Notario J, Gallardo F. Treatment with ustekinumab in a Spanish cohort of patients with psoriasis and psoriatic arthritis in daily clinical practice. Clin Rheumatol 2017;36:439–43.

[171] Ritchlin C, Rahman P, Kavanaugh A, McInnes IB, Puig L, Li S, et al. PSUMMIT 2 Study Group. Efficacy and safety of the anti-IL-12/23 p40 monoclonal antibody, ustekinumab, in patients with active psoriatic arthritis despite conventional non-biological and biological anti-tumour necrosis factor therapy: 6-month and 1-year results of the phase 3, multicentre, double-blind, placebo-controlled, randomised PSUMMIT 2 trial. Ann Rheum Dis 2014;73:990–9.

[172] McInnes IB, Kavanaugh A, Gottlieb AB, Puig L, Rahman P, Ritchlin C, et al. PSUMMIT 1 Study Group. Efficacy and safety of ustekinumab in patients with active psoriatic arthritis: 1 year results of the phase 3, multicentre, double-blind, placebo-controlled PSUMMIT 1 trial. Lancet 2013;382:780–9.

[173] Kavanaugh A, Puig L, Gottlieb AB, Ritchlin C, Li S, Wang Y, et al. PSUMMIT 1 study Group. Maintenance of clinical efficacy and radiographic benefit through two years of ustekinumab therapy in patients with active psoriatic arthritis: results from a randomized, placebo-controlled phase III trial. Arthritis Care Res (Hoboken) 2015;67:1739–49.

[174] Kavanaugh A, Ritchlin C, Rahman P, Puig L, Gottlieb AB, Li S, et al. PSUMMIT-1 and 2 Study Groups. Ustekinumab, an anti-IL-12/23 p40 monoclonal antibody, inhibits radiographic progression in patients with active psoriatic arthritis: results of an integrated analysis of radiographic data from the phase 3, multicentre, randomised, double-blind, placebo-controlled PSUMMIT-1 and PSUMMIT-2 trials. Ann Rheum Dis 2014;73:1000–6.

[175] Singh RP, Hasan S, Sharma S, Nagra S, Yamaguchi DT, Wong DT, et al. Th17 cells in inflammation and autoimmunity. Autoimmun Rev 2014;13:1174–81.

[176] Suzuki E, Mellins ED, Gershwin ME, Nestle FO, Adamopoulos IE. The IL-23/IL-17 axis in psoriatic arthritis. Autoimmun Rev 2014;13:496–502.

[177] McInnes IB, Sieper J, Braun J, Emery P, van der Heijde D, Isaacs JD, et al. Efficacy and safety of secukinumab, a fully human anti-interleukin-17A monoclonal antibody, in patients with moderate-to-severe psoriatic arthritis: a 24-week, randomised, double-blind, placebo-controlled, phase II proof-of-concept trial. Ann Rheum Dis 2014;73:349–56.

[178] McInnes IB, Mease PJ, Kirkham B, Kavanaugh A, Ritchlin CT, Rahman P, et al. FUTURE 2 Study Group. Secukinumab, a human anti-interleukin-17A monoclonal antibody, in patients with psoriatic arthritis (FUTURE 2): a randomised, double-blind, placebo-controlled, phase 3 trial. Lancet 2015;386:1137–46.

[179] Mease PJ, Genovese MC, Greenwald MW, Ritchlin CT, Beaulieu AD, Deodhar A, et al. Brodalumab, an anti-IL17RA monoclonal antibody, in psoriatic arthritis. N Engl J Med 2014;370:2295–306.

[180] Gottlieb AB, Langley RG, Philipp S, Sigurgeirsson B, Blauvelt A, Martin R, et al. Secukinumab improves physical function in subjects with plaque psoriasis and psoriatic arthritis: results from two randomized, phase 3 trials. J Drugs Dermatol August 2015;14(8):821–33.

[181] Gooderham M, Papp K. Apremilast in the treatment of psoriasis and psoriatic arthritis. Skin Therapy Lett 2015;20:1–6.

[182] McAndrew R, Levin E, Koo J. Emerging oral Immunomodulators for the treatment of psoriasis: a review of phase III clinical trials for apremilast and tofacitinib. J Drugs Dermatol 2015;14:786–92.

[183] Paul C, Cather J, Gooderham M, Poulin Y, Mrowietz U, Ferrandiz C, et al. Efficacy and safety of apremilast, an oral phosphodiesterase 4 inhibitor, in patients with moderate-to-severe plaque psoriasis over 52 weeks: a phase III, randomized controlled trial (ESTEEM 2). Br J Dermatol 2015;173:1387–99.

[184] Kavanaugh A, Mease PJ, Gomez-Reino JJ, Adebajo AO, Wollenhaupt J, Gladman DD, et al. Longterm (52-week) results of a phase III randomized, controlled trial of apremilast in patients with psoriatic arthritis. J Rheumatol 2015;42:479–88.

[185] O'Shea JJ, Plenge R. JAK and STAT signaling molecules in immunoregulation and immune-mediated disease. Immunity 2012;36:542–50.

[186] Gao W, McGarry T, Orr C, McCormick J, Veale DJ, Fearon U. Tofacitinib regulates synovial inflammation in psoriatic arthritis, inhibiting STAT activation and induction of negative feedback inhibitors. Ann Rheum Dis 2016;75:311–5.

[187] LaBranche TP, Jesson MI, Radi ZA, Storer CE, Guzova JA, Bonar SL, et al. JAK inhibition with tofacitinib suppresses arthritic joint structural damage through decreased RANKL production. Arthritis Rheum 2012;64:3531–42.

[188] Maeshima K, Yamaoka K, Kubo S, Nakano K, Iwata S, Saito K, et al. The JAK inhibitor tofacitinib regulates synovitis through inhibition of interferon-γ and interleukin-17 production by human CD4+ T cells. Arthritis Rheum 2012;64:1790–8.

[189] Hsu L, Armstrong AW. JAK inhibitors: treatment efficacy and safety profile in patients with psoriasis. J Immunol Res 2014;2014:283617.

[190] Mease P, Hall S, FitzGerald O, van der Heijde D, Merola JF, Avila-Zapata F, et al. Tofacitinib or adalimumab versus placebo for psoriatic arthritis. N Engl J Med 2017;377:1537–50.

[191] Gladman D, Rigby W, Azevedo VF, Behrens F, Blanco R, Kaszuba A, et al. Tofacitinib for psoriatic arthritis in patients with an inadequate response to TNF inhibitors. N Engl J Med 2017;377:1525–36.

[192] Caso F, Costa L, Del Puente A, Scarpa R. Psoriatic arthritis and TNF inhibitors: advances on effectiveness and toxicity. Expert Opin Biol Ther 2015;15:1–2.

[193] Scarpa R, Costa L, Atteno M, Del Puente A, Caso F, Moll JM. Psoriatic arthritis: advances in pharmacotherapy based on molecular target. Expert Opin Pharmacother December 2013;14(17):2311–3.

Chapter 48

Neurological Disorders

Tali Drori[1,2], Joab Chapman[1,2,3]

[1]*The Department of Neurology, Sheba Medical Center, Tel Hashomer, Ramat-Gan, Israel;* [2]*The Zabludovich Autoimmune Center, Sheba Medical Center, Tel Hashomer, Ramat-Gan, Israel;* [3]*Robert and Martha Harden Chair in Mental and Neurological Disease, Sackler Faculty of Medicine, Tel Aviv University, Tel Aviv, Israel*

PART A MYASTHENIA GRAVIS

INTRODUCTION

Myasthenia gravis (MG) is an autoimmune disease, characterized by defective transmission of nerve impulses to muscle. It usually affects ocular, bulbar, and proximal extremity muscles and causes weakness and fatigability [1]. The disease is relatively rare, with an annual incidence of 8–10 cases per 1 million persons and a prevalence of 150–300 per 1 million [2]. MG can occur at any age and either gender; however, early-onset (before age 50) MG is characterized by female predominance, whereas very late onset, after the age of 60, has a clear male majority [2,3]. The natural history of MG is unpredictable, though generally characterized by relapses, with 85% of patients reaching a peak in severity within 3 years. 20%–30% of patients will experience a severe course, with respiratory muscle involvement and swallowing difficulties. In contrast, the disease will remain mild in 25% of patients [4].

IMMUNOPATHOLOGY OF MYASTHENIA GRAVIS

MG is an archetype for B-cell-mediated autoimmune disorders, the antibodies specifically targeting components of the acetylcholine receptor (AChR), thus resulting in impaired neuromuscular transmission in the postsynaptic membrane. The specific end-plate abnormalities include disruption of receptor signaling and complement-mediated tissue damage [5]. This has been demonstrated most convincingly through passive transfer of patient-derived serum, which reproduces features of the disease in experimental animals [6].

Acetylcholine Receptor Autoantibodies

AChR antibodies are found in 80% of all MG patients [7]. They are predominantly IgG1 and IgG3, activating complement and causing postsynaptic membrane damage and blocking the signaling pathway [8]. AChR antibodies are present in generalized and ocular MG, both early- and late-onset disease. Total antibody concentration does not correlate with severity of disease, though an increase in concentration may indicate MG exacerbation [9].

Muscle-Specific Kinase (MuSK) Antibodies

Muscle-specific kinase (MuSK) is an AChR-related membrane protein necessary for neuromuscular junction formation [10]. MuSK antibody positive MG account for 1%–10% percent of cases, with a majority of females. The disease is characterized by more severe and generalized weakness, often with facial and bulbar muscles involvement. Limb and ocular weakness are less common [11].

Other Autoantibodies in Myasthenia Gravis

Recent studies of MG patients without AChR antibody and MuSK antibody revealed additional autoantibodies specific to other neuromuscular junction proteins, such as lipoprotein-related protein 4 (LRP4), agrin, and collagen Q [12–14]. LRP4 antibody account for 7% of this group and associated with less severe disease [15]. In about 10% of all MG patients no muscle antibodies have been detected.

Mosaic of Autoimmunity. https://doi.org/10.1016/B978-0-12-814307-0.00048-7

TABLE 48.1 Subtypes of Myasthenia Gravis and Its Features

Antibody	Thymus Pathology	Target Population	Severity	Weakness Pattern
Acetylcholine receptor (AChR)	Hyperplasia	Early onset <50 yrs F > M	All severity grades: generalized and ocular forms	Any
AChR	Atrophy	Late onset >50 yrs F = M		Any
AChR	Thymoma	40–60 yrs	Mainly severe	Any
Muscle-specific kinase	Normal	Any age	Mainly severe	Bulbar
Lipoprotein-related protein 4	Normal	Any age	Mainly mild	Generalized

Thymus in Myasthenia Gravis Autoimmunity

In 10%–15% of MG patients, a thymoma is present, and up to 50% of thymoma patients develop MG [16], constituting a paraneoplastic disease. The thymic epithelial cells express epitopes cross-reactive with skeletal muscle proteins such as the AChR, thus the immune response against an epitope expressed on thymoma cells spills over to neuromuscular junction components sharing the same epitope [17].

Thymic hyperplasia is usually associated with early-onset AChR antibody positive patients, whereas thymic atrophy is characteristic of late-onset MG (Table 48.1).

DIAGNOSIS

The diagnosis of MG relies on the combination of clinical signs and symptoms and positive autoantibodies. Suggestive signs of MG include a combination of diplopia, ptosis, facial and neck weakness, dysphonia, and proximal muscle weakness. The pattern of neurological dysfunction is purely muscular damage, without sensory or central nervous system (CNS) involvement. The symptoms will typically worsen in the evening and exacerbate by exercise.

In antibody-negative cases, neurophysiological tests and a characteristic response to therapy confirm the diagnosis [18]. If there is significant ptosis, the ice test (ice cubes applied on the eye lid for 1 min) corrects the drop lid for a few seconds. Thymic status should be assessed by CT scan of the mediastinum.

TREATMENT

Symptomatic Therapy

All subtypes of MG respond to acetylcholinesterase inhibition, pyridostigmine being the preferred drug [19]. The exception is MG with MuSK antibodies, which has a less favorable response to symptomatic drugs [11]. Dosage should be titrated as needed based on symptoms and tolerance to side effects. These mainly consist of cholinergic symptoms such as diarrhea, abdominal pain, increased salivation, and sweating. For patients with mild disease, achieving remission with symptomatic therapy alone, no other drug therapy is recommended.

Immunosuppressive Therapy

Corticosteroids should be used in all patients with MG who have not met treatment goals after an adequate trial of pyridostigmine [19]. The dose of prednisone is usually increased gradually, up to 60–80 mg (sometimes on alternate days), to avoid initial deterioration. After control of symptoms has been achieved, glucocorticoid dose should be slowly reduced to lowest effective dose, often 10–40 mg on alternate days [1]. A nonsteroidal immunosuppressant should be added when response to steroids is not adequate, when dosage cannot be reduced, or when significant side effects appear [19]. In most patients, azathioprine is added to prednisone, as the combination provides a better functional result than prednisone alone [20].

The effect of azathioprine often takes months to appear; however, long-term safety profile is very good [21]. Other therapeutic options include cyclosporine, mycophenolate mofetil, methotrexate, and tacrolimus [19].

The anti-CD20 monoclonal antibody rituximab represents a potentially potent treatment for refractory and MuSK positive MG [22]. Rituximab treatment was shown in several studies to achieve significant clinical improvement, allowing for discontinuation of other immunotherapies in AChR and MuSK MG patients [23]. Exact regimen of treatment has not been established, however, and a second case of progressive multifocal encephalopathy in MG patients has recently been reported [24]. Eculizumab, a C5 inhibitor, which prevents membrane attack complex formation, proved effective in a small trial in AChR MG patients [25] and is now being evaluated in a phase III study. Inebilizumab is an anti-CD19 antibody with enhanced antibody-dependent cell-mediated cytotoxicity against B-cell lineages. The drug is currently being evaluated in the treatment of neuromyelitis optica and might be considered for testing in rituximab-resistant MG patients in the future [26].

Thymectomy

In patients with a thymoma and MG, thymectomy should be performed to remove the tumor. A benefit is also reported for patients with early-onset MG without a thymoma. A recent randomized controlled trial of 126 patients identified benefit for early thymectomy in patients with generalized disease, aged less than 60 to 65 and disease duration less than 3–5 years, not responding to anticholinesterase drugs [27]. Thymectomy is usually not recommended in MuSK- or LRP4-positive MG patients, as well as in seronegative patients [19].

Immunoglobulins and Plasma Exchange

Immunoglobulins (IVIg) and plasma exchange are regarded as equally effective [28] and are mainly used as short-term treatment in MG with life-threatening signs, such as dysphagia or respiratory involvement. Other indications include preparation to surgery in patients with bulbar dysfunction and prior to beginning corticosteroids to avoid exacerbations. The use of IVIg as maintenance therapy can be considered for patients with refractory MG or those in whom other immunosuppressant medications are contraindicated [19].

FUTURE DIRECTIONS AND CONCLUSIONS

With specialized treatment, most patients with MG do well. However, only few have full remission and most continue to require pharmacologic therapy. Although the disease-inducing antibodies have been characterized, the treatment is far from immunospecific. Semiselective forms of immunosuppression, as in the use of biological monoclonal antibodies, are promising options in MG. Their efficacy and safety profile need to be further evaluated in randomized trials.

PART B MULTIPLE SCLEROSIS

INTRODUCTION

Multiple sclerosis (MS) is a chronic inflammatory disease of the CNS. Its prevalence accounts for over 2.5 million affected individuals and estimated to be over 100 per 100,000 in North America and across most of Europe [29]. MS is most commonly diagnosed between the third and fourth decade, with a ratio of about 2:1 women to men. Although usually not life-shortening, the chronicity and progression of the disease heavily impacts on patients' quality of life, interfering with life and career plans of an individual [30].

Although the etiology of MS is still uncertain, the current model for disease pathogenesis proposes the interplay between genetic and environmental factors. Viral infections, such as Epstein–Barr virus exposure, are a hypothesized trigger for the development of MS by means of molecular mimicry and infection of B cells which may mediate chronic inflammation in MS [31]. Vitamin D might be another important mediator of susceptibility, with growing evidence demonstrating a relationship between low vitamin D levels and disease relapses, progression [32], and MRI activity [33].

The genetic predisposition is evident by the 10-fold increased risk of MS in monozygotic twins, and mainly associated with major histocompatibility complex class II phenotype, human leukocyte antigen (HLA)-DR2, and HLA-DR4 [34].

MS may take several forms, primarily based on its clinical course. In 85%–90% of patients the onset is relapsing–remitting MS (RRMS), with new symptoms occurring in isolated attacks. Symptoms of relapses vary and may include long-tract symptoms (weakness, numbness, paresthesias), optic neuritis, brainstem dysfunction (intranuclear ophthalmoplegia or nystagmus), impaired balance, Lhermitte sign, and transverse myelitis.

Secondary progressive MS develops over time following diagnosis of RRMS, where permanent neurological disability accumulates and frequency of attacks declines. In this stage, chronic symptoms often accumulate, including fatigue, cognitive dysfunction, bowel/bladder dysfunction, affective disturbances, sleep disturbances, sexual dysfunction, and spasticity. Around 10% of patients will experience a primary progressive form (PPMS), described as gradual continuous neurological deterioration [35]. Overall the course of the disease is varied; some patients experience a rather mild course, whereas most (up to 60%) require a wheelchair 20 years from diagnosis [36].

The diagnosis of MS relies heavily on clinical basis, combined with the demonstration of lesions on MRI images of the brain and spinal cord [37]. MS lesions are commonly found in the periventricular white matter and corpus callosum although they are evident throughout the white matter. Cerebrospinal fluid analysis and specifically oligoclonal band testing is positive in 95% of patients with clinically definite MS and doubles risk of progression to MS among patients with clinically isolated syndrome [38].

IMMUNOPATHOLOGY OF MULTIPLE SCLEROSIS

The acute MS lesion is the pathophysiologic end result of a highly coordinated cascade of inflammatory activity. Active blood–brain barrier breakdown is mediated by the recruitment of perivascular inflammatory infiltrates comprised of myelin-reactive T cells, B cells, and macrophages [39].

One of the major pathophysiological mechanisms of MS involves autoreactive T cells, primarily T helper (Th)-1, CD4+ T cells, and Th17 cells leading to cytokine secretion and activation of an inflammatory cascade. The result is demyelination within the brain and spinal cord and axonal damage; autoreactive antibodies cannot be discounted. Demyelination increases the inflammatory activation processes leading to further damage of the blood–brain barrier and stimulation of macrophage activation and oxidative stress pathways [40].

It is therefore conceivable to target immune cells and their products to prevent tissue damage by modulating inflammation, while reducing potential side effects such as global immunosuppression.

CURRENT DRUG THERAPIES

Management of Acute Exacerbations

Acute MS exacerbations are treated with glucocorticoids, typically with a course of 3–5 days of intravenous methylprednisolone 1000 mg daily, usually without oral prednisone taper [41]. This regimen is usually associated with minimal side effects, though caution should be used in patients with recurrent infections, gastric reflux, or psychiatric history. For refractory flares, retreatment with steroids or plasmapheresis might be beneficial [42]. Though effective in reducing the duration of the relapse and patients recovery, there are no long-term neuroprotective benefits [43].

Maintenance Therapy

Management of MS has become increasingly complex as there are now 15 FDA-approved disease-modifying treatments for MS. MS medications can be broadly classified into three groups [1]: injectable medications (beta interferon and glatiramer acetate [GA]) [2], oral medications (fingolimod, dimethyl fumarate, teriflunomide, and cladribine), and [3] infusion therapy (natalizumab, ocrelizumab, and alemtuzumab).

Injectable Medications

Interferon-beta-1 (INFβ-1) was the first disease-modifying drug for RRMS. It is presumed to alter the autoreactive environment in MS, balancing the expression of pro- and antiinflammatory cytokines in the brain and decrease the number of inflammatory cells crossing the blood–brain barrier [44]. In clinical trials, reduction of relapse rate with high dose interferon-beta-1b treatment was 34% compared with placebo and the severity of attacks was also reduced [45]. Side effects range from local body aches, flu-like symptoms, and less commonly depression and heart and liver problems.

GA is mixture of amino acids with antigenic similarity to myelin basic protein that alters T-cell activation, diverting Th1 cells to Th2 cells that suppress inflammatory response and activate Treg in the periphery [46]. GA reduced relapse rates and development of new lesions by up to 30% in RRMS, although it showed no improvement on progression of disability [47].

Oral Medications

Oral medications offer easier administration but have unique side effect and safety profiles. Dimethyl fumarate is a twice daily oral pill that was approved by the FDA in 2013. It reduces the migration of inflammatory cells through the blood–brain barrier and was showed in vitro to protect neuronal cells from oxidative stress [48]. Side effects include gastrointestinal upset, facial flushing, and, rarely, progressive multifocal leukoencephalopathy (PML) [49].

Fingolimod was granted FDA approval in 2010 and was the first oral therapy available for patients with relapsing forms of MS. It is a sphingosine receptor modulator, reducing lymphocyte migration and causing their sequestration in the lymph nodes [50]. In phase III clinical trials, fingolimod was more effective compared to INFβ-1a and placebo in reducing relapse rate, disability progression, and MRI outcome measures [51,52]. Due to the presence of sphingosine receptors on cardiac myocytes and in the eye, bradycardia and macular edema can occur. Cases of PML were also reported [53].

Teriflunomide is an active metabolite of leflunomide (an immunosuppressive disease-modifying drug used for rheumatoid arthritis), which inhibits the enzyme dihydroorotate dehydrogenase [54] and inhibits the proliferation of B and T cells. Its efficacy is in line with the injectable medications (tier I), whereas dimethyl fumarate and fingolimod are considered a second tier of efficacy. Side effects include hair thinning, diarrhea, and abnormal liver function test [55], though usually well tolerated. It is known to be teratogenic in animals and is pregnancy category X, limiting use in women of childbearing age.

Cladribine is a synthetic analogue of deoxyadenosine that preferentially reduces circulating T and B lymphocytes. This produces moderate and discontinuous reductions in T and B cells with relatively minor and transient effects on innate immune cells, such as neutrophils and monocytes [56]. The dosing regimen of cladribine tablets involves very short treatment periods relative to the length of clinical effect—eight to 10 days annually. Phase III clinical trials of cladribine showed significant benefits in rate of relapse, disability progression, and MRI measures [57].

Infusion Therapy

Currently available FDA-approved infusions for MS treatment are in the highest (third) tier of efficacy.

Natalizumab is a humanized monoclonal antibody against the cellular adhesion molecule α4-integrin, thus inhibiting immune cell migration across the blood–brain barrier [58]. Natalizumab is given as a monthly infusion and has high efficacy in lowering annualized relapse rate and MRI activity in MS patients [59]. However, this comes with a significant risk of PML [60]. Duration of treatment (>24 months), prior exposure to immunosuppression, and a high JCV virus antibody index increase the risk [60].

Alemtuzumab is a humanized monoclonal antibody against CD52. It is infused in two separate courses, 12 months apart. Dosing of the drug can precipitate late autoimmune side effects, including thyroid disease, seen in 30% of patients at 5 years, immune thrombocytopenia (2%) and rarely kidney disease (0.5%). Other side effects include risk of infection, malignancy, and bone marrow suppression [61]. It was approved by the FDA in 2014 to be used in RRMS, but due to the severity of the adverse events, its use is usually reserved for aggressive or refractory MS.

A newly approved anti-CD20 antibody infusion, ocrelizumab, has been a source of optimism in the MS community. Phase 3 clinical trial data showed high efficacy in relapsing MS [62] and reduction in disability progression of 24% in PPMS versus placebo [63]. Ocrelizumab is administered every 6 months. Side effects include higher rates of infections and a slightly increased risk of breast cancer [62] (Table 48.2).

CONCLUSIONS

MS is an autoimmune disorder of the CNS with an array of immune cells being either activated or suppressed leading to demyelination and disease progression. Historically, limited therapy choices in MS resulted in an "escalation" treatment strategy. Patients were placed on injectable medications and failure resulted in cessation or use of strong immunosuppressants. As a wide variety of treatment options became available in recent years, in particular to those with active disease, an ongoing debate arose in the MS community as to whether an "escalation" or "induction" approach to treatment initiation is optimal. Thus, MS treatment in today requires not only careful risk–benefit calculation, consideration of immune side effects, and patient preference but also a willingness to treat early and aggressively if circumstances are appropriate.

TABLE 48.2 Disease-Modifying Drugs in the Treatment of Multiple Sclerosis

Mode of Action	Dosage Mode of Administration	Brand Name	Drug
Injectables			
Balances pro- and antiinflammatory cytokines	250 mcg 3/week	Betaferon	INF-β1b
Decreases Th-17 Decreases IL-17	30 mcg 1/week 22 mcg/44 mcg 3/week	Avonex Rebif	INF-β1a
	125 mcg 1/2 weeks	Plegridy	Peg–INF–β1a
Amino acid mixture with antigenic similarity to myelin basic protein, alters T-cell activation	20 mg 1/day 40 mg 3/week	Copaxone	Glatiramer acetate
Orals			
Inhibits pyrimidine-dependent lymphocyte activation	14 mg qd	Aubagio	Terflunamide
Activates nuclear-factor-like 2 modulation of oxidative stress and reduced activation of autoreactive T cells	240 mg bid	Tecfidera	Dimethyl fumarate
Binds sphingosine-1-phosphate receptors, alters lymphocyte migration into CNS	0.5 mg qd	Gilenya	Fingolimod
Analogue of deoxyadenosine reduces circulating T and B lymphocytes	Two treatment weeks annually for 2 years	Mavenclad	Cladribine
Monoclonal Antibody Infusions			
Binds integrin receptors on leukocyte cell wall and alters migration into CNS	300 mg every 28 days	Tysabri	Natalizumab
Binds CD52 surface antigen resulting in cell lysis	2 infusions; the 1st lasting 5 days and the 2nd lasting 3 days, separated by 12 months	Lemtrada	Alemtuzumab
Binds B lymphocyte CD20 surface antigen	600 mg every 6 months	Ocrevus	Ocrelizumab

REFERENCES

[1] Gilhus NE. Myasthenia gravis. N Engl J Med 2016;375:2570–81.

[2] Carr AS, Cardwell CR, McCarron PO, McConville J. A systematic review of population based epidemiological studies in myasthenia gravis. BMC Neurol 2010;10:46.

[3] Alkhawajah NM, Oger J. Late onset myasthenia gravis: a review when incidence in the older adults keeps increasing. Muscle Nerve 2013;48:705e10.

[4] Grob D, Brunner NG, Namba T. The natural course of myasthenia gravis and effect of therapeutic measures. Ann NY Acad Sci 1981;377:652e69.

[5] Vincent A, Beeson D, Lang B. Molecular targets for autoimmune and genetic disorders of neuromuscular transmission. Eur J Biochem 2000;267(23):6717–28.

[6] Lindstrom JM, Engel AG, Seybold ME, Lennon VA, Lambert EH. Pathological mechanisms in experimental autoimmune myasthenia gravis. II. Passive transfer of experimental autoimmune myasthenia gravis in rats with anti acetylcholine receptor antibodies. J Exp Med 1976;144(3):739–53.

[7] Gilhus NE, Skeie GO, Romi F, Lazaridis K, Zisimopoulou P, Tzartos S. Myasthenia gravis — autoantibody characteristics and their implications for therapy. Nat Rev Neurol 2016;12:259–68.

[8] Verschuuren JJ, Huijbers MG, Plomp JJ, Niks EH, Molenaar PC, Martinez-Martinez P, Gomez AM, De Baets MH, Losen M. Pathophysiology of myasthenia gravis with antibodies to the acetylcholine receptor, muscle-specific kinase, and low density lipoprotein receptor-related protein 4. Autoimmune Rev 2013;12:918–23.

[9] Heldal AT, Eide GE, Romi F, Owe JF, Gilhus NE. Repeated acetylcholine receptor antibody-concentrations and association to clinical myasthenia gravis development. PLoS One 2014;9. e114060.

[10] Messe´ ant J, Dobbertin A, Girard E, Delers P, Manuel M, Mangione F, Schmitt A, Le Denmat D, Molgo´ J, Zytnicki D, Schaeffer L, Legay C, Strochlic L. MuSK frizzled-like domain is critical for mammalian neuromuscular junction formation and maintenance. J Neurosci 2015;35:4926–41.

[11] Guptill JT, Sanders DB, Evoli A. Anti-MuSK antibody myasthenia gravis; clinical findings and response to treatment in two large cohorts. Muscle Nerve 2011;44:36–40.

[12] Zhang B, Tzartos JS, Belimezi M, Ragheb S, Bealmear B, Lewis RA, et al. Autoantibodies to lipoprotein-related protein 4 in patients with double-seronegative myasthenia gravis. Arch Neurol 2012;69(4):445–51. 97.

[13] Gasperi C, Melms A, Schoser B, Zhang Y, Meltoranta J, Risson V, et al. Anti-agrin autoantibodies in myasthenia gravis. Neurology 2014;82(22):1976–83.

[14] Zoltowska Katarzyna M, Belaya K, Leite M, Patrick W, Vincent A, Beeson D. Collagen Q—a potential target for autoantibodies in myasthenia gravis. J Neurol Sci 2015;348(1–2). 241–24.

[15] Pevzner A, Schoser B, Peters K, Cosma NC, Karakatsani A, Schalke B, Melms A, Kroger S. anti-LRP4 autoantibodies in AChR and MuSK-antibody negative myasthenia gravis. J Neurol 2012;259:427–35.

[16] Romi F. Thymoma in myasthenia gravis: from diagnosis to treatment. Autoimmune Dis 2011;2011. 474512 https://doi.org/10.4061/2011/474512.

[17] Marx A, Porubsky S, Belharazem D, Saruhan-Direskeneli G, Schalke B, Strobel P, Weis CA. Thymoma related myasthenia gravis in humans and potential animal models. Exp Neurol 2015;270:55–65.

[18] Chiou-Tan FY, Gilchrist JM. Repetitive nerve stimulation and single-fiber electromyography in the evaluation of patients with suspected myasthenia gravis or Lambert-Eaton myasthenic syndrome: review of recent literature. Muscle Nerve 2015;52:455–62.

[19] Sanders DB, Wolfe GI, Benatar M, et al. International consensus guidance for management of myasthenia gravis: executive summary. Neurology 2016;87:419–25.

[20] Rae W, Burke G, Pinto A. A study of the utility of azathioprine metabolite testing in myasthenia gravis. J Neuroimmunol 2016;293:82–5.

[21] Pedersen EG, Pottegård A, Hallas J, et al. Risk of non-melanoma skin cancer in myasthenia patients treated with azathioprine. Eur J Neurol 2014;21:454–8.

[22] Keung B, Robeson KR, DiCapua DB, et al. Long-term benefit of rituximab in MuSK autoantibody myasthenia gravis patients. J Neurol Neurosurg Psychiatry 2013;84:1407–9.

[23] Nowak RJ, Dicapua DB, Zebardast N, Goldstein JM. Response of patients with refractory myasthenia gravis to rituximab: a retrospective study. Ther Adv Neurol Disord 2011;4(5):259–66.

[24] Robeson KR, Kumar A, Keung B, et al. Durability of the rituximab response in acetylcholine receptor autoantibody-positive myasthenia gravis. JAMA Neurol 2017;74:60–6.

[25] Howard Jr JF, Barohn RJ, Cutter GR, et al. A randomized, double-blind, placebo-controlled phase II study of eculizumab in patients with refractory generalized myasthenia gravis. Muscle Nerve 2013;48:76–84.

[26] Yi JS, Guptill JT, Stathopoulos P, Nowak RJ, O'Connor KC. B cells in the pathophysiology of myasthenia gravis. Muscle Nerve 2018;57(2):172–84.

[27] Wolfe GI, Kaminski HJ, Aban IB, et al. Randomized trial of thymectomy in myasthenia gravis. N Engl J Med 2016;375:511–22.

[28] Barth D, Nabavi Nouri M, Ng E, Nwe P, Bril V. Comparison of IVIg and PLEX in patients with myasthenia gravis. Neurology 2011;76:2017–23.

[29] Multiple Sclerosis International Federation. Atlas of MS. 2013. [pdf] http://www.msif.org/wp-content/uploads/2014/09/Atlas-of-MS.

[30] Rieckmann P. Improving ms patient care. J Neurol Suppl 2004;251:v69–73.

[31] Fernandez-Menendez S, Fernandez-Moran M, Fernandez-Vega I, Perez-Alvarez A, Villafani-Echazu J. Epstein-Barr virus and multiple sclerosis. From evidence to therapeutic strategies. J Neurol Sci 2016;361:213–9. Sospedra M, Martin R. Immunology of multiple sclerosis. Annu Rev Immunol 2005;23:683–747.

[32] Ascherio A, Munger KL, White R, et al. Vitamin D as an early predictor of multiple sclerosis activity and progression. JAMA Neurol 2014;71(3):306–14.

[33] Mowry EM, Waubant E, McCulloch CE, et al. Vitamin D status predicts new brain magnetic resonance imaging activity in multiple sclerosis. Ann Neurol 2012;72(2):234–40.

[34] Lincoln MR, Montpetit A, Cader MZ, et al. A predominant role for the HLA class II region in the association of the MHC region with multiple sclerosis. Nat Genet 2005;37(10):1108–12.

[35] Lublin FD, Reingold SC. Defining the clinical course of multiple sclerosis: results of an international survey. Neurology 1996;46:907–11.

[36] Katsara M, Matsoukas J, Deraos G, Apostolopoulos V. Towards immunotherapeutic drugs and vaccines against multiple sclerosis. Acta Biochim Biophys Sin 2008;40:636–42.

[37] Polman CH, Reingold SC, Banwell B, Clanet M, Cohen JA, Filippi M, Fujihara K, Havrdova E, Hutchinson M, Kappos L, et al. Diagnostic criteria for multiple sclerosis: 2010 revisions to the mcdonald criteria. Ann Neurol 2011;69:292–302.

[38] Dobson R, Ramagopalan S, Davis A, Giovannoni G. Cerebrospinal fluid oligoclonal bands in multiple sclerosis and clinically isolated syndromes: a meta-analysis of prevalence, prognosis and effect of latitude. J Neurol Neurosurg Psychiatry 2013;84(8):909–14.

[39] Lucchinetti C, Brück W, Parisi J, Scheithauer B, Rodriguez M, Lassmann H. Heterogeneity of multiple sclerosis lesions: implications for the pathogenesis of demyelination. Ann Neurol 2000;47(6):707–17.

[40] Kallaur AP, Lopes J, Oliveira SR, Simão AN, Reiche EM, de Almeida ERD, Morimoto HK, de Pereira WL, Alfieri DF, Borelli SD, et al. Immune-inflammatory and oxidative and nitrosative stress biomarkers of depression symptoms in subjects with multiple sclerosis: increased peripheral inflammation but less acute neuroinflammation. Mol Neurobiol 2016;53:5191–202.

[41] Galea I, Ward-Abel N, Heesen C. Relapse in multiple sclerosis. BMJ 2015;350:h1765.

[42] Weinshenker BG, O'Brien PC, Petterson TM, et al. A randomized trial of plasma exchange in acute central nervous system inflammatory demyelinating disease. Ann Neurol 1999;46(6):878–86.

[43] Myhr KM, Mellgren SI. Corticosteroids in the treatment of multiple sclerosis. Acta Neurol Scand 2009;120:73–80.

[44] Mitsdoerffer M, Kuchroo V. New pieces in the puzzle: how does interferon-beta really work in multiple sclerosis? Ann Neurol 2009;65:487–8.

[45] The IFNB Multiple Sclerosis Study Group. Interferon beta-1b is effective in relapsing-remitting multiple sclerosis. I. Clinical results of a multicenter, randomized, double-blind, placebo-controlled trial. Neurology 1993;43:655–61.

[46] Haas J, Korporal M, Balint B, Fritzsching B, Schwarz A, Wildemann B. Glatiramer acetate improves regulatory t-cell function by expansion of naive CD4(+)CD25(+)Foxp3(+)CD31(+) t-cells in patients with multiple sclerosis. J Neuroimmunol 2009;216:113–7.

[47] Johnson KP, Brooks BR, Cohen JA, Ford CC, Goldstein J, Lisak RP, Myers LW, Panitch HS, Rose JW, Schiffer RB, et al. Copolymer 1 reduces relapse rate and improves disability in relapsing-remitting multiple sclerosis: results of a phase iii multicenter, double-blind placebo-controlled trial. Neurology 1995;45:1268–76.

[48] Albrecht P, Bouchachia I, Goebels N, Henke N, Hofstetter HH, Issberner A, Kovacs Z, Lewerenz J, Lisak D, Maher P, et al. Effects of dimethyl fumarate on neuroprotection and immunomodulation. J. Neuroinflamm 2012:9.

[49] Gold R, Kappos L, Arnold DL, et al. Placebo-controlled phase 3 study of oral BG-12 for relapsing multiple sclerosis. N Engl J Med 2012;367(12):1098–107.

[50] Mandala S, Hajdu R, Bergstrom J, Quackenbush E, Xie J, Milligan J, Thornton R, Shei GJ, Card D, Keohane C, et al. Alteration of lymphocyte trafficking by sphingosine-1-phosphate receptor agonists. Science 2002;296:346–9.

[51] Cohen JA, Barkhof F, Comi G, Hartung HP, Khatri BO, Montalban X, Pelletier J, Capra R, Gallo P, Izquierdo G, et al. Oral fingolimod or intramuscular interferon for relapsing multiple sclerosis. N Engl J Med 2010;362:402–15. 137.

[52] Kappos L, Radue EW, O'Connor P, Polman C, Hohlfeld R, Calabresi P, Selmaj K, Agoropoulou C, Leyk M, Zhang-Auberson L, et al. A placebo-controlled trial of oral fingolimod in relapsing multiple sclerosis. N Engl J Med 2010;362:387–401.

[53] Novartis. Novartis, 2016. Internal data on file. 2016.

[54] Palmer AM. Teriflunomide, an inhibitor of dihydroorotate dehydrogenase for the potential oral treatment of multiple sclerosis. Curr Opin Investig Drugs 2010;11:1313–23.

[55] Confavreux C, O'Connor P, Comi G, et al. Oral teriflunomide for patients with relapsing multiple sclerosis (TOWER): a randomised, double-blind, placebo-controlled, phase 3 trial. Lancet Neurol 2014;13(3):247–56.

[56] Beutler E. Cladribine (2-chlorodeoxyadenosine). Lancet 1992;340:952–6.

[57] Giovannoni G, Comi G, Cook S, et al. A placebo controlled trial of oral cladribine for relapsing multiple sclerosis. N Engl J Med 2010;362:416–26.

[58] Sheremata WA, Minagar A, Alexander JS, Vollmer T. The role of alpha-4 integrin in the aetiology of multiple sclerosis: Current knowledge and therapeutic implications. CNSDrugs 2005;19:909–22.

[59] Miller DH, Khan OA, Sheremata WA, Blumhardt LD, Rice GPA, Libonati MA, Willmer-Hulme AJ, Dalton CM, Miszkiel KA, O'Connor PWA. Controlled trial of natalizumab for relapsing multiple sclerosis. N Engl J Med 2003;348:15–23.

[60] Berger JR, Fox RJ. Reassessing the risk of natalizumab-associated PML. J Neurovirol 2016;22(4):533–5.

[61] Coles AJ, Fox E, Vladic A, et al. Alemtuzumab more effective than interferon β-1a at 5-year follow-up of CAMMS223 clinical trial. Neurology 2012;78(14):1069–78.

[62] Hauser SL, Bar-Or A, Comi G, et al. Ocrelizumab versus interferon Beta-1a in relapsing multiple sclerosis. N Engl J Med 2017;376(3):221–34.

[63] Montalban X, Hauser SL, Kappos L, Arnold DL, Bar-Or A, et al. Ocrelizumab versus placebo in primary progressive multiple sclerosis. N Engl J Med January 19, 2017;376(3):209–20.

Chapter 49

Systemic Sclerosis: An Autoimmune Disease Without a Known Pathology and to Be Conquered

Przemyslaw J. Kotyla

Department of Internal Medicine Rheumatology and Clinical Immunology, Medical University of Silesia Katowice, Poland

INTRODUCTION

Systemic sclerosis (SSc) also called scleroderma is a connective tissue disease of unknown origin, characterized by fibrosis, vasculopathy, inflammation, immune dysregulation that leads to widespread internal organs fibrosis, chronic ischemia, and subsequent end-stage organ failure [1,2]. Internal organ involvement including lung fibrosis, pulmonary arterial hypertension, renal crisis, upper and lower digestive tract dysmotility, and heart involvement contribute to generally poor prognosis [3–5]. Although skin fibrosis is a hallmark of the disease, it is not only a fibrosis but deep changes in immune system functioning are believed to be responsible for the initiation and disease progression. The cause of scleroderma is unknown, but similarly to the other autoimmune diseases, it is a combination of environmental factors and genetic predisposition [6–10]. SSc is recognized as an orphan disease with prevalence being as low as 7 per million in some geographic area reaching the value of 700 per million in the others suggesting nonrandom distribution of cases in some populations and a possible spatiotemporal clustering of a disease in particular areas [11,12]. SSc is definitely an autoimmune disease, and presence of antinuclear antibodies (ANAs) in sera of patients with disease is almost universal reaching a level of 90%. It is still a matter of controversy whether these antibodies are directly responsible for driving autoimmunity in patients [13]. It is also still unclear what is the role of genetic susceptibility in the development of the disease. Twin studies performed by Feghali-Bostwick et al. confirmed role of genetic predisposition; however, scanty data on twins with SSc limit the certainty of the final conclusion based on this model [14]. It is claimed that a positive family history may be the strongest risk factor identified for SSc. Although the absolute risk in individual family members is below 1%, in a small but significant proportion of families (1%–1.6%) more than one first-degree relative was affected. Unfortunately, SSc is a rare disease that makes difficult to draw meaningful genetic conclusions from family-based linkage studies [15]. More supporting data come from studies on HLA in SSc patients. Similarly to the other autoimmune diseases, HLA class II region represents the most important region associated with SSc [10]. Recent genetic studies pointed to the role of some gene polymorphisms of key cytokines and their receptors in promotion of SSc with IL-1, IL-12, TNF-α, and interferons being the most intensively studied [16]. Obviously cytokines alone are not responsible for the whole picture of disease. To get a more precise insight we have to recognize source and cells that orchestrate immune environment. Fibrosis is the hallmark of the disease that has attracted research activity toward fibroblasts in the past. Now it is recognized as a part of dysregulated immune response [13]. Overactivity of fibroblasts is, however, the result of intensive cross talk with the other immunocompetent cells (B cells, T cells, and their regulatory variants) [17,18]. Finally endothelial dysfunction, impaired angiogenesis, and vasculopathy are leading causes for premature mortality, rapid reduction of quality of life, and generally severe course of the disease [19].

We are still on the crossroads thinking which way to take to find a Holy Grail that enables us to understand the complex pathogenesis of SSc. This review summarizes all important steps in recognition and understanding the nature of the disease.

GENETICS AND EPIGENETICS

HLA Studies

The genetic background of SSc was initially confirmed by the candidate gene studies, chosen on the base of previous reported association with other autoimmune diseases. During recent years, a substantial progression in understanding the role of genetic factors in development of disease has been made, enabling to identify a role of several groups of genes and their polymorphism in pathogenesis of SSc. Introduction of genome-wide association studies (GWASs) provided an excellent platform to investigate the genetics components of complex diseases. As autoimmunity shares the similar pathophysiological mechanisms regardless of diseases, it is not surprising that majority of genes identified in pathogenesis of SSc already play a role in the other connective tissue diseases. A substantial battery of evidence exists regarding the association of genes of major histocompatibility complex (MHC) with SSc. With 12 different genes identified so far, the majority belong to HLA class II (*HLA-DRA, HLA-DRB1, HLA-DRB5, HLA-DQA1, HLA-DQB1, HLA-DMB, HLA-DOA, HLA-DPA1, HLA-DPB1, and HLA-DPB2*) and only two to class I (*HLA-B and HLA-C*). There is a strong linkage between genes/haplotypes of HLA and SSc clinical subtypes and autoantibody production. There is, however, also negative association, because some HLA haplotypes may exert a protective role (DQB1*03:01, DQB1*03:03, DRB1*04:06) [20–24]. What is also important is that the genetic heterogeneity between different population is observed as the same allele is linked with disease in one population but exerts a protective role in the another [25,26]. So far nine GWAS including five GWAS, three follow-up GWAS, and one pan-meta GWAS have been performed in SSc populations. The first GWAS published in 2003 identified microsatellite polymorphic markers associated with susceptibility to SSc. The weak point of this analysis was fact that the study was performed in a Choctaw Indian population, a population with the highest world SSc prevalence. On the other hand, associations of SSc with 17 markers loci (including one HLA-D6S422) have been subsequently confirmed many years later in pan-meta and follow-up GWASs [27–35]. Detailed analysis of SNPs in a wide range of examined genes revealed more than 100 SNPs. It is noteworthy that the polymorphism described is present mainly in key genes responsible for cytokine synthesis. Unfortunately, some associations were not confirmed by follow-up studies. The striking example is a study on SNP rs 3128965 that initially found association with ATA but showed protective role in a follow-up study [36]. Keeping in mind difficulties in interpretation, HLA genetic studies that may be at least partially affected by statistical and methodological bias as well as heterogeneity of populations studied, recent finding suggests that specific HLA alleles could be responsible or provide protective activity to the development of SSc [26].

Non-HLA Studies

Besides studies on HLA genes, a significant portion of research has been focused on non-HLA genes indicating that genes associated with SSc may have various biological functions and play a role in such a processes as apoptosis, DNA methylation, tissue fibrosis, and regulation of interferon activity [37–40]. In the majority of completed studies so far, some genes variants are associated with SSc, and their roles have been confirmed in replication studies. The most promising findings are variants in CD247, IRF5, and STAT4. These findings cannot be overestimated as they are directly linked to immune response and their impaired activity is a hallmark of autoimmunity [41]. The same is true as far as cluster molecule genes are concerned. Several variants were identified in CD 6, CD19, CD22, CD58, CD226, and CD247. These small molecules are responsible for such functions as T-cell interactions, B-cell signaling, B-cell–B-cell interaction, cell adhesion, adhesion of cytotoxic T and NK cells to target cells, and intracellular signaling. The other promising candidates establishing the genetic role in SSc autoimmunity are genes encoding interleukins and their receptors with IL-1, IL-2, IL-6, IL-10, IL-13, and IL-21 being the most widely studied [10,42,43]. In line with these signaling molecules, regulatory factors and ligand receptors as STAT4, CD247, CD226, PTPN22, and TNSF4 exhibit significant polymorphisms linked to the development of SSc [44].

STAT4 is a transcription factor stimulated by IL-12 and IL-23 that orchestrates T-cell differentiation toward Th1 and Th17 response. Initial studies on STAT polymorphism replicated in five subsequent independent Caucasian cohorts showed that several gene variants are strongly linked to SSc. In particular, the rs7574865 T allele has been associated with the limited variant of SSc [45,46]. Special attention is due to the two CD molecules, CD247 and CD226. The first one represents the zeta chain, a component of the T-cell receptor, the second is an accessory molecule responsible for T-cell costimulation. Both molecules are associated with development of SSc, as shown in a GWAS and replication study [47,48]. CD226 overexpression is noted in patients with SSc which is linked to overproduction of cytokines, endothelial damage, and lung fibrosis [49,50]. Taking into account the role of molecules in T-cell function (T-cell antigen recognition and costimulation), it is plausible that impaired antigen recognition and costimulation in SSc patients contributes at least partially to susceptibility to SSc and other autoimmune diseases [48,51].

The role of T-cell costimulation is supported by the other genetic studies focused on the tumor necrosis factor ligand superfamily member 4 (TNFSF4) encoding OX40L (CD 252). OX40-OX40L-mediated signaling is essential for the generation of effector and memory T cells, which may be linked to anti-TNF activity [52]. Unfortunately, this signaling pathway is also involved in generation of autoimmune responses that have already been shown in autoimmune diseases in humans [53]. Two candidate genes studies on SSc identified both protective and risk variants of TNFSF4 gene with minor alleles rs1234313, rs2205960, and rs844644 being associated with SSc risk, whereas rs844644 exerted protective effect [34,54]. Genetic studies indicate the association of genetic variants with limited rather than the diffuse form of the disease [55]. This finding may be of importance, because patients with SSc exhibit high serum concentration of soluble OX40 and blockade of OX40L is recognized as a promising target for treating SSc-related fibrosis [56,57].

PTPN22 encodes the protein tyrosine phosphatase which is one of the mechanisms of T-cell suppression activation. PTPN22 R620W variant is the result of switch-off mutation leading to enzymatic inactivity and downregulating of T-cell receptor function. Impaired T cell recognition, but also what is perhaps more important impaired function of regulatory T cells (Tregs) is observed. PTPN22 (rs2476601) leading to a R620W variant is strongly linked to SSc in different populations as excellently reviewed elsewhere [58]. Because B cells share similar receptor signaling, individuals carrying the RW620 variant may exhibit impaired B-cell receptor transmission leading to impaired B-cell function. This finding is important in the light of overproduction of autoantibodies in SSc.

PATHOGENESIS OF SYSTEMIC SCLEROSIS

Role of Innate Immunity

The innate immunity stays at the frontline, protecting against invasive microorganisms. The innate system is, however, the first to recognize antigens and autoantigens and to cooperate with adaptive immunity to mount an adequate immune response. For a long time, SSc was recognized as a disease with impaired adaptive immune response where impaired immune response of immunocompetent cells plays a role. Recent advantages in understanding the pathophysiological background of the diseases highlighted the role of innate immunity as a link between fibrosis, interferon activation, autoantibodies synthesis cytokine, overproduction, and B- and T-cells response [59]. The first step in this process is activation of a group of special surface or endosomal receptors pattern recognition receptor (PRR) that are able to recognize conserved molecular structures in microbes termed pathogen-associated molecular patterns [60]. They also can recognize many self-antigens and molecules named danger-associated molecular patterns (DAMPs) as they are widely generated in such processes as inflammation, necrosis, apoptosis, trauma, and cell injury. Toll-like receptors (TLRs) are a group of PRRs designed to recognize molecular patterns of invading microbes or internal DAMPs. Although the role of innate immunity in SSc is only partially understood, there is growing evidence that activation of immune system via TLR triggering has an infectious basis or is dependent on activation by DAMPS [61,62]. Less is known on infectious agents in this regard. Quite recently, the role of Epstein–Barr virus (EBV) as a trigger of immune response has been underlined. EBV is a potent trigger for TLR9 which is able to recognize unmethylated EBV viral genomes [63]. Moreover, patients with SSc showed aberrant antibody response against EBV lytic antigens, resulting in accumulation of lytic mRNA and proteins in PBMCs and skin [64]. Serological data on patients with SSc underline the possible role of other infections including Toxoplasma gondii, CMV, parvovirus B 19, and endogenous retrovirus [65–67]. The second players on this field are DAMPs—endogenous TLR ligands released from injured tissues, necrotic or apoptotic cells, or generated from tissues on injury and that these elicit signaling via TLRs to induce inflammation and direct immunity [68]. Among 11 TLRs identified in human so far, TLR4 seems to play a special role. TLR4 was initially recognized as a receptor for bacterial LPS and is directly involved in recognition of DAMPs released for injured tissues in patients with SSc. Endogenous ligands for TLR4 include heat shock proteins HSP22, HSP60, HSP70, HSP72, and GP96, fibronectin, tenascin, high-mobility group box 1 (HMGB1), low-molecular hyaluronic acid (LMWHA), and the others. Many TLR ligands have been identified in SSc, consisting of both endogenous and microbial origin. It may be speculated that some DAMPs are released from endothelial cells (ECs) as the result of primary injury, and it is the major stimulus for inflammation and wound healing resulting in fibrosis seen in the disease [69–71]. Obviously interaction with TLRs is only the first step in creating an immune response. Following activation signals from TLRs may be transmitted via two separate pathways—myeloid differentiation factor 88 (MyD88) dependent or MyD88 independent. Activation of both pathways results in activation of the transcription factor activator protein-1 (AP-1). AP-1 and NFκB working together activates the expression of proinflammatory cytokines, chemokines, and MHC costimulatory molecules (Fig. 49.1). The second pathway is responsible for activation of interferons and late synthesis of cytokines, as reviewed in detail elsewhere [59]. Innate immune response seems to be an important factor in pathogenesis of SSc with activation of TLR playing a pivotal role. There is still an open question whether there is a missing link between endothelial injury immune response and fibrosis.

Interferons

Regulation of interferons type I synthesis is dependent on TLR signaling and closely linked to innate immune response [72,73]. Recently, we accumulated many data suggesting that similarly to SLE, in SSc interferons may play a role creating a

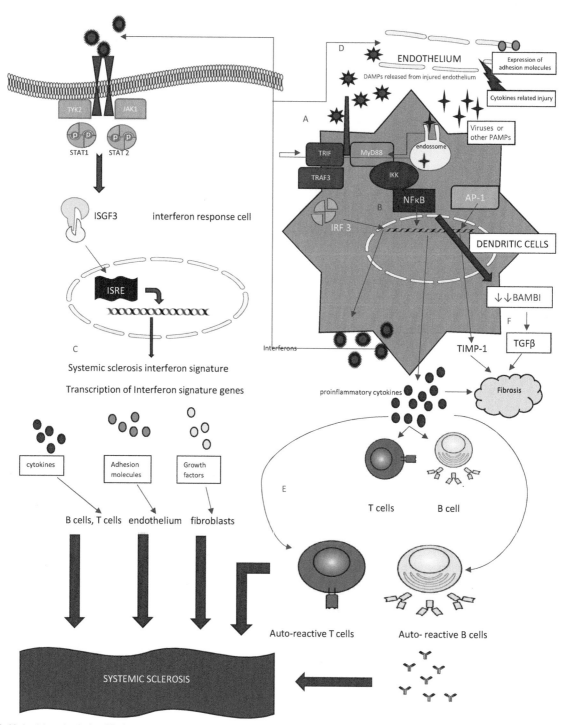

FIGURE 49.1 Mutual relationship between innate and adaptive immune system in systemic sclerosis. (A) Danger-associated molecular patterns (DAMPs) released from endothelium and other injured tissues are recognized by toll-like receptors (TLRs) located at dendritic cells. (B) TLR signaling resulted in activation of interferon response element, NFκB and Ap-1, resulting in interferon, inflammatory cytokine, and tissue inhibitor of metalloproteinases synthesis, respectively. (C) Released interferons than bind to their receptors and activate transcription of genes responsible for cytokines, growth factor, and adhesion molecules synthesis (systemic sclerosis gene signature). (D) Due to strong antiangiogenic properties, interferon contributes to impaired endothelium repair and subsequent vascular and endothelial damage. (E) Released cytokines dramatically change polarization of normal T and B cells toward autoreactive response resulting in autoantibodies synthesis that in turn facilitated vascular and tissue damage. (F) Signaling through a TLR4/MyD88/NF-κB pathway downregulates inhibitory receptor BAMBI that leads to sensitize cells to the relatively abundant levels of TGF-β1, promoting fibrosis. This process is augmented by activation of TIMP.

link between tissue injury and improper wound healing resulting in massive and uncontrolled fibrosis [74,75]. With striking similarity to SLE in SSc patients, interferon signature is observed that refers to interferon-dependent activation of several genes responsible for such processes as antigen-processing cell–cell cross talk, signaling proteins, adhesions angiogenesis, cell cycle immune modulation inflammation, and apoptosis (Fig. 49.1). Activation of IFN pathways in SSc brings many pathophysiological consequences. Firstly, IFNs are responsible for enhancement of expression of TLR which propagate recognition of DAMPs initially released from injured tissues. Secondly, IFN contributes to maturation of dendritic cells which in turn increases antigen uptake and their presentation to T cells. IFNs are potent antiangiogenic factors so in cases of overproduction of IFN angiogenesis is either stopped or at least impaired as it is observed in SSc. Finally, biological activities of IFN are associated with activation of several downstream proteins with NFκB being one of the most important. NFκB is a potent profibrotic factor working together with connective tissue growth factor to create a potent profibrotic milieu [76]. Signaling via NFκB-augmented profibrotic activity of TGF β by inhibition of expression TGF β pseudoreceptor BAMBI (bone morphogenetic protein and activin membrane-bound inhibitor), that create a link between tool signaling and TGF β activity [77]. On the other hand, NFκB plays the key role as a master of regulation of immune responses and components of NFκB interact with various cells regulating central and peripheral tolerance [78]. NFκB activity is responsible for such processes as cytokines synthesis (as TNF, IL-1, and IL-6) and upregulation of EC adhesion molecules, promoting cell migration into tissues.

Cytokines

With its 11 members, the family of IL-1 represents typical proinflammatory and profibrotic activity being involved in the nonspecific innate response to infection. The role of the IL-1 family, especially IL-1 and its receptor, has been addressed by many studies [79]. There are direct links between expressions of IL-1α and IL-1β in SSc fibroblasts, and their abnormal expression might contribute to the fibrosis SSc. IL-1α is a potent inducer of IL-6 and platelet-derived growth factor A (PDGF-A), which are strong stimulators of collagen production and proliferation in normal fibroblasts, which can be blocked by inhibition of endogenous IL-1α [80]. Moreover, by inhibition of IL-1 related IL-6 it is possible to stop procollagen type I synthesis in cultured SSc fibroblasts.

Since its discovery, the second member in the IL-1 family, IL-33 has attracted much attention, and many studies on the role of this interleukin have been conducted so far. IL-33 protein concentration is reduced in ECs and epidermis in skin biopsies from patients with SSc. On the other side, overexpression of ST2 (the receptor for Il-33) in ECs, mast cells, macrophages, T cells, B cells, and fibroblasts/myofibroblasts is seen. After activation, EC may release high amounts of IL-33 that may explain relatively low concentration of IL-33 in cells. IL-33 may provide strong profibrotic and proinflammatory signals through integration with its receptor ST2 in key profibrotic cells such as inflammatory/immune cells and fibroblasts/myofibroblasts [81]. Moreover, serum IL-33 was significantly increased in patients with SSc and was associated with early disease stage and early capillaroscopic changes. A German study on IL-33 did not reveal any relationship between serum concentration, SSc type, disease activity measured as Rodnan skin score, renal insufficiency, gastroesophageal involvement, and treatment administered. They, however, found a significant relationship between Il-33 and vascular changes—digital ulcers that may indicate more vascular than systemic activity IL-33 in SSc [82].

Less is known on the role of the third main interleukin from IL-1 family—IL-18. Serum levels of Il-18 are increased in SSc patients and strongly correlate with clinical stages of disease and formation of ANA [83]. However, not all studies confirmed that [84]. Other studies suggest that in fact IL-18 may exert antifibrotic potential, as it reduces collagen synthesis in SSc patients' dermal fibroblasts [85]. The possible explanation of these contradictory results is a role of IL-18-binding protein isoform (IL-18BPa) a soluble decoy receptor for Il-18 that may modulate biological activity of Il-18, resulting in pro- or antifibrotic activity [86]. Moreover, it was recently discovered that serum level of IL-18BPa correlates positively with vascular abnormalities and inflammatory status, but not with symptoms of skin and visceral involvement in SSc patients [87].

Interleukin 6

Interleukin 6 is a typical proinflammatory cytokine released from a wide variety of cells, and its role in development of many autoimmune diseases has been highlighted in many studies [88,89]. Patients with SSc show high IL-6 expression in fibroblasts, mononuclear cells, and ECs. Some studies link serum IL-6 levels with the extent of skin involvement, that may serve as a marker of disease and as a prognostic factor [90,91]. As a pleiotropic cytokine IL-6 affects key components of immune response being involved in such processes as immunoregulation, T-cell differentiation, angiogenesis, and osteoclast formation. Although dSSc fibroblasts express low levels of IL-6 receptor on their surface, elevation of fibrinogen synthesis may be mediated by so-called transsignaling which refers to cell that normally do not express IL-6R [92]. After interaction with IL-6R downstream signaling occurs with activation of Janus kinases with subsequent activation of signal transducers and activators of transcription 1 and 3 (STATs1/3), the RAS/Raf/MAPK, and also the PI-3 kinase pathways which may regulate such pathophysiological processes as cell–cell cross talk maturation of immunocompetent cell and fibrosis [93].

This pathophysiological finding makes IL-6 as an interesting target for therapeutic manipulation. Indeed, recently small controlled trails with tocilizumab showed improvement in patients outcome described as "patients' acceptable symptom state" as well as SSc-related arthritis and joint and skin score [94–96]. These are promising findings; however, as a preliminary data, the results should be confirmed in phase 3 trials.

IL-17

IL-17 is a family of cytokines (Il-17A-F), but the most studied one is IL-17A. The pathophysiological role of IL-17 is protection against infectious agents at sites of invasions and to coordinate a strong inflammatory response by activation of inflammatory response in IL-17-dependent cells including fibroblasts, epithelial and endothelial cells. As a potent inflammatory inducer IL-17 has been studied in the context of its role in SSc pathogenesis. Many studies, but not all, confirmed elevation of IL-17 levels in the sera of patients with SSc and confirmed a link between cytokine levels and clinical outcomes such as skin thickness, disease activity, and lung fibrosis [97,98]. Of special interest is the fact that in human studies IL-17 exerted antifibrotic potential and is negatively correlated with mRSS, but not with disease activity (Valentini score) [99].

Th1/Th2 Cytokines

The Th1/Th2 paradigm refers to the philosophy that Th1 cells secreting IFN-γ, TNF-α, and IL-2 are recognized as mainly proinflammatory cells and are involved in immune response. Polarization of Th cell toward Th2 response results in the synthesis of antiinflammatory cytokines not only IL-4, IL-10, and IL-13 but also IL-6 (with strong pleiotropic activity). So far there are no data pointing to a specific cytokine to be a key one, but most of studies completed suggest that Th1 response may play a role in early phase of the disease (inflammation) followed by Th2 response with fibrosis, repair, and activation of humoral response. The majority of studies indicate elevation of serum Th2 cytokines in SSc patients. Therefore, due to the complex of interaction between various cytokines, pointing to the pivotal one is not possible at the moment. Complex of interaction between Th cytokines has been reviewed in detail elsewhere [100].

B CELLS

In recent years, many studies underlined the role of B cells in the pathogenesis of SSc [101]. It is not surprising as autoantibody synthesis is seen nearly in 90% in SSc patients. On the other hand, B cells can promote fibrosis by cytokines, autoantibodies, and cell–cell contact and play a role as antigen-presenting cells [18]. B-cell infiltrates in affected skin are commonly seen in SSc. They may act in a paracrine manner releasing profibrotic cytokines to the surrounding tissues thus promoting fibrosis [102]. Of special importance is the fact that B cells in SSc are hyperactive. They overexpress the CD19 molecule, a crucial regulator of B-cell activation. Data from flow cytometry studies showed that B-cell surface density of CD19 is higher in SSc patients by 20% than in healthy individuals [103]. Keeping in mind the fact that CD19 overexpression reduces peripheral tolerance in B cells and facilitates autoantibody synthesis and autoimmunity, it is clear why patients with SSc develop autoimmunity with overproduction of autoantibodies being a hallmark of disease. CD 22 and CD35 inhibitory molecules expressed on the surface of B cell counteract stimulation mediated via CD19 and CD21. In SSc, however, function of both molecules is impaired [104]. Quite recently Odaka et al. proposed a functional role of antibodies against CD22 as a negative regulator of CD22 activity resulting in switch off their inhibitory function [105]. Blocking activity of anti-CD22 may superimpose on possible functional abnormalities in CD22, CD35 structure/function, as well as reflect intracellular abnormalities of intracellular pathways that transmit signals from B-cell receptors [106,107].

CONCLUSIONS

In spite of the progress in research in SSc, we are still far away from understanding the pathogenesis of the disease and why any drug tried in this indication failed to work. It is worth note that all immunologic alterations described in the paper are secondary to the activation of the innate immune system as the result of recognition of viral antigens or internal DAMPs followed by generation of interferon (interferon signature) activation of the adaptive immune system, B-cells and T-cells response, synthesis of antibodies cytokines, and chemokines. It is also not clear why the immune response is redirected toward fibrosis and vasculopathy. It is plausible that fibrosis may be a fatal coincidence, when many potentially profibrotic cytokine and other factors work together in patients genetically predisposed to hyper fibrotic response.

REFERENCES

[1] Elhai M, Avouac J, Kahan A, Allanore Y. Systemic sclerosis: recent insights. Joint Bone Spine 2015;82(3):148–53.

[2] Denton CP, Khanna D. Systemic sclerosis. Lancet 2017;10103(390):1685–99.

[3] Domsic RT, Nihtyanova SI, Wisniewski SR, Fine MJ, Lucas M, Kwoh CK, et al. Derivation and validation of a prediction rule for two-year mortality in early diffuse cutaneous systemic sclerosis. Arthritis Rheumatol 2014;66(6):1616–24.

[4] Allanore Y, Simms R, Distler O, Trojanowska M, Pope J, Denton CP, et al. Systemic sclerosis. Nat Rev Dis Primers 2015;1:15002.

[5] Kruszec A, Kotyla P. Heart involvement in systemic sclerosis. Pol Merkur Lekarski 2016;41(243):156–9.

[6] Elhai M, Avouac J, Kahan A, Allanore Y. Systemic sclerosis at the crossroad of polyautoimmunity. Autoimmun Rev 2013;12(11):1052–7.

[7] Marie I, Gehanno JF. Environmental risk factors of systemic sclerosis. Semin Immunopathol 2015;37(5):463–73.

[8] Marie I, Gehanno JF, Bubenheim M, Duval-Modeste AB, Joly P, Dominique S, et al. Systemic sclerosis and exposure to heavy metals: a case control study of 100 patients and 300 controls. Autoimmun Rev 2017;16(3):223–30.

[9] Marie I, Gehanno JF, Bubenheim M, Duval-Modeste AB, Joly P, Dominique S, et al. Prospective study to evaluate the association between systemic sclerosis and occupational exposure and review of the literature. Autoimmun Rev 2014;13(2):151–6.

[10] Murdaca G, Contatore M, Gulli R, Mandich P, Puppo F. Genetic factors and systemic sclerosis. Autoimmun Rev 2016;15(5):427–32.

[11] Chifflot H, Fautrel B, Sordet C, Chatelus E, Sibilia J. Incidence and prevalence of systemic sclerosis: a systematic literature review. Semin Arthritis Rheum 2008;37(4):223–35.

[12] Bernatsky S, Joseph L, Pineau CA, Belisle P, Hudson M, Clarke AE. Scleroderma prevalence: demographic variations in a population-based sample. Arthritis Rheum 2009;61(3):400–4.

[13] Chizzolini C, Brembilla NC, Montanari E, Truchetet ME. Fibrosis and immune dysregulation in systemic sclerosis. Autoimmun Rev 2011;10(5):276–81.

[14] Feghali-Bostwick C, Medsger Jr TA, Wright TM. Analysis of systemic sclerosis in twins reveals low concordance for disease and high concordance for the presence of antinuclear antibodies. Arthritis Rheum 2003;48(7):1956–63.

[15] Arnett FC, Cho M, Chatterjee S, Aguilar MB, Reveille JD, Mayes MD. Familial occurrence frequencies and relative risks for systemic sclerosis (scleroderma) in three United States cohorts. Arthritis Rheum 2001;44(6):1359–62.

[16] Mayes MD, Trojanowska M. Genetic factors in systemic sclerosis. Arthritis Res Ther 2007;9(Suppl. 2):S5.

[17] MacDonald KG, Dawson NA, Huang Q, Dunne JV, Levings MK, Broady R. Regulatory T cells produce profibrotic cytokines in the skin of patients with systemic sclerosis. J Allergy Clin Immunol 2015;135(4). 946–e9.

[18] Sakkas LI, Bogdanos DP. Systemic sclerosis: new evidence re-enforces the role of B cells. Autoimmun Rev 2016;15(2):155–61.

[19] Mostmans Y, Cutolo M, Giddelo C, Decuman S, Melsens K, Declercq H, et al. The role of endothelial cells in the vasculopathy of systemic sclerosis: a systematic review. Autoimmun Rev 2017;16(8):774–86.

[20] Kuwana M, Okano Y, Kaburaki J, Inoko H. HLA class II genes associated with anticentromere antibody in Japanese patients with systemic sclerosis (scleroderma). Ann Rheum Dis 1995;54(12):983–7.

[21] Kuwana M, Pandey JP, Silver RM, Kawakami Y, Kaburaki J. HLA class II alleles in systemic sclerosis patients with anti-RNA polymerase I/III antibody: associations with subunit reactivities. J Rheumatol 2003;30(11):2392–7.

[22] He D, Wang J, Yi L, Guo X, Guo S, Guo G, et al. Association of the HLA-DRB1 with scleroderma in Chinese population. PLoS One 2014;9(9):e106939.

[23] Wang J, Guo X, Yi L, Guo G, Tu W, Wu W, et al. Association of HLA-DPB1 with scleroderma and its clinical features in Chinese population. PLoS One 2014;9(1):e87363.

[24] Rodriguez-Reyna TS, Mercado-Velazquez P, Yu N, Alosco S, Ohashi M, Lebedeva T, et al. HLA class I and II blocks are associated to susceptibility, clinical subtypes and autoantibodies in Mexican systemic sclerosis (SSc) patients. PLoS One 2015;10(5):e0126727.

[25] Bossini-Castillo L, Lopez-Isac E, Martin J. Immunogenetics of systemic sclerosis: defining heritability, functional variants and shared-autoimmunity pathways. J Autoimmun 2015;64:53–65.

[26] Chairta P, Nicolaou P, Christodoulou K. Genomic and genetic studies of systemic sclerosis: a systematic review. Hum Immunol 2017;78(2):153–65.

[27] Broen JC, Coenen MJ, Radstake TR. Deciphering the genetic background of systemic sclerosis. Expert Rev Clin Immunol 2011;7(4):449–62.

[28] Gorlova O, Martin JE, Rueda B, Koeleman BP, Ying J, Teruel M, et al. Identification of novel genetic markers associated with clinical phenotypes of systemic sclerosis through a genome-wide association strategy. PLoS Genet 2011;7(7):e1002178.

[29] Lopez-Isac E, Bossini-Castillo L, Simeon CP, Egurbide MV, Alegre-Sancho JJ, Callejas JL, et al. A genome-wide association study follow-up suggests a possible role for PPARG in systemic sclerosis susceptibility. Arthritis Res Ther 2014;16(1):R6.

[30] Lopez-Isac E, Campillo-Davo D, Bossini-Castillo L, Guerra SG, Assassi S, Simeon CP, et al. Influence of TYK2 in systemic sclerosis susceptibility: a new locus in the IL-12 pathway. Ann Rheum Dis 2016;75(8):1521–6.

[31] Lopez-Isac E, Martin JE, Assassi S, Simeon CP, Carreira P, Ortego-Centeno N, et al. Brief report: IRF4 newly identified as a common susceptibility locus for systemic sclerosis and rheumatoid arthritis in a cross-disease meta-analysis of genome-wide association studies. Arthritis Rheumatol 2016;68(9):2338–44.

[32] Radstake TR, Gorlova O, Rueda B, Martin JE, Alizadeh BZ, Palomino-Morales R, et al. Genome-wide association study of systemic sclerosis identifies CD247 as a new susceptibility locus. Nat Genet 2010;42(5):426–9.

[33] Allanore Y, Saad M, Dieude P, Avouac J, Distler JH, Amouyel P, et al. Genome-wide scan identifies TNIP1, PSORS1C1, and RHOB as novel risk loci for systemic sclerosis. PLoS Genet 2011;7(7):e1002091.

[34] Bossini-Castillo L, Broen JC, Simeon CP, Beretta L, Vonk MC, Ortego-Centeno N, et al. A replication study confirms the association of TNFSF4 (OX40L) polymorphisms with systemic sclerosis in a large European cohort. Ann Rheum Dis 2011;70(4):638–41.

[35] Bossini-Castillo L, Martin JE, Broen J, Gorlova O, Simeon CP, Beretta L, et al. A GWAS follow-up study reveals the association of the IL12RB2 gene with systemic sclerosis in Caucasian populations. Hum Mol Genet 2012;21(4):926–33.

[36] Zhou X, Lee JE, Arnett FC, Xiong M, Park MY, Yoo YK, et al. HLA-DPB1 and DPB2 are genetic loci for systemic sclerosis: a genome-wide association study in Koreans with replication in North Americans. Arthritis Rheum 2009;60(12):3807–14.

[37] Carmona FD, Cenit MC, Diaz-Gallo LM, Broen JC, Simeon CP, Carreira PE, et al. New insight on the Xq28 association with systemic sclerosis. Ann Rheum Dis 2013;72(12):2032–8.

[38] Dieude P, Dawidowicz K, Guedj M, Legrain Y, Wipff J, Hachulla E, et al. Phenotype-haplotype correlation of IRF5 in systemic sclerosis: role of 2 haplotypes in disease severity. J Rheumatol 2010;37(5):987–92.

[39] Koumakis E, Wipff J, Dieude P, Ruiz B, Bouaziz M, Revillod L, et al. TGFbeta receptor gene variants in systemic sclerosis-related pulmonary arterial hypertension: results from a multicentre EUSTAR study of European Caucasian patients. Ann Rheum Dis 2012;71(11):1900–3.

[40] Wipff J, Dieude P, Avouac J, Tiev K, Hachulla E, Cracowski JL, et al. Association of metalloproteinase gene polymorphisms with systemic sclerosis in the European Caucasian population. J Rheumatol 2010;37(3):599–602.

[41] Dieude P, Boileau C, Allanore Y. Immunogenetics of systemic sclerosis. Autoimmun Rev 2011;10(5):282–90.

[42] Mayes MD, Bossini-Castillo L, Gorlova O, Martin JE, Zhou X, Chen WV, et al. Immunochip analysis identifies multiple susceptibility loci for systemic sclerosis. Am J Hum Genet 2014;94(1):47–61.

[43] Abtahi S, Farazmand A, Mahmoudi M, Ashraf-Ganjouei A, Javinani A, Nazari B, et al. IL-1A rs1800587, IL-1B rs1143634 and IL-1R1 rs2234650 polymorphisms in Iranian patients with systemic sclerosis. Int J Immunogenet 2015;42(6):423–7.

[44] Jin J, Chou C, Lima M, Zhou D, Zhou X. Systemic sclerosis is a complex disease associated mainly with immune regulatory and inflammatory genes. Open Rheumatol J 2014;8:29–42.

[45] Rueda B, Broen J, Simeon C, Hesselstrand R, Diaz B, Suarez H, et al. The STAT4 gene influences the genetic predisposition to systemic sclerosis phenotype. Hum Mol Genet 2009;18(11):2071–7.

[46] Gourh P, Agarwal SK, Divecha D, Assassi S, Paz G, Arora-Singh RK, et al. Polymorphisms in TBX21 and STAT4 increase the risk of systemic sclerosis: evidence of possible gene-gene interaction and alterations in Th1/Th2 cytokines. Arthritis Rheum 2009;60(12):3794–806.

[47] Dieude P, Boileau C, Guedj M, Avouac J, Ruiz B, Hachulla E, et al. Independent replication establishes the CD247 gene as a genetic systemic sclerosis susceptibility factor. Ann Rheum Dis 2011;70(9):1695–6.

[48] Dieude P, Guedj M, Truchetet ME, Wipff J, Revillod L, Riemekasten G, et al. Association of the CD226 Ser(307) variant with systemic sclerosis: evidence of a contribution of costimulation pathways in systemic sclerosis pathogenesis. Arthritis Rheum 2011;63(4):1097–105.

[49] Ayano M, Tsukamoto H, Kohno K, Ueda N, Tanaka A, Mitoma H, et al. Increased CD226 expression on CD8+ T cells is associated with upregulated cytokine production and endothelial cell injury in patients with systemic sclerosis. J Immunol 2015;195(3):892–900.

[50] Bossini-Castillo L, Simeon CP, Beretta L, Broen JC, Vonk MC, Rios-Fernandez R, et al. A multicenter study confirms CD226 gene association with systemic sclerosis-related pulmonary fibrosis. Arthritis Res Ther 2012;14(2):R85.

[51] Song G, Bae SC, Choi S, Ji J, Lee Y. Association between the CD226 rs763361 polymorphism and susceptibility to autoimmune diseases: a meta-analysis. Lupus 2012;21(14):1522–30.

[52] Buchan SL, Rogel A, Al-Shamkhani A. The immunobiology of CD27 and OX40 and their potential as targets for cancer immunotherapy. Blood 2017.

[53] Webb GJ, Hirschfield GM, Lane PJ. OX40, OX40L and autoimmunity: a comprehensive review. Clin Rev Allergy Immunol 2016;50(3):312–32.

[54] Gourh P, Arnett FC, Tan FK, Assassi S, Divecha D, Paz G, et al. Association of TNFSF4 (OX40L) polymorphisms with susceptibility to systemic sclerosis. Ann Rheum Dis 2010;69(3):550–5.

[55] Coustet B, Bouaziz M, Dieude P, Guedj M, Bossini-Castillo L, Agarwal S, et al. Independent replication and meta analysis of association studies establish TNFSF4 as a susceptibility gene preferentially associated with the subset of anticentromere-positive patients with systemic sclerosis. J Rheumatol 2012;39(5):997–1003.

[56] Komura K, Yoshizaki A, Kodera M, Iwata Y, Ogawa F, Shimizu K, et al. Increased serum soluble OX40 in patients with systemic sclerosis. J Rheumatol 2008;35(12):2359–62.

[57] Elhai M, Avouac J, Hoffmann-Vold AM, Ruzehaji N, Amiar O, Ruiz B, et al. OX40L blockade protects against inflammation-driven fibrosis. Proc Natl Acad Sci USA 2016;113(27):E3901–10.

[58] Lee YH, Choi SJ, Ji JD, Song GG. The association between the PTPN22 C1858T polymorphism and systemic sclerosis: a meta-analysis. Mol Biol Rep 2012;39(3):3103–8.

[59] Jimenez-Dalmaroni MJ, Gerswhin ME, Adamopoulos IE. The critical role of toll-like receptors–from microbial recognition to autoimmunity: a comprehensive review. Autoimmun Rev 2016;15(1):1–8.

[60] Gianchecchi E, Fierabracci A. Gene/environment interactions in the pathogenesis of autoimmunity: new insights on the role of Toll-like receptors. Autoimmun Rev 2015;14(11):971–83.

[61] Dowson C, Simpson N, Duffy L, O'Reilly S. Innate immunity in systemic sclerosis. Curr Rheumatol Rep 2017;19(1):2.

[62] Lafyatis R, Farina A. New insights into the mechanisms of innate immune receptor signalling in fibrosis. Open Rheumatol J 2012;6:72–9.

[63] Lunemann A, Rowe M, Nadal D. Innate immune recognition of EBV. Curr Top Microbiol Immunol 2015;391:265–87.

[64] Farina A, Cirone M, York M, Lenna S, Padilla C, McLaughlin S, et al. Epstein-Barr virus infection induces aberrant TLR activation pathway and fibroblast-myofibroblast conversion in scleroderma. J Invest Dermatol 2014;134(4):954–64.

[65] Grossman C, Dovrish Z, Shoenfeld Y, Amital H. Do infections facilitate the emergence of systemic sclerosis? Autoimmun Rev 2011;10(5):244–7.

[66] Randone SB, Guiducci S, Cerinic MM. Systemic sclerosis and infections. Autoimmun Rev 2008;8(1):36–40.

[67] Vaughan JH, Shaw PX, Nguyen MD, Medsger Jr TA, Wright TM, Metcalf JS, et al. Evidence of activation of 2 herpesviruses, Epstein-Barr virus and cytomegalovirus, in systemic sclerosis and normal skins. J Rheumatol 2000;27(3):821–3.

[68] Fullard N, O'Reilly S. Role of innate immune system in systemic sclerosis. Semin Immunopathol 2015;37(5):511–7.

[69] Bhattacharyya S, Midwood KS, Yin H, Varga J. Toll-like Receptor-4 signaling drives persistent fibroblast activation and rrevents fibrosis resolution in scleroderma. Adv Wound Care 2017;6(10):356–69.

[70] Bhattacharyya S, Varga J. Endogenous ligands of TLR4 promote unresolving tissue fibrosis: implications for systemic sclerosis and its targeted therapy. Immunol Lett 2017.

[71] Kahaleh B. The microvascular endothelium in scleroderma. Rheumatology (Oxford) 2008;47(Suppl. 5). v14-5.

[72] Santana-de Anda K, Gomez-Martin D, Diaz-Zamudio M, Alcocer-Varela J. Interferon regulatory factors: beyond the antiviral response and their link to the development of autoimmune pathology. Autoimmun Rev 2011;11(2):98–103.

[73] Chen K, Liu J, Cao X. Regulation of type I interferon signaling in immunity and inflammation: a comprehensive review. J Autoimmun 2017;83:1–11.

[74] Dantas AT, Goncalves SM, Pereira MC, de Almeida AR, Marques CD, Rego MJ, et al. Interferons and systemic sclerosis: correlation between interferon gamma and interferon-lambda 1 (IL-29). Autoimmunity 2015;48(7):429–33.

[75] Wu M, Assassi S. The role of type 1 interferon in systemic sclerosis. Front Immunol 2013;4:266.

[76] Mori T, Kawara S, Shinozaki M, Hayashi N, Kakinuma T, Igarashi A, et al. Role and interaction of connective tissue growth factor with transforming growth factor-beta in persistent fibrosis: a mouse fibrosis model. J Cell Physiol 1999;181(1):153–9.

[77] Sekiya T, Oda T, Matsuura K, Akiyama T. Transcriptional regulation of the TGF-beta pseudoreceptor BAMBI by TGF-beta signaling. Biochem Biophys Res Commun 2004;320(3):680–4.

[78] Pai S, Thomas R. Immune deficiency or hyperactivity-Nf-kappab illuminates autoimmunity. J Autoimmun 2008;31(3):245–51.

[79] Zhang L, Yan J-W, Wang Y-J, Wan Y-N, Wang B-X, Tao J-H, et al. Association of interleukin 1 family with systemic sclerosis. Inflammation 2014;37(4):1213–20.

[80] Kawaguchi Y, Hara M, Wright TM. Endogenous IL-1alpha from systemic sclerosis fibroblasts induces IL-6 and PDGF-A. J Clin Invest 1999;103(9):1253–60.

[81] Manetti M, Ibba-Manneschi L, Liakouli V, Guiducci S, Milia AF, Benelli G, et al. The IL1-like cytokine IL33 and its receptor ST2 are abnormally expressed in the affected skin and visceral organs of patients with systemic sclerosis. Ann Rheum Dis 2010;69(3):598–605.

[82] Terras S, Opitz E, Moritz RK, Hoxtermann S, Gambichler T, Kreuter A. Increased serum IL-33 levels may indicate vascular involvement in systemic sclerosis. Ann Rheum Dis 2013;72(1):144–5.

[83] Mosaad YM, Metwally SS, Auf FA, Abd ELSER, el-Deek B, Limon NI, et al. Proinflammatory cytokines (IL-12 and IL-18) in immune rheumatic diseases: relation with disease activity and autoantibodies production. Egypt J Immunol 2003;10(2):19–26.

[84] Scala E, Pallotta S, Frezzolini A, Abeni D, Barbieri C, Sampogna F, et al. Cytokine and chemokine levels in systemic sclerosis: relationship with cutaneous and internal organ involvement. Clin Exp Immunol 2004;138(3):540–6.

[85] Kim HJ, Song SB, Choi JM, Kim KM, Cho BK, Cho DH, et al. IL-18 downregulates collagen production in human dermal fibroblasts via the ERK pathway. J Invest Dermatol 2010;130(3):706–15.

[86] Dinarello CA, Novick D, Kim S, Kaplanski G. Interleukin-18 and IL-18 binding protein. Front Immunol 2013;4:289.

[87] Nakamura K, Asano Y, Taniguchi T, Minatsuki S, Inaba T, Maki H, et al. Serum levels of interleukin-18-binding protein isoform a: clinical association with inflammation and pulmonary hypertension in systemic sclerosis. J Dermatol 2016;43(8):912–8.

[88] Ishihara K, Hirano T. IL-6 in autoimmune disease and chronic inflammatory proliferative disease. Cytokine Growth Factor Rev 2002;13(4–5):357–68.

[89] Fonseca JE, Santos MJ, Canhao H, Choy E. Interleukin-6 as a key player in systemic inflammation and joint destruction. Autoimmun Rev 2009;8(7):538–42.

[90] Khan K, Xu S, Nihtyanova S, Derrett-Smith E, Abraham D, Denton CP, et al. Clinical and pathological significance of interleukin 6 overexpression in systemic sclerosis. Ann Rheum Dis 2012;71(7):1235–42.

[91] Sato S, Hasegawa M, Takehara K. Serum levels of interleukin-6 and interleukin-10 correlate with total skin thickness score in patients with systemic sclerosis. J Dermatol Sci 2001;27(2):140–6.

[92] Jones SA, Scheller J, Rose-John S. Therapeutic strategies for the clinical blockade of IL-6/gp130 signaling. J Clin Invest 2011;121(9):3375–83.

[93] O'Reilly S, Cant R, Ciechomska M, van Laar JM. Interleukin-6: a new therapeutic target in systemic sclerosis? Clin Transl Immunol 2013;2(4):e4.

[94] Arnold MB, Khanna D, Denton CP, van Laar JM, Frech TM, Anderson ME, et al. Patient acceptable symptom state in scleroderma: results from the tocilizumab compared with placebo trial in active diffuse cutaneous systemic sclerosis. Oxford: Rheumatology; 2017.

[95] Elhai M, Meunier M, Matucci-Cerinic M, Maurer B, Riemekasten G, Leturcq T, et al. Outcomes of patients with systemic sclerosis-associated polyarthritis and myopathy treated with tocilizumab or abatacept: a EUSTAR observational study. Ann Rheum Dis 2013;72(7):1217–20.

[96] Khanna D, Denton CP, Jahreis A, van Laar JM, Frech TM, Anderson ME, et al. Safety and efficacy of subcutaneous tocilizumab in adults with systemic sclerosis (faSScinate): a phase 2, randomised, controlled trial. Lancet 2016;387(10038):2630–40.

[97] Rolla G, Fusaro E, Nicola S, Bucca C, Peroni C, Parisi S, et al. Th-17 cytokines and interstitial lung involvement in systemic sclerosis. J Breath Res 2016;10(4):046013.

[98] Balanescu P, Balanescu E, Balanescu A. IL-17 and Th17 cells in systemic sclerosis: a comprehensive review. Rom J Intern Med 2017;55(4):198–204.

[99] Chizzolini C, Dufour AM, Brembilla NC. Is there a role for IL-17 in the pathogenesis of systemic sclerosis? Immunol Lett 2017.

[100] Baraut J, Michel L, Verrecchia F, Farge D. Relationship between cytokine profiles and clinical outcomes in patients with systemic sclerosis. Autoimmun Rev 2010;10(2):65–73.

[101] Sakkas LI, Bogdanos DP. The role of B cells in the pathogenesis of systemic sclerosis. Isr Med Assoc J 2016;18(9):516–9.

[102] O'Reilly S, Ciechomska M, Cant R, van Laar JM. Interleukin-6 (IL-6) trans signaling drives a STAT3-dependent pathway that leads to hyperactive transforming growth factor-beta (TGF-beta) signaling promoting SMAD3 activation and fibrosis via Gremlin protein. J Biol Chem 2014;289(14):9952–60.

[103] Sato S, Hasegawa M, Fujimoto M, Tedder TF, Takehara K. Quantitative genetic variation in CD19 expression correlates with autoimmunity. J Immunol (Baltimore Md 1950) 2000;165(11):6635–43.

[104] Soto L, Ferrier A, Aravena O, Fonseca E, Berendsen J, Biere A, et al. Systemic sclerosis patients present alterations in the expression of molecules involved in B-cell regulation. Front Immunol 2015;6:496.

[105] Odaka M, Hasegawa M, Hamaguchi Y, Ishiura N, Kumada S, Matsushita T, et al. Autoantibody-mediated regulation of B cell responses by functional anti-CD22 autoantibodies in patients with systemic sclerosis. Clin Exp Immunol 2010;159(2):176–84.

[106] Dawidowicz K, Dieude P, Avouac J, Wipff J, Hachulla E, Diot E, et al. Association study of B-cell marker gene polymorphisms in European Caucasian patients with systemic sclerosis. Clin Exp Rheumatol 2011;29(5):839–42.

[107] Hitomi Y, Tsuchiya N, Hasegawa M, Fujimoto M, Takehara K, Tokunaga K, et al. Association of CD22 gene polymorphism with susceptibility to limited cutaneous systemic sclerosis. Tissue Antigens 2007;69(3):242–9.

Chapter 50

Sjogren's Syndrome

Barone Francesca[1], Colafrancesco Serena[2]

[1]Centre for Translational Inflammation Research, Institute of Inflammation and Ageing, College of Medical & Dental Sciences, University of Birmingham Research Laboratories, Queen Elizabeth Hospital, Birmingham, United Kingdom; [2]Department of Internal Medicine and Medical Specialties, Rheumatology Unit, Sapienza University of Rome, Rome, Italy

Sjögren's syndrome (SS) is a chronic autoimmune condition characterized by autoantibody production, sicca syndrome, and intraglandular accumulation of immune cells in periepithelial lymphocytic lesions. Periductal aggregate formation is associated with glandular hypofunction and destruction of functional glandular epithelium leading to the development of the xerophthalmia or xerostomia. Patients with primary SS (pSS) are known to display altered peripheral blood B cells frequencies with the predominance of CD27- naive B cells and a progressive accumulation in the glands of memory B cells [1–3]. B cells accumulate in large aggregates characterized by the aberrant secretion of lymphoid chemokines, which is able to drive the formation of ectopic germinal centers (GCs).

Systemically, the disease is characterized by organ involvement and increased B cell activation, as demonstrated by increased level of immunoglobulins in the blood. In this chapter, an overview on the central pathogenic mechanisms in SS will be provided with a special focus on the role of epithelium, the development of ectopic lymphoid structures (ELS), and the possible therapeutic strategies for this condition.

PATHOGENESIS OVERVIEW

Chronic sialadenitis results in progressive tissue damage with loss of secretory gland function leading to the primary clinical features of keratoconjunctivitis sicca (dry eyes) and xerostomia (dry mouth). The inflammatory process can progress to involve almost any organ system resulting in systemic manifestations of disease [4,5]. In addition, patients with primary disease are at increased risk of B cell lymphomas compared with the general population [6].

The disorder was first described both clinically and histologically in 1933 by the Swedish ophthalmologist Henry Sjögren. The organ-specific pathology is caused by local inflammation and progressive loss of the glandular parenchyma [7]. In 50%–60% of cases, this disorder is associated with other systemic autoimmune diseases, such as rheumatoid arthritis (RA) or systemic lupus erythematous (SLE), where it is considered to be a secondary rather than primary disease process [7,8]. pSS, which occurs in the absence of other conditions, has a higher frequency in female patients (9:1) and a prevalence of 0.5% in the general population, making pSS one of the three most frequent autoimmune diseases [4,7,9].

Compelling evidence suggests that several biological processes are involved in pSS and contribute to the establishment of salivary gland pathology. Those encompass pathways of activation belonging to both the innate and acquired immune systems, such as interferon (IFN) activation [10], defective regulatory T cell activity [11], an increased number and function of Th17 cells [12], and excessive co-stimulation [13]. Lymphangiogenesis with GC formation and clonal expansion of malignant B cells is ascribed to the aberrant B cell activation that characterizes a subset of patients with high serum titers of autoantibodies and systemic manifestations of the disease.

PSS is clinically characterized by, but not limited to, secretory glandular dysfunction. One-third of patients exhibit systemic extraglandular manifestations, whose development and onset varies during the disease progression [8,14]. As a result, the clinical management of the disease requires a multidisciplinary approach including input from rheumatologists, ophthalmologists, and oral medicine specialists.

The extraglandular manifestations include cutaneous vasculitis (leukocytoclastic vasculitis), peripheral neuropathy, polyarthralgia and synovitis, fatigue, renal tubular acidosis, interstitial lung disease, lymphoproliferative disease, and immunological abnormalities, such as lymphopenia, anemia, or thrombocytopenia [5]. Immunological findings are also observed in pSS, such as the presence of anti–SS-related antigen A and B autoantibodies (anti-SSA/Ro and SSB/La), hypergammaglobulinemia and low complement levels (C4) [14].

Mosaic of Autoimmunity. https://doi.org/10.1016/B978-0-12-814307-0.00050-5

Approximately 5% of patients with pSS develop lymphoma, conferring a higher mortality risk as compared with the normal population [15]. Histologically, the malignancy is predominantly a mucosal associated lymphoid tissue (MALT) non-Hodgkin's lymphoma that predominantly arises in extranodal sites, in particular the parotid glands [6,16]. However, other forms of B cell lymphoma, such as diffuse large B cell lymphoma, are also observed. Patients displaying GC were suggested to be at higher risk to develop the malignancy [17].

AN "AUTOIMMUNE EPITHELITIS"

The definition "autoimmune epithelitis" was provided in 1994 with the aim to highlight the involvement of this cellular population in disease pathogenesis [8]. In pSS, glandular epithelial cells do not act as innocent bystander subjected to the lymphocytic toxic effect but have been shown able to produce chemokines and cytokines essential for the local migration and organization of immune cells and to act as antigen-presenting cells. Those include CXCL13 [18], known B cell chemoattractant, B-cell activating factor (BAFF), and IL-7, two key survival factors that, respectively, regulate B and T cell homeostasis, and CXCL12, a chemokine implicated in the migration of autoreactive B cells within the ducts during the process of lymphomagenesis [88].

Epithelial cells activation can be driven by several external stimuli, and the role of infections, mainly viruses, triggering this process and driving inflammation by different molecules, with special reference to the "IFN signature," is well known [19]. Indeed, an overexpression of IFN inducible genes, such as BAFF or IFN-induced transmembrane protein 1, has been demonstrated in ductal epithelial cells from pSS patients [20]. A prominent type I IFN signature in patients with pSS has been demonstrated both in gene expression profile in minor salivary glands [19] and in peripheral blood cells [21]. Moreover, plasmacytoid dendritic cells, which represent the main source of type I IFN, were found recruited within pSS salivary glands and reduced in the peripheral compartment suggesting an active recruitment for this population in the salivary glands (sg) [22].

Recently, a role for type II IFN (IFNγ) has also been demonstrated [23]. Type II IFN is predominantly produced by T and natural killer (NK) cells and seems to be able to promote antimicrobial protection, apoptosis, inflammation, and tissue damage by upregulation of IFN II genes [24]. In 2015, Nezos A et al. confirmed a predominance of the type I IFN signature in peripheral blood of SS patients but found a predominant type II IFN signature in pSS sg biopsies [24]. Similarly, biopsies from pSS lymphoma display a higher IFNγ and type II IFN-induced genes transcripts as compared with type I IFN [24].

While involved in the earliest phases of the disease as major provider of chemoattractant stimuli and expression of survival factors, the epithelium in pSS is also the ultimate target of the pathogenic process. Ductal and acini epithelial cells apoptosis has been associated to loss of function of the secretory tissue in pSS. High expression of FasR has been shown on pSS epithelial cells in proximity to inflammatory infiltrates and a contribution of addictive signals has been demonstrated by CD40 ligation by CD40L expressed on accumulated immune cells [25,26].

Aberrant expression of IFNγ and TNFα has been shown to promote upregulation of other proapoptotic molecules [27] and, more recently, the involvement of the intracellular cascade of the phosphatidylinositol 3-kinase/Akt [28] has been suggested to play a role in the deregulated survival of pSS epithelial cells and in the exposure of intracellular autoantigen [25] that contributes to the formation of local lymphocytic aggregates.

Next to apoptosis, the secretion of small exosomes containing autoantigenic proteins also appears to play a role in pSS pathogenesis [29]. Exosomes are small secreted endosomal vesicles useful in discharging redundant material and allowing intracellular communication. In pSS, activated epithelial cells are able to constitutively release exosomes being accountable for the extracellular exposition of different intracytoplasmic antigen including Ro/SSA and La/SSb [29]. This phenomenon, in turn, provides a continuous antigenic challenge for the incoming lymphocytes, supporting the local process of B cell affinity maturation observed in the large aggregates of severely affected pSS patients.

The reason for an impaired saliva secretion can be found in different aspects related to the epithelium involvement. Although nerve stimulation of minor sg appears not to be damaged, a reduced cytokine-mediated release of neurotransmitters seems to participate in salivary glands hypofunction [30]. In addition, autoantibodies directed against the muscarinic type 3 acetylcholine receptor have been demonstrated in pSS patient, which can reduce acinar secretion and impair the intracellular trafficking of the water transport protein aquaporin-5 [31]. These mechanisms provide a modulation in mucins production and trafficking, determining a saliva modification both in terms of quantity and quality [32].

These mechanisms, together with the direct epithelial damage and the progressive glandular fibrosis, contribute to the development of the *sicca*, clinical syndrome characterized by difficulties in swallowing dry foods, presence of multiple caries and oral infections in the mouth, and major risk to undergo corneal lesions or keratoconjunctivitis in the eyes.

AUTOANTIBODIES AND AUTOANTIGENS

Antibodies raise against Ro/SSA and La/SSB are the main specificities detectable in pSS patients, and they serve not only as disease markers but also appear to be directly involved in the local autoimmune response. Rheumatoid factor (RF) and cryoglobulins are also present in the blood and associate with significant clinical phenotypes. Other antibodies, such as the anticarbonic anhydrase II and the antimuscarinic type 3 receptor, exhibit a possible pathogenic role [33].

The Ro/La ribonucleoprotein are intracellular complexes formed by the association of the Ro52 kDa, Ro60 kDa, and La proteins with small cytoplasmic RNA [34]. Surface exposition on the cellular membrane is mediated by apoptosis and by exosomes release [35]. It is still debated whether in pSS, circulating autoantibodies binding to a plethora of organ and non–organ-specific autoantigens have a direct pathogenic role or represent just an epiphenomenon. However, it is clear that patients with positive anti-Ro/SSA and anti-La/SSB antibodies are more often characterized by systemic manifestation and more aggressive disease outcome. In seropositive patients, a major prevalence of extraglandular manifestations [5], as well as an earlier and longer disease duration with severe exocrine glands dysfunction, recurrent parotid enlargement, and more severe inflammatory infiltrates, has been described [36].

ECTOPIC LYMPHOID STRUCTURES

pSS is characterized by the formation of periepithelial mononuclear cell infiltrates, defined tertiary or ELS, which preferentially form in the exocrine glands: salivary glands (both minor and major), lachrymal glands, and exocrine pancreas. ELS formation, when characterized by the full maturation of ectopic and functional GCs, has been associated to systemic uncontrolled B cell proliferation and subsequent production of autoantibodies.

The large diffuse infiltrates display the tendency to spread into the parenchyma, resulting in the loss of tissue architecture and atrophic acini involution. Parenchymal and ductal alterations can be observed in the affected glands including atrophic involution of the acini and hyperplasia of the lining cells of the intraglandular ducts [7,37]. Accumulation of hyaline material is also found in the lumen of altered ducts and around blood vessels [37]. Small inflammatory foci consist predominantly of plasma cells with a smaller lymphocytic component that is evenly distributed throughout the aggregates. Larger foci are mainly composed of lymphocytes with fewer macrophages and plasma cells. A discrete plasma cell component can still be observed at the periphery of the larger foci [37].

Activated CD4+ T cells predominate in small aggregates and decrease in severe lesions; on the other hand, B cell infiltration predominates in the larger foci [38]. Accordingly, the T/B cell ratio is negatively associated with the degree of inflammation [38]. On the contrary, the percentage of CD8+ T cells and NK cells does not significantly change with lesion severity [38].

Higher numbers of regulatory T cells have been found in patients with pSS as compared with patients with secondary SS or connective tissue disease patients without pSS [39]. Sarigul et al. also described the presence of a higher percentage of FoxP3-expressing CD4+ T cells in the salivary glands of pSS patients, although similar numbers were found in peripheral blood of patients with either pSS or RA and healthy controls [40]. The frequency of regulatory T cell detection appears to correlate with lesion severity [40]. Plasmacytoid dendritic cells and CD123+BDCA-2+ cells are the main sources of IFN-α and have also been identified in all pSS salivary gland biopsies analyzed by Gottenberg et al. [20]. Circulatory plasmacytoid dendritic cells are more activated in pSS patients with a higher expression of CD40 [22].

Infiltrating lymphocytes in the ducts can give rise to the formation of lymphoepithelial sialadenitis (LESA) such that areas of lymphocytic infiltration (mainly B cells) can lead to atrophy of the columnar ductal epithelium and proliferation of the basal epithelial cells [41]. B cells represent the predominant infiltrating cell type, often acquiring monocytoid features or centrocyte-like morphology frequently accompanied by immunoblasts, plasmacytoid lymphocytes, and plasma cell differentiation [42]. In up to 50% of cases clonal intraepithelial B cell infiltration is present [41], and in some cases it is possible to observe, either by in situ hybridization or immunohistochemistry, kappa or lambda light chain excess production in the infiltrating cells [43].

ELS hub the process of affinity maturation (which include class switch recombination, CSR, and somatic hypermutation [SHM]) and clonal selection toward autoantigens, determining the selection and differentiation of autoreactive B cells into high-affinity plasma cells able to recognize autoantigens [44]. According to this background, it is not surprising that patients with positive GC in minor gs present with a worst disease outcome [17].

We and others have provided supporting evidence for the presence of a functional GC response in the salivary gland, in support of the concept that even if there are no clear evidences that ELS initiate the disease process they are involved in its progression. We demonstrated that the enzyme responsible for CSR, SHM, and AID (activation-induced cytidine deaminase) is expressed in pSS salivary gland in association with CD21+ networks of follicular dendritic cells [45]. This expression is retained in the large GCs found in parotid pSS-MALT lymphomas, whereas neoplastic marginal zone–like B cells are consistently AID negative [45]. Transplantation into SCID mice of ELS from SS salivary glands infected with Epstein–Barr virus (EBV) can support the production of anti-Ro 52/anti-La 48 and anti-EBV antibodies, while the survival and proliferation of B cells in the mice was shown to correlate with the overexpression of ectopic lymphoneogenesis genes [46].

Formation of ELS in SS is mediated by the release of several immune mediators released by epithelial, endothelial, and activated fibroblasts within the sg. Those include IL-1, TNF-α, LTα, BAFF, IL-8, IFN-β and -λ, CCL3, CCL4, CCL5, CXL12, CXL13, and CCL11 [47]. Nonhematopoietic cells are not only responsible for the release of proinflammatory mediators but also express co-stimulatory molecules, such as B7 and CD40, implicated in lymphocytic activation [48].

Among stromal cells within the ELS, we and others have described the formation of an activated fibroblastic network identified by the expression of gp38, ER-TR7, VCAM-1, and ICAM-1 and able to produce CCL21, CCL19, and CXCL13 [49] and the presence of follicular dendritic cells (FDCs), which produce CXCL13 and BAFF [50,51]. The role of CXCL12 has been also reported with evidence of its predominant expression in pSS epithelium and in areas of malignant B cell infiltration in patients with pSS and MALT lymphoma, suggesting a possible role of these cytokines in the process of lymphomagenesis [51].

GERMINAL CENTERS

ELS appear to play a role in disease progression, supporting the generation of memory B cells and long-lived plasma cells responsible for the production of autoantibodies [52].

A large proportion of B cell–rich ELS form ectopic GCs, complex structures composed of B lymphocytes, macrophages, DCs, FDCs, and T cells. DCs play a key role in ectopic GC formation and persistence supporting antigen presentation and producing key cytokines for B cell maturation and proliferation [50]. Structurally, within the GCs it is possible to identify a *dark zone*, inhabited by highly proliferating centroblasts and a *light zone*, populated by FDCs and centrocytes [53]. While the *dark zone* represents the area where the B cell clones undergo expansion, the *light zone* is the site of antigen presentation and affinity maturation of the B cell compartment [53], where B cells undergo SHM, the process that drives B cell receptor diversification and changes in antigen specificity and affinity. As mentioned above, SHM is regulated by AID, which introduces single base pair substitutions into the variable regions of antibody gene segments [54]. Considering that SHM is able to carry potential risks as the generation of pathogenic autoantibody specificities and unintended oncogenic mutations, the knowledge on the presence of these structures in ectopic sites is essential to understand autoimmune disease pathogenesis [54]. Accordingly, oligoclonal B cell expansion and SHM of Ig variable genes within GCs from SS salivary glands have been demonstrated [55].

Not surprisingly, the presence of histologically detectable GCs in approximately 25% of pSS patients has been associated with high titers of autoantibody in the serum, suggesting the direct contribution of ELS to disease progression [56], and found to correlate with the presence of a higher focus score (FS) (1.25 points higher) [57].

While there is evidence that the presence of GC in SS is associated with a negative prognosis and lymphoma development [17,57], the direct contribution of ELS to lymphoma development has been recently debated [58]. Higher prevalence of active systemic disease, lymphadenopathy, leucopenia, hypergammaglobulinemia, low C4 levels, positive anti-Ro/SSA, anti-La/SSB antibodies, positive ANA, and RF was observed in GC+ patients with pSS [56,59,60]. The presence of a FS > 1 has been also shown to associate with the presence of autoantibodies, keratoconjunctivitis sicca, and unstimulated whole salivary flow rates <0.1 mL per min and the formation of GCs [61]. Not surprisingly, patients with positive GCs display in the tissue higher expression of LTα, LTβ, BAFF, CXCR4, CXCL12, CXCR5, CXCL13, CCR7, CCL19, and CCL21 [62]. Increased local and systemic (serum and saliva) levels of CXCL13 correlate with xerostomia and in lymphoid aggregates the level of CXCL13 or CCL21 correlates with the degree of organization of the foci [18,45].

THERAPY IN SJÖGREN'S SYNDROME: "OLD" AND "NEW"
Conventional Therapies

To date the treatment of pSS is mainly symptomatic and aimed to alleviate the symptoms and consequences of the sicca. The use of topic saliva substitutes, lacrimal drops, and muscarinic agonists (pilocarpine or cevimeline) is recommended in the majority of pSS patients [63–65]. The use of artificial tears such as hypromellose and the use of oral gels/sprays/lozenges and careful dental hygiene is also recommended. In addition, a more severe ocular dryness can be managed through careful eyelid hygiene, regular use of preservative-free viscous artificial tears, and blockage of the tear (runoff) ducts.

The local administration of ciclosporin eye drops, under the guidance of the ophthalmologists, is useful tool to reduce ocular surface inflammation [66]. Humidification of the ambient increased intake of water, and possibility to use systemic muscarinic agonists is advisable in patients presenting with systemic sicca [67,68].

Hydroxychloroquine is one of the most common oral drugs for pSS. It has been used to treat fatigue and joint pain [69,70], and some small studies have also suggested a potential benefit in sicca symptoms and glandular function [71,72] and in the reduction of BAFF [73]. Unfortunately, the efficacy of Hydroxychloroquine (HQC) has not been proved in randomized clinical trials; however, revision of the data and patient stratification suggests the possibility to use this treatment in a selected population of pSS.

In case of important systemic features, classical disease-modifying antirheumatic drugs including methotrexate, azathioprine, ciclosporin, leflunomide, and mycophenolate may be helpful. In addition, in rare cases of severe manifestations, such as progressive sensorimotor neuropathy, immunosuppression may be required and the use of intravenous steroids and cyclophosphamide is recommended [74].

Biologic Therapies

The recent improved understanding of the mechanisms involved in pSS pathogenesis has prompted the development of new classes of drugs and, in this setting, the introduction of biologic treatments has led to a step change in pSS management.

There are no ongoing clinical trials on the use of anti-IFN agents in this condition. Recently, a trial aimed at determining the safety and efficacy of *rontalizumab*, a humanized IgG1 anti–IFN-α monoclonal antibody in patients with moderate-to-severe SLE, has been published. Efficacy was examined by an exploratory measure of IFN-regulated gene expression (interferon signature metric, ISM). This treatment was associated with improvements in disease activity, reduced flares, and decreased steroid use in patients with low IFN ISM. However, the primary and secondary end points were not met in patients with high ISM scores [75]. The ISM-low patients had higher mean trough concentrations (56.5 μg/mL) of rontalizumab compared with ISM-high patients (39.4 μg/mL), raising the possibility that differing rontalizumab exposure in the two groups may have contributed to the differential outcomes. In addition, *sifalimumab*, another anti–IFN-α monoclonal antibody, demonstrated safety/tolerability in SLE patients and a partial improvement in clinical activity profile was shown [76].

Given the key role of lymphotoxin in GC establishment and ectopic chemokine production in ELS, this molecule has been targeted in a randomized, double-blind, placebo-controlled phase 2 clinical trial by Lilly, with *baminercept*, a lymphotoxin beta receptor fusion protein. Although an improvement in ESSDAI calculation was demonstrated, baminercept did not provide evidence of superiority compared with placebo in increasing salivary flow or reducing ocular dryness [77].

Targeting co-stimulatory molecules is another possible therapeutic approach of pSS. Abatacept, a fusion protein of CTLA-4 linked to the Fc portion of IgG1, belongs to the T cell co-stimulation blockers and is able to inhibit T cell activation. It was first licensed for the treatment of rheumatoid arthritis [78] and in 2014 an open-label study evaluating the efficacy and safety of abatacept has been conducted in pSS patients too, showing promising results. Patients with pSS were treated with eight intravenous abatacept infusions on days 1, 15, and 29 and every 4 weeks thereafter. Abatacept demonstrated to be well tolerated and disease activity, laboratory parameters, and fatigue significantly improved during treatment [79]. Moreover, an open-label study on 15 patients aimed at determining efficacy and safety of abatacept in 15 pSS patients demonstrated how this drug is safe and well tolerated in pSS with evidence of a potential role in improving disease activity, laboratory parameters, fatigue, and health-related quality of life [79]. In all 15 pSS patients included in the open-label active Sjögren abatacept pilot study parotid gland biopsies were taken before treatment and at 24 weeks of follow-up. Abatacept proved to affect the formation of GCs and to inhibit local formation of (autoreactive) memory B cells [80]. Another study, with the aim to evaluate efficacy and safety of subcutaneous abatacept treatment in pSS in a larger and randomized double-blind phase 3 clinical trial, is currently recruiting patients.

ICOS is a CD28-like molecule that interacts with B7RP-1 and treatment with an anti-B7RP-1 antibody in two mouse models of SLE and collagen-induced arthritis, demonstrated to ameliorate disease manifestation leading to a decrease in follicular helper T cells and GC B cells as well as a decrease in the frequency of ICOS (+) T cells [81]. This finding supported the utility of this kind of therapy also in patients with pSS. A phase 2, randomized, placebo-controlled, clinical trial to evaluate the clinical and biologic efficacy, as well as the safety of SC doses of AMG 557/MEDI5872 in adult subjects with pSS, is currently active but still not recruiting patients.

Novel data have been recently made available for the direct blocking of the CD40 pathway. A multicenter, randomized, double-blind, placebo-controlled phase 2 clinical trial has shown for the first time in pSS a significant improvement of the treatment versus placebo with a positive impact on ESSDAI and CXCL13 serum levels [82].

Concerning B cells depleting therapies, a 6-month pilot double-blind randomized controlled trial of rituximab 1 g at time 0 and 15 days versus placebo in patients with pSS, not designed to evaluate salivary symptoms or function, has been performed. This study showed a significant improvement in the fatigue visual analog scale (VAS) between baseline and 6 months in patients who received active therapy [83]. A second double-blind randomized controlled trial has also been published with evidence of a significant improvement in stimulated salivary flow and oral dryness [84].

A randomized, placebo-controlled, parallel group trial conducted in France on 120 patients with pSS demonstrated no significant difference between groups in the primary end point (improvement of at least 30 mm in 2 of 4 VASs by week 24). An improvement in fatigue from baseline to week 24 was greater with rituximab (anti-CD20 antibody). Despite the low disease activity at baseline and a primary outcome probably insensitive to detect clinically important changes, the conclusion of this trial was that rituximab seems not to alleviate symptoms or disease activity in patients with pSS at week 24, although it alleviated some symptoms at earlier time points [85].

Soluble BLyS/BAFF is a member of the human TNF family, able to induce B cell proliferation and immunoglobulin secretion. A monoclonal antibody that recognizes soluble BlyS/BAFF, belimumab, has successfully completed clinical trials in SLE and is already in clinical use [86]. To evaluate the efficacy and safety of belimumab, in 30 patients with pSS, an open-label phase 2 trial has been completed. Patients received belimumab, 10 mg/kg, at weeks 0, 2, and 4 and then every 4 weeks to week 24. The primary end point (week 28) was the improvement in two of five items: reduction in $\geq$30% in dryness score on a VAS, $\geq$30% in fatigue VAS score, $\geq$30% in VAS pain score, $\geq$30% in systemic activity VAS assessed by the physician, and/or >25% improvement in any B cell activation biomarker values. The primary end point was achieved at 60%. The mean ESSDAI and ESSPRI both significantly decreased, as well as the mean dryness. Fatigue, pain VAS, salivary flow, and Schirmer's test did not significantly change [87]. The recruitment of patients into another trial aimed at determining the safety and efficacy of monoclonal antibody directed to BAFF-R (VAY736) is ongoing. In addition, a study on the use of subcutaneous belimumab and intravenous rituximab in co-administration in patients with pSS is currently recruiting patients.

A number of studies have identified raised IL-6 levels in the serum and salivary glands of patients with pSS. Tocilizumab is a humanized anti–IL-6 receptor monoclonal antibody, now in clinical use in rheumatoid arthritis. An academic lead clinical trial with anti–IL-6 is ongoing.

The large number of trials currently recruiting exemplifies the therapeutic interest around a disease that for long time has been neglected by the interest of Big Pharma. New initiative targeted at better understanding the potential for patient stratification and identification of biomarkers predictive of response is ongoing and hopes to shape in the next few years a brighter future for patients with pSS.

REFERENCES

[1] Bohnhorst JØ, Djørgan MD, Thoen JE, Jonsson R, Natvig JB, Thompson KM. Abnormal B cell differentiation in primary Sjögren's syndrome results in a depressed percentage of circulating memory B cells and elevated levels of soluble CD27 that correlate with Serum IgG concentration. Clin Immunol 2002;103(1):79–88.

[2] Bohnhorst JO, Thoen JE, Natvig JB, Thompson KM. Significantly depressed percentage of CD27+ (memory) B cells among peripheral blood B cells in patients with primary Sjögren's syndrome. Scand J Immunol 2001;54(4):421–7.

[3] Larsson A, Bredberg A, Henriksson G, Manthorpe R, Sallmyr A. Immunohistochemistry of the B-cell component in lower lip salivary glands of Sjögren's syndrome and healthy subjects. Scand J Immunol 2005;61(1):98–107.

[4] Fox RI. Sjögren's syndrome. Lancet 2005;366(9482):321–31.

[5] Ramos-Casals M, Solans R, Rosas J, Camps MT, Gil A, Del Pino-Montes J, Calvo-Alen J, Jiménez-Alonso J, Micó ML, Beltrán J, Belenguer R, Pallarés L, GEMESS Study Group. Primary Sjögren syndrome in Spain: clinical and immunologic expression in 1010 patients. Medicine (Baltim) 2008;87(4):210–9.

[6] Theander E, Henriksson G, Ljungberg O, Mandl T, Manthorpe R, Jacobsson LT. Lymphoma and other malignancies in primary Sjögren's syndrome: a cohort study on cancer incidence and lymphoma predictors. Ann Rheum Dis 2006;65(6):796–803.

[7] Chisholm DM, Mason DK. Labial salivary gland biopsy in Sjögren's disease. J Clin Pathol 1968;21(5):656–60.

[8] Moutsopoulos HM. Sjögren's syndrome: autoimmune epithelitis. Clin Immunol Immunopathol August 1994;72(2):162–5. Review.

[9] Pillemer SR, Matteson EL, Jacobsson LT, Martens PB, Melton 3rd LJ, O'Fallon WM, Fox PC. Incidence of physician-diagnosed primary Sjögren syndrome in residents of Olmsted County, Minnesota. Mayo Clin Proc 2001;76(6):593–9.

[10] Brkic Z, Maria NI, van Helden-Meeuwsen CG, van de Merwe JP, van Daele PL, Dalm VA, Wildenberg ME, Beumer W, Drexhage HA, Versnel MA. Prevalence of interferon type I signature in CD14 monocytes of patients with Sjogren's syndrome and association with disease activity and BAFF gene expression. Ann Rheum Dis 2013;72(5):728–35.

[11] Christodoulou MI, Kapsogeorgou EK, Moutsopoulos NM, Moutsopoulos HM. Foxp3+ T-regulatory cells in Sjogren's syndrome: correlation with the grade of the autoimmune lesion and certain adverse prognostic factors. Am J Pathol 2008;173(5):1389–96.

[12] Katsifis GE, Rekka S, Moutsopoulos NM, Pillemer S, Wahl SM. Systemic and local interleukin-17 and linked cytokines associated with Sjögren's syndrome immunopathogenesis. Am J Pathol September 2009;175(3):1167–77.

[13] Dimitriou ID, Kapsogeorgou EK, Moutsopoulos HM, Manoussakis MN. CD40 on salivary gland epithelial cells: high constitutive expression by cultured cells from Sjögren's syndrome patients indicating their intrinsic activation. Clin Exp Immunol 2002;127(2):386–92.

[14] Malladi AS, Sack KE, Shiboski SC, Shiboski CH, Baer AN, Banushree R, Dong Y, Helin P, Kirkham BW, Li M, Sugai S, Umehara H, Vivino FB, Vollenweider CF, Zhang W, Zhao Y, Greenspan JS, Daniels TE, Criswell LA. Primary Sjögren's syndrome as a systemic disease: a study of participants enrolled in an international Sjögren's syndrome registry. Arthritis Care Res (Hoboken) 2012;64(6):911–8.

[15] Moutsopoulos HM, Manoussakis MN. Lumping or splitting autoimmune rheumatic disorders? Lessons from Sjögren's syndrome. Br J Rheumatol 1998;37(12):1263–4.

[16] Voulgarelis M, Dafni UG, Isenberg DA, Moutsopoulos HM. Malignant lymphoma in primary Sjögren's syndrome: a multicenter, retrospective, clinical study by the European concerted action on Sjögren's syndrome. Arthritis Rheum 1999;42(8):1765–72.

[17] Theander E, Vasaitis L, Baecklund E, Nordmark G, Warfvinge G, Liedholm R, Brokstad K, Jonsson R, Jonsson MV. Lymphoid organisation in labial salivary gland biopsies is a possible predictor for the development of malignant lymphoma in primary Sjögren's syndrome. Ann Rheum Dis 2011;70(8):1363–8.

[18] Barone F, Bombardieri M, Manzo A, Blades MC, Morgan PR, Challacombe SJ, Valesini G, Pitzalis C. Association of CXCL13 and CCL21 expression with the progressive organization of lymphoid-like structures in Sjögren's syndrome. Arthritis Rheum 2005;52(6):1773–84.

[19] Hjelmervik TO, Petersen K, Jonassen I, Jonsson R, Bolstad AI. Gene expression profiling of minor salivary glands clearly distinguishes primary Sjögren's syndrome patients from healthy control subjects. Arthritis Rheum 2005;52(5):1534–44.

[20] Gottenberg JE, Cagnard N, Lucchesi C, Letourneur F, Mistou S, Lazure T, Jacques S, Ba N, Ittah M, Lepajolec C, Labetoulle M, Ardizzone M, Sibilia J, Fournier C, Chiocchia G, Mariette X. Activation of IFN pathways and plasmacytoid dendritic cell recruitment in target organs of primary Sjögren's syndrome. Proc Natl Acad Sci USA February 21, 2006;103(8):2770–5.

[21] Emamian ES, Leon JM, Lessard CJ, Grandits M, Baechler EC, Gaffney PM, Segal B, Rhodus NL, Moser KL. Peripheral blood gene expression profiling in Sjögren's syndrome. Genes Immun 2009;10(4):285–96.

[22] Wildenberg ME, van Helden-Meeuwsen CG, van de Merwe JP, Drexhage HA, Versnel MA. Systemic increase in type I interferon activity in Sjögren's syndrome: a putative role for plasmacytoid dendritic cells. Eur J Immunol 2008;38(7):2024–33.

[23] Hall JC, Casciola-Rosen L, Berger AE, Kapsogeorgou EK, Cheadle C, Tzioufas AG, Baer AN, Rosen A. Precise probes of type II interferon activity define the origin of interferon signatures in target tissues in rheumatic diseases. Proc Natl Acad Sci USA 2012;109(43):17609–14.

[24] Nezos A, Gravani F, Tassidou A, Kapsogeorgou EK, Voulgarelis M, Koutsilieris M, Crow MK, Mavragani CP. Type I and II interferon signatures in Sjögren's syndrome pathogenesis: contributions in distinct clinical phenotypes and Sjögren's related lymphomagenesis. J Autoimmun 2015;63:47–58.

[25] Abu-Helu RF, Dimitriou ID, Kapsogeorgou EK, Moutsopoulos HM, Manoussakis MN. Induction of salivary gland epithelial cell injury in Sjögren's syndrome: in vitro assessment of T cell-derived cytokines and Fas protein expression. J Autoimmun 2001;17(2):141–53.

[26] Ping L, Ogawa N, Sugai S. Novel role of CD40 in Fas-dependent apoptosis of cultured salivary epithelial cells from patients with Sjögren's syndrome. Arthritis Rheum 2005;52(2):573–81.

[27] Matsumura R, Umemiya K, Goto T, Nakazawa T, Ochiai K, Kagami M, Tomioka H, Tanabe E, Sugiyama T, Sueishi M. Interferon gamma and tumor necrosis factor alpha induce Fas expression and anti-Fas mediated apoptosis in a salivary ductal cell line. Clin Exp Rheumatol 2000;18(3):311–8.

[28] Ohlsson M, Szodoray P, Loro LL, Johannessen AC, Jonsson R. CD40, CD154, Bax and Bcl-2 expression in Sjögren's syndrome salivary glands: a putative anti-apoptotic role during its effector phases. Scand J Immunol 2002;56(6):561–71.

[29] Kapsogeorgou EK, Abu-Helu RF, Moutsopoulos HM, Manoussakis MN. Salivary gland epithelial cell exosomes: a source of autoantigenic ribonucleoproteins. Arthritis Rheum 2005;52(5):1517–21.

[30] Zoukhri D, Kublin CL. Impaired neurotransmission in lacrimal and salivary glands of a murine model of Sjögren's syndrome. Adv Exp Med Biol 2002;506(Pt B):1023–8.

[31] Dawson LJ, Stanbury J, Venn N, Hasdimir B, Rogers SN, Smith PM. Antimuscarinic antibodies in primary Sjögren's syndrome reversibly inhibit the mechanism of fluid secretion by human submandibular salivary acinar cells. Arthritis Rheum 2006;54(4):1165–73.

[32] Castro I, Sepúlveda D, Cortés J, Quest AF, Barrera MJ, Bahamondes V, Aguilera S, Urzúa U, Alliende C, Molina C, González S, Hermoso MA, Leyton C, González MJ. Oral dryness in Sjögren's syndrome patients. Not just a question of water. Autoimmun Rev 2013;12(5):567–74.

[33] Tzioufas AG, Tatouli IP, Moutsopoulos HM. Autoantibodies in Sjögren's syndrome: clinical presentation and regulatory mechanisms. Presse Med 2012;41(9 Pt 2):e451–60.

[34] Keene JD. Molecular structure of the La and Ro autoantigens and their use in autoimmune diagnostics. J Autoimmun 1989;2(4):329–34.

[35] Théry C, Zitvogel L, Amigorena S. Exosomes: composition, biogenesis and function. Nat Rev Immunol 2002;2(8):569–79. https://doi.org/10.1038/nri855.

[36] Mavragani CP, Tzioufas AG, Moutsopoulos HM. Sjögren's syndrome: autoantibodies to cellular antigens. Clinical and molecular aspects. Int Arch Allergy Immunol 2000;123(1):46–57.

[37] Greenspan JS, Daniels TE, Talal N, Sylvester RA. The histopathology of Sjögren's syndrome in labial salivary gland biopsies. Oral Surg Oral Med Oral Pathol 1974;37(2):217–29.

[38] Christodoulou MI, Kapsogeorgou EK, Moutsopoulos HM. Characteristics of the minor salivary gland infiltrates in Sjögren's syndrome. J Autoimmun 2010;34(4):400–7.

[39] Furuzawa-Carballeda J, Sánchez-Guerrero J, Betanzos JL, Enriquez AB, Avila-Casado C, Llorente L, Hernández-Molina G. Differential cytokine expression and regulatory cells in patients with primary and secondary Sjögren's syndrome. Scand J Immunol 2014;80(6):432–40.

[40] Sarigul M, Yazisiz V, Bassorgun CI, Ulker M, Avci AB, Erbasan F, Gelen T, Gorczynski RM, Terzioglu E. The numbers of Foxp3 + Treg cells are positively correlated with higher grade of infiltration at the salivary glands in primary Sjogren's syndrome. Lupus 2010;19(2):138–45.

[41] Carbone A, Gloghini A, Ferlito A. Pathological features of lymphoid proliferations of the salivary glands: lymphoepithelial sialadenitis versus low-grade B-cell lymphoma of the malt type. Ann Otol Rhinol Laryngol 2000;109(12 Pt 1):1170–5.

[42] Greaves WO, Wang SA. Selected topics on lymphoid lesions in the head and neck regions. Head Neck Pathol 2011;5(1):41–50.

[43] Harris NL. Lymphoid proliferations of the salivary glands. Am J Clin Pathol 1999;111(1 Suppl. 1):S94–103.

[44] Corsiero E, Nerviani A, Bombardieri M, Pitzalis C. Ectopic lymphoid structures: powerhouse of autoimmunity. Front Immunol 2016;7:430.

[45] Bombardieri M, Barone F, Humby F, Kelly S, McGurk M, Morgan P, Challacombe S, De Vita S, Valesini G, Spencer J, Pitzalis C. Activation-induced cytidine deaminase expression in follicular dendritic cell networks and interfollicular large B cells supports functionality of ectopic lymphoid neogenesis in autoimmune sialoadenitis and MALT lymphoma in Sjögren's syndrome. J Immunol 2007;179(7):4929–38.

[46] Croia C, Astorri E, Murray-Brown W, Willis A, Brokstad KA, Sutcliffe N, Piper K, Jonsson R, Tappuni AR, Pitzalis C, Bombardieri M. Implication of Epstein-Barr virus infection in disease-specific autoreactive B cell activation in ectopic lymphoid structures of Sjögren's syndrome. Arthritis Rheumatol 2014;66(9):2545–57.

[47] Goules AV, Kapsogeorgou EK, Tzioufas AG. Insight into pathogenesis of Sjögren's syndrome: dissection on autoimmune infiltrates and epithelial cells. Clin Immunol 2017;182:30–40.

[48] Manoussakis MN, Kapsogeorgou EK. The role of intrinsic epithelial activation in the pathogenesis of Sjögren's syndrome. J Autoimmun 2010;35(3):219–24.

[49] Barone F, Gardner DH, Nayar S, Steinthal N, Buckley CD, Luther SA. Stromal fibroblasts in tertiary lymphoid structures: a novel target in chronic inflammation. Front Immunol 2016;7:477.

[50] Aguzzi A, Kranich J, Krautler NJ. Follicular dendritic cells: origin, phenotype, and function in health and disease. Trends Immunol 2014;35(3):105–13.

[51] Barone F, Nayar S, Buckley CD. The role of non-hematopoietic stromal cells in the persistence of inflammation. Front Immunol 2013;3:416.

[52] Allen CD, Okada T, Cyster JG. Germinal-center organization and cellular dynamics. Immunity 2007;27(2):190–202.

[53] MacLennan IC. Somatic mutation. From the dark zone to the light. Curr Biol 1994;4(1):70–2.

[54] Gatto D, Brink R. The germinal center reaction. J Allergy Clin Immunol 2010;126(5):898–907.

[55] Stott DI, Hiepe F, Hummel M, Steinhauser G, Berek C. Antigen-driven clonal proliferation of B cells within the target tissue of an autoimmune disease. The salivary glands of patients with Sjögren's syndrome. J Clin Investig 1998;102(5):938–46.

[56] Salomonsson S, Jonsson MV, Skarstein K, Brokstad KA, Hjelmström P, Wahren-Herlenius M, Jonsson R. Cellular basis of ectopic germinal center formation and autoantibody production in the target organ of patients with Sjögren's syndrome. Arthritis Rheum 2003;48(11):3187–201.

[57] Risselada AP, Looije MF, Kruize AA, Bijlsma JW, van Roon JA. The role of ectopic germinal centers in the immunopathology of primary Sjögren's syndrome: a systematic review. Semin Arthritis Rheum 2013;42(4):368–76.

[58] Haacke EA, van der Vegt B, Vissink A, Spijkervet FKL, Bootsma H, Kroese FGM. Germinal centres in diagnostic labial gland biopsies of patients with primary Sjögren's syndrome are not predictive for parotid MALT lymphoma development. Ann Rheum Dis 2017;76(10):1781–4.

[59] Jonsson MV, Skarstein K, Jonsson R, Brun JG. Serological implications of germinal center-like structures in primary Sjögren's syndrome. J Rheumatol 2007;34(10):2044–9.

[60] He J, Jin Y, Zhang X, Zhou Y, Li R, Dai Y, Sun X, Zhao J, Guo J, Li Z. Characteristics of germinal center-like structures in patients with Sjögren's syndrome. Int J Rheum Dis 2017;20(2):245–51.

[61] Daniels TE, Cox D, Shiboski CH, Schiødt M, Wu A, Lanfranchi H, Umehara H, Zhao Y, Challacombe S, Lam MY, De Souza Y, Schiødt J, Holm H, Bisio PA, Gandolfo MS, Sawaki T, Li M, Zhang W, Varghese-Jacob B, Ibsen P, Keszler A, Kurose N, Nojima T, Odell E, Criswell LA, Jordan R, Greenspan JS, Sjögren's International Collaborative Clinical Alliance Research Groups. Associations between salivary gland histopathologic diagnoses and phenotypic features of Sjögren's syndrome among 1,726 registry participants. Arthritis Rheum 2011;63(7):2021–30.

[62] Carubbi F, Alunno A, Cipriani P, Di Benedetto P, Ruscitti P, Berardicurti O, Bartoloni E, Bistoni O, Caterbi S, Ciccia F, Triolo G, Gerli R, Giacomelli R. Is minor salivary gland biopsy more than a diagnostic tool in primary Sjögren's syndrome? Association between clinical, histopathological, and molecular features: a retrospective study. Semin Arthritis Rheum 2014;44(3):314–24.

[63] Plemons JM, Al-Hashimi I, Marek CL, American Dental Association Council on Scientific Affairs. Managing xerostomia and salivary gland hypofunction: executive summary of a report from the American Dental Association Council on Scientific Affairs. J Am Dent Assoc 2014;145(8):867–73.

[64] Papas AS, Sherrer YS, Charney M, Golden HE, Medsger Jr TA, Walsh BT, Trivedi M, Goldlust B, Gallagher SC. Successful treatment of dry mouth and dry eye symptoms in Sjögren's syndrome patients with oral pilocarpine: a randomized, placebo-controlled, dose-adjustment study. J Clin Rheumatol 2004;10(4):169–77.

[65] Petrone D, Condemi JJ, Fife R, Gluck O, Cohen S, Dalgin P. A double-blind, randomized, placebo-controlled study of cevimeline in Sjögren's syndrome patients with xerostomia and keratoconjunctivitis sicca. Arthritis Rheum 2002;46(3):748–54.

[66] Sall K, Stevenson OD, Mundorf TK, Reis BL. Two multicenter, randomized studies of the efficacy and safety of cyclosporine ophthalmic emulsion in moderate to severe dry eye disease. CsA Phase 3 Study Group. Ophthalmology 2000;107(4):631–9.

[67] Vivino FB, Al-Hashimi I, Khan Z, LeVeque FG, Salisbury 3rd PL, Tran-Johnson TK, Muscoplat CC, Trivedi M, Goldlust B, Gallagher SC. Pilocarpine tablets for the treatment of dry mouth and dry eye symptoms in patients with Sjögren syndrome: a randomized, placebo-controlled, fixed-dose, multicenter trial. P92-01 Study Group. Arch Intern Med 1999;159(2):174–81.

[68] Fife RS, Chase WF, Dore RK, Wiesenhutter CW, Lockhart PB, Tindall E, Suen JY. Cevimeline for the treatment of xerostomia in patients with Sjögren syndrome: a randomized trial. Arch Intern Med 2002;162(11):1293–300.

[69] Kruize AA, Hené RJ, Kallenberg CG, van Bijsterveld OP, van der Heide A, Kater L, Bijlsma JW. Hydroxychloroquine treatment for primary Sjögren's syndrome: a two year double blind crossover trial. Ann Rheum Dis 1993;52(5):360–4.

[70] Tishler M, Yaron I, Shirazi I, Yaron M. Hydroxychloroquine treatment for primary Sjögren's syndrome: its effect on salivary and serum inflammatory markers. Ann Rheum Dis 1999;58(4):253–6.

[71] Fox RI, Dixon R, Guarrasi V, Krubel S. Treatment of primary Sjögren's syndrome with hydroxychloroquine: a retrospective, open-label study. Lupus 1996;5(Suppl. 1):S31–6.

[72] Rihl M, Ulbricht K, Schmidt RE, Witte T. Treatment of sicca symptoms with hydroxychloroquine in patients with Sjögren's syndrome. Rheumatology (Oxf) 2009;48(7):796–9.

[73] Yavuz S, Asfuroğlu E, Bicakcigil M, Toker E. Hydroxychloroquine improves dry eye symptoms of patients with primary Sjögren's syndrome. Rheumatol Int 2011;31(8):1045–9.

[74] Delalande S, de Seze J, Fauchais AL, Hachulla E, Stojkovic T, Ferriby D, Dubucquoi S, Pruvo JP, Vermersch P, Hatron PY. Neurologic manifestations in primary Sjögren syndrome: a study of 82 patients. Medicine (Baltim) 2004;83(5):280–91.

[75] Kalunian KC, Merrill JT, Maciuca R, McBride JM, Townsend MJ, Wei X, Davis Jr JC, Kennedy WP. A Phase II study of the efficacy and safety of rontalizumab (rhuMAb interferon-α) in patients with systemic lupus erythematosus (ROSE). Ann Rheum Dis 2016;75(1):196–202.

[76] Petri M, Wallace DJ, Spindler A, Chindalore V, Kalunian K, Mysler E, Neuwelt CM, Robbie G, White WI, Higgs BW, Yao Y, Wang L, Ethgen D, Greth W. Sifalimumab, a human anti-interferon-α monoclonal antibody, in systemic lupus erythematosus: a phase I randomized, controlled, dose-escalation study. Arthritis Rheum 2013;65(4):1011–21.

[77] St Clair EW, et al. The clinical efficacy and safety of Baminercept, a lymphotoxin-beta receptor fusion protein, in primary Sjögren's syndrome: results from a randomized, double-blind, placebo-controlled phase II trial. Abstract 3203. In: ACR/ARHP annual meeting. 2015.

[78] Westhovens R, Kremer JM, Moreland LW, Emery P, Russell AS, Li T, Aranda R, Becker JC, Qi K, Dougados M. Safety and efficacy of the selective costimulation modulator abatacept in patients with rheumatoid arthritis receiving background methotrexate: a 5-year extended phase IIB study. J Rheumatol 2009;36(4):736–42.

[79] Meiners PM, Vissink A, Kroese FG, Spijkervet FK, Smitt-Kamminga NS, Abdulahad WH, Bulthuis-Kuiper J, Brouwer E, Arends S, Bootsma H. Abatacept treatment reduces disease activity in early primary Sjögren's syndrome (open-label proof of concept ASAP study). Ann Rheum Dis 2014;73(7):1393–6.

[80] Haacke EA, van der Vegt B, Meiners PM, Vissink A, Spijkervet FK, Bootsma H, Kroese FG. Abatacept treatment of patients with primary Sjögren's syndrome results in a decrease of germinal centres in salivary gland tissue. Clin Exp Rheumatol 2017;35(2):317–20.

[81] Hu YL, Metz DP, Chung J, Siu G, Zhang M. B7RP-1 blockade ameliorates autoimmunity through regulation of follicular helper T cells. J Immunol 2009;182(3):1421–8.

[82] Fisher B, et al. The novel anti-CD40 monoclonal antibody CFZ533 shows beneficial effects in patients with primary Sjögren's syndrome: a phase IIa double-blind, placebo-controlled randomized trial. Abstract. In: ACR/ARHP annual meeting. 2017.

[83] Dass S, Bowman SJ, Vital EM, Ikeda K, Pease CT, Hamburger J, Richards A, Rauz S, Emery P. Reduction of fatigue in Sjögren syndrome with rituximab: results of a randomised, double-blind, placebo-controlled pilot study. Ann Rheum Dis 2008;67(11):1541–4.

[84] Meijer JM, Meiners PM, Vissink A, Spijkervet FK, Abdulahad W, Kamminga N, Brouwer E, Kallenberg CG, Bootsma H. Effectiveness of rituximab treatment in primary Sjögren's syndrome: a randomized, double-blind, placebo-controlled trial. Arthritis Rheum 2010;62(4):960–8. https://doi.org/10.1002/art.27314.

[85] Devauchelle-Pensec V, Mariette X, Jousse-Joulin S, Berthelot JM, Perdriger A, Puéchal X, Le Guern V, Sibilia J, Gottenberg JE, Chiche L, Hachulla E, Hatron PY, Goeb V, Hayem G, Morel J, Zarnitsky C, Dubost JJ, Pers JO, Nowak E, Saraux A. Treatment of primary Sjögren syndrome with rituximab: a randomized trial. Ann Intern Med 2014;160(4):233–42.

[86] van Vollenhoven RF, Petri MA, Cervera R, Roth DA, Ji BN, Kleoudis CS, Zhong ZJ, Freimuth W. Belimumab in the treatment of systemic lupus erythematosus: high disease activity predictors of response. Ann Rheum Dis 2012;71(8):1343–9.

[87] Mariette X, Seror R, Quartuccio L, Baron G, Salvin S, Fabris M, Desmoulins F, Nocturne G, Ravaud P, De Vita S. Efficacy and safety of belimumab in primary Sjögren's syndrome: results of the BELISS open-label phase II study. Ann Rheum Dis 2015;74(3):526–31.

[88] Barone F, Bombardieri M, Rosado MM, Morgan PR, Challacombe SJ, De Vita S, Carsetti R, Spencer J, Valesini G, Pitzalis C. CXCL13, CCL21, and CXCL12 expression in salivary glands of patients with Sjögren's syndrome and MALT lymphoma: association with reactive and malignant areas of lymphoid organization. J Immunol 2008;180(7):5130–40.

Chapter 51

Autoimmune/Inflammatory Syndrome Induced by Adjuvants (Shoenfeld's Syndrome)

Luis J. Jara[1,5], Olga Vera-Lastra[2,5], Gabriela Medina[3,5], María del Pilar Cruz-Domínguez[4,5], Michel A. Martínez-Bencomo[4,5], Grettel García-Collinot[4,6], Rosa A. Carranza-Muleiro[4,6]

[1]*Direction of Education and Research, Hospital de Especialidades Centro Médico Nacional La Raza, IMSS, Mexico City, Mexico;* [2]*Internal Medicine Department, Hospital de Especialidades Centro Médico Nacional La Raza, IMSS, Mexico City, Mexico;* [3]*Clinical Research Unit, Hospital de Especialidades Centro Médico Nacional La Raza, IMSS, Mexico City, Mexico;* [4]*Research Division, Hospital de Especialidades Centro Médico Nacional La Raza, IMSS, Mexico City, Mexico;* [5]*Universidad Nacional Autónoma de México, Mexico City, Mexico;* [6]*Instituto Politécnico Nacional, Mexico City, Mexico*

INTRODUCTION

In 2011, Shoenfeld and Agmon-Levin described five medical conditions with similar complex of symptoms and signs and a common pathogenesis, namely siliconosis, the Gulf War syndrome (GWS), the macrophagic myofasciitis syndrome (MMF), post vaccination phenomena, and the sick building syndrome, linked with previous exposure to an adjuvant substance. The authors proposed to gather these five entities under a common syndrome denominated "autoimmune/inflammatory syndrome induced by adjuvants" (ASIA) and suggested a set of diagnostic criteria for this new entity [1].

Environmental factors and genetic predisposition have been shown to play a pivotal role in the pathogenesis of immune-mediated diseases, being systemic lupus erythematosus (SLE) the best example of interaction between them. Epidemiologic evidences strongly suggest an increased risk of SLE associated with exposure to crystalline silica, current cigarette smoking, oral contraceptives, postmenopausal hormone replacement therapy, solvents, agricultural pesticides, heavy metals, air pollution, ultraviolet light, infections, and vaccinations. These factors interact with susceptible family members and individuals with genetic risk profiles [2]. Therefore, it is possible that in genetically predisposed individuals, the exposure to environmental factors or "innocuous" adjuvant with immune activity, such as silicone, aluminum salts, and Freund's adjuvant contained in vaccines, mineral oils, collagen, and hyaluronic acid used in cosmetic fillers and metal implants, may induce the well-defined and nondefined immune-mediated diseases, a prerequisite to the appearance of ASIA [3–5].

From its initial presentation in 2011–16, more than 4000 ASIA cases have been identified, varying from mild to severe clinical manifestations, with the majority of severe cases related to vaccines, silicone implants, and mineral oil fillers [6]. Recently, more than 300 ASIA cases have been documented in the ASIA syndrome registry established and managed by the Zabludowicz Center for Autoimmune Diseases at the Chaim Sheba Medical Center [7].

The aim of this chapter is to summarize the knowledge about ASIA syndrome to analyze the epidemiology, basic and clinical aspects, and treatment, supporting the relationship between the exposure to adjuvant agents and clinical manifestations of ASIA.

HISTORICAL ASPECTS

An adjuvant is defined as a substance that enhances antigen-specific immune response preferably without triggering one on its own. However, for many years, many studies in animal models and humans have shown the ability of adjuvants to trigger autoimmune phenomena [8,9].

Mosaic of Autoimmunity. https://doi.org/10.1016/B978-0-12-814307-0.00051-7

Complete Freund's Adjuvant

In the 60s of the last century, the scientific community was interested in the clinical and immunological effect of the injection of mycobacterial adjuvant (complete Freund's adjuvant, CFA). A generalized disease was induced experimentally in the rat by administration of CFA. The primary clinical and pathologic lesions were arthritis, periarthritis, peritendinitis, and periostitis in the joints of the extremities and tail. Other specific tissue lesions such as iridocyclitis, nodular lesions in the glabrous skin (ear, genitalia, feet, tail), transient rashes, a chronic skin disease, genitourinary lesions, and diarrhea were observed. Histologically, the basic lesion was a lymphocytic, histiocytic infiltration, proliferation of mesenchymal cells, especially fibroblasts, fibrinoid necrosis in the articular and nodular lesions, and destructive lesions of the joints. This experimental disease presented similarities with Reiter's syndrome for reactive arthritis (RA) (is the current denomination), and other autoimmune disorders in humans [10].

Later on, sheep immunized with human lung basement membranes and CFA developed progressive glomerulonephritis with deposition of autoantibodies and complement in the glomerular basement membrane, possibly being the first autoimmune disease (AID) induced by non–organ-specific antigens. By clinical and immunopathologic criteria, this nephritis was notably resembling human nephritides like in Goodpasture's disease [11].

In the 70s, guinea pigs were sensitized to tuberculin with CFA and were challenged in the central and peripheral nervous system either with live or killed sonicated tubercle bacilli, old tuberculin, or tuberculin purified protein derivative. Local inflammatory reactions were invariably produced, and primary demyelination was a constant feature of the lesions. The morphological picture was rather similar to that observed in human neurotuberculosis and early tuberculoid leprosy, as well as in experimental allergic encephalomyelitis. The cell-mediated immune reactions could be responsible for a component of the demyelination seen in some inflammatory demyelinating conditions [12]. These studies in animal models demonstrate a direct relationship between the adjuvant, the interaction with infectious agents, and development of ASIA.

In the early 80s, a study demonstrated that in vivo administration of a monoclonal antibody that recognizes a specific I-A haplotype in a heterozygous F1 mouse can exert a potent, relatively specific suppression of a humoral response controlled by an Ir gene in the I-A subregion. However, specificity of the suppression was decreased when the antigen was administered in CFA. Because antigenic stimulation has been reported to increase expression of I-A on splenic macrophages, one possibility is that CFA immunization makes macrophages more susceptible to the effects of an anti–I-A antibody [13].

Silicone

The human adjuvant disease related to silicone is known since the 60s and until 1979 about 30 cases of adjuvant disease in humans were published. In 1964, Miyoshi reported two cases of connective tissue disease-like disorders on patients who had undergone the procedure several years previously. One of the patients had a dramatic improvement in the disease symptoms after removal of the foreign substances by bilateral mastectomy. In 1979, nine cases of human adjuvant disease and four cases of scleroderma (three progressive systemic sclerosis [SSc] and one localized morphea) were published. 7–19 years after injection of foreign substances into the breasts or nose for cosmetic purposes, these patients developed human adjuvant disease. Histopathologic findings of the removed breasts demonstrated foreign body granulomas with calcification. The injected substance was identified as a mixture of liquid and solid paraffin. These clinical observations show that human adjuvant disease might be caused by prolonged hypersensitization activated by the injected foreign materials that act as an adjuvant, similar to what happens in the experimental models mentioned previously [14].

After these clinical observations, great efforts were made to clarify the mechanisms by which the silicone stimulates the immune response. Most studies conclude that silicones are chemically stable compounds, which, however, are often capable of eliciting a chronic inflammatory response. Experimental studies on commercial breast implants have indicated that silicone gel is a potent humoral (antibody) adjuvant and are capable to elicit inflammatory and fibroproliferative response. These properties of silicone gel and clinical descriptions support the hypothesis that silicone-breast implants may participate to the development of AIDs [15,16].

Vaccines

Since the 60s, the side effects of vaccines have been of interest to a part of the scientific community. Vaccines have favored millions of people in the world, and it is important to stress that reporting these potential adverse events does not mean going against vaccines. Moreover, we are in the opinion that the benefits of the vaccines largely overwhelm the potential risks of the vaccines. The purpose of these reports is to alert the population about its application and its potential adverse effects and to alert vaccine manufacturers to identify molecules that can cause harm and improve vaccines and thus protect the healthy individual. The incidence and severity of the complications of smallpox vaccination were reviewed in the year 1968. Over 14 million vaccinations were performed during the year and 572 patients were treated for complications such as postvaccinal encephalitis, vaccinia necrosum, eczema vaccinatum, erythema multiforme, and 143 cases of generalized vaccinia. The majority of these complications were minor, but 238 patients required in-patient treatment, 9 died, and several had neurological sequelae after encephalitis [17–19]. From 1976 National Swine Influenza Immunization Program in the United States, a large number of cases of Guillain-Barre syndrome and other demyelinating autoimmune neuropathies were described: involvement of the brain, cerebellum, optic nerve, cranial nerves, and spinal cord occurred. Of interest, these neuropathies were observed up to 10 months after vaccination [20,21].

Macrophagic Myofasciitis Syndrome

In France in 1998, Gherardi RK described for first time the MMF. This new syndrome is defined by the presence of diffuse and severe myalgias and arthralgias after aluminum hydroxide administration in the absence of a clearly cause. The deltoid muscle biopsy demonstrated immunologically active lesion. It was demonstrated that this lesion is the consequence of long-term persistence of the immunologic adjuvant aluminum hydroxide within the cytoplasm of macrophages at the site of previous intramuscular injection [22]. Aluminum adjuvants, or "alum," are the most commonly used adjuvants in human and animal vaccines worldwide. In relation with the mechanism underlying the stimulation of the immune system by alum, it has been demonstrated that alum induce the production of proinflammatory cytokines in vitro without intact Toll-like receptor signaling to activate the immune system. Eisenbarth SC [23] et al. demonstrated that aluminum adjuvants activate an intracellular innate immune response system called the Nalp3 or inflammasome. Production of the proinflammatory cytokines IL-1β and IL-18 by macrophages in response to alum in vitro required inflammasome signaling. Therefore, the Nalp3 inflammasome is a crucial element in the adjuvant effect of aluminum adjuvants. These findings will allow to prepare safer and effective adjuvants in the future.

Gulf War Syndrome

Squalene-based adjuvants have been included in influenza vaccines since 1997 and it is another adjuvant that stimulates Th2 immune response. GWS is a multisystemic illness afflicting many Gulf War era veterans. A study determined the presence of antibodies to squalene and signs and symptoms of 144 Gulf War era veterans or 58 military employees immunized for service in Desert Shield/Desert Storm Operation during 1990–91. Blood donors, SLE patients, silicone breast implant recipients, and chronic fatigue syndrome patients were included under a control group. Serum antibodies to squalene were found in 95% of GWS patients. All (100%) GWS patients immunized (deploy or not deploy) for service in Desert Shield/Desert Storm had the same signs and symptoms and antibodies to squalene. In contrast, none (0%) patients with idiopathic AID or healthy controls had detectable serum antibodies to squalene [24].

These are part of the background that served as the basis for the proposal of the new ASIA. Next, we will develop the epidemiological, basic, and clinical aspects of ASIA to support the existence of this new entity.

EPIDEMIOLOGY

AIDs affect from 3% to 10% of the general population [25,26]. Due to the relative rarity of this condition and its recent identification, as well as to collect data of the disease features, the ASIA syndrome registry was created in 2011. It consists in internationally published case reports and newly diagnosed cases of ASIA syndrome reported in the first instance by rheumatologists. As mentioned before, more than 4000 ASIA cases have been reported. The worldwide distribution of the reported cases can be seen on Table 51.1 and Fig. 51.1 [27–47].

According to the main condition previously identified as part of ASIA, the epidemiological characteristics tend to change. In this autoimmune entity, the most commonly affected demographic group is represented by young women. Another important variation besides sex is the severity; women have worse outcomes than men [29,32].

Pellegrino et al. reported an analysis of 26,508 patients with adverse events after human papillomavirus (HPV) vaccination. From the original population, 15% of the patients presented diagnostic criteria for ASIA because of the presence of typical clinical manifestation or at least two minor criteria. An incidence of ASIA related with HPV vaccination of 3.6 cases per 100,000 vaccinated patients was found [29]. Vaccines seem to be the most significant ASIA potential trigger [48].

In a descriptive analysis of 300 patients from the international ASIA syndrome registry, adjuvant foreign materials were identified in one-third of the subjects. Cosmetic fillers such as mineral oil, hyaluronic acid, and collagen were recognized in 38.8% of the patients; metal implants were recognized in 43.7% and breast implants in 17.5%. Metal implants, especially

TABLE 51.1 Autoimmune/Inflammatory Syndrome Induced by Adjuvants Case Reports by Country From 2011 to 2017

United States	3939
Israel	421
The Netherlands	315
Mexico	219
Spain	65
France	44
Japan	40
Italy	36
Denmark	21
Sweden	5
Australia	4
Brazil	4
Colombia	4
Serbia	3
Portugal	2
Canada	2

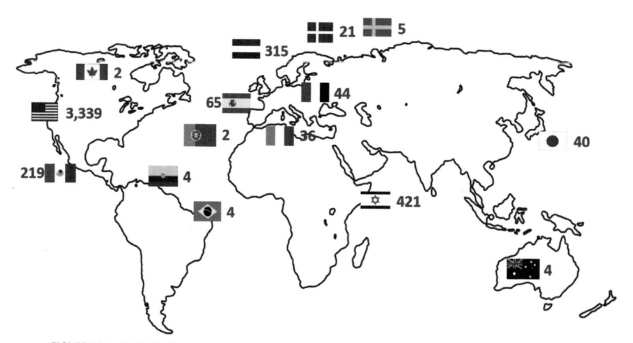

FIGURE 51.1 Worldwide distribution of autoimmune/inflammatory syndrome induced by adjuvants cases from 2011 to 2017.

those used in dentistry, seem to be the most common foreign adjuvant in ASIA. The undifferentiated connective tissue disorder is the most prevalent presentation, following fibromyalgia and lupus-like syndrome [32]. MMF is a rare entity, and its prevalence is not exactly known. Its presence has been related to vaccines containing aluminum as adjuvant. In addition, it has been associated with the human leukocyte antigen (HLA) class II allele DRB1*01 [39,49]. At last, results from some epidemiologic studies suggest that GWS is more common in Gulf War veteran women and that they may have differences in the biomarkers expression [50]. ASIA seems to have a relatively high frequency and a causal relationship between adjuvant materials. According to the map presented in Table 51.1 and Fig. 51.1, ASIA is evolving to a global distribution and in some areas such as Latin America, Serbia, Portugal, and Canada, and there seems to be an underreporting of this entity.

CLINICAL MANIFESTATIONS OF ASIA

Clinical criteria proposed by Shoelfeld et al. [1] included a combination of major and minor criteria. Major: External stimulus exposure before clinical signs, development of manifestations such as myalgia, myositis or muscle weakness, arthralgia and or arthritis, chronic fatigue or sleep disturbances, neurological manifestations, cognitive impairment, memory loss, pyrexia, dry mouth, typical biopsy of the organs involved, and improvement of symptoms after removal of the foreign agent. Minor: Appearance of autoantibodies, other clinical symptoms (for example, irritable bowel disease), specific HLA, or development of an AID (multiple sclerosis, SSc, etc.). Recently, the clinical spectrum of ASIA has been expanded, varying from mild to life-threatening conditions.

In a comparative study of 30 years including 200 cases of ASIA syndrome after the use of silicone implants in the Maastricht cohort consisting of 99 female patients and 1 transgender, the median latency period from silicone implant until onset of clinical symptoms was 4 years (range 1–39 years), being arthralgia and chronic fatigue the most common symptoms. Other manifestations observed were Raynaud's phenomenon, irritable bowel syndrome, recurrent respiratory tract infections, recurrent cystitis, livedo reticularis, and allergies with similar findings in the Baylor College cohort, concluding that silicone-related disease has not changed during the last 30 years [27]. Data obtained from ASIA syndrome registry up to December 2016 analyzed 300 cases of this syndrome and found that arthralgia, myalgia, and chronic fatigue were the most frequent symptoms with a mean latency period of 16.8 months, ranging from 3 days to 5 years [29]. In the same way, clinical manifestations of ASIA due to postvaccination phenomena includes neurologic diseases, such as multiple sclerosis and Guillain-Barré syndrome, other manifestations such as vasculitides, SLE, inflammatory myopathies and arthropathies, autoimmune thrombocytopenia, inflammatory bowel diseases, and organ-specific autoimmune manifestations [51]. Postvaccine diseases reported in pediatric patients are the acute disseminated encephalomyelitis after measles, rabies, mumps, hepatitis B, rubella, influenza, and human papillomavirus vaccinations, as well as narcolepsy and Henoch–Schonlein purpura. Well-defined AIDs such as lupus erythematosus, RA, mixed connective tissue disease, Sjogren's syndrome, dermatomyositis, and SSc have also been reported in adolescents after vaccination [52]. In a systematic review by our group of 4479 ASIA cases identified from 2011 to 2016, 305 were classified as severe, with the majority of them developing after vaccination. The most common symptoms reported were arthralgia, arthritis, chronic fatigue, myalgia, sleep disturbances, generalized weakness, dryness of mucosa, fever, and neurological manifestations. Another aspect of the clinical spectrum of ASIA is the development of clear-cut diagnosis that was reported in 267 patients (89%), namely undifferentiated connective tissue disease, fibromyalgia and/or chronic fatigue syndrome, SLE, and other connective tissue disorders, as well as neurologic autoinflammatory diseases, as seen on Fig. 51.2 [6]. Other rare manifestations of ASIA are systemic autoimmune or granulomatous disorders which have been reported in association to biomaterials of human use. A recent study found inflammatory features at the site of implant preceding distant or systemic manifestations such as localized inflammatory nodules and panniculitis evolving to diverse disorders comprised in ASIA such as primary biliary cirrhosis, Sjögren's syndrome, sarcoidosis, vasculitis, inflammatory bowel syndrome, and inflammatory polyradiculopathy [28]. Siliconosis, calcinosis cutis with hypercalcemia, and chronic kidney disease have also been described in association with silicone injection [53].

Some endocrinopathies have also been observed after exposure to adjuvants contained in vaccines and silicone implants; for example, cases of Hashimoto thyroiditis, subacute thyroiditis, and primary ovarian failure were observed [54]. Recently it has been published in the first case of a seasonal influenza vaccine–induced ASIA in a previously healthy male who presented to hospital with simultaneous rhabdomyolysis and myocarditis, 5 days postinfluenza vaccine which contain the MF59 adjuvant. He responded well to conservative management and did not require immune suppressive therapy [55]. It has been reported that silicone can induce lymphoproliferative disorders such as the anaplastic large B cell lymphoma. Therefore, silicone may cause a chronic activation of B cells and eventually lead to the development of lymphoproliferative disorders [56,57]. A summary of the main diseases associated to ASIA are described in Table 51.2 [1,6,7,28,29,40,45,52–57].

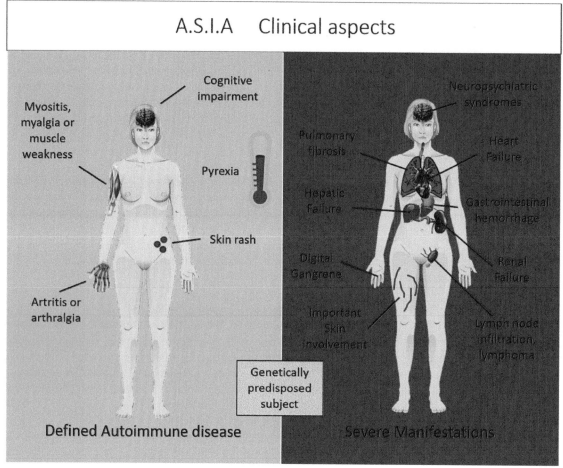

FIGURE 51.2 Autoimmune/inflammatory syndrome induced by adjuvants clinical spectrum from defined autoimmune disease to severe manifestations.

TABLE 51.2 The Wide Spectrum of Diseases Associated to Autoimmune/Inflammatory Syndrome Induced by Adjuvants

Neurologic manifestations	Acute disseminated encephalomyelitis, Guillain-Barré syndrome, multiple sclerosis, narcolepsy, transverse myelitis, inflammatory polyradiculopathy, memory loss, peripheral neuropathy, epilepsy, cerebral vascular disease
Well-defined rheumatic diseases	Systemic lupus erythematosus, rheumatoid arthritis, mixed connective tissue disease, Sjogren's syndrome, dermatomyositis, systemic sclerosis, giant cell arteritis, polyarteritis nodosa, inflammatory myopathy, Still's disease, Kawasaki disease, severe cutaneous small-vessel vasculitis, fibromyalgia, psoriatic arthritis
Gastroenterologic manifestations	Inflammatory bowel disease, primary biliary cirrhosis, autoimmune hepatitis, antiphospholipid syndrome, ulcerative colitis, Crohn's disease, pancreatitis
Endocrine manifestations	Hashimoto thyroiditis, subacute thyroiditis, primary ovarian failure
Hematologic manifestations	Hemolytic anemia, autoimmune thrombocytopenia, pseudolymphoma, lymphoma
Renal manifestations	Chronic kidney disease
Psychiatric manifestations	Depression, obsessive compulsive disorder, sleep disorders
Cardiac manifestations	Postural orthostatic tachycardia, myocarditis, pericarditis
Other	Sarcoidosis, sicca syndrome, angioedema

For all that mentioned above, we can conclude that because of the broadness of clinical manifestations that may be related to ASIA, physicians of different medical specialties should be aware of the causal relationship that exists between adjuvant molecules and AIDs. Personalized medicine is a guarantee to avoid unnecessary exposures to adjuvants such as silicone, vaccines, mineral oils, and metals in healthy individuals but at high risk of developing an AID and other entities such as lymphoma.

ETIOPATHOGENESIS OF ASIA

Any substance that acts to accelerate, prolong, or enhance antigen-specific immune response is an adjuvant and fundamental for the successful vaccination. However, enhancing the body's immune reactions also could conduce to adverse autoimmune reactions. The question is why some individuals have more susceptibility to develop adverse reactions from minimal to lethal severities. Some options had been analyzed for some subtype of substances that acts as an adjuvant: (1) genetically predisposed individuals, (2) ambient pollution leading to epigenetic modifications, (3) possible toxicity because of its vast homology with human proteins, and (4) innate and adaptive response in each individual [1].

Genetic predisposition has been mentioned in ASIA, but there is little investigation in these specific patients. DNA methylation, histone modifications, and chromatin remodeling are the most important on control and modulate gene expression and phenotypic variation present between individuals and ethnicities. Epigenetic differences between ethnicities are an important consideration when investigating autoimmune disorders with a pattern of heterogeneous risk [58].

Epigenetic means any process that alters gene activity without changes genetic sequence (deoxyribonucleic acid sequence). These modifications in gene activity can be transmitted by decades and the changes have some linking with cancers, cognitive dysfunction, respiratory, cardiovascular, reproductive, neurobehavioral disease, and systemic autoimmune/inflammatory illness. Actually, many agents are under the suspect to be promoter of gene dysfunction, including heavy metals, pesticides, diesel exhaust, tobacco smoke, polycyclic aromatic hydrocarbons, hormones, radioactivity, viruses, bacteria, basic nutrients, and adjuvants substance (silicone, squalene, aluminum hydroxide, mineral oil, guaiacol, iodine gadital, mercury, and titanium among others), as seen in Fig. 51.3. In most cases the environmental exposure is related to lifestyle, so it can be modified to prevent or attenuate the risk of developing disease [6,59].

In ASIA syndrome there is a previous exposition to an adjuvant that changes the normal local environment and could be an inductor for epigenetic mild or severe variation. The epigenetic variations had led to aberrant cellular gene expression, dysfunction of T cells, incapacity to recognize self-antigens, inflammation, and eventually autoimmunity and tissue damage [60] as seen on Fig. 51.4.

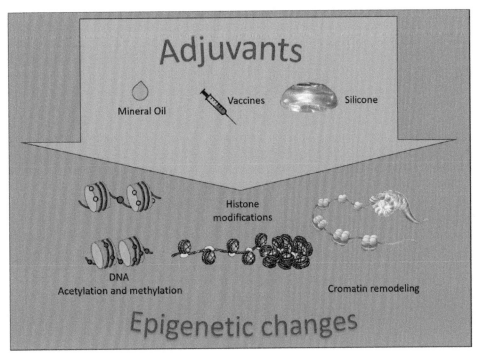

FIGURE 51.3   The different described adjuvants may have the capacity to produce epigenetic changes in susceptible subjects.

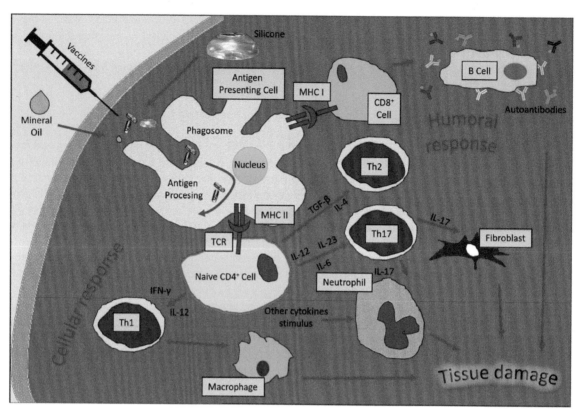

FIGURE 51.4 Mechanisms of adjuvants. Adjuvants may generate depots that trap antigens at the injection site, continually stimulating of the immune system. The downstream signaling pathways lead to the activation of transcription factors. As a consequence, the induction of cytokines and chemokines is started. They play a key role in the priming, expansion, and polarization of the immune responses. *MHC I*, type I major histocompatibility complex; *MHC II*, type II major histocompatibility complex; *TCR*, T-cell receptor; *TFG-β*, transforming growth factor beta.

Destruction and dysfunction of self-tissues results of misbalance between effector T cells and negative regulators Tregs of the immune system drive the production of autoantibodies [58]. The adjuvant must improve the immune response to antigens or haptens; but if they contain molecular patterns associated with pathogens or lead to mild tissue injury that exposes some molecular patterns associated with damage, they will be recognized by the innate immune system through specific pattern recognition receptors. The adaptive cross-reactivity response occurs with both the antigenic and adjuvant components of the vaccine at the injection site, in the afferent lymph nodes, and distant organs including the central nervous system [61]. On the other hand, antigens such as silicon lead to a local immune response that involves activated Th1/Th17 lymphocytes and synthesis of interleukins and growth factors [62].

There are two main sources of air pollution related to the traffic (TRAP) of automotive vehicles and biomass fuel (BMF); however, consequences for autoimmune/inflammatory had been few investigated. TRAP effects on the regulation of the inflammatory cascade and oxidative stress also act as adjuvants inducing the synthesis of specific IgE and up to 50 times more Th2 profile in some cases [63]. It has importance because in a cohort of patients who developed silicone-induced ASIA, 75% reported preexisting allergic conditions after silicone implantation [62]. Fine particles with aerodynamic diameter ≤ 2.5 μm easily reach alveoli; they are then phagocyted by alveolar macrophages and transported by circulation to other organs, producing a systemic inflammatory response [63]. Some metals are essential for metabolism, but both the excess of these and the accumulation in tissues of nonessential metals can alter the structure of DNA causing mutations, cellular dysfunction, or favoring autoimmunity [34,64]. High and continuous exposition to toxic environment could conduce to DNA methylation; as an example of their impact, very high levels of methylation (~90%) within the IL-4 locus contribute to the restrained Th2 cytokine expression in naïve T cells [58].

In conclusion, in the course of life, humans are exposed to interact with adjuvants such as silicone, aluminum, pristane, mineral oils, metals, etc. These molecules can produce epigenetic changes and modify the innate and adaptive immune response. However, the development of an adjuvant disease is rare. Therefore, exposure to an adjuvant is necessary but not sufficient to develop an AID. Additional genetic and environmental factors are needed to develop an autoimmune/inflammatory disease induced by adjuvant.

TREATMENT

Treatment of ASIA is focused on the nonspecific and specific manifestations of autoimmunity. In relation to nonspecific manifestations of ASIA such as fatigue, cognitive disorders, sleep disorders, memory loss, myalgia, arthralgias, or arthritis, treatment with analgesics, nonsteroidal antiinflammatories (NSAIDs), and steroids should be given. In case of specific AIDs such as SLE, RA, SSc, dermatomyositis, and fibromyalgia, the treatment should be given according to established guidelines. The removal of the adjuvant substances is necessary, although it does not always improve the clinical picture [34,49]. ASIA postimmunization diseases caused by autoimmune phenomena such as small-, medium-, and large caliber vasculitis require treatment with steroids and immunosuppressants. In cases of RA, treatment with disease-modifying drugs such as methotrexate, sulfasalazine, hydroxychloroquine, and biologic therapy is indicated. In patients with SLE, the treatment will be focused according to the involvement of the major organ with intravenous steroids and immunosuppressants. In cases of Guillain-Barré syndrome, the administration of immunoglobulin or plasmapheresis is necessary [40,49].

With respect to MMF syndrome in which the manifestations of inflammatory myopathy are predominate, steroids and immunosuppressants must also be given [49]. Regarding of siliconosis and silicone breast implants, it is mandatory to remove the breast prostheses and give specific treatment for the predominant autoimmune rheumatic disease or for the nonspecific symptoms of the connective tissue. If patients had Still disease, SSc, or RA, the treatment is according to the main disease [49,65,66].

Because smoking is linked to autoimmunity and a predisposing factor for worsening clinical course of some diseases such as SLE, it is advisable to recommend stop smoking in patients with ASIA–MO and these features. Another factor that contributes to both initiation and progression of AID is obesity; therefore a program to control overweight should be included in the management of these patients [67,68].

It has been postulated that vitamin D deficiency and adjuvants is associated with autoimmunity in ASIA patients in relation to silicone implant incompatibility. On the other hand, an inverse correlation between serum vitamin D levels and the presence of autoantibodies in several AIDs has been observed. Therefore, patients with ASIA–MO and D hypovitaminosis could be benefited with supplementation of vitamin D to prevent the development of autoantibodies and possibly ASIA syndrome. Likewise, it is important to take advantage of its effects as antifibrotic treatment [69,70].

Regarding ASIA by mineral oil, treatment should be focused on local or systemic clinical manifestations and depend on the involved areas such as breast, buttocks, lower extremities, face, and genitalia. In general, treatment is divided into medical and surgical and may represent a great challenge, and the results can be frustrating [47].

Medical treatment of patients with ASIA should be multidisciplinary, owing to the diverse reactions the patient may have. The team attending the patient should include a rheumatologist, internist, psychiatrist, dermatologist, angiologist, plastic surgeon, neurologist, psychologist, and a rehabilitation specialist, among others [47,49,71]. Because chronic pain and inflammation are important manifestations, the use of analgesics, NSAIDs, and steroids is the cornerstone in the treatment of this syndrome. On the other hand, because of the presence of emotional problems such as depression or anxiety, management with antidepressants is essential. If patients meet criteria for fibromyalgia, they should be treated accordingly. Another important treatment is the management of chronic ulcers, which frequently are infected, thus making necessary the use of antibiotics and in some cases hospitalization. If the ASIA–MO patients develop systemic AID, for example, nephropathy, thrombocytopenia, and vasculitis, they may receive methylprednisolone pulses or prednisone plus immunosuppressant therapy [47,49].

If patients meet criteria for some AIDs such as RA, SLE, SSc, etc., they should be treated according to established guidelines for these diseases. When patients have a defined autoimmune rheumatic disease such as RA, they may be treated with low doses of prednisone and disease-modifying antirheumatic drugs or even biological therapy. Patients with severe SLE may be treated with oral or intravenous doses of corticoids plus intravenous cyclophosphamide or other immunosuppressants. Those with SSc need antifibrotic treatment or immunosuppressants to improve skin thickening. Management of vasculature involvement as Raynaud's phenomenon and pulmonary arterial hypertension requires vasodilators, phosphodiesterase inhibitors, and antagonists of endothelin. Treatment of gastrointestinal affections is also necessary. Those with nonspecific Autoimmune Rheumatic Disease (ARD) manifestations could receive nonsteroid antiinflammatory drugs, analgesics, and low to moderate doses of prednisone, chloroquine or hydroxychloroquine or immunosuppressant drugs, for example, azathioprine, with the aim of improving chronic inflammation [47,49].

Several local treatments have been used in cases with ulceration at the application site, for example, in a case with penile paraffinoma that improved with topical application of potassium permanganate soaks. Conservative local treatment depending on the type of wound includes control of inflammation or infections and moisture balance with adequate dressings. In a case, dermabrasion was used to treat silicone granuloma in a patient who received silicone injections on her hips for cosmetic purposes. Due to the chronicity of lesions in some cases, it would be possible to use negative pressure wound therapy (vacuum-assisted closure) that accelerates wound healing by promoting angiogenesis [72]. Ultimately, patients with ASIA–MO require a holistic and multidisciplinary treatment. In cases of ASIA by MO, the surgical treatment is necessary. Biological behavior of the modeling substances is complex and will depend on the quantity, frequency, and type of oily substance and site infiltrated, so the treatment represents a challenge [73,74].

The objective of surgical treatment is to remove the injected material in skin and muscles and deep tissues to improve clinical manifestations. Most patients with ASIA–MO will develop chronic relapses and the treatment is disheartening, requiring many surgeries. Treatment of ASIA–MO constitutes a great challenge for the physician and an ominous outlook for the patients [47].

PERSPECTIVES AND CONCLUSIONS

- In relation to the epidemiology of ASIA, it is necessary to increase the international database because it is possible that there is underreporting.
- In relation to the clinical picture, it is necessary to identify other risk factors, in addition to the adjuvant exposure.
- The immunogenetic, epigenetic, and inflammatory mechanisms of each adjuvant should continue to be studied.
- ASIA is a defined entity of worldwide distribution that needs to be studied in each country and region to know the natural history of ASIA and propose new therapeutic targets.
- It is important to remind that benefits of the vaccines are largely more than the potential adverse events, and that nowadays there is no specific test to understand the predisposition to the development of an abnormal reaction to vaccines.

REFERENCES

[1] Shoenfeld Y, Agmon-Levin N. "ASIA" – autoimmune/inflammatorysyndrome induced by adjuvants. J Autoimmun 2011;36:4–8.

[2] Parks CG, de Souza Espindola Santos A, Barbhaiya M, Costenbader KH. Understanding the role of environmental factors in the development of systemic lupus erythematosus. Best Pract Res Clin Rheumatol 2017;31:306–20.

[3] Israeli E, Agmon-Levin N, Blank M, Shoenfeld Y. Adjuvants and autoimmunity. Lupus 2009;18:1217–25.

[4] Guimaraes LE, Baker B, Perricone C, Shoenfeld Y. Vaccines, adjuvants and autoimmunity. Pharmacol Res 2015;100:190–209.

[5] Arango MT, Perricone C, Kivity S, Cipriano E, Ceccarelli F, Valesini G, Shoenfeld Y. HLA-DRB1 the notorious gene in the mosaic of autoimmunity. Immunol Res 2017;65:82–98.

[6] Jara LJ, Garcia-Collinot G, Medina G, Cruz-DominguezMDP, Vera-Lastra O, Carranza-Muleiro RA, Saavedra MA. Severe manifestations of autoimmune syndrome induced by adjuvants(Shoenfeld's syndrome). Immunol Res 2017;65:8–16.

[7] Watad A, Quaresma M, Brown S, Cohen Tervaert JW, Rodríguez-Pint I, Cervera R, Perricone C, ShoenfeldY. Autoimmune/inflammatory syndrome induced by adjuvants (Shoenfeld's syndrome) - an update. Lupus 2017;26:675–81.

[8] Agmon-Levin N, Arango MT, Kivity S, Katzav A, GilburdB, Blank M, Tomer N, Volkov A, Barshack I, Chapman J, ShoenfeldY. Immunization with hepatitis B vaccine accelerates SLE like disease in a murine model. J Autoimmun 2014;54:21–32.

[9] Ruiz JT, Lujan L, Blank M, Shoenfeld Y. Adjuvants- andvaccines-induced autoimmunity: animal models. Immunol Res 2017;65(1):55–65.

[10] Pearson CM, Waksman BH, Sharp JT. Studies of arthritis, and other lessions in rats by injection of mycobacterial adjuvant.V. Changes affecting the skin and mucous membranes. Comparison of the experimental process with human disease. J Exp Med 1961;113:485–510.

[11] Steblay RW, Rudofsky U. Autoimmune glomerulonephritis induced in sheep by injections of human lung and Freund's adjuvant. Science 1968;160(3824):204–6.

[12] Wisniewski HM, Bloom BR. Primary demyelination as a nonspecific consequence of a cell-mediated immune reaction. J Exp Med 1975;141:346–59.

[13] Rosenbaum JT, Adelman NE, McDevitt HO. In vivo effects of antibodies to immune response gene products. I. Haplotype-specific suppression of humoral immune responses with a monoclonal anti-I-A. J Exp Med 1981;54:1694–702.

[14] Kumagai Y, Abe C, Shiokawa Y. Scleroderma after cosmetic surgery: four cases of human adjuvant disease. Arthritis Rheum 1979;22:532–7.

[15] Naim JO, Lanzafame RJ, van Oss CJ. The effect of silicone-gel on the immune response. J Biomater Sci Polym Ed 1995;7:123–32.

[16] Spiera RF, Gibofsky A, Spiera H. Silicone gel filled breast implants and connective tissue disease: an overview. J Rheumatol 1994;21:239–45.

[17] For and against smallpox vaccination. Br Med J 1970;2(5705):311–2.

[18] Neff JM, Lane JM, Pert JH, Moore R, Millar JD. Henderson DA Complications of smallpox vaccination. I. National survey in the United States, 1963. N Engl J Med 1967;276:125–32.

[19] Neff JM, Levine RH, Lane JM, Ager EA, Moore H, Rosenstein BJ, Millar JD. Henderson DA Complications of smallpox vaccination United States 1963. II. Results obtained by four state wide surveys. Pediatrics 1967;39:916–23.

[20] Poser CM. Neurological complications of swine influenza vaccination. Acta Neurol Scand 1982;66:413–31.

[21] Poser CM, Behan PO. Late onset of Guillain-Barré syndrome. J Neuroimmunol 1982;3:27–41.

[22] Gherardi RK, Coquet M, Chérin P, Authier F-J, Laforêt P, Belec L, et al. Macrophagic myofasciitis: an emerging entity. Lancet 1998;352:347–52.

[23] Eisenbarth SC, Colegio OR, O'Connor W, Sutterwala FS, Flavell RA. Crucial role for the Nalp3 inflammasome in the immunostimulatory properties of aluminium adjuvants. Nature 2008;453(7198):1122–6.

[24] Asa PB, Cao Y, Garry RF. Antibodies to squalene in Gulf war syndrome. Exp Mol Pathol 2000;68:55–64.

[25] Cooper G, Stroehla B. The epidemiology of autoimmune diseases. Autoimmun Rev 2003;2:119–25.

[26] Cooper G, Bynum M, Somers E. Recent insights in the epidemiology of autoimmune diseases: improved prevalence estimates and understanding of clustering of diseases. J Autoimmun 2009;33:197–207.

[27] Colaris MJL, de Boer M, van der Hulst RR, Cohen Tervaert JW. Two hundreds cases of ASIA syndrome following silicone implants: a comparative study of 30 years and a review of current literature. Immunol Res 2017;65:120–8.

[28] Alijotas-Reig J, Esteve-Valverde E, Gil-Aliberas N, Garcia-Gimenez V. Autoimmune/inflammatory syndrome induced by adjuvants-ASIA-related to biomaterials: analysis of 45 cases and comprehensive review of the literatura. Immunol Res December 3, 2017. https://doi.org/10.1007/s12026-017-8980-5.

[29] Watad A, Quaresma M, Bragazzi N, Cervera R, Tervaert J, Amital H. The autoimmune/inflammatory syndrome induced by adjuvants (ASIA)/Shoenfeld's syndrome: descriptive analysis of 300 patients from the international ASIA syndrome registry. Clin Rheumatol 2017. https://doi.org/10.1007/s10067-017-3748-9.

[30] Palmieri B, Poddighe D, Vadalà M, Laurino C, Carnovale C, Clementi E. Severe somatoform and dysautonomic syndromes after HPV vaccination: case series and review of literature. Immunol Res 2017;65:106–16.

[31] Brinth LS, Pors K, Theibel AC, Mehlsen J. Orthostatic intolerance and postural tachycardia syndrome as suspected adverse effects of vaccination against human papilloma virus. Vaccine May 21, 2015;33:2602–5.

[32] Pellegrino P, Perrone V, Pozzi M, Carnovale C, Perrota C, Clementi E, et al. The epidemiological profile of ASIA síndrome after HPV vaccination: an evaluation based on the Vaccine Adverse Event Reporting Systems. Immunol Res 2015;61(1–2):90–6.

[33] Martínez-Lavín M, Martínez-Martínez LA, Reyes-Loyola P. HPV vaccination syndrome. A questionnaire-based study. Clin Rheumatol 2015;34:1981–3.

[34] Stejskal V. Metals as a common trigger of inflammation resulting in non-specific symptoms: diagnosis and treatment. Isr Med Assoc J 2014;16:753–8.

[35] Agmon-Levin N, Zafrir Y, Kivity S, Balofsky A, Amital H, Shoenfeld Y. Chronic fatigue syndrome and fibromyalgia following immunization with the hepatitis B vaccine: another angle of the 'autoimmune (auto-inflammatory) syndrome induced by adjuvants' (ASIA). Immunol Res 2014;60:376–83.

[36] Blitshteyn S. Postural tachycardia syndrome following human papillomavirus vaccination. Eur J Neurol 2014;21:135–9.

[37] Kinoshita T, Abe RT, Hineno A, Tsunekawa K, Nakane S, Ikeda S. Peripheral sympathetic nerve dysfunction in adolescent Japanese girls following immunization with the human papillomavirus vaccine. Intern Med 2014;53:2185–200.

[38] Little DT, Ward HR. Adolescent premature ovarian insufficiency following human papillomavirus vaccination: a case series seen in general practice. J Investig Med High Impact Case Rep 2014;2:1–12.

[39] Cadusseau J, Ragunathan-Thangarajah N, Surenaud M, Hue S, Authier FJ, Gherardi RK. Selective elevation of circulating CCL2/MCP1 levels in patients with longstanding post-vaccinal macrophagic myofasciitis and ASIA. Curr Med Chem 2014;21:511–7.

[40] Cerpa-Cruz S, Paredes-Casillas P, Landeros Navarro E, Bernard-Medina AG, Martínez-Bonilla G, Gutiérrez-Ureña S. Adverse events following immunization with vaccines containing adjuvants. Immunol Res 2013;56:299–303.

[41] Maijers MC, de Blok CJ, Niessen FB, van derVeldt AA, Ritt MJ, Winters HA, et al. Women with silicone breast implants and unexplained systemic symptoms: a descriptive cohort study. Neth J Med 2013;71:534–40.

[42] Gatto M, Agmon-Levin N, Soriano A, Manna R, Maoz-Segal R, Kivity S, et al. Human papillomavirus vaccine and systemic lupus erythematosus. Clin Rheumatol 2013;32:1301–7.

[43] Cohen Tervaert JW, Kappel RM. Silicone implant incompatibility syndrome (SIIS): a frequent cause of ASIA (Shoenfeld's syndrome). Immunol Res 2013;56:293–8.

[44] Zafrir Y, Agmon-Levin N, Paz Z, Shilton T, Shoenfeld Y. Autoimmunity following hepatitis B vaccine as part of the spectrum of 'Autoimmune (Auto-inflammatory) Syndrome induced by Adjuvants' (ASIA): analysis of 93 cases. Lupus 2012;21:146–52.

[45] Alijotas-Reig J, Garcia-Gimenez V, Llurba E, Vilardell-Tarrés M. Autoimmune/inflammatory syndrome (ASIA) induced by biomaterials injection other than silicone medical grade. Lupus 2012;21:1326–34.

[46] Soriano A, Verrecchia E, Marinaro A, Giovinale M, Fonnesu C, Landolfi R. Giant cell arteritis and polymyalgia rheumatica after influenza vaccination: report of 10 cases and review of the literature. Lupus 2012;21:153–7.

[47] Vera-Lastra O, Medina G, Cruz-DominguezMdel P, Ramirez P, Gayosso-Rivera JA, Anduaga-Dominguez H, et al. Human adjuvant disease induced by foreign substances: a new model of ASIA (Shoenfeld's syndrome). Lupus 2012;21:128–35.

[48] Scanzi F, Andreoli M, Martinelli M, Taraborelli M, Cavazzana I, Carabellese N, et al. Are the autoimmune/inflammatory syndrome induced by adjuvants (ASIA) and the undifferentiated connective tissue disease (UCTD) related to each other? A case-control study of environmental exposures. Immunol Res 2017;65:150–6.

[49] Vera-Lastra O, Medina G, Cruz-Dominguez Mdel P, Jara LJ, Shoenfeld Y. Autoimmune/inflammatory syndrome induced by adjuvants (Shoenfeld's syndrome): clinical and immunological spectrum. Expert Rev Clin Immunol 2013;9:361–73.

[50] Coughlin SS, Krengel M, Sullivan K, Pierce PF, Heboyan V, Wilson LCC. A review of epidemiologic studies of the health of Gulf war women veterans. J Environ Health Sci 2017;3(2).

[51] Molina V, Shoenfeld Y. Infection, vaccines and other environmental triggers of autoimmunity. Autoimmunity 2005;38:235–45.

[52] Esposito S, Prada E, Mastrolia MV, Tarantino G, Codecà C, Rigante D. Autoimmune/inflammatory syndrome induced by adjuvants (ASIA): clues and pitfalls in the pediatric background. Immunol Res 2014;60:366–75.

[53] Barilaro G, Spaziani Testa C, Cacciani A, Donato G, Dimko M, Mariotti A. ASIA syndrome, calcinosis cutis and chronic kidney disease following silicone injections. A case-based review. Immunol Res 2016;64:1142–9.

[54] Watad A, David P, Brown S, Shoenfeld Y. Autoimmune/inflammatory syndrome induced by adjuvants and thyroid autoimmunity. Front Endocrinol (Lausanne) 2017;7:150. https://doi.org/10.3389/fendo.2016.00150. eCollection 2016.

[55] Cheng MP, Kozoriz MG, Ahmadi AA, Kelsall J, Paquette K, Onrot JM. Post-vaccination myositis and myocarditis in a previously healthy male. Allergy Asthma Clin Immunol 2016;12:6. https://doi.org/10.1186/s13223-016-0114-4. eCollection 2016.

[56] Luigi Bragazzi N, Watad A, Adawi M, Amital H, Aljadeff G, Shoenfeld Y. Adjuvants and autoimmunity: why do we develop autoantibodies, autoimmune diseases and lymphomas. Isr Med Assoc J 2017 l;19:403–5.

[57] Bizjak M, Selmi C, Praprotnik S, et al. Silicone implants and lymphoma: the role of inflammation. J Autoimmun 2015;65:64–73.

[58] Coit P, Ognenovski M, Gensterblum E, Maksimowicz-McKinnon K, Wren JD, Amr H. Sawalha Ethnicity-specific epigenetic variation in naïve CD4+ T cells and the susceptibility to autoimmunity. Epigenet Chromatin 2015;8:49.

[59] Klein K, Gay S. Epigenetics in rheumatoid arthritis. Curr Opin Rheumatol January 2015;27(1):76–82. https://doi.org/10.1097/BOR.0000000000000128.

[60] Nielsen HM, Tost J. Epigenetic changes in inflammatory and autoimmune diseases. Epigenet Chromatin 2015;8:49.

[61] Pellegrino P, Clementi E, Radice S. Review on vaccine's adjuvants and autoimmunity: current evidence and future perspectives. Autoimmun Rev 2015;14(10):880–8.

[62] Goren I, Segal G, Shoenfeld Y. Autoimmune/inflammatory syndrome induced by adjuvant (ASIA) evolution after silicone implants. Who is at risk? Clin Rheumatol 2015;34(10):1661–6. https://doi.org/10.1007/s10067-015-2931-0.

[63] Laumbach R, Kipen H. Respiratory health effects of air pollution: update on biomass smoke and traffic pollution. J Allergy Clin Immunol 2012;129(1):3–13.

[64] Cruz-Domínguez MP, Vera-Lastra O, Deras-Quiñones A, Jandete-Rivera F, Grajeda-Lopez P, Montes-Cortes DH, Medina G, Jara LJ. Mercury tissue deposits: a new adjuvant in autoimmune/inflammatory syndrome. Isr Med Assoc J 2013;15(11):716–9.

[65] Jara LJ, Medina G, Gómez-Bañuelos E, Saavedra MA, Vera-Lastra O. Still's disease, lupus-like syndrome, and silicone breast implants. A case of 'ASIA' (Shoenfeld's syndrome). Lupus 2012;21:140–5.

[66] Kappel RM, Cohen Tervaert JW, Pruijn GJ. Autoimmune/inflammatory syndrome induced by adjuvants (ASIA) due to silicone implant incompatibility syndrome in three sisters. Clin Exp Rheumatol 2014;32:256–8.

[67] Harel-MeirM, Sherer Y, Shoenfeld Y. Tobacco smoking and autoimmune rheumatic diseases. Nat Clin Pract Rheumatol 2007;3:707–15.

[68] Arnson Y, Shoenfeld Y, Amital H. Effects of tobacco smoke on immunity, inflammation and autoimmunity. J Autoimmun 2010;34:J258–65.

[69] Versini M, Aljadeff G, Jeandel PY, et al. Obesity: an additional piece in the mosaic of autoimmunity. Isr Med Assoc J 2014;16:619–21.

[70] Colaris MJL, van derHulst RR, Tervaert JWC. Vitamin D deficiency as a risk factor for the development of autoantibodies in patients with ASIA and silicone breast implants: a cohort study and review of the literature. Clin Rheumatol 2017;36:981–93.

[71] Martínez-Villarreal AA, Asz-Sigall D, Gutiérrez-Mendoza D, et al. A case series and a review of the literature on foreign modelling agent reaction: an emerging problem. Int Wound J 2017;14:546–54.

[72] Ma Z, Li Z, Shou K, Jian C, Li P, Niu Y, Qi B, Yu A. Negative pressure wound therapy: regulating blood flow perfusion and microvessel maturation through microvascular pericytes. Int J Mol Med September 13, 2017. https://doi.org/10.3892/ijmm.2017.3131.

[73] Hage J, Kanhai CJ, Oen AL, et al. The devastating outcome of massive subcutaneous injection of highly viscous fluids in male-to-female transsexuals. Plast Reconstr Surg 2001;107:734–41.

[74] Behar T, Anderson EE, Barwick WJ. Sclerosing lipogranulomatosis: a case report of scrotal injection of automobile transmission fluid and literature review of subcutaneous injection of oils. Plast Reconstr Surg 1993;91:352–61.

Chapter 52

Reproductive Failure

Caterina De Carolis, Paola Triggianese, Roberto Perricone

Rheumatology, Allergy and Clinical Immunology – University of Rome "Tor Vergata", Rome, Italy

Reproduction is crucial for evolution of species, and implantation represents an event depending on several steps. The immunology of pregnancy is not only an intriguing phenomenon but also an interesting model for transplantation. The survival of the allogeneic concepts has long been an "immunological paradox," and definition of pregnancy as a semiallograft is the most basic building stone in discussing autoimmunity and reproduction [1]. Evidence supports the idea that the fetal–maternal immune interaction is more complex than a transplant allograft [2]. An uncomplicated acceptance by the mother of the immunological foreign semiallogenic fetus is one of the enigmas of human reproduction [3]. Normal pregnancy consists of special hormonal changes and immunologic challenges [4]. Therefore, it seems plausible to suggest that these changes might contribute to the development of autoimmune diseases in healthy women. The basic features of the fetal–maternal communication system comprise two arms: placental and paracrine. The placental arm consists of the extravillous trophoblast (EVT), the fetal tissue of the anatomic interface, whereas the fetal membranes are the tissues of the paracrine arm of this system [5]. A communication link is established by way of the placental arm; the placenta connects the fetus to the uterine wall and establishes a vascular connection between mother and child. Decidua is a newly formed tissue on the maternal side of human placenta and is characterized by active angiogenesis and structural modifications of the spiral arteries in the early phase of pregnancy. These changes are essential to create vessels of low resistance unresponsive to vasoconstrictive agents, allowing continuous blood flow in the intervillous space. The site where the placenta comes in direct contact with the maternal decidua is called the fetal–maternal interface [6]. During pregnancy, there is a bidirectional flow of fetal and maternal cells; in the mother immunological and neuroendocrine dysfunctions and remodulation of the composition and function of the immunocompetent cells protect the fetus against maternal attacks and the fetus promote tolerance against paternal antigens throughout the migration of the fetal cells in the maternal blood. This phenomenon creates a state of "maternal" microchimerism. In 1992, Starzl et al. discovered that long-term cell chimerism in donor organs and recipients is essential for graft success as well as the integration of maternal cells with the fetal immune and organ systems [7]. The "fetal" microchimerism is acquired by the mother during pregnancy where immunocompetent fetal cells cross the placental barrier; it is known as the persistence of immunocompetent fetal cells in the mother's circulation after pregnancy. These fetal cells increase in frequency in the maternal body with increasing gestational age and have been identified in maternal tissues for decades following birth [8]. Similarly, maternal microchimerism is acquired by an infant during the pregnancy [9]. Cellular fetal microchimerism has been hypothesized to play a role in the female predominance of certain autoimmune diseases [10,11], as well as with pregnancy complications [12], whereas the persistence of fetal cells has been associated with paradoxical effects, both positive and negative, on maternal health [13]. The cooperation and conflict theory can elucidate the paradoxical role that fetal cell microchimerism plays in maternal health. Tissues involved in resource allocation, such as brain, thyroid, and breast, would likely be reservoirs for fetal cells [14]. Additionally, the maternal immune system is likely to play an active role in fetal–maternal interactions. Within these tissues, the outcomes of these fetal–maternal negotiations (mother–offspring "tug–of–war") are important in maternal health and well-being [14]. At every step, there is a continuous embryo–uterus interaction against the fetus, and rejection is avoided due to the presence of the trophoblast. Trophoblast does not represent a wall that "protects" the fetus as an immune-favored site, but it is an immune-regulation site of active tolerance. The integration and the balance of immune factors lead to an environment that enables the fetus to escape rejection by the maternal immune system [15]. Innate immune responses against microorganisms at the maternal–fetal interface may have a significant impact on the success of pregnancy, as intrauterine infections have been shown to be strongly associated with certain complications of pregnancy [16]. Among several possible protective mechanisms that may be involved, the extraordinary human leukocyte antigen (HLA) class I expression on trophoblast seems to be relevant to explain why pregnancy should not be considered an "immunologic paradox." Human trophoblast cells express an unusual HLA repertoire of molecules as identified by Ellis et al. [17]. Only EVT expresses selective HLA class I molecules, whereas other trophoblast cells do not express HLA. EVT expresses maternal and paternal HLA-C allotypes [18], HLA-E, HLA-G, and

Mosaic of Autoimmunity. https://doi.org/10.1016/B978-0-12-814307-0.00052-9

possibly HLA-F [19–21]. In particular, the EVT does not express polymorphic HLA-A and HLA-B, but only the highly polymorphic HLA-C. The interaction at maternal–fetal interface between HLA molecules and natural killer (NK) cells is the checkpoint of the local immune regulation. Both maternal and fetal HLA may influence pregnancy outcome; because of the variability of HLA genes, every pregnancy will have a unique interaction between HLA-C and killer-cell immunoglobulin-like receptors (KIRs) on NK cells [22]. Differences in cell expression, binding strength, and signaling functions of individual KIR alleles as well as functional differences among HLA-C alleles confer the variability of challenges and the outcome of pregnancy [23]. Three different immunologic phases can be characterized during reproduction: a proinflammatory environment during embryo implantation, placentation and early stage of pregnancy; an antiinflammatory milieu during midpregnancy; and a proinflammatory environment at third trimester and at the end of pregnancy [16]. The discovery of the implantation window and the emergence of the concept of uterine receptivity led to the intriguing idea that many immunological factors could be central to a such process [15]. Reproduction has been associated with placental expression of immunologic and inflammatory factors such as toll-like receptors (TLRs), placental inflammatory cytokines, heat-shock proteins (Hsps), complement system (CS), reactive oxygen species (ROS), anti-angiogenic soluble vascular endothelial growth factor receptor-1 (sFlt-1), NK cells, monocytes, and proinflammatory cytokines producing macrophages (M1-like MQs) [24–27]. Moreover, also the amniotic sac, composed of a tight junction-interconnected epithelial layer secreting the amniotic fluid, is equipped with hormones with immune-regulatory capacities (human chorionic gonadotropin, α-fetoprotein, and others) and several immunologic and inflammatory factors (KIRs, complement regulatory proteins, NK cells, and others) [28]. Placenta serves as an active barrier between the embryo and the surrounding environment, and different pattern recognition receptors are involved in this interaction including the TLRs and nod-like receptors [29,30]. Placental expression of TLRs seems to be regulated in both temporal and spatial manner being for the TLR4 expression higher at term compared with the first-trimester placenta [31,32]. Hsp such as Hsp60, Hsp70, Hs90, and others have been reported to act on TLRs [33,34]. Evidence reports that placental Hsps expression represents a part of the physiological pregnancy process and circulating Hsps show positive correlation with gestational age and inverse correlation with maternal age [35,36]. Moreover, extracellular Hsp70 can stimulate proinflammatory cytokine production by antigen-presenting cells and can also activate the classical pathway of CS [37]. During normal pregnancy, the CS is activated at the maternal–fetal interface through the relative hypoxia as well as the presence of externalized phosphatidylserine on the outer leaflets of trophoblast. Complement dysregulation has an essential and causative role in damage to the fetal–placental unit [38]. It has been documented that MQs mediate the anti-angiogenic activity of CS including the upregulation of the secretion of the anti-angiogenic sFlt-1 [39]. The interrelationship of complement activation fragments Bb, C3a, and sC5b-9, and placental growth factor (PlGF), sFlt-1, and soluble endoglin, in early pregnancy and their association with pregnancy syndromes, have been described [40,41] (Fig. 52.1). Defective receptivity, implantation, and/or decidualization can lead to infertility (Fig. 52.2). Deferred implantation past the window of receptivity can lead to misguided embryo placement and implantation, resulting in placenta *previa*, ectopic placentation (placenta *accreta*), or placental insufficiency resulting in intrauterine growth restriction and/or preeclampsia (PE) [42]. Implantation beyond the normal window can also give rise to recurrent spontaneous abortion (RSA) and miscarriage, leading to infertility [43,44]. Premature decidual senescence can lead to preterm birth and intrauterine fetal death, whereas shallow trophoblast invasion into maternal decidua and/or blood vessels can lead to HELLP syndrome or PE [45,46] (Fig. 52.2). During pregnancy hormonal changes that play a critical role in determining the effector T cell cytokine profile at feto–maternal interface could explain why in some conditions pregnant women are more prone to develop T helper (h)2 type autoimmune diseases, whereas in other cases the Th1 and Th17 type autoimmune and inflammatory diseases are improved [47]. Successful pregnancy is characterized by a Th17/Th1–Th17/Th2 and T regulatory cells cooperation phenomenon, with a predominantly Th2 type immune response. Mechanisms of RSA and other obstetrical syndromes involve immune-mediated pathways including the presence of a predominant Th1 type immunity during

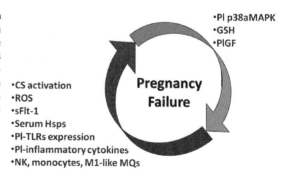

FIGURE 52.1 The imbalance of inflammation and innate immune system in pregnancy failure. Pregnancy failure has been associated with an increase of activation of complement system (CS), reactive oxygen species (ROS), anti-angiogenic soluble vascular endothelial growth factor receptor-1 (sFlt-1), serum heat-shock proteins (Hsp), placental (PL) expression of toll-like receptors (TLRs), placental (PL) inflammatory cytokines, natural killer (NK) cells, monocytes, and proinflammatory cytokines producing macrophages (M1-like MQs). On the other hand, pregnancy failure has been associated with a decrease of placental p38MAPK, glutathione (GSH), and pro-angiogenic placental growth factor (PlGF).

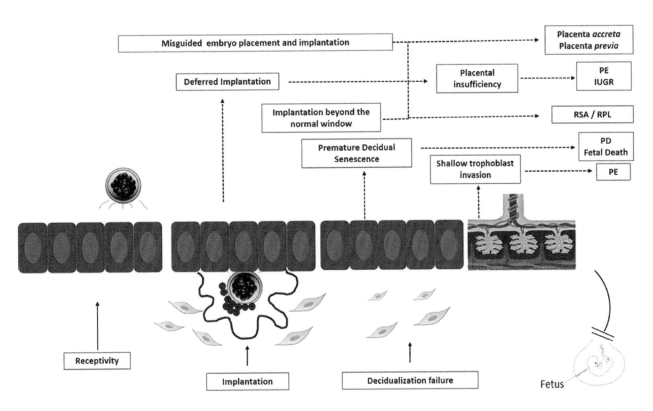

FIGURE 52.2 **Mechanisms of implantation.** Defective receptivity, implantation, and/or decidualization can lead to infertility and pregnancy syndromes. *IUGR*, intrauterine growth restriction; *PD*, preterm birth; *PE*, preeclampsia; *RPL*, recurrent pregnancy loss; *RSA*, recurrent spontaneous abortion.

pregnancy, a decrease in Foxp3+ regulatory T cells and an increase in NK cells [48–50]. These phenomena can occur at the site of implant, and they are often reflected in the peripheral blood. NK cells are the predominant leukocyte population in the endometrium at the time of implantation and in early pregnancy [51,52]. The role of NK cells has been reported to be immune-surveillance; these cells may also mediate the angiogenesis processes occurring in pregnancy and in the remodeling of the spiral arteries to uteroplacental arteries [53]. In normal pregnancy, the major role of NK cells is to provide benefit by secreting a number of cytokines/chemokines and angiogenic factors rather than to exert a cytotoxic activity [54]. However, the origin of decidual NK cells is still debated remaining unclear whether they can derive from peripheral blood NK cell populations or from self-renewal of NK cell progenitors [54]. Evidence suggests that peripheral blood NK recruitment to the uterus contributes to the accumulation of NK cells during early pregnancy, and progesterone seems to play a crucial role in this event [55]. Evolution of NK cells adjusting to an appropriate status is essential to protect pregnant women from any complication [56,57]. Because peripheral NK cells downregulate decidual NK under the influence of estrogen and progesterone levels, both the hormonal status and the NK cytokines contribute to the shift toward a Th2 response that characterizes normal pregnancy. Interactions between immune system (NK cells in particular) and hormonal factors (thyroid function and prolactin—PRL) are well established. Both thyroid autoimmunity and hypothyroidism have been associated with infertility and miscarriages [58–61]. Moreover, elevated peripheral NK cell have been reported in association with thyroid autoimmunity in women with reproductive failures [56,62]. The thyroid-stimulating hormone (TSH) may act as direct stimulator of the immune system due to the TSH receptors localization and to the ability owned by bone marrow hematopoietic cells, splenic dendritic cells, T and B cells to produce TSH. Evidence suggests that thyroid hormones act on migration and proliferation of dendritic cells, NK cells, and T cells [63–66]. PRL, a peptide hormone mainly secreted from the anterior pituitary gland and regulated by tonic inhibition of the hypothalamus via dopamine, has been primarily identified as a major stimulating factor for lactation in the postpartum period [67]. The extrapituitary synthesis includes deciduas and cells of immune system and PRL-receptors (PRL-Rs) are distributed throughout monocytes, macrophages, T and mainly B cells, NK cells, granulocytes, and thymus epithelial cells [68–70]. An association between serum PRL and peripheral blood NK cells has been described in both healthy and infertile women [71]. Data from the literature may suggest that hyperprolactinemia in women with reproductive failure could represent an epiphenomenon of preexisting immune disorder and/or a direct stimulator on the immune cells resulting in modifications of NK cells [71]. Concerning the hormonal factors interacting with the immune system, also vitamin D exhibits a plethora of regulatory effects on immune cells in addition to its actions on calcium and bone metabolism [72]. It is well reported that vitamin D can modulate the innate and adaptive immune responses by acting in an autocrine manner in a local immunologic milieu: vitamin D receptor is expressed on immune cells (B cells, T cells, and antigen-presenting cells) and these immunologic cells are all capable of synthesizing the active vitamin D metabolite [73]. Immunoregulatory effects of vitamin D have been reported not only on T cells but also on innate immune cells [74,75]. In addition, vitamin D receptors are expressed on the reproductive system including ovary, uterus, and placenta [76]. Low levels of vitamin D have been reported extensively to be associated with autoimmune diseases as well as with increased risk of pregnancy complications such as gestational diabetes and fetus growth abnormality [77–81].

Reproductive failure recognizes a common link with autoimmunity. In this context, an important role is represented by NK cell abnormalities that may characterize women with both primary infertility and RSA according to "alloimmune" mechanisms of the pregnancy failure [56,82–84]. Also women with early-onset severe PE show an increased NK cell function related to cytokine production, cytotoxicity, and expression of lectin-like receptors such as NKG2 [85]. CS dysregulation occurs in particular in the early severe forms of PE [40,86]. Accumulation of "waste products" in the placenta related to an abnormal CS activity together with insufficient repair functions could be related to the pathophysiology of PE [87]. The cross talk between CS receptors and the B-cell receptor strongly influences humoral immunity and thus autoimmune mechanisms [88]. In this view, elevated serum levels of IgG and reduced complement components can be considered as markers of enhanced autoimmune reactivity in women with reproductive failure [89].

Taken together all these considerations, we can assume that female reproduction, first of all the pregnancy, induces a selective state of immune tolerance but may stimulate several autoimmune pathogenic mechanisms. How these pathways may impact on reproductive failure as well as on specific pregnancy syndromes is well documented and is still under investigations. The knowledge of the underlying mechanisms of the reproduction in the context of the "mosaic of autoimmunity" remains a crucial tool for a deep and correct management of pregnancy syndromes and for the development of effective and targeted therapies.

REFERENCES

[1] Moffett A, Loke YW. The immunological paradox of pregnancy: a reappraisal. Placenta 2004;25:1–8.

[2] Mor G, Cardenas I, Abrahams V, Guller S. Inflammation and pregnancy: the role of the immune system at the implantation site. Ann N Y Acad Sci 2011;1221:80–7.

[3] Scherjon S, Lashley L, van der Hoorn ML, Claas F. Fetus specific T cell modulation during fertilization, implantation and pregnancy. Placenta 2011;32:S291–7.

[4] Wegmann TG, Lin H, Guilbert L, Mosmann TR. Bidirectional cytokine interactions in the maternal-fetal relationship: is successful pregnancy a TH2 phenomenon? Immunol Today 1993;14:353–6.

[5] De Carolis C, Perricone C, Perricone R. War and peace at the feto-placental front line: recurrent spontaneous abortion. Isr Med Assoc J 2014;16:667–8.

[6] Vazquez J, Chavarria M, Li Y, Lopez GE, Stanic AK. Computational flow cytometry analysis reveals a unique immune signature of the human maternal-fetal interface. Am J Reprod Immunol 2018;79(1).

[7] Starzl TE, Demetris AJ, Murase N, Ildstad S, Ricordi C, Trucco M. Cell migration, chimerism, and graft acceptance. Lancet 1992;339:1579–82.

[8] Adams Waldorf KM, Gammill HS, Lucas J, Aydelotte TM, Leisenring WM, Lambert NC, Nelson JL. Dynamic changes in fetal microchimerism in maternal peripheral blood mononuclear cells, CD4+ and CD8+ cells in normal pregnancy. Placenta 2010;31:589–94.

[9] Østensen M, Villiger PM, Förger F. Interaction of pregnancy and autoimmune rheumatic disease. Autoimmun Rev 2012;11:A437–46.

[10] Fugazzola I, Cirello V, Beck-Peccoz P. Fetal microchimerism as an explanation of disease. Nat Rev Endocrinol 2011;7:89–97.

[11] Østensen M, Andreoli L, Brucato A, Cetin I, Chambers C, Clowse ME, Costedoat-Chalumeau N, Cutolo M, Dolhain R, Fenstad MH, Förger F, Wahren-Herlenius M, Ruiz-Irastorza G, Koksvik H, Nelson-Piercy C, Shoenfeld Y, Tincani A, Villiger PM, Wallenius M, von Wolff M. State of the art: reproduction and pregnancy in rheumatic diseases. Autoimmun Rev 2015;14:376–86.

[12] Gammill HS, Stephenson MD, Aydelotte TM, Nelson JL. Microchimerism in women with recurrent miscarriage. Chimerism 2014;5:103–5.

[13] Stevens AM. Maternal microchimerism in health and disease. Best Pract Res Clin Obstet Gynaecol 2016;31:121–30.

[14] Boddy AM, Fortunato A, Wilson Sayres M, Aktipis A. Fetal microchimerism and maternal health: a review and evolutionary analysis of cooperation and conflict beyond the womb. Bioessays 2015;37:1106–18.

[15] Triggianese P, Perricone C, Chimenti MS, De Carolis C, Perricone R. Innate immune system at the maternal-fetal interface: mechanisms of disease and targets of therapy in pregnancy syndromes. Am J Reprod Immunol 2016;76:245–57.

[16] Mor G. Inflammation and pregnancy: the role of toll-like receptors in trophoblast-immune interaction. Ann N Y Acad Sci 2008;1127:121–8.

[17] Ellis SA, Sargent IL, Redman WC, McMichael AJ. Evidence for a novel HLA antigen found on human extravillous trophoblast and a choriocarcinoma cell line. Immunology 1986;59:595–601.

[18] King A, King A, Burrows TD, Hiby SE, Bowen JM, Joseph S, Verma S, Lim PB, Gardner L, Le Bouteiller P, Ziegler A, Uchanska-Ziegler B, Loke YW. Surface expression of HLA-C antigen by human extravillous trophoblast. Placenta 2000;21:376–87.

[19] Apps R, Murphy SP, Fernando R, Gardner L, Ahad T, Moffett A. Human leucocyte antigen (HLA) expression of primary trophoblast cells and placental cell lines, determined using single antigen beads to characterize allotype specificities of anti-HLA antibodies. Immunology 2009;127:26–39.

[20] Apps R, Gardner L, Traherne J, Male V, Moffett A. Natural-killer cell ligands at the maternal-fetal interface: UL-16 binding proteins, MHC class-I chain related molecules, HLA-F and CD48. Hum Reprod 2008;23:2535–48.

[21] Hackmon R, Pinnaduwage L, Zhang J, Lye SJ, Geraghty DE, Dunk CE. Definitive class I human leukocyte antigen expression in gestational placentation: HLA-F, HLA-E, HLA-C, and HLA-G in extravillous trophoblast invasion on placentation, pregnancy, and parturition. Am J Reprod Immunol 2017;77(6).

[22] Colucci F. The role of KIR and HLA interactions in pregnancy complications. Immunogenetics 2017;69:557–65.

[23] Chazara O, Xiong S, Moffett A. Maternal KIR and fetal HLA-C: a fine balance. J Leukoc Biol 2011;90:703–16.

[24] Saito S, Nakashima A, Shima T, Ito M. Th1/Th2/Th17 and regulatory T-cell paradigm in pregnancy. Am J Reprod Immunol 2010;63:601–10.

[25] Ito M, Nakashima A, Hidaka T, Okabe M, Bac ND, Ina S, Yoneda S, Shiozaki A, Sumi S, Tsuneyama K, Nikaido T, Saito S. A role for IL-17 in induction of an inflammation at the fetomaternal interface in preterm labour. J Reprod Immunol 2010;84:75–85.

[26] Colucci F, Boulenouar S, Kieckbusch J, Moffett A. How does variability of immune system genes affect placentation? Placenta 2011;32:539–45.

[27] Weghofer A, Himaya E, Kushnir VA, Barad DH, Lazzaroni-Tealdi E, Yu Y, et al. Some aspects of interactivity between endocrine and immune systems required for successful reproduction. Reprod Biol Endocrinol 2015;11:13–29.

[28] Velicky P, Knöfler M, Pollheimer J. Function and control of human invasive trophoblast subtypes: intrinsic vs. maternal control. Cell Adhes Migr 2016;10:154–62.

[29] Lavieri R, Piccioli P, Carta S, Delfino L, Castellani P, Rubartelli A. TLR costimulation causes oxidative stress with unbalance of proinflammatory and anti-inflammatory cytokine production. J Immunol 2014;192:5373–81.

[30] Abrahams VM. The role of the Nod-like receptor family in trophoblast innate immune responses. J Reprod Immunol 2011;88:112–7.

[31] Beijar EC, Mallard C, Powell TL. Expression and subcellular localization of TLR-4 in term and first trimester human placenta. Placenta 2006;27:322–6.

[32] Koga K, Cardenas I, Aldo P, Abrahams VM, Peng B, Fill S, Romero R, Mor G. Activation of TLR3 in the trophoblast is associated with preterm delivery. Am J Reprod Immunol 2009;61:196–212.

[33] Asea A, Rehli M, Kabingu E, Boch JA, Bare O, Auron PE, Stevenson MA, Calderwood SK. Novel signal transduction pathway utilized by extracellular HSP70: role of toll-like receptor (TLR) 2 and TLR4. J Biol Chem 2002;277:15028–34.

[34] Zeytun A, Chaudhary A, Pardington P, Cary R, Gupta G. Induction of cytokines and chemokines by Toll-like receptor signaling: strategies for control of inflammation. Crit Rev Immunol 2010;30:53–67.

[35] Molvarec A, Tamási L, Losonczy G, Madách K, Prohászka Z, Rigó Jr J. Circulating heat shock protein 70 (HSPA1A) in normal and pathological pregnancies. Cell Stress Chaperones 2010;15:237–47.

[36] Pockley AG, Shepherd J, Corton JM. Detection of heat shock protein 70 (Hsp70) and anti-Hsp70 antibodies in the serum of normal individuals. Immunol Invest 1998;27:367–77.

[37] Prohászka Z, Singh M, Nagy K, Kiss E, Lakos G, Duba J, Füst G. Heat shock protein 70 is a potent activator of the human complement system. Cell Stress Chaperones 2002;7:17–22.

[38] Perricone C, De Carolis C, Giacomelli R, Greco E, Cipriani P, Ballanti E, Novelli L, Perricone R. Inhibition of the complement system by glutathione: molecular mechanisms and potential therapeutic implications. Int J Immunopathol Pharmacol 2011;24:63–8.

[39] Langer HF, Chung KJ, Orlova VV, Choi EY, Kaul S, Kruhlak MJ, Alatsatianos M, DeAngelis RA, Roche PA, Magotti P, Li X, Economopoulou M, Rafail S, Lambris JD, Chavakis T. Complement-mediated inhibition of neovascularization reveals a point of convergence between innate immunity and angiogenesis. Blood 2010;116:4395–403.

[40] Lynch AM, Murphy JR, Gibbs RS, Levine RJ, Giclas PC, Salmon JE, Holers VM. The interrelationship of complement-activation fragments and angiogenesis-related factors in early pregnancy and their association with pre-eclampsia. BJOG 2010;117:456–62.

[41] Zeisler H, Llurba E, Chantraine F, Vatish M, Staff AC, Sennström M, Olovsson M, Brennecke SP, Stepan H, Allegranza D, Dilba P, Schoedl M, Hund M, Verlohren S. Predictive value of the sFlt-1:PlGF ratio in women with suspected preeclampsia. N Engl J Med 2016;374:13–22.

[42] Leeman L, Dresang LT, Fontaine P. Hypertensive disorders of pregnancy. Am Fam Physician 2016;93:121–7.

[43] Practice Committee of the American Society for Reproductive Medicine. Evaluation and treatment of recurrent pregnancy loss: a committee opinion. Fertil Steril 2012;98:1103–11.

[44] Rai R, Regan L. Recurrent miscarriage. Lancet 2006;368:601–11.

[45] Audibert F, Friedman SA, Frangieh AY, Sibai BM. Clinical utility of strict diagnostic criteria for the HELLP (hemolysis, elevated liver enzymes, and low platelets) syndrome. Am J Obstet Gynecol 1996;175:460–4.

[46] Triggianese P, Perricone C, Perricone R, De Carolis C. HELLP syndrome: a complication or a new autoimmune syndrome? Reumatologia 2014;52:377–83.

[47] Piccinni MP, Lombardelli L, Logiodice F, Kullolli O, Parronchi P, Romagnani S. How pregnancy can affect autoimmune diseases progression? Clin Mol Allergy 2016;14:11.

[48] Saito S, Nakashima A, Myojo-Higuma S, Shiozaki A. The balance between cytotoxic NK cells and regulatory NK cells in human pregnancy. J Reprod Immunol 2008;77:14–22.

[49] Bansal AS. Joining the immunological dots in recurrent miscarriage. Am J Reprod Immunol 2010;64:307–15.

[50] Liu S, Diao L, Huang C, Li Y, Zeng Y, Kwak-Kim JYH. The role of decidual immune cells on human pregnancy. J Reprod Immunol 2017;124:44–53.

[51] Perricone R, De Carolis C, Perricone C, Shoenfeld Y. NK cells in autoimmunity: a two-edg'd weapon of the immune system. Autoimmun Rev 2008;7:384–90.

[52] Konova E. The role of NK cells in the autoimmune thyroid disease-associated pregnancy loss. Clin Rev Allergy Immunol 2010;39:176–84.

[53] Perricone C, De Carolis C, Perricone R. Pregnancy and autoimmunity: a common problem. Best Pract Res Clin Rheumatol 2012;26:47–60.

[54] Santoni A, Carlino C, Stabile H, Gismondi A. Mechanisms underlying recruitment and accumulation of decidual NK cells in uterus during pregnancy. Am J Reprod Immunol 2008;59:417–24.

[55] Carlino C, Stabile H, Morrone S, Bulla R, Soriani A, Agostinis C, et al. Recruitment of circulating NK cells through decidual tissues: a possible mechanism controlling NK cell accumulation in the uterus during early pregnancy. Blood 2008;111:3108–15.

[56] Triggianese P, Perricone C, Conigliaro P, Chimenti MS, Perricone R, De Carolis C. Peripheral blood Natural Killer cells and mild thyroid abnormalities in women with reproductive failure. Int J Immunopathol Pharmacol 2016;29:65–75.

[57] Loewendorf AI, Nguyen TA, Yesayan MN, Kahn DA. Preeclampsia is characterized by fetal NK cell activation and a reduction in regulatory T cells. Am J Reprod Immunol 2015;74:258–67.

[58] De Carolis C, Greco E, Guarino MD, Perricone C, Dal Lago A, Giacomelli R, Fontana L, Perricone R. Anti-thyroid antibodies and antiphospholipid syndrome: evidence of reduced fecundity and poor pregnancy outcome in recurrent spontaneous aborters. Am J Reprod Immunol 2004;52:263–6.

[59] Negro R, Schwartz A, Gismondi R, Tinelli A, Mangieri T, Stagnaro-Green A. Thyroid antibody positivity in the first trimester of pregnancy is associated with negative pregnancy outcomes. J Clin Endocrinol Metab 2011;96:920–4.

[60] Thangaratinam S, Tan A, Knox E, Kilby MD, Franklyn J, Coomarasamy A. Association between thyroid autoantibodies and miscarriage and preterm birth: meta-analysis of evidence. BMJ 2011;342:d2616.

[61] Dal Lago A, Vaquero E, Pasqualetti P, Lazzarin N, De Carolis C, Perricone R, Moretti C. Prediction of early pregnancy maternal thyroid impairment in women affected with unexplained recurrent miscarriage. Hum Reprod 2011;26:1324–30.

[62] Kim NY, Cho HJ, Kim HY, Yang KM, Ahn HK, Thornton S, Park JC, Beaman K, Gilman-Sachs A, Kwak-Kim J. Thyroid autoimmunity and its association with cellular and humoral immunity in women with reproductive failures. Am J Reprod Immunol 2011;65:78–87.

[63] Fabris N, Mocchegiani E, Provinciali M. Pituitary-thyroid axis and immune system: a reciprocal neuroendocrine-immune interaction. Horm Res 1995;43:29–38.

[64] Klecha AJ, Genaro AM, Gorelik J, Barreiro Arcos ML, Silberman DM, Schuman M, Garcia SI, Pirola C, Cremaschi GA. Integrative study of hypothalamus-pituitary-thyroid-immune system interaction: thyroid hormone-mediated modulation of lymphocyte activity through the protein kinase C signaling pathway. J Endocrinol 2006;189:45–55.

[65] De Vito P, Balducci V, Leone S, Percario Z, Mangino G, Davis PJ, Nongenomic effects of Montesinos, Mdel M, Alamino VA, Mascanfroni ID, Susperreguy S, Gigena N, Masini-Repiso AM, Rabinovich GA, Pellizas CG, et al. Dexamethasone counteracts the immunostimulatory effects of triiodothyronine (T3) on dendritic cells. Steroids 2012;77:67–76.

[66] Mascanfroni I, Montesinos Mdel M, Susperreguy S, Ilarrequi JM, Ramseyer VD, Masini-Repiso AM, Targovnik HM, Rabinovich GA, Pellizas CG. Control of dendritic cell maturation and function by triiodothyronine. FASEB J 2008;22:1032–42.

[67] Freeman ME, Kanyicska B, Lenart A, Nagy G. Prolactin: structure, function and regulation of secretion. Physiol Rev 2000;80:1523–631.

[68] Yang L, Hu Y, Li X, Zhao J, Hou Y. Prolactin modulates the functions of murine spleen CD11c-positive dendritic cells. Int Immunopharmacol 2006;6:1478–86.

[69] Tomio A, Schust DJ, Kawana K, Yasugi T, Kawana Y, Mahalingaiah S, Fujii T, Taketani Y. Prolactin can modulate CD4+ T-cell response through receptor-mediated alterations in expression of T-bet. Immunol Cell Biol 2008;86:616–21.

[70] Xu D, Lin L, Lin X, Huang Z, Lei Z. Immunoregulation of autocrine prolactin: suppressing the expression of costimulatory molecules and cytokines in T lymphocytes by prolactin receptor knockdown. Cell Immunol 2010;263:71–8.

[71] Triggianese P, Perricone C, Perricone R, De Carolis C. Prolactin and natural killer cells: evaluating the neuroendocrine-immune axis in women with primary infertility and recurrent spontaneous abortion. Am J Reprod Immunol 2015;73:56–65.

[72] Orbach H, Zandman-Goddard G, Amital H, Barak V, Szekanecz Z, Szucs G, Danko K, Nagy E, Csepany T, Carvalho JF, Doria A, Shoenfeld Y. Novel biomarkers in autoimmune diseases: prolactin, ferritin, vitamin D, andTPA levels in autoimmune diseases. Ann N Y Acad Sci 2007;1109:385–400.

[73] Aranow C. Vitamin D and the immune system. J Investig Med 2011;59:881–6.

[74] Evans KN, Nguyen L, Chan J, Innes BA, Bulmer JN, Kilby MD, Hewison M. Effects of 25-hydroxyvitamin D3 and 1,25-dihydroxyvitamin D3 on cytokine production by human decidual cells. Biol Reprod 2006;75:816–22.

[75] Hornsby E, Pfeffer PE, Laranjo N, Cruikshank W, Tuzova M, Litonjua AA, Weiss ST, Carey VJ, O'Connor G, Hawrylowicz C. Vitamin D supplementation during pregnancy: effect on the neonatal immune system in a randomized controlled trial. J Allergy Clin Immunol 2018;141:269–78.

[76] Lerchbaum E, Obermayer-Pietsch B. Vitamin D and fertility: a systematic review. Eur J Endocrinol 2012;166:765–78.

[77] Orbach H, Shoenfeld Y. Hyperprolactinemia and autoimmune diseases. Autoimmun Rev 2007;6:537–42.

[78] Perricone C, Shoenfeld N, Agmon-Levin N, de Carolis C, Perricone R, Shoenfeld Y. Smell and autoimmunity: a comprehensive review. Clin Rev Allergy Immunol 2013;45:87–96.

[79] Pludowski P, Holick MF, Pilz S, Wagner CL, Hollis BW, Grant WB, Shoenfeld Y, Lerchbaum E, Llewellyn DJ, Kienreich K, Soni M. Vitamin D effects on musculoskeletal health, immunity, autoimmunity, cardiovascular disease, cancer, fertility, pregnancy, dementia and mortality-a review of recent evidence. Autoimmun Rev 2013;12:976–89.

[80] Anagnostis P, Karras S, Goulis DG. Vitamin D in human reproduction: a narrative review. Int J Clin Pract 2013;67:225–35.

[81] Triggianese P, Watad A, Cedola F, Perricone C, Amital H, Giambini I, Perricone R, Shoenfeld Y, De Carolis C. Vitamin D deficiency in an Italian cohort of infertile women. Am J Reprod Immunol 2017;78(4).

[82] Aoki K, Kajiura S, Matsumoto Y, Ogasawara M, Okada S, Yagami Y, Gleicher N. Pre-conceptional natural-killer-cell activity as a predictor of miscarriage. Lancet 1995;345:1340–2.

[83] Perricone R, Di Muzio G, Perricone C, Giacomelli R, De Nardo D, Fontana L, De Carolis C. High levels of peripheral blood NK cells in women suffering from recurrent spontaneous abortion are reverted from high-dose intravenous immunoglobulins. Am J Reprod Immunol 2006;55:232–9.

[84] Perricone C, De Carolis C, Giacomelli R, Zaccari G, Cipriani P, Bizzi E, Perricone R. High levels of NK cells in the peripheral blood of patients affected with anti-phospholipid syndrome and recurrent spontaneous abortion: a potential new hypothesis. Rheumatology 2007;46:1574–8.

[85] Bueno-Sánchez JC, Agudelo-Jaramillo B, Escobar-Aguilerae LF, Lopera A, Cadavid-Jaramillo AP, Chaouat G, Maldonado-Estrada JG. Cytokine production by non-stimulated peripheral blood NK cells and lymphocytes in early-onset severe pre-eclampsia without HELLP. J Reprod Immunol 2013;97:223–31.

[86] Hoffman MC, Rumer KK, Kramer A, Lynch AM, Winn VD. Maternal and fetal alternative complement pathway activation in early severe pre-eclampsia. Am J Reprod Immunol 2014;71:55–60.

[87] Lokki AI, Heikkinen-Eloranta J, Jarva H, Saisto T, Lokki ML, Laivuori H, Meri S. Complement activation and regulation in preeclamptic placenta. Front Immunol 2014;5:312.

[88] Del Nagro CJ, Kolla RV, Rickert RC. A critical role for complement C3d and the B cell coreceptor (CD19/CD21) complex in the initiation of inflammatory arthritis. J Immunol 2005;175:5379.

[89] Carvalheiras G, Faria R, Braga J, Vasconcelos C. Fetal outcome in autoimmune diseases. Autoimmun Rev 2012;11:A520–30.

Chapter 53

Atherosclerosis in Systemic Autoimmune Rheumatic Diseases

Katarzyna Fischer[1], Iwona Brzosko[1], Marek Brzosko[2]

[1]*Independent Laboratory for Rheumatologic Diagnostics, Pomeranian Medical University in Szczecin, Szczecin, Poland;* [2]*Department of Rheumatology, Internal Medicine and Geriatrics, Pomeranian Medical University in Szczecin, Szczecin, Poland*

BACKGROUND

Atherosclerosis (ATS) is a multifactorial disease which may be considered an immune/inflammatory response of intima to tissue damage. Indeed, an involvement of both innate and adaptive immunity as well as a low-grade inflammatory component in ATS pathogenesis is well documented. The presence of monocytes/macrophages transformed into lipid-loaded foam cells, natural killer cells, dendritic cells, mast cells, activated lymphocytes, and immunoglobulins within the plaque has been documented.

Systemic autoimmune rheumatic diseases (SARDs) are a heterogeneous group of disorders characterized by an immune response against self-antigens based on the interaction between genetic predisposition, dysregulation of the immune system, and environmental factors. Various SARDs, including rheumatoid arthritis (RA), systemic lupus erythematosus (SLE), and spondyloarthritis, are associated with accelerated and often premature ATS. Traditional risk factors alone fail to fully account for this phenomenon, thus it has been attributed to complex interactions between traditional risk factors and factors associated with the disease process and its treatment. Accelerated atherosclerotic vessel wall damage has been regarded as the main pathogenetic mechanism leading to the enhanced cardiovascular risk in SARDs patients. As cardiovascular disease (CVD) still remains the leading cause of morbidity and mortality in SARDs, there is an immense need for an improved CVD prevention in this patients group. Noninvasive imaging assessment of vascular pathophysiology as well as selected biomarkers can help to improve risk assessment.

BIOMARKERS OF ACCELERATED ATHEROSCLEROSIS IN SYSTEMIC AUTOIMMUNE RHEUMATIC DISEASES

Inflammatory Biomarkers

Chronic inflammation is considered a major contributor to early stages of ATS damage. Endothelial activation and dysfunction constitute the earliest stage in the development of atherosclerotic lesions. Proinflammatory cytokines such as tumor necrosis factor alpha (TNFα) and interleukin (IL)-6 play a crucial role in this process. Particularly, TNFα shows a wide-ranging effect through dyslipidemia and insulin resistance increase, prothrombotic state induction, upregulation of other proinflammatory mediators, and endothelial activation markers such as IL-1, IL-6, IL-8, matrix metalloproteinases (MMPs), prostaglandins, and adhesion molecules.

The next stages of atherosclerotic plaque formation and progression also are controlled by inflammatory factors. Adhesion molecules such as E-selectin, vascular cell adhesion molecule 1, and intercellular adhesion molecule 1 are crucial in monocytes/macrophages and T-cells recruitment to the endothelial surface. Their levels are increased in SARDs and associated with both subclinical ATS and CVD in particular in RA, SLE and vasculitis. Cells migration into the intima, the next step in plaque development, is influenced by several inflammatory markers including monocyte chemotactic protein 1 and its elevated levels correlate with CVD even in the general population.

Moreover, CD40–CD40 ligand interaction is implicated in ATS and plaque rupture in RA and SLE. Similarly, complement activation might contribute to endothelial damage, plaque formation, and a condition favoring its instability and rupture.

Endothelial activation facilitates low-density lipoprotein (LDL) accumulation and their subsequent oxidation in the sub-endothelial space. Oxidized LDL (ox-LDL) is phagocyted by monocytes/macrophages which results in foam cell formation, main component of atherosclerotic plaque's lipid core. Chronic inflammatory process increases oxidative stress and highly immunogenic ox-LDL production. In SLE and RA patients with CVD, elevated concentrations of circulating ox-LDL were confirmed. Especially, in SLE ox-LDL tends to form complexes with beta-2 glycoprotein I (β2GPI) that increase arterial thrombosis and foam cell formation. Inflammation also promotes dysfunctional high-density lipoprotein (HDL) increase. This form of HDL is unable to prevent LDL oxidation, and significantly higher concentrations of proinflammatory HDL were found in SARDs patients, especially in SLE and RA with the frequency of 45% and 20%, respectively. Additionally, dysfunctional HDL might play a role in subclinical ATS development as association with carotid intima-media thickness (cIMT) and plaque formation in SLE patients was demonstrated.

Furthermore, proteolytic enzymes such as MMPs also are involved in ATS development and plaque stability reduction.

The adipose tissue releases proteins termed adipokines that also play a role in atherogenesis. Resistin is considered a biomarker of insulin resistance, ATS, and CVD. Leptin stimulates T-cell activation, selected cytokines production, and endothelial dysfunction. Chemerin, a novel chemoattractant adipokine, was shown in arthritides to regulate both inflammation and cardiometabolic comorbidities.

Finally, classical acute phase reactants have been implicated in accelerated ATS in SARDs with a potential of both systemic and local effects in this process.

Selected Autoimmune Biomarkers

An involvement of both innate and adaptive immunity in ATS pathogenesis is well documented, and the data clearly characterize ATS as an inflammatory and autoimmune disease which is of great importance in SARDs such as SLE. There are findings that mechanisms involved in antibody formation may play a role in early ATS damage, and the main target for antibodies could be endothelial cells.

Circulating anti-ox-LDL and anti-ox-LDL/β2GPI complexes have been found in SLE, vasculitis, and RA; but their role in ATS might be dual. On the one hand, they may downregulate atherosclerotic process. On the other hand, they may be associated with ATS perpetuation. Some studies in RA patients have confirmed their correlation with unstable angina and plaque destabilization. In addition, the cross-reactivity between anti-ox-LDL and antiphospholipid antibodies (aPLs) was suggested to be involved in atherothrombotic events development in SLE and antiphospholipid syndrome (APS). Moreover, aPLs have been demonstrated to be an independent predictor of the first cardiovascular event in SLE and involved in subclinical development of ATS in RA patients.

Anti-citrullinated protein antibodies (ACPAs) are the main pathogenic, diagnostic, and prognostic markers in RA. They reveal proinflammatory and proatherogenic properties and might be detected in atherosclerotic plaque. ACPAs seropositive patients are at increased risk of cardiovascular mortality. Furthermore, periodontitis and *Porphyromonas gingivalis* infections are involved in both RA and ATS pathogenesis. It was shown that ACPAs produced against *P. gingivalis* α-enolase protein might be a link between these two disease states.

Antinuclear antibodies (ANAs) have been shown to predict cardiovascular events and mortality in patients with and without rheumatic diseases. The study in young women without clinically evident SLE and ATS documented that ANAs have been also associated with impaired carotid elasticity.

All these observations suggest that autoantibodies might be directly involved in structural changes of the arterial wall and ATS development in SARDs patients, but their exact role is still a matter of debate.

Imaging Biomarkers

Various noninvasive imaging techniques might be used for detection of atherosclerotic changes at different stages of their development, from endothelial dysfunction and reduced vascular elasticity, through morphological changes in the arterial wall, to advanced plaque formation.

The earliest stage of ATS presented as endothelial dysfunction is commonly detected by brachial artery flow-mediated vasodilation (FMD) determined using B-mode ultrasound. Impaired FMD was confirmed even in young patients with RA and SLE. Additionally, in SARDs patients, the presence of subclinical coronary artery disease (CAD) was shown by coronary flow velocity reserve reduction.

Measurement of pulse wave velocity (PWV) is used to assess arterial stiffness caused by structural and functional arterial alterations. Significantly increased PWV values are often found in SARDs patients and correlate with endothelial dysfunction and carotid ATS.

cIMT and plaque detection with B-mode ultrasound is a well-established marker of generalized ATS and is widely recommended for cardiovascular risk assessment. Increased cIMT values are commonly detected in SARDs patients and reflect subclinical ATS even in those with negative history for vascular disease.

Ankle–brachial index (ABI) measurement is a simple and useful method for lower extremities arteries assessment. Emphasis is put on a significant correlation between ABI and CVD in SARDs patients. In addition, high resistance index measurements might be helpful in subclinical vascular lesions in SLE patients detection, especially those with APS coexistence.

EPIDEMIOLOGY AND SPECTRUM OF CARDIOVASCULAR DISEASE IN SYSTEMIC AUTOIMMUNE RHEUMATIC DISEASES

CVD is considered a major mortality cause in SARDs. The data in RA report a broad spectrum of cardiovascular manifestations including stroke, hypertension, ischemic heart disease (IHD), cIMT, CAD, myocardial infarction (MI), peripheral vascular disease (PVD), thrombosis, and left ventricular diastolic dysfunction (LVDD), and their frequency ranges from 30% to 50% of RA patients.

Similarly, in SLE cardiovascular involvement is frequent, and CVD is at least doubled among SLE patients compared with other populations, and the mortality rate is significantly increased. The risk of IHD is more than 6 times higher in this patient group and even 50 times higher in women aged from 35 to 44 years than in the controls. Of note, while clinical symptoms of CAD occur in 6%–10% of SLE patients, subclinical ATS can be documented in 21% of patients under age 35 and in up to 100% of those over 65.

The prevalence of CVD in APS patients ranges from 1.7% to 14%. It was shown in Euro-Phospholipid cohort that MI affects 2.8% of patients and it appeared during the evolution of the disease in 5.5% of the cohort. Cardiac manifestations are described in up to 40% with the significant morbidity in 4%–6% of patients. Most of these manifestations (either coronary or on the valves) are related to thrombotic lesions.

Cardiovascular events in Sjögren's syndrome are reported in 5%–7.7% of patients. CVD burden includes stroke, MI, cerebrovascular accidents, deep vein thrombosis, arrhythmias, valvular involvement, pulmonary hypertension, and increased left ventricular mass.

Mortality in systemic sclerosis caused by CVD is between 20% and 30% and occurs about 10 years earlier compared to the general population. Cardiovascular manifestations are found in 10% of patients. On the other hand, asymptomatic coronary artery calcification ranges from 33% to 40% of patients with diffuse and limited form of the disease, respectively, and carotid stenosis might affect up to 64% of systemic sclerosis patients. Moreover, arrhythmias, coronary spasm, cerebrovascular accidents, PVD, CAD, MI, LVDD, and myocardial fibrosis are reported in this patient group.

PREVENTION AND THERAPY

The ATS etiopathology in SARDs is multifactorial; thus, the prophylactic approach should be comprehensive. The medical and family history, social situation, lifestyle, and laboratory/imaging results need to be taken into account. Of note, the traditional risk factors must be fully identified and treated aggressively. Cardiovascular risk scoring calculators such as Framingham score or Systemic Coronary Risk Evaluation (SCORE) based on selected traditional risk factors are incorporated into CVD risk management in rheumatologic patients.

It is generally desirable to include healthy diet, proper physical activity, smoking cessation, regular control of blood sugar and blood pressure, optimal treatment of dyslipidemia, depression, hyperuricemia, hypothyroidism, sleep apnea and vitamin supplementation (especially vitamin D and folate), dental hygiene, pneumococcus, and influenza vaccination, as well as minimizing the use of drugs that might increase cardiovascular risk.

Indeed, a number of medications used in SARDs may play a role in risk profile. Corticosteroids and nonsteroidal antiinflammatory drugs (NSAIDS) promote hypertension development. Moreover, corticosteroids can cause weight gain, insulin resistance, and dyslipidemia. Use of steroid monotherapy has been linked to a 50% increased risk of cardiovascular event. On the other hand, use of methotrexate and other disease-modifying drugs have been associated with decreased cardiovascular risk in RA patients. Similarly, hydroxychloroquine in SLE patients is associated with improved survival and vascular events reduction. There is also a growing bulk of evidence on the beneficial effect of anti-TNFα therapy use. In fact, these agents are related to the decrease in systemic inflammation, and thus they can inhibit the formation and destabilization of atherosclerotic lesions; however, their exact role in cardiovascular risk still remains unclear.

The use of statins therapy is associated with lipid-lowering effects and inflammatory process inhibition. Statins have positive effects on endothelial progenitor cells and prevent endothelial dysfunction. Indeed, their beneficial effects were

TABLE 53.1 The European League Against Rheumatism Recommendations for CVD Risk Management in RA and Other Forms of Inflammatory Joint Disorders

1. Disease activity should be controlled optimally in order to lower CVD risk.
2. CVD risk assessment is recommended at least once every 5 years and should be reconsidered following major changes in antirheumatic therapy.
3. CVD risk estimation should be performed according to national guidelines and the SCORE CVD risk prediction model should be used if no national guideline is available.
4. Total cholesterol and HDL cholesterol should be used in CVD risk assessment, and lipids should be measured when disease activity is stable or in remission. Nonfasting lipids measurements are also acceptable.
5. CVD risk models should be adapted for patients with RA by a 1.5 multiplication factor.
6. Screening for asymptomatic atherosclerotic plaques by use of carotid ultrasound may be considered as part of the CVD risk evaluation in RA patients.
7. Lifestyle recommendations should emphasize the benefits of a healthy diet, regular exercise, and smoking cessation.
8. CVD risk management should be carried out according to national guidelines, antihypertensive and statins may be used as in the general population.
9. Prescription of NSAIDs in RA and PsA should be with caution, especially for patients with documented CVD or in the presence of CVD risk factors.
10. Corticosteroids: for prolonged treatment, the glucocorticoid dosage should be kept to a minimum and a glucocorticoid taper should be attempted in case of remission or low disease activity; the reason to continue glucocorticoid therapy should be regularly checked.

CVD, cardiovascular disease; *HDL*, high-density lipoprotein; *NSAIDs*, nonsteroid anti-inflammatory drugs; *PsA*, psoriatic arthritis; *RA*, rheumatoid arthritis; *SCORE*, Systemic Coronary Risk Evaluation.
Adapted from Agca R, Heslinga SC, Rollefstad S, et al. EULAR recommendations for cardiovascular disease risk management in patients with rheumatoid arthritis and other forms of inflammatory joint disorders: 2015/2016 update. Ann Rheum Dis 2017;76:17–28.

documented in SARDs. Trial on atorvastatin in RA study showed that after 6 months therapy the disease activity score improved significantly in the atorvastatin-treated group versus the placebo group. There was also the decrease in inflammatory markers levels.

The updated European League Against Rheumatism (EULAR) recommendations for CVD risk management in RA, ankylosing spondylitis, and psoriatic arthritis patients are summarized in Table 53.1.

FURTHER READING

[1] Bartoloni E, Shoenfeld Y, Gerli R. Inflammatory and autoimmune mechanisms in the induction of atheroscleritc damage in systemic rheumatic diseases: two faces of the same coin. Arthritis Care Res 2011;63(2):178–83.
[2] Ronda N, Meroni PL. Accelerated atherosclerosis in autoimmune diseases. In: Shoenfeld Y, Cervera R, Gershwin ME, editors. Diagnostic criteria in autoimmune diseases. Totowa, NJ: Humana Press; 2008. p. 383–7.
[3] Szekanecz Z, Kerekes G, Vegh E, et al. Autoimmune atherosclerosis in 3D: how it develops, how to diagnose and what to do. Autoimmun Rev 2016;15:756–69.
[4] Fischer K, Brzosko M. Diagnosis of early atherosclerotic lesions, and selected atherosclerotic risk factors, in patients with systemic lupus erythematosus. Pol Arch Med Wewn 2009;119(11):736–41.
[5] Hollan I, Meroni PL, Ahearn JM, et al. Cardiovascular disease in autoimmune rheumatic diseases. Autoimmun Rev 2013;12:1004–15.
[6] Mankad R. Atherosclerotic vascular disease in the autoimmune rheumatologic patients. Curr Atheroscler Rep 2015;17:21.
[7] Amaya-Amaya J, Montoya-Sanchez L, Rojas-Villarraga A. Cardiovascular involvement in autoimmune diseases. BioMed Res Int 2014:31 pages. ID 367359.
[8] Agca R, Heslinga SC, Rollefstad S, et al. EULAR recommendations for cardiovascular disease risk management in patients with rheumatoid arthritis and other forms of inflammatory joint disorders: 2015/2016 update. Ann Rheum Dis 2017;76:17–28.

Chapter 54

A to Z of Some New Autoimmune Diseases: From Alzheimer's to Zinc Deficiency

Zoltán Szekanecz

Division of Rheumatology, Institute of Internal Medicine, Faculty of Medicine, University of Debrecen, Debrecen, Hungary

This chapter may be rather controversial. Here we include a real "mosaic" of different diseases. Some of them may be autoimmune, others may not. However, each of them carry some characteristics of autoimmunity.

ALZHEIMER'S DISEASE

Alzheimer's disease (AD) has been associated with aging; however, autoimmunity, inflammation, and the disruption of blood–brain barrier have emerged as potential mechanisms. Amyloid β protein (Aβ) plaques induce brain inflammation, whereas oligomeric Aβ exerts synaptotoxicity. T cells, complement and various cytokines have been implicated in AD. Microglial activation is a major feature of AD contributing to neuroinflammation. Autoimmunity in AD is a double-edged sword; it is a defensive mechanism but also a harmful process. On one hand, the presence of natural autoantibodies and the apparently good outcome after immunotherapy as seen in animal model and in a few patients. On the other hand, antibodies to Aβ isolated from AD patients actually stimulated Aβ production. Natural Aβ antibodies present in the serum from healthy humans can decrease the levels of Aβ in cerebrospinal fluid. With respect to therapy, while active immunization caused serious side effects such as sterile encephalitis and mobilization of neurotoxic soluble Aβ oligomers, passive immunization seems to be a useful therapeutic goal. Furthermore, enhancing the clearance of Aβ has been tried using various strategies such as peripheral sequestration or targeting the toxic domain of Aβ. Yet, trials using solanezumab used to induce Aβ clearance failed [1–5].

ATHEROSCLEROSIS

Numerous autoimmune-inflammatory mechanisms have been implicated in the pathogenesis of atherosclerosis, primarily accelerated (autoimmune) atherosclerosis associated with autoimmune diseases. In addition to immune cells, cytokines, chemokines, adhesion molecules, and other factors, some autoantibodies may also play a role. Endothelial cells may be the main target for these antibodies. Rheumatoid factor levels were associated with endothelial dysfunction and carotid atherosclerosis in rheumatoid arthritis (RA). Citrullination of some proteins, primarily fibrinogen, has been detected in atherosclerotic plaques and anti-citrullinated peptide/protein antibodies, which are crucial markers of RA, have been associated with increased cardiovascular risk. In addition, numerous other antibodies, such as anti-oxLDL, anti-β2GPI, anti-oxLDL/β2GPI complex, anti-cardiolipin, and others may play a role in autoimmune atherosclerosis [6–13].

AUTOIMMUNE HEMATOLOGICAL DISEASES

In thrombotic thrombocytopenic purpura, anti-ADAMTS13 autoantibodies inhibit the metalloproteinase function of ADAMTS13. This enzyme is unable to cleave von Willebrand factor (vWF) leading to the persistence of ultra-large vWF multimers, increased platelet aggregation, and vascular occlusion. Inhibitory antibodies bind to the domain of ADAMTS13 that interacts with vWF. Anti-ADAMTS13 antibodies are detected in >95% of patients with severely low (<10% of normal) ADAMTS13 levels. The autoimmune mechanism is supported by the successful use of plasmapheresis to remove inhibitors and replace functional ADAMTS13. Currently, plasmapheresis is standard first-line therapy and B-cell depletion is recommended in patients refractory to corticosteroids and plasmapheresis [14–18].

Mosaic of Autoimmunity. https://doi.org/10.1016/B978-0-12-814307-0.00054-2

Immune thrombocytopenic purpura (ITP) results from autoantibodies against multiple platelet surface antigens, including glycoproteins gpIb/IX and gpIIb/IIIa, leading to platelet destruction. These antibodies bind complement and inhibit megakaryocytopoiesis. These autoantibodies are pathogenic as plasma transfer from ITP patients induced thrombocytopenia in human recipients. Rituximab exerts high efficacy in ITP [19–21].

In autoimmune hemolytic anemia (AIHA), the binding of autoantibodies to different erythrocyte antigens leads to red blood cell agglutination and lysis. Antibodies in warm AIHA are predominantly IgG, act at body temperature, and lead to both complement-mediated and Fc-dependent erythrocyte destruction. In contrast, cold agglutinin disease (CAD) involves mainly IgM antibodies that bind at low temperature and result in complement-mediated hemolysis. These antibodies are highly sensitive and pathogenic. In CAD, plasma exchange is a reasonable second-line option in cases of severe hemolysis. B-cell depletion by rituximab may also be a promising approach [22–25].

AUTOIMMUNE ENCEPHALITIS AND EPILEPSY

In the last 10–15 years, new forms of encephalitis associated with antibodies to cell surface or synaptic proteins have been discovered and characterized. Anti-NMDAR (N-methyl-D-aspartate receptor) encephalitis is the most common type of autoimmune encephalitis. In addition, several subtypes of limbic encephalitis have been associated with various antibodies, primarily anti-AMPAR (α-amino-3-hydroxy-5-methyl-4-isoxazol-propionic acid receptor), anti-GABAbR (γ-aminobutyric acid B-receptor), anti-LGI1 (leucine-rich, glioma-inactivated 1), anti-Caspr2 (contactin-associated protein-like 2), and others. The clinical picture is characterized by seizures, amnesia, movement disorders, catatonia, and psychiatric symptoms. Sometimes autoimmune encephalitis may overlap with other neuroimmunologic disorders, such as neuromyelitis optica (NMO) (see later). Treatment is difficult; IVIg is less effective than in myasthenia gravis [26–29].

BULLOUS SKIN DISEASES

Pemphigus has been associated with autoantibodies to desmoglein (Dsg) dermal cell adhesion molecules. These autoantibodies cause epithelial blistering, which may lead to potentially severe malnutrition, dehydration, and infection. There are two major subtypes of pemphigus: pemphigus vulgaris and foliaceus characterized by autoantibodies to Dsg3 and Dsg1, respectively. Anti-Dsg antibodies are pathogenic. Pemphigus does not occur in the absence of these antibodies, and disease activity correlates with serum autoantibody levels. Autoimmunity against other antigens in pemphigus has also been described. Autoantibody-producing B cells play a major role in the development of pemphigus. B-cell targeting by rituximab is highly effective in this disease [18,30,31].

Epidermolysis bullosa acquisita (EBA) and bullous pemphigoid (BP) are subepithelial blistering diseases caused by autoantibodies against different epithelial basement membrane antigens. EBA and BP have been associated with pathogenic antibodies against type VII collagen (COL7) and against BP antigens (BP180 or BP230), respectively. Autoantibody levels correlate with disease activity in both diseases. The pathogenicity of these antibodies is supported by the efficacy of immunoadsorption or rituximab in these diseases [32–36].

NEUROMYELITIS OPTICA DEVIC

NMO is characterized by inflammation, demyelination, and axonal injury of the spinal cord and optic nerve. NMO patients have antibodies against the astrocyte water channel aquaporin-4 (AQP4). Anti-AQP4, which is almost 100% specific for the disease, differentiates NMO and multiple sclerosis. Correlation between antibody levels and disease activity or relapse risk is rather controversial. On the other hand, anti-AQP4 antibodies may have prognostic value. Antibody levels have been correlated with the extent of transverse myelitis. Furthermore, increasing levels may predict relapse. The pathogenicity of this antibody was confirmed by passive transfer studies; however, antibodies themselves may not be sufficient to trigger the disease. Corticosteroids, plasma exchange, and rituximab may be effective [37–41].

OTOSCLEROSIS

Idiopathic sensorineural hearing disorders including otosclerosis have been associated with immune-inflammatory mechanisms. The cause of otosclerosis is unknown. Genetic, viral, hormonal factors, as well as autoimmunity have been implicated in the pathogenesis of the disease. Autoimmune reaction against the otic capsule has been suggested as a possible etiologic factor in otosclerosis; however, data are somewhat conflicting. Autoantibodies against type II and IX collagens have been detected in the sera of patients with otosclerosis. Collagen-specific autoimmune reaction induced in rats may cause lytic bone lesions in the otic capsule that highly resemble otosclerosis [42–47].

PARKINSON'S DISEASE

Parkinson's disease (PD) is also a multifactorial disease. Recently, autoimmune and inflammatory mechanisms have been implicated in the pathogenesis of the disease. Both innate and adaptive immune mechanisms may play a role in the development of PD. Several autoantibodies including those against melanin, α-synuclein, or GM1 ganglioside have been detected in PD patients. PD-associated antibodies have been found in the plasma and brain. One target of autoimmunity is the pigment neuromelanin (NM) found in dopaminergic neurons. NM may trigger dendritic cell maturation and activation. Activated DCs may migrate to the cervical lymph nodes and present potential autoantigens to T- and B cells. Anti-NM autoimmunity against NM-rich cells may lead to the death of dopaminergic cells. NM may also activate microglia leading to the amplification of autoimmunity against NM. Experimental studies suggest that transfer of antibodies isolated from PD patients to the substantia nigra of rats may induce the loss of dopaminergic neurons. Recent studies also suggest that immune activation in PD may be the cause of, rather than a response to, neuronal loss. Finally, gut microbiota have recently been implicated in PD, as well as other neurological diseases. Some immunosuppressive agents, such as minocycline, are investigated in clinical trials [48–50].

ZIKA

Zika virus (ZIKV), an arbovirus, is transmitted by the bite of female Aedes mosquitoes, sexual contact, and blood transfusions. For many years, human ZIKV infection was sporadic; however, major ZIKV outbreaks occurred in 2007 and 2013. ZIKV infection has been associated with the development of some autoimmune diseases, such as Guillain-Barré syndrome and ITP. Until now, more than 20 cases of ITP in patients with ZIKV disease have been published. Only a few fatal cases have been published. Most ZIKV-induced ITP patients responded well to immunomodulatory therapy. On the other hand, no rheumatic or thyroid autoimmunity could be observed in association with ZIKV infection. Molecular mimicry may be the most important mechanism by which *Flaviviruses*, such as ZIKV, may induce autoimmunity [51].

ZINC DEFICIENCY

Early studies in the 1980s suggested that zinc deprivation can retard the development of autoimmunity in young mice. Later studies found that zinc restriction does not improve autoimmunity in adult animals. Zinc deficiency may exert marked effects on most components of the immune system. Strong epidemiological data support that zinc deficiency is a major factor underlying immune dysfunction in some humans. Zinc is essential for proper immune function and zinc deficiency has been accompanied by allergies, autoimmunity, and an increased presence of transplant rejection. Zinc is able to induce regulatory T cells (Treg) and attenuate inflammatory responses. In the murine EAE model for multiple sclerosis, zinc administration diminished EAE scores, reduced Th17 and increased Treg cell numbers. Thus, zinc supplementation may be able to restore immune tolerance and may be a tool for treating autoimmune diseases [52–56].

REFERENCES

[1] Sardi F, Fassina L, Venturini L, Inguscio M, Guerriero F, Rolfo E, Ricevuti G. Alzheimer's disease, autoimmunity and inflammation. The good, the bad and the ugly. Autoimmun Rev 2011;11(2):149–53.

[2] Hawkes CA, McLaurin J. Immunotherapy as treatment for Alzheimer's disease. Expert Rev Neurother 2007;7(11):1535–48.

[3] Moir RD, Tseitlin KA, Soscia S, Hyman BT, Irizarry MC, Tanzi RE. Autoantibodies to redox-modified oligomeric Abeta are attenuated in the plasma of Alzheimer's disease patients. J Biol Chem 2005;280(17):17458–63.

[4] Monsonego A, Nemirovsky A, Harpaz I. CD4 T cells in immunity and immunotherapy of Alzheimer's disease. Immunology 2013;139(4):438–46.

[5] Liu YH, Giunta B, Zhou HD, Tan J, Wang YJ. Immunotherapy for Alzheimer disease: the challenge of adverse effects. Nat Rev Neurol 2012;8(8):465–9.

[6] Montecucco F, Mach F. Common inflammatory mediators orchestrate pathophysiological processes in rheumatoid arthritis and atherosclerosis. Rheumatol (Oxf) 2009;48(1):11–22.

[7] Shoenfeld Y, Gerli R, Doria A, Matsuura E, Cerinic MM, Ronda N, Jara LJ, Abu-Shakra M, Meroni PL, Sherer Y. Accelerated atherosclerosis in autoimmune rheumatic diseases. Circulation 2005;112(21):3337–47.

[8] Matsuura E, Kobayashi K, Kasahara J, Yasuda T, Makino H, Koike T, Shoenfeld Y. Anti-beta 2-glycoprotein I autoantibodies and atherosclerosis. Int Rev Immunol 2002;21(1):51–66.

[9] Matsuura E, Kobayashi K, Koike T, Shoenfeld Y. Autoantibody-mediated atherosclerosis. Autoimmun Rev 2002;1(6):348–53.

[10] Matsuura E, Kobayashi K, Inoue K, Lopez LR, Shoenfeld Y. Oxidized LDL/beta2-glycoprotein I complexes: new aspects in atherosclerosis. Lupus 2005;14(9):736–41.

[11] Kerekes G, Szekanecz Z, Der H, Sandor Z, Lakos G, Muszbek L, Csipo I, Sipka S, Seres I, Paragh G, et al. Endothelial dysfunction and atherosclerosis in rheumatoid arthritis: a multiparametric analysis using imaging techniques and laboratory markers of inflammation and autoimmunity. J Rheumatol 2008;35(3):398–406.

[12] Sokolove J, Brennan MJ, Sharpe O, Lahey LJ, Kao AH, Krishnan E, Edmundowicz D, Lepus CM, Wasko MC, Robinson WH. Brief report: citrullination within the atherosclerotic plaque: a potential target for the anti-citrullinated protein antibody response in rheumatoid arthritis. Arthritis Rheum 2013;65(7):1719–24.

[13] Soltesz P, Veres K, Laczik R, Der H, Csipo I, Timar O, Szomjak E, Szegedi G, Szodoray P. Evaluation of antibodies to oxidized low-density lipoprotein and assessment of C-reactive protein in acute coronary syndrome and stable coronary artery disease. Thromb Haemost 2007;98(2):413–9.

[14] Tsai HM, Lian EC. Antibodies to von Willebrand factor-cleaving protease in acute thrombotic thrombocytopenic purpura. N Engl J Med 1998;339(22):1585–94.

[15] Rieger M, Mannucci PM, Kremer Hovinga JA, Herzog A, Gerstenbauer G, Konetschny C, Zimmermann K, Scharrer I, Peyvandi F, Galbusera M, et al. ADAMTS13 autoantibodies in patients with thrombotic microangiopathies and other immunomediated diseases. Blood 2005;106(4):1262–7.

[16] Rock GA, Shumak KH, Buskard NA, Blanchette VS, Kelton JG, Nair RC, Spasoff RA. Comparison of plasma exchange with plasma infusion in the treatment of thrombotic thrombocytopenic purpura. Canadian Apheresis Study Group. N Engl J Med 1991;325(6):393–7.

[17] Lim W, Vesely SK, George JN. The role of rituximab in the management of patients with acquired thrombotic thrombocytopenic purpura. Blood 2015;125(10):1526–31.

[18] Ran NA, Payne AS. Rituximab therapy in pemphigus and other autoantibody-mediated diseases. F1000Res 2017;6:83.

[19] van Leeuwen EF, van der Ven JT, Engelfriet CP. Von dem Borne AE: specificity of autoantibodies in autoimmune thrombocytopenia. Blood 1982;59(1):23–6.

[20] Harrington WJ, Sprague CC, Minnich V, Moore CV, Aulvin RC, Dubach R. Immunologic mechanisms in idiopathic and neonatal thrombocytopenic purpura. Ann Intern Med 1953;38(3):433–69.

[21] Arnold DM, Dentali F, Crowther MA, Meyer RM, Cook RJ, Sigouin C, Fraser GA, Lim W, Kelton JG. Systematic review: efficacy and safety of rituximab for adults with idiopathic thrombocytopenic purpura. Ann Intern Med 2007;146(1):25–33.

[22] Jandl JH, Jones AR, Castle WB. The destruction of red cells by antibodies in man. I. Observations of the sequestration and lysis of red cells altered by immune mechanisms. J Clin Invest 1957;36(10):1428–59.

[23] Atkinson JP, Frank MM. Studies on the in vivo effects of antibody. Interaction of IgM antibody and complement in the immune clearance and destruction of erythrocytes in man. J Clin Invest 1974;54(2):339–48.

[24] Schwartz J, Padmanabhan A, Aqui N, Balogun RA, Connelly-Smith L, Delaney M, Dunbar NM, Witt V, Wu Y, Shaz BH. Guidelines on the use of therapeutic apheresis in clinical practice-evidence-based approach from the writing committee of the American Society for Apheresis: the Seventh special issue. J Clin Apher 2016;31(3):149–62.

[25] Birgens H, Frederiksen H, Hasselbalch HC, Rasmussen IH, Nielsen OJ, Kjeldsen L, Larsen H, Mourits-Andersen T, Plesner T, Ronnov-Jessen D, et al. A phase III randomized trial comparing glucocorticoid monotherapy versus glucocorticoid and rituximab in patients with autoimmune haemolytic anaemia. Br J Haematol 2013;163(3):393–9.

[26] Leypoldt F, Armangue T, Dalmau J. Autoimmune encephalopathies. Ann NY Acad Sci 2015;1338:94–114.

[27] Oldham M. Autoimmune encephalopathy for psychiatrists: when to suspect autoimmunity and what to do next. Psychosomatics 2017;58(3):228–44.

[28] Vincent A. Developments in autoimmune channelopathies. Autoimmun Rev 2013;12(6):678–81.

[29] Gaspard N. Autoimmune epilepsy. Continuum 2016;22(1 Epilepsy):227–45.

[30] Amagai M, Komai A, Hashimoto T, Shirakata Y, Hashimoto K, Yamada T, Kitajima Y, Ohya K, Iwanami H, Nishikawa T. Usefulness of enzyme-linked immunosorbent assay using recombinant desmogleins 1 and 3 for serodiagnosis of pemphigus. Br J Dermatol 1999;140(2):351–7.

[31] Schmidt E, Dahnrich C, Rosemann A, Probst C, Komorowski L, Saschenbrecker S, Schlumberger W, Stocker W, Hashimoto T, Brocker EB, et al. Novel ELISA systems for antibodies to desmoglein 1 and 3: correlation of disease activity with serum autoantibody levels in individual pemphigus patients. Exp Dermatol 2010;19(5):458–63.

[32] Woodley DT, Briggaman RA, O'Keefe EJ, Inman AO, Queen LL, Gammon WR. Identification of the skin basement-membrane autoantigen in epidermolysis bullosa acquisita. N Engl J Med 1984;310(16):1007–13.

[33] Schmidt E, Obe K, Brocker EB, Zillikens D. Serum levels of autoantibodies to BP180 correlate with disease activity in patients with bullous pemphigoid. Arch Dermatol 2000;136(2):174–8.

[34] Niedermeier A, Eming R, Pfutze M, Neumann CR, Happel C, Reich K, Hertl M. Clinical response of severe mechanobullous epidermolysis bullosa acquisita to combined treatment with immunoadsorption and rituximab (anti-CD20 monoclonal antibodies). Arch Dermatol 2007;143(2):192–8.

[35] Ahmed AR, Shetty S, Kaveri S, Spigelman ZS. Treatment of recalcitrant bullous pemphigoid (BP) with a novel protocol: a retrospective study with a 6-year follow-up. J Am Acad Dermatol 2016;74(4). 700–708 e703.

[36] Schmidt E, Benoit S, Brocker EB, Zillikens D, Goebeler M. Successful adjuvant treatment of recalcitrant epidermolysis bullosa acquisita with anti-CD20 antibody rituximab. Arch Dermatol 2006;142(2):147–50.

[37] Lennon VA, Wingerchuk DM, Kryzer TJ, Pittock SJ, Lucchinetti CF, Fujihara K, Nakashima I, Weinshenker BG. A serum autoantibody marker of neuromyelitis optica: distinction from multiple sclerosis. Lancet 2004;364(9451):2106–12.

[38] Weinshenker BG, Wingerchuk DM, Vukusic S, Linbo L, Pittock SJ, Lucchinetti CF, Lennon VA. Neuromyelitis optica IgG predicts relapse after longitudinally extensive transverse myelitis. Ann Neurol 2006;59(3):566–9.

[39] Takahashi T, Fujihara K, Nakashima I, Misu T, Miyazawa I, Nakamura M, Watanabe S, Shiga Y, Kanaoka C, Fujimori J, et al. Anti-aquaporin-4 antibody is involved in the pathogenesis of NMO: a study on antibody titre. Brain 2007;130(Pt 5):1235–43.

[40] Abboud H, Petrak A, Mealy M, Sasidharan S, Siddique L, Levy M. Treatment of acute relapses in neuromyelitis optica: steroids alone versus steroids plus plasma exchange. Mult Scler 2016;22(2):185–92.

[41] Zephir H, Bernard-Valnet R, Lebrun C, Outteryck O, Audoin B, Bourre B, Pittion S, Wiertlewski S, Ouallet JC, Neau JP, et al. Rituximab as first-line therapy in neuromyelitis optica: efficiency and tolerability. J Neurol 2015;262(10):2329–35.

[42] Karosi T, Szekanecz Z, Sziklai I. Otosclerosis: an autoimmune disease? Autoimmun Rev 2009;9(2):95–101.

[43] Liktor B, Szekanecz Z, Batta TJ, Sziklai I, Karosi T. Perspectives of pharmacological treatment in otosclerosis. Eur Arch Otol Rhinol Laryngol 2012;270(3):793–804.

[44] Szekanecz Z, Szekanecz E, Morvai K, Racz T, Szegedi G, Sziklai I. [Current aspects of the pathogenesis and clinical characteristics of otosclerosis: possibilities of drug therapy]. Orv Hetil 1999;140(44):2435–40.

[45] Yoo TJ. Etiopathogenesis of otosclerosis: a hypothesis. Ann Otol Rhinol Laryngol 1984;93(1 Pt 1):28–33.

[46] Joliat T, Seyer J, Bernstein J, Krug M, Ye XJ, Cho JS, Fujiyoshi T, Yoo TJ. Antibodies against a 30 kilodalton cochlear protein and type II and IX collagens in the serum of patients with inner ear diseases. Ann Otol Rhinol Laryngol 1992;101(12):1000–6.

[47] Van Wijk F, Staecker H, Keithley E, Lefebvre PP. Local perfusion of the tumor necrosis factor alpha blocker infliximab to the inner ear improves autoimmune neurosensory hearing loss. Audiol Neurotol 2006;11(6):357–65.

[48] De Virgilio A, Greco A, Fabbrini G, Inghilleri M, Rizzo MI, Gallo A, Conte M, Rosato C, Ciniglio Appiani M, de Vincentiis M. Parkinson's disease: autoimmunity and neuroinflammation. Autoimmun Rev 2016;15(10):1005–11.

[49] Benkler M, Agmon-Levin N, Shoenfeld Y. Parkinson's disease, autoimmunity, and olfaction. Int J Neurosci 2009;119(12):2133–43.

[50] Wekerle H. Brain autoimmunity and intestinal microbiota: 100 trillion game changers. Trends Immunol 2017;38(7):483–97.

[51] Monsalve DM, Pacheco Y, Acosta-Ampudia Y, Rodriguez Y, Ramirez-Santana C, Anaya JM. Zika virus and autoimmunity. One-step forward. Autoimmun Rev 2017;16(12):1237–45.

[52] Beach RS, Gershwin ME, Hurley LS. Nutritional factors and autoimmunity. III. Zinc deprivation versus restricted food intake in MRL/1 mice–the distinction between interacting dietary influences. J Immunol 1982;129(6):2686–92.

[53] Vruwink KG, Keen CL, Gershwin ME, Hurley LS. Studies of nutrition and autoimmunity. Failure of zinc deprivation to alter autoantibody production when initiated in disease-established mice. J Nutr 1987;117(1):177–82.

[54] Keen CL, Gershwin ME. Zinc deficiency and immune function. Annu Rev Nutr 1990;10:415–31.

[55] Rosenkranz E, Maywald M, Hilgers RD, Brieger A, Clarner T, Kipp M, Plumakers B, Meyer S, Schwerdtle T, Rink L. Induction of regulatory T cells in Th1-/Th17-driven experimental autoimmune encephalomyelitis by zinc administration. J Nutr Biochem 2016;29:116–23.

[56] Maywald M, Rink L. Zinc supplementation induces CD4(+)CD25(+)Foxp3(+) antigen-specific regulatory T cells and suppresses IFN-gamma production by upregulation of Foxp3 and KLF-10 and downregulation of IRF-1. Eur J Nutr 2017;56(5):1859–69.

Treatment of Autoimmune Diseases

Chapter 55

Neuroimmunology

Maurizio Cutolo, Amelia Chiara Trombetta
Research Laboratory and Academic Division of Clinical Rheumatology, Department of Internal Medicine, University of Genova, Polyclinic San Martino Hospital, Genoa, Italy

INTRODUCTION

Central (CNS) and peripheral nervous systems (PNS) integrate and coordinate the functions of all structures of the living organism and, among those, also of immune system and immune response [1,2].

Several evidences have shown from long time that, at the same time, immune system cells and products have an afferent arm through which they communicate to CNS, with effects on behavior, thermoregulation (microvascular system), and sleep [3].

In this chapter, the most relevant and recent acquisitions showing how CNS and PNS exercise a mutual influence with immune system in health and disease will be exposed.

CENTRAL NERVOUS SYSTEM

CNS control on immune system functions takes place through hormones and nerves fibers (Fig. 55.1). One of the most important effects of CNS is exercised though the modulation of hypothalamic–pituitary–adrenal (HPA) axis functions and especially through the regulation of production and release of steroidal hormones. HPA axis in fact comprise paraventricular nucleus of the hypothalamus, secreting corticotrophin-releasing hormone (CRH), anterior pituitary gland, secreting adrenocorticotropic hormone (ACTH), and adrenal glands, secreting steroidal hormones: cortisol and adrenal androgens like dehydroepiandrosterone, dehydroepiandrosterone sulfate, and androstenedione [4].

Neuroimmune connections were recognized soon after the discovery of steroidal hormones immune-suppressive functions, through the description of the role of HPA axis (Fig. 55.1) [5]. Subsequently, these acquisitions were confirmed in pathological conditions, on animal models, where alterations in the HPA axis function determined the development of inflammatory disorders [6].

Numerous cells belonging to innate or adaptive immune system such as neutrophils, macrophages, dendritic cells, innate lymphoid cells, and T cells and B cells express receptors for neurotransmitters, such as glutamate, dopamine, acetylcholine (ACh), and serotonin (5-HT) (Table 55.1) [7]. Receptors number and activity change with different states of activation of the cell. For instance, higher exposition of β-adrenergic receptors is observed on activated T lymphocytes compared with lymphocytes in resting state [8,9].

On the other hand, receptors for immune system products such as tumor necrosis factor (TNF)-α and interleukin (IL)-1, IL-2, IL-6 were demonstrated in healthy CNS tissues (Table 55.2) [10–14].

IL-1 receptors in the brain showed similar characteristics to IL-1 receptors in immune and endocrine tissues, providing support for a physiological role of cytokines in regulating CNS activity [15]. A study performed in healthy subjects showed that cytokines like IL-6, administered subcutaneously, determined a dose-dependent increase in the resting metabolic rate and stimulated HPA axis, with consequent higher cortisol or plasma ACTH secretion, suggesting that hypothalamic CRH may mediate these functions in humans [16].

In immune-mediated rheumatic diseases, the discovery of a reduced cortisol and adrenal androgen secretion, in comparison to the very high cytokine levels, leads to the hypothesis of a "relative adrenal insufficiency." In fact, during acute inflammation, a robust activation of HPA axis is observed, with consequent high circulating concentrations of ACTH and cortisol. With the time, cytokine high levels determine a reduced HPA axis hormones production [17].

Remarkably, HPA axis circulating hormones concentrations are lower than expected in autoimmune/inflammatory diseases not only for a cytokine-induced block of their production but also for an increased peripheral catabolism, in inflamed tissues [4,18]. From supplementary studies, corroborating the hypothesis that inflammatory cytokines alter

Mosaic of Autoimmunity. https://doi.org/10.1016/B978-0-12-814307-0.00055-4

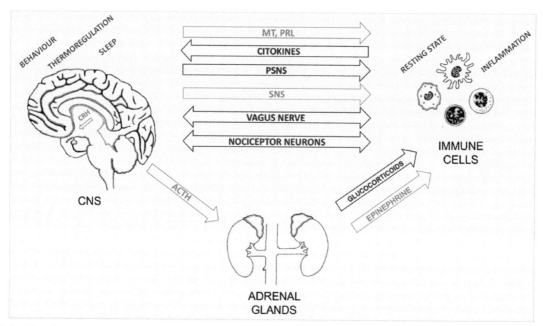

FIGURE 55.1 Neuroimmune interactions cited in the text are resumed. In green are indicated activation functions. In orange, substances or structures having both activation and inhibitory functions on target cells are shown. In red, substances or structures with inhibitory functions are shown. *ACTH*, adrenocorticotropic hormone; *CNS*, central nervous system; *CRH*, corticotrophin-releasing hormone; *MT*, melatonin; *PRL*, prolactin; *PSNS*, parasympathetic nervous system; *SNS*, sympathetic nervous system.

TABLE 55.1 Nervous System Cell Products Cited in the Text and Implicated in Neuroimmune Connections are Summarized, Together With Organs or Cells of Production

Nervous System Cell Products Implicated in Neuroimmune Connections	
Producing Cells	**Neurotransmitters or Hormones**
HPA axis	CRH—ACTH—Cortisol and adrenal androgens
Pineal gland	Melatonin
Pituitary gland	Prolactin
CNS neurons	Glutamate
CNS neurons	Dopamine
CNS neurons Autonomic nervous system cells Sympathetic nervous system cells Motor neurons	Acetylcholine
CNS neurons	Serotonin
Adrenal glands Sympathetic nervous system cells	Epinephrine
Sympathetic nervous system cells	Norepinephrine
Sensory neurons	SP
Sensory neurons	VIP
Sensory neurons	CGRP

ACTH, adrenocorticotropic hormone; *CGRP*, calcitonin gene-related peptide; *CNS*, central nervous system; *CRH*, corticotrophin-releasing hormone; *HPA*, hypothalamic–pituitary–adrenal; *SP*, substance P; *VIP*, vasoactive intestinal peptide.

TABLE 55.2 Immune System Cell Products Cited in the Text and Implicated in Neuroimmune Connections are Summarized, Together With Producing Cells

Immune System Cell Products Implicated in Neuroimmune Connections	
Producing Cells	**Products**
Macrophages, NK cells, neutrophils, mast cells, eosinophils, CD4+ T lymphocytes	TNF
Macrophages, monocytes, fibroblasts, dendritic cells, B lymphocytes, NK cells, microglia, epithelial cells	IL-1
CD4+ T-helper cells CD8+ T-helper cells	IL-2
T cells and macrophages	IL-6
T helper 17 cell	IL-17
Plasma cells	Ig
Macrophages, fibroblasts	Semaphorin
Macrophages, fibroblasts	Neuropilin

Ig, immunoglobulins; *IL*, interleukin; *NK*, natural killer cells; *TNF*, tumor necrosis factor.

antiinflammatory hormones secretion, it was possible to demonstrate that biologic drugs against TNF and IL-6 were able to restore HPA axis functions and adrenal hormones secretion [19,20].

Further supporting a possible direct effect of cytokines like TNF on CNS, studies on animal models of rheumatic diseases like experimental arthritis demonstrated that the anti-TNF agent etanercept, administered intrathecally, reduced peripheral inflammation and hyperalgesia [21].

In CNS, the suprachiasmatic nucleus of the ventral hypothalamus constitutes the pacemaker that determines the daily rhythmicity of pituitary, gonadal, adrenal hormones but also cytokines and growth factors secretion [22].

In fact, light impulse gets to SCN through the retinohypothalamic nerve, subsequently determining humoral and neuronal communications to other peripheral quasiautonomous pacemakers, located within organs, tissues, and cells [23]. The coordination of central and peripheral pacemakers is determinant for all organism functions, from sleep/wake cycle to mechanisms of inflammation [24].

As a matter of fact, bidirectional interactions occur between immune system and the circadian clock, being an inflammatory reaction able to directly alter cellular expression of clock genes [25].

In animals, inflammatory stimuli or experimental administration of lipopolysaccharide (LPS) or TNFα was demonstrated to induce or suppress particular clock genes [26,27].

Furthermore, effects on SCN of proinflammatory factors seem to be age-dependent and are thought to mediate the age changes in circadian timekeeping [28].

Night hormones are known to be predominantly proinflammatory. Melatonin and prolactin have a 24-h daily cycle and are able to determine an increased release of cytokines from immune cells, whereas cortisol exerts its antiinflammatory function from the early hours of the day [29].

It was shown that cytokines such as TNF-α or IL-6 reach higher concentrations at late night and on the contrary their levels are very low after 12 a.m. [30].

It appears that, in pathological conditions, IL-6 can reach serum levels 10 times higher than the normal and loose its regular secretion rhythmicity, whereas the circadian rhythm of serum cortisol has a similar amplitude and period in healthy controls and RA patients [31]. As a consequence, during rheumatologic diseases as rheumatoid arthritis or polymyalgia rheumatica, the reactivation of inflammatory symptoms, such as joint pain or stiffness, occurs mainly in the morning [32,33].

PERIPHERAL NERVOUS SYSTEM

Autonomous nervous system modulates immune/inflammatory phenomena through sympathetic branch, with mixed pro- and antiinflammatory functions, and parasympathetic branch, with mainly antiinflammatory activities (Table 55.1).

However, the function of the two branches adapts depending on different phases of resting state and inflammatory reactions and on different receptors for each neurotransmitter.

Moreover, at the local level, direct interactions are known to occur between nervous and immune systems cells, in healthy and diseased tissues [34,35].

THE PARASYMPATHETIC NERVOUS SYSTEM

The parasympathetic nervous system (PSNS) relation with immune system is less studied, compared to that of sympathetic branch. However, a relatively recent discovery showed that PSNS exerts its antiinflammatory and immunosuppressive function mainly through a nicotinic receptor characterized by α7 subunits [36].

The principal neurotransmitter is ACh. ACh binds to α7 nicotinic receptors on macrophages, activating the JAK2/STAT3 and suppressing of NF-kB nuclear translocation, reducing cytokine production and inflammasome activation [37–39].

VAGUS NERVE

Vagus nerve sensory fibers detect and transmit the information about peripheral immune responses to CNS. In fact, vagal stimulation was demonstrated to constitute the fundamental component of an afferent loop that activates HPA axis responses after systemic endotoxaemia and cytokinaemia [40,41].

It was demonstrated that electrical stimulation of the vagus nerve decreases TNF synthesis in the liver after LPS administration, whereas vagotomy is associated with higher TNF production. These data demonstrated the existence of an efferent vagus nerve signaling participating in the regulation of TNF production in vivo [42].

Efferent vagal signal arrives to celiac ganglia and activates the splenic nerve. Adrenergic splenic neurons secrete norepinephrine (NE) and determine the release of ACh by a group of T cells in the spleen [43].

Vagus nerve antiinflammatory function was demonstrated in disease models including arthritis, pancreatitis, inflammatory bowel disease, and autoimmune myocarditis [44–47].

Interestingly, studies on bioelectronic devices stimulation demonstrated efficacy of vagal inflammatory reflex activation in attenuating disease severity in inflammatory and autoimmune diseases such as rheumatoid arthritis and Crohn's disease [48].

THE SYMPATHETIC NERVOUS SYSTEM

The main neurotransmitters for sympathetic nervous system (SNS) are epinephrine, NE, adenosine triphosphate, neuropeptide Y, and endogenous opioids. Epinephrine is also secreted by adrenal medulla (Table 55.1).

In course of inflammations, a simultaneous activation of SNS and HPA axis, with maximal mediator secretion in the early morning, is observed [49]. SNS activity increases as a consequence of hypothalamic function alterations and of a shift from production of CRH to vasopressin [50].

The connexion between HPA axis and SNS seems to be important for several cooperative effects and for efficient regulation of the inflammatory processes [51].

The role of SNS in relation to immune reactions has been more extensively studied and schematized according to the different phases of the immune/inflammatory reaction: acute, intermediate, and chronic.

In the acute phase, a predominantly proinflammatory effect is exercised by SNS, through mobilization of leukocytes to inflammation sites, plasma extravasation, induction of matrix metalloproteinases, stimulation of nociceptors via α2-adrenergic and prostaglandin cross signaling, and supply of glucose and free fatty acids to the immune system [4]. Intermediate phase of inflammation is characterized by loss of SNS fibers in inflamed tissues. Interestingly, a higher nerve growth factor (NGF) serum concentration and autoantibodies against NGF were found in serum and synovial fluid in inflammatory conditions like spondyloarthropathy, RA, calcium pyrophosphate dihydrate crystal deposition disease, and osteoarthritis [52,53].

NGFs are nonspecific chemoattractants, but definite repellent factors such as semaphorins seem to determine the specific loss of sympathetic nerve fibers [54]. Nerve-repellent factors such as semaphorin and neuropilin seem to be produced by macrophages and fibroblasts in inflamed tissues (Table 55.2) [55]. The specific reduction of SNS fibers is complemented by sensory nerve fibers increase, a process-defined inflammation-induced sensory hyperinnervation [56].

In the chronic phase, SNS appears to exercise antiinflammatory functions. In fact, in animal studies on collagen-induced arthritis, late sympathectomy leads to increased levels of TNFα and interferon (IFN)γ [57].

Additionally, increased SNS activity is associated in rheumatic and autoimmune diseases to production of insufficient cortisol in relation to the inflammatory reaction, with the purpose of maintaining homeostatic status. This phenomenon was described in several rheumatic diseases and defined as HPA axis and SNS uncoupling [58].

It was demonstrated, in the treatment of asthma, that topical adrenergic agonists and corticosteroids have an additive effect if compared with each agent alone [59]. In fact, besides the direct broncho-dilation effect, an increase of receptors for glucocorticoids and of intracellular cAMP was demonstrated if both agents were administered together [60,61].

A similar antiinflammatory cooperative effect of cortisol and NE was demonstrated in vivo and in vitro in patients with RA. In fact, RA patients who undergo prednisolone treatment and present more synovial sympathetic innervation (SSI) show significantly lower inflammation compared with patients without prednisolone treatment, or with patients with prior prednisolone treatment but with less SSI [51].

The parallel raising and the cooperation of cortisol and NE at a molecular level causes stabilization of cyclic AMP (cAMP)/protein kinase A/cAMP responsive element-binding protein signaling pathway [62].

On the contrary, this effect is lost and cAMP concentration is reduced through catecholamine binding to $\alpha 2$ receptor. Similar function is that of adenosine, in fact if it binds to A2 receptor, it determines high cAMP levels, whereas low levels of cAMP result from binding with A1 receptor [63,64].

Furthermore, cortisol induces the production of synthesizing enzymes for NE and epinephrine from sympathetic nerve terminals and adrenal gland [65].

Higher cAMP concentrations were demonstrated to reduce the levels of several inflammation mediators: TNF, IL1, IL6, IL12, IL17, IFNγ, while increasing antiinflammatory factors like IL-10 and TGFβ [66–71].

$\beta 2$ adrenergic receptors were classically thought to exert an inhibitory action through induction of cAMP and protein kinase A. However, several studies testified that $\beta 2$ receptors, like other G protein-coupled receptors, have much more complex functions and can activate multiple signal transduction pathways to exert also enhancing effects on immune system. Alterations of β-adrenergic cross talk between SNS fibers and immune cells were reported in rheumatic diseases [72].

In patients with chronic rheumatic diseases, such as RA, a decreased density of $\beta 2$ receptors was observed on peripheral blood mononuclear cells, with a consequent impairment of cAMP regulation mechanism and dysfunction of G protein antiinflammatory signaling [73].

SENSORY NERVOUS SYSTEM

Nociceptor fibers have an essential function in modulation of immune system activity. In nociceptor nerve terminals, vesicles containing neuropeptides such as substance P (SP), vasoactive intestinal peptide, and calcitonin gene-related peptide are stored (Table 55.1 and Fig. 55.1).

Pain stimulus determines the release of neuropeptides that have a potent stimulating effect on vasculature and immune system, a process termed "neurogenic inflammation" [74].

Proinflammatory substance P positive (SP+) sensory nerve fibers are known to increase, whereas sympathetic nerve fibers density reduces in inflammatory conditions [75,76].

The terminal portion of nociceptive sensory neurons expresses receptors for TNFα, IL-1 β, IL-6, and IL-17 so that it is believable that these cytokines at least contribute to persistence of hyperalgesia in inflammatory articular diseases [77].

Moreover, immunoglobulins have Fc gamma receptors on nociceptive nerve fiber terminals (Table 55.2) [78].

The comprehension of mechanisms connecting nervous and immune systems favored the development of chronobiology and chronotherapy. Treatments synchronized with the endogenous rhythms of the disease were developed, such as low dose night-time steroidal therapy, with a release between 2 and 3 a.m., before the rise of cytokines concentrations and consequently of proinflammatory activity and during the increase of endogenous cortisol, accordingly to when they could best exert their effect. The long-term efficacy and safety of this treatment was proven not to alter HPA axis function, giving a new necessary treatment option to rheumatologic patients [79–81].

CONCLUSIONS

The extending knowledge on neuroimmune interactions could determine a better relation between therapeutic choices and understanding of individual patients' characteristics and disease stage classification. The consequent acquisitions could be used, for instance, to recognize which patients and at which disease phase could benefit more from a specific therapy and with a better risk/benefit profile. To this purpose, for instance, the study of a possible presence of adrenocortical insufficiency through baseline dynamic testing of adrenal function, adrenal glucocorticoids, and steroids evaluation could be performed, together with monitoring of inflammatory biomarkers [82–84].

Finally, new therapeutic strategies are now possible, following the discovery of neuroimmune connections and inflammatory reflexes, devices that regulate immune cell functions and cytokine production were successfully applied in rheumatic diseases like RA, targeting neural pathway, deriving the techniques acquired in the treatment of neurological diseases like epilepsy, and giving rise to the concept of "bioelectronic medicine" [48].

REFERENCES

[1] Masi A, Bijlsma J, Chikanza I, Pitzalis C, Cutolo M. Neuroendocrine, immunologic, and microvascular systems interactions in rheumatoid arthritis: physiopathogenetic and therapeutic perspectives. Semin Arthritis Rheum 1999;29(2):65–81.

[2] Cutolo M, Bijlsma JW, Lahita RG, Masi AT, Straub RH, Bradlow HL. Altered neuroendocrine immune (NEI) networks in rheumatology. Ann NY Acad Sci 2002;966:xiii–viii.

[3] Besedovsky H. Immune-neuro-endocrine interactions: facts and hypotheses. Endocr Rev 1996;17:64–102.

[4] Straub R, Bijlsma J, Masi A, Cutolo M. Role of neuroendocrine and neuroimmune mechanisms in chronic inflammatory rheumatic diseases—the 10-year update. Semin Arthritis Rheum 2013;43:392–404.

[5] Gisler R, Schenkel-Hulliger L. Hormonal regulation of the immune response. Cell Immunol 1971;2:646–65.

[6] Sternberg E, Hill J, Chrousos G, Kamilaris T, Listwak S, Gold P, et al. Inflammatory mediator-induced hypothalamic-pituitary-adrenal axis activation is defective in streptococcal cell wall arthritis-susceptible Lewis rats. Proc Natl Acad Sci USA 1989;86:2374–8.

[7] Chavan SS, Pavlov VA, Tracey KJ. Mechanisms and therapeutic relevance of neuro-immune communication. Immunity 2017;46:927–42.

[8] Helderman JH, Strom T. Specific insulin binding site on T and B lymphocytes as a marker of cell activation. Nature 1978;274:62–3.

[9] Dailey MO, Schreurs J, Schulman H. Hormone receptors on cloned T lymphocytes. Increased responsiveness to histamine, prostaglandins and β-adrenergic agents as a late stage in T cell activation. J Immunol 1988;140:2931–6.

[10] Kinouchi K, Brown G, Pasternak G, Donner D. Identification and characterization of receptors for tumor necrosis factor-α in the brain. Biochem Biophys Res Commun 1991;181:1532–8.

[11] Souza E. Corticotropin-releasing factor and Interleukin-1 receptors in the brain-endocrine-immune axis role in stress response and infection. Ann NY Acad Sci 1993;697:9–27.

[12] Smith L, Brown S, Blalock J. Interleukin-2 induction of ACTH secretion: presence of an interleukin-2 receptor α-chain-like molecule on pituitary cells. J Neuroimmunol 1989;21:249–54.

[13] Ohmichi M, Hirota K, Koike K, Kurachi H, Ohtsuka S, Matsuzaki N, et al. Binding sites for interleukin-6 in the anterior pituitary gland. Neuroendocrinology 1992;55:199–203.

[14] Chang Y, Albright S, Lee F. Cytokines in the central nervous system: expression of macrophage colony stimulating factor and its receptor during development. J Neuroimmunol 1994;52:9–17.

[15] Takao T, Tracey D, Mitchell W, De E. Interleukin-1 receptors in mouse brain: characterization and neuronal localization. Endocrinology 1990;127:3070–8.

[16] Tsigos C, Papanicolaou DA, Defensor R, Mitsiadis CS, Kyrou I, Chrousos GP. Dose effects of recombinant human interleukin-6 on pituitary hormone secretion and energy expenditure. Neuroendocrinology 1997;66:54–62.

[17] Cutolo M, Sulli A, Pizzorni C, Craviotto C, Straub RH. Hypothalamic-pituitary-adrenocortical and gonadal functions in rheumatoid arthritis. Ann NY Acad Sci 2003;992:107–17.

[18] Cutolo M, Foppiani L, Prete C, Ballarino P, Sulli A, Villaggio B, et al. Hypothalamic-pituitary-adrenocortical axis function in premenopausal women with rheumatoid arthritis not treated with glucocorticoids. J Rheumatol 1999;26:282–8.

[19] Straub RH, Pongratz G, Scho¨lmerich J, Kees F, Schaible TF, Antoni C, et al. Long-term anti-tumor necrosis factor antibody therapy in rheumatoid arthritis patients sensitizes the pituitary gland and favors adrenal androgen secretion. Arthritis Rheumatol 2003;48:1504–12.

[20] Ernestam S, Hafstrom I, Werner S, Carlstrom K, Tengstrand B. Increased DHEAS levels in patients with rheumatoid arthritis after treatment with tumor necrosis factor antagonists: evidence for improved adrenal function. J Rheumatol 2007;34:1451–8.

[21] Boettger M, Weber K, Grossmann D, Gajda M, Bauer R, Bär K, et al. Spinal tumor necrosis factor α neutralization reduces peripheral inflammation and hyperalgesia and suppresses autonomic responses in experimental arthritis: a role for spinal tumor necrosis factor α during induction and maintenance of peripheral inflammation. Arthritis Rheum 2010;62:1308–18.

[22] Albrecht U. Timing to perfection: the biology of central and peripheral circadian clocks. Neuron 2012;74:246–60.

[23] Guilding C, Piggins H. Challenging the omnipotence of the suprachiasmatic timekeeper: are circadian oscillators present throughout the mammalian brain? Eur J Neurosci 2007;25:3195–216.

[24] Cutolo M, Villaggio B, Otsa K, Aakre O, Sulli A, Seriolo B. Altered circadian rhythms in rheumatoid arthritis patients play a role in the disease's symptoms. Autoimmun Rev 2005;4:497–502.

[25] Coogan A, Wyse C. Neuroimmunology of the circadian clock. Brain Res 2008;1232:104–12.

[26] Takahashi S. Physical and inflammatory stressors elevate circadian clock gene mPer1 mRNA levels in the paraventricular nucleus of the mouse. Endocrinology 2001;142:4910–7.

[27] Okada K, Yano M, Doki Y, Azama T, Iwanaga H, Miki H, et al. Injection of LPS causes transient suppression of biological clock genes in rats. J Surg Res 2008;145:5–12.

[28] Godbout J, Johnson R. Age and neuroinflammation: a lifetime of psychoneuroimmune consequences. Neurol Clin 2006;24:521–38.

[29] Bijlsma J, Cutolo M, Masi A, Chikanza I. The neuroendocrine immune basis of rheumatic diseases. Immunol Today 1999;20:298–301.

[30] Cutolo M. Circadian rhythms in RA. Ann Rheum Dis 2003;62:593–6.

[31] Crofford L. Circadian relationships between interleukin (IL)-6 and hypothalamic-pituitary-adrenal axis hormones: failure of IL-6 to cause sustained hypercortisolism in patients with early untreated rheumatoid arthritis. J Clin Endocrinol Metab 1997;82:1279–83.

[32] Straub R, Cutolo M. Circadian rhythms in rheumatoid arthritis: implications for pathophysiology and therapeutic management. Arthritis Rheum 2007;56:399–408.

[33] Spies C, Cutolo M, Straub R, Burmester G, Buttgereit F. More night than day – circadian rhythms in polymyalgia rheumatica and ankylosing spondylitis. J Rheumatol 2010;37:894–9.

[34] Herxheimer H, Rosa L. The protective effect of sympathomimetic amines and of aminophylline in the anaphylactic microshock of the guinea-pig. Br J Pharmacol Chemother 1953;8:177–80.

[35] Galant SP, Remo RA. Beta-adrenergic inhibition of human T lymphocyte rosettes. J Immunol 1975;114:512–3.

[36] Wang H, Yu M, Ochani M, Amella CA, Tanovic M, Susarla S, et al. Nicotinic acetylcholine receptor alpha7 subunit is an essential regulator of inflammation. Nature 2003;421:384–8.

[37] de Jonge W, van der Zanden E, The F, Bijlsma M, van Westerloo D, Bennink R, et al. Stimulation of the vagus nerve attenuates macrophage activation by activating the Jak2-STAT3 signaling pathway. Nat Immunol 2005;6:844–51.

[38] Guarini S, Altavilla D, Cainazzo MM, Giuliani D, Bigiani A, Marini H, et al. Efferent vagal fibre stimulation blunts nuclear factor-kappaB activation and protects against hypovolemic hemorrhagic shock. Circulation 2003;107:1189–94.

[39] Lu B, Kwan K, Levine YA, Olofsson PS, Yang H, Li J, et al. alpha7 nicotinic acetylcholine receptor signaling inhibits inflammasome activation by preventing mitochondrial DNA release. Mol Med 2014;20:350–8.

[40] Milligan E, McGorry M, Fleshner M, Gaykema R, Goehler L, Watkins L, et al. Subdiaphragmatic vagotomy does not prevent fever following intracerebroventricular prostaglandin E2: further evidence for the importance of vagal afferents in immune-to-brain communication. Brain Res 1997;766:240–3.

[41] Watkins LR, Goehler LE, Relton JK, Tartaglia N, Silbert L, Martin D, et al. Blockade of interleukin-1 induced hyperthermia by subdiaphragmatic vagotomy: evidence for vagal mediation of immune-brain communication. Neurosci Lett 1995;183:27–31.

[42] Borovikova LV, Ivanova S, Zhang M, Yang H, Botchkina GI, Watkins LR, et al. Vagus nerve stimulation attenuates the systemic inflammatory response to endotoxin. Nature 2000;405:458–62.

[43] Rosas-Ballina M, Olofsson PS, Ochani M, Valdes-Ferrer SI, Levine YA, Reardon C, et al. Acetylcholine-synthesizing T cells relay neural signals in a vagus nerve circuit. Science 2011;334:98–101.

[44] Levine YA, Koopman FA, Faltys M, Caravaca A, Bendele A, Zitnik R, et al. Neurostimulation of the cholinergic anti-inflammatory pathway ameliorates disease in rat collagen-induced arthritis. PLoS One 2014;9:e104530.

[45] van Westerloo DJ, Giebelen IA, Florquin S, Bruno MJ, Larosa GJ, Ulloa L, et al. The vagus nerve and nicotinic receptors modulate experimental pancreatitis severity in mice. Gastroenterology 2006;130:1822–30.

[46] Ghia JE, Blennerhassett P, Kumar-Ondiveeran H, Verdu EF, Collins SM. The vagus nerve: a tonic inhibitory influence associated with inflammatory bowel disease in a murine model. Gastroenterology 2006;131:1122–30.

[47] Leib C, Goser S, Luthje D, Ottl R, Tretter T, Lasitschka F, et al. Role of the cholinergic antiinflammatory pathway in murine autoimmune myocarditis. Circ Res 2011;109:130–40.

[48] Koopman F, Chavan S, Miljko S, Grazio S, Sokolovic S, Schuurman P, et al. Vagus nerve stimulation inhibits cytokine production and attenuates disease severity in rheumatoid arthritis. Proc Natl Acad Sci USA 2016;113:8284–9.

[49] del Rey A, Besedovsky H. Sympathetic nervous system-immune interactions in autoimmune lymphoproliferative diseases. Neuroimmunomodulation 2008;15:29–36.

[50] Harbuz MS, Rees RG, Eckland D, Jessop DS, Brewerton D, Lightman SL. Paradoxical responses of hypothalamic corticotropin-releasing factor (CRF) messenger ribonucleic acid (mRNA) and CRF-41 peptide and adeno-hypophysial propiomelanocortin mRNA during chronic inflammatory stress. Endocrinology 1992;130:1394–400.

[51] Straub RH, Günzler C, Miller LE, Cutolo M, Schölmerich J, Schill S. Anti-inflammatory cooperativity of corticosteroids and norepinephrine in rheumatoid arthritis synovial tissue in vivo and in vitro. FASEB J 2002;16:993–1000.

[52] Dicou E, Perrot S, Menkes CJ, Masson C, Nerriere V. Nerve growth factor (NGF) autoantibodies and NGF in the synovial fluid: implications in spondylarthropathies. Autoimmunity 1996;24:1–9.

[53] Weidler C, Holzer C, Harbuz M, Hofbauer R, Angele P, Schölmerich J, et al. Low density of sympathetic nerve fibres and increased density of brain derived neurotrophic factor positive cells in RA synovium. Ann Rheum Dis 2005;64:13–20.

[54] Miller L, Weidler C, Falk W, Angele P, Schaumburger J, Schölmerich J, et al. Increased prevalence of semaphorin 3C, a repellent of sympathetic nerve fibers, in the synovial tissue of patients with rheumatoid arthritis. Arthritis Rheum 2004;50:1156–63.

[55] Fassold A, Falk W, Anders S, Hirsch T, Mirsky V, Straub R. Soluble neuropilin-2, a nerve repellent receptor, is increased in rheumatoid arthritis synovium and aggravates sympathetic fiber repulsion and arthritis. Arthritis Rheum 2009;60:2892–901.

[56] Pongratz G, Straub R. Role of peripheral nerve fibres in acute and chronic inflammation in arthritis. Nat Rev Rheumatol 2012;9:117–26.

[57] Härle P, Möbius D, Carr D, Schölmerich J, Straub R. An opposing time-dependent immune-modulating effect of the sympathetic nervous system conferred by altering the cytokine profile in the local lymph nodes and spleen of mice with type II collagen-induced arthritis. Arthritis Rheum 2005;52:1305–13.

[58] Härle P, Straub RH, Wiest R, Maier A, Schölmerich J, Atzeni F, et al. Increase of sympathetic outflow measured by neuropeptide Y and decrease of the hypothalamic-pituitary-adrenal axis tone in patients with systemic lupus erythematosus and rheumatoid arthritis: another example of uncoupling of response systems. Ann Rheum Dis 2005;65:51–6.

[59] Pauwels R, Löfdahl C, Postma D, Tattersfield A, O'Byrne P, Barnes P, et al. Effect of inhaled formoterol and budesonide on exacerbations of asthma. N Engl J Med 1997;337:1405–11.

[60] Oikarinen J, Hämäläinen L, Oikarinen A. Modulation of glucocorticoid receptor activity by cyclic nucleotides and its implications on the regulation of human skin fibroblast growth and protein synthesis. Biochim Biophys Acta Gen Subj 1984;799:158–65.

[61] Eickelberg O, Roth M, Lörx R, Bruce V, Rüdiger J, Johnson M, et al. Ligand-independent activation of the glucocorticoid receptor by β2-adrenergic receptor agonists in primary human lung fibroblasts and vascular smooth muscle cells. J Biol Chem 1999;274:1005–10.

[62] Schmidt P, Holsboer F, Spengler D. beta(2)-Adrenergic receptors potentiate glucocorticoid receptor transactivation via g protein betagamma-subunits and the phosphoinositide 3-kinase pathway. Mol Endocrinol 2001;15:553–64.

[63] Guirao X, Kumar A, Katz J, Smith M, Lin E, Keogh C, et al. Catecholamines increase monocyte TNF receptors and inhibit TNF through β2-adrenoreceptor activation. Am J Physiol Endocrinol Metab 1997;273(6):E1203–8.

[64] Le Moine O, Stordeur P, Schandene L, Marchant A, De Groote D, Goldman M, et al. Adenosine enhances IL-10 secretion by human monocytes. J Immunol 1996;156:4408–14.

[65] Schubert D, LaCorbiere M, Klier FG, Steinbach JH. The modulation of neurotransmitter synthesis by steroid hormones and insulin. Brain Res 1980;190:67–79.

[66] Verghese MW, McConnell RT, Strickland AB, Gooding RC, Stimpson SA, Yarnall DP, et al. Differential regulation of human monocyte-derived TNF alpha and IL-1 beta by type IV cAMP-phosphodiesterase (cAMP-PDE) inhibitors. J Pharmacol Exp Ther 1995;72:1313–20.

[67] Severn A, Rapson NT, Hunter CA, Liew FY. Regulation of tumor necrosis factor production by adrenaline and beta-adrenergic agonists. J Immunol 1992;148:3441–5.

[68] Szabo G, Girouard L, Mandrekar P, Catalano D. Regulation of monocyte IL-12 production: augmentation by lymphocyte contact and acute ethanol treatment, inhibition by elevated intracellular cAMP. Int J Immunopharmacol 1998;20:491–503.

[69] Bosmann M, Meta F, Ruemmler R, Haggadone MD, Sarma JV, Zetoune FS, et al. Regulation of IL-17 family members by adrenal hormones during experimental sepsis in mice. Am J Pathol 2013;182:1124–30. Int Immunol April 1995;7:517–23.

[70] Platzer C, Meisel C, Vogt K, Platzer M, Volk H. Up-regulation of monocytic IL-10 by tumor necrosis factor-α and cAMP elevating drugs. Int Immunol 1995;7:517–23.

[71] Bailly S, Ferrua B, Fay M, Gougerot-Pocidalo M. Differential regulation of IL 6, IL 1 A, IL 1β and TNFα production in LPS-stimulated human monocytes: role of cyclic AMP. Cytokine 1990;2:205–10.

[72] Lorton D, Bellinger D. Molecular mechanisms underlying β-adrenergic receptor-mediated cross-talk between sympathetic neurons and immune cells. Int J Mol Sci 2015;16:5635–65.

[73] Baerwald C, Wahle M, Ulrichs T, Jonas D, von Bierbrauer A, von Wichert P, et al. Reduced catecholarnine response of lymphocytes from patients with rheumatoid arthritis. Immunobiology 1999;200:77–91.

[74] (a) Chiu IM, Heesters BA, Ghasemlou N, Von Hehn CA, Zhao F, Tran J, et al. Bacteria activate sensory neurons that modulate pain and inflammation. Nature 2013;501:52–7.
(b) Pereira da Silva JA, Carmo-Fonseca M. Peptide containing nerves in human synovium: immunehistochemical evidence for decreased innervation in rheumatoid arthritis. J Rheumatol 1990;17:1592–9.

[75] Miller LE, Jüsten HP, Schölmerich J, Straub RH. The loss of sympathetic nerve fibers in the synovial tissue of patients with rheumatoid arthritis is accompanied by increased norepinephrine release from synovial macrophages. FASEB J 2000;14:2097–107.

[76] Miller LE, Grifka J, Schölmerich J, Straub RH. Norepinephrine from synovial tyrosine hydroxylase positive cells is a strong indicator of synovial inflammation in rheumatoid arthritis. J Rheumatol 2002;29:427–35.

[77] Schaible H. Nociceptive neurons detect cytokines in arthritis. Arthritis Res Ther 2014;16:470.

[78] Jiang H, Shen X, Chen Z, Liu F, Wang T, Xie Y, et al. Nociceptive neuronal Fc-gamma receptor I is involved in IgG immune complex induced pain in the rat. Brain Behav Immun 2017;62:351–61.

[79] Cutolo M, Sulli A, Pincus T. Circadian use of glucocorticoids in rheumatoid arthritis. Neuroimmunomodulation 2015;22:33–9.

[80] Cutolo M. Chronobiology and the treatment of rheumatoid arthritis. Curr Opin Rheumatol 2012;24:312–8.

[81] Alten R, Doring G, Cutolo M, Gromnica-Ihle E, Witte S, Straub R, et al. Hypothalamus-pituitary-adrenal axis function in patients with rheumatoid arthritis treated with nighttime-release prednisone. J Rheumatol 2010;37:2025–31.

[82] Straub RH, Cutolo M. Glucocorticoids and chronic inflammation. Rheumatology (Oxf) 2016;55:ii6–14.

[83] Masi A, Imrich R, Cutolo M. Hypothesis: can neuroendocrine immune (NEI) testing of individual RA patients guide benefits to harms ratio in glucocorticoid therapy?. Arthritis Care Res 2017. https://doi.org/10.1002/acr.23453. [Epub ahead of print].

[84] Cutolo M, Straub R. Insights into endocrine-immunological disturbances in autoimmunity and their impact on treatment. Arthritis Res Ther 2009;11:218.

Chapter 56

Large-Vessel Vasculitis

Francesco Muratore[1,3], Stefania Croci[2], Alessandra Soriano[2], Nicolò Pipitone[1], Carlo Salvarani[1,3]

[1]Rheumatology Unit, Azienda USL-IRCCS di Reggio Emilia, Reggio Emilia, Italy; [2]Unit of Clinical Immunology, Allergy and Advanced Biotechnologies, Azienda USL-IRCCS di Reggio Emilia, Reggio Emilia, Italy; [3]Università di Modena e Reggio Emilia, Modena, Italy

CLASSIFICATION CRITERIA OF LARGE-VESSEL VASCULITIS

The large-vessel vasculitides (LVV) giant cell arteritis (GCA) (Table 56.1) and Takayasu arteritis (TAK) (Table 56.2) are currently classified using the 1990 American College of Rheumatology (ACR) criteria [1,2]. These criteria included as comparators other vasculitides; therefore, they were meant to distinguish patients affected by various forms of vasculitides but not to differentiate vasculitis from other disorders. Hence, these criteria should be used to classify, rather than diagnose, patients, although in practice they are also used to support a clinical diagnosis.

Even for the purpose of classification there are some inadequacies about these criteria. The ACR criteria for GCA focus on the subset of patients with predominant cranial manifestations, but some patients with GCA have prevalent or exclusive manifestations of large-vessel involvement and/or systemic manifestations. In particular, patients with LVV have less frequently cranial symptoms and a positive temporal artery biopsy (TAB); therefore, they are more likely not be identified by these criteria [3,4]. In addition, even patients with predominant features of cranial arteritis and a positive TAB may not show the classical histological features of transmural granulomatous inflammation contemplated in the 1990 ACR criteria. However, in the appropriate clinical context, inflammation restricted to the advential or periadvential arteries can be consistent with GCA and carries the same risk of visual loss as transmural inflammation [5,6].

With regard to the ACR criteria for TAK, these criteria emphasize clinical manifestations of large-vessel disease, but do not include vascular imaging techniques except for conventional angiography, which is not able to show the vessel wall inflammatory changes that precede clinical symptoms and signs [7]. From this point of view, the OMERACT has underscored the need to consider imaging findings in diagnosing patients with LVV and imaging findings should be included in new classification criteria [8].

To overcome the limitations of the ACR criteria, a diagnostic algorithm has been proposed that includes both biopsy and ultrasonography findings, although this algorithm remains to be validated [9]. Furthermore, a multicentric project, the Diagnostic and Classification in Vasculitis Study is being conducted with the aim to substitute the ACR with new criteria [10].

PORTRAIT OF THE PATHOGENESIS OF GIANT CELL ARTERITIS

GCA is the most common systemic vasculitis in people older than 50 years of age. Inflammation affects mainly the extracranial branches of the carotid artery, particularly the temporal arteries. Clinical features of GCA are generally the result of ischemic events caused by luminal occlusion subsequent to arterial remodeling and intima hyperplasia fueled by inflammation [11]. The most feared complication is blindness. The gold standard for the diagnosis of GCA is a TAB showing infiltration of immune cells [12].

The causes (etiology) of GCA are currently unknown, but the understanding of mechanisms involved in GCA pathogenesis is constantly growing. GCA development involves a breakdown of arterial immunoprivilege. Age-related immune alterations, in genetically predisposed subjects, seem essential for the development of the disease. The evidence that identical CD4+ T-cell clones are present in different arteries affected by inflammation and the strong association between GCA and the class II human leukocyte antigen (HLA), particularly with the HLA-DRB1*04 alleles, suggest that GCA is likely driven by T cell (and possibly also B cell) responses to specific antigens [13]. The development and the growing of myofibroblasts represent a critical step in the disease because it can favor arterial occlusion.

Mosaic of Autoimmunity. https://doi.org/10.1016/B978-0-12-814307-0.00056-6

TABLE 56.1 1990 ACR Criteria for the Classification of Giant Cell (Temporal) Arteritis

1. Age at disease onset ≥50 years—Development of symptoms or findings beginning at age 50 or older
2. New headache—New onset of or new type of localized pain in the head
3. Temporal artery abnormality—Temporal artery tenderness to palpation or decreased pulsation, unrelated to atherosclerosis of cervical arteries
4. Elevated Erythrocyte sedimentation rate ≥50 mm per h by the Westergren method
5. Abnormal artery biopsy—Biopsy specimen with artery showing vasculitis characterized by a predominance of mononuclear cell infiltration or granulomatous inflammation, usually with multinucleated giant cells

For purposes of classification, a patient shall be said to have giant cell (temporal) arteritis if at least three of the five criteria are present. The presence of any three or more criteria yields a sensitivity of 93.5% and a specificity of 91.2%.

TABLE 56.2 1990 Criteria for the Classification of Takayasu Arteritis

1. Age at disease onset <40 years—Development of symptoms or findings related to Takayasu arteritis at age equal to or greater than 40 years
2. Claudication of extremities—Development and worsening of fatigue and discomfort in muscles of one or more extremity while in use, especially the upper extremities
3. Decreased brachial artery pulse—Decreased pulsation of one or both brachial arteries
4. BP difference >10 mm Hg—Difference of >10 mm Hg in systolic blood pressure between arms
5. Bruit over subclavian arteries or aorta—Bruit audible on auscultation over one or both subclavian arteries or abdominal aorta
6. Arteriogram abnormality—Arteriographic narrowing or occlusion of the entire aorta, its primary branches, or large arteries in the proximal upper or lower extremities, not due to arteriosclerosis, fibromuscular dysplasia, or similar causes; changes usually focal or segmental

For purposes of classification, a patient shall be said to have Takayasu arteritis if at least three of these six criteria are present. The presence of any three or more criteria yields a sensitivity of 90.5% and a specificity of 97.8%. *BP*, blood pressure (systolic; difference between arms).

CURRENT MODEL OF GIANT CELL ARTERITIS IMMUNOPATHOGENESIS

A model of GCA pathogenesis based on four phases has been outlined [13]:

Phase 1: activation of dendritic cells (DCs) in the adventitia. Immature myeloid DCs localized in the adventitia act as immune sentinels. After sensing danger signals by means of toll-like receptors (TLRs), particularly TLR-2, TLR-4, and TLR-5, they can trigger and shape adaptive immune responses through chemokine and cytokine production and antigen presentation.

Phase 2: recruitment, activation, and polarization of CD4+ T lymphocytes. The cytokine milieu recruits, activates, and retains CD4+ T lymphocytes in the arterial wall and polarizes CD4+ T lymphocytes toward T helper (Th)1, Th9, Th17, Th21, and Th22 subsets.

Phase 3: recruitment of CD8+ T cells and monocytes. Interleukins produced by CD4+ T lymphocytes, particularly IFN-γ, induce the production of downstream chemokines and cytokines that attract monocytes and CD8+ T lymphocytes. Monocytes differentiate in macrophages and form granulomas in the media. Macrophages can secrete matrix metalloproteinases (e.g., MMP-2, MMP-9), reactive oxygen species, and nitric oxide leading to lipid peroxidation and the destruction of elastic laminae. Besides, CD8+ T lymphocytes can produce further cytokines and cytotoxic molecules (granzymes and perforin).

Phase 4: vascular remodeling. Feedback mechanisms are induced to restore homeostasis. Several growth factors including PDGF, VEGF, FGF, ET-1, and TGF-β are produced, which can favor the transition of vascular smooth muscle cells (VSMC) from a contractile to a secretory phenotype and their migration to the intima. The formation of a neo-intima made of myofibroblasts and extra cellular matrix proteins can lead to the occlusion of the arterial lumen.

ARTERIAL INFLAMMATION AND REMODELING

Arteries of GCA patients become infiltrated by DCs, T lymphocytes (mainly CD4+), macrophages, and multinucleated giant cells (hence, the name). Giant cells are present in about half of the TABs. B lymphocytes and neutrophils are sometimes present in TABs, whereas NK cells have not been reported to date [13]. The classic histologic picture of GCA is a transmural lymphomononuclear inflammatory cell infiltrate crossing all layers, with or without giant cells. However, inflammation can also be restricted to the adventitial vasa vasorum and/or to the periadventitial small vessels [5,6].

Dendritic cells. It has been proposed that the initiating immunological event in GCA pathogenesis is the activation of adventitial DCs through TLRs. DCs remain in the arteries where they can release several chemokines and cytokines such as IL-6, IL-18, IL-23, IL-32, IL-33, CCL18, CCL19, CCL20, CCL21, which attract and activate pathogenic T lymphocytes [14].

T lymphocytes. The majority of arterial-residing lymphocytes are CD4+. Compared with TABs from control subjects, TABs from patients with GCA are infiltrated by IFN-γ–secreting Th1, IL-9–secreting Th9, IL-17–secreting Th17, IL-21–secreting Th21 and, recently detected by our group, IL-22–secreting Th22 lymphocytes [15,16]. To date, two main pathogenic pathways have been characterized in GCA: a IL-6/IL-17/Th17 pathway sensitive to the glucocorticoid (GC) therapy and a IL-12/IFN-γ/Th1 pathway that persists despite treatment with GCs and thus underlies the chronic phase of the disease [17]. The Notch signaling pathway is activated in GCA and is emerging as a key pathogenic hit. Multiple CD4+ T lymphocyte subsets express Notch1 receptor in TABs from GCA patients and Notch1 ligands are expressed by tissue cells, particularly endothelial cells (ECs) [18]. CD8+ T lymphocytes can also infiltrate the arteries. A strong percentage of CD8+ T lymphocyte in TAB is associated with a more severe disease supporting their pathogenic role [19]. Moreover, in patients with GCA, a defect in the immunoprotective PD-1/PD-L1 immune checkpoint has recently been reported. Inflamed temporal arteries show a lower expression of PD-L1 by DCs and a higher expression of PD-1 receptor by T cells compared to normal arteries. This can lead to unrestricted T-cell activation and cytokine production [20].

B lymphocytes. B lymphocytes can be detected in TABs from GCA patients but at a lower degree than T lymphocytes. In addition, several types of autoantibodies have been documented in patients with GCA [13]. Recently, tertiary lymphoid organs (TLOs) structures have been detected in TABs from GCA patients. These TLOs are formed by B cell aggregates with a follicular DC network, loosely surrounded by T cells and with the extensive formation of high endothelial venules [21]. TLOs in GCA arteries might have a role in the disruption of the arterial immune privilege, possibly representing the immune sites where immune responses toward unknown arterial wall–derived antigens start. Overall these data support a possible contribution of the humoral immune responses in the pathogenesis of GCA.

Macrophages. CD68+ macrophages constitute a major subset of the inflammatory cells forming the granuloma and can orchestrate both immune cell functions and tissue remodeling. CD68+ macrophages are heterogeneous: some can secrete proinflammatory cytokines such as IL-1β and IL-6; others can secrete tissue-degrading metalloproteinases and collagenases. Recently it has been demonstrated that most macrophages in TABs of GCA patients have the phenotype of nonclassical monocytes being CD68+CD16+CXCR1+CCR2^{neg} [22].

Cytokines, chemokines, and growth factors. Several proinflammatory cytokines, chemokines, and growth factors have been detected upregulated in the inflamed arteries of patients with GCA compared to normal arteries: IL-1β, IL-6, IL-7, IL-9, IL-12, IL-17, IL-18, IL-21, IL-22, IL-23, IL-32, IL-33, IFN-γ, TNF-α, PTX-3, CCL2, CCL18, CCL19, CCL20, CCL21, CX3CL1, CXCL13, BAFF, APRIL, LT-β, VEGF, FGF, PDGF, ET-1. They can promote the recruitment of immune cells and shape not only the polarization of lymphocyte and monocytes/macrophages but also the phenotype of VSMCs and ECs thus contributing to GCA pathogenesis [13,14].

Endothelial cells and vascular smooth muscle cells. Arterial resident ECs and VSMC are indeed key effectors in GCA pathogenesis being the actors of tissue remodeling. ECs and VSMCs can respond to the inflammatory mediators acquiring proinflammatory properties (e.g., expression of adhesion molecules and homing chemokines for leukocytes) and new phenotypes (e.g., enhanced proliferation and migratory abilities). ECs of adventitial microvessels and neovessels from TAB of GCA patients express high levels of adhesion molecules such as ICAM-1, ICAM-2, PECAM-1, P-selectin, E-selectin, and VCAM-1, all of which are involved in the recruitment of immune cells [13]. In addition, microvascular ECs in the adventitial vasa vasorum but not ECs lining the lumen, express Jagged1, the Notch ligand [18], which can lead to CD4+ T lymphocyte recruitment and lineage differentiation. VSMCs can acquire a proliferative potential and can migrate toward the intima, thus resulting in intimal hyperplasia. MiR-21, a small noncoding RNA, has been detected in spindle-shaped cells of the medial layer and stellate fibroblasts-like cells of the intimal layer in inflamed TABs from GCA patients thus emerging as a potential marker of the phenotypic transition of VSMCs [23].

SYSTEMIC DEREGULATION OF THE IMMUNE SYSTEM

GCA has two components: arterial and systemic inflammation. The laboratory hallmarks of active disease are increased levels of erythrocyte sedimentation rate and/or C-reactive protein. Some cytokines have been detected at higher concentration in plasma or serum samples from GCA patients compared to healthy subjects: IL-6, sIL-6R, IL-10, IL-22, VEGF, PTX-3, BAFF, CXCL9, sIL-2R, granzymes A and B. GCA patients with very recent optic nerve ischemia have significantly higher PTX3 and VEGF levels compared to other GCA patients and controls suggesting a role for PTX3 and VEGF [24].

Levels of IL-6 and BAFF seem associated with disease activity [25,26]. BAFF and IL-22 might be involved in B-cell responses [16]. Changes in the percentage and/or absolute numbers of some immune subsets in the blood have also been detected in patients with GCA. The percentages of circulating Th17 and Th21 lymphocytes are increased in GCA patients compared with healthy controls. The percentage of Th22 lymphocytes is similar, whereas data on differences in the percentage Th1 lymphocytes between GCA patients and healthy subjects are controversial [15,27]. Besides, GCA patients have a decreased frequency of circulating antiinflammatory regulatory CD4+ and CD8+ T cells [27,28] indicating an imbalance between pathogenic and regulatory T cells, which is likely involved in disease pathogenesis. Higher percentages of circulating cytotoxic CD8 T lymphocytes, Tc17 and CD63+CD8+ T cells [19] and a decreased numbers of circulating B cells have been detected in the peripheral blood of GCA patients [29]. Finally a higher number of circulating neutrophils with a classically activated phenotype ($CD16^{hi}AnxA1^{hi}CD62L^{lo}CD11b^{hi}$) has been found in GCA patients, suggesting neutrophil involvement in GCA pathogenesis. Interestingly, therapy with GCs can dampen neutrophil activation but after 24 weeks of therapy neutrophils can display again an activated phenotype and might thus be involved in GCA flares [30].

EPIGENETICS

Differences in DNA methylation in temporal arteries from GCA patients versus control subjects have been recently reported suggesting a role for the calcineurin/nuclear factor of activated T cells signaling pathway in GCA [31].

miRNA

MiRNAs are small noncoding RNAs that can inhibit expression of multiple genes posttranscription. Six miRNAs have been found overexpressed in inflamed TABs from GCA patients compared to noninflamed TABs: miR-146b-5p, -146a, -21, -150, -155, -299, -5p. They might be biomarkers of specific infiltrating immune cell subsets and activated pathways in inflamed TABs and/or have a functional role in GCA pathogenesis. MiR-146a, -21, -155 and -150 can be expressed by specific immune cell subsets as well as by arterial cells such as VSMCs, ECs, and fibroblasts. MiR-155 is mainly a proinflammatory miRNA. MiR-21 can have both pro- and antiinflammatory activities, whereas miR-146a and miR-150 mainly counteract inflammation by negative feedback loops. Noteworthy such miRNAs can be induced by cellular senescence. MiR-21 is the only miRNA overexpressed in GCA that has documented pathogenic effects on VSMCs, ECs, and adventitial fibroblasts, thus emerging as a promising target for the development of novel gene-therapy approaches for GCA [23].

FUNCTIONAL ANALYSES

To discover and confirm which pathways are crucial in GCA pathogenesis two preclinical models have been and are mainly used: a mouse model in which human temporal arteries are engrafted into severe combined-immunodeficiency mice and an *ex vivo* model in which human temporal arteries are cultured in vitro for few days. Using the mouse model it was shown that the depletion of DC and CD4+ T cells and the inhibition of the Notch pathway can reduce vasculitis, whereas the activation of TLR4 and TLR5 and the inhibition of PD-1 checkpoint can induce arteritis, thus demonstrating the essential role of these pathways in GCA pathogenesis [20,32–35]. Using the ex vivo model the pathogenic role of IFN-γ and ET-1 has recently been elucidated [36,37]. Moreover, a potential role for VEGF (in activating the Notch pathway) [18] and PDGF (in inducing VSMCs proliferation and migration) have been demonstrated [38]. Finally, treatment of GCA patients with the IL-6 pathway inhibitor tocilizumab (TCZ) and the IL-12/IL-23 pathway inhibitor ustekinumab have proven effective and indicated a key role of these pathways in disease pathogenesis [39,40].

IMAGING OF VASCULITIS

The increasing availability and improvement of imaging techniques are making a profound impact in the evaluation of patients with vasculitis, particularly for those with LVV, which include GCA and TAK, and will most likely play an ever more important role in the future [7,41]. Deep, large vessels can be examined by computed tomography (CT) and magnetic resonance imaging (MRI), whereas ultrasound is the method of choice for the evaluation of superficial vessels (such as temporal, carotid, and axillary arteries). ^{18}F-Fluorodeoxyglucose (FDG) positron emission tomography (PET), often coregistered with computerized tomography (PET/CT), is very sensitive in detecting large vessel inflammation, but it does not delineate the vessel wall. Except for the detection of the characteristic microaneurysms alternating with stenoses in medium-sized vessel vasculitis, digital subtraction angiography (DSA) has become a therapeutic procedure for endovascular intervention in LVV rather than a diagnostic method. Imaging studies can also be used to monitor the disease course and the development of late vascular complication. Finally, in small vessel vasculitis imaging modalities are usually required to document internal organs involvement [42].

Computed Tomography

CT and CT angiography (CTA) are well suited to detect inflammatory changes in large, deep arteries because of their good spacial resolution and convenient scanning time. CT can measure aortic diameter and detect mural calcifications. CTA can evaluate both the vessel wall and the lumen of the large vessels, but cannot visualize relatively small vessels.

CTA has a role in diagnosing early and advanced LVV. In early LVV, CT may show arterial wall thickening with mural enhancement and low-attenuation ring on delayed images. In late LVV the arterial wall is slightly thickened with high attenuation or calcifications. Furthermore, CTA may show LVV complications such as arterial stenosis, occlusion, and dilatation. The role of CTA in monitoring disease activity in LVV patients is still unclear. The main disadvantage of CT/CTA is the exposure to a significant amount of ionizing radiation, which limits its repeated use. Furthermore, it is contraindicated in patients with impaired renal function and in those allergic to iodine [7,41].

Magnetic Resonance Imaging

Similarly to CT, MRI is particularly indicated to examine the aorta and the other deep, large vessels without the use of ionizing radiation or ioniodated contrast. Increased vessel wall thickness (usually with a diffuse circumferential pattern), associated with vessel wall oedema on T2 and fat-suppressed sequences, and mural contrast enhancement on T1 sequences are early signs of vascular inflammation. Postcontrast T1 images are superior to T2 or fat-suppressed images to detect early large vessel inflammation. Moreover, MRI angiography (MRA) provides luminal information, such as arterial stenosis, occlusion, and dilatation. The role of MRI in monitoring disease activity in LVV patients is still unclear [7,41].

MRI is the key screening test for primary central nervous system vasculitis (PCNSV), a vasculitis affecting the brain and rarely the spinal cord because its sensitivity is close to 100% [42]. However, MRI changes are largely nonspecific. Infarctions are the most common type of lesion and are bilateral in the majority of cases. Both the cortex and subcortex are involved. Gadolinium-enhanced intracranial lesions and meningeal gadolinium–enhanced lesions occur in about one-fourth of patients [43]. MRA is less sensitive than conventional angiography to detect vessel abnormalities in PCNSV, particularly in detecting lesions involving the posterior circulation and distal vessels [43]. Advances in neuroimaging techniques used to study the wall of large intracranial vessels could improve detection of inflammation. Vessel wall thickening and intramural enhancement of large arteries are considered specific to cerebral vasculitis [44]. Occasionally enhancement can extend into the adjacent leptomeningeal tissue (perivascular enhancement) [45].

Limitations of MRI/MRA include poor visualization of calcifications and falsely accentuated stenoses. Disadvantages include poor visualization of medium and small vessels, high cost of the procedure, and long acquisition time. Furthermore, it is contraindicated in patients with impaired renal function, claustrophobia, and in those with some metal devices [7,41].

Conventional Angiography

DSA clearly depicts vessel luminal changes in LVV. The commonest angiographic findings are long, smooth vascular stenoses and sometimes occlusions and aneurysm [46]. However, DSA cannot demonstrate earlier vasculitic inflammatory changes such as thickening of the vessel wall and mural enhancement and is not useful for early diagnosis. Disadvantages of DSA include its invasive nature and the exposition to ionizing radiation. Furthermore, it is contraindicated in patients with impaired renal function and in those allergic to iodine. For all these reasons, DSA has become a therapeutic procedure for endovascular intervention rather than a diagnostic method in LVV [7,41].

DSA has a sensitivity of 40%–90% and specificity of 30% for PCNSV [47]. Changes suggestive of vasculitis are alternating areas of smooth-wall narrowing and dilatation of cerebral arteries or arterial occlusion affecting many cerebral vessels in the absence of proximal vascular atherosclerosis or other recognized abnormalities. In contrast, single abnormalities in several arteries or several abnormalities in one artery are less consistent with PCNSV [42].

Positron Emission Tomography

In active LVV, PET shows increased FDG uptake by the vessel wall, typically with a smooth linear pattern [48]. PET is able to visualize virtually all vessels larger than 4 mm in diameter, but not arteries of smaller caliber such as the temporal or the renal arteries [7]. There is no generally accepted way of interpreting PET scans in vasculitis. A time-honored approach is to use the so-called Meller scale, a semiquantitative four-point scale, which includes the following grades: no vascular uptake (grade 0), vascular uptake less than liver uptake (grade 1), similar to liver uptake (grade 2), and higher than liver uptake (grade 3) [49]. In untreated patients, grade 2 and 3 are considered relatively specific for active vasculitis, whereas grade 1 uptake (less commonly grade 2) can also be observed in arteries affected by atherosclerosis in the absence of vasculitis [50]. Further clues pointing to vasculitis and away from atherosclerosis are the involvement of arteries usually spared by atherosclerosis and a linear pattern of FGD uptake over long vascular segments (in contrast to the irregular and patchy FDG uptake seen in atherosclerosis) [7]. The diagnostic performance of PET declines by nearly 50% shortly after the onset of corticosteroid and immunosuppressive treatment [51]. After effective treatment, vascular FDG uptake decreases or normalizes, often in parallel with a reduction in serum inflammatory markers [52–54]. However, low-grade vascular FDG uptake may persist in a sizeable number of patients [55]. The role of PET is less well established in predicting the course of the disease and its complications [7,41].

Ultrasound

Ultrasound depicts inflammatory artery wall thickening in LVV similar to MRI and CT. Furthermore, it can easily asses the temporal arteries [41]. The wall thickening is most commonly concentric in axial views and appears hypoechoic compared to the surrounding tissue. This phenomenon has been described as "halo sign" [56]. According to a metaanalysis, the presence of a halo in the temporal arteries has a sensitivity of 75% and a specificity of 83% for the diagnosis of GCA using the histologic criteria as reference standard [57], and a sensitivity of 68% and specificity of 91% for GCA diagnosed according to the ACR criteria [58]. The specificity of the halo sign increases to nearly 100% when the sign is bilateral [58]. However, the halo sign is infrequently found in GCA characterized by a histological pattern of periadventitial small vessel vasculitis or adventitial vasa vasorum vasculitis [59]. Therefore, while a positive halo sign strongly supports a diagnosis of GCA in the presence of compatible clinical manifestations, the absence of a halo at ultrasonography does not rule out the diagnosis of GCA. The temporal artery wall swelling disappears after 2–3 weeks with corticosteroid treatment in most patients, with a wide range (from 2 days to 6 months) in some cases [60,61]. Therefore patients with suspected GCA should be seen as early as possible.

The halo sign can also be noted in inflamed large vessels in both GCA and TAK. In clinical practice ultrasound of the epiaortic (carotid, subclavian, and axillary) arteries is a valuable screening test for suspected LV-GCA and TAK [41]. Furthermore, ultrasound may also detect large vessel stenoses, occlusions, and dilatations. The wall swelling of extracranial arteries remains longer compared to temporal arteries, so that the diagnosis of LVV can be established also after months and years of treatment in many patients. Advantages of ultrasound include its limited cost, the relatively short time required, and the absence of radiation. However, ultrasound has a number of limitations. It is operator-dependent and cannot image well some arterial segments, such as proximal subclavian arteries and the thoracic aorta because of overlying structures, while abdominal vessels may be obscured by bowel gases and fat [7,41].

TREATMENT OF LARGE-VESSEL VASCULITIS

GCA and TAK are the two major forms of idiopathic LVV. Both diseases are chronic idiopathic granulomatous vasculitides that affect the large- and medium-sized arteries (the aorta and/or its major branches) [62]. Both diseases share pathogenetic, clinical, radiographic, and histological features and have thus been proposed to represent different phenotypes on a spectrum of a single disorder [63–65]. As a result, the therapeutic approach to GCA and TAK has generally been similar. Both GCA and TAK are rare conditions, and most information on the treatment of these diseases comes from retrospective case series and small open-label trials. High doses of GCs are effective in inducing remission in both conditions, and remain the cornerstone first-line treatment for both GCA and TAK [66]. However, relapses during GC tapering and recurrences after GC discontinuation are common, requiring prolonged GC treatment with ensuing GC-related adverse events. These findings have prompted the search for alternative treatments including biological agents.

Giant Cell Arteritis

The immediate initiation of high-dose GC treatment is recommended after a clinical suspicion of GCA is raised. TAB should be obtained to determine the diagnosis of GCA with high certainly, but it should not delay treatment initiation. An initial dose of 40–60 mg daily of oral prednisone (or its equivalent) is suggested in uncomplicated GCA [66,67]. Suspected GCA with transient or permanent visual loss should be treated immediately with 1 mg/kg per day of oral prednisone or 500–1000 mg per day of intravenous methylprednisolone daily for 3 days (followed by oral prednisone at 1 mg/kg per day), according to the regimen that can be most rapidly initiated [68]. The initial dose of GC is usually given for 4 weeks until all reversible signs and symptoms have resolved and acute phase reactants are back to normal. The prednisone dose is then reduced by 10 mg every 2 weeks to 20 mg, then by 2.5 mg every 2–4 weeks to 10 mg, and then by 1 mg every 1–2 months if no flare occurs [67]. The taper should not be in the form of alternate day therapy, as this is more likely to lead to a relapse of vasculitis [66]. Even with gradual reduction of doses of GC, clinical flares occur in more than 50% of patients, particularly during the first 12–16 months, when the prednisone dose is reduced to about 10 mg per day [12]. Adverse events related to GC are very common and are related to the age of patients and the cumulative dose of GC [69].

Adjunctive MTX treatment reduces the risk of relapses and the cumulative exposure to GC. However, the advantage of the treatment effect of MTX appears only after 24–36 weeks and does not reduce the occurrence of adverse events [70]. The results of treatment trials with other conventional immunosuppressive (IS) agents have overall been disappointing in that no reduction in GC-related side effects could be demonstrated [71].

TNF-α blockers are ineffective or at best have only a marginal beneficial effect in new-onset GCA and may be associated with safety concerns and are therefore not recommended in this setting. However, the role of TNF-α blockers in refractory GCA needs further investigation [71].

Two RCTs recently showed the efficacy of the IL-6 receptors inhibitor monoclonal antibody TCZ for the induction and maintenance of remission in patients with new-onset and relapsing GCA. Furthermore, the addition of TCZ to prednisone led to a substantial reduction in the cumulative prednisone doses required to control GCA. The profile of adverse events was balanced across treatment groups and no safety concerns raised during the trial [39,72]. However, about half of patients with refractory GCA who showed an adequate response to TCZ relapsed after its discontinuation, suggesting that long-term therapy may be required [73]. In clinical practice, subcutaneous TCZ at a dosage of 162 mg weekly or intravenous TCZ at a dosage of 8 mg/kg per 4 weeks may be used in patients with multiple relapses or recurrences, or in those with GC-dependent GCA. Early introduction of TCZ in addition to GC may also be considered in selected patients with newly diagnosed GCA at high risk for serious side effects from GCs [71]. The addition of abatacept, a selective T cells costimulation modulator, to a treatment regimen with prednisone moderately reduced the GCA risk of relapse in a recent RCT [74].

Several retrospective studies have evaluated the effect of low-dose aspirin on the risk of ischemic events in newly diagnosed GCA patients, with conflicting results. To date, low-dose aspirin use should follow the current recommendations for preventing complications of atherosclerosis [71]. Calcium, vitamin D, and bisphosphonates should be started together with GCs in all newly diagnosed GCA patients to prevent GC-induced osteoporosis.

Takayasu Arteritis

As in GCA, GC is still the mainstay of treatment for TAK, with a suggested initial prednisone dosage of 0.5–1 mg/kg per day (maximum 60 mg per day). Initial high-dose GC should be maintained for a month, and then tapered gradually [75,76]. Although most patients initially achieve disease remission, relapses and GC dependence is seen in more than two thirds of patients during GC tapering, and between 46% and 84% of patients will need a second IS agent to achieve remission with acceptable GC dosages [77]. In TAK, no RCTs are available for traditional IS agents so far, and all information on the treatment of this disease comes from retrospective case series and small open-label trials. In clinical practice, first-line IS agents include MTX at a dosage of 15–20 mg per week, AZA at a dosage of 2–2.5 mg/kg per day, and MMF at a dosage of 2 g per day [71].

Retrospective open-label studies have provided strong evidence in favor of the use of anti-TNF-α agents in TAK patients with relapsing disease. Infliximab, associated with MTX in the majority of cases, is the most commonly used anti-TNF agent. Over 40% of patients are able to reduce and discontinue GC, but relapses occur in about 40% of patients, and approximately one-half of patients require an increased dose or switch to another anti-TNF-α to maintain remission over time [78].

Case reports and small case series have shown efficacy and safety of TCZ in the treatment of patients with relapsing/refractory TAK. Overall TCZ appeared to be effective for treating difficult-to-control TAK patients refractory to both non-biologic IS agents and anti-TNF-α agents [77–79]. A clinical response allowing taper of GC is observed and follow-up imaging parameters improve in most patients. However, the effect of TCZ on vascular inflammation is still unclear, and worsening of vascular lesions on imaging despite a favorable clinical and laboratory response has been reported. Because TCZ suppresses serum inflammatory markers (which are strongly IL-6-dependent) even in the absence of a significant clinical response, assessment of disease activity in TAK patients on TCZ should preferentially rely on a combination of clinical assessments and serial imaging studies [71]. Recently the results of the first randomized, double-blind, placebo-controlled, phase 3 trial evaluating the efficacy and safety of TCZ in patients with refractory TAK have been reported. Although the primary endpoint was not met (time to first relapse in the intent-to-treat population), the results suggest favor for TCZ over placebo for time to relapse of TAK without new safety concerns [80]. In clinical practice biological agents may be prescribed to patients with relapsing or GC-dependent TAK in case of synthetic IS failure. Both anti-TNF-α agents and TCZ seem equally effective and safe in TAK patients with relapsing disease. In case of a relapse under biological therapy, a switch to another biologic agent should be considered [71]. Large RCTs are required to generate convincing evidence of efficacy for both anti-TNF-α and anti-IL-6 (-receptor) therapies in TAK.

A recent RCT showed that abatacept is not an effective treatment for TAK. In this study the addition of abatacept to a treatment regimen with prednisone did not reduce the risk of relapse [81].

To date the data on the efficacy of ustekinumab and rituximab in both GCA and TAK are too preliminary to advocate their routine use in clinical practice [40,82]. Different RCTs assessing the efficacy and safety of biological agents in the treatment of GCA and TAK have been recently completed, and others are ongoing. Therefore, in the near future we will probably face a wider use of biological agents as second-line treatment for relapsing LVV and maybe as a first-line in patients with more severe prognosis or replacing GC treatment. The possible indications for biological treatment in patients with LVV should be better defined.

REFERENCES

[1] Hunder GG, Bloch DA, Michel BA, Stevens MB, Arend WP, Calabrese LH, et al. The American College of Rheumatology 1990 criteria for the classification of giant cell arteritis. Arthritis Rheum 1990;33:1122–8.

[2] Arend WP, Michel BA, Bloch DA, Hunder GG, Calabrese LH, Edworthy SM, et al. The American College of Rheumatology 1990 criteria for the classification of Takayasu arteritis. Arthritis Rheum 1990;33:1129–34.

[3] Brack A, Martinez-Taboada V, Stanson A, Goronzy JJ, Weyand CM. Disease pattern in cranial and large-vessel giant cell arteritis. Arthritis Rheum 1999;42:311–7.

[4] Muratore F, Kermani TA, Crowson CS, Green AB, Salvarani C, Matteson EL, et al. Large-vessel giant cell arteritis: a cohort study. Rheumatology (Oxf) 2015;54:463–70.

[5] Restuccia G, Cavazza A, Boiardi L, Pipitone N, Macchioni P, Bajocchi G, et al. Small-vessel vasculitis surrounding an uninflamed temporal artery and isolated vasa vasorum vasculitis of the temporal artery: two subsets of giant cell arteritis. Arthritis Rheum 2012;64:549–56.

[6] Cavazza A, Muratore F, Boiardi L, Restuccia G, Pipitone N, Pazzola G, et al. Inflamed temporal artery: histologic findings in 354 biopsies, with clinical correlations. Am J Surg Pathol 2014;38:1360–70.

[7] Pipitone N, Versari A, Salvarani C. Role of imaging studies in the diagnosis and follow-up of large-vessel vasculitis: an update. Rheumatology (Oxf) 2008;47:403–8.

[8] Direskeneli H, Aydin SZ, Kermani TA, Matteson EL, Boers M, Herlyn K, et al. Development of outcome measures for large-vessel vasculitis for use in clinical trials: opportunities, challenges, and research agenda. J Rheumatol 2011;38:1471–9.

[9] Karahaliou M, Vaiopoulos G, Papaspyrou S, Kanakis MA, Revenas K, Sfikakis PP. Colour duplex sonography of temporal arteries before decision for biopsy: a prospective study in 55 patients with suspected giant cell arteritis. Arthritis Res Ther 2006;8:R116.

[10] Craven A, Robson J, Ponte C, Grayson PC, Suppiah R, Judge A, et al. ACR/EULAR-endorsed study to develop diagnostic and classification criteria for vasculitis (DCVAS). Clin Exp Nephrol 2013;17:619–21.

[11] Salvarani C, Pipitone N, Versari A, Hunder GG. Clinical features of polymyalgia rheumatica and giant cell arteritis. Nat Rev Rheumatol 2012;8:509–21.

[12] Salvarani C, Cantini F, Hunder GG. Polymyalgia rheumatica and giant-cell arteritis. Lancet 2008;372:234–45.

[13] Samson M, Corbera-Bellalta M, Audia S, Planas-Rigol E, Martin L, Cid MC, et al. Recent advances in our understanding of giant cell arteritis pathogenesis. Autoimmun Rev 2017;16:833–44.

[14] Ciccia F, Rizzo A, Ferrante A, Guggino G, Croci S, Cavazza A, et al. New insights into the pathogenesis of giant cell arteritis. Autoimmun Rev 2017;16:675–83.

[15] Watanabe R, Hosgur E, Zhang H, Wen Z, Berry G, Goronzy JJ, et al. Pro-inflammatory and anti-inflammatory T cells in giant cell arteritis. Joint Bone Spine 2017;84:421–6.

[16] Zerbini A, Muratore F, Boiardi L, Ciccia F, Bonacini M, Belloni L, et al. Increased expression of interleukin-22 in patients with giant cell arteritis. Rheumatology (Oxf) 2018;57:64–72.

[17] Weyand CM, Goronzy JJ. Immune mechanisms in medium and large-vessel vasculitis. Nat Rev Rheumatol 2013;9:731–40.

[18] Wen Z, Shen Y, Berry G, Shahram F, Li Y, Watanabe R, et al. The microvascular niche instructs T cells in large vessel vasculitis via the VEGF-Jagged1-Notch pathway. Sci Transl Med 2017;9(399).

[19] Samson M, Ly KH, Tournier B, Janikashvili N, Trad M, Ciudad M, et al. Involvement and prognosis value of CD8(+) T cells in giant cell arteritis. J Autoimmun 2016;72:73–83.

[20] Zhang H, Watanabe R, Berry GJ, Vaglio A, Liao YJ, Warrington KJ, et al. Immunoinhibitory checkpoint deficiency in medium and large vessel vasculitis. Proc Natl Acad Sci USA 2017;114:E970–9.

[21] Ciccia F, Rizzo A, Maugeri R, Alessandro R, Croci S, Guggino G, et al. Ectopic expression of CXCL13, BAFF, APRIL and LT-β is associated with artery tertiary lymphoid organs in giant cell arteritis. Ann Rheum Dis 2017;76:235–43.

[22] van Sleen Y, Wang Q, van der Geest KSM, Westra J, Abdulahad WH, Heeringa P, et al. Involvement of monocyte subsets in the immunopathology of giant cell arteritis. Sci Rep 2017;7:6553.

[23] Croci S, Zerbini A, Boiardi L, Muratore F, Bisagni A, Nicoli D, et al. MicroRNA markers of inflammation and remodelling in temporal arteries from patients with giant cell arteritis. Ann Rheum Dis 2016;75:1527–33.

[24] Baldini M, Maugeri N, Ramirez GA, Giacomassi C, Castiglioni A, Prieto-González S, et al. Selective up-regulation of the soluble pattern-recognition receptor pentraxin 3 and of vascular endothelial growth factor in giant cell arteritis: relevance for recent optic nerve ischemia. Arthritis Rheum 2012;64:854–65.

[25] Pulsatelli L, Boiardi L, Assirelli E, Pazzola G, Muratore F, Addimanda O, et al. Interleukin-6 and soluble interleukin-6 receptor are elevated in large-vessel vasculitis: a cross-sectional and longitudinal study. Clin Exp Rheumatol 2017;35(Suppl. 103):102–10.

[26] van der Geest KS, Abdulahad WH, Rutgers A, Horst G, Bijzet J, Arends S, Roffel MP, et al. Serum markers associated with disease activity in giant cell arteritis and polymyalgia rheumatica. Rheumatology (Oxf) 2015;54:1397–402.

[27] Samson M, Audia S, Fraszczak J, Trad M, Ornetti P, Lakomy D, et al. Th1 and Th17 lymphocytes expressing CD161 are implicated in giant cell arteritis and polymyalgia rheumatica pathogenesis. Arthritis Rheum November 2012;64(11):3788–98.

[28] Wen Z, Shimojima Y, Shirai T, Li Y, Ju J, Yang Z, et al. NADPH oxidase deficiency underlies dysfunction of aged CD8+ Tregs. J Clin Investig 2016;126:1953–67.

[29] van der Geest KS, Abdulahad WH, Chalan P, Rutgers A, Horst G, Huitema MG, et al. Disturbed B cell homeostasis in newly diagnosed giant cell arteritis and polymyalgia rheumatica. Arthritis Rheumatol 2014;66:1927–38.

[30] Nadkarni S, Dalli J, Hollywood J, Mason JC, Dasgupta B, Perretti M. Investigational analysis reveals a potential role for neutrophils in giant-cell arteritis disease progression. Circ Res 2014;114:242–8.

[31] Coit P, De Lott LB, Nan B, Elner VM, Sawalha AH. DNA methylation analysis of the temporal artery microenvironment in giant cell arteritis. Ann Rheum Dis 2016;75:1196–202.

[32] Brack A, Geisler A, Martinez-Taboada VM, Younge BR, Goronzy JJ, Weyand CM. Giant cell vasculitis is a T cell-dependent disease. Mol Med 1997;3:530–43.

[33] Ma-Krupa W, Jeon MS, Spoerl S, Tedder TF, Goronzy JJ, Weyand CM. Activation of arterial wall dendritic cells and breakdown of self-tolerance in giant cell arteritis. J Exp Med 2004;199:173–83.

[34] Piggott K, Deng J, Warrington K, Younge B, Kubo JT, Desai M, et al. Blocking the NOTCH pathway inhibits vascular inflammation in large-vessel vasculitis. Circulation 2011;123:309–18.

[35] Deng J, Ma-Krupa W, Gewirtz AT, Younge BR, Goronzy JJ, Weyand CM. Toll-like receptors 4 and 5 induce distinct types of vasculitis. Circ Res 2009;104:488–95.

[36] Corbera-Bellalta M, Planas-Rigol E, Lozano E, Terrades-García N, Alba MA, Prieto-González S, et al. Blocking interferon γ reduces expression of chemokines CXCL9, CXCL10 and CXCL11 and decreases macrophage infiltration in ex vivo cultured arteries from patients with giant cell arteritis. Ann Rheum Dis 2016;75:1177–86.

[37] Planas-Rigol E, Terrades-Garcia N, Corbera-Bellalta M, Lozano E, Alba MA, Segarra M, et al. Endothelin-1 promotes vascular smooth muscle cell migration across the artery wall: a mechanism contributing to vascular remodelling and intimal hyperplasia in giant-cell arteritis. Ann Rheum Dis 2017;76:1624–34.

[38] Lozano E, Segarra M, García-Martínez A, Hernández-Rodríguez J, Cid MC. Imatinib mesylate inhibits in vitro and ex vivo biological responses related to vascular occlusion in giant cell arteritis. Ann Rheum Dis 2008;67:1581–8.

[39] Stone JH, Tuckwell K, Dimonaco S, Klearman M, Aringer M, Blockmans D, et al. Trial of tocilizumab in giant-cell arteritis. N Engl J Med 2017;377:317–28.

[40] Conway R, O'Neill L, O'Flynn E, Gallagher P, McCarthy GM, Murphy CC, et al. Ustekinumab for the treatment of refractory giant cell arteritis. Ann Rheum Dis 2016;75:1578–9.

[41] Muratore F, Pipitone N, Salvarani C, Schmidt WA. Imaging of vasculitis: state of the art. Best Pract Res Clin Rheumatol 2016;30:688–706.

[42] Salvarani C, Brown Jr RD, Hunder GG. Adult primary central nervous system vasculitis. Lancet 2012;380:767–77.

[43] Salvarani C, Brown Jr RD, Christianson T, Miller DV, Giannini C, Huston 3rd J, et al. An update of the Mayo Clinic cohort of patients with adult primary central nervous system vasculitis: description of 163 patients. Medicine (Baltim) 2015;94:e738.

[44] Salvarani C, Brown Jr RD, Huston 3rd J, Hunder GG. Prominent perivascular enhancement in primary central nervous system vasculitis. Clin Exp Rheumatol 2008;26(3 Suppl. 49):S111.

[45] Zuccoli G, Pipitone N, Haldipur A, Brown Jr RD, Hunder G, Salvarani C. Imaging findings in primary central nervous system vasculitis. Clin Exp Rheumatol 2011;29(1 Suppl. 64):S104–9.

[46] Stanson AW. Imaging findings in extracranial (giant cell) temporal arteritis. Clin Exp Rheumatol 2000;18:S43–8.

[47] Salvarani C, Brown Jr RD, Hunder GG. Adult primary central nervous system vasculitis: an update. Curr Opin Rheumatol 2012;24:46–52.

[48] Besson FL, Parienti JJ, Bienvenu B, Prior JO, Costo S, Bouvard G, et al. Diagnostic performance of (1)(8)F-fluorodeoxyglucose positron emission tomography in giant cell arteritis: a systematic review and meta-analysis. Eur J Nucl Med Mol Imaging 2011;38:1764–72.

[49] Meller J, Strutz F, Siefker U, Scheel A, Sahlmann CO, Lehmann K, et al. Early diagnosis and follow-up of aortitis with [(18)F]FDG PET and MRI. Eur J Nucl Med Mol Imaging 2003;30:730–6.

[50] Belhocine T, Blockmans D, Hustinx R, Vandevivere J, Mortelmans L. Imaging of large vessel vasculitis with (18)FDG PET: illusion or reality? A critical review of the literature data. Eur J Nucl Med Mol Imaging 2003;30:1305–13.

[51] Fuchs M, Briel M, Daikeler T, Walker UA, Rasch H, Berg S, et al. The impact of 18F-FDG PET on the management of patients with suspected large vessel vasculitis. Eur J Nucl Med Mol Imaging 2012;39:344–53.

[52] Iwabu M, Yamamoto Y, Dobashi H, Kameda T, Kittaka K, Nishiyama Y. F-18 FDG PET findings of Takayasu arteritis before and after immunosuppressive therapy. Clin Nucl Med 2008;33:872–3.

[53] Henes JC, Mueller M, Pfannenberg C, Kanz L, Koetter I. Cyclophosphamide for large vessel vasculitis: assessment of response by PET/CT. Clin Exp Rheumatol 2011;29:S43–8.

[54] de Leeuw K, Bijl M, Jager PL. Additional value of positron emission tomography in diagnosis and follow-up of patients with large vessel vasculitides. Clin Exp Rheumatol 2004;22:S21–6.

[55] Blockmans D, Bley T, Schmidt W. Imaging for large-vessel vasculitis. Curr Opin Rheumatol 2009;21:19–28.

[56] Schmidt WA, Kraft HE, Vorpahl K, Völker L, Gromnica-Ihle EJ. Color duplex ultrasonography in the diagnosis of temporal arteritis. N Engl J Med 1997;337:1336–42.

[57] Ball EL, Walsh SR, Tang TY, Gohil R, Clarke JM. Role of ultrasonography in the diagnosis of temporal arteritis. Br J Surg 2010;97:1765–71.

[58] Arida A, Kyprianou M, Kanakis M, Sfikakis PP. The diagnostic value of ultrasonography-derived edema of the temporal artery wall in giant cell arteritis: a second meta-analysis. BMC Musculoskelet Disord 2010;11:44.

[59] Muratore F, Boiardi L, Restuccia G, Macchioni P, Pazzola G, Nicolini A, et al. Comparison between colour duplex sonography findings and different histological patterns of temporal artery. Rheumatology (Oxf) 2013;52:2268–74.

[60] Hauenstein C, Reinhard M, Geiger J, Markl M, Hetzel A, Treszl A, et al. Effects of early corticosteroid treatment on magnetic resonance imaging and ultrasonography findings in giant cell arteritis. Rheumatology (Oxf) 2012;51:1999–2003.

[61] Diamantopoulos AP, Myklebust G. Long-term inflammation in the temporal artery of a giant cell arteritis patient as detected by ultrasound. Ther Adv Musculoskelet Dis 2014;6:102–3.

[62] Jennette JC, Falk RJ, Bacon PA, Basu N, Cid MC, Ferrario F, et al. 2012 revised international Chapel Hill consensus conference nomenclature of vasculitides. Arthritis Rheum 2013;65:1–11.

[63] Maksimowicz-McKinnon K, Clark TM, Hoffman GS. Takayasu arteritis and giant cell arteritis: a spectrum within the same disease? Medicine (Baltim) 2009;88:221–6.

[64] Polachek A, Pauzner R, Levartovsky D, Rosen G, Nesher G, Breuer G, et al. The fine line between Takayasu arteritis and giant cell arteritis. Clin Rheumatol 2015;34:721–7.

[65] Grayson PC, Maksimowicz-McKinnon K, Clark TM, Tomasson G, Cuthbertson D, Carette S, et al. Distribution of arterial lesions in Takayasu's arteritis and giant cell arteritis. Ann Rheum Dis 2012;71:1329–34.

[66] Mukhtyar C, Guillevin L, Cid MC, Dasgupta B, de Groot K, Gross W, et al. EULAR recommendations for the management of large vessel vasculitis. Ann Rheum Dis 2009;68:318–23.

[67] Dasgupta B, Borg FA, Hassan N, Alexander L, Barraclough K, Bourke B, et al. BSR and BHPR guidelines for the management of giant cell arteritis. Rheumatology (Oxf) 2010;49:1594–7.

[68] Soriano A, Muratore F, Pipitone N, Boiardi L, Cimino L, Salvarani C. Visual loss and other cranial ischaemic complications in giant cell arteritis. Nat Rev Rheumatol 2017;13:476–84.

[69] Proven A, Gabriel SE, Orces C, O'Fallon WM, Hunder GG. Glucocorticoid therapy in giant cell arteritis: duration and adverse outcomes. Arthritis Rheum 2003;49:703–8.

[70] Mahr AD, Jover JA, Spiera RF, Hernández-García C, Fernández-Gutiérrez B, Lavalley MP, et al. Adjunctive methotrexate for treatment of giant cell arteritis: an individual patient data meta-analysis. Arthritis Rheum 2007;56:2789–97.

[71] Muratore F, Pipitone N, Salvarani C. Standard and biological treatment in large vessel vasculitis: guidelines and current approaches. Expert Rev Clin Immunol 2017;13:345–60.

[72] Villiger PM, Adler S, Kuchen S, Wermelinger F, Dan D, Fiege V, et al. Tocilizumab for induction and maintenance of remission in giant cell arteritis: a phase 2, randomised, double-blind, placebo-controlled trial. Lancet 2016;387:1921–7.

[73] Adler S, Reichenbach S, Kuchen S, Wermelinger F, Dan D, Seitz M, et al. Termination of tocilizumab-treatment in giant cell arteritis: follow-up of patients after the RCT (ClinicalTrials.gov registration number: NCT01450137) [abstract]. Arthritis Rheumatol 2016;68(Suppl. 10).

[74] Langford CA, Cuthbertson D, Ytterberg SR, Khalidi N, Monach PA, Carette S, et al. A randomized, double-blind trial of abatacept (CTLA-4Ig) for the treatment of giant cell arteritis. Arthritis Rheumatol 2017;69:837–45.

[75] Kerr GS, Hallahan CW, Giordano J, Leavitt RY, Fauci AS, Rottem M, et al. Takayasu arteritis. Ann Intern Med 1994;120:919–29.

[76] Liang P, Hoffman GS. Advances in the medical and surgical treatment of Takayasu arteritis. Curr Opin Rheumatol 2005;17:16–24.

[77] Ferfar Y, Mirault T, Desbois AC, Comarmond C, Messas E, Savey L, et al. Biotherapies in large vessel vasculitis. Autoimmun Rev 2016;15:544–51.

[78] Clifford A, Hoffman GS. Recent advances in the medical management of Takayasu arteritis: an update on use of biologic therapies. Curr Opin Rheumatol 2014;26:7–15.

[79] Mekinian A, Comarmond C, Resche-Rigon M, Mirault T, Kahn JE, Lambert M, et al. Efficacy of biological-targeted treatments in Takayasu arteritis: multicenter, retrospective study of 49 patients. Circulation 2015;132:1693–700.

[80] Nakaoka Y, Isobe M, Takei S, Tanaka Y, Ishii T, Yokota S, et al. Efficacy and safety of tocilizumab in patients with refractory Takayasu arteritis: results from a randomised, double-blind, placebo-controlled, phase 3 trial in Japan (the TAKT study). Ann Rheum Dis November 30, 2017. pii: annrheumdis-2017–211878. [Epub ahead of print].

[81] Langford CA, Cuthbertson D, Ytterberg SR, Khalidi N, Monach PA, Carette S, et al. A randomized, double-blind trial of abatacept (CTLA-4Ig) for the treatment of Takayasu arteritis. Arthritis Rheumatol 2017;69:846–53.

[82] Pazzola G, Muratore F, Pipitone N, Crescentini F, Cacoub P, Boiardi L, et al. Rituximab therapy for Takayasu arteritis: a seven patients experience and a review of the literature. Rheumatology (Oxf) July 18, 2017. https://doi.org/10.1093/rheumatology/kex249. [Epub ahead of print].

Chapter 57

Personalized Medicine in Autoimmunity: Rheumatoid Arthritis as a Paradigm

Pier Luigi Meroni[1], Roberta Gualtierotti[2,3]

[1]Immunorheumatology Research Laboratory, IRCCS Istituto Auxologico Italiano, Milan, Italy; [2]Lupus Clinic, Department of Clinical Rheumatology and Medical Sciences, ASST Pini-CTO, Milan, Italy; [3]Department of Clinical Sciences and Community Health, University of Milan, Milan, Italy

INTRODUCTION

Personalized Medicine

It is widely accepted that a significant proportion of patients do not respond to treatments in an appropriate manner even when they are prescribed correctly. The most used drugs can help between 1 in 25 and 1 in 4 of the people who take them (imprecision medicine). Moreover, these treatments may also display severe side effects that make the drugs even harmful [1].

The main reason for that is linked to the individual variability, which in turn can be related to ethnicity, genetic/epigenetic, or environmental causes. The best example is represented by drugs that are not beneficial or even harmful for a given ethnic group because of the bias toward white Western participants in classical clinical trials used for the registration of the drug.

In contrast to "imprecision medicine," in which disease treatment and prevention strategies are developed for the average person with less consideration for the individual differences, there is the emerging approach for the "precision medicine." Such an approach is intended to use/predict more accurately which treatment and prevention strategies for a particular disease will work in a given group of patients. To do this, individual variability in genes, environment, and lifestyle is taken into account for tailoring the best treatment/prevention [1,2].

Although the term "precision medicine" is relatively new, the concept is old and has been a part of our daily life. For example, a person who needs a blood transfusion is not given blood from a randomly selected donor; instead, the donor's blood type is matched to the recipient to reduce the risk of adverse reactions. The most recent application of precision medicine is in oncology, where it focuses on matching the most accurate and effective treatment to each individual cancer patient based on the genetic profile of the cancer and the individual [3].

The role of precision medicine in day-to-day health care is relatively limited, being a young and growing field. Many of the needed technologies are in the early stages of development or have not yet been developed or are not easily available on a large scale (e.g., genetic biomarkers). For example, researchers will need to collect a huge series of genetic, serological, biochemical, and diagnostic imaging data ("big data") to set up new tools for health stakeholders to put in practice personalized medicine. Other issues are costs of the techniques used for precision medicine as well as the need to teach doctors and other health-care providers how to use these tools appropriately. Additionally, drugs that are developed to target a person's genetic or molecular characteristics are likely to be expensive, and their reimbursement from third-party payers is also likely to become an issue.

Autoimmune Diseases and Personalized Medicine

Autoimmune diseases represent a large and heterogeneous group of disorders, in which the loss of tolerance against a self-antigen triggers an autoimmune-mediated inflammatory tissue damage that is responsible of variegated clinical manifestations depending on the involved tissue/organ. Despite such heterogeneity, autoimmune patients have been treated for many years with a limited panel of immunosuppressive drugs aimed at downregulating the immune response and the consequent inflammation in a nonspecific manner [4]. Following the emergence of different biological drugs that target some specific pathogenic mediators and/or signaling pathways (e.g., monoclonal antibodies, intracellular signaling), autoimmune patients have been treated in a more precise manner [5]. Nevertheless, most of the patients are receiving these drugs in a relatively blind manner. Tumor necrosis factor (TNF) inhibitors represent the best example. In fact, TNF plays a pathogenic role in several chronic inflammatory autoimmune disorders, but its blocking by means of TNF inhibitors has been reported to be associated with inadequate response or intolerance in some patients with certain types of autoimmune diseases [6]. The same is also true for rituximab, an anti-CD20 monoclonal antibody that depletes B cells. It has been used in several systemic autoimmune conditions in which a B-lymphocyte response is thought to play a key role, but with contrasting results [7,8]. This suggests once more that different pathogenic pathways are taking place at the same time or in sequence, and that we still are not able to "personalize" our treatments. In addition, we do not have sound evidence for biomarkers that can predict the response for a given treatment.

On the other hand, we have useful biomarkers for the diagnosis and subgrouping of autoimmune diseases. This is the case of serum autoantibodies, which in several cases are actually formal classification/diagnostic tools [9]. Moreover, some autoantibodies are associated with disease activity or specific organ damage being quite useful in the clinical practice for subgrouping the patients and also for monitoring the response to the treatment [9]. Certain autoantibodies can be detected even years before the full-blown disease appears, and their value in predicting the risk of developing a given disease is emerging [10].

Additional biomarkers such as single nucleotide polymorphisms of different genes, noncoding RNAs, and epigenetic biomarkers are under active investigation, but sound evidence for their use in the clinical practice is still a matter of study [11–15].

RHEUMATOID ARTHRITIS AS A GOOD EXAMPLE FOR PERSONALIZED MEDICINE

Rheumatoid arthritis (RA) is an autoimmune chronic inflammatory systemic disorder characterized by destructive synovitis. RA affects approximately 1% of the adult population, with a higher prevalence in women and increasing with the age. Left untreated, RA patients experience progressive, destructive joint disease leading to reduced physical function, impaired quality of life, and increased risk for comorbidity and premature death disease (e.g., accelerated atherosclerosis and cardiovascular events) [16]. The economic and social impact of the disease is huge because of the high direct and indirect costs [17].

Recent guidelines recommend an early diagnosis to start the treatment as soon as possible. In addition, a close monitoring to reach and maintain a low disease activity is strongly suggested. Such an approach was found to prevent tissue damage/disability and cardiovascular comorbidities [18]. On the other hand, the clinical course and outcome vary widely among individuals, as well as the response to the available therapies. Clinical trials are mandatory for evaluating the efficacy/safety of the new therapies, but the results are frequently far from the clinical real life because of the heterogeneity of the patients linked to ethnic and geopolitical differences [19].

The main unmet needs in RA are still represented by the requirement of an early diagnosis and by the choice of the most appropriate therapy. Efforts are made nowadays to identify new tools (biomarkers) that can be useful to meet such needs in a "personalized" manner (Fig. 57.1) [6,16].

Serological Rheumatoid Arthritis Markers

The diagnosis of RA is made on the basis of clinical symptoms, imaging, and laboratory parameters [20]. The detection of autoantibodies associated with the disorder in 50%–80% of RA patients represents a useful diagnostic/classification tool. According to their presence or absence, subgroups of patients have been identified with more homogeneous characteristics regarding the disease aggressivity [21].

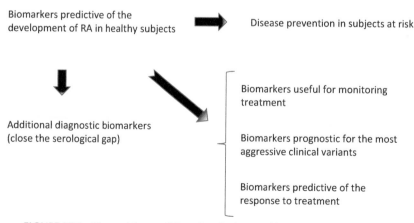

FIGURE 57.1 The need for novel biomarkers in rheumatoid arthritis (RA) management.

Rheumatoid factor (RF) is the first autoantibody reported in RA; it is directed against the Fc part of human IgG and can be detected in autoimmune conditions other than RA, in infectious disorders and in healthy elderlies. Despite its low specificity, it was included in the 1987 ACR classification criteria for RA. Anti-citrullinated protein antibodies (ACPA) were then described to be more-specifically associated with RA [22,23]. Both RF and ACPA have been included in the recent ACR-EULAR 2010 classification criteria for RA as the serological classification/diagnostic biomarkers. The detection of ACPA in patients negative for RF represents an important diagnostic help; in addition, the presence of ACPA may help in particular cases when the occurrence of RF could be due to causes unrelated to RA (e.g., in elderly patients or hepatitis B and C infection). Besides the diagnostic utility, the presence of RF and/or ACPA is associated with increased radiographic progression and joint damage [24]. Altogether, these findings may explain why these two biomarkers offer a better chance for an early diagnosis and a more personalized RA treatment.

However, a significant proportion of RA patients is negative for RF and ACPA, making the diagnosis more difficult or delayed. Because of the need of an early diagnosis and a prompt treatment to avoid tissue damage (i.e., window of opportunity), new diagnostic biomarkers have been recently described.

In addition to citrullination, another posttranslational modification of proteins has been described in RA: carbamylation. Anti-carbamylated protein antibodies (Anti-CarP) antibodies have been described in RA. Carbamylation is a chemical reaction mediated by cyanide in which a lysine is converted into a homocitrulline. Inflammation as well as renal disease and smoking can increase cyanide levels and thus carbamylation [25]. However, the increase of carbamylation by itself does not seem to be responsible for the occurrence of anti-CarP response, because these autoantibodies are much more frequent in RA than in patients with renal disorders [26]. Despite the similarity between citrullination and carbamylation, ACPA and anti-CarP antibodies are different non–cross-reacting autoantibodies, being anti-CarP present in both ACPA-positive and ACPA-negative patients [27]. While anti-CarP testing does not seem to improve our diagnostic power for RA, there is preliminary evidence that anti-CarP autoantibodies are associated with radiographic progression in patients negative for RF and ACPA. The last finding suggests a more aggressive treatment in these patients [27–29]. In addition, anti-CarP antibodies have been described in EORA even in the absence of RF or ACPA, being useful in making the correct diagnosis especially in patients with polymyalgia rheumatica overlapping manifestations [30]. Table 57.1 reports the main take-home messages on anti-CarP autoantibodies as an additional biomarker that may be useful in RA-personalized medicine.

Antibodies against peptidyl-arginine deiminase (PAD) antigens have been also reported in RA patients [33,34]. PAD proteins are calcium-dependent enzymes that catalyze the production of citrullinated proteins which represent key antigenic targets in RA. A recent study described a subset of autoantibodies cross-reacting between PAD3 and PAD4; these autoantibodies induce a gain of function of the enzymatic proteins thereby increasing the catalytic efficiency of PAD4 and consequently the production of citrullinated proteins [33]. Besides their potential pathogenic role, these antibodies are also associated with higher baseline radiographic damage and a higher risk of disease progression [34] In conclusion, antibodies cross-reacting with PAD3/PAD3 molecules might represent promising markers to predict joint damage in RA and to be used for tuning our therapeutic approach to the disease.

Furthermore, there is preliminary evidence that the profile of conjoined autoantibodies might be relevant for characterizing distinct phenotypes of RA patients [35]. It is tempting to speculate that such autoantibody profiles will be investigated in the future for their predictive role for disease activity and response to therapy.

RF, ACPA, and anti-CarP antibodies have been also evaluated for their predictive value for RA development in asymptomatic positive subjects. Although with some differences among them, basically all these biomarkers have been shown to predict the development of the disease [36,37]. Consequently, these autoantibodies together with genetic markers (e.g., shared epitope) and cigarette smoking have been included among the markers to identify subjects at risk for RA and potentially eligible for preventive treatment [38].

TABLE 57.1 Anti-Carbamylated Protein Antibodies (anti-CarP) Autoantibodies: Take-Home Messages

- Anti-CarP autoantibodies are distinct Abs from ACPA
- Anti-CarP can be found in ACPA neg RA patients
- Diagnostic classification of RA patients did not improve by adding anti-CarP testing, as RF and ACPA are already good predictors for disease
- Anti-CarP autoantibodies can predict joint damage independently from ACPA
- Anti-CarP are frequent in EORA
- Anti-CarP autoantibodies can be found in JIA [31]
- Anti-CarP autoantibodies can be associated with erosions in SLE and primary SS [32]

Personalized Treatment in Rheumatoid Arthritis

Disease-modifying antirheumatic drugs (DMARDs) target inflammatory mechanisms and have been shown to reduce tissue damage particularly in the joints. DMARDs are divided into two classes: synthetic and biological. Synthetic DMARDs are further defined as conventional or targeted drugs [16]. Whereas conventional synthetic DMARDs have been empirically used in RA because of their effect on the immune-mediated inflammatory responses, by contrast, targeted synthetic DMARDs have been developed to target inflammatory pathways involved in RA pathogenesis (e.g., JAK inhibitors). In addition, biological DMARDs have been developed in the last decade targeting proinflammatory mediators (e.g., TNF, IL-6) and T or B cells, via T-cell costimulation blockade or cell depletion, that have been shown to play a pathogenic role in RA. However, irrespective of their targets, all DMARDs achieve similar therapeutic effects in RA patients suggesting that their use is still empiric as the conventional immunosuppressive therapy [6,16]. Although there is evidence that rituximab and abatacept therapy is more effective in RA patients positive for RF and ACPA, the choice of the biological DMARD is still based on the safety profile rather than on the predictive efficacy of the molecule [6,16].

Patients may never respond to treatment (primary failure) or display loss of response after an initial efficacy of the treatment (secondary failure). The reason(s) of the primary failure is still matter of debate and only in part due to the "pathotype" of the patient. In other words, a given biological DMARD is targeting a pathogenic pathway that is not actually responsible for the disease. This issue has been more investigated regarding the TNF inhibitors. A primary failure to TNF blocking was related to the fact that non-TNF-mediated pathogenic pathways are taking place in the nonresponder patient, suggesting a switch to molecules affecting different pathways (e.g., IL-6 or T- or B-cell blockade). A lack of response defined as a reduction of DAS 28 < 1.2 within 16 weeks in a patient treated with a TNF inhibitor for the first time is considered a primary failure. Effectiveness of TNF inhibitor can also disappear after the initial response; an increase of DAS20 > 0.6 or of the EULAR disease activity score suggests a secondary treatment failure [39]. There is evidence that the production of ADA is mainly responsible for the secondary failure by blocking the binding activity of the TNF inhibitors (neutralizing antibodies) or enhancing their clearance as immune complexes [40]. In other words, the occurrence of ADA is associated with a reduced plasma level of the TNF inhibitor and at the same time with a poorer clinical response. Consequently, the detection of ADA and at the same time the measurement of the drug plasma levels have been suggested as useful tools for identifying patients at risk for a secondary failure due to the presence of ADA. Fig. 57.2 reports algorithms that have been suggested to "personalize" the treatment with TNF inhibitors as a recent example of personalized medicine in RA.

Notably, a therapeutic unresponsiveness has been reported also for methotrexate (MTX), the first-line conventional synthetic DMARD for RA. In addition to its antifolate effect, MTX also reduces inflammation by maintaining high levels of extracellular adenosine (ADO). The extracellular ADO production mediated by CD39/CD73 is highly expressed on the Treg surface and was thought to be pivotal for their suppressive activity. A recent study showed that low expression of CD39 on regulatory T cells may be a useful biomarker predicting the resistance to MTX [41]. If confirmed, this finding may suggest that the detection of low CD39 expression on peripheral Tregs could be a noninvasive biomarker for identifying/predicting MTX-resistant RA patients.

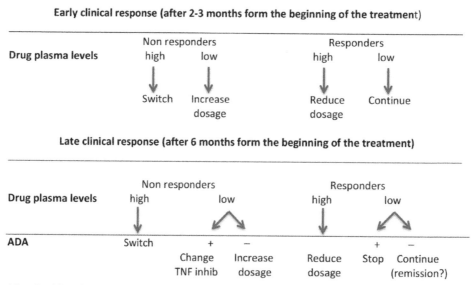

FIGURE 57.2   Decision algorithm of tumor necrosis factor (TNF) inhibitor therapy based on drug and antidrug antibodies (ADA) plasma levels.

CONCLUSIONS

Personalized medicine aimed at treating and preventing the diseases is the current trend in all the medical branches.

Efforts in putting personalized medicine in practice in patients suffering from autoimmune disorders are recent and still lacking appropriate tools. Nevertheless, preliminary results with the available biomarkers are promising. We reported in this article the evidence for personalized medicine in RA as a prototype example.

LIST OF ABBREVIATIONS

ACPA Anti-citrullinated protein antibodies
ADA Antidrug antibodies
ADO Adenosine
anti-CarP Anti-carbamylated protein antibodies
DAS 28 Disease activity score 28
DMARDs Disease-modifying antirheumatic drugs
EORA Elderly-onset RA
IL Interleukin
JIA Juvenile idiopathic arthritis
MTX Methotrexate
PAD Peptidyl-arginine deiminase
RA Rheumatoid arthritis
RF Rheumatoid factor
SLE Systemic lupus erythematosus
SS Sjögren syndrome
TNF Tumor necrosis factor

REFERENCES

[1] Schork NJ. Personalized medicine: time for one-person trials. Nature 2015;520(7549):609–11.

[2] Tavakolpour S. Towards personalized medicine for patients with autoimmune diseases: opportunities and challenges. Immunol Lett 2017;190:130–8.

[3] Maciejko L, Smalley M, Goldman A. Cancer immunotherapy and personalized medicine: emerging technologies and biomarker-based approaches. J Mol Biomark Diagn 2017;8(5).

[4] Pozsgay J, Szekanecz Z, Sarmay G. Antigen-specific immunotherapies in rheumatic diseases. Nat Rev Rheumatol 2017;13(9):525–37.

[5] Wolfe RM, Ang DC. Biologic therapies for autoimmune and connective tissue diseases. Immunol Allergy Clin N Am 2017;37(2):283–99.

[6] Smolen JS, Aletaha D. Rheumatoid arthritis therapy reappraisal: strategies, opportunities and challenges. Nat Rev Rheumatol 2015;11(5):276–89.

[7] Buch MH. Sequential use of biologic therapy in rheumatoid arthritis. Curr Opin Rheumatol 2010;22(3):321–9.

[8] Looney RJ, Anolik J, Sanz I. B cells as therapeutic targets for rheumatic diseases. Curr Opin Rheumatol 2004;16(3):180–5.

[9] Meroni PL, Biggioggero M, Pierangeli SS, Sheldon J, Zegers I, Borghi MO. Standardization of autoantibody testing: a paradigm for serology in rheumatic diseases. Nat Rev Rheumatol 2014;10(1):35–43.

[10] Arbuckle MR, McClain MT, Rubertone MV, Scofield RH, Dennis GJ, James JA, et al. Development of autoantibodies before the clinical onset of systemic lupus erythematosus. N Engl J Med 2003;349(16):1526–33.

[11] Deng Y, Tsao BP. Advances in lupus genetics and epigenetics. Curr Opin Rheumatol 2014;26(5):482–92.

[12] Hedrich CM, Tsokos GC. Epigenetic mechanisms in systemic lupus erythematosus and other autoimmune diseases. Trends Mol Med 2011;17(12):714–24.

[13] Hammaker D, Firestein GS. Epigenetics of inflammatory arthritis. Curr Opin Rheumatol 2018 Mar;30(2):188–96.

[14] Richardson BC, Patel DR. Epigenetics in 2013. DNA methylation and miRNA: key roles in systemic autoimmunity. Nat Rev Rheumatol 2014;10(2):72–4.

[15] Kolarz B, Majdan M. Epigenetic aspects of rheumatoid arthritis: contribution of non-coding RNAs. Semin Arthritis Rheum 2017;46(6):724–31.

[16] Smolen JS, Aletaha D, McInnes IB. Rheumatoid arthritis. Lancet 2016;388(10055):2023–38.

[17] Furneri G, Mantovani LG, Belisari A, Mosca M, Cristiani M, Bellelli S, et al. Systematic literature review on economic implications and pharmacoeconomic issues of rheumatoid arthritis. Clin Exp Rheumatol 2012;30(4 Suppl. 73):S72–84.

[18] Smolen JS, Landewe R, Bijlsma J, Burmester G, Chatzidionysiou K, Dougados M, et al. EULAR recommendations for the management of rheumatoid arthritis with synthetic and biological disease-modifying antirheumatic drugs: 2016 update. Ann Rheum Dis 2017;76(6):960–77.

[19] Currie GP, Lee DK, Lipworth BJ. Long-acting beta2-agonists in asthma: not so SMART? Drug Saf 2006;29(8):647–56.

[20] Aletaha D, Neogi T, Silman AJ, Funovits J, Felson DT, Bingham 3rd CO, et al. 2010 rheumatoid arthritis classification criteria: an American College of Rheumatology/European League against Rheumatism collaborative initiative. Ann Rheum Dis 2010;69(9):1580–8.

[21] Derksen V, Huizinga TWJ, van der Woude D. The role of autoantibodies in the pathophysiology of rheumatoid arthritis. Semin Immunopathol 2017;39(4):437–46.

[22] Schellekens GA, de Jong BA, van den Hoogen FH, van de Putte LB, van Venrooij WJ. Citrulline is an essential constituent of antigenic determinants recognized by rheumatoid arthritis-specific autoantibodies. J Clin Invest 1998;101(1):273–81.

[23] Schellekens GA, Visser H, de Jong BA, van den Hoogen FH, Hazes JM, Breedveld FC, et al. The diagnostic properties of rheumatoid arthritis antibodies recognizing a cyclic citrullinated peptide. Arthritis Rheum 2000;43(1):155–63.

[24] van der Helm-van Mil AH, Verpoort KN, Breedveld FC, Toes RE, Huizinga TW. Antibodies to citrullinated proteins and differences in clinical progression of rheumatoid arthritis. Arthritis Res Ther 2005;7(5):R949–58.

[25] Wang Z, Nicholls SJ, Rodriguez ER, Kummu O, Horkko S, Barnard J, et al. Protein carbamylation links inflammation, smoking, uremia and atherogenesis. Nat Med 2007;13(10):1176–84.

[26] Verheul MK, van Erp SJ, van der Woude D, Levarht EW, Mallat MJ, Verspaget HW, et al. Anti-carbamylated protein antibodies: a specific hallmark for rheumatoid arthritis. Comparison to conditions known for enhanced carbamylation; renal failure, smoking and chronic inflammation. Ann Rheum Dis 2016;75(8):1575–6.

[27] Shi J, Knevel R, Suwannalai P, van der Linden MP, Janssen GM, van Veelen PA, et al. Autoantibodies recognizing carbamylated proteins are present in sera of patients with rheumatoid arthritis and predict joint damage. Proc Natl Acad Sci USA 2011;108(42):17372–7.

[28] Ajeganova S, van Steenbergen HW, Verheul MK, Forslind K, Hafstrom I, Toes RE, et al. The association between anti-carbamylated protein (anti-CarP) antibodies and radiographic progression in early rheumatoid arthritis: a study exploring replication and the added value to ACPA and rheumatoid factor. Ann Rheum Dis 2017;76(1):112–8.

[29] Yee A, Webb T, Seaman A, Infantino M, Meacci F, Manfredi M, et al. Anti-CarP antibodies as promising marker to measure joint damage and disease activity in patients with rheumatoid arthritis. Immunol Res 2015;61(1–2):24–30.

[30] Lopez-Hoyos M, Alvarez-Rodriguez L, Mahler M, Torices S, Calvo-Alen J, Villa I, et al. Anti-carbamylated protein antibodies in patients with ageing associated inflammatory chronic disorders. Rheumatology (Oxford) 2016;55(4):764–6.

[31] Muller PC, Anink J, Shi J, Levarht EW, Reinards TH, Otten MH, et al. Anticarbamylated protein (anti-CarP) antibodies are present in sera of juvenile idiopathic arthritis (JIA) patients. Ann Rheum Dis 2013;72(12):2053–5.

[32] Bergum B, Koro C, Delaleu N, Solheim M, Hellvard A, Binder V, et al. Antibodies against carbamylated proteins are present in primary Sjogren's syndrome and are associated with disease severity. Ann Rheum Dis 2016;75(8):1494–500.

[33] Auger I, Martin M, Balandraud N, Roudier J. Rheumatoid arthritis-specific autoantibodies to peptidyl arginine deiminase type 4 inhibit citrullination of fibrinogen. Arthritis Rheum 2010;62(1):126–31.

[34] Auger I, Charpin C, Balandraud N, Martin M, Roudier J. Autoantibodies to PAD4 and BRAF in rheumatoid arthritis. Autoimmun Rev 2012;11(11):801–3.

[35] Derksen VF, Ajeganova S, Trouw LA, van der Helm-van Mil AH, Hafstrom I, Huizinga TW, et al. Rheumatoid arthritis phenotype at presentation differs depending on the number of autoantibodies present. Ann Rheum Dis 2017;76(4):716–20.

[36] Shi J, van de Stadt LA, Levarht EW, Huizinga TW, Hamann D, van Schaardenburg D, et al. Anti-carbamylated protein (anti-CarP) antibodies precede the onset of rheumatoid arthritis. Ann Rheum Dis 2014;73(4):780–3.

[37] Brink M, Verheul MK, Ronnelid J, Berglin E, Holmdahl R, Toes RE, et al. Anti-carbamylated protein antibodies in the pre-symptomatic phase of rheumatoid arthritis, their relationship with multiple anti-citrulline peptide antibodies and association with radiological damage. Arthritis Res Ther 2015;17:25.

[38] van Steenbergen HW, da Silva JAP, Huizinga TWJ, van der Helm-van Mil AHM. Preventing progression from arthralgia to arthritis: targeting the right patients. Nat Rev Rheumatol 2018;14(1):32–41.

[39] Kalden JR, Schulze-Koops H. Immunogenicity and loss of response to TNF inhibitors: implications for rheumatoid arthritis treatment. Nat Rev Rheumatol 2017;13(12):707–18.

[40] Prado MS, Bendtzen K, Andrade LEC. Biological anti-TNF drugs: immunogenicity underlying treatment failure and adverse events. Expert Opin Drug Metab Toxicol 2017;13(9):985–95.

[41] Peres RS, Liew FY, Talbot J, Carregaro V, Oliveira RD, Almeida SL, et al. Low expression of CD39 on regulatory T cells as a biomarker for resistance to methotrexate therapy in rheumatoid arthritis. Proc Natl Acad Sci USA 2015;112(8):2509–14.

Chapter 58

Biologics and Biosimilars

Fabiola Atzeni[1], Giuseppe Barilaro[2], Piercarlo Sarzi-Puttini[3]

[1]*Rheumatology Unit, Department of Clinical and Experimental Medicine, University of Messina, Messina, Italy;* [2]*Department of Internal Medicine, ASST Rhodense, Milan, Italy;* [3]*Rheumatology Unit, L. Sacco University Hospital, Milan, Italy*

INTRODUCTION

Biological drugs have greatly improved the outcomes of patients with chronic inflammatory diseases, but access to them is limited by their high cost [1], which means that many patients are unlikely to receive them even as second-line treatment. To make them more widely available, cheaper biosimilar versions of the products that are no longer protected by a patent have been developed. Biosimilars of adalimumab, etanercept, infliximab, and rituximab have been approved and are now marketed in the European Union (EU), the United States, Japan, and other countries.

In some countries, the health-care system is overseen by the government, which acts as a single payer of the costs of medical treatment for its citizens; others (such as the United States) have a variety of systems aimed at ensuring public access to health care: some patients are covered by government-supported insurance plans, others purchase private insurance policies, and some have no health insurance at all. These differences need to be borne in mind when selecting the most appropriate drugs for individual patients.

The aim of this chapter is to consider the advantages and disadvantages of using biosimilars to treat rheumatoid arthritis (RA) and spondyloarthritis (SpA).

DEFINITION OF A BIOSIMILAR

A biosimilar is a replicate of a biopharmaceutical that meets the biosimilarity criteria of equivalent pharmacokinetics (PK) and pharmacodynamics (PD), as well as comparable efficacy, safety, and immunogenicity, and is approved by a regulatory authority. Many regulatory agencies are members of the International Council for Harmonisation of Technical Requirements for Pharmaceuticals for Human Use [2], which has the aim of recommending guidelines and requirements for the approval of pharmaceutical products to ensure harmonization worldwide.

The European Medicines Agency (EMA) defines a biosimilar as "a biological medicinal product that contains a version of the active substance of an already authorized" bio-originator, for which "similarity to the reference product in terms of quality characteristics, biological activity, safety and efficacy" has been demonstrated [3]. In the United States, a biosimilar is defined in the Biologics Price Competition and Innovation Act of 2009 as a biological product that is "highly similar to the reference product notwithstanding minor differences in clinically inactive components" and that "there are no clinically meaningful differences between the reference product and the biologic product in terms of the safety, purity and potency of the product" [4].

There are slight differences in the procedures for obtaining regulatory approval of a biosimilar between the EMA and the American Food and Drug Agency (FDA), but both require extensive analytical tests followed by clinical studies comparing the PK, PD, immunogenicity, efficacy, and safety of the proposed biosimilar with its bio-originator to confirm that there are "no clinical meaningful differences" between them. Many other countries have adopted a similar approach.

BIOSIMILARS: CLINICAL AND NONCLINICAL DATA

The first biosimilar approved in the United States was filgrastim-sndz, a biosimilar of the filgrastim granulocyte colony-stimulating factor, which is currently the only biosimilar specifically approved for oncological indications, although a proposed biosimilar of epoetin alfa is being reviewed by the FDA. Since then, the United States has approved four biosimilar monoclonal antibodies. The first was infliximab-dyyb, a biosimilar of the tumor necrosis factor alpha (TNF-α) inhibitor infliximab, which was approved on the basis of the findings of the phase I PLANETAS study of patients with ankylosing spondylitis (AS)

Mosaic of Autoimmunity. https://doi.org/10.1016/B978-0-12-814307-0.00058-X

and the phase III PLANETRA trial of patients with RA. The three other approved anti–TNF-α biosimilars (etanercept-szzs, adalimumab-atto, and infliximab-abda) are not yet available in the United States because of ongoing patent litigation.

EU regulators have licensed three biosimilars to treat rheumatic diseases: two infliximab (Remicade) biosimilars, CT-P13 (Remsima [5] and Inflectra [6]) and SB2 (Flixabi [7]), and one etanercept (Enbrel) biosimilar, SB4 (Benepali [8]), and a number of other biosimilars are under development. The next milestone in this therapeutic area will be the projected expiry of the EU adalimumab patent in April 2018. The aim of the next generation of biologics (sometimes referred to as biobetter agents) will be to improve the PK and PD of the available biologic agents.

Typical nonclinical studies of biosimilars are in vitro receptor-binding or cell-based assays to establish comparable reactivity but, if these fail to demonstrate comparability, additional animal studies to investigate the questions that were not answered by the nonclinical studies are required.

Biosimilarity is established by means of a series of comparative studies. It must be analytically demonstrated that a biosimilar and its bio-originator have the same primary amino acid sequence, and multiple batches of the two molecules must be tested over time to ensure that there are no significant differences in charge isoforms and glycosylation or other posttranslational modifications or impurities (there may be minor differences, but these must not affect the critical quality attributes of the biologic). In the case of therapeutic monoclonal antibodies, the essential functional properties include Fc receptor binding and both complement-dependent and antibody-dependent cytotoxicity. Subsequent clinical studies must demonstrate that the biosimilar is equivalent in terms of PK and PD, has equivalently efficacious effects on at least one disease for which the bio-originator has been approved, is comparably safe, and is not more immunogenic.

As the clinical data collected for the approval of a bio-originator can also be used for its biosimilar, the approval of the latter takes less time in the EU, United States, and most other countries. PK is usually tested by comparing single doses of the biosimilar and its bio-originator in healthy subjects [9–11], followed by multiple doses in patients [12]. Most regulatory agencies assume PK equivalence when 90% of the confidence intervals (CIs) of the ratios between the geometric mean area under the curve and maximum concentration of the biosimilar and its bio-originator fall within the log-transformed range of 80%–125% (±20%).

Phase III randomized controlled trials (RCTs) comparing the efficacy of a candidate biosimilar with that of its bio-originator should involve patients with a disease that is capable of potential differences between the two drugs. The EMA accepts two-sided therapeutic equivalence in comparative RCTs when the 95% CI of the mean absolute difference in the primary endpoint between the biosimilar and its bio-originator falls within the predefined margin of equivalence [3], but the FDA prefers the use of the narrower 90% CI [9].

Safety evaluations are also essential in the prelicensing assessment of biosimilars, and it is necessary to collect enough patient data to allow comparison with the reference product [13].

A biosimilar that has obtained regulatory approval is neither more nor less efficacious and at least as safe as its bio-originator.

IMMUNOGENICITY

Antidrug antibodies (ADAs) are frequently found in patients who have received biological treatment for a long time, and almost all monoclonal antibodies induce an immune response stimulating the production of often antiidiotype antibodies [14]. The binding of ADAs to therapeutic monoclonal antibodies may lead to the formation of immune complexes that, after being cleared by the reticuloendothelial system, lower trough drug concentrations and potentially decrease efficacy [15]. ADA assays have gradually become more sensitive and specific but, although trough drug concentrations are usually not routinely measured by rheumatologists in everyday clinical practice, they allow a more relevant indirect comparison of the immunogenicity of a biosimilar and its bio-originator than the detection of ADAs.

There is general concern that there may be differences in the immunogenicity of original drugs and their biosimilars because it may be affected by any posttranslational change. However, according to the EMA guidelines, an immunogenic response to biologics in humans cannot be predicted on the basis of nonclinical immunogenicity findings. ADAs to biosimilars do not need to be measured in clinical practice because no clinically significant difference in immunogenicity has been detected between biosimilars and their bio-originators [16,17]; however, assessing immunogenicity is useful for purposes of drug surveillance. Evaluating the comparative immunogenicity data acquired in the clinical and postmarketing studies may also increase the confidence of health-care providers in using biosimilars.

Biosimilars have only recently become available, and so many patients and health-care providers are not familiar with the concept underlying them, and some even think that their usually lower price raises questions concerning their quality. This is a misconception that can be corrected by providing more information not only about the nature of biosimilars but also the rigorous approval procedures they have to go through, and the fact that approved biosimilars are as safe and efficacious as their bio-originators.

A biosimilar that is authorized for marketing on the grounds that it is structurally highly similar and clinically equivalent to its bio-originator in a sensitive population can essentially be considered the same as a new batch of the original drug. However, it has been questioned whether its demonstrated similar efficacy and safety in one indication is sufficient to support its licensing for other diseases. On the basis of the extensive clinical experience acquired in each of the licensed indications of a biosimilar's bio-originator, regulatory agencies allow the efficacy and safety data to be extrapolated from one approved indication to others only if the mechanism(s) of action of the reference product is consistent in its different indications; otherwise, further evidence is required. Once it has been demonstrated that the efficacy and safety of a biosimilar is equivalent to that of its bio-originator in at least one RCT involving patients with a disease for which the bio-originator is authorized, its manufacturer is permitted to apply for a license in any or all of the indications for which the bio-originator has already been authorized without the need to further separate RCTs.

However, unlike nonbiological products, biosimilars have to undergo additional postmarketing safety monitoring because their shortened approval pathway may not have allowed the collection of sufficient long-term safety data. For example, one of the licensing conditions of Remsima in Europe was that it be entered in a mandatory postmarketing program that would monitor multiple registries until 2026 [18].

SWITCHING FROM A BIO-ORIGINATOR TO A BIOSIMILAR AND VICE VERSA

Switching patients from a bio-originator to its biosimilar, and from one biosimilar to another, needs to be based on evidence. A recent, government-funded, multicentre, randomized, double-blind, phase IV study carried out in Norway (NOR-SWITCH) assessed the safety and efficacy of switching patients from reference infliximab (Remicade) to Remsima. Four hundred and ninety-eight patients with various stable chronic inflammatory diseases who had been treated with Remicade for at least 6 months were randomized 1:1 to switch to Remsima or continue treatment with Remicade for 52 weeks. It was found that the incidence of ADAs and adverse events and the values of generic and specific disease measures were similar in the groups and the fact that there was no statistically significant difference in disease worsening between the groups confirmed the noninferiority of Remsima.

We have carried out a small study involving 41 patients with a previous diagnosis of SpA and clinically inactive or moderate disease activity who had been treated with innovator INX in accordance with the ASAS/EULAR guidelines for more than 6 months. They were switched to biosimilar INX for pharmacoeconomic reasons (Tuscany Law No. 450 of 7 April 2015), and the results showed that the switch was not associated with any statistically significant difference in efficacy, adverse events, or ADA levels [19].

The albeit small number of switching studies carried out so far has shown that switching a reference product and approved biosimilar does not affect treatment efficacy or safety as either should lead to comparable results. However, the efficacy and safety of switching between two biosimilars of the same bio-originator has not yet been studied, although crucial real-world data should come from national and regional registries and postmarketing studies.

The competition arising the introduction of infliximab and etanercept biosimilars in the EU has reduced the prices of their reference products and those of other original TNF inhibitors [19]. Patients with even still active rheumatological diseases may hesitate when it is suggested that they should change their treatment because they are afraid that their disease may worsen or they may develop an unfamiliar adverse effect, but the data published so far suggest that neither of these fears is founded when switching from a bio-originator to its biosimilar. However, until appropriate studies have been carried, it is not recommended to switch from one biosimilar to another or to make repeated switches between a bio-originator and its biosimilar.

CONCLUSIONS

Biosimilars extend access to effective medications by increasing the range of available choices and helping to limit currently increasing drug expenditure, and it is expected that this will allow patients to receive effective biological treatment at appropriate times during the course of their disease. The effectiveness and safety of biosimilars in clinical practice is being monitored, and there is growing evidence that patients can be safely switched to them. One important question to be answered by future research is how to approach multiple switching as the number of biosimilars increases.

REFERENCES

[1] Kay J. Biosimilars: a regulatory perspective from America. Arthritis Res Ther 2011;13(3):112.

[2] The international council for harmonisation of technical requirements for pharmaceuticals for human use. ICH official website. 2017. http://www.ich.org/. [Internet].

[3] Committee for Medicinal Products for Human Use. Guideline on similar biological medicinal products. 2014. http://www.ema.europa.eu/docs/en_GB/document_library/Scientific_guideline/2014/10/WC500176768.pdf. [Internet].

[4] Biologics price competition and innovation act of 2009. In: United States code. 111th congress. 2nd session edn. United States. 2010. p. 804–21.

[5] Remsima summary of product characteristics. www.ema.europa.eu/docs/en_GB/document_library/EPAR_-_Product_Information/human/002576/. [Internet].

[6] Inflectra summary of product characteristics. http://wwwema.europa.eu/docs/en_GB/document_library/EPAR_-_Product_Information/human/002778/WC500151489.pdf. [Internet].

[7] European Medicines Agency. Summary of opinion (initial authorization). Flixabi; April 1, 2016. http://www.ema.europa.eu/docs/en_GB/document_library/Summary_of_opinion_-_Initial_authorisation/human/004020/WC500203991.pdf.

[8] Benepali Summary of Product Characteristics. www.medicines.org.uk/emc/medicine/31511. [Internet].

[9] Gu N, Yi S, Kim TE, Kim J, Shin SG, Jang IJ, et al. Comparative pharmacokinetics and tolerability of branded etanercept (25 mg) and its biosimilar (25 mg): a randomized, open-label, single-dose, two-sequence, crossover study in healthy Korean male volunteers. Clin Ther 2011;33(12):2029–37.

[10] Park W, Lee SJ, Yun J, Yoo DH. Comparison of the pharmacokinetics and safety of three formulations of infliximab (CT-P13, EU-approved reference infliximab and the US-licensed reference infliximab) in healthy subjects: a randomized, double-blind, three-arm, parallel-group, single-dose, Phase I study. Expert Rev Clin Immunol 2015;11(Suppl. 1):S25–31.

[11] Yi S, Kim SE, Park MK, Yoon SH, Cho JY, Lim KS, et al. Comparative pharmacokinetics of HD203, a biosimilar of etanercept, with marketed etanercept (Enbrel(R)): a double-blind, single-dose, crossover study in healthy volunteers. BioDrugs 2012;26(3):177–84.

[12] Park W, Hrycaj P, Jeka S, Kovalenko V, Lysenko G, Miranda P, et al. A randomised, double-blind, multicentre, parallel-group, prospective study comparing the pharmacokinetics, safety, and efficacy of CT-P13 and innovator infliximab in patients with ankylosing spondylitis: the PLANETAS study. Ann Rheum Dis 2013;72(10):1605–12.

[13] Calvo B, Zuniga L. EU's new pharmacovigilance legislation: considerations for biosimilars. Drug Saf 2014;37(1):9–18.

[14] van Schouwenburg PA, van de Stadt LA, de Jong RN, van Buren EE, Kruithof S, de Groot E, et al. Adalimumab elicits a restricted anti-idiotypic antibody response in autoimmune patients resulting in functional neutralisation. Ann Rheum Dis 2013;72(1):104–9.

[15] van Schouwenburg PA, Rispens T, Wolbink GJ. Immunogenicity of anti-TNF biologic therapies for rheumatoid arthritis. Nat Rev Rheumatol 2013;9(3):164–72.

[16] Ben-Horin S, Yavzori M, Benhar I, Fudim E, Picard O, Ungar B, et al. Cross-immunogenicity: antibodies to infliximab in Remicade-treated patients with IBD similarly recognise the biosimilar Remsima. Gut 2016;65(7):1132–8.

[17] Ruiz-Arguello MB, Maguregui A, Ruiz Del Agua A, Pascual-Salcedo D, Martinez-Feito A, Jurado T, et al. Antibodies to infliximab in Remicade-treated rheumatic patients show identical reactivity towards biosimilars. Ann Rheum Dis 2016;75(9):1693–6.

[18] Isaacs JD, Cutolo M, Keystone EC, Park W, Braun J. Biosimilars in immune-mediated inflammatory diseases: initial lessons from the first approved biosimilar anti-tumour necrosis factor monoclonal antibody. J Intern Med 2016;279(1):41–59.

[19] Benucci M, Gobbi FL, Bandinelli F, Damiani A, Infantino M, Grossi V, et al. Safety, efficacy and immunogenicity of switching from innovator to biosimilar infliximab in patients with spondyloarthritis: a 6-month real-life observational study. Immunol Res 2017;65(1):419–22.

FURTHER READING

[1] IMS Health. The impact of biosimilar competition. London, UK: IMS Health Inc. 2016. p. 1–30.

Chapter 59

Small Molecules

Yoshiya Tanaka

The First Department of Internal Medicine, School of Medicine, University of Occupational and Environmental Health, Japan, Kitakyushu, Japan

Rheumatoid arthritis (RA) is a representative systemic autoimmune disease characterized with chronic and destructive inflammatory synovitis and multiple organ manifestations that cause severe disability and mortality. Autoreactive T cells and inflammatory cytokines play a pivotal role during the pathological processes of RA through the accumulation of inflammatory cells, the self-perpetuation of inflammation, and production of matrix metalloproteinase and induction and/or activation of osteoclasts, leading to destruction of cartilage and bone. Because such a joint damage derived from synovial inflammation is apparent in the early stage of the disease, it is required to treat patients at a stage when the evolution of joint destruction can still be prevented. However, the combined use of methotrexate (MTX), a standard synthetic disease-modifying antirheumatic drug (DMARD) and a biological DMARD targeting TNF, IL-6, and T cells has revolutionized treatment of RA, producing significant improvements in clinical, structural, and functional outcomes that were not previously observed. Clinical remission is perceived as an appropriate and realistic primary goal in many patients, and its maintenance leads to structural and functional remission (Fig. 59.1) [1–4].

However, biological DMARDs are limited to intravenous or subcutaneous uses because of their size, 90,000–150,000 Da. Orally available small molecules targeting key molecules in the disease processes, therefore, currently attract particular attention because they enter into cytoplasm and directly regulate intracellular signals. Among them, products targeting kinase proteins have been emerging because multiple signaling kinases are involved in the pathological processes of RA. We here review recent progress in the development of kinase inhibitors for the treatment of RA, shedding light on a small molecule inhibitor of the Janus kinase (JAK) [5–10].

CYTOKINE-MEDIATED KINASE

Cytokines have critical roles in the pathogenesis of immune- and inflammation-driven diseases and can be targeted therapeutically. Type I and Type II cytokine receptors, a family of receptors employed by over 50 cytokines, interleukins, interferons, colony-stimulating factors, and hormones, are all related by their mode of intracellular signaling, resulting in the activation of various signaling, including phosphorylation of kinase proteins. Protein kinases are key regulators of cell function that constitute one of the largest and most functionally diverse gene families, and 518 genes encoding kinases have been identified from human genome-wide studies. By adding phosphate groups to substrate proteins, they direct the activity, localization, and overall function of many proteins and serve to orchestrate the activity of almost all cellular processes. Kinases are particularly prominent in signal transduction and coordination of complex functions.

Among them, the tyrosine kinase is phosphorylated following cytokine receptor binding and is involved in multiple cellular functions during pathological processes of various inflammatory diseases such as RA. Therefore, tyrosine kinases have been emerging as the target for the treatment of these diseases. More than 80 genes encoding tyrosine kinases have been identified from human genome-wide studies and nine receptor tyrosine kinases and five nonreceptor tyrosine kinases are known to be involved in synovial inflammation in patients with RA, compared to those with osteoarthritis [11]. Spleen tyrosine kinase (Syk), Bruton's tyrosine kinase (Btk), lymphocyte-specific protein tyrosine kinase, Src, and JAK are known to be involved in the synovial inflammation. Btk is a key intracellular kinase to regulate B-cell function, and Syk is widely expressed in immunocompetent cells, such as mast cells, macrophages, neutrophils, and B cells and is activated via multichain immune receptors, such as B-cell receptor and Fc receptor.

Members of JAK family are essential for the signaling pathways of multiple cytokines, growth factors, and hormones and are implicated in the pathogenesis of RA. These molecules consist of homodimer or heterodimer of JAK1, JAK2, JAK3, and TYK2. After the engagement of cytokines receptors constitutively bound to JAK, JAK is activated by a conformational change and phosphorylated. These in turn phosphorylate the cytokine receptors, resulting in phosphorylation of the signal transducers and activators of transcription (STAT) that subsequently translocate into the nucleus, where they regulate gene expression (Fig. 59.2). More than 40 different cytokines and growth factors have been shown to activate

Mosaic of Autoimmunity. https://doi.org/10.1016/B978-0-12-814307-0.00059-1

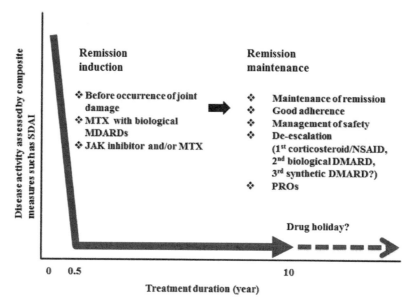

FIGURE 59.1 **Current treatment strategy for rheumatoid arthritis to stop joint damage.** After diagnosed as rheumatoid arthritis the treatment with methotrexate (MTX) should be initiated prior to occurrence of joint damage. However, if patients failed to achieve remission by MTX, any biological disease-modifying antirheumatic drug (DMARD) or JAK inhibitor should be added to the conventional DMARD, aiming at >50% improvement within 3 and target attainment within 6 months is recommended. After achieving remission, long-term maintenance of remission is required with good adherence of the drugs and appropriate management of safety and efficacy. After the maintenance of remission, de-escalation of used treatment may be considered.

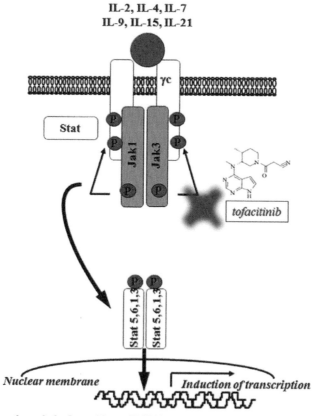

FIGURE 59.2 **Signaling mechanisms through the Janus kinase (JAK)/signal transducers and activators of transcription (STAT) pathway and action point of a JAK inhibitor tofacitinib.** After the engagement of cytokines receptors constitutively bound to JAK, JAK is phosphorylated. These in turn phosphorylate the cytokine receptors, resulting in phosphorylation of the STAT that subsequently translocate into the nucleus, where they regulate gene expression.

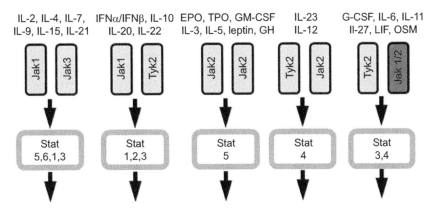

FIGURE 59.3   Janus kinase (JAK)/signal transducers and activators of transcription (STAT) pathway of different cytokine receptor family. Members of JAK family consist of homodimer or heterodimer of JAK1, JAK2, JAK3, and TYK2. More than 40 different cytokines and growth factors have been shown to activate specific combination of JAKs and STATs. The use of homodimer or heterodimer of JAK1, JAK2, JAK3, and TYK2 is different dependently on the use of cytokine receptor families.

specific combination of JAKs and STATs. The use of homodimer or heterodimer of JAK1, JAK2, JAK3, and TYK2 is different dependently on the use of cytokine receptor families. For instance, the common γ-chain constitutively binds to JAK1/JAK3 (Fig. 59.3). Reflecting the involvement of multiple inflammatory cytokines in the pathological processes of RA, both JAKs and STATs were increased in the synovium from RA patients compared with osteoarthritis patients, and the expression of JAK-STAT was diminished following treatment with synthetic DMARDs [12].

MECHANISMS OF ACTION OF SMALL MOLECULES TARGETING JANUS KINASE

A variety of small molecules targeting JAK have been investigated in clinical trials at different phases with promising outcomes in RA. Tofacitinib was approved for RA in 2012 in United States (US) and Japan and baricitinib was in 2017 in European Union (EU) and Japan.

Among members of a JAK family, the expression of JAK3 is limited to lymphocytes and constitutively binds to the common γ-chain for IL-2, IL-4, IL-7, IL-9, IL-15, and IL-21 [13]. Because the expression of JAK3 was known to be limited on hematopoietic cells, the lack of JAK3 was supposed to marginally affect other organs. Thus, selective inhibition of JAK3 was considered as a potential target for the treatment of RA without affecting other organ systems. Changelian et al. found tofacitinib by screening for inhibitors of in vitro JAK3 kinase activity from the Pfizer chemical library and extensive chemical modification by the company [14,15]. Tofacitinib is an orally available compound that binds to the ATP-binding pocket of JAK3 and its molecular weight is 504.49 Da with nitrile citrate. However, recent kinome-binding maps showed that tofacitinib inhibits not only JAK3 but also JAK2 and is also able to bind to the ATP pocket in both JAK1 and JAK2 [16]. Ghoreschi et al. reported that tofacitinib potentially inhibited signaling by IFN-γ and IL-6 and to a lesser extent IL-12 and IL-23 [17]. Therefore, tofacitinib is currently categorized as a JAK inhibitor preferentially inhibiting JAK1 and JAK3 and, to a lesser extent, JAK2 with minimum effect on TYK2.

We assessed the effects of tofacitinib on CD4+ T cells purified from synovium and peripheral blood in patients with active RA [18]. The addition of tofacitinib to the CD4+ T cells stimulated with anti-CD3 and anti-CD28 antibodies inhibited the transcription of IL-17 and IFN-γ, but not IL-6, IL-8, and TNF, as well as the proliferation in a dose-dependent manner. Although tofacitinib did not affect synovial fibroblasts and CD14+ monocytes derived from synovium in patients with RA, conditioned medium from CD4+ T cells cultured with tofacitinib inhibited IL-6 production from synovial fibroblasts and IL-8 production from CD14+ monocytes, indicating the indirect effect of tofacitinib on monocytes and fibroblasts in synovium. These results support that the primary targets of tofacitinib appear limited on lymphocytes. Tofacitinib also suppressed production and stimulation loop of a type-I IFN through JAK1/JAK3, decreased CD80/CD86 expression, and suppressed T-cell stimulatory capacity in monocyte-derived dendritic cells, which leads to its immunomodulatory effects [19]. Furthermore, tofacitinib suppresses B-cell activation, differentiation, and class switching, whereas it maintains B-cell regulatory function [20]. Taken together, the primary targets of tofacitinib appear dendritic cells, CD4+ T cells, and activated B cells that lead to multi-cytokine targeting beyond simply a JAK3 inhibitor.

The deficiency or dysfunction of JAK3 is synonymous with impairment in these cytokines that impaired lymphocyte development and function and leads to severe combined immunodeficiency (SCID) in both human and mouse. In vivo

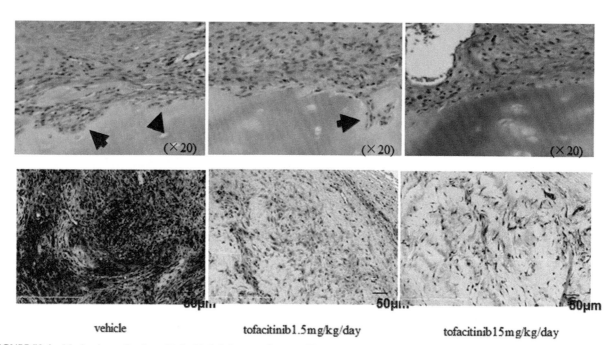

FIGURE 59.4 **Mechanisms of action of tofacitinib in human rheumatoid arthritis (RA) transgenic severe combined immunodeficiency (SCID) mice.** RA animal model utilizing SCID mice implanted with synovium and cartilage from patients with RA and tofacitinib was continuously given to the mice by the osmotic mini-pump [18]. Treatment of SCID-HuRAg mice with tofacitinib suppressed synovial inflammation, cartilage destruction (above) and the production of human matrix metalloproteinase-3 from implanted synovium (below).

efficacies of tofacitinib were initially demonstrated by its prevention of transplant rejection in a murine heterotropic heart transplantation model and in a nonhuman primate renal transplant model with prolongation of graft survival by tofacitinib monotherapy [13]. Additional studies with rodent aorta transplantation model and nonhuman primate kidney transplantation model treated with tofacitinib also showed significantly enhanced graft survival [21,22]. Besides them, when tofacitinib was administered into an established murine collagen-induced arthritis, arthritis and inflammation were rapidly ameliorated through the inhibition of the JAK1 and JAK3 signaling pathways and the suppression of Stat1-dependent gene expression in the joint [17]. These results indicate that tofacitinib efficiently inhibits JAK1 and JAK3, subsequent STAT1, and transcription of Stat1-inducible genes.

We also assessed the in vivo effects of tofacitinib using the SCID-HuRAg mice, an RA animal model utilizing SCID mice implanted with synovium and cartilage from patients with RA, and tofacitinib was continuously given to the mice by the osmotic mini-pump (Fig. 59.4) [18]. Treatment of SCID-HuRAg mice with tofacitinib suppressed synovial inflammation, cartilage destruction, and the production of human IL-6, IL-8, and matrix metalloproteinase-3 from implanted synovium. Tofacitinib also directly suppressed the production of IL-17 and IFN-γ and the proliferation of CD4+ T cells, resulting in inhibition of IL-6 and IL-8 production by synovial fibroblasts and CD14+ cells as well as cartilage destruction. Thus, JAK plays a crucial role in CD4+ T cells, Th-1 and Th-17 cells during RA synovial inflammation.

Baricitinib is a low-molecule weight compound (371.42 Da) that binds to the ATP-binding cleft and inhibits JAK1 and JAK2, with good selectivity, relative to JAK3. In peripheral blood mononuclear cells, baricitinib inhibited IL-6-stimulated STAT3 phosphorylation within 1–2 h and subsequent MCP-1 production [23]. However, precise mechanisms of action of baricitinib in vivo and in vitro remain unclear.

CLINICAL EFFICACY AND SAFETY OF SMALL MOLECULES TARGETING JANUS KINASE

Subsequently, multiple phase 3 studies were completed to investigate the efficacy and safety of tofacitinib and published ORAL start, ORAL solo, ORAL standard, ORAL sync, ORAL scan, and ORAL step, and all reported the efficacy of oral administration of tofacitinib at 5 and 10 mg twice a day [24–29]. Briefly, tofacitinib was significantly effective than placebo with or without MTX in RA patients with MTX-naïve, inadequately responsive to MTX or inadequately responsive to TNF inhibitors. The efficacy occurred rapidly and strongly. It is noteworthy there was not significant difference between tofacitinib and adalimumab, a TNF inhibitor. In addition, significant improvement in 6 months changes of modified total Sharp score, bone erosion score, and joint space narrowing score was observed in patients treated with

10 mg of tofacitinib, compared to placebo, indicating that tofacitinib has a potential to inhibit progress in joint destruction in patients with RA.

The most commonly reported adverse events were infections such as nasopharyngitis, increases in total cholesterol, elevation of transaminase and serum creatinine, decreases in neutrophil counts, and anemia. Although the majority of the adverse events have been tolerable and managed, opportunistic infections such as herpes zoster disseminated, pulmonary tuberculosis, cryptococcal pneumonia, and pneumocystis pneumonitis were reported. We also reported that receiver operating characteristic analysis identified a CD8[+] T-cell count <211 per μL at baseline as a significant predictor of clinically significant infectious adverse events [30]. Although tofacitinib has not been shown to increase the incidence of malignancies, collection of evidence regarding long-term safety is warranted and careful posttreatment follow-up is necessary for early diagnosis of any infection or malignancy [31,32].

Multiple phase 3 trials using baricitinib have recently completed. Oral administration of 2 or 4 mg once a day of baricitinib was significantly effective than placebo with or without MTX in RA patients with MTX-naïve, inadequately responsive to MTX or inadequately responsive to TNF inhibitors [33–35]. The clinical efficacy of baricitinib was observed from as early as week 1, and in DMARDs-naïve patients the efficacy of baricitinib monotherapy was higher than that of MTX. It is noteworthy that baricitinib with MTX was superior to placebo or adalimumab with MTX in virtually all clinical outcomes assessed by several composite measures as well as patient-related outcomes with similar inhibition of radiographic progression [34]. Thus, baricitinib is the first orally available small molecules which has better efficacy than biological DMARDs such as adalimumab in patients with active RA.

Baricitinib shows similar safety profiles to those of tofacitinib. Adverse infectious events occur at a higher frequency during treatment with baricitinib than MTX. The most commonly observed adverse events are related to infection, hematologic, hepatic, and renal disorders, and the association of baricitinib with carcinogenicity is under debate. The incidence rate of herpes zoster observed in baricitinib studies is also increased, especially in Japan. Increases in serum levels of total cholesterol, LDL, HDL, and triglycerides have also been reported in patients treated with baricitinib. Further long-term investigation of these findings with correlation to cardiovascular risk needs to be assessed. However, the US government claimed the incidence of serious adverse events associated with venous thromboembolism and pulmonary embolism. Postmarketing surveillance is required following approval of baricitinib for safety evaluation with a large patient population and a long observation period.

The results from clinical trials above have accelerated the development of other JAK inhibitors, such as decernotinib, peficitinib, filgotinib, and upadacitinib. Decernotinib (Vertex VX-509) is a selective JAK3 inhibitor under the phase 3 trial. In phase 2b study, the efficacy and safety of oral administration of decernotinib 100, 150, and 200 mg once a day in RA patients with inadequate response to MTX was similar to those of tofacitinib [36]. Peficitinib (ASP015K), a JAK1/JAK3 inhibitor, is under the phase 3 trial in east Asia and its efficacy and safety reported in phase 2b study held in Japan was similar to those of tofacitinib [37]. Filgotinib (GLPG0634) is a novel oral selective JAK1 inhibitor. In two different phase 2b studies, efficacy of its monotherapy or combination with MTX was superior to placebo and phase 3 trials are globally undertaken [38,39]. Upadacitinib (ABT-494) was engineered to enhance selectivity for JAK1 by exploiting interactions outside the ATP-binding site. The features of efficacy and safety of upadacitinib reported in phase 2b studies were similar to those of baricitinib and it is undergoing evaluation in phase 3 trials [40,41]. In addition to JAK inhibitors, small molecules targeting Syk and Btk are also in a development stage (Fig. 59.5).

CLINICAL USE OF SMALL MOLECULES TARGETING JANUS KINASE

Tofacitinib was approved for RA in the US in 2012 and Japan in 2013 and it is now used in many countries. In the US and Japan, oral administration of 5 mg twice a day of tofacitinib is used in RA patients with inadequate response to at least one synthetic DMARD such as MTX. Baricitinib was approved for RA in the EU and Japan in 2017, and 4 mg once a day of baricitinib is used in RA patients with inadequate response to DMARD such as MTX.

In 2015 ACR guideline for the treatment of RA, tofacitinib has been included as an option when the disease remains uncontrolled after failing initial conventional DMARDs in established RA [42]. The use of combination conventional DMARDs or addition of a TNF inhibitor or a non-TNF biologic or tofacitinib to patients with RA with moderate or high disease activity despite DMARD monotherapy is strongly recommended. However, the recommendation is conditional despite the published positive tofacitinib efficacy data because the balance of benefit (tofacitinib slightly more efficacious), risk (long-term safety of tofacitinib is currently not well known vs. the well-known long-term safety of MTX), and cost considerations (MTX is less expensive than tofacitinib) favored MTX overall. In addition, there is not enough difference in efficacy between biological DMARDs and tofacitinib to outweigh the longer-term safety data and greater amount of experience with biological DMARDs, compared to tofacitinib.

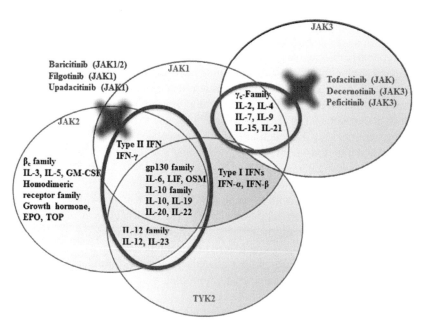

FIGURE 59.5 The development of small molecules targeting Janus kinase (JAK). The successful results from clinical trials of a JAK1/3 inhibitor tofacitinib and a JAK1/2 inhibitor baricitinib have accelerated the development of other JAK inhibitors, such as JAK3 inhibitors decernotinib and peficitinib and JAK1 inhibitors filgotinib and upadacitinib.

In the 2016 updated EULAR recommendation for the management of RA, MTX (rapid escalation to 25 mg per week), aiming at >50% improvement within 3 and target attainment within 6 months is recommended as the first strategy (phase I) [43]. If patients failed the phase I and have unfavorable prognostic markers (autoantibodies, high disease activity, early erosions, failure of 2 conventional DMARDs), any biological DMARD or JAK inhibitor should be added to the conventional DMARD at the phase II. If this fails, any other biological DMARD or JAK inhibitor is recommended. Thus, this recommendation is expanded to include the JAK inhibitor tofacitinib and further JAK inhibitors, such as baricitinib. Since previous revision of the recommendation in 2013, more data on tofacitinib, especially regarding long-term safety aspects, and new data for baricitinib have been published. However, biological DMARDs have been given a slight preference over JAK inhibitors due to availability of long-term registry data for the former but not the latter. This notion on current practice is an expert opinion and not based on solid evidence.

The successful results from clinical trials in RA have accelerated its application for other diseases such as inflammatory bowel disease (IBD) that encompasses two diseases, ulcerative colitis and Crohn's disease. Ulcerative colitis is typically restricted to the colon and primarily affects the mucosa, whereas Crohn's disease is characterized by transmural inflammation, skip lesions, and inflammation throughout the gastrointestinal tract. Despite the success of biologics including TNF inhibitors, ustekinumab and vedolizumab, current IBD therapies are ineffective for many patients. Tofacitinib 10 mg twice daily has proven an effective induction treatment for both moderate or severe ulcerative colitis, inducing remission and mucosal healing in a significant proportion of patients [44]. A subsequent ulcerative colitis trial has demonstrated that both 5 and 10 mg doses of tofacitinib are effective in maintaining remission for up to 1 year. By contrast, results in Crohn's disease have been less consistent, with the most recent data suggesting a very modest treatment effect of tofacitinib. However, filgotinib displays clinically significant efficacy in Crohn's disease, with a twofold increase in clinical remission compared with placebo and rates similar to those seen with the standard-of-care therapy infliximab. Multiple phase 3 trials of small molecules including upadacitinib are currently ongoing for both ulcerative colitis and ulcerative colitis.

Psoriasis is an autoimmune skin disorder, which is responsive to targeting multiple cytokines including TNF, IL-17, IL-12, and IL-23. Given the JAK dependence of multiple cytokines, tofacitinib has been tested extensively in clinical trials for the treatment of this disease [45]. Patients treated with tofacitinib experienced clinically significant improvements in the skin scores at both 5 and 10 mg twice daily doses. However, in a trial directly comparing tofacitinib to standard-of-care treatment with etanercept, only the 10 mg dose of tofacitinib showed noninferiority. The US would not be able to approve tofacitinib for psoriasis, unless the 10 mg dose provides an appropriate safety/benefit ratio, which was the reason why only the 5 mg dose was approved for RA. Baricitinib was also found to be efficacious in a phase 2 study testing its effect in patients with moderate-to-severe psoriasis, but responses were seen predominantly at the higher, 8 and 10 mg, daily doses and baricitinib has been compared with neither TNF inhibitors nor IL-17 inhibitors. Additional safety data will be warranted if it can be approved in US and EU. Currently, a phase 2 trial of TYK2 inhibitors is ongoing for the treatment of psoriasis.

Small molecules targeting JAK are also being used to treat other diseases associated with an interferon signature, namely systemic lupus erythematosus, dermatomyositis, scleroderma, and Sjogren's syndrome. A phase 3 baricitinib study is currently under the investigation. Furthermore, early phase clinical trials and large retrospective studies indicate that tofacitinib, baricitinib, and topical use of another JAK1/2 inhibitor ruxolitinib are effective for the spectrum of autoimmune forms of alopecia. However, symptoms recur on drug discontinuation, and tofacitinib may lose efficacy in some patients. A clinical trial using baricitinib to treat allergic dermatitis is ongoing. Balancing efficacy and safety is always a priority, especially in these diseases where morbidity may be high but mortality is low, so topical formulations of small molecules targeting JAK are desirable if efficacious [46].

CONCLUSION

Small molecules targeting intracellular signaling kinase or kinase inhibitors have been emerging for the treatment of RA and other autoimmune diseases. Oral administration of a small molecule targeting JAK tofacitinib was significantly effective than placebo with or without MTX in active RA patients with MTX-naïve, inadequately responsive to MTX or TNF inhibitors in multiple phase 3 studies. Therapeutic efficacy of tofacitinib was observed in a short term after administration and was as strong as adalimumab, a TNF inhibitor. It is noteworthy that baricitinib with MTX was superior to placebo or adalimumab with MTX in virtually all clinical outcomes assessed by several composite measures as well as patient-related outcomes with similar inhibition of radiographic progression. Multiple small molecules targeting JAK are now emerging for the development. Thus, orally available small molecules targeting specific kinase could represent a valuable addition to the conventional DMARDs and biological DMARDs and these small molecules targeting JAK would take in the therapeutic armamentarium in RA and multiple autoimmune diseases.

The most commonly observed adverse events of JAK inhibitors are related to infection, hematologic, hepatic, and renal disorders, and the association of tofacitinib with carcinogenicity is under debate. Most recently the occurrence of venous thromboembolism and pulmonary embolism has been reported in patients treated with baricitinib and upadacitinib. The risks and benefits of JAK isoform selectivity in different rheumatic diseases will become increasingly clear and will perhaps contribute to our understanding of disease pathogenesis. The development of small molecules targeting JAK is an example to encourage the translation from bench to bedside, shedding light on basic research regarding intracellular signaling mechanisms and their relevance to pathological processes, but their safety concerns also have brought about the significance of translational research from bedside to bench.

ACKNOWLEDGMENTS

The authors thank all medical staff in all institutions for providing the data. This work was supported in part by a Grant-In-Aid for Scientific Research from the Ministry of Health, Labor and Welfare of Japan, the Ministry of Education, Culture, Sports, Science and Technology of Japan, and the University of Occupational and Environmental Health, Japan, through UOEH Grant for Advanced Research.

COMPETING INTERESTS

Y. Tanaka has received speaking fees and/or honoraria from Daiichi-Sankyo, Astellas, Pfizer, Mitsubishi-Tanabe, Bristol-Myers, Chugai, YL Biologics, Eli Lilly, Sanofi, Janssen, UCB and has received research grants from Mitsubishi-Tanabe, Takeda, Bristol-Myers, Chugai, Astellas, Abbvie, MSD, Daiichi-Sankyo, Pfizer, Kyowa-Kirin, Eisai, Ono.

REFERENCES

[1] Smolen JS, Aletaha D, McInnes IB. Rheumatoid arthritis. Lancet 2016;388:2023–38.

[2] McInnes IB, Schett G. Pathogenetic insights from the treatment of rheumatoid arthritis. Lancet 2017;389:2328–37.

[3] Smolen JS, Breedveld FC, Burmester GR, et al. Treating rheumatoid arthritis to target: 2014 update of the recommendations of an international task force. Ann Rheum Dis 2016;75:3–15.

[4] Tanaka Y. Current concepts in the management of rheumatoid arthritis. Korean J Intern Med 2016;31:210–8.

[5] O'Shea JJ, Kontzias A, Yamaoka K, Tanaka Y, Laurence A. Janus kinase inhibitors in autoimmune diseases. Ann Rheum Dis 2013;72:ii111–5.

[6] Nakayamada S, Kubo S, Iwata S, Tanaka Y. Chemical JAK inhibitors for the treatment of rheumatoid arthritis. Expert Opin Pharmacother 2016;17:2215–25.

[7] Nakayamada S, Kubo S, Iwata S, Tanaka Y. Recent progress in JAK inhibitors for the treatment of rheumatoid arthritis. BioDrugs 2016;30:407–19.

[8] Kubo S, Nakayamada S, Tanaka Y. Baricitinib for the treatment of rheumatoid arthritis. Expert Rev Clin Immunol 2016;12:911–9.

[9] Tanaka Y. Recent progress and perspective in JAK inhibitors for rheumatoid arthritis: from bench to bedside. J Biochem 2015;158:173–9.

[10] Winthrop KL. The emerging safety profile of JAK inhibitors in rheumatic disease. Nat Rev Rheumatol 2017;13:234–43.

[11] D'Aura Swanson C, Paniagua RT, Lindstrom TM, Robinson WH. Tyrosine kinases as targets for the treatment of rheumatoid arthritis. Nat Rev Rheumatol 2009;5:317–24.

[12] Walker JG, Ahern MJ, Coleman M, Weedon H, Papangelis V, Beroukas D, Roberts-Thomson PJ, Smith MD. Characterisation of a dendritic cell subset in synovial tissue which strongly expresses Jak/STAT transcription factors from patients with rheumatoid arthritis. Ann Rheum Dis 2007;66:992–9.

[13] Macchi P, Villa A, Giliani S, Sacco MG, Frattini A, Porta F, Ugazio AG, Johnston JA, Candotti F, O'Shea JJ, et al. Mutations of Jak-3 gene in patients with autosomal severe combined immune deficiency (SCID). Nature 1995;377:65–8.

[14] Changelian PS, Flanagan ME, Ball DJ, Kent CR, Magnuson KS, Martin WH, Rizzuti BJ, Sawyer PS, Perry BD, Brissette WH, McCurdy SP, Kudlacz EM, Conklyn MJ, Elliott EA, Koslov ER, Fisher MB, Strelevitz TJ, Yoon K, Whipple DA, Sun J, Munchhof MJ, Doty JL, Casavant JM, Blumenkopf TA, Hines M, Brown MF, Lillie BM, Subramanyam C, Shang-Poa C, Milici AJ, Beckius GE, Moyer JD, Su C, Woodworth TG, Gaweco AS, Beals CR, Littman BH, Fisher DA, Smith JF, Zagouras P, Magna HA, Saltarelli MJ, Johnson KS, Nelms LF, Des Etages SG, Hayes LS, Kawabata TT, Finco-Kent D, Baker DL, Larson M, Si MS, Paniagua R, Higgins J, Holm B, Reitz B, Zhou YJ, Morris RE, O'Shea JJ, Borie DC. Prevention of organ allograft rejection by a specific Janus kinase 3 inhibitor. Science (New York NY) 2003;302:875–8.

[15] Flanagan ME, Blumenkopf TA, Brissette WH, Brown MF, Casavant JM, Shang-Poa C, Doty JL, Elliott EA, Fisher MB, Hines M, Kent C, Kudlacz EM, Lillie BM, Magnuson KS, McCurdy SP, Munchhof MJ, Perry BD, Sawyer PS, Strelevitz TJ, Subramanyam C, Sun J, Whipple DA, Changelian PS. Discovery of CP-690,550: a potent and selective Janus kinase (JAK) inhibitor for the treatment of autoimmune diseases and organ transplant rejection. J Med Chem 2010;53:8468–84.

[16] Karaman MW, Herrgard S, Treiber DK, Gallant P, Atteridge CE, Campbell BT, Chan KW, Ciceri P, Davis MI, Edeen PT, Faraoni R, Floyd M, Hunt JP, Lockhart DJ, Milanov ZV, Morrison MJ, Pallares G, Patel HK, Pritchard S, Wodicka LM, Zarrinkar PP. A quantitative analysis of kinase inhibitor selectivity. Nat Biotechnol 2008;26:127–32.

[17] Ghoreschi K, Jesson MI, Li X, Lee JL, Ghosh S, Alsup JW, Warner JD, Tanaka M, Steward-Tharp SM, Gadina M, Thomas CJ, Minnerly JC, Storer CE, LaBranche TP, Radi ZA, Dowty ME, Head RD, Meyer DM, Kishore N, O'Shea JJ. Modulation of innate and adaptive immune responses by tofacitinib (CP-690,550). J Immunol 2011;186:4234–43.

[18] Maeshima K, Yamaoka K, Kubo S, Nakano K, Iwata S, Saito K, Ohishi M, Miyahara H, Tanaka S, Ishii K, Yoshimatsu H, Tanaka Y. The JAK inhibitor tofacitinib regulates synovitis through inhibition of interferon-gamma and interleukin-17 production by human CD4+ T cells. Arthritis Rheum 2012;64:1790–8.

[19] Kubo S, Yamaoka K, Kondo M, Yamagata K, Zhao J, Iwata S, Tanaka Y. The JAK inhibitor, tofacitinib, reduces the T cell stimulatory capacity of human monocyte-derived dendritic cells. Ann Rheum Dis 2014;73:2192–8.

[20] Wang S-P, Iwata S, Nakayamada S, Sakata K, Yamaoka K, Tanaka Y. Tofacitinib, a Jak inhibitor, inhibits human B cell activation in vitro. Ann Rheum Dis 2014;73:2213–5.

[21] Borie DC, Larson MJ, Flores MG, Campbell A, Rousvoal G, Zhang S, Higgins JP, Ball DJ, Kudlacz EM, Brissette WH, Elliott EA, Reitz BA, Changelian PS. Combined use of the JAK3 inhibitor CP-690,550 with mycophenolate mofetil to prevent kidney allograft rejection in nonhuman primates. Transplantation 2005;80:1756–64.

[22] Rousvoal G, Si MS, Lau M, Zhang S, Berry GJ, Flores MG, Changelian PS, Reitz BA, Borie DC. Janus kinase 3 inhibition with CP-690,550 prevents allograft vasculopathy. Transpl Int 2006;19:1014–21.

[23] Shi JG, Chen X, Lee F, et al. The pharmacokinetics, pharmacodynamics, and safety of baricitinib, an oral JAK 1/2 inhibitor, in healthy volunteers. J Clin Pharmacol 2014;54(12):1354–61.

[24] Fleischmann R, Kremer J, Cush J, Schulze-Koops H, Connell CA, Bradley JD, et al. Placebo-controlled trial of tofacitinib monotherapy in rheumatoid arthritis. N Engl J Med 2012;367(6):495–507.

[25] Kremer J, Li ZG, Hall S, Fleischmann R, Genovese M, Martin-Mola E, et al. Tofacitinib in combination with nonbiologic disease-modifying antirheumatic drugs in patients with active rheumatoid arthritis: a randomized trial. Ann Intern Med 2013;159(4):253–61.

[26] Lee EB, Fleischmann R, Hall S, Wilkinson B, Bradley JD, Gruben D, et al. Tofacitinib versus methotrexate in rheumatoid arthritis. N Engl J Med 2014;370(25):2377–86.

[27] van Vollenhoven RF, Fleischmann R, Cohen S, Lee EB, Garcia Meijide JA, Wagner S, et al. Tofacitinib or adalimumab versus placebo in rheumatoid arthritis. N Engl J Med 2012;367(6):508–19.

[28] van der Heijde D, Tanaka Y, Fleischmann R, Keystone E, Kremer J, Zerbini C, et al. Tofacitinib (CP-690,550) in patients with rheumatoid arthritis receiving methotrexate: twelve-month data from a twenty-four-month phase III randomized radiographic study. Arthritis Rheum 2013;65(3):559–70.

[29] Burmester GR, Blanco R, Charles-Schoeman C, Wollenhaupt J, Zerbini C, Benda B, et al. Tofacitinib (CP-690,550) in combination with methotrexate in patients with active rheumatoid arthritis with an inadequate response to tumour necrosis factor inhibitors: a randomised phase 3 trial. Lancet 2013;381(9865):451–60.

[30] Sonomoto K, Yamaoka K, Kubo S, Hirata S, Fukuyo S, Maeshima K, Suzuki K, Saito K, Tanaka Y. Effects of tofacitinib on lymphocytes in rheumatoid arthritis: relation to efficacy and infectious adverse events. Rheumatology (Oxf Engl) 2014;53:914–8.

[31] Winthrop KL, Park SH, Gul A, et al. Tuberculosis and other opportunistic infections in tofacitinib-treated patients with rheumatoid arthritis. Ann Rheum Dis 2016;75:1133–8.

[32] Curtis JR, Lee EB, Kaplan IV, Kwok K, Geier J, Benda B, et al. Tofacitinib, an oral Janus kinase inhibitor: analysis of malignancies across the rheumatoid arthritis clinical development programme. Ann Rheum Dis 2016;75(5):831–41.

[33] Genovese MC, Kremer J, Zamani O, Ludivico C, Krogulec M, Xie L, et al. Baricitinib in patients with refractory rheumatoid arthritis. N Engl J Med 2016;374(13):1243–52.

[34] Taylor PC, Keystone EC, van der Heijde D, et al. Baricitinib versus placebo or adalimumab in rheumatoid arthritis. N Engl J Med 2017;376:652–62.

[35] Dougados M, van der Heijde D, Chen YC, Greenwald M, Drescher E, Liu J, Beattie S, Witt S, de la Torre I, Gaich C, Rooney T, Schlichting D, de Bono S, Emery P. Baricitinib in patients with inadequate response or intolerance to conventional synthetic DMARDs: results from the RA-BUILD study. Ann Rheum Dis 2017;76:88–95.

[36] Genovese MC, van Vollenhoven RF, Pacheco-Tena C, et al. VX-509 (Decernotinib), an oral selective JAK-3 Inhibitor, in combination with methotrexate in patients with rheumatoid arthritis. Arthritis Rheumatol 2016;68:46–55.

[37] Takeuchi T, Tanaka Y, Iwasaki M, Ishikura H, Saeki S, Kaneko Y. Efficacy and safety of the oral Janus kinase inhibitor peficitinib (ASP015K) monotherapy in patients with moderate to severe rheumatoid arthritis in Japan: a 12-week, randomised, double-blind, placebo-controlled phase IIb study. Ann Rheum Dis 2016;75:1057–64.

[38] Westhovens R, Taylor PC, Alten R, Pavlova D, Enríquez-Sosa F, Mazur M, Greenwald M, Van der Aa A, Vanhoutte F, Tasset C, Harrison P. Filgotinib (GLPG0634/GS-6034), an oral JAK1 selective inhibitor, is effective in combination with methotrexate (MTX) in patients with active rheumatoid arthritis and insufficient response to MTX: results from a randomised, dose-finding study (DARWIN 1). Ann Rheum Dis June 2017;76(6):998–1008.

[39] Kavanaugh A, Kremer J, Ponce L, Cseuz R, Reshetko OV, Stanislavchuk M, Greenwald M, Van der Aa A, Vanhoutte F, Tasset C, Harrison P. Filgotinib (GLPG0634/GS-6034), an oral selective JAK1 inhibitor, is effective as monotherapy in patients with active rheumatoid arthritis: results from a randomised, dose-finding study (DARWIN 2). Ann Rheum Dis June 2017;76(6):1009–19.

[40] Genovese MC, Smolen JS, Weinblatt ME, Burmester GR, Meerwein S, Camp HS, Wang L, Othman AA, Khan N, Pangan AL, Jungerwirth S. Efficacy and safety of ABT-494, a selective JAK-1 inhibitor, in a phase IIb study in patients with rheumatoid arthritis and an inadequate response to methotrexate. Arthritis Rheumatol 2016;68:2857–66.

[41] Kremer JM, Emery P, Camp HS, Friedman A, Wang L, Othman AA, Khan N, Pangan AL, Jungerwirth S, Keystone EC. A phase IIb study of ABT-494, a selective JAK-1 inhibitor, in patients with rheumatoid arthritis and an inadequate response to anti-tumor necrosis factor therapy. Arthritis Rheumatol 2016;68:2867–77.

[42] Singh JA, Saag KG, Bridges Jr SL, et al. 2015 American College of Rheumatology guideline for the treatment of rheumatoid arthritis. Arthritis Rheum 2016;68:1–26.

[43] Smolen JS, Landewé R, Bijlsma J, et al. EULAR recommendations for the management of rheumatoid arthritis with synthetic and biological disease-modifying antirheumatic drugs. 2016 update. Ann Rheum Dis 2017;76:960–78.

[44] Sandborn WJ, Su C, Sands BE, et al. Tofacitinib as induction and maintenance therapy for ulcerative colitis. N Engl J Med 2017;376:1723–36.

[45] Tan KW, Griffiths CE. Novel systemic therapies for the treatment of psoriasis. Expert Opin Pharmacother 2016;17:79–92.

[46] Damsky W, King BA. JAK inhibitors in dermatology: the promise of a new drug class. J Am Acad Dermatol 2017;76:736–44.

Chapter 60

Helminthes and Autoimmunity, a Love Story

Sharon Slomovich[1], Hanan Guzner-Gur[1,2], Miri Blank[3], Yehuda Shoenfeld[3,4]

[1]Zabludowicz Center for Autoimmune Diseases, Sheba Medical Center, Tel-Hashomer, Israel; [2]Sackler Faculty of Medicine, Tel Aviv University, Tel Aviv, Israel; [3]Zabludowicz Center for Autoimmune Diseases, Sheba Medical Center, affiliated to Sackler Faculty of Medicine, Tel Aviv University, Tel Aviv, Israel; [4]Laboratory of the Mosaics of Autoimmunity, Saint-Petersburg University, Saint-Petersburg, Russian Federation

INTRODUCTION

The frequency of autoimmune diseases (AID) in Western countries has been increasing dramatically in the last decades. In North America and Europe alone, 5%–10% of the population has been diagnosed with an AID [1]. One of the major hypotheses to explain this trend is the hygiene theory, first described in 1989, as children of large families in the United Kingdom were observed to have a significantly lower incidence of hay fever and eczema, when compared with smaller families [2]. According to this theory, early and repeated exposure to infections matures the immune system, whereas improved sanitary conditions increase autoimmunity [3,4]. In addition, geographic locations with a higher prevalence of parasitic worms further alter the host immune response and confer protection from autoimmune conditions [5].

Experimental treatments with helminthes in animal models of AID such as multiple sclerosis (MS), type 1 diabetes mellitus (TIDM), rheumatoid arthritis (RA), and inflammatory bowel diseases prove the ability of the parasitic worms to prevent and even reverse inflammation [6]. Furthermore, helminth infection is associated with reduced reactivity to allergens and autoantigens, both in animal model systems [7,8] and in human studies [9,10]. Ingestion of parasitic worms ameliorated experimental AID via several mechanisms, mostly by induction of FoxP3+ Tregs expression and stimulation of regulatory cytokine production (e.g., IL-4, IL-10, TGFβ), and inhibition of IFN-γ and IL-17 inflammatory cytokine release by T cell, macrophages, and dendritic cells (DCs) [11]. For example, in a colitis mice model, helminthes reduced activation of DCs of the small bowel [12], by altering MHC antigen-presenting complex (e.g., CD40, CD80, CD86, H2), and downmodulation of Jak1/2 and MAP kinase signaling pathway, affecting antigen presentation and T-cell activation [12].

Current treatment options for AIDs include corticosteroids and immunosuppressive drugs, associated with wide-ranging side effects. Corticosteroid adverse effects include, among others, the development of osteoporosis, cardiovascular disease, infections, and cancer [13]. Alternative immunosuppressive drugs, such as methotrexate, azathioprine, and cyclophosphamide, are used as steroid-sparing agents but can cause severe, life-threatening symptoms [14]. There is a need, therefore, for a more specific and less toxic treatment for AID.

Helminthes are not innocent across all species. Some constitute a public health risk and are associated with a high incidence of morbidity and mortality. For example, *Schistosoma*, a parasitic flatworm, causes schistosomiasis, a disease that affects the intestines and urinary tract, leading to suffering and death. This condition is close to malaria and tuberculosis in disability-adjusted life year units [15]. World Health Organization characterizes schistosomiasis as the second-most socioeconomically devastating disease [16]. In contrast, most helminth species colonize their human hosts with little to no health consequences [17]. In addition, the colonization of helminthes might modulate the host immune system and thus confer protection and even reverse AID. Understanding the mechanisms, by which helminthes affect the human host immune system, might help us to derive specific treatments and produce investigational drugs for patients with autoimmune conditions.

Phosphorylcholine (PC) is a small molecule found in secretions of helminthes, attached to a glycoprotein, and is considered as the moiety responsible for the immunosuppressive activity of helminthes [18,19]. For example, filarial nematode, *Acanthocheilonema vitae*, secretes ES-62, a 62 KDa glycoprotein molecule, shown to modulate B-cell activity, by selectively targeting B-cell antigen receptor signaling and as a result disrupting B-cell activation [18]. Additionally, ES-62 affects T-cell response indirectly by modulating function of DCs, macrophage, and APCs [18,]. Thus, exposure of macrophages and DCs to ES-62, significantly reduced LPS-induced Th1 proinflammatory cytokine response [19]. It is suggested that PC mediates its effects by a TLR4-dependent manner [19].

Mosaic of Autoimmunity. https://doi.org/10.1016/B978-0-12-814307-0.00060-8

While preliminary studies with ES-62 was proven to be very effective in the treatment of autoimmune experimental models such as arthritis, lupus and in asthma [20–23]. A major challenge is to take advantage of the unique properties of PC and to develop a small molecule drug [24].

Preliminary experiments with injection of PC to attenuate murine lupus were not successful (unpublished data. Blank, M.), probably related to the nonimmunogenicity of PC by itself. In an effort to create an immunogenic, biologically active compound, that could be utilized as a small-molecule drug, Shoenfeld and Blank et al. conjugated the PC moiety to tuftsin, thus forming tuftsin-phosphorylcholine (TPC) [25].

Tuftsin is a natural immunomodulator, which was described in 1970 as an endogenous four amino acid peptide, with a Thr-Lys-Pro-Arg amino acid sequence. It is derived from the Fc domain of the heavy chain of IgG via enzymatic cleavage in the spleen [26]. The biological activities of tuftsin include binding to polymorphonuclear cells and enhancing their chemotaxis and phagocytosis ability, as well as augmenting their bactericidal activity and tumor cell cytotoxicity by inducing mitogenic activity and formation of reactive oxygen species [26,27].

The stimulating qualities of tuftsin make it a natural adjuvant and an immunomodulator. Therefore, it was assumed that combining tuftsin with PC might induce the expected immunomodulation in vivo, not achieved in preliminary experiments by PC alone.

Indeed, studies using TPC treatment in murine models of autoimmunity such as colitis, lupus nephritis, and collagen-induced arthritis (CIA) showed favorable results [25,33]. The effects of TPC and its promise as a new treatment in various AID will be detailed and discussed herein, in the context of the experimental data known to date about the successful treatment of AID with helminthes and helminth products.

CLINICAL EXPERIMENTAL THERAPY IN ANIMAL AND HUMAN MODELS WITH HELMINTH DERIVATIVES

As discussed, helminthes and their derivatives have been proven successful in treating AID in animals and humans. For example, in one study, development of TIDM, a chronic AID involving inflammation of insulin-producing β cells, was evaluated in a mice model experiment. In this experiment, 6-week-old-NOD mice were infected with *Litomosoides sigmodontis*, a filarial nematode [28]. The experiment included 15 filarial-infected NOD mice and 11 controls. Of the 15 infected NOD mice, 3 received filarial larvae, 5 received adult filarial male worms, and 7 received adult filarial female worms [28]. Blood glucose levels >230 mg/dL were considered diabetes. Filarial nematodes treatment completely prevented the development of diabetes, compared with 63% in infected NOD mice [28]. Moreover, the infected NOD mice had more total pancreatic islet cells on histology compared to the control group [28]. In addition, *L. sigmodontis*-infected NOD mice developed a Th2 shift, shown by isolating spleen cells from infected and noninfected NOD mice and cultured them in the presence of α-CD3/α-CD28 or without stimulant [28].

Another study investigated the protective effect of *Schistosoma japonicum*, a human blood fluke, in murine collagen induced arthritis (CIA). CIA, a murine model of RA, is a disease thought to mediate predominately a Th1 response and the release of IFN-γ, TNF-α, and lymphotoxin β resulting in joint inflammation and destruction [29]. DBA/1 mice were infected with *S. japonicum* 2 weeks prior to bovine type II collagen (CII) immunization. A significant reduction in CIA severity was seen in mice infected with the blood fluke, with reduction Th1 cells and proinflammatory cytokines (IFN-γ, TNF-α, IL-1β, and IL-6), and upregulation of Th2 cells and antiinflammatory cytokines IL-10 [29].

Successful experiments in murine models treated with helminthes drove investigational studies in humans. *Trichuris suis*, a whipworm, was tested in Crohn's disease. Disease activity was measured via the active Crohn's disease activity index (CDAI). 29 patients with active Crohn's disease, (CDAI)≥220, ingested 2500 live *T. suis* ova every 3 weeks, for 24 weeks [30]. Remission was classified as <150 CDIA. The remission rate was 21/29 (72.4%) without any adverse events [30]. In a randomized, double blind, placebo-controlled trial, in ulcerative colitis (UC), 54 UC patients were randomly assigned to ingest pig whipworm *T. suis* ova or placebo. The treatment group received 2500 live *T. suis* ova every 2 weeks, for 12 weeks. Remission was achieved in 13/30 (43.3%) of treated patients, compared with 4/24 (16.7%) of placebo-treated patients [31].

MS is an inflammatory and demyelinating disease affecting the central nervous system. Like RA, MS is also believed to be mediated via a Th1-predominant immune mechanism, and therefore it was assumed that MS patients could benefit from helminthes by inducing a Th2 shift [10]. A prospective, double blind study of 12 MS patients who presented with eosinophilia and positive parasitic infection with *Hymenolepis nana*, *Trichuris trichiura*, *Ascaris lumbricoides*, *Strongyloides stercoralis*, *or Enterobius vermicularis*. Infected patients had significant improvement in clinical MS manifestations, as well as increased myelin basic protein-specific T-cells secretion of antiinflammatory cytokines (IL-10 and TGF-β) and reduction in inflammatory cytokines (IL-12 and IFN-γ). In addition, Treg cells, CD4+, CD25+, FoxP+, were increased [10].

TUFTSIN-PHOSPHORYLCHOLINE, A NOVEL TREATMENT FOR AUTOIMMUNE DISEASES

As discussed above, the unique feature of the combined molecule of PC and tuftsin, designated TPC, enabled enhancing the immunomodulating effect of PC, while still keeping the drug a small molecule. First, TPC was studied in Dextransulfate-Sodium-Salt (DSS)–induced experimental model of murine colitis [25]. The experiment included 30 mice, classified into three groups. 10 DSS colitis mice were treated with TPC, 10 DSS colitis mice were treated with a control PBS, and 10 healthy, nontreated mice were used as another control. DSS colitis disease activity index (DAI) was measured based on weight loss, rectal bleeding, stool consistency, and survival. 10 days after disease induction, the mice were sacrificed and their colon was sent for histological and cytokine expression evaluation. Colitis-untreated mice had a maximal average DAI score of 2.59, compared to a significantly lower DAI score of 1.16, in PBS controls. In addition, histological assessment of the colon showed that DSS-treated mice had scant leukocyte infiltrations, similar to the control noncolitis mice. The TPC-treated mice showed reduction in proinflammatory cytokines (TNFa, IL-17, IL-1b) and an increased expression of the antiinflammatory cytokine IL-10, in colon lysates [25].

Next, the effects of TPC were examined in a model of lupus prone (NZBxW) F1 murine lupus nephritis. 60 female lupus prone mice (14–15 weeks old) were split into 4 groups, each with 15 mice, and received either TPC subcutaneously, or PC alone, or tuftsin, or PBS. Treatment was given at week 14 prior to the onset of proteinuria. At 30 weeks of age, 72% of the PBS-injected mice had proteinuria compared with 21% of the TPC-treated group. In addition, TPC-treated mice had a reduced evidence of immune complex (IC) deposition in the mesangium, and thus exhibiting class-II nephritis as compared to class-IV in PC- and PBS-treated groups. Tuftsin had a moderate effect on IC deposition. TPC was able to inhibit mRNA expression of proinflammatory cytokines (IFN-γ, IL-17) and to increase expression of antiinflammatory cytokines (TGF-β, IL-10), as well as to increase Tregs in splenocytes derived from TPC-treated mice compared with PBS- or PC-treated control mice. Of note, treatment with Tuftsin increased IL-10 secretion by splenocytes, though less significant compared with TPC ($P < .01$). In addition, no significant change was found in circulating serum anti-dsDNA between groups. Importantly, TPC, PC, and tuftsin were shown to prolong survival in female mice with lupus nephritis compared to PBS controls. However, TPC was significantly superior to tuftsin or PC alone [32].

More recently, TPC was evaluated in the treatment of murine CIA. The mice were classified into four groups of treatment: TPC or PBS and oral or subcutaneous, all initiated 6 weeks prior to CIA induction [33]. Assessment of arthritis was via observation and corresponding arthritis score, histology, anticollagen type II antibodies, and analysis of cytokine production, Tregs, and Bregs. In both TPC-treated groups (oral and subcutaneous), a mean arthritis score of 1.5 was found, significantly lower than PBS-treated groups with a mean arthritis score of 11.8. While histology in PBS-treated mice showed noteworthy inflammation with neutrophil and leukocyte infiltration, fibrosis, necrosis, and cartilage erosion, TPC-treated mice showed much less synovial hyperplasia, with normal fat tissue without any inflammation, and preserved cartilage and bone. Anticollagen type II antibody levels were significantly lower in both TPC-treated groups, compared with PBS. Furthermore, both TPC-treated groups enhanced Tregs (CD4+, CD25+, FoxP3+) and Bregs (CD19+IL-10+TIM-1+ and IL-10^{high}CD25^{high}CD1d^{high}) expansion. Similarly, there was a significant preferential increase in antiinflammatory cytokines and a decrease in inflammatory cytokines produced by splenocytes in TPC-treated mice [33].

CONCLUSION

AIDs are a group of inflammatory disabling and chronic disorders, often resulting in agony, comorbidities, and shortened survival. Available treatment options are mostly not curative, and unfortunately associated with significant adverse effects, which contribute to morbidity and mortality. Research for better treatments has been a central topic of autoimmune experiments for decades.

Helminthes, long considered deleterious to health, were recently found to have beneficial effects on AID. The PC moiety, which is a part of a glycoprotein produced by helminthes, carries important antiinflammatory effects. The novel constructed molecule, combined of PC and tuftsin, a natural adjuvant produced by spleen, designated TPC, demonstrated a significant efficacy in several murine models of autoimmunity. Hence, TPC might prove to be an important small molecule drug, in combating human AID.

REFERENCES

[1] Ahmed SS, Lambert PH. Autoimmune diseases: the role for vaccines. In: The autoimmune diseases. 5th ed. 2014. p. 275–82.

[2] Strachan DP. Hay fever, hygiene, and household size. BMJ Br Med J (Clin Res Ed) November 18, 1989;299(6710):1259.

[3] Lambrecht BN, Hammad H. The immunology of the allergy epidemic and the hygiene hypothesis. Nat Immunol October 2017;18(10):1076.

[4] Okada H, Kuhn C, Feillet H, Bach JF. The 'hygiene hypothesis' for autoimmune and allergic diseases: an update. Clin Exp Immunol April 1, 2010;160(1):1–9.

[5] Kuijk LM, van Die I. Worms to the rescue: can worm glycans protect from autoimmune diseases? IUBMB Life April 1, 2010;62(4):303–12.

[6] Fleming JO, Weinstock JV. Clinical trials of helminth therapy in autoimmune diseases: rationale and findings. Parasite Immunol June 1, 2015;37(6):277–92.

[7] Elliott DE, Summers RW, Weinstock JV. Helminths as governors of immune-mediated inflammation. Int J Parasitol 2007;37:457–64.

[8] Wilson MS, Taylor M, Balic A, Finney CAM, Lamb JR, Maizels RM. Suppression of allergic airway inflammation by helminth-induced regulatory T cells. J Exp Med 2005;202:1199–212.

[9] van den Biggelaar A, van Ree R, Roderigues LC. Decreased atopy in children infected with Schistosoma haematobium: a role for parasite-induced interleukin-10. Lancet 2000;356:1723–7.

[10] Correale J, Farez M. Association between parasite infection and immune responses in multiple sclerosis. Ann Neurol 2007;61:97–108.

[11] Weinstock JV, Elliott DE. Helminth infections decrease host susceptibility to immune-mediated diseases. J Immunol October 1, 2014;193(7):3239–47.

[12] Hang L, Setiawan T, Blum AM, Urban J, Stoyanoff K, Arihiro S, Reinecker HC, Weinstock JV. Heligmosomoides polygyrus infection can inhibit colitis through direct interaction with innate immunity. J Immunol September 15, 2010;185(6):3184–9.

[13] Seguro LP, Rosario C, Shoenfeld Y. Long-term complications of past glucocorticoid use. Autoimmun Rev March 31, 2013;12(5):629–32.

[14] Watad A, Amital H, Shoenfeld Y. Intravenous immunoglobulin: a biological corticosteroid-sparing agent in some autoimmune conditions. Lupus January 1, 2017. 0961203317696589.

[15] Olds GR. Deworming the world. Trans Am Clin Climatol Assoc 2013;124:265.

[16] Schistosomiasis. Centers for Disease Control and Prevention. 2011.

[17] Weinstock JV. Autoimmunity: the worm returns. Nature November 8, 2012;491(7423):183–5.

[18] Goodridge HS, McGuiness S, Houston KM, Egan CA, Al-Riyami L, Alcocer MJ, Harnett MM, Harnett W. Phosphorylcholine mimics the effects of ES-62 on macrophages and dendritic cells. Parasite Immunol March 1, 2007;29(3):127–37.

[19] Goodridge HS, Marshall FA, Else KJ, Houston KM, Egan C, Al-Riyami L, Liew FY, Harnett W, Harnett MM. Immunomodulation via novel use of TLR4 by the filarial nematode phosphorylcholine-containing secreted product, ES-62. J Immunol January 1, 2005;174(1):284–93.

[20] Colthord JC, Rodgers DT, Lawrie RE, Al-Riyami L, Suckling CJ, Harnett W, Harnett MM. The parasitic worm-derived immunomodulator, ES-62 and its drug-like small molecule analogues exhibit therapeutic potential in a model of chronic asthma. Sci Rep January 14, 2016;6:19224.

[21] Aprahamian TR, Zhong X, Amir S, Binder CJ, Chiang LK, Al-Riyami L, Gharakhanian R, Harnett MM, Harnett W, Rifkin IR. The immunomodulatory parasitic worm product ES-62 reduces lupus-associated accelerated atherosclerosis in a mouse model. Int J Parasitol March 31, 2015;45(4):203–7.

[22] Rodgers DT, Pineda MA, Suckling CJ, Harnett W, Harnett MM. Drug-like analogues of the parasitic worm-derived immunomodulator ES-62 are therapeutic in the MRL/Lpr model of systemic lupus erythematosus. Lupus November 2015;24(13):1437–42.

[23] Pineda MA, Rodgers DT, Al-Riyami L, Harnett W, Harnett MM. ES-62 protects against collagen-induced arthritis by resetting Interleukin-22 toward resolution of inflammation in the joints. Arthritis Rheumatol June 1, 2014;66(6):1492–503.

[24] Harnett W, Harnett MM. Inhibition of murine B cell proliferation and down-regulation of protein kinase C levels by a phosphorylcholine-containing filarial excretory-secretory product. J Immunol November 1, 1993;151(9):4829–37.

[25] Shor DB, Bashi T, Lachnish J, Fridkin M, Bizzaro G, Barshak I, Blank M, Shoenfeld Y. Phosphorylcholine-tuftsin compound prevents development of dextransulfate-sodium-salt induced murine colitis: implications for the treatment of human inflammatory bowel disease. J Autoimmun January 31, 2015;56:111–7.

[26] Najjar VA, Nishioka K. 'Tuftsin': a natural phagocytosis stimulating peptide. Nature November 14, 1970;228(5272):672–3.

[27] Fridkin M, Najjar VA. Tuftsin: its chemistry, biology, and clinical potentia. Crit Rev Biochem Mol Biol January 1, 1989;24(1):1–40.

[28] Hübner MP, Thomas Stocker J, Mitre E. Inhibition of type 1 diabetes in filaria-infected non-obese diabetic mice is associated with a T helper type 2 shift and induction of FoxP3+ regulatory T cells. Immunology August 1, 2009;127(4):512–22.

[29] Song X, Shen J, Wen H, Zhong Z, Luo Q, Chu D, Qi Y, Xu Y, Wei W. Impact of Schistosoma japonicum infection on collagen-induced arthritis in DBA/1 mice: a murine model of human rheumatoid arthritis. PLoS One August 8, 2011;6(8):e23453.

[30] Summers RW, Elliott DE, Urban JF, Thompson R, Weinstock JV. Trichuris suis therapy in Crohn's disease. Gut January 1, 2005;54(1):87–90.

[31] Summers RW, Elliott DE, Urban JF, Thompson RA, Weinstock JV. Trichuris suis therapy for active ulcerative colitis: a randomized controlled trial. Gastroenterology April 30, 2005;128(4):825–32.

[32] Bashi T, Blank M, Shor DB, Fridkin M, Versini M, Gendelman O, Volkov A, Barshak I, Shoenfeld Y. Successful modulation of murine lupus nephritis with tuftsin-phosphorylcholine. J Autoimmun May 31, 2015;59:1–7.

[33] Bashi T, Shovman O, Fridkin M, Volkov A, Barshack I, Blank M, Shoenfeld Y. Novel therapeutic compound tuftsin–phosphorylcholine attenuates collagen-induced arthritis. Clin Exp Immunol April 1, 2016;184(1):19–28.

Chapter 61

Intravenous Immunoglobulin Treatment in Rheumatic Diseases

Antonella Fioravanti[1], Sara Tenti[2]

[1]*Rheumatology Unit, Azienda Ospedaliera Universitaria Senese, Siena, Italy;* [2]*Department of Medicine, Surgery and Neuroscience, Rheumatology Unit, University of Siena, Policlinico Le Scotte, Siena, Italy*

INTRODUCTION

Intravenous immunoglobulin (IVIG) is a therapeutic preparation of human polyspecific IgG, derived from the plasma of healthy donors [1]. IVIG was initially administered, in the early 1980s, as a replacement therapy in patients with primary or secondary immunodeficiencies. Since then, IVIG was used in a larger spectrum of autoimmune and systemic inflammatory disorders, thanks to its properties to modulate different pathways of the immune system [2,3].

There are actually several commercially available IVIG preparations that vary in composition and preparations methods with consecutive different efficacy and safety profile [4].

Firstly, in accordance with the World Health Organization (WHO) recommendations, the IVIG manufacturing process includes the purification of pooled donor plasma through fractioning and chromatography to obtain viral inactivation and removal. As a consequence of multiple methods, IVIG differs in the quantity of IgG, IgM, and IgA component, distribution of IgG subclasses, structure and function of Fc portion of IgG, and presence of aggregates. The optimal IVIG formulation should contain at least 80% of intact IgG with a normal IgG subclasses distribution, as little IgA as possible, and no fragments or aggregates [5,6].

Furthermore, IVIG products differ for concentration with higher concentrated formulation requiring smaller infusion volume loads and for the type of stabilizer, as glycine, L-proline, L-isoleucine or glucose, maltose, sucrose, or sorbitol. The use of IVIG preparation containing sucrose could arise some concerns in diabetic patients and is more likely associated to some adverse events, such as acute renal failure.

In addition, the sodium content, the osmolarity, and the osmolality vary from an IVIG formulation to another with a greater incidence of adverse effects as renal complications or thromboembolic events associated to hyperosmolar solutions [7].

Finally, other differences in the IVIG group lie in the levels of IgA and in the pH with pH close to neutral able to reduce the risk of injection site reaction [8].

MECHANISMS OF ACTION

The exact mechanism in which IVIG exerts its immunomodulatory and antiinflammatory effects remains not fully understood, but different pathways targeting the innate and adaptive immune systems are involved [9].

The action of high-dose IVIG administration was modulated either by the $F(ab')_2$ or the Fc segment. The saturation of the Fc receptors on phagocytic and vascular endothelial cells accelerates the degradation of circulating pathogenic autoantibodies and decreases phagocytosis and the release of inflammatory mediators. In addition, genetic and functional variations in Fc receptors as well as the differential IgG-Fc glycosylation patterns could play a role in modulating an inflammatory response [9].

The supraphysiologic doses of IgG induce the inhibition of the differentiation of the dendritic cells from monocytes with a consequent decrease of the cytokines and chemokines production. Other mechanisms involve the downregulation of B cells receptors and decrease of B cell proliferation and differentiation leading to a consequent reduction of their antibody production and the increase of the number and function of regulatory T cells. Additional IVIG effects include the modulation of pro/antiinflammatory cytokines and of metalloproteinases [9,10].

Furthermore, it was showed that sialic acid–enriched IVIG preparations have a greater antiinflammatory activity [11].

Mosaic of Autoimmunity. https://doi.org/10.1016/B978-0-12-814307-0.00061-X

INTRAVENOUS IMMUNOGLOBULIN THERAPY AND RHEUMATOLOGICAL CONDITIONS

The Food and Drug Administration–approved indications for IVIG therapy are, actually, limited (Table 61.1) and restricted in the rheumatologic field to the Kawasaki disease (KD); however, several reports demonstrated the beneficial effect of IVIG in a wide variety of other rheumatologic diseases, such as idiopathic inflammatory myopathies (IIM), systemic lupus erythematosus (SLE), antiphospholipid syndrome (APS), antineutrophil cytoplasm antibody (ANCA) vasculitis, and systemic sclerosis (SSc) [12,13] (Table 61.2).

TABLE 61.1 The Food and Drug Administration–Approved Indications for Intravenous Immunoglobulin Therapy (https://www.fda.go)

- Allogenic bone marrow transplantation
- Chronic lymphocytic leukemia
- Common variable immunodeficiency
- Chronic inflammatory demyelinating polyneuropathy
- Kidney transplantation with a high antibody recipient or with an "ABO" incompatible donor
- Primary immunodeficiency disorders associated with defects in humoral immunity
- Immune-mediated thrombocytopenia
- Kawasaki disease
- Hematopoietic stem cell transplantation in patients older than 20 years
- Chronic B cell lymphocytic leukemia
- Pediatric HIV type 1 infection

TABLE 61.2 Summary of the Scientific Evidence on Intravenous Immunoglobulin (IVIG) Therapy in Rheumatic Diseases

Indications	Literature Data
DM/PM	IVIG therapy is usually recommended in idiopathic inflammatory myopathies, especially in cases of steroid resistance and aggressive forms.
IBM	Controversial data. There is not sufficient evidence to support or refute the use of IVIG in IBM.
Lupus nephritis	IVIG resulted as effective as CYC in maintaining remission, after an induction therapy.
Refractory SLE	IVIG resulted effective in improving the disease activity scores and some clinical manifestations, when other treatments have failed.
SLE-associated autoimmune hemolytic anemia	The use of IVIG is only reserved to severe life-threatening conditions.
Cutaneous lupus erythematosus	Encouraging, but not sufficient evidence.
Obstetric APS	IVIG therapy should be reserved to patients not responsive to the conventional treatment or in case of association of other autoimmune manifestations such as thrombocytopenia or when concomitant infections exist or in patients in whom anticoagulation is contraindicated.
Nonobstetric APS	Additional therapy with IVIG could be useful to prevent recurrent thrombosis in patients refractory to conventional anticoagulant treatment.
CAPS	The international consensus guidelines recommend a combination therapy with anticoagulants plus corticosteroids, plasma exchange, and/or IVIG.
ANCA vasculitis	IVIG is considered an alternative therapy in particular conditions, as in immunocompromised patients with remittent infections, those with frequent relapses, or with refractory disease.
Systemic sclerosis	IVIG resulted effective in improving muscle and joint involvement, gastrointestinal symptoms, and skin fibrosis.

ANCA, antineutrophil cytoplasm antibody; *APS*, antiphospholipid syndrome; *CAPS*, catastrophic APS; *CYC*, cyclophosphamide; *DM*, dermatomyositis; *IBM*, inclusion body myositis; *PM*, polymyositis; *s*, systemic lupus erythematosus.

Kawasaki Disease

KD is the most common systemic vasculitis in children that leads to coronary artery aneurysms in a quarter of untreated cases. The efficacy of IVIG therapy in this disease was firstly described in 1984 by Furusho et al. [14] who observed a reduction of coronary abnormalities in KD patients treated with high-dose IVIG (400 mg/kg/die for four consecutive days). Consecutive randomized controlled trials (RCTs) confirmed the efficacy of IVIG in preventing the coronary aneurysms and a Cochrane review on 59 trials concluded that KD patients should be treated with a single high dose of IVIG (2 g/kg) and aspirin within 10 days of onset [15]. Previous metanalyses clearly stated that the efficacy of IVIG in preventing the coronary aneurysms is dose-dependent, so it is recommended to repeat the IVIG infusion 36 h after the first administration in patients with recurrent or persistent fever [16,17]. Different factors were found to affect the response to IVIG therapy in KD, such as high neutrophil count, high C-reactive protein and erythrocyte sedimentation rate, low hemoglobin and albumin levels, high aspartate and alanine aminotransferase levels, low sodium levels, and high total bilirubin and gamma-glutamyltransferase levels [13]. The RCTs to assess immunoglobulin plus steroid efficacy for KD (RAISE study) showed that the combination therapy of IVIG and prednisolone could be a very useful tool to overcome the IVIG resistance [18].

Idiopathic Inflammatory Myopathies

The term IIM refers to a heterogeneous group of acquired muscle disorders characterized by muscular weakness and signs of inflammation on muscle biopsy, such as dermatomyositis (DM), polymyositis (PM), and inclusion body myositis (IBM). Despite the scientific evidence on this topic is limited by the rarity of the disease and by the heterogeneity of the published studies, experts usually recommend IVIG in IIM, especially in cases of steroid resistance and aggressive disorder [13,19]. The IVIG therapy is supported by two RCTs and some uncontrolled trials. The first study was published in 1993 by Dalakas et al. [20] and reported a significant improvement in muscle strength and cutaneous rash in patients treated with IVIG at the dosage of 2 g/kg (divided over 2 days) monthly for 3 months, in comparison with placebo. The more recent RCT compared a single course of IVIG (2 g/kg divided over 5 days) with placebo in DM/PM patients refractory to high-dose corticosteroids, reporting no significant difference between the two groups in the primary outcomes, although IVIG resulted significantly superior to the placebo concerning the time to normalization of serum creatine kinase (CK) level and score of swallowing action [21]. The role of IVIG therapy as first-line therapy has been less investigated and only a RCT was published. This study described 60 DM patients who were randomized to receive IVIG (at the dosage of 400 mg/kg per day for 3 days, monthly for 3 times) in association to corticosteroids or steroids alone, reporting a major efficacy of IVIG concerning both clinical and biochemical outcomes at the end of month 3 [22]. However, the real efficacy of IVIG in the short term as first-line therapy in DM/PM population remains not clear because the other open-label studies rarely showed clinical effectiveness of IVIG [23,24]. On the contrary, there is more evidence of a relevant benefit on survival of IVIG in the long term, as demonstrated by studies reporting the maintenance of disease remission at different follow-up times (4–6 months in one study, 4 years in another one, and yet up 28 years in another study, respectively) [25–27].

The role of IVIG in IBM is still controversial and based on few trials showing only modest improvements and not significant differences with placebo [28–30]. In 2011, the American Academy of Neurology clearly stated that there is not sufficient evidence to support or refute the use of IVIG in IBM [31].

Finally, there are some reports showing encouraging results about the use of IVIG in certain subset of IIM, such as juvenile DM, anti-HMGCR antibody-associated autoimmune myopathies or for specific manifestations, such as rash and dysphagia [19].

Systemic Lupus Erythematosus

Although the increasing use of IVIG therapy in several different manifestations of SLE, the evidence supporting its efficacy mainly derived from small clinical trials, case series, and case reports. Only one small RCT was published to compare the utility of IVIG with cyclophosphamide (CYC) in 14 patients affected by lupus nephritis [32]. In this study, all patients were initially treated with intravenous (i.v.) CYC to induce the disease remission and then randomized to IVIG therapy (400 mg/kg monthly) or i.v. CYC (1 g/m² every 2 months for 6 months). At the end of the 18 months follow-up, a significant improvement of renal function was observed in both groups and IVIG resulted as effective as CYC in maintaining remission.

Other encouraging results derived from not controlled open trials, as that one of Francioni et al. [33] who evaluated the IVIG treatment (400 mg/kg for 5 days, monthly, for 6–24 months) in patients with chronically active lupus, observing a clinical and serological improvement in 11 of 12 studied subjects.

Furthermore, IVIG seems to significantly improve the disease activity scores, as demonstrated by Schroeder et al. [34] in 12 patients treated with two courses of high-dose IVIG and by Levy et al. [35] in 17 of 20 individuals treated monthly with IVIG (400 mg/kg per day for 5 consecutive days). In the first study the improvement was observed within 6 weeks from the treatment and lasted 5–12 months; in the second study, 80% of patients presented improvements of disease activity score, hypocomplementemia, and autoantibody titer after one to eight IVIG courses.

IVIG may also have a steroid-sparing effect, as showed by Zandman-Goddard et al. [36] who observed that 9 of 11 SLE patients treated with IVIG (400 mg/kg/die for 5 days) monthly for 6 months presented a full or partial remission, measured by SLEDAI score and a reduction of steroids consumption.

Finally, promising results derived from a large retrospective study [37] in which 62 SLE patients received low-dose IVIG (500 mg/kg in a single administration every 5±2 weeks). Good responses for many clinical manifestations were observed, as well as consistent reduction of SLEDAI score. However, some manifestations, such as thrombocytopenia, alopecia, vasculitis, and proteinuria, failed to respond to IVIG, pointing out the importance of the appropriate IVIG dosage.

Actually, IVIG in SLE is indicated in refractory disease where other therapies have failed, in acute severe flares, and in lupus nephritis as maintenance therapy or when SLE can be controlled only with high-dose steroids [36,38].

Particular Clinical Manifestations Associated to Systemic Lupus Erythematosus

Autoimmune hemolytic anemia is frequently associated with SLE and is in first line managed with corticosteroids; the use of IVIG is reserved to severe life-threatening conditions. On this respect, the available data are in fact controversial, mainly because the evidence is limited to small case series and the only retrospective study on 73 patients reported a significative response of hemoglobin levels in 40% of cases [39].

Some encouraging, but still limited, data on the use of IVIG were published in SLE patients with skin lesions. A prospective study was conducted to investigate the efficacy of IVIG, administered for the first two times at the dosage of 1 g/kg over 2 days and followed by 400 mg/kg monthly for no more than 6 months in 12 patients with cutaneous lupus erythematosus (LE). The authors observed a full remission in 40% patients, a partial remission in 20%, and no or limited response in 40% [40]. Good results with IVIG therapy were also obtained in case series of patients with chronic discoid LE and in lupus panniculitis resistant to other treatments [41,42]. However, contrasting results were described by De Pita et al. [43] who reported SLE and cutaneous LE patients with no improvement or even with exacerbation after IVIG and by Wollina et al. [44] who observed no response in patients with SLE.

Antiphospholipid Syndrome

APS is recognized as the most common cause of acquired thrombophilia in the general population, presenting as early pregnancy loss or arteriovenous thrombosis.

Obstetric APS should be treated by a multidisciplinary team of specialists with experience in this field. In this contest, secondary thromboprophylaxis with low-dose aspirin (LDA) and heparin is the mainstay of treatment, and hydroxychloroquine is usually added for patients suffering from SLE [45]. Although an optimal therapeutic target was not often reached, several new emerging therapies have been implemented in the last years. Among these IVIG showed a beneficial effect in some case reports/series and observational or randomized trials [46].

The literature data seem controversial; indeed, while some studies demonstrated a decrease of pregnancy complications or of the abortion rate, other trials concluded that no benefits derived from the use of IVIG in association with LDA and low molecular weight heparin (LMWH) compared with LDA and LMWH alone [47–50]. At the moment, IVIG therapy in obstetric APS seems to be reserved to selected situations, such as patients not responsive to the conventional treatment or in case of association of other autoimmune manifestations such as thrombocytopenia or when concomitant infections exist or in patients in whom anticoagulation is contraindicated. It's noteworthy to underline that the IVIG dosage and the schedule of the treatment were different in each study varying from 200 mg/kg per day until 32 week of gestation to 1 g/kg per day for 2 consecutive days each month until week 36.

The evidence about the efficacy and safety of IVIG therapy in not-pregnant APS patients is scarce; in particular the use of IVIG in the primary or secondary thromboprophylaxis was described only in two prospective open studies and in few case reports. According to these data, it seems that an additional therapy with IVIG could be useful to prevent recurrent thrombosis in APS patients refractory to conventional anticoagulant treatment [51,52].

Catastrophic APS (CAPS) is a severe subset of APS characterized by multiorgan failure originated by widespread thrombotic disease, which usually affects small vessels over a short period and is associated with high mortality rates [53]. Combination therapy with anticoagulants plus corticosteroids, plasma exchange (PE), and/or IVIG ("triple therapy") was the most commonly used treatment for CAPS, in agreement with the international consensus guidelines [54]. IVIG is used in a dose of 0.4 g/d/kg for 5 days and should be administered after the last day of PE, when planned, to prevent their removal. IVIG is well tolerated, but they should be used with caution in case of thrombosis, particularly in those patients whose anticoagulation was discontinued because of bleeding. Avoiding products with high osmolality, reducing the rate of IVIG infusion, hydration, and using nonsucrose IVIG products (especially in patients with renal failure) are strategies that can reduce thrombosis risk [55]. Elderly patients with diabetes, hypertension, or hypercholesterolemia should also be infused with care, with a reduced rate of IVIG infusion. IVIG is strongly recommended in CAPS patients with severe thrombocytopenia refractory to high-dose steroid therapy or when a concomitant infection exists [56]. As there were no metanalyses or RCTs, most of the scientific evidence derives from the online available "CAPS Registry" that includes the description of 342 cases of CAPS and their treatments. The analysis of this registry confirms that the "triple therapy" strategy improves the survival rate (around 70%) [56,57].

Antineutrophil Cytoplasm Antibody–Associated Vasculitis

ANCA vasculitis is a group of systemic small vessel vasculitis associated with circulating ANCA that includes granulomatosis with polyangiitis, microscopic polyangiitis, and eosinophilic granulomatosis with polyangiitis. The therapeutic strategy usually comprises high-dose corticosteroids often associated to immunosuppressive agents, such as CYC, rituximab, azathioprine (AZT), methotrexate, or leflunomide. Considering the possible toxicity of these treatments, IVIG was studied as adjuvant or alternative therapy. Also the British Society for Rheumatology, in 2007, regarding ANCA vasculitis described IVIG as "an alternative therapy in patients with refractory disease or in patients for whom conventional therapy is contra-indicated, for example, in the presence of infection, in the severely ill patient or in pregnancy" [58]. A 2009 Cochrane review (recently updated) [59] identified only a RCT with 34 participants who were equally and randomly assigned to receive IVIG (a single course of 400 mg/kg daily for 5 days) or placebo in addition to AZT and corticosteroids for remission maintenance. There were no significant differences between adjuvant IVIG and adjuvant placebo in mortality, serious adverse events, time to relapse, and infection rates. The authors demonstrated that a single course of high-dose IVIG reduces disease activity in ANCA vasculitis where active disease persists, but the benefit of IVIG was not maintained beyond 3 months [60]. A recent French multicentre retrospective study was published on 92 ANCA vasculitis patients and it showed that 83% of individuals treated with IVIG for relapsing disease for a median of 6 months were more likely to go into remission and required less corticosteroid [61].

Other studies demonstrated the usefulness of IVIG therapy during the acute flares of vasculitis in patients with concomitant infection and at high risks for immunosuppressive treatment [62,63]. Based on this evidence, we can consider IVIG not a first-line therapy in clinical practice but a good option in particular conditions, as in immunocompromised patients with remittent infections, those with frequent relapses, or with refractory disease.

Systemic Sclerosis

Considering both immunomodulatory and antifibrotic properties of IVIG, it was studied as a potential promising therapy in SSc. IVIG resulted effective in improving muscle involvement in SSc, as demonstrated by a reduction of muscle pain, Medical Research Council test, and CK serum levels [64], confirming the good results of IVIG in IIM. A significant decrease of tender and swollen counts with recovery of joint function was also observed in an open-label trial of seven SSc patients [65]. Promising data derive from IVIG therapy for gastrointestinal involvement in SSc, as reported by a not controlled study [64] and a case series [66]. In both papers, the authors described a reduction of frequency and severity of Gastroesophageal reflux disease (GERD) and gastrointestinal symptoms.

Regarding skin involvement several studies reported a benefit of IVIG therapy in reducing skin score and fibrosis. In 2015, Poelman et al. [67] presented their experience with 30 patients with severe, refractory, active diffuse cutaneous scleroderma treated with adjunctive IVIG (2 g/kg per month for 6 months). The authors observed a significant reduction of skin thickening, and the improvement of modified Rodnan skin score (mRSS) was greater in IVIG-treated patients at 12 months follow-up compared with data from historical controls from negative trials. Furthermore, the only RCT study conducted on IVIG therapy in SSc patients reported no significant difference in the mRSS score between the group of participants treated with IVIG (400 mg/kg per day for 5 consecutive days in a single course) compared with patients who had received placebo, but when a second cycle of IVIG was administered skin sclerosis significantly ameliorated in the IVIG group [68].

More recently, a French nationwide cohort study analyzed the data of 46 SSc patients treated with at least an infusion of IVIG (at a dosage >1 g/kg/cycle) reporting a significant improvement of musculoskeletal and gastrointestinal involvement, systemic inflammation, and a reduction of steroid consumption, but it failed to demonstrate a benefit in skin and lung fibrosis [69].

Other Rheumatic Diseases

Many other rheumatological conditions were successfully treated with IVIG, such as peripheral neuropathy associated to Sjogren syndrome (SS). Over the years, 10 case reports showed the benefit of IVIG therapy in SS patients with peripheral nervous system involvement. At this regard, the largest study dated back to 2011, when Rist et al. [70] retrospectively evaluated the efficacy and tolerability of at least an infusion of IVIG in 19 patients with SS complicated with peripheral neuropathy. The authors observed an improvement or at least a stabilization of the clinical symptoms, measured by the disability Modified Rankin Scale and the global evaluation of the physician, in most cases. Particularly, IVIG resulted more useful in patients with sensorimotor or nonataxic sensory neuropathy without necrotizing vasculitis.

Furthermore, considering the ability of IVIG to counteract the placental transport of autoantibodies and to exert an antiidiotype regulation, this therapy was employed in the treatment of fetal congenital heart block (CHB), a severe complication in pregnant women anti-Ro or anti-La positive. The use of IVIG alone or in association to steroids failed to prevent CHB occurrence at the dosages used (usually one single IVIG course during pregnancy) [71–74]. More recently, IVIG was administered in association to weekly sessions of plasmapheresis and betamethasone (4 mg/day) in 12 pregnant women positive to anti-SSA/Ro and/or anti-SSB/La in whom CHB was diagnosed. Of six fetuses who presented atrioventricular block of second type, two returned to a first-type block and one to a normal conduction, whereas the six fetuses with block of third type remained stable during the pregnancy and no fetal complications or neonatal deaths were reported. On these basis, a combination therapy including IVIG seems effective in the management of the second-type CHB [75].

The beneficial effect of IVIG therapy was also described in case series or reports on patients affected by Behcet's disease.

TOLERABILITY

IVIG is usually well tolerated with mild and transient side effects. The majority of the adverse reactions are related to the infusion rate and include headache, nausea, malaise, myalgia, arthralgia, and fewer. Other side effects depend on the use of different formulations in certain at risk patients. For example, patients at risk of renal failure should avoid IVIG stabilized with sucrose, which is shown to cause osmotic nephrosis. In these patients, also formulations with high content of sodium or with high osmolality/osmolarity should be avoided and reduced and fractionated doses should be preferred. In patients with cardiovascular disease or at risk of thromboembolic events, the appropriate IVIG preparation should have low osmolarity with a concentration of 5%–10% and should be administered in more days' course and at slow rate infusion. Furthermore, high-dose treatment was demonstrated to be related to the onset of hemolysis or to aseptic meningitis, particularly in case of rapid infusion. Finally, the content of IgA is another property to be considered because of the described severe anaphylactic or anaphylactoid reactions in patients with IgA deficiency.

To minimize the risk of side effects, the prescription of IVIG therapy and the choice of the product should be individualized according to the medical history and the patient's comorbidities, such as diabetes, obesity, hypercholesterolemia, cardiovascular and renal diseases, and thrombotic events.

Before the infusion, the patients need a proper hydration.

The rate of the infusion depends on the different IVIG formulation, and during the first administration, a low rate of infusion with gradual increases is recommended; in case of adverse events, the rate of infusion has to be decreased [6,7].

SUBCUTANEOUS IMMUNOGLOBULIN THERAPY

Although the subcutaneous (SC) route of administration of immunoglobulin (IG) was employed from the 1940s in primary immunodeficiencies, there has recently been an increased interest in this kind of IG. Several studies demonstrated that there is no difference between SCIG and IVIG in terms of efficacy and that SC formulation resulted to be well tolerated. Indeed, the fractionating of the dosage into smaller but more frequent portions prevents the systemic adverse events described with IVIG, and the adverse reactions usually described with SCIG are mild, mostly consisting in localized injection site reactions. SCIG presents the undoubted advantage to permit a better quality of life to the patients, assuring them to preserve their independence and to save missed working days. Furthermore, the therapy with SCIG is associated to reduced costs in comparison with IVIG and there are no reports of renal failure with this formulation of IG. On the other side, SCIG treatment requires an appropriate education and training of the patients, a more frequent administration and some patients continue to prefer IVIG to SCIG [76].

The scientific evidence on SCIG derives mainly from studies on primary and secondary immunodeficiency diseases. In 2011, Danieli et al. [77] firstly reported the efficacy and tolerability of SCIG in PM and DM patients and then some data were collected also in IBM. The above-mentioned trials confirmed the equivalence in efficacy between SCIG and IVIG but pointed out the problem to administer a large amount of IgG, as requested in autoimmune disorders. Recently, the feasibility of SCIG in IIM was demonstrated by Cherin et al. [78] who described 19 patients with long-standing PM, DM, and IBM treated with SCIG (at the median dosage of 1.9 g/kg per month, with a frequency of two infusions per week). The authors observed significant improvement in muscle strength and disability in the majority of the patients and a good tolerability of this therapy in the long term.

REFERENCES

[1] Kivity S, Katz U, Daniel N, Nussinovitch U, Papageorgiou N, Shoenfeld Y. Evidence for the use of intravenous immunoglobulins–a review of the literature. Clin Rev Allergy Immunol 2010;38:201–69.

[2] Katz U, Shoenfeld Y, Zandman-Goddard G. Update on intravenous immunoglobulins (IVIg) mechanisms of action and off- label use in autoimmune diseases. Curr Pharm Des 2011;17:3166–75.

[3] Zandman-Goddard G, Krauthammer A, Levy Y, Langevitz P, Shoenfeld Y. Long-term therapy with intravenous immunoglobulin is beneficial in patients with autoimmune diseases. Clin Rev Allergy Immunol 2012;42:247–55.

[4] Hooper JA. Intravenous immunoglobulins: evolution of commercial IVIG preparations. Immunol Allergy Clin North Am 2008;28:765–78.

[5] Martin TD. IGIV: contents, properties, and methods of industrial production–evolving closer to a more physiologic product. Int Immunopharmacol 2006;6:517–22.

[6] Cherin P, Marie I, Michallet M, Pelus E, Dantal J, Crave JC, et al. Management of adverse events in the treatment of patients with immunoglobulin therapy: a review of evidence. Autoimmun Rev 2016;15:71–81.

[7] Chérin P, Cabane J. Relevant criteria for selecting an intravenous immunoglobulin preparation for clinical use. BioDrugs 2010;24:211–23.

[8] Lemm G. Composition and properties of IVIg preparations that affect tolerability and therapeutic efficacy. Neurology 2002;59:S28–32.

[9] Gelfand EW. Intravenous immune globulin in autoimmune and inflammatory diseases. N Engl J Med 2012;367:2015–25.

[10] Basyreva LY, Brodsky IB, Gusev AA, Zhapparova ON, Mikhalchik EV, Gusev SA, et al. The effect of Intravenous Immunoglobulin (IVIG) on \ textit{ex vivo} activation of human leukocytes. Hum Antibodies 2016;24:39–44.

[11] von Gunten S, Shoenfeld Y, Blank M, Branch DR, Vassilev T, Käsermann F, et al. IVIG pluripotency and the concept of Fc-sialylation: challenges to the scientist. Nat Rev Immunol 2014;14:349.

[12] Mulhearn B, Bruce IN. Indications for IVIG in rheumatic diseases. Rheumatology (Oxf) 2015;54:383–91.

[13] Bayry J, Negi VS, Kaveri SV. Intravenous immunoglobulin therapy in rheumatic diseases. Nat Rev Rheumatol 2011;7:349–59.

[14] Furusho K, Kamiya T, Nakano H, Kiyosawa N, Shinomiya K, Hayashidera T, et al. High-dose intravenous gammaglobulin for Kawasaki disease. Lancet 1984;2:1055–8.

[15] Oates-Whitehead RM, Baumer JH, Haines L, Love S, Maconochie IK, Gupta A, et al. Intravenous immunoglobulin for the treatment of Kawasaki disease in children. Cochrane Database Syst Rev 2003;4:CD004000.

[16] Terai M, Shulman ST. Prevalence of coronary artery abnormalities in Kawasaki disease is highly dependent on gamma globulin dose but independent of salicylate dose. J Pediatr 1997;131:888–93.

[17] Shulman ST. Intravenous immunoglobulin for the treatment of Kawasaki disease. Pediatr Ann 2017;46:e25–8.

[18] Kobayashi T, Saji T, Otani T, Takeuchi K, Nakamura T, Arakawa H, et al. Efficacy of immunoglobulin plus prednisolone for prevention of coronary artery abnormalities in severe Kawasaki disease (RAISE study): a randomised, open-label, blinded-endpoints trial. Lancet 2012;379:1613–20.

[19] Anh-Tu Hoa S, Hudson M. Critical review of the role of intravenous immunoglobulins in idiopathic inflammatory myopathies. Semin Arthritis Rheum 2017;46:488–508.

[20] Dalakas MC, Illa I, Dambrosia JM, Soueidan SA, Stein DP, Otero C, Dinsmore ST, McCrosky S. A controlled trial of high-dose intravenous immune globulin infusions as treatment for dermatomyositis. N Engl J Med 1993;329:1993–2000.

[21] Miyasaka N, Hara M, Koike T, Saito E, Yamada M, Tanaka Y. GB-0998 Study Group. Effects of intravenous immunoglobulin therapy in Japanese patients with polymyositis and dermatomyositis resistant to corticosteroids: a randomized double-blind placebo-controlled trial. Mod Rheumatol 2012;22:382–93.

[22] Tian J, Gao JS, Chen JW, Li F, Xie X, Du JF. Efficacy and safety of the combined treatment with intravenous immunoglobulin and oral glucocorticoid in the elderly with dermatomyositis. Chin J Geriatr 2008;27:588–90.

[23] Cherin P, Piette JC, Wechsler B, Bletry O, Ziza JM, Laraki R, et al. Intravenous gamma globulin as first line therapy in polymyositis and dermatomyositis: an open study in 11 adult patients. J Rheumatol 1994;21:1092–7.

[24] Göttfried I, Seeber A, Anegg B, Rieger A, Stingl G, Volc-Platzer B. High dose intravenous immunoglobulin (IVIG) in dermatomyositis: clinical responses and effect on sIL-2R levels. Eur J Dermatol 2000;10:29–35.

[25] Cherin P, Pelletier S, Teixeira A, Laforet P, Genereau T, Simon A, et al. Results and long-term followup of intravenous immunoglobulin infusions in chronic, refractory polymyositis: an open study with thirty-five adult patients. Arthritis Rheum 2002;46:467–74.

[26] Danieli MG, Malcangi G, Palmieri C, Logullo F, Salvi A, Piani M, et al. Cyclosporin A and intravenous immunoglobulin treatment in polymyositis/dermatomyositis. Ann Rheum Dis 2002;61:37–41.

[27] Danieli MG, Gambini S, Pettinari L, Logullo F, Veronesi G, Gabrielli A. Impact of treatment on survival in polymyositis and dermatomyositis. A single-centre long-term follow-up study. Autoimmun Rev 2014;13:1048–54.

[28] Dalakas MC, Sonies B, Dambrosia J, Sekul E, Cupler E, Sivakumar K. Treatment of inclusion-body myositis with IVIg: a double-blind, placebo-controlled study. Neurology 1997;48:712–6.

[29] Walter MC, Lochmüller H, Toepfer M, Schlotter B, Reilich P, Schröder M, et al. High-dose immunoglobulin therapy in sporadic inclusion body myositis: a double-blind, placebo-controlled study. J Neurol 2000;247:22–8.

[30] Dalakas MC, Koffman B, Fujii M, Spector S, Sivakumar K, Cupler E. A controlled study of intravenous immunoglobulin combined with prednisone in the treatment of IBM. Neurology 2001;56:323–7.

[31] Patwa HS, Chaudhry V, Katzberg H, Rae-Grant AD, So YT. Evidence-based guideline: intravenous immunoglobulin in the treatment of neuro-muscular disorders: report of the Therapeutics and Technology Assessment Subcommittee of the American Academy of Neurology. Neurology 2012;78:1009–15.

[32] Boletis JN, Ioannidis JP, Boki KA, Moutsopoulos HM. Intravenous immunoglobulin compared with cyclophosphamide for proliferative lupus nephritis. Lancet 1999;354:569–70.

[33] Francioni C, Galeazzi M, Fioravanti A, Gelli R, Megale F, Marcolongo R. Long-term i.v. Ig treatment in systemic lupus erythematosus. Clin Exp Rheumatol 1994;12:163–8.

[34] Schroeder JO, Zeuner RA, Euler HH, Löffler H. High dose intravenous immunoglobulins in systemic lupus erythematosus: clinical and serological results of a pilot study. J Rheumatol 1996;23:71–5.

[35] Levy Y, Sherer Y, Ahmed A, Langevitz P, George J, Fabbrizzi F, et al. A study of 20 SLE patients with intravenous immunoglobulin–clinical and serologic response. Lupus 1999;8:705–12.

[36] Zandman-Goddard G, Blank M, Shoenfeld Y. Intravenous immunoglobulins in systemic lupus erythematosus: from the bench to the bedside. Lupus 2009;18:884–8.

[37] Sherer Y, Kuechler S, Jose Scali J, Rovensky J, Levy Y, Zandman-Goddard G, et al. Low dose intravenous immunoglobulin in systemic lupus erythematosus: analysis of 62 cases. Isr Med Assoc J 2008;10:55–7.

[38] Watad A, Amital H, Shoenfeld Y. Intravenous immunoglobulin: a biological corticosteroid-sparing agent in some autoimmune conditions. Lupus 2017;26:1015–22.

[39] Flores G, Cunningham-Rundles C, Newland AC, Bussel JB. Efficacy of intravenous immunoglobulin in the treatment of autoimmune hemolytic anemia: results in 73 patients. Am J Hematol 1993;44:237–42.

[40] Goodfield M, Davison K, Bowden K. Intravenous immunoglobulin (IVIg) for therapy-resistant cutaneous lupus erythematosus (LE). J Dermatol Treat 2004;15:46–50.

[41] Piette JC, Frances C, Roy S, et al. High-dose immunoglobulins in the treatment of refractory kg/day for five consecutive days each month for a 12-cutaneous lupus erythematosus: open trial in 5 patients. Arthritis Rheum 1995;38(Suppl. 9):304.

[42] Espírito Santo J, Gomes MF, Gomes MJ, Peixoto L, Pereira SC, Acabado A, et al. Intravenous immunoglobulin in lupus panniculitis. Clin Rev Allergy Immunol 2010;38:307–18.

[43] De Pità O, Bellucci AM, Ruffelli M, Girardelli CR, Puddu P. Intravenous immunoglobulin therapy is not able to efficiently control cutaneous manifestations in patients with lupus erythematosus. Lupus 1997;6:415–7.

[44] Wollina U, Looks A, Kammler H-J. Intravenous immunoglobulin therapy in dermatology: overview and center experience. An Bras Dermatol 1998;73:255–9.

[45] Alijotas-Reig J. Treatment of refractory obstetric antiphospholipid syndrome: the state of the art and new trends in the therapeutic management. Lupus 2013;22:6–17.

[46] Tenti S, Cheleschi S, Guidelli GM, Galeazzi M, Fioravanti A. Intravenous immunoglobulins and antiphospholipid syndrome: how, when and why? A review of the literature. Autoimmun Rev 2016;15:226–35.

[47] Branch DW, Peaceman AM, Druzin M, Silver RK, El-Sayed Y, Silver RM, et al. A multicenter, placebo-controlled pilot study of intravenous immune globulin treatment of antiphospholipid syndrome during pregnancy. The Pregnancy Loss Study Group. Am J Obstet Gynecol 2000;182:122–7.

[48] Triolo G, Ferrante A, Ciccia F, Accardo-Palumbo A, Perino A, Castelli A, et al. Randomized study of subcutaneous low molecular weight heparin plus aspirin versus intravenous immunoglobulin in the treatment of recurrent fetal loss associated with antiphospholipid antibodies. Arthritis Rheum 2003;48:728–31.

[49] Jeremić K, Pervulov M, Gojnić M, Dukanac J, Ljubić A, Stojnić J. Comparison of two therapeutic protocols in patients with antiphospholipid antibodies and recurrent miscarriages. Vojnosanit Pregl 2005;62:435–9.

[50] Dendrinos S, Sakkas E, Makrakis E. Low-molecular-weight heparin versus intravenous immunoglobulin for recurrent abortion associated with antiphospholipid antibody syndrome. Int J Gynaecol Obstet 2009;104:223–5.

[51] Sciascia S, Giachino O, Roccatello D. Prevention of thrombosis relapse in antiphospholipid syndrome patients refractory to conventional therapy using intravenous immunoglobulin. Clin Exp Rheumatol 2012;30:409–13.

[52] Tenti S, Guidelli GM, Bellisai F, Galeazzi M, Fioravanti A. Long-term treatment of antiphospholipid syndrome with intravenous immunoglobulin in addition to conventional therapy. Clin Exp Rheumatol 2013;31:877–82.

[53] Cervera R, Bucciarelli S, Plasín MA, Gómez-Puerta JA, Plaza J, Pons-Estel G, et al. Catastrophic antiphospholipid syndrome (CAPS) registry project group (European forum on antiphospholipid antibodies). Catastrophic antiphospholipid syndrome (CAPS): descriptive analysis of a series of 280 patients from the "CAPS Registry". J Autoimmun 2009;32:240–5.

[54] Asherson RA, Cervera R, de Groot PG, Erkan D, Boffa MC, Piette JC, et al. Catastrophic Antiphospholipid Syndrome Registry Project Group. Catastrophic antiphospholipid syndrome: international consensus statement on classification criteria and treatment guidelines. Lupus 2003;12:530–4.

[55] Cervera R. Update on the diagnosis, treatment, and prognosis of the catastrophic antiphospholipid syndrome. Curr Rheumatol Rep 2010;12:70–6.

[56] Cervera R, Rodríguez-Pintó I, Colafrancesco S, Conti F, Valesini G, Rosário C, et al. 14th international congress on antiphospholipid antibodies task force report on catastrophic antiphospholipid syndrome. Autoimmun Rev 2014;13:699–707.

[57] Bucciarelli S, Cervera R, Espinosa G, Gómez-Puerta JA, Ramos-Casals M, Font J. Mortalityn in the catastrophic antiphospholipid syndrome: causes of death and prognostic factors. Autoimmun Rev 2006;6:72–5.

[58] Lapraik C, Watts R, Bacon P, Carruthers D, Chakravarty K, D'Cruz D, et al. BSR and BHPR guidelines for the management of adults with ANCA associated vasculitis. Rheumatology (Oxf) 2007;46:1615–6.

[59] Fortin PM, Tejani AM, Bassett K, Musini VM. Intravenous immunoglobulin as adjuvant therapy for Wegener's granulomatosis. Cochrane Database Syst Rev 2013;1:CD007057.

[60] Jayne DR, Chapel H, Adu D, Misbah S, O'Donoghue D, Scott D, et al. Intravenous immunoglobulin for ANCA-associated systemic vasculitis with persistent disease activity. Q J Med 2000;93:433–9.

[61] Crickx E, Machelart I, Lazaro E, Kahn JE, Cohen-Aubart F, Martin T, et al. Intravenous immunoglobulin as an immunomodulating agent in anti-neutrophil cytoplasmic antibody-associated vasculitides: a French nationwide study of ninety-two patients. French Vasculitis Study Group. Arthritis Rheumatol 2016;68:702–12.

[62] Simoes J, Sciascia S, Camara I, Baldovino S, Karim Y, Roccatello D, et al. Use of intravenous immunoglobulin in patients with active vasculitis associated with concomitant infection. J Clin Rheumatol 2015;21:35–7.

[63] Guidelli GM, Tenti S, Pascarelli NA, Galeazzi M, Fioravanti A. Granulomatosis with polyangiitis and intravenous immunoglobulins: a case series and review of the literature. Autoimmun Rev 2015;14:659–64.

[64] Raja J, Nihtyanova SI, Murray CD, Denton CP, Ong VH. Sustained benefit from intravenous immunoglobulin therapy for gastrointestinal involvement in systemic sclerosis. Rheumatology (Oxf) 2016;55:115–9.

[65] Nacci F, Righi A, Conforti ML, Miniati I, Fiori G, Martinovic D, et al. Intravenous immunoglobulins improve the function and ameliorate joint involvement in systemic sclerosis: a pilot study. Ann Rheum Dis 2007;66:977–9.

[66] Clark KE, Etomi O, Denton CP, Ong VH, Murray CD. Intravenous immunoglobulin therapy for severe gastrointestinal involvement in systemic sclerosis. Clin Exp Rheumatol 2015;33(4 Suppl. 91):S168–70.

[67] Poelman CL, Hummers LK, Wigley FM, Anderson C, Boin F, Shah AA. Intravenous immunoglobulin may be an effective therapy for refractory, active diffuse cutaneous systemic sclerosis. J Rheumatol 2015;42:236–42.

[68] Takehara K, Ihn H, Sato S. A randomized, double-blind, placebo-controlled trial: intravenous immunoglobulin treatment in patients with diffuse cutaneous systemic sclerosis. Clin Exp Rheumatol 2013;31:151–6.

[69] Sanges S, Rivière S, Mekinian A, Martin T, Le Quellec A, Chatelus E, et al. Intravenous immunoglobulins in systemic sclerosis: data from a French nationwide cohort of 46 patients and review of the literature. Autoimmun Rev 2017;16:377–84.

[70] Rist S, Sellam J, Hachulla E, Sordet C, Puéchal X, Hatron PY, et al. Experience of intravenous immunoglobulin therapy in neuropathy associated with primary Sjögren's syndrome: a national multicentric retrospective study. Arthritis Care Res (Hoboken) 2011;63:1339–44.

[71] Friedman DM, Llanos C, Izmirly PM, Brock B, Byron J, Copel J, et al. Evaluation of fetuses in a study of intravenous immunoglobulin as preventive therapy for congenital heart block: results of a multicenter, prospective, open-label clinical trial. Arthritis Rheum 2010;62:1138–46.

[72] Pisoni CN, Brucato A, Ruffatti A, Espinosa G, Cervera R, Belmonte-Serrano M, et al. Failure of intravenous immunoglobulin to prevent congenital heart block: findings of a multicenter, prospective, observational study. Arthritis Rheum 2010;62:1147–52.

[73] Brucato A, Cimaz R, Caporali R, Ramoni V, Buyon J. Pregnancy outcomes in patients with autoimmune diseases and anti-Ro/SSA antibodies. Clin Rev Allergy Immunol 2011;40:27–41.

[74] Brucato A, Ramoni V, Gerosa M, Pisoni MP. Congenital fetal heart block: a potential therapeutic role for intravenous immunoglobulin. Obstet Gynecol 2011;117:177.

[75] Ruffatti A, Cerutti A, Favaro M, Del Ross T, Calligaro A, Hoxha A, Marson P, Leoni L, Milanesi O. Plasmapheresis, intravenous immunoglobulins and bethametasone - a combined protocol to treat autoimmune congenital heart block: a prospective cohort study. Clin Exp Rheumatol 2016;344:706–13.

[76] Perez EE, Orange JS, Bonilla F, Chinen J, Chinn IK, Dorsey M, et al. Update on the use of immunoglobulin in human disease: a review of evidence. J Allergy Clin Immunol 2017;139:S1–46.

[77] Danieli MG, Pettinari L, Moretti R, Logullo F, Gabrielli A. Subcutaneous immunoglobulin in polymyositis and dermatomyositis: a novel application. Autoimmun Rev 2011;10:144–9.

[78] Cherin P, Belizna C, Cartry O, Lascu-Dubos G, de Jaeger C, Delain JC, Crave JC, Hachulla E. Long-term subcutaneous immunoglobulin use in inflammatory myopathies: a retrospective review of 19 cases. Autoimmun Rev 2016;15:281–6.

Chapter 62

Autoimmunity and Allergic Diseases*

Matilde Leon-Ponte[1], Eyal Grunebaum[1,2]

[1]*Developmental and Stem Cell Biology Program, Research Institute, Food Allergy and Anaphylaxis Program, Hospital for Sick Children, Toronto, ON, Canada;* [2]*University of Toronto, Toronto, ON, Canada*

Allergic, also known as atopic, diseases are a large group of conditions often involving IgE-mediated immune responses to environmental antigens (allergens), which commonly present as allergic rhinitis, atopic dermatitis, or asthma. In addition, IgE-mediated allergic reactions can occur following exposure to exogenous triggers such as food, medications, and venoms. The allergen–IgE complex can signal through the high- and low-affinity receptors (known as the FcεRI and FcεRII, respectively) on mast cells and basophils. Activation of these cells leads to release of inflammatory mediators such as biogenic amines, lipid mediators, proteases, and cytokines. These secondary allergic mediators affect multiple target cells, tissues, and organs leading to variety of symptoms that can culminate in anaphylaxis and death. Allergic diseases have traditionally been considered as type II immune responses, directed by T-helper (Th) -2 cells and identified by a cytokine signature that included interleukin (IL) -4, -5 and -13. A subset of allergic responses can develop also without identifiable IgE involvement. In contrast, autoimmune diseases are considered as type I responses, directed by Th-1 and characterized by presence of interferon gamma. The hypothesis that immune responses could be either type I or type II suggested that autoimmune and allergic diseases would be mutually exclusive. Indeed, initial studies supported this hypothesis, yet in recent years accumulating epidemiological data, advances in the understanding the complexities of the Th-1 and Th-2 immune responses, as well as lessons from primary and acquired immune abnormalities indicate that allergies and autoimmunity can coexist. Appreciation of the overlap in pathogenesis of allergies and autoimmunity suggests that lessons in the management of one disorder might also be applicable to the other.

EPIDEMIOLOGICAL STUDIES OF ALLERGY AND AUTOIMMUNITY

The occurrence of allergies with rheumatoid arthritis has been investigated extensively and results have been controversial. Swedish and French patients with rheumatoid arthritis questioned about their allergies identified an inverse relationship between the conditions [1,2]. Similarly, a questioner of 487 German patients with rheumatoid arthritis revealed that 8.6%, 2.9%, and 4.3% suffered from allergic rhinitis, atopic dermatitis, and asthma, respectively, which were lower than controls [3]. A Dutch retrospective cohort study of 304 patients with rheumatoid arthritis identified significant decrease in the risk to develop allergic rhinitis compared with controls [4]. Moreover, subjects with both rheumatoid arthritis and allergic rhinitis had lower rheumatoid arthritis clinical scores and inflammatory markers. However, other studies did not find difference in the incidence of allergic diseases in patients with rheumatoid arthritis [5]. Moreover, a recent nationwide population-based cohort study from Taiwan found that the incidence of rheumatoid arthritis was directly related with the presence of asthma and allergic rhinitis [6]. In addition, patients with more than one allergic manifestation had an increased risk of developing rheumatoid arthritis. Similarly, a Finish birth registry showed that the frequency of asthma was significantly higher among children with rheumatoid arthritis [7].

The correlation between multiple sclerosis and allergies has also been studied extensively, although the number of patients included has been typically lower than in rheumatoid arthritis studies. Among 35 patients with multiple sclerosis followed at Stanford, allergy symptoms scores were significantly lower when compared with controls, and patients also had lower allergen-specific IgE levels to 36 different allergens [8]. Analysis of hospital records of 320 Welsh patients with multiple sclerosis and matched controls revealed a lower prevalence of asthma, although not of atopic dermatitis [9]. A questioner-based study demonstrated that the frequency of asthma and allergic rhinitis was reduced in 610 French, 20–44 years old, patients with multiple sclerosis when compared with age matched controls [10]. However, there were no differences in the concentrations of specific IgE to fish, eggs, or cow's milk among patients with multiple sclerosis [11,12].

* This work was supported in part by the Food Allergy and Anaphylaxis Program.

Moreover, in contrast to adults with multiple sclerosis, a recent survey of in patients younger than 18 years old found no difference in prevalence of allergies or asthma between cases and controls [13]. Thus, the reciprocal and possibly "protective" effects of multiple sclerosis in the development of allergies might not exist in all multiple sclerosis and allergies subgroups.

Comparison of 157 patients with insulin-dependent diabetes mellitus with 173 unaffected siblings indicated that fewer patients wheezed during the 12 months of the study or had multiple episodes of wheezing, a surrogate for asthma [14]. A retrospective case–controlled comparison of 928 Danish children with insulin-dependent diabetes mellitus with 10,000 controls found a significant lower cumulative incidence of atopic dermatitis in the diabetics, however, only if atopic dermatitis occurred prior to the insulin-dependent diabetes mellitus onset [15]. A large European multicenter study found decreased atopic dermatitis and asthma among patients with insulin-dependent diabetes mellitus [16]. However, this inverse relationship was evident predominantly in Western Europe and not in Eastern Europe. Moreover, a Finish registry query [7], a Swedish case–control study [17], a Dutch cross-sectional survey [18], and a British nutritional report [19] did not find differences in asthma incidence between children suffering from insulin-dependent diabetes mellitus and controls.

Patients with systemic lupus erythematosus (SLE) have often, although not uniformly, been found to have increased risk for diverse allergies. A study of 27 SLE patients indicated greater risk of allergic rhinitis, drug-induced urticaria, as well as angioedema and anaphylaxis compared with age- and sex-matched healthy controls [20]. Similarly, 44 of 60 SLE patients had one or more allergic disorder such as conjunctivitis, rhinitis, asthma, and skin eruptions related to food or drugs [21]. Another study identified increased frequency of allergy to medications, particularly to antibiotics among patients with SLE, as well as weaker associations with asthma and food allergies [22]. Patients with active SLE were found to have higher IgE concentrations in comparison to periods of remission [23]. The increased IgE concentrations were not associated with elevated total serum IgG concentrations. More recently, a population-based case study of 1673 SLE patients in Taiwan found increased allergic disease comorbidities in the SLE group when compared with controls, including allergic rhinitis, atopic dermatitis, and asthma [24].

Among 4725 patients from Taiwan with primary Sjögren's syndrome, the prevalence of allergic rhinitis and atopic dermatitis was significantly increased, as was the cumulative incidence of asthma after 12-year follow-up [25]. These results further support earlier reports of increased respiratory disorders, including asthma, among patients with Sjögren's syndrome [26–29].

Ankylosing spondylitis patients were found to have a higher prevalence of allergic rhinitis and a trend for higher prevalence of asthma relative to controls who suffered from disc prolapse [30]. Similarly, patients with ankylosing spondylitis from Taiwan had increased risk of asthma, atopic dermatitis, and allergic rhinitis over 10 years [31].

Increased frequency of allergic rhinitis, asthma, positive skin prick test, and total IgE was found among 59 patients suffering from vitiligo [32]. Similarly, a prospective online questionnaire of over 2500 patients with physicians-based diagnosis of Vitiligo revealed allergic rhinitis in 48.2%, atopic dermatitis in 24.0%, food allergy in 18.2%, and asthma in 17.8% of patients, which were higher than levels found in a general adult population [33].

Allergies are more frequent in patients with celiac disease, whereas asthma incidence is increased in patients with celiac disease diagnosed in childhood [7,34]. Another large study in adult patients with recently diagnosed celiac disease found increased prevalence of atopic dermatitis but not of other allergies [35]. Celiac disease was also found to be increased among patients with allergies [36].

Several studies have also investigated the occurrence of autoimmunity among patients with allergic diseases. Allergies were identified as a risk factor for thyroid autoimmunity in a small group of children affected with atopic dermatitis [37]. Autoimmune diseases occurred more common ($P < .001$) among 8112 Danish adults with atopic dermatitis, than among 40,560 matched controls [38]. These autoimmune diseases included alopecia areata, ankylosing spondylitis, celiac disease, inflammatory bowel disease, vitiligo, SLE, systemic sclerosis, Sjögren's syndrome, and rheumatoid arthritis. Interestingly, insulin-dependent diabetes mellitus and multiple sclerosis were not increased. Another large study that included 49,847 German adults, younger than 40 years of age, who had atopic dermatitis, also found increased risk for rheumatoid arthritis and inflammatory bowel disease, but not insulin-dependent diabetes mellitus [39]. Also recently a population-based cohort study in Taiwan found an overall 2.52 greater incidence of Juvenile SLE among children with asthma when compared with controls [40].

Taken together, these studies suggest that the occurrence of most autoimmune diseases, including rheumatoid arthritis, SLE, Sjögren's syndrome, ankylosing spondylitis, vitiligo, and celiac disease, do not seem to prevent development of some allergies, albeit not all. In other autoimmune conditions, such as multiple sclerosis and insulin-dependent diabetes mellitus, some protection from allergies could be provided.

PATHOPHYSIOLOGY OF ALLERGY AND AUTOIMMUNITY

Advances in the understanding of the mechanisms contributing to the development of allergy and autoimmunity suggest plasticity that allows transition, either directly or indirectly between Th-1- and Th-2-mediated inflammatory processes. Differentiation into Th-1 and Th-2 cells is controlled by key DNA-binding proteins transcription factors, T-bet, and GATA3 respectively, and involves epigenetic mechanisms that drive subset-specific differentiation and restriction of alternative fates. Because IL-12, interferon gamma, and T-bet have the capacity to repress Th-2 polarization and, conversely, the IL-4 and GATA3 axis represses Th-1 differentiation, it appeared that Th-1 and Th-2 cells represented mutually exclusive and stable, self-reinforcing, terminally differentiated subsets. This dichotomous Th-1/Th-2 division paradigm was challenged by the identification of highly stable T-bet/GATA3 expressing bifunctional Th-1/Th-1 hybrid cells that coproduced interferon gamma and IL-4 at the single-cell level [41]. Subsequently, it was shown that Th cells can also differentiate into many additional subtypes, including regulatory T cells (Treg), Th-9, Th-17, Th-22, follicular T helper (Tf-h), and follicular Treg (Tf-r), each with its unique cytokine and transcription expression pattern [42]. Initially, Th subset differentiation was thought to rely predominantly on single "master" factors that enforced lineage commitment and engaged in positive autoregulatory feedback loops and reciprocal cross regulation. However, accumulating data suggest that complex regulatory networks that allow for shared transcriptional programs and plasticity across T-cell subsets orchestrate Th subset differentiation. For example, it was shown that Th-17 may lose IL-17 expression while producing interferon gamma thereby adopting a type I phenotype. Moreover, exposure of CD4+ T cells in vitro to numerous combinations of cytokines resulted in a continuum of cell fates, rather than a limited number of distinct phenotypes [43], while mass cytometry demonstrated that human Th cells could not easily be separated into distinct lineages [44]. Hence, the dogma that Th subsets are mutually exclusive may not be as strict as previously thought. Moreover, since the identification of the critical role of Treg in modulating effector T cells, it has become evident that presence of Th is not the only factor that determines the phenotype of the immune response. Treg are a very heterogeneous population of CD4+ T cells with suppressive functions. FOXP3+ Treg are primarily generated in the thymus and are often referred to as tTreg. In addition, induced Treg (iTreg) can also be generated at peripheral sites. The precise mechanism by which Treg exert their suppressive effects in vivo are not clear, although secretion of IL-10 or expression of CTLA-4 that may sequester ligands from CD28 and prevent T-cell costimulation have been suggested [42]. Importantly, Treg have been shown to maintain both tolerance to food/self-antigens and prevent autoimmune disease, and dysfunction of Treg might contribute to the development of both conditions. Indeed, as detailed further in this review, patients with defects in Treg, caused by mutations in IPEX or Dock8, have been shown to suffer simultaneously from autoimmunity and allergies.

Another major development in the area of allergies and autoimmunity has been the appreciation that IgE might actively contribute to the pathogenesis of autoimmune disease. IgE was extensively studied in patients with SLE, where it was shown to be particularly prevalent and to correlate with disease activity. Moreover, some of the IgE was specific to self-antigens binding directly or indirectly to nucleic acids, as is also the case for the most important IgG autoantibodies found in this disease [45]. Indeed, several groups found that the level of anti-dsDNA IgE in circulation is a risk factor for SLE activity, independent of the concentration of the dsDNA-specific IgG counterpart [46,47]. Further evidence supporting the notion that IgE had a pathogenic role was the presence of IgE precipitates in kidney biopsy specimens from patients with lupus nephritis [45]. The mechanisms by which IgE exerts its effects in SLE is still not known, yet emerging data suggest that it could be through modulation of interferon responses [48]. A potential role of IgE was also extensively studied in bullous pemphigoid, a skin blistering disease that results from an autoimmune attack against hemidesmosomal proteins situated in the dermal–epidermal junction. IgE autoantibodies against the hemidesmosomal protein BP180 were found in 70%–90% of patients with bullous pemphigoid, often with IgG antibodies against the same antigens [49,50]. Additionally, IgE deposits were found at the dermal–epidermal junction of patients [48], and injecting serum from patients containing IgE autoantibodies into an animal model of bullous pemphigoid was able to induce skin changes similar to the ones associated with the disease [51]. IgE autoantibodies have also been identified in other autoimmune diseases. These include the anti-GAS65 antibodies in insulin-dependent diabetes mellitus [52], anti-TSH receptor antibodies in Grave's disease [53], and anti-myeloid peptides in multiple sclerosis [52]. However, the mechanisms and significance are less well studied [48]. Finally, a metaanalysis of genome-wide association studies on self-reported allergies and sensitization identified significant enrichment for single nucleotide polymorphisms previously associated with autoimmune diseases, as well as commonalities in pathways, further suggesting shared disease mechanisms [54].

INHERITED AND ACQUIRED IMMUNE ABNORMALITIES WITH ALLERGY AND AUTOIMMUNITY

In addition to the mechanistic and genetic data described above, inherited and acquired immune defects have been described where patients are affected by both allergies and autoimmunity.

Immune dysregulation, polyendocrinopathy, enteropathy, X linked (IPEX) syndrome is characterized by diverse autoimmune manifestations including neonatal insulin-dependent diabetes mellitus, enterocolitis, and thyroiditis. Autoimmune hematological cytopenia, hepatitis, and nephritis are frequent. Atopic dermatitis and food allergies are also common with extremely elevated IgE levels, eosinophilia, and evidence of overt Th-2 skewing [55]. IPEX syndrome is caused by mutations in the X-chromosome transcription factor FOXP3 that is important for the generation and function of regulatory T cells [56].

Hyper IgE syndrome is attributed to a growing number of gene abnormalities. Among them, patients with autosomal recessive defects in DOCK8 have been reported to suffer from increased susceptibility to infections and autoimmunity [57]. Additionally, patients might suffer from atopic dermatitis, asthma, food allergies vasculitis, enterocolitis, autoimmune hepatitis, and hematological cytopenia similar to those observed in IPEX syndrome. Patients with DOCK8 deficiency exhibit elevated IgE to allergic foods and similar to IPEX syndrome they have abnormalities in the function of Treg [58].

CARD11 is required for B- and T-cell receptors signaling through the nuclear factor-kappa B transcription factor, which controls genes important for the differentiation, proliferation, and survival of lymphocytes. Autosomal dominant CARD11 mutations were identified among family members suffering from food allergies and autoimmunity, including severe atopic dermatitis, lichen sclerosis, and primary infertility [59]. In addition, the patients experienced increased frequency of infections, whereas laboratory evaluations demonstrated impaired humoral and cellular responses.

Loeys–Dietz syndrome is characterized by spine deformity and arterial tortuosity with predisposition for aneurysm and dissection, similar to Marfan's syndrome, and is caused by autosomal dominant mutations in the TGF-beta receptor subunits. Food allergies occur among more than 50% of patients, with many also suffering from other allergic disorders such as asthma and eosinophilic gastrointestinal disorders [60]. In addition, few affected children had severe inflammatory colitis and autoimmune thyroiditis [61].

Recently, among 273 children who received liver, kidney, heart, or multivisceral transplants, 34% developed de novo allergy including atopic dermatitis, food allergy, eosinophilic gastrointestinal disease, or autoimmune diseases such as hematologic cytopenia [62]. Food allergies and autoimmunity were more common after liver and heart than kidney transplantations, a discrepancy noted also previously [63]. The differences in frequency might reflect the earlier age that liver and heart transplants are performed, when Th-2 responses dominate or the common use of calcineurin inhibitors to prevent rejection, which suppresses Treg [64].

THE IMPORTANCE OF COEXISTENCE OF ALLERGY AND AUTOIMMUNITY

Importantly, recognizing the overlap between both pathogenesis has led to the use of treatments shown to be effective in allergic diseases as well as in patients with autoimmune disorders. Administration of omalizumab, a monoclonal antibody that binds to the Fc portion of IgE and blocks its interaction with FcεR in patients with chronic autoimmune urticaria, led to significant improvement in their mean disease activity score and use of rescue medications [65]. Similar success has also been shown in patients with bullous pemphigoid [66], and a clinical trial is underway assessing the benefits of omalizumab for patients with SLE (NCT01716312). Whether additional strategies used in allergies, such as "tolerance induction" by gradual exposure to increasing amount of the antigen, or other methods to enhance regulatory immune cells would be beneficial also for autoimmunity is still not known. Nevertheless, advances in the understanding of immune dysregulation have clear implications and promise for the comprehension of both allergic and autoimmune diseases.

REFERENCES

[1] Olsson AR, Wingren G, Skogh T, Svernell O, Ernerudh J. Allergic manifestations in patients with rheumatoid arthritis. APMIS October 2003;111(10):940–4. PubMed PMID: 14616545.

[2] Hilliquin P, Allanore Y, Coste J, Renoux M, Kahan A, Menkès CJ. Reduced incidence and prevalence of atopy in rheumatoid arthritis. Results of a case-control study. Rheumatology (Oxf) September 2000;39(9):1020–6. PubMed PMID: 10986309.

[3] Rudwaleit M, Andermann B, Alten R, Sörensen H, Listing J, Zink A, Sieper J, Braun J. Atopic disorders in ankylosing spondylitis and rheumatoid arthritis. Ann Rheum Dis November 2002;61(11):968–74. PubMed PMID: 12379517; PubMed Central PMCID: PMC1753933.

[4] Verhoef CM, van Roon JA, Vianen ME, Bruijnzeel-Koomen CA, Lafeber FP, Bijlsma JW. Mutual antagonism of rheumatoid arthritis and hay fever; a role for type 1/type 2 T cell balance. Ann Rheum Dis May 1998;57(5):275–80. PubMed PMID: 9741310; PubMed Central PMCID: PMC1752592.

[5] O'Driscoll BR, Milburn HJ, Kemeny DM, Cochrane GM, Panayi GS. Atopy and rheumatoid arthritis. Clin Allergy November 1985;15(6):547–53. PubMed PMID: 3907887.

[6] Lai NS, Tsai TY, Koo M, Lu MC. Association of rheumatoid arthritis with allergic diseases: a nationwide population-based cohort study. Allergy Asthma Proc 2015 Sep-Oct;36(5):99–103. https://doi.org/10.2500/aap.2015.36.3871. PubMed PMID: 26314811.

[7] Kero J, Gissler M, Hemminki E, Isolauri E. Could TH1 and TH2 diseases coexist? Evaluation of asthma incidence in children with coeliac disease, type 1 diabetes, or rheumatoid arthritis: a register study. J Allergy Clin Immunol November 2001;108(5):781–3. PubMed PMID: 11692104.

[8] Oro AS, Guarino TJ, Driver R, Steinman L, Umetsu DT. Regulation of disease susceptibility: decreased prevalence of IgE-mediated allergic disease in patients with multiple sclerosis. J Allergy Clin Immunol June 1996;97(6):1402–8. PubMed PMID: 8648038.

[9] Tremlett HL, Evans J, Wiles CM, Luscombe DK. Asthma and multiple sclerosis: an inverse association in a case-control general practice population. QJM November 2002;95(11):753–6. PubMed PMID: 12391388.

[10] Neukirch F, Lyon-Caen O, Clanet M, Bousquet J, Feingold J, Druet P. Asthma, nasal allergies, and multiple sclerosis. J Allergy Clin Immunol February 1997;99(2):270–1. PubMed PMID: 9042063.

[11] Ashtari F, Jamshidi F, Shoormasti RS, Pourpak Z, Akbari M. Cow's milk allergy in multiple sclerosis patients. J Res Med Sci March 2013;18(Suppl. 1):S62–5. PubMed PMID: 23961290; PubMed Central PMCID: PMC3743324.

[12] Ashtari F, Jamshidi F, Shoormasti RS, Pourpak Z, Akbari M, Zandieh F. Fish and egg specific immunoglobin E in multiple sclerosis patients. Int J Prev Med May 2013;4(Suppl. 2):S185–8. PubMed PMID: 23776721; PubMed Central PMCID: PMC3678215.

[13] Bourne T, Waltz M, Casper TC, Kavak K, Aaen G, Belman A, Benson L, Candee M, Chitnis T, Graves J, Greenberg B, Gorman M, Harris Y, Krupp L, Lotze T, Mar S, Ness J, Olsen C, Roalstad S, Rodriguez M, Rose J, Rubin J, Schreiner T, Tillema JM, Kahn I, Waldman A, Barcellos L, Waubant E, Weinstock-Guttman B. US Network of Pediatric MS Centers. Evaluating the association of allergies with multiple sclerosis susceptibility risk and disease activity in a pediatric population. J Neurol Sci April 15, 2017;375:371–5. https://doi.org/10.1016/j.jns.2017.02.041. Epub 2017 Feb 20. PubMed PMID: 28320170; PubMed Central PMCID: PMC5606138.

[14] Douek IF, Leech NJ, Gillmor HA, Bingley PJ, Gale EA. Children with type-1 diabetes and their unaffected siblings have fewer symptoms of asthma. Lancet May 29, 1999;353(9167):1850. PubMed PMID: 10359413.

[15] EURODIAB. Decreased prevalence of atopic diseases in children with diabetes. The EURODIAB Substudy 2 Study Group. J Pediatr October 2000;137(4):470–4. PubMed PMID: 11035823.

[16] Strömberg LG, Ludvigsson GJ, Björkstén B. Atopic allergy and delayed hypersensitivity in children with diabetes. J Allergy Clin Immunol August 1995;96(2):188–92. PubMed PMID: 7636056.

[17] Meerwaldt R, Odink RJ, Landaeta R, Aarts F, Brunekreef B, Gerritsen J, Van Aalderen WM, Hoekstra MO. A lower prevalence of atopy symptoms in children with type 1 diabetes mellitus. Clin Exp Allergy February 2002;32(2):254–5. PubMed PMID: 11929490.

[18] Sheikh A, Smeeth L, Hubbard R. There is no evidence of an inverse relationship between TH2-mediated atopy and TH1-mediated autoimmune disorders: lack of support for the hygiene hypothesis. J Allergy Clin Immunol January 2003;111(1):131–5. PubMed PMID: 12532108.

[19] Olesen AB, Juul S, Birkebaek N, Thestrup-Pedersen K. Association between atopic dermatitis and insulin-dependent diabetes mellitus: a case-control study. Lancet June 2, 2001;357(9270):1749–52. PubMed PMID: 11403811.

[20] Goldman JA, Klimek GA, Ali R. Allergy in systemic lupus erythematosus. IgE levels and reaginic phenomenon. Arthritis Rheum 1976 Jul-Aug;19(4):669–76. PubMed PMID: 942498.

[21] Shahar E, Lorber M. Allergy and SLE: common and variable. Isr J Med Sci February 1997;33(2):147–9. PubMed PMID: 9254878.

[22] Cooper GS, Dooley MA, Treadwell EL, St Clair EW, Gilkeson GS. Risk factors for development of systemic lupus erythematosus: allergies, infections, and family history. J Clin Epidemiol October 2002;55(10):982–9. PubMed PMID: 12464374.

[23] Elkayam O, Tamir R, Pick AI, Wysenbeek A. Serum IgE concentrations, disease activity, and atopic disorders in systemic lupus erythematosus. Allergy January 1995;50(1):94–6. PubMed PMID: 7741196.

[24] Hsiao YP, Tsai JD, Muo CH, Tsai CH, Sung FC, Liao YT, Chang YJ, Yang JH. Atopic diseases and systemic lupus erythematosus: an epidemiological study of the risks and correlations. Int J Environ Res Public Health August 8, 2014;11(8):8112–22. https://doi.org/10.3390/ijerph110808112. PubMed PMID: 25111878; PubMed Central PMCID: PMC4143852.

[25] Shen TC, Chen HJ, Wei CC, Chen CH, Tu CY, Hsia TC, Shih CM, Hsu WH, Sung FC, Bau DT. Risk of asthma in patients with primary Sjögren's syndrome: a retrospective cohort study. BMC Pulm Med November 16, 2016;16(1):152. PubMed PMID: 27852248; PubMed Central PMCID: PMC5112692.

[26] Potena A, La Corte R, Fabbri LM, Papi A, Trotta F, Ciaccia A. Increased bronchial responsiveness in primary and secondary Sjögren's syndrome. Eur Respir J May 1990;3(5):548–53. PubMed PMID: 2198166.

[27] Gudbjörnsson B, Hedenström H, Stålenheim G, Hällgren R. Bronchial hyperresponsiveness to methacholine in patients with primary Sjögren's syndrome. Ann Rheum Dis January 1991;50(1):36–40. PubMed PMID: 1994866; PubMed Central PMCID: PMC1004322.

[28] Lúdvíksdóttir D, Janson C, Björnsson E, Stålenheim G, Boman G, Hedenström H, Venge P, Gudbjörnsson B, Valtysdóttir S. Different airway responsiveness profiles in atopic asthma, nonatopic asthma, and Sjögren's syndrome. BHR Study Group. Bronchial hyperresponsiveness. Allergy March 2000;55(3):259–65. PubMed PMID: 10753017.

[29] Kang JH, Lin HC. Comorbidities in patients with primary Sjogren's syndrome: a registry-based case-control study. J Rheumatol June 2010;37(6):1188–94. https://doi.org/10.3899/jrheum.090942. Epub 2010 Apr 1. PubMed PMID: 20360180.

[30] Zochling J, Bohl-Bühler MH, Baraliakos X, Feldtkeller E, Braun J. The high prevalence of infections and allergic symptoms in patients with ankylosing spondylitis is associated with clinical symptoms. Clin Rheumatol September 2006;25(5):648–58. Epub 2005 Dec 23.

[31] Chang WP, Kuo CN, Kuo LN, Wang YT, Perng WT, Kuo HC, Wei JC. Increase risk of allergic diseases in patients with ankylosing spondylitis: a 10-year follow-up population-based study in Taiwan. Medicine (Baltim) November 2016;95(45):e5172. PubMed PMID: 27828843; PubMed Central PMCID: PMC5106049.

[32] Perfetti L, Cespa M, Nume A, Orecchia G. Prevalence of atopy in vitiligo. A preliminary report. Dermatologica 1991;182(4):218–20. PubMed PMID: 1884856.

[33] Silverberg JI, Silverberg NB. Association between vitiligo and atopic disorders: a pilot study. JAMA Dermatol August 2013;149(8):983–6. https://doi.org/10.1001/jamadermatol.2013.4228. PubMed PMID: 23740223.

[34] Williams AJ. Coeliac disease and allergic manifestations. Lancet April 4, 1987;1(8536):808. PubMed PMID: 2882213.

[35] Ciacci C, Cavallaro R, Iovino P, Sabbatini F, Palumbo A, Amoruso D, Tortora R, Mazzacca G. Allergy prevalence in adult celiac disease. J Allergy Clin Immunol June 2004;113(6):1199–203. PubMed PMID: 15208605.

[36] Zauli D, Grassi A, Granito A, Foderaro S, De Franceschi L, Ballardini G, Bianchi FB, Volta U. Prevalence of silent coeliac disease in atopics. Dig Liver Dis December 2000;32(9):775–9. PubMed PMID: 11215557.

[37] Pedullá M, Fierro V, Papacciuolo V, Alfano R, Ruocco E. Atopy as a risk factor for thyroid autoimmunity in children affected with atopic dermatitis. J Eur Acad Dermatol Venereol August 2014;28(8):1057–60. https://doi.org/10.1111/jdv.12281. PubMed PMID: 24118567.

[38] Andersen YM, Egeberg A, Gislason GH, Skov L, Thyssen JP. Autoimmune diseases in adults with atopic dermatitis. J Am Acad Dermatol February 2017;76(2):274–80.e1. https://doi.org/10.1016/j.jaad.2016.08.047. Epub 2016 Oct 11. PubMed PMID: 27742171.

[39] Schmitt J, Schwarz K, Baurecht H, Hotze M, Fölster-Holst R, Rodríguez E, Lee YAE, Franke A, Degenhardt F, Lieb W, Gieger C, Kabesch M, Nöthen MM, Irvine AD, McLean WHI, Deckert S, Stephan V, Schwarz P, Aringer M, Novak N, Weidinger S. Atopic dermatitis is associated with an increased risk for rheumatoid arthritis and inflammatory bowel disease, and a decreased risk for type 1 diabetes. J Allergy Clin Immunol January 2016;137(1):130–6. https://doi.org/10.1016/j.jaci.2015.06.029. Epub 2015 Aug 4. PubMed PMID: 26253344.

[40] Wei CC, Lin CL, Shen TC, Tsai JD, Chung CJ, Li TC. Increased incidence of juvenile-onset systemic lupus erythematosus among children with asthma. Pediatr Allergy Immunol June 2014;25(4):374–9. https://doi.org/10.1111/pai.12228. PubMed PMID: 24953297.

[41] Peine M, Rausch S, Helmstetter C, Fröhlich A, Hegazy AN, Kühl AA, Grevelding CG, Höfer T, Hartmann S, Löhning M. Stable T-bet(+)GATA-3(+) Th1/Th2 hybrid cells arise in vivo, can develop directly from naive precursors, and limit immunopathologic inflammation. PLoS Biol 2013;11(8):e1001633. https://doi.org/10.1371/journal.pbio.1001633. Epub 2013 Aug 20. PubMed PMID: 23976880; PubMed Central PMCID: PMC3747991.

[42] Stadhouders R, Lubberts E, Hendriks RW. A cellular and molecular view of T helper 17 cell plasticity in autoimmunity. J Autoimmun December 21, 2017. https://doi.org/10.1016/j.jaut.2017.12.007. pii: S0896–8411(17)30803-X. PubMed PMID: 29275836.

[43] Eizenberg-Magar I, Rimer J, Zaretsky I, Lara-Astiaso D, Reich-Zeliger S, Friedman N. Diverse continuum of CD4(+) T-cell states is determined by hierarchical additive integration of cytokine signals. Proc Natl Acad Sci USA August 1, 2017;114(31):E6447–56. https://doi.org/10.1073/pnas.1615590114. Epub 2017 Jul 17. PubMed PMID: 28716917; PubMed Central PMCID: PMC5547583.

[44] Wong MT, Ong DE, Lim FS, Teng KW, McGovern N, Narayanan S, Ho WQ, Cerny D, Tan HK, Anicete R, Tan BK, Lim TK, Chan CY, Cheow PC, Lee SY, Takano A, Tan EH, Tam JK, Tan EY, Chan JK, Fink K, Bertoletti A, Ginhoux F, Curotto de Lafaille MA, Newell EW. A high-dimensional atlas of human T cell diversity reveals tissue-specific trafficking and cytokine signatures. Immunity August 16, 2016;45(2):442–56. https://doi.org/10.1016/j.immuni.2016.07.007. Epub 2016 Aug 9. PubMed PMID: 27521270.

[45] Zhu H, Luo H, Yan M, Zuo X, Li QZ. Autoantigen microarray for high-throughput autoantibody profiling in systemic lupus erythematosus. Genomics Proteomics Bioinformatics August 2015;13(4):210–8. https://doi.org/10.1016/j.gpb.2015.09.001. Epub 2015 Sep 28. Review. PubMed PMID: 26415621; PubMed Central PMCID: PMC4610965.

[46] Dema B, Pellefigues C, Hasni S, Gault N, Jiang C, Ricks TK, Bonelli MM, Scheffel J, Sacré K, Jablonski M, Gobert D, Papo T, Daugas E, Illei G, Charles N, Rivera J. Autoreactive IgE is prevalent in systemic lupus erythematosus and is associated with increased disease activity and nephritis. PLoS One February 28, 2014;9(2):e90424. https://doi.org/10.1371/journal.pone.0090424. eCollection 2014. PubMed PMID: 24587356; PubMed Central PMCID: PMC3938730.

[47] Henault J, Riggs JM, Karnell JL, Liarski VM, Li J, Shirinian L, Xu L, Casey KA, Smith MA, Khatry DB, Izhak L, Clarke L, Herbst R, Ettinger R, Petri M, Clark MR, Mustelin T, Kolbeck R, Sanjuan MA. Self-reactive IgE exacerbates interferon responses associated with autoimmunity. Nat Immunol February 2016;17(2):196–203. https://doi.org/10.1038/ni. 3326. Epub 2015 Dec 21. PubMed PMID: 26692173; PubMed Central PMCID: PMC4718782.

[48] Sanjuan MA, Sagar D, Kolbeck R. Role of IgE in autoimmunity. J Allergy Clin Immunol June 2016;137(6):1651–61. https://doi.org/10.1016/j.jaci.2016.04.007. Epub 2016 Apr 27. Review. PubMed PMID: 27264000.

[49] Dimson OG, Giudice GJ, Fu CL, Van den Bergh F, Warren SJ, Janson MM, Fairley JA. Identification of a potential effector function for IgE auto-antibodies in the organ-specific autoimmune disease bullous pemphigoid. J Investig Dermatol May 2003;120(5):784–8. PubMed PMID: 12713582.

[50] Messingham KA, Holahan HM, Fairley JA. Unraveling the significance of IgE autoantibodies in organ-specific autoimmunity: lessons learned from bullous pemphigoid. Immunol Res August 2014;59(1–3):273–8. https://doi.org/10.1007/s12026-014-8547-7. Review. PubMed PMID: 24845463.

[51] Fairley JA, Burnett CT, Fu CL, Larson DL, Fleming MG, Giudice GJ. A pathogenic role for IgE in autoimmunity: bullous pemphigoid IgE reproduces the early phase of lesion development in human skin grafted to nu/nu mice. J Investig Dermatol November 2007;127(11):2605–11. Epub 2007 Jul 5. PubMed PMID: 17611576.

[52] Hoppu S, Ronkainen MS, Kulmala P, Akerblom HK, Knip M, Childhood Diabetes in Finland Study Group. GAD65 antibody isotypes and epitope recognition during the prediabetic process in siblings of children with type I diabetes. Clin Exp Immunol April 2004;136(1):120–8. PubMed PMID: 15030523; PubMed Central PMCID: PMC1809002.

[53] Metcalfe R, Jordan N, Watson P, Gullu S, Wiltshire M, Crisp M, Evans C, Weetman A, Ludgate M. Demonstration of immunoglobulin G, A, and E autoantibodies to the human thyrotropin receptor using flow cytometry. J Clin Endocrinol Metab April 2002;87(4):1754–61. PubMed PMID: 11932312.

[54] Kreiner E, Waage J, Standl M, Brix S, Pers TH, Couto Alves A, Warrington NM, Tiesler CMT, Fuertes E, Franke L, Hirschhorn JN, James A, Simpson A, Tung JY, Koppelman GH, Postma DS, Pennell CE, Jarvelin MR, Custovic A, Timpson N, Ferreira MA, Strachan DP, Henderson J, Hinds D, Bisgaard H, Bønnelykke K. Shared genetic variants suggest common pathways in allergy and autoimmune diseases. J Allergy Clin Immunol September 2017;140(3):771–81. https://doi.org/10.1016/j.jaci.2016.10.055. Epub 2017 Feb 8. PubMed PMID: 28188724.

[55] Barzaghi F, Amaya Hernandez LC, Neven B, Ricci S, Kucuk ZY, Bleesing J, Nademi Z, Slatter MA, Ulloa ER, Shcherbina A, Roppelt A, Worth A, Silva J, Aiuti A, Murguia-Favela L, Speckmann C, Carneiro-Sampaio M, Fernandes JF, Baris S, Ozen A, Karakoc-Aydiner E, Kiykim A, Schulz A, Steinmann S, Notarangelo LD, Gambineri E, Lionetti P, Shearer WT, Forbes L, Martinez C, Moshous D, Blanche S, Fisher A, Ruemmele FM, Tissandier C, Ouachee-Chardin M, Rieux-Laucat F, Cavazzana M, Qasim W, Lucarelli B, Albert MH, Kobayashi I, Alonso L, Diaz De Heredia C, Kanegane H, Lawitschka A, Seo JJ, Gonzalez-Vicent M, Diaz MA, Goyal RK, Sauer MG, Yesilipek A, Kim M, Yilmaz-Demirdag Y, Bhatia M, Khlevner J, Richmond Padilla EJ, Martino S, Montin D, Neth O, Molinos-Quintana A, Valverde-Fernandez J, Broides A, Pinsk V, Ballauf A, Haerynck F, Bordon V, Dhooge C, Garcia-Lloret ML, Bredius RG, Kałwak K, Haddad E, Seidel MG, Duckers G, Pai SY, Dvorak CC, Ehl S, Locatelli F, Goldman F, Gennery AR, Cowan MJ, Roncarolo MG, Bacchetta R, PIDTC, IEWP of EBMT. Long-term follow up of IPEX syndrome patients after different therapeutic strategies: an international multicenter retrospective study. J Allergy Clin Immunol December 11, 2017. https://doi.org/10.1016/j.jaci.2017.10.041. pii: S0091–6749(17)31893-6. PubMed PMID: 29241729.

[56] Torgerson TR, Linane A, Moes N, Anover S, Mateo V, Rieux-Laucat F, Hermine O, Vijay S, Gambineri E, Cerf-Bensussan N, Fischer A, Ochs HD, Goulet O, Ruemmele FM. Severe food allergy as a variant of IPEX syndrome caused by a deletion in a noncoding region of the FOXP3 gene. Gastroenterology May 2007;132(5):1705–17. Epub 2007 Feb 23. PubMed PMID: 17484868.

[57] Aydin SE, Kilic SS, Aytekin C, Kumar A, Porras O, Kainulainen L, Kostyuchenko L, Genel F, Kütükcüler N, Karaca N, Gonzalez-Granado L, Abbott J, Al-Zahrani D, Rezaei N, Baz Z, Thiel J, Ehl S, Marodi L, Orange JS, Sawalle-Belohradsky J, Keles S, Holland SM, Sanal Ö, Ayvaz DC, Tezcan I, Al-Mousa H, Alsum Z, Hawwari A, Metin A, Matthes-Martin S, Hönig M, Schulz A, Picard C, Barlogis V, Gennery A, Ifversen M, van Montfrans J, Kuijpers T, Bredius R, Dückers G, Al-Herz W, Pai SY, Geha R, Notheis G, Schwarze CP, Tavil B, Azik F, Bienemann K, Grimbacher B, Heinz V, Gaspar HB, Aydin R, Hagl B, Gathmann B, Belohradsky BH, Ochs HD, Chatila T, Renner ED, Su H, Freeman AF, Engelhardt K, Albert MH, inborn errors working party of EBMT. DOCK8 deficiency: clinical and immunological phenotype and treatment options - a review of 136 patients. J Clin Immunol February 2015;35(2):189–98. https://doi.org/10.1007/s10875-014-0126-0. Epub 2015 Jan 28. PubMed PMID: 25627830.

[58] Alroqi FJ, Charbonnier LM, Keles S, Ghandour F, Mouawad P, Sabouneh R, Mohammed R, Almutairi A, Chou J, Massaad MJ, Geha RS, Baz Z, Chatila TA. DOCK8 deficiency presenting as an IPEX-like disorder. J Clin Immunol November 2017;37(8):811–9. https://doi.org/10.1007/s10875-017-0451-1. Epub 2017 Oct 23. PubMed PMID: 29058101; PubMed Central PMCID: PMC5691358.

[59] Dadi H, Jones TA, Merico D, Sharfe N, Ovadia A, Schejter Y, Reid B, Sun M, Vong L, Atkinson A, Lavi S, Pomerantz JL, Roifman CM. Combined immunodeficiency and atopy caused by a dominant negative mutation in caspase activation and recruitment domain family member 11 (CARD11). J Allergy Clin Immunol August 19, 2017. https://doi.org/10.1016/j.jaci.2017.06.047. pii: S0091–6749(17)31281-2. PubMed PMID: 28826773.

[60] Frischmeyer-Guerrerio PA, Guerrerio AL, Oswald G, Chichester K, Myers L, Halushka MK, Oliva-Hemker M, Wood RA, Dietz HC. TGFβ receptor mutations impose a strong predisposition for human allergic disease. Sci Transl Med July 24, 2013;5(195):195ra94. https://doi.org/10.1126/scitranslmed.3006448. PubMed PMID: 23884466; PubMed Central PMCID: PMC3905327.

[61] Naviglio S, Arrigo S, Martelossi S, Villanacci V, Tommasini A, Loganes C, Fabretto A, Vignola S, Lonardi S, Ventura A. Severe inflammatory bowel disease associated with congenital alteration of transforming growth factor beta signaling. J Crohns Colitis August 2014;8(8):770–4. https://doi.org/10.1016/j.crohns.2014.01.013. Epub 2014 Jan 31. PubMed PMID: 24486179.

[62] Marcus N, Amir AZ, Grunebaum E, Dipchand A, Hebert D, Ng VL, Walters T, Avitzur Y. De-novo allergy and immune mediated disorders following solid organ transplantation - prevalence, natural history and risk factors. J Pediatr 2018 May;196:154–160.e2. https://doi.org/10.1016/j.jpeds.2017.11.026. Epub 2018 Feb 1. PubMed PMID: 29395171.

[63] Levy Y, Davidovits M, Cleper R, Shapiro R. New-onset post-transplantation food allergy in children–is it attributable only to the immunosuppressive protocol? Pediatr Transplant February 2009;13(1):63–9. https://doi.org/10.1111/j.1399-3046.2007.00883.x. Epub 2007 Dec 30. PubMed PMID: 18179638.

[64] Hosakoppal SS, Bryce PJ. Transplant-acquired food allergy: current perspectives. J Asthma Allergy December 1, 2017;10:307–15. https://doi.org/10.2147/JAA.S136319. eCollection 2017. Review. PubMed PMID: 29238209; PubMed Central PMCID: PMC5716392.

[65] Kaplan AP, Joseph K, Maykut RJ, Geba GP, Zeldin RK. Treatment of chronic autoimmune urticaria with omalizumab. J Allergy Clin Immunol September 2008;122(3):569–73. https://doi.org/10.1016/j.jaci.2008.07.006. PubMed PMID: 18774392.

[66] Fairley JA, Baum CL, Brandt DS, Messingham KA. Pathogenicity of IgE in autoimmunity: successful treatment of bullous pemphigoid with omalizumab. J Allergy Clin Immunol March 2009;123(3):704–5. https://doi.org/10.1016/j.jaci.2008.11.035. Epub 2009 Jan 18. PubMed PMID: 19152970; PubMed Central PMCID: PMC4784096.

FURTHER READING

[1] Mikol DD, Ditlow C, Usatin D, Biswas P, Kalbfleisch J, Milner A, Calenoff E. Serum IgE reactive against small myelin protein-derived peptides is increased in multiple sclerosis patients. J Neuroimmunol November 2006;180(1–2):40–9. Epub 2006 Sep 20. PubMed PMID: 16996143.

Chapter 63

Proteomic "Molecular Fingerprints" Using an Epstein Barr Virus-Derived Microarray as a Diagnostic Method in Autoimmune Disease

David H. Dreyfus[1], Antonella Farina[2], Giuseppina Alessandra Farina[3]

[1]Keren LLC, New Haven CT, United States; [2]Department of Experimental Medicine, Sapienza University, Rome, Italy; [3]Rheumatology, Boston University School of Medicine, Arthritis Center, Boston, MA, United States

INTRODUCTION

Infectious agents such as EBV (Epstein Barr Virus) have been associated with numerous autoimmune syndromes in epidemiologic studies but the specific role of infection remains unresolved [1–3]. Conventional serologic testing for EBV is available using specific Immunoglobulin G (IgG) binding to viral proteins such as EBNA-1 (Epstein Barr Virus Nuclear Antigen-1), VCA (Viral Capsid Antigen), and EA (viral components termed Early Antigen). A correlation between antigen specific IgG levels to specific EBV proteins has been reported in SLE, MS (multiple sclerosis), and other autoimmune syndromes [4–9]. Because the vast majority of the adult population is positive for EBV, it would be useful to have additional laboratory analysis for clinical evaluation and monitoring of autoimmune disease in patients based on response to past EBV infection [10–13].

Recent developments in proteomic analysis and technology have dramatically increased the power and lowered the cost of many immunological tests [14]. Presently, the standard of diagnosis for many autoimmune diseases is based on ANA (antinuclear antibody) assays in which Immunoglobulin binding is characterized against the cell cytoplasm and nucleus, and related IgG binding assays. Although ANA and immunoassay technology can in principle be automated, a more recent approach is the use of specific antigenic host and viral proteins printed in a microarray with sensitivity similar or great than that of the ANA [15,16]. Using proteomic technology, hundreds or even thousands of epitopes can be analyzed simultaneously with a single serum sample. Detailed mapping of autoreactive viral epitopes could suggest epitopes capable of differentiating healthy patients versus patients with autoimmune syndromes such as SLE and scleroderma in which EBV reactivation and EBNA-1 and ZEBRA expressions are evident [17–19].

Viral proteins trigger autoreactive IgG is "molecular mimicry" in which short regions of similarity between viral and host proteins are proposed to cross react and through "epitope spreading" lead to IgG against host proteins in the presence of viral inflammation and defects in host suppressor cells [20–24]. EBV-encoded proteins such as ZEBRA (BZLF-1 protein) share regions with host transcription factors in the fos/jun family and also to host ankyrin proteins that anchor the cytoskeleton and regulate host transcription factors such as p53 and NF-kB important in the immune response [25]. A well-characterized example of "molecular mimicry" between EBV and host protein is the similarity between regions of EBNA-1 and the "Smith Antigen" in SLE [26,27]. EBNA-1 and other proteins including the viral-encoded recombinase BALF-2 protein share a DNA-binding domain termed an A/T hook with both vertebrate and invertebrate transcription factors and DNA-binding proteins such as histones and recombinases [28]. Chronic viruses also encode "virokines" similar to host cytokines [29].

It would therefore be useful to have a sensitive and inexpensive method to generate a "molecular fingerprint" of IgG binding to shared regions of viral and host proteins to compare between healthy patients with autoimmune disease or at risk in addition to available more labor-intensive and costly technology such as the ANA. Using "PEPperprint" technology the authors characterized peptide epitopes that might provide a sensitive and inexpensive method to generate a proteomic "molecular fingerprint" of IgG binding to shared regions of viral and host proteins [30]. Proteomic technology appears to be highly flexible and inexpensive relative to previous whole protein–based technologies and also permits localization of binding to precise intervals of the viral proteins. A limitation of the technology is that some epitopes that require complex folding and tertiary interactions of viral proteins, or secondary modifications evident in ELISA binding assays will not be detected [12,31]. Conclusions regarding clinical utility therefore must await confirmation in additional studies based on direct comparison with other diagnostic systems [14].

METHODS

Molecular images of "A/T hook" DNA-binding domains in figures shown were generated by the authors from published public access coordinates of X-ray crystallography coordinates from crystallized RAG-1 nonamer (pdb file 3GNA) and Herpes Simplex ICP8 (pdb file 1URJ). The "pymol" program was used through license from the author. IgG response to immunologically important viral proteins containing regions shared with human immune response proteins were characterized. Serum from a healthy EBV positive donor was obtained with consent for research as part of an ongoing research study of SLE and Scleroderma [32,33].

Using proprietary technology (PEPerprint,com, Heidelberg, Germany), overlapping arrays of 15 amino acid long peptides were synthesized on a microchip [30]. Each peptide was progressively printed across the region of interest with 13 amino acid overlap between each peptide or a progression of two amino acids per peptide. Chips were incubated with serum, developed, and analyzed with antibodies specific for IgG. Analysis of the immunoglobulin binding was provided by the chip manufacturer (PEPperprint.com) and data were presented using 1–100 and 1–500 dilutions of serum. Results are presented for both serum dilutions. Results shown in this work suggested that both dilutions of serum gave similar results. The 1–100 dilution of serum appears to have more specificity and lower background although results from both serum dilutions are presented.

In the tables shown in this work, the actual sequence of each printed peptide is shown with the corresponding location on the chip to the left of the peptide, followed to the right by the actual peptide sequence, followed to the right by the corrected binding intensity donor IgG at 1/500 and 1/100 dilutions of serum. In each 15 amino acid sequence the approximate position of amino acids with maximal IgG detected binding is underlined. Background binding was essentially 0 at the 1/500 dilution of serum and increased to more than 1000 arbitrary units for some peptides. Background binding was higher, approximately 2000 arbitrary units using the 1/100 dilution of serum but showed a similar absolute increase in arbitrary units to specific peptides. A similar profile or "fingerprint" of response to defined viral peptides could be defined for patients with EBV-related syndromes as well as syndromes associated with reactivation of other herpes viruses such as herpes simplex (an alpha herpes virus latent in neuronal tissues) and CMV or HHV-6 (beta herpes virus latent in hematopoietic stem cells).

RESULTS

Immunoglobulin G Response to ZEBRA Protein

EBV-encoded ZEBRA protein is a component of the molecular switch between latency and lytic cycles, and IgG response to ZEBRA is present in many autoimmune syndromes. For example, a high level of ZEBRA protein expression is also evident in SLE and scleroderma [32,33]. As shown in Fig. 63.1, ZEBRA has a modular structure with three regions each shared with a different host immune response protein. The amino terminus of ZEBRA is a transcription-activating domain

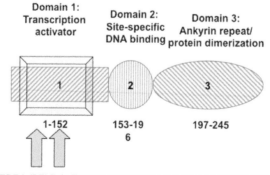

ZEBRA (BZLF-1) Epitopes TPDPYQV (15-21) and PTGSWFP (70-76)

FIGURE 63.1 A schematic diagram of EBV-encoded ZEBRA switch protein with IgG-binding peptide regions shown.

similar to host immune response transcription-activating domains, the central region is a DNA-binding domain similar to the fos/jun DNA-binding proteins that regulate the host immune response, and the terminal region is related to host-anchoring proteins regulating NF-kB and innate immune activation, resulting in potential antigen sharing with multiple host DNA–binding proteins including the p53 tumor suppressor [34,35].

IgG binding in a healthy EBV positive donor to the entire approximately 220 amino acid long ZEBRA amino acid sequence was analyzed using a laser-printed peptide chip using most of the laboratory strain B95-8 and a more virulent human strain of EBV termed "Akata." Data are shown for the Akata-based peptides, similar or identical to those obtained with B95-8 peptides (B95-8 data not shown). As shown in Table 63.1, IgG response in a healthy donor was confined to two epitopes both located in the amino terminal response of the ZEBRA protein. No IgG response was evident to the DNA binding or ZANK (Zebra ANKyrin-like regions) of ZEBRA in either B95-8 or Akata protein sequences suggesting that this region of ZEBRA is not the source of autoantiboides to p53 and related protein in SLE [36,37]. Similar IgG-binding epitopes in ZEBRA were evident in a patient with scleroderma, as will be discussed in more detail elsewhere (data not shown). IgG-binding regions of ZEBRA could be used as a part of a molecular fingerprint of IgG binding to regions of EBV shared with host genes (see discussion).

Immunoglobulin G Response to EBNA-1 Peptide Regions Shared With Host Smith Antigen and P53/TRAF Binding Domains

EBNA-1 protein is the primary protein expressed during EBV latency and is highly antigenic for the lifetime of the host due to periodic viral reactivation and cell lysis releasing small amounts of EBNA-1 into the circulation [38]. Despite the nuclear

TABLE 63.1 IgG Binding to ZEBRA (BZLF-1) Peptides TPDPYQV (aa 15-21) and PTGSWFP (aa 70-76). IgG Binding to Two Regions of the Highly Antigenic ZEBRA Protein is Shown. These Regions of ZEBRA are Identical in the Akata and B-958 EBV Strains. IgG Binding to (BZLF-1) Peptides TPDPYQV (aa 15-21) was Approximately 10 Times Greater Than PTGSWFP (aa 70-76)

10	6	GMMDPNSTSEDVKFT	BZLF1 Akata	0.0	2000.0
10	7	MDPNSTSEDVKFTPD	BZLF1 Akata	0.0	2000.0
10	8	PNSTSEDVKFTPDPY	BZLF1 Akata	0.0	2000.0
10	9	STSEDVKFTPDPYQV	BZLF1 Akata	164.5	2380.0
10	10	SEDVKFTPDPYQVPF	BZLF1 Akata	210.0	2456.5
10	11	DVKFTPDPYQVPFVQ	BZLF1 Akata	68.0	2167.0
10	12	KFTPDPYQVPFVQAF	BZLF1 Akata	45.0	2072.0
10	13	TPDPYQVPFVQAFDQ	BZLF1 Akata	0.0	2000.0
10	14	DPYQVPFVQAFDQAT	BZLF1 Akata	0.0	2044.0
10	15	YQVPFVQAFDQATRV	BZLF1 Akata	0.0	2000.0
10	34	LPQGQLTAYHVSMP	BZLF1 Akata	0.0	2000.0
10	35	QGQLTAYHVSMPTG	BZLF1 Akata	0.0	2000.0
10	36	QLTAYHVSAAPTGSW	BZLF1 Akata	0.0	2000.0
10	37	TAYHVSAAPTGSWFP	BZLF1 Akata	15.0	2023.0
10	38	YHVSAAPTGSWFPAP	BZLF1 Akata	9.0	2032.5
10	39	VSAAPTGSWFPAPQP	BZLF1 Akata	29.5	2074.0
10	40	AAPTGSWFPAPQPAP	BZLF1 Akata	61.0	2213.0
10	41	PTGSWFPAPQPAPEN	BZLF1 Akata	0.0	2013.0
10	42	GSWFPAPQPAPENAY	BZLF1 Akata	0.0	2000.0
10	43	WFPAPQPAPENAYQA	BZLF1 Akata	0.0	2017.0

TABLE 63.2 IgG Response was Present to the Region of EBNA-1 Protein PPPGRRPF (aa 391-398) Corresponding to the Smith Autoantigen PPPGMRPP (Shown Highlighted in Color). A Region of the EBNA-1 Protein is Similar to the Smith Antigen, an Early Autoantigen in Some but Not all SLE Patients. IgG Binding to the EBNA-1 Smith Ag-Like Peptide is Approximately Three Times Greater Than Maximal Binding to ZEBRA Epitope TPDPYQV (aa 15-21)

2	7	PSSQSSSSGSPPRRP	EBNA-1 region 1 (smithag)	0.0	2000.0
2	8	SQSSSSGSPPRRPPP	EBNA-1 region 1 (smithag)	0.0	2000.0
2	9	SSSSGSPPRRPPPGR	EBNA-1 region 1 (smithag)	0.0	2000.0
2	10	SSGSPPRRPPPGRRP	EBNA-1 region 1 (smithag)	24.0	2000.0
2	11	GSPPRRPPPGRRPFF	EBNA-1 region 1 (smithag)	109.0	2457.0
2	12	PPRRPPPGRRPFFHP	EBNA-1 region 1 (smithag)	613.5	3549.0
2	13	RRPPPGRRPFFHPVG	EBNA-1 region 1 (smithag)	839.0	4501.5
2	14	PPPGRRPFFHPVGEA	EBNA-1 region 1 (smithag)	44.0	2000.0
2	15	PGRRPFFHPVGEADY	EBNA-1 region 1 (smithag)	244.0	2976.0
2	16	RRPFFHPVGEADYFE	EBNA-1 region 1 (smithag)	145.0	2713.5
2	17	PFFHPVGEADYFEYH	EBNA-1 region 1 (smithag)	77.5	2345.0
2	18	FHPVGEADYFEYHQE	EBNA-1 region 1 (smithag)	38.0	2227.0
2	19	PVGEADYFEYHQEGG	EBNA-1 region 1 (smithag)	0.0	2000.0
2	20	GEADYFEYHQEGGPD	EBNA-1 region 1 (smithag)	0.0	2015.0
2	21	ADYFEYHQEGGPDGE	EBNA-1 region 1 (smithag)	0.0	2000.0

localization of EBNA-1 as suggested by the name "Epstein–Barr virus nuclear antigen" the EBNA-1 generates a persistent IgG response in both healthy patients and patients with autoimmune syndromes. The unique role of EBNA-1 in viral latency and persistence has decades of research on both the humoral and cellular immune response to EBNA-1 as a tool for viral diagnosis and potentially a tool for antiviral therapy and vaccines [7,17,19]. Because of the highly repetitive sequences of certain EBNA-1 regions and the large size of the protein, only specific defined regions of EBNA-1 were analyzed in this work, in contrast to the entire amino acid sequence of ZEBRA protein from two different EBV strains (Table 63.1).

Research has confirmed that suppressor mechanisms in healthy patients normally limit "epitope spreading" the similar regions of EBNA-1 and host antigens [26,27,39]. Several decades ago molecular mimicry between EBNA-1 and the SLE Smith antigen was observed and subsequently validated in animal models as a mechanism of viral pathogenesis. To facilitate comparison with previous studies, the PEPperprint microchip was applied to a well-characterized EBNA-1 protein epitope similar to the Smith antigen (Table 63.2). As shown in Table 63.3, another region of EBNA-1 unrelated to the Smith Antigen-like regions that bind to host transcription factors P53 and TRAF also generated a significant host IgG response [40]. This region of EBNA-1 is not related to ankyrin-like regions of ZEBRA and is also unlike regions of p53-binding autoantibodies described in SLE and related syndromes [36,37].

As with the ZEBRA protein regions, specific IgG-binding epitopes of EBNA-1 protein might be a useful diagnostic marker for characterizing a normal response to EBV infection and also for identifying defects in immune suppression in a variety of EBV-related syndromes. Remarkably, a peak of IgG binding was evident overlapping the EBNA-1 smith antigen-like sequence, which also colocalizes to a longer peptide: "PPRRPPPGRRPFFHPVGEADYFEYHQE (EBNA-1 391-420)" previously shown by ELISA assay to correlate with diagnosis of MS [18]. Similar results correlating IgG binding and also T-lymphocyte responses progression of MS and ELISA using EBNA-1 peptide region 400–641 containing the Smith Ag-like region with both T-lymphocyte and IgG binding were reported by another MS case control study [7,17,19].

Immunoglobulin G Response to A/T Hook Region Peptides of EBNA-1 Shared With Viral Recombinases and Host RAG-1 Recombinase

The "A/T hook" domain is a family of conserved DNA-binding proteins that bind A/T-rich regions of DNA such as the immunoglobulin nonamer region (Fig. 63.2). A/T hook domains are also present in host histone proteins as well as both

TABLE 63.3 IgG Response was Present to the Region of EBNA-1 Protein EBNA-1 P53/TRAF Binding Region DVPPGAIE (aa 421-428). IgG Binding to the EBNA-1 P5/TRAF Binding Region Peptide is Approximately Two Times Greater Than Maximal Binding to ZEBRA Epitope TPDPYQV (aa 15-21)

2	31	SGSGSGGGPDGEPDV	EBNA-1 region 2 (p53traf)	0.0	2000.0
2	32	SGSGGGPDGEPDVPP	EBNA-1 region 2 (p53traf)	0.0	2000.0
2	33	SGGGPDGEPDVPPGA	EBNA-1 region 2 (p53traf)	0.0	2000.0
2	34	GGPDGEPDVPPGAIE	EBNA-1 region 2 (p53traf)	926.5	4538.0
2	35	PDGEPDVPPGAIEQG	EBNA-1 region 2 (p53traf)	450.5	3394.5
2	36	GEPDVPPGAIEQGPA	EBNA-1 region 2 (p53traf)	171.5	2810.0
2	37	PDVPPGAIEQGPADD	EBNA-1 region 2 (p53traf)	314.0	3300.5
2	38	VPPGAIEQGPADDPG	EBNA-1 region 2 (p53traf)	9.0	2034.0
2	39	PGAIEQGPADDPGEG	EBNA-1 region 2 (p53traf)	0.0	2000.0
2	40	AIEQGPADDPGEGPS	EBNA-1 region 2 (p53traf)	0.0	2000.0

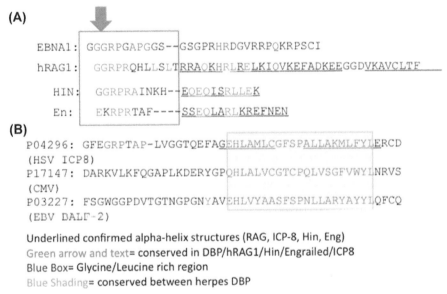

FIGURE 63.2 Amino acid similarities of A/T hook regions in EBNA-1-1, RAG-1, and herpes virus recombinases. Top Panel: An A/T hook region IgG-binding epitope in the amino terminus of EBNA-1 protein is similar in amino acid sequence a conserved region of both the RAG-1 A/T hook and to widely distributed invertebrate A/T hook proteins hin and engrailed. Bottom Panel: Herpes viruses also contain an A/T hook (Swissprot accession numbers provided for ICP8 from herpes simplex, CMV, and EBV BALF-2). Viral A/T hooks are significantly different in primary amino acid sequence but have a similar antigenic structure and thus could be useful in quantifying host response both to herpes viruses and related host proteins such as RAG-1 and histones.

vertebrate and invertebrate DNA-binding proteins including the RAG-1 recombinase [41,42]. The vertebrate RAG-1 protein is required for generation of the host immune repertoire and binds A/T-rich regions of immunoglobulin and T-cell receptor genes with an A/T hook domain shared with a conserved herpes virus recombinase [43]. Two different amino terminal EBNA-1 A/T hook regions are required for viral replication during genome latency probably by linking the host DNA replication and transcription process to specific regions of the viral episome [28]. Comparison between the EBNA-1 A/T hook 1 region of RAG-1, EBNA-1, EBV-encoded BALF-2, and of other BALF-2–like proteins in Herpes Simplex (ICP8) and CMV and EBV (BALF-2) are shown in Fig. 63.2. The crystal structure of herpes simplex ICP8 A/T hook is similar to the RAG-1 A/T hook, although little primary amino acid homology is evident (Fig. 63.3).

As shown in Fig. 63.3, the A/T hook is exposed on the surface of DNA-binding proteins (published data from host RAG-1 and unpublished data derived from viral ICP8 proteins shown) and therefore would presumably provoke a strong

RAG-1 AT hook region GGRPRQHL   ICP-8 AT hook region <u>EGRPTAPL</u>

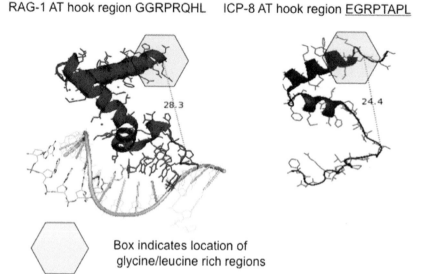

Box indicates location of
glycine/leucine rich regions

FIGURE 63.3 A/T hook domain from host RAG-1 and herpes simplex virus ICP8. IgG-binding regions of Herpes ICP-8 and corresponding regions of RAG-1 are shown (box). The human RAG-1 protein (recombination-activating gene-encoded protein) A/T hook has been crystallized bound to the A/T Rich nonamer region of immunoglobulin and T-cell receptor genes, and the corresponding region of the herpes simplex ICP-8 protein has also been crystallized although not bound to DNA. Very similar structures are evident in A/T hook proteins despite divergent amino acid sequences.

immunoglobulin response if presented to the host immune system. As shown in Table 63.4, a high level of IgG response is present to the first A/T hook region of EBNA-1, and a significantly lower response to the second hook region of EBNA-1. The difference in response to these two similar EBNA-1 structural regions of specificity is present favoring recognition of the first EBNA-1 hook region over the second hook region despite similar protein tertiary structure. Preliminary data suggest that a much lower response A/T hook regions of EBNA-1 is present in a patient with scleroderma relative to the data shown from a healthy control patient, suggesting that A/T hook regions could be useful to categorize normal and abnormal response to EBNA-1 (unpublished observations).

A/T hook regions described could provide a molecular fingerprint for diagnosis and evaluation of autoimmune syndromes as well as a specific marker for previous EBV and related herpes virus infection. As shown in Table 63.5, the A/T hook region of herpes simplex ICP8 protein is highly antigenic in a healthy donor. IgG response to the BALF-2 A/T hook was present but at a much decreased level to the A/T hooks of EBNA-1 or ICP-8 (data not shown). No IgG response was evident to the host RAG-1 A/T hook region presumably because RAG-1 is normally not present outside of the nucleus; however, the lack of response to BALF-2 A/T hook is not established. The authors suggest that in pathologic inflammation EBNA-1, related virus A/T hooks could serve as autoantigens, as the A/T hook is highly immunogenic in EBNA-1 and other herpes viruses.

Immunoglobulin G Response to Epstein Barr Virus–Encoded "Virokine" BCRF-1–Encoded Protein

Many viral pathogens including EBV encode cytokine-like molecules termed "virokines," and also viral-encoded cytokine receptors [44–46]. Virokines may also be reduced or masked as targets of the host immune response because of their small size and secondary modifications such as carboxylation [29]. Virokines could interfere with host-encoded cytokines through a variety of mechanisms. Preliminary results obtained with a healthy EBV positive donor suggest that most of the IgG response against virokine IL-10 is to regions of the BCRF-1 protein that are identical to the host IL-10. However, some unique epitopes are also present in the BCRF-1–encoded virokine not present in host IL-10 (data not shown). These preliminary results are consistent with previous studies demonstrating that most of the IgG response to virokines is directed at shared epitopes between virokine and host cytokine (Fig. 63.4). The authors suggest that characterization of IgG response to virokines, viral-encoded cytokine receptors, and host cytokines such as IL-10 is a novel use of proteomic molecular fingerprinting that could also help to distinguish between healthy controls and patients with autoimmune syndromes. A more extensive characterization of IgG immune response to virokines and viral-encoded cytokine receptors is in progress and will be reported elsewhere.

TABLE 63.4 IgG Response was Present to EBNA-1 Protein A/T Hook Region GRPGAPGG (aa 51-57). A Second A/T Hook Region of EBNA-1 AGAGGGAG (aa 103-110) Also Bound IgG at Lower Levels. Binding to the EBNA-1 A/T Hook Peptide GRPGAPGG is Approximately 10 Times Greater Than Maximal Binding to ZEBRA Epitope TPDPYQV (aa 15-21)

4	15	NHGRGRGRGRGRGGG	EBNA-1 region 3 (AThookI)	0.0	2000.0
4	16	GRGRGRGRGRGGGRP	EBNA-1 region 3 (AThookI)	0.0	2000.0
4	17	GRGRGRGRGGGRPGA	EBNA-1 region 3 (AThookI)	0.0	2000.0
4	18	GRGRGRGGGRPGAPG	EBNA-1 region 3 (AThookI)	1176.5	6843.0
4	19	GRGRGGGRPGAPGGS	EBNA-1 region 3 (AThookI)	300.0	3236.0
4	20	GRGGGRPGAPGGSGS	EBNA-1 region 3 (AThookI)	157.0	3064.5
4	21	GGGRPGAPGGSGSGP	EBNA-1 region 3 (AThookI)	135.0	2894.0
4	22	GRPGAPGGSGSGPRH	EBNA-1 region 3 (AThookI)	386.0	3401.0
4	23	PGAPGGSGSGPRHRD	EBNA-1 region 3 (AThookI)	0.0	2149.5
4	24	APGGSGSGPRHRDGV	EBNA-1 region 3 (AThookI)	0.0	2000.0
4	25	GGSGSGPRHRDGVRR	EBNA-1 region 3 (AThookI)	0.0	2000.0
4	39	SGGGAGAGGAGGAGA	EBNA-1 region 4 (AThook2)	0.0	2000.0
4	40	GGAGAGGAGGAGAGG	EBNA-1 region 4 (AThook2)	0.0	2000.0
4	41	AGAGGAGGAGAGGGA	EBNA-1 region 4 (AThook2)	0.0	2023.0
4	42	AGGAGGAGAGGGAGA	EBNA-1 region 4 (AThook2)	28.0	2000.0
4	43	GAGGAGAGGGAGAGG	EBNA-1 region 4 (AThook2)	11.0	2018.0
4	44	GGAGAGGGAGAGGAG	EBNA-1 region 4 (AThook2)	0.0	2005.0
4	45	AGAGGGAGAGGAGAG	EBNA-1 region 4 (AThook2)	5.0	2000.0
4	46	AGGGAGAGGAGAGGG	EBNA-1 region 4 (AThook2)	0.0	2000.0

TABLE 63.5 IgG Response to Herpes Simplex ICP-8 A/T Hook Region EGRPTAPL. Binding to the EBNA-1–Like Peptide GRPGAPGG is Less Than to EBNA-1 Protein A/T Hook Region GRPGAPGG and Similar to Maximal Binding to ZEBRA Epitope TPDPYQV (aa 15-21)

24	53	SGVDREGHWPGFEG	RAG1 AT hook region IA-1	0.0	2000.0
24	54	VDREGHVVPGFEGRP	RAG1 AT hook region IA-1	0.0	2000.0
24	55	REGHWPGFEGRPTA	RAG1 AT hook region IA-1	0.0	2000.0
24	56	GHWPGFEGRPTAPI	RAG1 AT hook region IA-1	226.0	2865.5
24	57	WPGFEGRPTAPLVG	RAG1 AT hook region IA-1	264.0	2906.5
24	58	PGFEGRPTAPLVGGT	RAG1 AT hook region IA-1	27.0	2112.5
24	59	FEGRPTAPLVGGTQE	RAG1 AT hook region IA-1	0.0	2028.0
24	60	GRPTAPLVGGTQEFA	RAG1 AT hook region IA-1	69.5	2219.5
24	61	PTAPLVGGTQEFAGE	RAG1 AT hook region IA-1	6.0	2000.0
24	62	APLVGGTQEFAGEHL	RAG1 AT hook region IA-1	0.0	2000.0
24	63	LVGGTQEFAGEHLAM	RAG1 AT hook region IA-1	0.0	2000.0
24	64	GGTQEFAGEHLAMLC	RAG1 AT hook region IA-1	0.0	2000.0

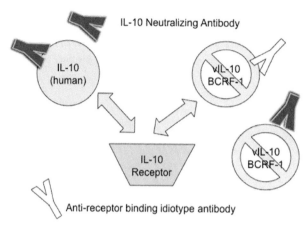

FIGURE 63.4 Virokines and viral-encoded cytokine receptors as targets for host IgG response. A schematic diagram illustrates several mechanisms through which host IgG against viral proteins similar to host cytokines (virokines) and cytokine receptors could interfere with endogenous regulation of suppressor cell regulatory cytokines such as IL-10. EBV encoded IL-10 like BCRF-1 is approximately 90% identical to host IL-10.

DISCUSSION

Our preliminary results with defined IgG-binding regions of the ZEBRA and EBNA-1 protein in a healthy donor suggest that related epitopes will prove to be a useful diagnostic tool significantly lowering the cost and time required for analysis. Further population-based studies would be useful to compare between healthy patients with autoimmune disease or at risk in addition to available more labor-intensive and costly technology such as the ANA. Proteomic assays could potentially be used both for diagnosis and also to monitor response to therapy. In particular using inexpensive and highly automated "molecular fingerprints" it might be possible in the future to identify patients at risk of autoimmune syndromes prior to development of symptoms based solely on their response to specific epitopes in viral proteins and shared host proteins. Targeting therapy prior to onset of disease would limit disease progression and therapy-related adverse events.

Published data from an FDA-approved protein microarray showed that levels of IgG response to host proteins and EBV-encoded EBNA-1 protein and other viral proteins could diagnosis both SLE and scleroderma with sensitivity and specificity similar or greater to conventional ANA testing [15]. Addition of viral protein antigens in this assay significantly improved the sensitivity and specificity although the specific IgG-binding epitopes recognized by IgG were not disclosed [15,16]. In this work IgG-binding results are presented, which are derived from a proprietary laser-printed peptide microchip containing overlapping peptides from immunologically important EBV proteins to illustrate the potential of this new technology.

Although abnormal immune response to EBV-specific proteins such as EBNA-1 has been described in autoimmune syndromes, specific short epitopes described in the work could facilitate proteomic "molecular fingerprints in autoimmune disease" [7,17–19]. The A/T hook region of EBNA-1 and many herpes virus and host proteins, as well as short IgG-binding regions in the lytic ZEBRA switch protein described in this work also appear to be a promising antigen for "molecular footprints" of other inflammatory and autoimmune syndromes. Viral proteins such as the viral recombinase BALF-2 protein in Epstein–Barr virus and its homologue ICP8 in herpes simplex and other alpha, beta, and gamma herpesviridae could also provide epitopes-defining parameters such as viral reactivation and molecular mimicry with host proteins [25,43]. The A/T hook regions of viral and host proteins is shared between both eukaryotic and prokaryotic DNA-binding proteins such as the RAG-1 recombinase and as histones in both vertebrates and invertebrates including the developmentally regulated "hin" and "engrailed" families [41].

Another interesting topic that can be studied with "proteomic molecular fingerprinting" technology is the antigenic response to "virokines" and "virokine receptors" in healthy and autoimmune patients [46]. The authors suggest that antibodies generated against "virokines" could interfere with important host cytokines through a variety of mechanisms. For example EBV-encoded virokines such as the IL-10 homologue BCRF-1 could trigger blocking antibodies or interfere in other ways with host IL-10 function contributing to "immunologic chaos [47]." In conclusion, proteomic "molecular fingerprints" of EBV and related herpes virus infection has the potential to facilitate diagnosis and management of numerous autoimmune syndromes.

ACKNOWLEDGMENTS

The author acknowledges Yehuda Shoenfeld, MD and his research group (Tel Shomer, Sheba Medical Center, Israel, and Erwin Gelfand (retired), National Jewish Medical And Research Center, Denver CO) for their contributions to mentoring of DHD and helpful comments. Also, the authors acknowledge Eugenia Spanopoulou (deceased) for her unique and enduring contributions to the study of RAG protein A/T hooks and RAG function. Data processing and IgG-binding analysis shown were provided on a complementary basis to Dr. Dreyfus, Keren LLC, New Haven CT by PEPperprint.com. All other Analysis of the data was self-funded by the authors.

REFERENCES

[1] Dreyfus DH. Autoimmune disease: a role for new anti-viral therapies? Autoimmun Rev 2011;11(2):88–97.

[2] Farina A, Farina GA. Fresh insights into disease etiology and the role of microbial pathogens. Curr Rheumatol Rep 2015;18(1):1.

[3] Shoenfeld Y. Everything is autoimmune until proven otherwise. Clin Rev Allergy Immunol 2013;45(2):149–51.

[4] Csuka D, Banati M, Rozsa C, Fust G, Illes Z. High anti-EBNA-1 IgG levels are associated with early-onset myasthenia gravis. Eur J Neurol 2012;19(6):842–6.

[5] Csuka D, Varga L, Farkas H, Fust G. Strong correlation of high EBNA-1-IgG levels with edematous attacks involving upper airway mucosa in hereditary angioedema due to C1-inhibitor deficiency. Mol Immunol 2012;49(4):649–54.

[6] Lassmann H, Niedobitek G, Aloisi F, Middeldorp JM, NeuroproMiSe EBVWG. Epstein-Barr virus in the multiple sclerosis brain: a controversial issue–report on a focused workshop held in the Centre for Brain Research of the Medical University of Vienna, Austria. Brain 2011;134(Pt 9):2772–86.

[7] Lunemann JD, Tintore M, Messmer B, Strowig T, Rovira A, Perkal H, et al. Elevated Epstein-Barr virus-encoded nuclear antigen-1 immune responses predict conversion to multiple sclerosis. Ann Neurol 2010;67(2):159–69.

[8] Mameli G, Cossu D, Cocco E, Masala S, Frau J, Marrosu MG, et al. EBNA-1 IgG titers in Sardinian multiple sclerosis patients and controls. J Neuroimmunol 2013;264(1–2):120–2.

[9] Sundar K, Jacques S, Gottlieb P, Villars R, Benito ME, Taylor DK, et al. Expression of the Epstein-Barr virus nuclear antigen-1 (EBNA-1) in the mouse can elicit the production of anti-dsDNA and anti-Sm antibodies. J Autoimmun 2004;23(2):127–40.

[10] Ingram G, Bugert JJ, Loveless S, Robertson NP. Anti-EBNA-1 IgG is not a reliable marker of multiple sclerosis clinical disease activity. Eur J Neurol 2010;17(11):1386–9.

[11] Middeldorp JM, Herbrink P. Epstein-Barr virus specific marker molecules for early diagnosis of infectious mononucleosis. J Virol Methods 1988;21(1–4):133–46.

[12] Schenk BI, Michel PO, Enders G, Thilo N, Radtke M, Oker-Blom C, et al. Evaluation of a new ELISA for the detection of specific IgG to the Epstein-Barr nuclear antigen 1 (EBNA-1). Clin Lab 2007;53(3–4):151–5.

[13] Yadav P, Carr MT, Yu R, Mumbey-Wafula A, Spatz LA. Mapping an epitope in EBNA-1 that is recognized by monoclonal antibodies to EBNA-1 that cross-react with dsDNA. Immun Inflamm Dis 2016;4(3):362–75.

[14] Davies JM, Mackay IR, Rowley MJ. Rheumatoid arthritis sera react with a phage-displayed peptide selected by a monoclonal antibody to type II collagen that has homology to EBNA-1. Autoimmunity 1999;30(1):53–9.

[15] Fattal I, Shental N, Molad Y, Gabrielli A, Pokroy-Shapira E, Oren S, et al. Epstein-Barr virus antibodies mark systemic lupus erythematosus and scleroderma patients negative for anti-DNA. Immunology 2014;141(2):276–85.

[16] Putterman C, Wu A, Reiner-Benaim A, Batty Jr DS, Sanz I, Oates J, et al. SLE-key((R)) rule-out serologic test for excluding the diagnosis of systemic lupus erythematosus: developing the ImmunArray iCHIP((R)). J Immunol Methods 2016;429:1–6

[17] Comabella M, Montalban X, Horga A, Messmer B, Kakalacheva K, Strowig T, et al. Antiviral immune response in patients with multiple sclerosis and healthy siblings. Mult Scler 2010;16(3):355–8.

[18] Jafari N, van Nierop GP, Verjans GM, Osterhaus AD, Middeldorp JM, Hintzen RQ. No evidence for intrathecal IgG synthesis to Epstein Barr virus nuclear antigen-1 in multiple sclerosis. J Clin Virol 2010;49(1):26–31.

[19] Kakalacheva K, Regenass S, Wiesmayr S, Azzi T, Berger C, Dale RC, et al. Infectious mononucleosis triggers generation of IgG auto-antibodies against native myelin oligodendrocyte glycoprotein. Viruses 2016;8(2).

[20] Mackay IR, Leskovsek NV, Rose NR. The odd couple: a fresh look at autoimmunity and immunodeficiency. J Autoimmun 2010;35(3):199–205.

[21] Rose NR. Molecular mimicry and clonal deletion: a fresh look. J Theor Biol 2015;375:71–6.

[22] Wucherpfennig KW. Structural basis of molecular mimicry. J Autoimmun 2001;16(3):293–302.

[23] Yadav P, Tran H, Ebegbe R, Gottlieb P, Wei H, Lewis RH, et al. Antibodies elicited in response to EBNA-1 may cross-react with dsDNA. PLoS One 2011;6(1):e14488.

[24] Yaniv G, Twig G, Shor DB, Furer A, Sherer Y, Mozes O, et al. A volcanic explosion of autoantibodies in systemic lupus erythematosus: a diversity of 180 different antibodies found in SLE patients. Autoimmun Rev 2015;14(1):75–9.

[25] Dreyfus DH. Gene sharing between Epstein-Barr virus and human immune response genes. Immunol Res 2017;65(1):37–45.

[26] Poole BD, Gross T, Maier S, Harley JB, James JA. Lupus-like autoantibody development in rabbits and mice after immunization with EBNA-1 fragments. J Autoimmun 2008;31(4):362–71.

[27] Poole BD, Templeton AK, Guthridge JM, Brown EJ, Harley JB, James JA. Aberrant Epstein-Barr viral infection in systemic lupus erythematosus. Autoimmun Rev 2009;8(4):337–42.

[28] Sears J, Ujihara M, Wong S, Ott C, Middeldorp J, Aiyar A. The amino terminus of Epstein-Barr Virus (EBV) nuclear antigen 1 contains AT hooks that facilitate the replication and partitioning of latent EBV genomes by tethering them to cellular chromosomes. J Virol 2004;78(21):11487–505.

[29] Dower SK. Cytokines, virokines and the evolution of immunity. Nat Immunol 2000;1(5):367–8.

[30] Mock A, Warta R, Geisenberger C, Bischoff R, Schulte A, Lamszus K, et al. Printed peptide arrays identify prognostic TNC serumantibodies in glioblastoma patients. Oncotarget 2015;6(15):13579–90.

[31] Maylin S, Feghoul L, Salmona M, Herda A, Mercier-Delarue S, Simon F, et al. Evaluation the Architect EBV VCA IgM, VCA IgG, and EBNA-1 IgG chemiluminescent immunoassays to assess EBV serostatus prior transplantation. J Med Virol 2017;89(11):2003–10.

[32] Farina A, Cirone M, York M, Lenna S, Padilla C, McLaughlin S, et al. Epstein-Barr virus infection induces aberrant TLR activation pathway and fibroblast-myofibroblast conversion in scleroderma. J Invest Dermatol 2014;134(4):954–64.

[33] Farina A, Peruzzi G, Lacconi V, Lenna S, Quarta S, Rosato E, et al. Epstein-Barr virus lytic infection promotes activation of Toll-like receptor 8 innate immune response in systemic sclerosis monocytes. Arthritis Res Ther 2017;19(1):39.

[34] Dreyfus DH, Liu Y, Ghoda LY, Chang JT. Analysis of an ankyrin-like region in Epstein Barr Virus encoded (EBV) BZLF-1 (ZEBRA) protein: implications for interactions with NF-kappaB and p53. Virol J 2011;8:422.

[35] Dreyfus DH, Nagasawa M, Gelfand EW, Ghoda LY. Modulation of p53 activity by IkappaBalpha: evidence suggesting a common phylogeny between NF-kappaB and p53 transcription factors. BMC Immunol 2005;6:12.

[36] Herkel J, Mimran A, Erez N, Kam N, Lohse AW, Marker-Hermann E, et al. Autoimmunity to the p53 protein is a feature of systemic lupus erythematosus (SLE) related to anti-DNA antibodies. J Autoimmun 2001;17(1):63–9.

[37] Herkel J, Modrow JP, Bamberger S, Kanzler S, Rotter V, Cohen IR, et al. Prevalence of autoantibodies to the p53 protein in autoimmune hepatitis. Autoimmunity 2002;35(8):493–6.

[38] Leskowitz RM, Zhou XY, Villinger F, Fogg MH, Kaur A, Lieberman PM, et al. CD4+ and CD8+ T-cell responses to latent antigen EBNA-1 and lytic antigen BZLF-1 during persistent lymphocryptovirus infection of rhesus macaques. J Virol 2013;87(15):8351–62.

[39] Rubicz R, Yolken R, Drigalenko E, Carless MA, Dyer TD, Bauman L, et al. A genome-wide integrative genomic study localizes genetic factors influencing antibodies against Epstein-Barr virus nuclear antigen 1 (EBNA-1). PLoS Genet 2013;9(1):e1003147.

[40] Sheng Y, Saridakis V, Sarkari F, Duan S, Wu T, Arrowsmith CH, et al. Molecular recognition of p53 and MDM2 by USP7/HAUSP. Nat Struct Mol Biol 2006;13(3):285–91.

[41] Spanopoulou E, Zaitseva F, Wang FH, Santagata S, Baltimore D, Panayotou G. The homeodomain region of Rag-1 reveals the parallel mechanisms of bacterial and V(D)J recombination. Cell 1996;87(2):263–76.

[42] Yin FF, Bailey S, Innis CA, Ciubotaru M, Kamtekar S, Steitz TA, et al. Structure of the RAG1 nonamer binding domain with DNA reveals a dimer that mediates DNA synapsis. Nat Struct Mol Biol 2009;16(5):499–508.

[43] Dreyfus DH. Paleo-immunology: evidence consistent with insertion of a primordial herpes virus-like element in the origins of acquired immunity. PLoS One 2009;4(6):e5778.

[44] Hoebe EK, Hutajulu SH, van Beek J, Stevens SJ, Paramita DK, Greijer AE, et al. Purified hexameric Epstein-Barr virus-encoded BARF1 protein for measuring anti-BARF1 antibody responses in nasopharyngeal carcinoma patients. Clin Vaccine Immunol 2011;18(2):298–304.

[45] Kis LL, Takahara M, Nagy N, Klein G, Klein E. IL-10 can induce the expression of EBV-encoded latent membrane protein-1 (LMP-1) in the absence of EBNA-2 in B lymphocytes and in Burkitt lymphoma- and NK lymphoma-derived cell lines. Blood 2006;107(7):2928–35.

[46] Ouyang P, Rakus K, van Beurden SJ, Westphal AH, Davison AJ, Gatherer D, et al. IL-10 encoded by viruses: a remarkable example of independent acquisition of a cellular gene by viruses and its subsequent evolution in the viral genome. J Gen Virol 2014;95(Pt 2):245–62.

[47] Dreyfus DH, editor. Anti-viral therapy, Epstein–Barr virus, autoimmunity, and chaos (the butterfly effect). 2015.

Chapter 64

Drug-Induced Autoimmunity: Statin-Induced Autoimmune Myositis as an Example

Sharon Slomovich[1], Hanan Guzner-Gur[1,2], Yehuda Shoenfeld[3,4]

[1]Zabludowicz Center for Autoimmune Diseases, Sheba Medical Center, Tel-Hashomer, Israel; [2]Sackler Faculty of Medicine, Tel Aviv University, Tel Aviv, Israel; [3]Zabludowicz Center for Autoimmune Diseases, Sheba Medical Center, affiliated to Sackler Faculty of Medicine, Tel Aviv University, Tel Aviv, Israel; [4]Laboratory of the Mosaics of Autoimmunity, Saint-Petersburg University, Saint-Petersburg, Russian Federation

INTRODUCTION

Drug-induced autoimmunity is well described in a variety of diseases such as systemic lupus erythematous, myasthenia gravis, vasculitis, arthritis, drug-induced liver injury with features of autoimmunity, and necrotizing myositis [1–3]. By and large, most cases of drug-induced autoimmunity are reversed following cessation of the drug. For example, both clinical and serological features of drug-induced lupus resolve after discontinuation of the drug [4]. In contrast, statin-induced autoimmune myositis (SIAM), a necrotizing autoimmune myositis triggered by statin exposure, differs. It is distinguished by autoimmunity that persists even after the cessation of the drug and requires immunosuppression [5].

Statins, 3-hydroxy-3-methylglutaryl-coenzyme A reductase (HMGCR) inhibitors, competitively inhibit HMGCR, a key enzyme in the biosynthesis of cholesterol. These drugs are one of the most frequently prescribed medications for the treatment of dyslipidemia with over a billion people taking the drug globally [6]. Statins contribute to both primary and secondary prevention of cardiovascular disease, the leading cause of morbidity and mortality worldwide [6].

However, statins are associated with adverse effects, mostly muscular symptoms. For example, among statin users, 20% will suffer from mild musculoskeletal side effects such as nonspecific myalgias, asymptomatic creatine kinase (CK) elevations, exercise intolerance, rhabdomyolysis, and reversible toxic necrotizing myositis [7,8].

Specifically, statin-induced myopathy spectrum includes statin-induced myalgias, statin-induced myositis, and statin-induced rhabdomyolysis. Patients with statin-induced myalgias have muscle symptoms without elevations in CK. Statin-induced myositis includes muscle symptoms with CK elevations. Statin-induced rhabdomyolysis includes muscle pain, CK elevation ≥10 times the upper limit of normal and intermittent myoglobinuria [9]. Most cases of statin-induced myopathies are self-limited and resolve after discontinuation of the drug [10].

In contrast, SIAM is a specific, rare, and severe complication of statin treatment. It is characterized by proximal muscle weakness, increased serum CK levels, and histological evidence of myonecrosis. No inflammatory cell infiltration is evident [9]. Another distinctive feature of SIAM is the presence of an **autoantibody directed against the HMGCR enzyme**. It was first described in 2010, as a 200/100 kDa-directed autoantibody in patients with necrotizing myositis, most of whom were statin users [11,12]. Statin-exposed patients who have this autoantibody are now classified as statin-induced necrotizing myositis or SIAM. The incidence of SIAM is estimated at 2 or 3 out of 100,000 people treated with statins [5]. Unlike other statin-induced myopathies, where most symptoms are reversible, SIAM requires immunosuppression therapy [13].

SIAM is part of the wide-spectrum autoimmune myositis, also designated idiopathic inflammatory myopathies (IIM), which includes a group of diseases that target skeletal muscle as a result of an autoimmune dysfunction [14]. The classic Bohan and Peter criteria for IIM are polymyositis (PM), dermatomyositis (DM), myositis-associated connective tissue disease, and cancer-associated myositis [14]. DM and PM are uncommon diseases with a prevalence of 22 in 100,000 [15]. These are two well-known autoimmune myopathies that result in symmetrical and proximal muscle weakness and elevated CK levels [16]. SIAM is an even more rare disease with a prevalence of 1 in 100,000 [12]. SIAM is more common after the age of 50 and less predominant in women [11].

Other immune-mediated myopathies have been recently described and are associated with specific autoantibodies. Examples are antisynthetase syndrome (Jo-1, histidyl transfer RNA (tRNA) synthetase), anti-MI-1, anti-signal recognition

Mosaic of Autoimmunity. https://doi.org/10.1016/B978-0-12-814307-0.00064-5

particle (SRP), anti-MI-2, and some other cancer related such as TIF1-γ [2,17,18]. Anti-SRP is associated with necrotizing myositis, histologically similar to SIAM [19]. However, in contradistinction with the abovementioned autoimmune myositis, in SIAM, extramuscular manifestations are generally absent.

PATHOPHYSIOLOGY OF STATIN-INDUCED AUTOIMMUNE MYOSITIS

The mechanism related to the development of SIAM remains unknown. HMGCR was identified as the 100 kd autoantigen in cultured cells with induced expression under exposure to statins. The presence of an anti-HMGCR autoantibody on exposure to statins suggests that statins may play a role in the pathogenesis of this condition. HMGCR is needed and found in high concentrations in regenerating muscle tissue [20]. The need for upregulation of this enzyme in regenerating muscle tissue proposes a possible stimulus for an antigen-driven immune process [21]. Statins may affect the HMGCR protein confirmation resulting in a protein unrecognized by the immune system, inducing autoimmunity [5].

Class II HLA allele DRB1*11:01 is strongly associated with development of anti-HMGCR autoantibodies in those patients with and without exposure to statins [22,23]. As a result, there may be a group of individuals who are more susceptible to developing SIAM.

The cause of muscle damage in SIAM is unknown. On biopsy, muscular tissue from these patients shows a predominance of macrophage cells most likely related to repair and lacks the expected inflammatory lymphocytic infiltrate. As a result, some may consider the anti-HMGCR autoantibody to be the pathogenic component of this disease. The finding of a correlation between autoantibody levels, CK levels, and muscular symptoms supports the theory that anti-HMGCR autoantibodies may be the pathogenic culprit [24].

Muscle biopsies from patients with SIAM show evidence of muscle cell necrosis, predominance of macrophage infiltration, and regeneration [5]. The cellular infiltrates on histology include macrophages as the leading group of cells but also small quantities of CD4+ lymphocytes, CD8+ lymphocytes, and CD123+ plasmacytoid dendritic cells. Major histocompatibility complex class I upregulation is also seen [25]. Macrophages most likely play a part of tissue repair [26]. The combinations of all mentioned histological features are reliable for the diagnosis of immune-mediated necrotizing myositis [5]. Nevertheless, it should be noted that in most causes of SIAM, the inflammatory infiltrate is scant if any [27].

CLINICAL FEATURES OF STATIN-INDUCED AUTOIMMUNE MYOSITIS

SIAM has a similar presentation to other autoimmune-related myopathies. Attention to medications, symptom onset, and extramuscular manifestations should be considered in making the diagnosis.

Clinical features are variable but usually comprise of myalgias, severe symmetric muscle weakness, and difficulty rising from a chair or lifting heavy objects. The severity of symptoms correlates with CK, especially in patients with a CK level >1000 [11]. However, extramuscular manifestations such as fever, skin rashes, arthritis, and Raynaud's phenomenon are generally absent or low [19].

Statin exposure, including dose and length, and its relationship to the onset of clinical features remain unclear. However, it is reported that in most cases, statin exposure of at least several months is required [28]. Nevertheless, cases of early or years of exposure have been reported [5]. Most patient will have progressive symptoms in spite of cessation of statins in contrasts to other statin-induced myopathies [13]. Moreover, patients with SIAM can have evidence of active necrotizing myopathy months and even years after the onset of myositis. In one study, patients showed active myopathic electromyography up to 11 years following the discontinuation of statins [8].

DIAGNOSIS OF STATIN-INDUCED AUTOIMMUNE MYOSITIS

SIAM should be part of the differential diagnosis of any patient with myositis, especially but not exclusively in statin users. The hallmark diagnostic test is the presence of autoantibodies. **Identification of the autoantibodies via enzyme-linked immunosorbent assay for anti-HMGCR autoantibodies can support the diagnosis of SIAM and was proven to be a highly specific biomarker for the condition** [29]. However, the presence of autoantibodies alone does not confirm the diagnosis. The anti-HMGCR antibody can be found in patients without prior exposure to statins but with a similar clinical presentation [9]. This subgroup of patients is generally younger and less responsive to treatment when compared to SIAM [24]. Additionally, these autoantibodies are found in much less numbers in patients with other muscle conditions [5]. Moreover, the anti-HMGCR autoantibodies are specific in SIAM patients, and not found in asymptomatic statin users in cases of self-limited statin-related myopathy. As a result, the presence of this autoantibody in statin-exposed patients with myopathy and elevated CK ≥ 10 times the upper limit of normal strongly suggests the diagnosis of SIAM. The false positive result of the enzyme-linked immunosorbent assay for anti-HMGCR antibodies is estimated at 0.7% only [22]. However, to avoid misdiagnosis, only those patients with markedly elevated CK levels should be tested for the presence of the autoantibody [5]. Of note, elevated CK levels above 2000 IU per liter (normal range 0–15 IU per liter varied with sex and race) have been observed in almost 90% of cases [5]. Moreover, the presumptive diagnosis of SIAM might be supported by EMG, MRI, and finding of muscle biopsy. Electromyography can show small amplitude motor-unit potentials with increased spontaneous activity, an irritable myopathy pattern as seen in other inflammatory myopathies [9]. MRI will show evidence of muscle edema [5]. The diagnosis is made after ruling out exposure to other drugs, toxins, other immune myositis, and genetic diseases, such as muscular dystrophies.

TREATMENT

Statin treatment should be promptly discontinued. Some cases of HMGCR-associated myositis have gone into spontaneous and complete remission [30]. However, most patients require treatment with immunosuppressive drugs. No clinical trials have been performed to conclude the optimal treatment regiment for SIAM patients. Management is derived from other autoimmune muscular diseases [5] and includes corticosteroids, usually 1 mg/kg followed by long-term immunosuppression such as methotrexate, mycophenolate mofetil, or azathioprine [9]. In addition, IVIG can be added to resistant cases or those who develop severe muscle weakness [5]. Moreover, IVIG has been used as part of a triple therapy (corticosteroid + immunosuppressant + IVIG) or as a monotherapy. Thus, IVIG has been successful as a monoimmunotherapy treatment and may be useful for certain subsets of patients with comorbid conditions in which certain immunosuppressive drugs can lead to serious complications [5].

Patients treated with immunosuppressive drugs should be carefully followed for adverse effects and medications tapered according to clinical symptoms. A relapse should be promptly retreated. While antibody levels do correlate with disease activity, it is important to keep in mind that even in patients who reach clinical remission, anti-HMGCR levels do not always return to normal [24]. The actual number of complete remission is unknown and long-term prognosis remains unknown [9].

CONCLUSION

Statins are crucially important in the treatment of dyslipidemia and complications of cardiovascular disease. The majority of patients taking statins do not suffer from any adverse effects. Still, statin-associated myopathies do exist on a spectrum of severity. An autoimmune connection has been well established in patients with myalgias, muscle weakness, elevated CK levels, and the presence of anti-HMGCR antibodies. While still a rare disease, SIAM has clinical implications and warrants accurate diagnosis and appropriate treatment. The presence of anti-HMGCR autoantibody should prompt immediate discontinuation of statins and initiation of immunosuppressive drugs. With the correct treatment, prognosis is generally well with significant improvement in muscle strength and function.

REFERENCES

[1] Xiao X, Chang C. Diagnosis and classification of drug-induced autoimmunity (DIA). J Autoimmun March 31, 2014;48:66–72.

[2] Foureau DM, Jacobs C, Ahrens W, Russo MW, Bonkovsky HL. Drug-induced liver injury with autoimmune features. Semin Liver Dis May 2014;34(2):194–204. Thieme Medical Publishers.

[3] Gale J, Danesh-Meyer HV. Statins can induce myasthenia gravis. J Clin Neurosci February 28, 2014;21(2):195–7.

[4] Rubin RL. Drug-induced lupus. Toxicology April 15, 2005;209(2):135–47.

[5] Mammen AL. Statin-associated autoimmune myopathy. N Engl J Med February 18, 2016;374(7):664–9.

[6] Ioannidis JP. More than a billion people taking statins?: Potential implications of the new cardiovascular guidelines. JAMA February 5, 2014;311(5):463–4.

[7] Franc S, Dejager S, Bruckert E, Chauvenet M, Giral P, Turpin G. A comprehensive description of muscle symptoms associated with lipid-lowering drugs. Cardiovasc Drugs Ther September 1, 2003;17(5–6):459–65.

[8] Ramanathan S, Langguth D, Hardy TA, Garg N, Bundell C, Rojana-Udomsart A, Dale RC, Robertson T, Mammen AL, Reddel SW. Clinical course and treatment of anti-HMGCR antibody–associated necrotizing autoimmune myopathy. Neurol Neuroimmunol Neuroinflamm June 1, 2015;2(3):e96.

[9] Hamann PD, Cooper RG, McHugh NJ, Chinoy H. Statin-induced necrotizing myositis–A discrete autoimmune entity within the "statin-induced myopathy spectrum". Autoimmun Rev October 31, 2013;12(12):1177–81.

[10] Soininen K, Niemi M, Kilkki E, Strandberg T, Kivist KT. Muscle symptoms associated with statins: a series of twenty patients. Basic Clin Pharmacol Toxicol January 1, 2006;98(1):51–4.

[11] Christopher-Stine L, Casciola-Rosen LA, Hong G, Chung T, Corse AM, Mammen AL. A novel autoantibody recognizing 200-kd and 100-kd proteins is associated with an immune-mediated necrotizing myopathy. Arthritis Rheumatol September 1, 2010;62(9):2757–66.

[12] Mammen AL, Chung T, Christopher-Stine L, Rosen P, Rosen A, Doering KR, Casciola-Rosen LA. Autoantibodies against 3-hydroxy-3-methylglutaryl-coenzyme A reductase in patients with statin-associated autoimmune myopathy. Arthritis Rheumatol March 1, 2011;63(3):713–21.

[13] Liang C, Needham M. Necrotizing autoimmune myopathy. Curr Opin Rheumatol November 1, 2011;23(6):612–9.

[14] Basharat P. Idiopathic Inflammatory myopathies: association with overlap myositis and syndromes: classification, clinical characteristics, and associated autoantibodies. Eur Med J Rheumatol July 1, 2016;3(1):128–35.

[15] Bernatsky S, Joseph L, Pineau CA, Bélisle P, Boivin JF, Banerjee D, Clarke AE. Estimating the prevalence of polymyositis and dermatomyositis from administrative data: age, sex and regional differences. Ann Rheum Dis July 1, 2009;68(7):1192–6.

[16] Bohan A, Peter JB. Polymyositis and dermatomyositis. N Engl J Med February 20, 1975;292(8):403–7.

[17] Thompson C, Piguet V, Choy E. The pathogenesis of dermatomyositis. Br J Dermatol May 24, 2017.

[18] Satoh M, Tanaka S, Ceribelli A, Calise SJ, Chan EK. A comprehensive overview on myositis-specific antibodies: new and old biomarkers in idiopathic inflammatory myopathy. Clin Rev Allergy Immunol February 1, 2017;52(1):1–9.

[19] Watanabe Y, Uruha A, Suzuki S, Nakahara J, Hamanaka K, Takayama K, Suzuki N, Nishino I. Clinical features and prognosis in anti-SRP and anti-HMGCR necrotising myopathy. J Neurol Neurosurg Psychiatry May 4, 2016. https://doi.org/10.1136/jnnp-2016-313166.

[20] Trapani L, Segatto M, La Rosa P, Fanelli F, Moreno S, Marino M, Pallottini V. 3-hydroxy 3-methylglutaryl coenzyme a reductase inhibition impairs muscle regeneration. J Cell Biochem June 1, 2012;113(6):2057–63.

[21] Casciola-Rosen L, Mammen AL. Myositis autoantibodies. Curr Opin Rheumatol November 2012;24(6).

[22] Mammen AL, Pak K, Williams EK, Brisson D, Coresh J, Selvin E, Gaudet D. Rarity of anti-3-hydroxy-3-methylglutaryl-coenzyme A reductase antibodies in statin users, including those with self-limited musculoskeletal side effects. Arthritis Care Res February 1, 2012;64(2):269–72.

[23] Tiniakou E, Christopher-Stine L. Immune-mediated necrotizing myopathy associated with statins: history and recent developments. Curr Opin Rheumatol November 1, 2017;29(6):604–11.

[24] Werner JL, Christopher-Stine L, Ghazarian SR, Pak KS, Kus JE, Daya NR, Lloyd TE, Mammen AL. Antibody levels correlate with creatine kinase levels and strength in anti-HMG-CoA reductase-associated autoimmune myopathy. Arthritis Rheum December 2012;64(12):4087.

[25] Needham M, Fabian V, Knezevic W, Panegyres P, Zilko P, Mastaglia FL. Progressive myopathy with up-regulation of MHC-I associated with statin therapy. Neuromuscul Disord February 28, 2007;17(2):194–200.

[26] Chung T, Christopher-Stine L, Paik JJ, Corse A, Mammen AL. The composition of cellular infiltrates in anti-HMG-CoA reductase-associated myopathy. Muscle Nerve August 1, 2015;52(2):189–95.

[27] Davies EJ, Newton L, Filer C. 021. a rare case of anti-3-hydroxy-3-methylglutaryl-coenzyme-a reductase-positive statin-induced autoimmune necrotizing myositis. Rheumatology April 1, 2017;56(Suppl. 2).

[28] Gunawardena H, Betteridge ZE, McHugh NJ. Myositis-specific autoantibodies: their clinical and pathogenic significance in disease expression. Rheumatology May 12, 2009;48(6):607–12.

[29] Shovman O, Gilburd B, Chayat C, Lazar AD, Amital H, Blank M, Bentow C, Mahler M, Shoenfeld Y. Anti-HMGCR antibodies demonstrate high diagnostic value in the diagnosis of immune-mediated necrotizing myopathy following statin exposure. Immunol Res February 1, 2017;65(1):276–81.

[30] Allenbach Y, Drouot L, Rigolet A, Charuel JL, Jouen F, Romero NB, Maisonobe T, Dubourg O, Behin A, Laforet P, Stojkovic T. Anti-HMGCR autoantibodies in European patients with autoimmune necrotizing myopathies: inconstant exposure to statin. Medicine May 2014;93(3).

Chapter 65

Autoimmunity and Primary Immunodeficiency

Raz Somech[1], Eyal Grunebaum[2,3]

[1]Department of Pediatrics, The Edmond and Lily Safra Children's Hospital, Sheba Medical Center, Tel Hashomer and the Sackler School of Medicine, Tel Aviv University, Tel Aviv, Israel; [2]Developmental and Stem Cell Biology Program, Research Institute, Food Allergy and Anaphylaxis Program, Hospital for Sick Children, Toronto, ON, Canada; [3]University of Toronto, Toronto, ON, Canada

Autoimmunity (AI), the breakdown of immune tolerance to self, and immunodeficiency, failure of immune reactivity to non-self have been traditionally considered as mutually exclusive conditions; however, astute clinical observations, advances in genetics, and better understanding of the immune mechanisms involved in these immune abnormalities have led to a paradigm shift. In a recent retrospective analysis of the records of 2183 French patients with primary immunodeficiency diseases (PIDD), 26.2% had at least one AI or inflammatory, which was 3–14 times relative risk increase compared with the general population in Western Europe [1]. Similarly, AI manifestations were reported among 22% of 247 Slovenian patients with PIDD [2] and 19.3% of 168 Mexican children with PIDD [3].

Single-gene defects can cause primary immune deficiencies that predispose individuals to recurrent infections and immune dysregulation and AI. Importantly, lessons learned from rare monogenic immunodeficiency diseases are being utilized in the understanding and management of the more common polygenic and multifactorial rheumatologic conditions. Over 300 distinct single-gene inborn errors of immunity have been identified, which can be categorized by the dominant affected immune cell or the disrupted mechanism [4]. These include defects in cellular and humoral immunity with or without associated nonimmune features, defects in the number and function of neutrophils and phagocytes, and intrinsic and innate immunity or complement deficiencies. An alternative characterization of primary immunodeficiency disease that incorporates the potential mechanisms involved in the development of AI [5] with some modifications will serve as the backbone for this chapter. For demonstrative purposes, diseases will be described within a specific subgroup; however, many conditions may involve multiple mechanisms acting simultaneously or concurrently.

BREAKDOWN OF T LINEAGE CENTRAL TOLERANCE

T lineage development requires positive and negative selection in the thymus, where thymocytes expressing receptors with high affinity to self-antigens are eliminated. Defects in the thymocytes or thymic epithelial cells in the cortical or medullary areas can lead to breakdown in this process and development of primary immune deficiency and AI.

1. Abnormalities in many genes, critical for the development of thymocytes, have been identified [6]. Many of these can lead to tolerance breakdown and AI at different frequencies and with diverse clinical and laboratory manifestations. Ineffective V(D)J recombination and impaired T cell receptor generation caused by defects in the recombinant activating genes −1 and −2, DNA ligase IV, artemis and DNA-PKs have been associated with failure of central tolerance. When these defects are severe, yet allow generation of few abnormal thymocytes and T cells, patients may suffer from severe combined immune deficiency complicated by Omenn syndrome phenotype [7,8]. Skin erythroderma and alopecia, colitis and hepatitis, enlarged lymph nodes spleen and liver, and AI cytopenia characterize Omenn syndrome. Clonally expanded T cells often infiltrate the tissues and secrete T helper (Th) type 2 cytokines, interleukin (IL) 4, −5, and −13, leading to severe inflammatory responses with eosinophilia and elevated IgE [9]. Importantly, it is now recognized that practically all profound T lineage abnormalities can be associated with Omenn syndrome, including defects in the IL2-JAK-STAT pathway [10], CD3 complex molecules [11], and many more. In some patients with hypomorphic mutations in these genes, a less severe immune deficiency might lead to AI and granulomatous disease later in life [12].

2. In recent years, there is better appreciation of the role of thymus antigen-presenting cells to central tolerance. DiGeorge syndrome is often caused by heterozygous of 22q11.2 microdeletion, an area containing genes involved in the development of the third and fourth branchial pouches, including thymus formation. DiGeorge syndrome is the most common cause of T lineage abnormalities in humans, affecting 1:4000 live births [13]. Most patients with DiGeorge syndrome present in infancy with hypocalcemia, cardiac, and facial malformations. Among adult patients, schizophrenia has been frequently reported. Patients have a wide range of T lineage dysfunction. In the majority of patients, the abnormalities in T cells are asymptomatic and tend to improve in the first years of life. In less than 0.5% of the cases, total absence of the thymus occurs with practically no generation of T cells, a condition known as complete DiGeorge syndrome. Additionally, up to 10% of the patients may suffer from diverse AI manifestations, including arthritis, hypothyroidism, and hematological cytopenia [14]. The reasons for the AI are not completely clear but might be related to incomplete negative selection by the defective thymus or compromised autoimmune regulator expression, described below. Impaired peripheral tolerance, possibly related to defective T cell production, as discussed below, has also been suggested to account for the increased AI observed among patients with DiGeorge syndrome [15].

3. Impaired central tolerance due to abnormalities in thymus antigen-presenting cells frequently occurs among patients with inherited defects in autoimmune regulator. The clinical condition has received several names, emphasizing different clinical features, including autoimmune polyendocrinopathy–candidiasis–ectodermal dysplasia, autoimmune polyendocrine syndrome type 1, and chronic mucocutaneous candidiasis syndrome. The autoimmune regulator gene encodes a transcription factor expressed in medullary thymus epithelial cells, which acts as co-activator in a large transcriptional complex, thereby controlling expression of tissue-specific antigens and negative selection of the autoreactive T lymphocytes. More than 70 autosomal recessive mutations in autoimmune regulator have been identified. Many organs and tissues can be affected by the AI associated with autoimmune regulator deficiency, with the most common being the parathyroid and adrenal, followed by the gonads, pancreas, mucus membranes, skin, and its appendices, liver, and gastrointestinal track. Hematological cytopenia is also common. The cause for the increased frequency of noninvasive candida has been attributed to autoantibodies against IL-22, IL-17F, and myosin-9 [16].

BREAKDOWN OF T LINEAGE PERIPHERAL TOLERANCE

The identification of autoreactive T cells in the peripheral blood and tissues of healthy individuals indicates that T cells can often escape central tolerance, yet remain quiescent because of peripheral regulation. Breakdown of peripheral tolerance can be caused by several mechanisms. These include impaired function of regulatory T cells (Tregs), proliferation of autoreactive lymphocytes, altered apoptosis of reactive lymphocytes, and decreased clearance of self-antigens overwhelming the regulatory capacity.

1. Tregs are characterized by the expression of CD4, CD25, and the FOXP3 transcription factor. Natural Tregs are generated in the thymus. In addition, peripheral CD4+ T lymphocytes can convert into induced Treg, particularly in the gut mucosa and sites of inflammation [17]. Inherited defects in the formation and function of Treg can cause peripheral tolerance breakdown. For example, deficiency of CD25 was shown to cause susceptibility to viral and opportunistic infections, as well as infiltration of T cells into tissues including the skin and gastrointestinal tract [18]. It is hypothesized that the lack of CD25 surface expression hinders the development of effective antigen-specific T cell responses while cytokine-driven T cells proliferate and mediate tissue damage [19]. Moreover, the dysfunction of CD25-deficient dendritic cells could contribute to ineffective antigen presentation and T cell activation.

2. A phenotype similar to CD25 deficiency is commonly identified among patients with immunodysregulation, polyendocrinopathy, enteropathy, and X-linked (IPEX syndrome), which is caused by inherited mutations in FOXP3. Affected patients suffer from multiorgan AI that can present at infancy with insulin-dependent diabetes mellitus, hypothyroidism, eczema, severe enteropathy, glomerulonephritis, and AI cytopenia. Some patients have also been identified later in life or with food allergies [20]. In contrast to CD25 deficiency, the defects in FOXP3 itself does not increase susceptibility to pathogens, although the frequent need for immune suppressive medication might be responsible for increased frequency of infections [21]. Tregs in patients with IPEX syndrome are severely reduced or absent and there is overproduction of inflammatory cytokines and autoantibodies [22].

3. Tregs exert their effect in part by secretion of various cytokines, such as IL-10, which help regulate innate and adaptive immune cells expressing the IL-10 receptor. The important role of IL-10 was emphasized by identifying patients suffering from early-onset AI and inflammatory bowel disease with inherited defects in IL-10 and its receptors [23]. Patients often presented with colitis and perianal disease including abscesses, fistulas, and/or deep fissures, as well as arthritis and folliculitis. IL-10 signaling is critical in regulating intestinal immune homeostasis, the interactions of innate

immune cells with T cells, and the generation and function of antiinflammatory macrophages. IL-10–dependent signals are also required for regulatory and effector CD4+ T cell function and Th-17–mediated responses [24].

4. The important role of Treg in maintaining tolerance was further emphasized by the identification of inherited mutations in the CTLA-4 pathway. CTLA-4 is one of the growing lists of important immune checkpoints [25]. Patients with heterozygous mutations in the CTLA-4 gene or with biallelic mutations in (lipopolysaccharide-responsive and beige-like anchor protein (LRBA), which is important for trafficking of proteins including CTLA-4) often display AI and impaired production of immunoglobulins. AI cytopenia, early-onset enteropathy, lymphoproliferation, and lymphocytic infiltration into nonlymphoid organs are common. Although features of both defects are similar, CTLA-4 deficiency is not fully penetrant and patients tend to present in older childhood or young adolescence, in contrast to the almost universal penetration and preschool presentation of deficiency. In both conditions, reduction in Treg number and function is commonly observed together with hypogammaglobulinemia. CTLA-4, which is constitutively expressed on Treg, can capture and remove it's ligands from antigen-presenting cells by a process known as trans-endocytosis [26].

BREAKDOWN OF B LINEAGE TOLERANCE

To prevent production of self-reactive B cells expressing autoantibodies, cells undergo "central selection" in the bone marrow. High-affinity autoreactive B cell receptors initially undergo receptor editing and if the receptor remains autoreactive, the cells will be destined to undergo apoptosis. Accordingly, molecular defects that impair B cell receptor signaling or V(D)J recombination in B cells, either combined with T defects (described above) or as an isolated B cell abnormality, can lead to AI.

1. Inherited defects in CD19 and CD81, which are co-receptor molecules important for B cell receptor signaling, have been associated with rare cases of immunodeficiency and AI [27,28]. The transmembrane activator and calcium-modulator and cyclophilin ligand interactor is a molecule important for class-switch recombination. Patients with inherited defects in transmembrane activator and calcium-modulator and cyclophilin ligand interactor suffer from increased frequency of infections and AI [28]. A similar phenotype is also common among patients with inherited defects in activation-induced cytidine deaminase, an RNA-editing enzyme important in immunoglobulin class-switch recombination and somatic hypermutation [29]. Patients typically suffer from recurrent bacterial infections, lymphadenopathy with enlarged germinal centers and AI cytopenias, Crohn's disease, or systemic lupus erythematosus. Laboratory evaluations reveal increased or normal serum IgM with reduced IgG and IgA.

2. Common variable immunodeficiency (CVID) is the most frequent symptomatic primary immune deficiency worldwide, with an estimated prevalence of 1 in 25,000–50,000. Patients with CVID have low levels of serum immunoglobulin and impaired production of antibodies, which lead to recurrent bacterial and viral infections. Additionally, more than one-third of patients develop hematologic or organ-specific AI, gastrointestinal and hepatic inflammatory disease, granulomatous disease, and lymphoproliferation. CVID is caused by diverse unidentified mono- or polygenetic etiologies. In some patients with CVID, defective T cells were identified [30,31], yet in the majority of patients with CVID and immune dysregulation, reduced numbers of switched memory B cells were found [32]. The breakdown of self-tolerance and enhanced autoreactivity in CVID may be caused by loss of the homeostatic immunologic regulatory network for B cells. In addition, defective antigen clearance may result in end organ deposition of complexes, leading to inflammation and perhaps the formation of antitissue antibodies. Impaired differentiation, maturation, and function of dendritic cells were also reported to be involved in the pathology of CVID and AI [33].

3. Wiskott–Aldrich syndrome (WAS), caused by defects in WAS protein, is characterized by thrombocytopenia with dysfunctional small platelets, recurrent bacterial invasive infections, and atopic dermatitis. Patients with WAS defects produce autoantibodies and exhibit high prevalence of AI complications. Up to 70% of patients suffer from at least one AI disorder such as hemolytic anemia, neutropenia, arthritis, vasculitis, glomerulonephritis, or inflammatory bowel disease. Multiple immunological mechanisms have been implicated in the development of the AI in WAS-deficient patients and mice [34]. These include (1) hyperresponsiveness of WAS-deficient B cells to stimulation via the B cell receptors and Toll-like receptors; (2) accumulation of CD21lowCD38low B lymphocytes indicative of type 1 interferon (IFN) signature and a marker of self-reactivity; (3) preferential usage of immunoglobulin variable genes that are enriched in patients with AI disease and decreased somatic hypermutation; (4) increased release of immature B cells from the bone marrow to the periphery; (5) elevated B cell activating factor (BAFF) serum levels; and (6) defects in IL-10–producing regulatory B cells [35]. Reduced number and decreased suppressive capacity of Tregs were also demonstrated in many patients with WAS. In addition, abnormalities in the diversity of T and B lymphocytes as well as the function of T and natural killer cells result in impaired clearance of pathogens and persistent inflammation. Moreover, WAS-deficient

plasmacytoid dendritic cells are hyperresponsive to Toll-like receptor 9 stimulation and produce high amounts of type 1 IFN, which may also contribute to AI [36,37]. Recent data from mice with conditional WAS deficiency restricted to platelets while sparing immune cells demonstrated that the platelets could be immune stimulatory and trigger the generation of antiplatelets antibodies [38].

HYPERACTIVATION OF LYMPHOCYTES AND FAILURE TO TERMINATE AN IMMUNE RESPONSE

Following activation of the immune system, an immune response must also be downregulated and eventually terminated when the offending threat has been neutralized and the immune response after it had run its course. Defects in this process, possibly because of abnormalities in apoptosis pathways, can lead to uncontrolled lymphoproliferation, with lymphadenopathy, hepatosplenomegaly, AI, and increased risk of lymphoma.

1. Autoimmune lymphoproliferative syndrome is characterized by lifelong spleen and lymph nodes lymphoproliferation with intermittent AI directed mainly toward blood cells. Increased percentages of CD3+, alpha/beta+, CD4-CD8-, known as double-negative T cells, elevated serum FAS-ligand, vitamin B12, and IL-10 as well as defective FAS-ligand–induced apoptosis are typically found. Autosomal dominant mutations in FAS are the most common cause for autoimmune lymphoproliferative syndrome, followed by defects in FAS-ligand and caspase-10. Somatic mutations in these genes have also been identified in patients with autoimmune lymphoproliferative syndrome. Somatic mutations in NRAS and KRAS can lead to a similar phenotype designated RAS-associated lymphoproliferative disease [39]. The reduced apoptosis is attributed in autoimmune lymphoproliferative syndrome to malfunction of the FAS–FAS ligand and caspase pathways, whereas in RAS-related defects, it is due to resistance to IL-2 depletion-dependent apoptosis.

2. Less common disorders associated with hyperactivation of immune cells include activating mutations in PIK3CD, which encodes p110 delta, and PIK3R1, which encodes the regulatory subunits p85alpha, p55alpha, and p50alpha as alternative splicing products. These defects compose the "activated phosphoinositide 3-kinase deficiency syndrome". Affected patients suffer from recurrent upper and lower respiratory infections that may lead to bronchiectasis, indicative of humoral defects. Patients also experience recurrent and severe herpes virus infections including Epstein–Barr Virus, cytomegalovirus, Herpes simplex virus, and varicella zoster virus; however, opportunistic infections typical of profound T cell deficits are rare. In addition, there is increased incidence of abscess formation, lymphadenitis, and cellulitis with Gram-positive bacteria suggestive of a mild deficit in innate immunity. Lymphadenopathy, hepatosplenomegaly, and focal nodular lymphoid hyperplasia are common features. There is a high frequency of lymphoma associated with activated phosphoinositide 3-kinase deficiency syndrome. Laboratory evaluations typically reveal low IgG and reduced or absent antibodies following vaccines or natural infections. Elevated IgM has also been reported. There is an increase in effector-type T cells with a severe reduction in naïve T cell numbers. There is impaired apoptosis of T cells on restimulation of the cells together with senescence [40]. AI cytopenias, arthritis, glomerulonephritis, thyroiditis, and sclerosing cholangitis have also been reported in 17%–34% of patients with activated phosphoinositide 3-kinase deficiency syndrome [41,42]. Autosomal recessive mutations in PIK3R1 leading to loss of function have also been reported and are typically associated with a more profound immunodeficiency [43].

3. Few patients with hyperactivation of immune cells have been described with autosomal recessive mutations in *PKCD*, encoding protein kinase C (PKC) delta [44]. The clinical picture included antibody deficiency with respiratory tract infections from the first year of life and immune dysregulation reminiscent of a CVID-like disease. Laboratory evaluations showed progressive reduction of CD19+ cells, impaired class switch, and reduced numbers of memory B cells. Patients also suffered from lymphoproliferation and early onset of AI that manifested in membranous glomerulonephritis, relapsing polychondritis, and antiphospholipid syndrome. Autoreactive antibodies including antinuclear antibodies could be detected, helping establish PKC delta deficiency as a monogenic cause for systemic lupus erythematosus. Evidence from mice models suggests that the phenotype is due to the important role of PKC delta in controlling B cell activation, differentiation, and apoptosis.

INCREASED ACTIVATION OF INTERFERON PATHWAYS

Signal transducer and activator of transcription (STAT) family members are transcription factors with key roles in the regulation of cellular response to IFNs, cytokines, growth factors, and hormones. After extracellular stimulation, Janus kinase activation leads to tyrosine phosphorylation of cytoplasmic STAT proteins, followed by dimerization with other phosphorylated STAT family members. STAT molecules then translocate into the nucleus where they bind to promoters of genes and activate complex transcription programs. Patients with autosomal dominant STAT1 gain of function mutations typically suffer from chronic mucocutaneous candidiasis and recurrent respiratory tract infections. AI, inflammatory, and vascular diseases are also common. Patients' cells demonstrate enhanced STAT1 phosphorylation following stimulation with IFN, including type I (IFN alpha and beta) and type II (IFN gamma) [45]. The abnormal response to IFN might be contributing to the impaired development of Th-17 cells that are important in controlling mucosal candida infections. While loss of dominant negative mutations in STAT3 causes hyper IgE syndrome, germline STAT3 gain of function mutations can result in increased susceptibility to infections and AI [46]. The immune dysregulation can manifest with early-onset enteropathy, insulin-dependent diabetes mellitus, interstitial lung disease and cytopenias, and lymphoproliferation with recurrent infections. The activating STAT3 mutations are associated with increased responses following type I IFN stimulation and are thought to cause increased transcriptional activity [47]. Few patients with autosomal recessive STAT5b defects have been described with increased susceptibility to infections, including Pneumocystis jirovecii pneumonia with severe growth hormone–resistant growth failure and diverse AI and lymphoproliferation [48]. In addition to increased IFN pathway activations, patients with STAT defects also often have abnormal Treg number or function, which might also contribute to the AI.

Recently defects in additional molecules involved in type I IFN-mediated inflammation have been identified among patients suffering from early-onset AI and infections. These include DNA polymerase alpha [49] and DNAse II and III [50].

DEFECTIVE REMOVAL OF CELL DEBRIS

Inherited defects in innate immune cells, such as neutrophils and macrophages, important for removal of pathogens and cell debris can also be associated with increased susceptibility to infections and AI.

1. Chronic granulomatous disease, a condition characterized by abnormal granulocyte bactericidal activity, is caused by hemizygous mutations in gp91phox and autosomal recessive defects in p47phox, p67phox, and p22phox. These molecules are important for the nicotinamide adenine dinucleotide phosphate oxidase complex and the production of reactive oxygen species superoxide [51]. Patients typically present with recurrent abscesses, osteomyelitis, pneumonia, lymphadenitis, and granuloma formation. More than 50% of patients with chronic granulomatous disease suffer from AI that commonly includes colitis, sarcoidosis, immune thrombocytopenia, arthritis, and celiac disease [52]. Carriers, such as mothers of patients with X-linked chronic granulomatous disease, have recently been reported to also have an increased incidence of AI [53]. The AI has been attributed to enhanced cellular activation and inflammation triggered by persistence of the pathogen or to failure of development of peripheral tolerance mechanisms, as reactive oxygen species is important for development of Tregs [54].

2. The complement system includes many plasma proteins that are activated consecutively and eventually form a membrane attack complex that can create a pore in the cell membrane of pathogens. Defects in any of these proteins therefore lead to increased susceptibility to infections, such as *Streptococcus pneumoniae*, *Neisseria meningitidis*, and *Haemophilus influenzae*. In addition, defects in the early components of the complement cascade are associated with systemic lupus erythematosus. Up to 90% of patients with C1q deficiency, 75% of patients with C4 complete deficiency, 50%–65% of patients with C1r/s deficiencies, and 10%–30% of patients with homozygous C2 deficiency suffer from systemic lupus erythematosus. Each of these components is important in the clearance of immune complexes and other apoptotic bodies. If this debris is not cleared, there is an increased exposure of intranuclear antigens, including DNA leading to the formation of antinuclear antibodies [55].

3. Similar to defects in early complement components, defects in phagocyte Fc-gamma-RII and Fc-gamma-RIII Fc receptors, variants in C-reactive protein, and defects in the receptor for C3bi on monocytes, all impair normal removal of cell debris and apoptotic cells by phagocytes and may contribute to the development of systemic lupus erythematosus [56].

CONCLUSIONS

Recent years have been marked by increase in the number of gene defects identified among patients with primary immunodeficiency disease and better appreciation of the mechanisms responsible for immune regulation. These advances can be translated into better identification of many other immune abnormalities, where polygenic and nongenetic factors might also contribute to the phenotype. Indeed, some of these advances are already being used to generate novel immune checkpoint inhibitors and are likely to influence the development of additional immune modifiers that will assist in patients' management.

ACKNOWLEDGMENTS

Dr. Somech is supported in part by the Jeffery Modell Foundation. Dr. Grunebaum is supported in part by the Donald and Audrey Campbell Chair for Immunology.

LIST OF ABBREVIATIONS

AI Autoimmunity
CVID Common variable immunodeficiency
IFN Interferon
IL Interleukin
IPEX Immunodysregulation, polyendocrinopathy, enteropathy, X-linked
STAT Signal transducer and activator of transcription
Treg Regulatory T cells
WAS Wiskott–Aldrich syndrome

REFERENCES

[1] Fischer A, Provot J, Jais JP, Alcais A, Mahlaoui N. Members of the CEREDIH French PID study group. Autoimmune and inflammatory manifestations occur frequently in patients with primary immunodeficiencies. J Allergy Clin Immunol November 2017;140(5):1388–93.e8. https://doi.org/10.1016/j.jaci.2016.12.978. Epub 2017 Feb 10. PubMed PMID: 28192146.

[2] Blazina Š, Markelj G, Jeverica AK, Toplak N, Bratanič N, Jazbec J, Kopač P, Debeljak M, Ihan A, Avčin T. Autoimmune and inflammatory manifestations in 247 patients with primary immunodeficiency-a report from the slovenian national registry. J Clin Immunol November 2016;36(8):764–73. Epub 2016 Aug 31. PubMed PMID: 27582173.

[3] Lugo Reyes SO, Ramirez-Vazquez G, Cruz Hernández A, Medina-Torres EA, Ramirez-Lopez AB, España-Cabrera C, Hernandez-Lopez CA, Yamazaki-Nakashimada MA, Espinosa-Rosales FJ, Espinosa-Padilla SE, Murata C. Clinical features, non-infectious manifestations and survival analysis of 161 children with primary immunodeficiency in Mexico: a single center experience over two decades. J Clin Immunol January 2016;36(1):56–65. https://doi.org/10.1007/s10875-015-0226-5. Epub 2015 Dec 28. PubMed PMID: 26707787.

[4] Picard C, Bobby Gaspar H, Al-Herz W, Bousfiha A, Casanova JL, Chatila T, Crow YJ, Cunningham-Rundles C, Etzioni A, Franco JL, Holland SM, Klein C, Morio T, Ochs HD, Oksenhendler E, Puck J, Tang MLK, Tangye SG, Torgerson TR, Sullivan KE. International union of immunological societies: 2017 primary immunodeficiency diseases committee report on inborn errors of immunity. J Clin Immunol January 2018;38(1):96–128. https://doi.org/10.1007/s10875-017-0464-9. Epub 2017 Dec 11. PubMed PMID: 29226302; PubMed Central PMCID: PMC5742601.

[5] Grimbacher B, Warnatz K, Yong PFK, Korganow AS, Peter HH. The crossroads of autoimmunity and immunodeficiency: lessons from polygenic traits and monogenic defects. J Allergy Clin Immunol January 2016;137(1):3–17. https://doi.org/10.1016/j.jaci.2015.11.004. Review. PubMed PMID: 26768758.

[6] Fischer A, Notarangelo LD, Neven B, Cavazzana M, Puck JM. Severe combined immunodeficiencies and related disorders. Nat Rev Dis Primers October 29, 2015;1:15061. https://doi.org/10.1038/nrdp.2015.61. Review. PubMed PMID: 27189259.

[7] Grunebaum E, Bates A, Roifman CM. Omenn syndrome is associated with mutations in DNA ligase IV. J Allergy Clin Immunol December 2008;122(6):1219–20. https://doi.org/10.1016/j.jaci.2008.08.031. Epub 2008 Oct 9. PubMed PMID: 18845326.

[8] Villa A, Notarangelo LD, Roifman CM. Omenn syndrome: inflammation in leaky severe combined immunodeficiency. J Allergy Clin Immunol December 2008;122(6):1082–6. https://doi.org/10.1016/j.jaci.2008.09.037. Epub 2008 Nov 6. Review. PubMed PMID: 18992930.

[9] Somech R, Simon AJ, Lev A, Dalal I, Spirer Z, Goldstein I, Nagar M, Amariglio N, Rechavi G, Roifman CM. Reduced central tolerance in Omenn syndrome leads to immature self-reactive oligoclonal T cells. J Allergy Clin Immunol October 2009;124(4):793–800. https://doi.org/10.1016/j.jaci.2009.06.048. Epub 2009 Sep 19. PubMed PMID: 19767069.

[10] Wada T, Yasui M, Toma T, Nakayama Y, Nishida M, Shimizu M, Okajima M, Kasahara Y, Koizumi S, Inoue M, Kawa K, Yachie A. Detection of T lymphocytes with a second-site mutation in skin lesions of atypical X-linked severe combined immunodeficiency mimicking Omenn syndrome. Blood September 1, 2008;112(5):1872–5. https://doi.org/10.1182/blood-2008-04-149708. Epub 2008 Jun 16. PubMed PMID: 18559672.

[11] Marcus N, Takada H, Law J, Cowan MJ, Gil J, Regueiro JR, Plaza Lopez de Sabando D, Lopez-Granados E, Dalal J, Friedrich W, Manfred H, Hanson IC, Grunebaum E, Shearer WT, Roifman CM. Hematopoietic stem cell transplantation for CD3δ deficiency. J Allergy Clin Immunol November 2011;128(5):1050–7. https://doi.org/10.1016/j.jaci.2011.05.031. Epub 2011 Jul 16.

[12] Lee YN, Frugoni F, Dobbs K, Tirosh I, Du L, Ververs FA, Ru H, Ott de Bruin L, Adeli M, Bleesing JH, Buchbinder D, Butte MJ, Cancrini C, Chen K, Choo S, Elfeky RA, Finocchi A, Fuleihan RL, Gennery AR, El-Ghoneimy DH, Henderson LA, Al-Herz W, Hossny E, Nelson RP, Pai SY, Patel NC, Reda SM, Soler-Palacin P, Somech R, Palma P, Wu H, Giliani S, Walter JE, Notarangelo LD. Characterization of T and B cell repertoire diversity in patients with RAG deficiency. Sci Immunol December 16, 2016;1(6). https://doi.org/10.1126/sciimmunol.aah6109. pii: eaah6109. Epub 2016 Dec 16. PubMed PMID: 28783691.

[13] McDonald-McGinn DM, Sullivan KE. Chromosome 22q11.2 deletion syndrome (DiGeorge syndrome/velocardiofacial syndrome). Medicine (Baltim) January 2011;90(1):1–18. https://doi.org/10.1097/MD.0b013e3182060469. Review. PubMed PMID: 21200182.

[14] McLean-Tooke A, Spickett GP, Gennery AR. Immunodeficiency and autoimmunity in 22q11.2 deletion syndrome. Scand J Immunol July 2007;66(1):1–7. https://doi.org/10.1111/j.1365-3083.2007.01949.x. Review. PubMed PMID: 17587340.

[15] Di Cesare S, Puliafito P, Ariganello P, Marcovecchio GE, Mandolesi M, Capolino R, Digilio MC, Aiuti A, Rossi P, Cancrini C. Autoimmunity and regulatory T cells in 22q11.2 deletion syndrome patients. Pediatr Allergy Immunol September 2015;26(6):591–4. https://doi.org/10.1111/pai.12420. PubMed PMID: 26058917.

[16] Guo CJ, Leung PSC, Zhang W, Ma X, Gershwin ME. The immunobiology and clinical features of type 1 autoimmune polyglandular syndrome (APS-1). Autoimmun Rev January 2018;17(1):78–85. https://doi.org/10.1016/j.autrev.2017.11.012. Epub 2017 Nov 4. Review. PubMed PMID: 29108822.

[17] Yuan X, Malek TR. Cellular and molecular determinants for the development of natural and induced regulatory T cells. Hum Immunol August 2012;73(8):773–82. https://doi.org/10.1016/j.humimm.2012.05.010. Epub 2012 Jun 1. Review. PubMed PMID: 22659217; PubMed Central PMCID: PMC3410644.

[18] Sharfe N, Dadi HK, Shahar M, Roifman CM. Human immune disorder arising from mutation of the alpha chain of the interleukin-2 receptor. Proc Natl Acad Sci USA April 1, 1997;94(7):3168–71. PubMed PMID: 9096364; PubMed Central PMCID: PMC20340.

[19] Goudy K, Aydin D, Barzaghi F, Gambineri E, Vignoli M, Ciullini Mannurita S, Doglioni C, Ponzoni M, Cicalese MP, Assanelli A, Tommasini A, Brigida I, Dellepiane RM, Martino S, Olek S, Aiuti A, Ciceri F, Roncarolo MG, Bacchetta R. Human IL2RA null mutation mediates immunodeficiency with lymphoproliferation and autoimmunity. Clin Immunol March 2013;146(3):248–61. https://doi.org/10.1016/j.clim.2013.01.004. Epub 2013 Jan 24. PubMed PMID: 23416241; PubMed Central PMCID: PMC3594590.

[20] Torgerson TR, Linane A, Moes N, Anover S, Mateo V, Rieux-Laucat F, Hermine O, Vijay S, Gambineri E, Cerf-Bensussan N, Fischer A, Ochs HD, Goulet O, Ruemmele FM. Severe food allergy as a variant of IPEX syndrome caused by a deletion in a noncoding region of the FOXP3 gene. Gastroenterology May 2007;132(5):1705–17. Epub 2007 Feb 23. PubMed PMID: 17484868.

[21] Barzaghi F, Amaya Hernandez LC, Neven B, Ricci S, Kucuk ZY, Bleesing JJ, Nademi Z, Slatter MA, Ulloa ER, Shcherbina A, Roppelt A, Worth A, Silva J, Aiuti A, Murguia-Favela L, Speckmann C, Carneiro-Sampaio M, Fernandes JF, Baris S, Ozen A, Karakoc-Aydiner E, Kiykim A, Schulz A, Steinmann S, Notarangelo LD, Gambineri E, Lionetti P, Shearer WT, Forbes LR, Martinez C, Moshous D, Blanche S, Fisher A, Ruemmele FM, Tissandier C, Ouachee-Chardin M, Rieux-Laucat F, Cavazzana M, Qasim W, Lucarelli B, Albert MH, Kobayashi I, Alonso L, Diaz De Heredia C, Kanegane H, Lawitschka A, Seo JJ, Gonzalez-Vicent M, Diaz MA, Goyal RK, Sauer MG, Yesilipek A, Kim M, Yilmaz-Demirdag Y, Bhatia M, Khlevner J, Richmond Padilla EJ, Martino S, Montin D, Neth O, Molinos-Quintana A, Valverde-Fernandez J, Broides A, Pinsk V, Ballauf A, Haerynck F, Bordon V, Dhooge C, Garcia-Lloret ML, Bredius RG, Kałwak K, Haddad E, Seidel MG, Duckers G, Pai SY, Dvorak CC, Ehl S, Locatelli F, Goldman F, Gennery AR, Cowan MJ, Roncarolo MG, Bacchetta R. Primary immune deficiency treatment consortium (PIDTC) and the inborn errors working party (IEWP) of the European society for blood and marrow transplantation (EBMT). Long-term follow-up of IPEX syndrome patients after different therapeutic strategies: an international multicenter retrospective study. J Allergy Clin Immunol December 11, 2017. https://doi.org/10.1016/j.jaci.2017.10.041. pii: S0091–6749(17)31893-6. [Epub ahead of print] PubMed PMID: 29241729.

[22] Tsuda M, Torgerson TR, Selmi C, Gambineri E, Carneiro-Sampaio M, Mannurita SC, Leung PS, Norman GL, Gershwin ME. The spectrum of autoantibodies in IPEX syndrome is broad and includes anti-mitochondrial autoantibodies. J Autoimmun November 2010;35(3):265–8. https://doi.org/10.1016/j.jaut.2010.06.017. Epub 2010 Jul 22. PubMed PMID: 20650610.

[23] Glocker EO, Kotlarz D, Boztug K, Gertz EM, Schäffer AA, Noyan F, Perro M, Diestelhorst J, Allroth A, Murugan D, Hätscher N, Pfeifer D, Sykora KW, Sauer M, Kreipe H, Lacher M, Nustede R, Woellner C, Baumann U, Salzer U, Koletzko S, Shah N, Segal AW, Sauerbrey A, Buderus S, Snapper SB, Grimbacher B, Klein C. Inflammatory bowel disease and mutations affecting the interleukin-10 receptor. N Engl J Med November 19, 2009;361(21):2033–45. https://doi.org/10.1056/NEJMoa0907206. Epub 2009 Nov 4. PubMed PMID: 19890111; PubMed Central PMCID: PMC2787406.

[24] Shouval DS, Konnikova L, Griffith AE, Wall SM, Biswas A, Werner L, Nunberg M, Kammermeier J, Goettel JA, Anand R, Chen H, Weiss B, Li J, Loizides A, Yerushalmi B, Yanagi T, Beier R, Conklin LS, Ebens CL, Santos FGMS, Sherlock M, Goldsmith JD, Kotlarz D, Glover SC, Shah N, Bousvaros A, Uhlig HH, Muise AM, Klein C, Snapper SB. Enhanced TH17 responses in patients with IL10 receptor deficiency and infantile-onset IBD. Inflamm Bowel Dis November 2017;23(11):1950–61. https://doi.org/10.1097/MIB.0000000000001270. PubMed PMID: 29023267.

[25] van der Vlist M, Kuball J, Radstake TR, Meyaard L. Immune checkpoints and rheumatic diseases: what can cancer immunotherapy teach us?. Nat Rev Rheumatol October 2016;12(10):593–604. https://doi.org/10.1038/nrrheum.2016.131. Epub 2016 Aug 19. Review. PubMed PMID: 27539666.

[26] Rowshanravan B, Halliday N, Sansom DM. CTLA-4: a moving target in immunotherapy. Blood January 4, 2018;131(1):58–67. https://doi.org/10.1182/blood-2017-06-741033. Epub 2017 Nov 8. Review. PubMed PMID: 29118008.

[27] Vince N, Boutboul D, Mouillot G, Just N, Peralta M, Casanova JL, Conley ME, Bories JC, Oksenhendler E, Malphettes M, Fieschi C. DEFI Study Group. Defects in the CD19 complex predispose to glomerulonephritis, as well as IgG1 subclass deficiency. J Allergy Clin Immunol February 2011;127(2):538–41.e1-5. https://doi.org/10.1016/j.jaci.2010.10.019. Epub 2010 Dec 14. PubMed PMID: 21159371.

[28] Warnatz K, Voll RE. Pathogenesis of autoimmunity in common variable immunodeficiency. Front Immunol July 18, 2012;3:210. https://doi.org/10.3389/fimmu.2012.00210. eCollection 2012. PubMed PMID: 22826712; PubMed Central PMCID: PMC3399211.

[29] Durandy A, Cantaert T, Kracker S, Meffre E. Potential roles of activation-induced cytidine deaminase in promotion or prevention of autoimmunity in humans. Autoimmunity March 2013;46(2):148–56. https://doi.org/10.3109/08916934.2012.750299. Epub 2013 Jan 10. Review. PubMed PMID: 23215867; PubMed Central PMCID: PMC4077434.

[30] Taraldsrud E, Fevang B, Jørgensen SF, Moltu K, Hilden V, Taskén K, Aukrust P, Myklebust JH, Olweus J. Defective IL-4 signaling in T cells defines severe common variable immunodeficiency. J Autoimmun July 2017;81:110–9. https://doi.org/10.1016/j.jaut.2017.04.004. Epub 2017 May 3. PubMed PMID: 28476239.

[31] Wong GK, Heather JM, Barmettler S, Cobbold M. Immune dysregulation in immunodeficiency disorders: the role of T-cell receptor sequencing. J Autoimmun June 2017;80:1–9. https://doi.org/10.1016/j.jaut.2017.04.002. Epub 2017 Apr 8. Review. PubMed PMID: 28400082.

[32] Sánchez-Ramón S, Radigan L, Yu JE, Bard S, Cunningham-Rundles C. Memory B cells in common variable immunodeficiency: clinical associations and sex differences. Clin Immunol September 2008;128(3):314–21. https://doi.org/10.1016/j.clim.2008.02.013. Epub 2008 Jul 11. PubMed PMID: 18620909; PubMed Central PMCID: PMC2692232.

[33] Xiao X, Miao Q, Chang C, Gershwin ME, Ma X. Common variable immunodeficiency and autoimmunity–an inconvenient truth. Autoimmun Rev 2014;13(8):858–64. https://doi.org/10.1016/j.autrev.2014.04.006. Epub 2014 Apr 18. Review. PubMed PMID: 24747700.

[34] Crestani E, Volpi S, Candotti F, Giliani S, Notarangelo LD, Chu J, Aldave Becerra JC, Buchbinder D, Chou J, Geha RS, Kanariou M, King A, Mazza C, Moratto D, Sokolic R, Garabedian E, Porta F, Putti MC, Wakim RH, Tsitsikov E, Pai SY, Notarangelo LD. Broad spectrum of autoantibodies in patients with Wiskott-Aldrich syndrome and X-linked thrombocytopenia. J Allergy Clin Immunol November 2015;136(5):1401–4.e1-3. https://doi.org/10.1016/j.jaci.2015.08.010. Epub 2015 Sep 26. PubMed PMID: 26409660; PubMed Central PMCID: PMC4640933.

[35] Yokoyama T, Yoshizaki A, Simon KL, Kirby MR, Anderson SM, Candotti F. Age-dependent defects of regulatory B cells in Wiskott-Aldrich syndrome gene knockout mice. PLoS One October 8, 2015;10(10):e0139729. https://doi.org/10.1371/journal.pone.0139729. eCollection 2015. PubMed PMID: 26448644; PubMed Central PMCID: PMC4598155.

[36] Prete F, Catucci M, Labrada M, Gobessi S, Castiello MC, Bonomi E, Aiuti A, Vermi W, Cancrini C, Metin A, Hambleton S, Bredius R, Notarangelo LD, van der Burg M, Kalinke U, Villa A, Benvenuti F. Wiskott-Aldrich syndrome protein-mediated actin dynamics control type-I interferon production in plasmacytoid dendritic cells. J Exp Med February 11, 2013;210(2):355–74. https://doi.org/10.1084/jem.20120363. Epub 2013 Jan 21. PubMed PMID: 23337808; PubMed Central PMCID: PMC3570108.

[37] Rawlings DJ, Metzler G, Wray-Dutra M, Jackson SW. Altered B cell signalling in autoimmunity. Nat Rev Immunol July 2017;17(7):421–36. https://doi.org/10.1038/nri.2017.24. Epub 2017 Apr 10. Review. PubMed PMID: 28393923; PubMed Central PMCID: PMC5523822.

[38] Sereni L, Castiello MC, Marangoni F, Anselmo A, di Silvestre D, Motta S, Draghici E, Mantero S, Thrasher AJ, Giliani S, Aiuti A, Mauri P, Notarangelo LD, Bosticardo M, Villa A. Autonomous role of Wiskott-Aldrich Syndrome platelet deficiency in inducing autoimmunity and inflammation. J Allergy Clin Immunol February 5, 2018. https://doi.org/10.1016/j.jaci.2017.12.1000. pii: S0091–6749(18)30201-X. [Epub ahead of print] PubMed PMID: 29421274.

[39] Levy-Mendelovich S, Lev A, Rechavi E, Barel O, Golan H, Bielorai B, Neumann Y, Simon AJ, Somech R. T and B cell clonal expansion in Ras-associated lymphoproliferative disease (RALD) as revealed by next-generation sequencing. Clin Exp Immunol September 2017;189(3):310–7. https://doi.org/10.1111/cei.12986. Epub 2017 Jun 5. PubMed PMID: 28500641; PubMed Central PMCID: PMC5543497.

[40] Lucas CL, Chandra A, Nejentsev S, Condliffe AM, Okkenhaug K. PI3Kδ and primary immunodeficiencies. Nat Rev Immunol November 2016;16(11):702–14. https://doi.org/10.1038/nri.2016.93. Epub 2016 Sep 12. Review. PubMed PMID: 27616589; PubMed Central PMCID: PMC5291318.

[41] Coulter TI, Chandra A, Bacon CM, Babar J, Curtis J, Screaton N, Goodlad JR, Farmer G, Steele CL, Leahy TR, Doffinger R, Baxendale H, Bernatoniene J, Edgar JD, Longhurst HJ, Ehl S, Speckmann C, Grimbacher B, Sediva A, Milota T, Faust SN, Williams AP, Hayman G, Kucuk ZY, Hague R, French P, Brooker R, Forsyth P, Herriot R, Cancrini C, Palma P, Ariganello P, Conlon N, Feighery C, Gavin PJ, Jones A, Imai K, Ibrahim MA, Markelj G, Abinun M, Rieux-Laucat F, Latour S, Pellier I, Fischer A, Touzot F, Casanova JL, Durandy A, Burns SO, Savic S, Kumararatne DS, Moshous D, Kracker S, Vanhaesebroeck B, Okkenhaug K, Picard C, Nejentsev S, Condliffe AM, Cant AJ. Clinical spectrum and features of activated phosphoinositide 3-kinase δ syndrome: a large patient cohort study. J Allergy Clin Immunol February 2017;139(2):597–606.e4. https://doi.org/10.1016/j.jaci.2016.06.021. Epub 2016 Jul 16. PubMed PMID: 27555459; PubMed Central PMCID: PMC5292996.

[42] Elkaim E, Neven B, Bruneau J, Mitsui-Sekinaka K, Stanislas A, Heurtier L, Lucas CL, Matthews H, Deau MC, Sharapova S, Curtis J, Reichenbach J, Glastre C, Parry DA, Arumugakani G, McDermott E, Kilic SS, Yamashita M, Moshous D, Lamrini H, Otremba B, Gennery A, Coulter T, Quinti I, Stephan JL, Lougaris V, Brodszki N, Barlogis V, Asano T, Galicier L, Boutboul D, Nonoyama S, Cant A, Imai K, Picard C, Nejentsev S, Molina TJ, Lenardo M, Savic S, Cavazzana M, Fischer A, Durandy A, Kracker S. Clinical and immunologic phenotype associated with activated phosphoinositide 3-kinase δ syndrome 2: a cohort study. J Allergy Clin Immunol July 2016;138(1):210–8.e9. https://doi.org/10.1016/j.jaci.2016.03.022. Epub 2016 Apr 21. PubMed PMID: 27221134.

[43] Tang P, Upton JEM, Barton-Forbes MA, Salvadori MI, Clynick MP, Price AK, Goobie SL. Autosomal recessive agammaglobulinemia due to a homozygous mutation in PIK3R1. J Clin Immunol January 2018;38(1):88–95. https://doi.org/10.1007/s10875-017-0462-y. Epub 2017 Nov 25. PubMed PMID: 29178053.

[44] Salzer E, Santos-Valente E, Klaver S, Ban SA, Emminger W, Prengemann NK, Garncarz W, Müllauer L, Kain R, Boztug H, Heitger A, Arbeiter K, Eitelberger F, Seidel MG, Holter W, Pollak A, Pickl WF, Förster-Waldl E, Boztug K. B-cell deficiency and severe autoimmunity caused by deficiency of protein kinase C δ. Blood April 18, 2013;121(16):3112–6. https://doi.org/10.1182/blood-2012-10-460741. Epub 2013 Jan 14. PubMed PMID: 23319571; PubMed Central PMCID: PMC3630826.

[45] Liu L, Okada S, Kong XF, Kreins AY, Cypowyj S, Abhyankar A, Toubiana J, Itan Y, Audry M, Nitschke P, Masson C, Toth B, Flatot J, Migaud M, Chrabieh M, Kochetkov T, Bolze A, Borghesi A, Toulon A, Hiller J, Eyerich S, Eyerich K, Gulácsy V, Chernyshova L, Chernyshov V, Bondarenko A, Grimaldo RM, Blancas-Galicia L, Beas IM, Roesler J, Magdorf K, Engelhard D, Thumerelle C, Burgel PR, Hoernes M, Drexel B, Seger R, Kusuma T, Jansson AF, Sawalle-Belohradsky J, Belohradsky B, Jouanguy E, Bustamante J, Bué M, Karin N, Wildbaum G, Bodemer C, Lortholary O, Fischer A, Blanche S, Al-Muhsen S, Reichenbach J, Kobayashi M, Rosales FE, Lozano CT, Kilic SS, Oleastro M, Etzioni A, Traidl-Hoffmann C, Renner ED, Abel L, Picard C, Maródi L, Boisson-Dupuis S, Puel A, Casanova JL. Gain-of-function human STAT1 mutations impair IL-17 immunity and underlie chronic mucocutaneous candidiasis. J Exp Med August 1, 2011;208(8):1635–48. https://doi.org/10.1084/jem.20110958. Epub 2011 Jul 4. PubMed PMID: 21727188; PubMed Central PMCID: PMC3149226.

[46] Milner JD, Vogel TP, Forbes L, Ma CA, Stray-Pedersen A, Niemela JE, Lyons JJ, Engelhardt KR, Zhang Y, Topcagic N, Roberson ED, Matthews H, Verbsky JW, Dasu T, Vargas-Hernandez A, Varghese N, McClain KL, Karam LB, Nahmod K, Makedonas G, Mace EM, Sorte HS, Perminow G, Rao VK, O'Connell MP, Price S, Su HC, Butrick M, McElwee J, Hughes JD, Willet J, Swan D, Xu Y, Santibanez-Koref M, Slowik V, Dinwiddie DL, Ciaccio CE, Saunders CJ, Septer S, Kingsmore SF, White AJ, Cant AJ, Hambleton S, Cooper MA. Early-onset lymphoproliferation and autoimmunity caused by germline STAT3 gain-of-function mutations. Blood January 22, 2015;125(4):591–9. https://doi.org/10.1182/blood-2014-09-602763. Epub 2014 Oct 30. PubMed PMID: 25359994; PubMed Central PMCID: PMC4304103.

[47] Consonni F, Dotta L, Todaro F, Vairo D, Badolato R. Signal transducer and activator of transcription gain-of-function primary immunodeficiency/immunodysregulation disorders. Curr Opin Pediatr December 2017;29(6):711–7. https://doi.org/10.1097/MOP.0000000000000551. [PubMed PMID].

[48] Kanai T, Jenks J, Nadeau KC. The STAT5b pathway defect and autoimmunity. Front Immunol August 14, 2012;3:234. https://doi.org/10.3389/fimmu.2012.00234. eCollection 2012. PubMed PMID: 22912632; PubMed Central PMCID: PMC3418548.

[49] Starokadomskyy P, Gemelli T, Rios JJ, Xing C, Wang RC, Li H, Pokatayev V, Dozmorov I, Khan S, Miyata N, Fraile G, Raj P, Xu Z, Xu Z, Ma L, Lin Z, Wang H, Yang Y, Ben-Amitai D, Orenstein N, Mussaffi H, Baselga E, Tadini G, Grunebaum E, Sarajlija A, Krzewski K, Wakeland EK, Yan N, de la Morena MT, Zinn AR, Burstein E. DNA polymerase-α regulates the activation of type I interferons through cytosolic RNA: DNA synthesis. Nat Immunol May 2016;17(5):495–504. https://doi.org/10.1038/ni. 3409. Epub 2016 Mar 28. PubMed PMID: 27019227; PubMed Central PMCID: PMC4836962.

[50] Rodero MP, Tesser A, Bartok E, Rice GI, Della Mina E, Depp M, Beitz B, Bondet V, Cagnard N, Duffy D, Dussiot M, Frémond ML, Gattorno M, Guillem F, Kitabayashi N, Porcheray F, Rieux-Laucat F, Seabra L, Uggenti C, Volpi S, Zeef LAH, Alyanakian MA, Beltrand J, Bianco AM, Boddaert N, Brouzes C, Candon S, Caorsi R, Charbit M, Fabre M, Faletra F, Girard M, Harroche A, Hartmann E, Lasne D, Marcuzzi A, Neven B, Nitschke P, Pascreau T, Pastore S, Picard C, Picco P, Piscianz E, Polak M, Quartier P, Rabant M, Stocco G, Taddio A, Uettwiller F, Valencic E, Vozzi D, Hartmann G, Barchet W, Hermine O, Bader-Meunier B, Tommasini A, Crow YJ. Type I interferon-mediated autoinflammation due to DNase II deficiency. Nat Commun December 19, 2017;8(1):2176. https://doi.org/10.1038/s41467-017-01932-3. PubMed PMID: 29259162; PubMed Central PMCID: PMC5736616.

[51] Kang EM, Marciano BE, DeRavin S, Zarember KA, Holland SM, Malech HL. Chronic granulomatous disease: overview and hematopoietic stem cell transplantation. J Allergy Clin Immunol June 2011;127(6):1319–26. https://doi.org/10.1016/j.jaci.2011.03.028. quiz 1327-8. Epub 2011 Apr 17. Review. PubMed PMID: 21497887; PubMed Central PMCID: PMC3133927.

[52] Magnani A, Brosselin P, Beauté J, de Vergnes N, Mouy R, Debré M, Suarez F, Hermine O, Lortholary O, Blanche S, Fischer A, Mahlaoui N. Inflammatory manifestations in a single-center cohort of patients with chronic granulomatous disease. J Allergy Clin Immunol September 2014;134(3):655–62.e8. https://doi.org/10.1016/j.jaci.2014.04.014. Epub 2014 Jun 27. PubMed PMID: 24985400.

[53] Marciano BE, Zerbe CS, Falcone EL, Ding L, DeRavin SS, Daub J, Kreuzburg S, Yockey L, Hunsberger S, Foruraghi L, Barnhart LA, Matharu K, Anderson V, Darnell DN, Frein C, Fink DL, Lau KP, Long Priel DA, Gallin JI, Malech HL, Uzel G, Freeman AF, Kuhns DB, Rosenzweig SD, Holland SM. X-linked carriers of chronic granulomatous disease: illness, lyonization, and stability. J Allergy Clin Immunol January 2018;141(1):365–71. https://doi.org/10.1016/j.jaci.2017.04.035. Epub 2017 May 18. PubMed PMID: 28528201.

[54] Kraaij MD, Savage ND, van der Kooij SW, Koekkoek K, Wang J, van den Berg JM, Ottenhoff TH, Kuijpers TW, Holmdahl R, van Kooten C, Gelderman KA. Induction of regulatory T cells by macrophages is dependent on production of reactive oxygen species. Proc Natl Acad Sci USA October 12, 2010;107(41):17686–91. https://doi.org/10.1073/pnas.1012016107. Epub 2010 Sep 22. PubMed PMID: 20861446; PubMed Central PMCID: PMC2955141.

[55] Macedo AC, Isaac L. Systemic lupus erythematosus and deficiencies of early components of the complement classical pathway. Front Immunol February 24, 2016;7:55. https://doi.org/10.3389/fimmu.2016.00055. eCollection 2016. Review. PubMed PMID: 26941740; PubMed Central PMCID: PMC4764694.

[56] Martin M, Blom AM. Complement in removal of the dead - balancing inflammation. Immunol Rev November 2016;274(1):218–32. https://doi.org/10.1111/imr.12462. Review. PubMed PMID: 27782329.

Index

Note: 'Page numbers followed by "f" indicate figures, "t" indicate tables and "b" indicate boxes.'